PEDIATRIC ALLERGY

Commissioning Editor: Claire Bonnett
Development Editor: Joanne Scott
Editorial Assistant: Kirsten Lowson
Project Manager: Joannah Duncan
Design: Stewart Larking
Illustration Manager: Bruce Hogarth
Illustrator: Robert Britton
Marketing Manager: Helena Mutak/Richard Jones

SECOND EDITION
PEDIATRIC ALLERGY
PRINCIPLES AND PRACTICE

DONALD Y. M. LEUNG, MD PHD FAAAAI
Edelstein Family Chair of Pediatric Allergy-Clinical Immunology
National Jewish Health
Professor of Pediatrics
University of Colorado Denver School of Medicine
Denver, CO, USA

HUGH A. SAMPSON, MD
Kurt Hirschhorn Professor of Pediatrics
Dean for Clinical and Translational Biomedical Sciences
Mount Sinai School of Medicine
New York, NY, USA

RAIF GEHA, MD
Chief, Division of Immunology
Children's Hospital
James L. Gamble Professor of Pediatrics
Harvard Medical School
Boston, MA, USA

STANLEY J. SZEFLER, MD
Helen Wohlberg and Herman Lambert Chair in Pharmacokinetics
Head, Pediatric Clinical Pharmacology
Department of Pediatrics
National Jewish Health
Professor of Pediatrics and Pharmacology
University of Colorado Denver School of Medicine
Denver, CO, USA

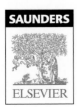

SAUNDERS

ELSEVIER

For additional online content visit
expertconsult.com

Edinburgh, London, New York, Oxford, Philadelphia, St Louis, Sydney, Toronto

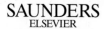

SAUNDERS an imprint of Elsevier Inc.

First edition 2003
Second edition 2010

Notices

Knowledge and best practice in this field are constantly changing. As new research and experience broaden our understanding, changes in research methods, professional practices, or medical treatment may become necessary. Practitioners and researchers must always rely on their own experience and knowledge in evaluating and using any information, methods, compounds, or experiments described herein. In using such information or methods they should be mindful of their own safety and the safety of others, including parties for whom they have a professional responsibility.

With respect to any drug or pharmaceutical products identified, readers are advised to check the most current information provided (i) on procedures featured or (ii) by the manufacturer of each product to be administered, to verify the recommended dose or formula, the method and duration of administration, and contraindications. It is the responsibility of practitioners, relying on their own experience and knowledge of their patients, to make diagnoses, to determine dosages and the best treatment for each individual patient, and to take all appropriate safety precautions.

To the fullest extent of the law, neither the Publisher nor the authors, contributors, or editors, assumes any liability for any injury and/or damage to persons or property as a matter of products liability, negligence or otherwise, or from any use or operation of any methods, products, instructions, or ideas contained in the material herein.

British Library Cataloguing in Publication Data
A catalogue record for this book is available from the British Library
Saunders

Pediatric allergy: principles and practice. – 2nd ed.
  1. Allergy in children. 2. Immunologic diseases in children.
  I. Leung, Donald Y M, 1949-
618.9'297–dc22

ISBN-13: 9781437702712

Library of Congress Cataloging in Publication Data
A catalog record for this book is available from the Library of Congress

ELSEVIER your source for books,
journals and multimedia
in the health sciences

www.elsevierhealth.com

Working together to grow
libraries in developing countries

www.elsevier.com | www.bookaid.org | www.sabre.org

ELSEVIER   BOOK AID
International   Sabre Foundation

The
publisher's
policy is to use
**paper manufactured
from sustainable forests**

Printed in China
Last digit is the print number: 9 8 7 6 5 4 3 2 1

CONTENTS

Contents

Contents

PREFACE

These are exciting times for physicians who treat children and investigators interested in mechanisms underlying diseases in the area of pediatric allergy, asthma and clinical immunology. There has been a well-documented rise in prevalence of this group of diseases during the past three decades. Protection against microbial infection and treatment of hypersensitivity reactions to environmental triggers have become primary goals for the practicing pediatrician. As a result, investigators at academic centers and in the pharmaceutical industry have partnered to understand mechanisms underlying these diseases and have developed evidence- and mechanism-based approaches for management and treatment of these illnesses. In addition, the National Institutes of Health through the National Institutes of Allergy and Infectious diseases and the National Heart, Lung and Blood Institute have formed networks and collaborative studies to study allergic/immunologic diseases, such as food allergy and asthma. The need to document and summarize this recent remarkable increase in information justifies this new textbook in the field of pediatric allergy and clinical immunology for practicing physicians and investigators interested in this area.

It is often said, 'Children are not simply small adults.' In no other subspecialty is this more true than in pediatric allergy and immunology, where the immune system and allergic responses are developing in different host organs. This early age of onset of disease offers special opportunities for prevention and intervention, which cannot be carried out once disease processes have been established in the older child and adult. Indeed, many diseases that pediatricians see in clinical practice are complex diseases thought to result from a multigene predisposition in combination with exposure to an unknown environmental agent. However, the age at which the host is exposed to a particular environmental agent and the resultant immune response are increasingly being recognized as important factors. Furthermore, determining the appropriate time for intervention will be important in defining a window of opportunity to induce disease remission. For example, endotoxin is a known trigger of established asthma in adults but the 'hygiene hypothesis' in children suggests that early exposure to endotoxin prior to the onset of allergies may actually prevent allergic responses and thus account for the low prevalence of allergic disease in children living on farms. New information is available on controlling asthma in early childhood but our current treatment does not alter the natural history of the disease.

Pediatric Allergy: Principles and Practice is aimed at updating the reader on the pathophysiology of allergic responses and the atopic triad (asthma, allergic rhinitis, and atopic dermatitis), the mechanisms underlying specific allergic and immunologic diseases, and their socioeconomic impact and new treatment approaches that take advantage of emerging concepts of the pathobiology of these diseases. An outstanding group of authors who are acknowledged leaders in their fields has been assembled because of their personal knowledge, expertise, and involvement with their subject matter in children. Every effort has been made to achieve prompt publication of this book, thus ensuring that the content of each chapter is 'state of the art.'

Section A presents general concepts critical to an understanding of the impact and causes of allergic diseases. These include reviews of the epidemiology and natural history of allergic disease, genetics of allergic disease and asthma, biology of inflammatory-effector cells, regulation of IgE synthesis, and the developing immune system and allergy. Section B reviews an approach to the child with recurrent infection and specific immunodeficiency and autoimmune diseases that pediatricians frequently encounter. Section C updates the reader on a number of important and emerging immune-directed therapies including immunoglobulin therapy, bone marrow transplantation, immunizations, gene therapy, and stem cell therapy. Section D examines the diagnosis and treatment of allergic disease. The remainder of the book is devoted to the management and treatment of asthma and a number of specific allergic diseases such as upper airway disease, food allergy, allergic skin and eye diseases, drug allergy, latex allergy, insect hypersensitivity, and anaphylaxis. In each chapter, the disease is discussed in the context of its differential diagnoses, key concepts, evaluations, environmental triggers, and concepts of emerging and established treatments.

Major advances in this second edition include updates on new genetic advances in allergic diseases, inflammatory conditions and immunodeficiencies, new biomarkers to monitor allergic diseases, recent revisions in asthma guidelines emphasizing a step-care approach to control asthma, appropriate evaluation of drug allergy and a better understanding of drug cross-reactivity to eliminate the difficulty prescribing antibiotics in the pediatric population, the role of new biologics and immunomodulatory therapy in the treatment of inflammatory diseases and emerging evidence that barrier dysfunction can drive allergic disease.

We would like to thank each of the contributors for their time and invaluable expertise, which were vital to the success of this book. The editors are also grateful to Joanne Scott (Deputy Head of Development), Claire Bonnett (Acquisitions Editor), Joannah Duncan (Project Manager) and Kirsten Lowson (Senior Editorial Assistant), who have played a major role in editing and organizing this textbook, as well as the production staff at Elsevier Ltd for their help in the preparation of this book.

Donald Y. M. Leung, MD PhD FAAAAI
Hugh A. Sampson, MD
Raif Geha, MD
Stanley J. Szefler, MD
2010

LIST OF CONTRIBUTORS

Leonard B. Bacharier MD
Associate Professor of Pediatrics
Clinical Director
Division of Pediatric Allergy, Immunology and
Pulmonary Medicine
Washington University School of Medicine
St. Louis Children's Hospital
St. Louis, MO, USA

Mark Ballow MD
Professor of Pediatrics
Chief, Division of Allergy, Immunology and Pediatric
Rheumatology
State University of New York at Buffalo
Women's and Children's Hospital of Buffalo
Buffalo, NY, USA

Bruce G. Bender PhD
Head, Division of Pediatric Behavioral Health
National Jewish Health
Professor of Psychiatry
University of Colorado Medical School
Denver, CO, USA

M. Cecilia Berin PhD
Assistant Professor of Pediatrics
Mount Sinai School of Medicine
New York, NY, USA

Leonard Bielory MD FACAAI FAAAAI FACP
Professor, Rutgers University
STARx Allergy and Asthma Center, LLC
Springfield, NJ, USA

S. Allan Bock MD
Clinical Professor
Department of Pediatrics
University of Colorado Denver, School of Medicine
Research Affiliate
National Jewish Health
Denver, CO, USA

Mark Boguniewicz MD
Professor, Division of Pediatric Allergy-Immunology
Department of Pediatrics
National Jewish Health
University of Colorado School of Medicine
Denver, CO, USA

Catherine M. Bollard MBChB MD FRACP FRCPA
Associate Professor of Pediatrics, Medicine and
Immunology
Center for Cell and Gene Therapy
Baylor College of Medicine
Houston, TX, USA

Francisco A. Bonilla MD PhD
Assistant Professor of Pediatrics
Harvard Medical School
Division of Immunology, Children's Hospital Boston
Boston, MA, USA

Malcolm K. Brenner MB PhD FRCP FRCPath
Professor of Medicine and of Pediatrics
Director, Center for Cell and Gene Therapy
Baylor College of Medicine
Houston, TX, USA

Wesley Burks MD
Professor and Chief
Pediatric Allergy and Immunology
Duke University Medical Center
Durham, NC, USA

Martin D. Chapman PhD
President
Indoor Biotechnologies Inc.
Charlottesville, VA, USA

Mirna Chehade MD MPH
Assistant Professor of Pediatrics and Medicine
Pediatric Gastroenterology and Allergy
Adult Gastroenterology
Mount Sinai School of Medicine
New York, NY, USA

Loran T. Clement MD
Professor and Chairman
Department of Pediatrics
University of South Alabama College of Medicine
Mobile, AL, USA

Ronina A. Covar MD
Associate Professor
Department of Pediatrics
National Jewish Health
Denver, CO, USA

Conrad Russell Y. Cruz MD
Research Associate
Center for Cell and Gene Therapy
Baylor College of Medicine
Houston, TX, USA

Shelley A. Davis BSc (Hons) MRes
Postgraduate Research Student
Respiratory Genetics Group
Infection, Inflammation and Immunity Division
School of Medicine
University of Southampton
Southampton, UK

Charles W. DeBrosse MD
Allergy and Immunology Fellow
Division of Allergy and Immunology
Cincinnati Children's Hospital Medical Center
Cincinnati, OH, USA

Fatma Dedeoglu MD
Instructor of Pediatrics
Harvard Medical School
Children's Hospital Boston
Boston, MA, USA

Rosemarie DeKruyff PhD
Associate Professor
Division of Immunology
Children's Hospital Boston
Harvard Medical School
Boston, MA, USA

Peyton A. Eggleston MD
Professor Emeritus of Pediatrics
Department of Pediatrics
The Johns Hopkins Hospital
Baltimore, MD, USA

Harold J. Farber MD MSPH FAAP FCCP
Associate Professor of Pediatrics
Pediatric Pulmonary Section
Baylor College of Medicine
Texas Children's Hospital
Houston, TX, USA

Thomas A. Fleisher MD
Chief, Department of Laboratory Medicine
NIH Clinical Center
National Institutes of Health
Bethesda, MD, USA

Luz Fonacier MD FAAAAI FACAAI
Professor of Clinical Medicine
SUNY at Stony Brook
Head of Allergy and Immunology
Training Program Director
Winthrop University Hospital
Mineola, NY, USA

Noah J. Friedman MD FAAAAI
Staff Allergist
Southern California Permanente Medical Group
Assistant Clinical Professor of Pediatrics
University of California San Diego
San Diego, CA, USA

Erwin W. Gelfand MD
Chairman, Department of Pediatrics
National Jewish Health
Denver, CO, USA

Deborah A. Gentile MD
Director of Research
Division of Allergy, Asthma and Immunology
Allegheny General Hospital
Associate Professor of Pediatrics
Drexel University School of Medicine
Philadelphia, PA, USA

James E. Gern MD
Professor of Pediatrics and Medicine
Divisions of Allergy and Immunology
University of Wisconsin School of Medicine and Public Health
Madison, WI, USA

Marion Groetch MS RD CDN
Senior Dietitian
Jaffe Food Allergy Institute
Division of Pediatric Allergy and Immunology
Mount Sinai School of Medicine
New York, NY, USA

Theresa Guilbert MD MS
Assistant Professor of Pediatrics
Division of Pediatric Pulmonary Medicine
University of Wisconsin School of Medicine and Public Health
Madison, WI, USA

Susanne Halken MD DMSci
Associate Professor
University of Southern Denmark Consultant in Pediatrics
Department of Paediatrics
Hans Christian Andersen Children's Hospital
Odense University Hospital
Odense, Denmark

Robert G. Hamilton PhD DABMLI FAAAAI
Professor of Medicine and Pathology
Division of Allergy and Clinical Immunology
Departments of Medicine and Pathology
Johns Hopkins University School of Medicine
Baltimore, MD, USA

Ronald J. Harbeck PhD
Medical Director, Advanced Diagnostic Laboratories
Professor, Departments of Medicine and Immunology
National Jewish Health
Denver, CO, USA

Stephen T. Holgate MD DSc FRCP FMed Sci MRC
Clinical Professor of Immunopharmacology
School of Medicine
University of Southampton
Southampton, UK

Elysia M. Hollams PhD
Senior Research Officer
Division of Cell Biology
Telethon Institute for Child Health Research
Centre for Child Health Research
The University of Western Australia
Perth, WA, Australia

Steven M. Holland MD
Chief, Laboratory of Clinical Infectious Diseases
National Institute of Allergy and Infectious Disease
National Institutes of Health
Bethesda, MD, USA

J. Roger Hollister MD
Chief
Department of Rheumatology
The Children's Hospital
Aurora, CO, USA

List of Contributors

John W. Holloway PhD
Reader
Division of Infection, Inflammation and Immunity
School of Medicine
University of Southampton
Southampton, UK

Patrick G. Holt DSc FAA
Professor and Head, Division of Cell Biology
Telethon Institute for Child Health Research
Professor
Centre for Child Health Research
University of Western Australia
Perth, WA, Australia

Arne Høst MD DMSci
Associate Professor and Head
Department of Paediatrics
Hans Christian Andersen Children's Hospital
Odense University Hospital
Odense, Denmark

Alan K. Ikeda MD
Assistant Professor of Pediatrics
David Geffen School of Medicine
Associate Director of Pediatric Blood and Marrow
Transplant
Mattel Children's Hospital
University of California
Los Angeles, CA, USA

John M. James, MD
Private Clinical Practice
Colorado Allergy and Asthma Centers, PC
Fort Collins, CO, USA

Erin Janssen MD PhD
Clinical Fellow in Rheumatology
Division of Immunology, Department of Medicine
Children's Hospital Boston
Department of Pediatrics, Harvard Medical School
Boston, MA, USA

Craig A. Jones MD
Director, Vermont Blueprint for Health
Vermont Department of Health
Burlington, VT, USA

James F. Jones MD
Research Medical Officer
Chronic Viral Diseases Branch
Division of Viral and Rickettsial Diseases
Centers for Disease Control and Prevention
Atlanta, GA, USA

Stacie M. Jones MD
Professor of Pediatrics
Chief, Division of Allergy and Immunology
University of Arkansas for Medical Sciences
Arkansas Children's Hospital
Little Rock, AR, USA

Kevin J. Kelly MD
Professor of Pediatrics and Medicine
Division of Allergy and Immunology
Children's Corporate Center
Medical College of Wisconsin
Milwaukee, WI, USA

Susan Kim MD MMSc
Instructor of Pediatrics
Division of Immunology
Rheumatology Program
Harvard University
Boston, Children's Hospital
Boston, MA, USA

Donald B. Kohn MD
Professor
Departments of Microbiology, Immunology and
Molecular Genetics and Pediatrics
University of California, Los Angeles
Los Angeles, CA, USA

Gary L. Larsen MD
Professor and Head
Division of Pediatric Pulmonary Medicine
National Jewish Health
Denver, CO, USA

Howard M. Lederman MD PhD
Professor of Pediatrics, Medicine and Pathology
Division of Pediatric Allergy and Immunology
The Johns Hopkins Hospital
Baltimore, MD, USA

Heather K. Lehman MD
Research Assistant
Professor of Pediatrics
University of Buffalo Medicine and Biomedical Sciences
Division of Allergy, Immunology and Pediatric
Rheumatology
Women and Children's Hospital of Buffalo
Buffalo, NY, USA

Robert F. Lemanske Jr MD
Professor of Pediatrics and Medicine
Head, Division of Pediatric Allergy, Immunology and
Rheumatology
University of Wisconsin School of Medicine and Public
Health
Madison, WI, USA

Donald Y. M. Leung MD PhD FAAAAI
Edelstein Family Chair of Pediatric Allergy-Clinical
Immunology
National Jewish Health
Professor of Pediatrics
University of Colorado Denver School of Medicine
Denver, CO, USA

Chris A. Liacouras MD
Professor of Pediatric Gastroenterology
University of Pennsylvania School of Medicine
Director, Center for Pediatric Eosinophilic Diseases
The Children's Hospital of Philadelphia
Philadelphia, PA, USA

Andrew H. Liu MD
Associate Professor
Division of Allergy and Clinical Immunology
Department of Pediatrics
National Jewish Health
University of Colorado School of Medicine
Denver, CO, USA

Claudia Macaubas PhD
Research Associate
Department of Pediatrics
Stanford University School of Medicine
Stanford, CA, USA

Jonathan E. Markowitz MD MSCE
Chief, Pediatric Gastroenterology
Greenville Hospital System University Medical Center
Associate Professor of Clinical Pediatrics
University of South Carolina School of Medicine
Greenville, SC, USA

Fernando D. Martinez MD
Regents' Professor
Director, Arizona Respiratory Center
Director, BIO5 Institute
Swift-McNear Professor of Pediatrics
University of Arizona
Tucson, AZ, USA

Elizabeth C. Matsui MD MHS
Associate Professor of Pediatrics, Epidemiology, and Environmental Health Sciences
Johns Hopkins University
Baltimore, MD, USA

Bruce D. Mazer MD
Associate Professor of Pediatrics, McGill University
Division Head
Pediatric Allergy and Immunology
McGill University Health Center
Montreal Children's Hospital
Montreal, QC, Canada

Evelina Mazzolari MD
Assistant Professor of Pediatrics
Department of Pediatrics
University of Brescia
Brescia, Italy

Louis M. Mendelson MD
Clinical Professor of Pediatrics
University of Connecticut Health Center
Allergist/Immunologist
Connecticut Asthma and Allergy Center, LLC
West Hartford, CT, USA

Henry Milgrom MD
Professor of Pediatrics and Clinical Science
National Jewish Health
School of Medicine
University of Colorado
Denver, CO, USA

Harold S. Nelson MD
Professor of Medicine
Division of Allergy and Clinical Immunology
National Jewish Health
University of Colorado Health Sciences Center
Denver, CO, USA

David P. Nichols MD
Assistant Professor of Pediatric Pulmonology
Department of Pediatrics, Medicine
National Jewish Health
University of Colorado Health Sciences Center
Denver, CO, USA

Luigi D. Notarangelo MD
Professor of Pediatrics and Pathology
Harvard Medical School
Boston, MA, USA

Natalija Novak MD
Professor of Dermatology
Department of Dermatology and Allergy
University of Bonn
Bonn, Germany

Hans C. Oettgen MD PhD
Associate Chief, Division of Immunology, Children's Hospital, Boston
Associate Professor of Pediatrics
Harvard Medical School
Boston, MA, USA

Joao Bosco Oliveira MD PhD
Assistant Director, Immunology Service
Department of Laboratory Medicine
Clinical Center, National Institutes of Health
Bethesda, MD, USA

Catherine Origlieri MD
Resident
Institute of Ophthalmology and Visual Science
University of Medicine and Dentistry of New Jersey – New Jersey Medical School
Newark, NJ, USA

Mary E. Paul MD
Associate Professor of Pediatrics
Department of Pediatrics-Allergy/Immunology
Baylor College of Medicine
Texas Children's Hospital
Houston, TX, USA

Robert E. Reisman MD
Clinical Professor
Departments of Medicine and Pediatrics
State University of New York at Buffalo School of Medicine
Buffalo, NY, USA

Matthew J. Rose-Zerilli BSc (Hons)
Postgraduate Research Student
Respiratory Genetics Group
Infection, Inflammation and Immunity Division
School of Medicine
University of Southampton
Southampton, UK

Sergio D. Rosenzweig MD
Chief
Infectious Diseases Susceptibility Unit
Laboratory of Host Defenses
National Institute of Allergy and Infectious Diseases
National Institutes of Health
Bethesda, MD, USA

Marc E. Rothenberg MD PhD
Director, Cincinnati Center for Eosinophilic Disorders
Professor of Pediatrics
Cincinnati Children's Hospital Medical Center
University of Cincinnati College of Medicine
Cincinnati, OH, USA

Julie Rowe PhD
Senior Research Officer
Division of Cell Biology
Telethon Institute for Child Research
Centre for Child Health Research
The University of Western Australia
Perth, WA, Australia

Hugh A. Sampson MD
Kurt Hirschhorn Professor of Pediatrics
Dean for Clinical and Translational Biomedical Sciences
Mount Sinai School of Medicine
New York, NY, USA

Filiz O. Seeborg, MD
Assistant Professor of Pediatrics
Department of Pediatrics – Allergy and Immunology
Baylor College of Medicine
Houston, TX, USA

Lauren M. Segal MDCM
Fellow in Pediatric Allergy and Immunology
Department of Allergy and Clinical Immunology
Montreal Children's Hospital
Montreal, QC, Canada

William T. Shearer MD PhD
Professor of Pediatrics and Immunology
Baylor College of Medicine
Chief, Allergy and Immunology Service
Texas Children's Hospital
Houston, TX, USA

Andrew I. Shulman MD PhD
Fellow in Rheumatology
Division of Immunology
Children's Hospital Boston
Department of Pediatrics
Harvard Medical School
Boston, MA, USA

Scott H. Sicherer MD
Clinical Professor of Pediatrics
Department of Pediatrics
Division of Allergy and Immunology
Mount Sinai Hospital
New York, NY, USA

F. Estelle R. Simons MD FRCPC
Professor of Pediatrics and Immunology
Faculty of Medicine
University of Manitoba
Winnipeg, MB, Canada

David P. Skoner MD
Professor of Pediatrics, Drexel University College of Medicine
Clinical Professor of Pediatrics, West Virginia University School of Medicine, Morgantown, WV, USA
Director, Allergy, Asthma and Immunology
Department of Pediatrics
Allegheny General Hospital
Pittsburgh, PA, USA

Roland Solensky MD
Allergist/Immunologist
The Corvallis Clinic
Corvallis, OR, USA

Joseph D. Spahn MD
Associate Professor
Department of Pediatrics
National Jewish Health
Denver, CO, USA

David A. Stempel MD
Director
Respiratory Clinical Development
GlaxoSmithKline
Research Triangle Park, NC, USA

Philippe Stock MD
Assistant Professor in Pediatrics
Pediatric Pneumology and Immunology
Charité University of Medicine
Berlin, Germany

Robert C. Strunk MD
Professor of Pediatrics
Washington University School of Medicine
Member, Division of Allergy, Immunology, and Pulmonary Medicine
St. Louis Children's Hospital
St. Louis, MO, USA

Kathleen E. Sullivan MD PhD
Professor of Pediatrics
Division of Allergy Immunology
The University of Pennsylvania School of Medicine
The Children's Hospital of Philadelphia
Philadelphia, PA, USA

Robert P. Sundel MD
Associate Professor of Pediatrics
Harvard Medical School
Director of Rheumatology
Children's Hospital
Boston, MA, USA

Stanley J. Szefler MD
Helen Wohlberg and Herman Lambert Chair in Pharmacokinetics
Head, Pediatric Clinical Pharmacology
Department of Pediatrics
National Jewish Health
Professor of Pediatrics and Pharmacology
University of Colorado Denver School of Medicine
Denver, CO, USA

Lynn M. Taussig MD
Special Advisor to the Provost, University of Denver
Formerly President and CEO (Retired), National Jewish
Medical and Research Center
Professor of Pediatrics
University of Colorado Health Sciences Center
Denver, CO, USA

Troy R. Torgerson MD PhD
Assistant Professor
Pediatric Immunology and Rheumatology
Seattle Children's Research Institute
Seattle, WA, USA

Dale T. Umetsu MD PhD
The Prince Turki bin Abdul Aziz al Saud Professor of
Pediatrics, Harvard Medical School
Division of Immunology and Allergy
Boston Children's Hospital
Boston, MA, USA

Erika von Mutius MD MSc
Professor of Pediatrics
Division of Pediatrics
Munich University Children's Hospital
University of Munich
Munich, Germany

Rudolph S. Wagner MD
Clinical Associate Professor of Ophthalmology
Director of Pediatric Ophthalmology
Institute of Ophthalmology and Visual Science
University of Medicine and Dentistry of New Jersey –
New Jersey Medical School
Newark, NJ, USA

Richard W. Weber MD
Professor of Medicine
National Jewish Health
University of Colorado School of Medicine
Denver, CO, USA

Sandra R. Wilson PhD
Senior Staff Scientist and Chair
Department of Health Services Research
Palo Alto Medical Foundation Research Institute
Palo Alto, CA
Adjunct Clinical Professor of Medicine
Department of Medicine, Division of Pulmonary and
Critical Care Medicine
Stanford University School of Medicine
Stanford, CA, USA

Robert A. Wood MD
Professor of Pediatrics
Director, Pediatric Allergy and Immunology
Johns Hopkins University School of Medicine
Baltimore, MD, USA

Bruce L. Zuraw MD
Professor of Medicine in Residence
University of California San Diego
Staff Physician
San Diego VA Healthcare
San Diego, CA, USA

To our families and patients who have supported our efforts to advance the care of asthma, allergy, and immunology treatment for children

CHAPTER 1

Epidemiology of Allergic Diseases

Erika von Mutius

Introduction

A large proportion of the population in affluent countries reports allergic reactions to a wide range of environmental stimuli. Many of the so-called allergic reactions are nonspecific, vague adverse effects of ingestion, inhalation or other contact to environmental factors and should not be confused with atopic illnesses which are characterized by the presence of immunoglobulin E (IgE) antibodies in affected subjects. Traditionally, asthma, allergic rhinitis and hay fever, as well as atopic dermatitis, have been categorized as atopic diseases. Yet, the relation between clinical manifestations of these diseases and the production of IgE antibodies has not been fully clarified. Although in many patients with severe enough symptoms to seek medical advice in tertiary referral centers high levels of total and specific IgE antibodies are found, many individuals in the general population will not show any signs of illness despite elevated IgE levels. Not surprisingly, risk factors and determinants of atopy, defined in the following as the presence of IgE antibodies, differ from those associated with asthma, atopic dermatitis and hay fever. Moreover, in some individuals various atopic illnesses can be co-expressed, whereas in other subjects only one manifestation of an atopic illness is present. The prevalence of these four atopic entities therefore only partially overlaps in the general population (Figure 1-1).

Whereas asthma had already been described in ancient times, hay fever, an easy and obvious to recognize clinical syndrome, was virtually unknown in Europe and North America until the late 19th century when it was regarded as a rare disease entity.[1] In that time the main causes of infant and adult morbidity were infectious diseases such as tuberculosis, smallpox, dysentery, pneumonia, typhoid fever and diphtheria. Since the beginning of the 20th century, improvements in housing conditions, sanitation, water supply, nutrition and medical treatment have drastically reduced infectious diseases as major causes of death in developed countries such as the USA, and increased the average life expectancy from about 50 years in 1900 to nearly 74 years in 1984. But many other environmental exposures have changed over the last decades and it has been impossible to firmly relate any changes in environmental exposures to time trends of allergic diseases.

Asthma, atopic dermatitis and hay fever are complex diseases and their incidence is determined by an intricate interplay of genetic and environmental factors. Environmental exposures may affect susceptible individuals during certain time windows in which particular organ systems are vulnerable to extrinsic influences, and these windows of opportunity are likely to differ between types of atopic conditions. Moreover, most allergic illnesses are likely to represent syndromes with many different phenotypes rather than single disease entities. The search for determinants of allergic illnesses must therefore take phenotypes, genes, environmental exposures and the timing of these exposures into account.

Prevalence of Childhood Asthma and Allergies

Asthma is a complex syndrome rather than a single disease entity. Different phenotypes with varying prognosis and determinants have been described, particularly over childhood years[2] and will be discussed in detail in the following chapter. For example, transient early wheezing is characterized by the occurrence of wheezing in infants up to the age of 2 to 3 years which disappears thereafter. The main predictor of these wheezing illnesses is premorbid reduced lung function before the manifestation of any wheeze.[2,3] These decrements in pulmonary function are in part determined by passive smoke exposure in utero[4] and result in symptoms of airway obstruction when infants get infected with respiratory viruses. Atopy and a family history of asthma and atopy do not influence the incidence of this wheezing phenotype.

Wheeze among school-aged children can be classified into an atopic and nonatopic phenotype.[5] This differentiation has clinical implications as nonatopic children with wheeze at school age outgrow their symptoms rapidly and retain normal lung function. In turn, among atopic wheezy children, the time of new onset of atopic sensitization and the severity of airway responsiveness determine the progression of this wheezing phenotype over school and adolescent years.[6]

Most epidemiological studies have used cross-sectional designs and therefore do not allow disentanglement of the different wheezing phenotypes. Only prospective studies following infants from birth up to school age and adolescence will identify different wheezing phenotypes and enable the differential analysis of risk factors and determinants for certain wheezing phenotypes. These limitations must be borne in mind when discussing and interpreting findings from cross-sectional surveys. The relative proportion of different wheezing phenotypes is likely to vary among age groups and therefore the strength of association between different risk factors and wheeze is also likely to vary across age groups.

Similarly, limitations apply with respect to the epidemiology of atopic dermatitis.[7] The definition of atopic eczema varies

©2010 Elsevier Ltd, Inc, BV
DOI: 10.1016/B978-1-4377-0271-2.00001-8

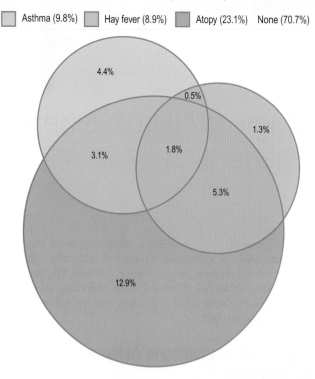

GERMAN 9- TO 11-YEAR-OLD CHILDREN IN MUNICH (N = 2612)
VENN DIAGRAM FOR ASTHMA, HAY FEVER, AND ATOPY

Asthma (9.8%)   Hay fever (8.9%)   Atopy (23.1%)   None (70.7%)

Percentages calculated for all non-missing cases (N = 1729)

Figure 1-1 The prevalence of asthma, hay fever and atopic sensitization only partially overlaps on a population level. Description of findings from the ISAAC Phase II study in Munich, of German children aged 9 to 11 years. (From The International Study of Asthma and Allergies in Childhood [ISAAC]. Lancet 1998;351:1225.)

from study to study and validations of questionnaire-based estimates have been few. Skin examinations by trained field workers that can add an objective parameter to questionnaire-based data do reflect a point prevalence of skin symptoms at the time of examination and can therefore, only in limited ways, corroborate estimates of lifetime prevalence, for example if assessed by questions inquiring about a doctor's diagnosis of eczema ever. In all cross-sectional surveys, identified risk factors relate to the prevalence of the condition, i.e. the incidence and persistence of the disease. It is therefore often difficult to disentangle aggravating from causal factors in such studies. There are very few prospective surveys aimed at identifying environmental exposures prior to the onset of clinical manifestations of atopic dermatitis.

Western versus Developing Countries

In general, reported rates of asthma, hay fever and atopic dermatitis are higher in affluent, western countries than in developing countries. The worldwide prevalence of allergic diseases was assessed in the 1990s by the large scale International Study of Asthma and Allergy in Childhood (ISAAC).[8] A total of 463 801 children in 155 collaborating centers in 56 countries were studied. Children self-reported, through one-page questionnaires, symptoms of these three atopic disorders. Between 20-fold and 60-fold differences were found between centers in the prevalence of symptoms of asthma, allergic rhinoconjunctivitis, and atopic eczema. The highest 12-month prevalence of asthma symptoms was reported from centers in the UK, Australia, New Zealand, and the Republic of Ireland (Figure 1-2). These were followed by most centers in North, Central, and South America. The lowest prevalence was reported by centers in several Eastern European

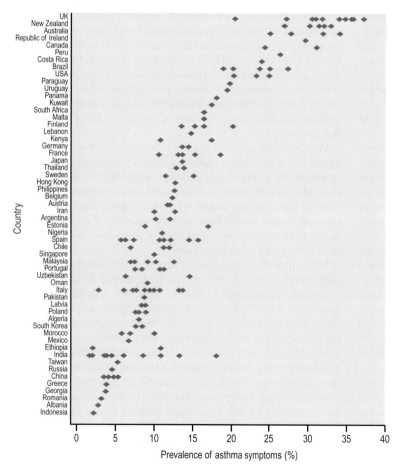

Figure 1-2 Prevalence of allergic conditions worldwide according to the ISAAC Phase I study. (From The International Study of Asthma and Allergies in Childhood [ISAAC]. Lancet 1998;351:1225.)

countries, Indonesia, Greece, China, Taiwan, Uzbekistan, India and Ethiopia. In general, centers with low asthma rates also showed low levels of other atopic diseases. However, countries with the highest prevalence of allergic rhinitis and atopic eczema were not identical to those with the highest asthma rates.

The European Community Respiratory Health Survey (ECRHS) studied young adults aged 20 to 44 years.[9] A highly standardized and comprehensive study instrument including questionnaires, lung function and allergy testing was used by 35 to 48 centers in 22 countries, predominantly in Western Europe, but also included centers in Australia, New Zealand and the USA. The ECRHS has shown large geographical differences in the prevalence of respiratory symptoms, asthma, bronchial responsiveness and atopic sensitization with high prevalence in English speaking countries and low prevalence rates in the Mediterranean region and Eastern Europe.[10] The geographical pattern emerging from questionnaire findings was consistent with the distribution of atopy and bronchial hyperresponsiveness supporting the conclusion that the geographical variation in asthma is true and not attributable to methodological factors such as the questionnaire phrasing, the skin testing technique or the type of assay for the measurement of specific IgE.

Moreover, a strong correlation was found between the findings from children as assessed by the ISAAC Study and the rates in adults as reported by the ECRHS questionnaire.[11] Sixty-four percent of the variation at the country level, and 74% of the variation at the center level in the prevalence of 'wheeze in the last 12 months' in the ECRHS data, was explained by the variation rates reported for children in the ISAAC Study. Thus, although there were differences in the absolute prevalences observed in the two surveys, there was good overall agreement adding support to the validity of both studies.

Within this global perspective some comparisons seem particularly informative. For example, studies of populations with comparable ethnic backgrounds but striking differences in environmental exposures were performed in China among children living in Hong Kong and mainland China, namely Beijing and Urumqui.[12] Beijing children reported significantly more asthma symptoms than those living in Urumqui. But Hong Kong children had the highest prevalence of asthma and other allergic symptoms of all. Urumqui, Beijing and Hong Kong represent communities at increasing stages of affluence and westernization, and the findings from these three cities can be interpreted as a reflection of a worldwide trend for increasing prevalence of asthma and allergies as westernization intensifies.

The prevalence of symptoms, diagnosis and management of asthma in school-aged children in Australia was furthermore compared to rates of Nigerian children, using another standardized methodology.[13] Wheeze, asthma and asthma medication use were less prevalent in Nigeria in comparison to Australia. No significant difference was found in the overall prevalence of atopy between the two countries, although atopy was a strong risk factor for asthma in both countries. Dissociations between the prevalence of asthma and atopy have been documented in other developing countries such as in Ethiopia[14,15] In these areas a high prevalence of atopy has been found despite low rates of asthma. Infestation with parasites has been proposed as a potential explanation, but further work must confirm or refute these hypotheses. The findings, however, suggest that 'asthma' and 'atopy' are only loosely linked phenotypes and that the strength of association between these traits is dependent on the environmental conditions individuals live in. This notion has been further investigated in the ISAAC Phase II Study with respect to a measure of affluence, i.e. the gross national income per capita (GNI).[16] Across all centers, there were no correlations between current wheeze and atopic sensitization, and only weak correlations of both with GNI. However, the fractions and prevalence rates of wheeze attributable to skin test reactivity correlated strongly with GNI. These findings suggest that the strength of association between atopy and asthma across the world is determined by affluence and factors relating to affluence.

Migration Studies

As proposed above, the timing of exposure to certain environments may play a crucial role in the development of allergic diseases, particularly for asthma. Therefore, the relation between the prevalence of respiratory symptoms and time since arrival in Australia was studied in immigrant teenagers living in Melbourne. In subjects born outside Australia, residence for 5 to 9 years in Australia was associated with a 2-fold increase in the odds of self-reported wheeze; after 10 to 14 years, this risk increased 3-fold. This 'time-dose' effect on the prevalence of symptoms in subjects born outside Australia and living in Melbourne was independent of age and country of birth.[17] The findings can be interpreted as suggestive of duration of exposure being the important determinant of incidence of illness. Alternatively, the results indicate that exposure early in life is more important than exposure thereafter.

Likewise, in children migrating from the Pacific Islands of Tokelau to New Zealand a large increase in the prevalence of atopic eczema as compared to children of similar ethnic groups in their country of origin has been documented.[18] Furthermore, Asian children born in Australia have been reported to be at higher risk of atopic eczema than those who recently immigrated to Australia.[19]

The East-West Gradient across Europe

A number of reports have been published demonstrating, in part, large differences in the prevalence of asthma, airway hyperresponsiveness, hay fever and atopy in children and adults between east and west European areas.[20,21,22,23,24] The prevalence of asthma was significantly lower in all study areas in eastern Europe in comparison to western Europe. Furthermore, all, except one investigator, reported significantly lower prevalences of hay fever, nasal allergies and atopy, either measured by skin prick tests or specific serum IgE antibodies towards environmental allergens, among children and adults living in east European areas in comparison to subjects living in western Europe.

Data from the East European ISAAC studies have corroborated these notions and expanded findings to areas such as Georgia and Uzbekistan.[21] Among the older age group of 13- to 14-year-old children, the prevalence of wheezing was 11.2% to 19.7% in Finland and Sweden, 7.6% to 8.5% in Estonia, Latvia and Poland and 2.6% to 5.9% in Albania, Romania, Russia, Georgia and Uzbekistan (except Samarkand). The prevalence of itching eyes and flexural dermatitis varied in similar manner between the three regions.

In contrast to hay fever, atopy, asthma and airway hyperresponsiveness, the prevalence of atopic dermatitis is likely to be higher in East Germany in comparison to West Germany. In the preschool studies[24] in which children also underwent skin examination by trained dermatologists the prevalence of atopic eczema was 17.5% in the East German area in comparison to 5.7% to 15.3% in the West German regions. Furthermore, Schäfer and colleagues recently reported that the excess of atopic eczema in East Germany is likely to be related to an intrinsic, nonatopic phenotype of the disease.[24] Whereas half of the West German children with atopic eczema were sensitized according to skin prick test results, only one third of the East German children had positive skin prick test reactions. A nationwide study of asthma, allergic illnesses and atopic sensitization enrolling 17 641 one to seventeen-year-old German children and adolescents in 2003–2006 no longer observed differences in the prevalence rates between East and West Germany. The causes underlying the increase in the prevalence in East Germany are not fully understood. The drastic decrease in family size after reunification, changes in dietary habits or indoor exposures may have contributed to this trend.

Differences between Rural and Urban Populations

The prevalence of asthma and allergies is not only increasing with westernization and affluence, but also with urbanization. The rates of asthma and atopy among children living in Hong Kong are similar to European figures, whereas much lower rates have been found among children living in Beijing and Urumqui in mainland China. In rural China, asthma is almost nonexistent with a prevalence of less than 1%.[25] In Mongolia, a country in transition from rural, farming lifestyles to an industrial society, marked differences in the prevalence of asthma, allergic rhinoconjunctivitis and atopy exist.[26] Inhabitants of small rural villages are least affected, whereas residents of the capital Ulaanbaatar city have high rates of allergic diseases comparable to affluent western countries.

Across Europe, differences between urban and rural areas are less clear. However, strong contrasts exist on a lower spatial scale, i.e. among children raised on a farm in comparison to their neighbors living in the same rural area but not on a farm.[27] Since 1999, 15 studies have corroborated these findings in rural areas of Europe (Switzerland, Germany, Austria, France, Sweden, Denmark, Finland and Britain). Studies from Canada and New Zealand have further substantiated these observations. Children raised on farms retain their protection from allergy at least into adulthood.[28,29,30]

The timing and duration of exposure seem to play a critical role. The largest reduction in risk of developing respiratory allergies is seen among those who are exposed prenatally and continue to be exposed throughout their life.[31] The protective factors in these farming environments have not been completely unraveled. There is indication that the contact with farm animals, particularly cattle, confers protection. Also the consumption of milk directly produced on the farm has been shown to be beneficiary with respect to childhood asthma and allergies. Increased levels of microbial substances may at least, in part, contribute to the protective effects. Yet, only few measures of microbial exposures have been performed in these environments and results suggest that the underlying protective microbial exposure(s) await further elucidation.

Inner City Areas of the USA

In contrast to the protective factors encountered in pediatric farming populations of rural areas, living conditions of inner city areas in the USA are associated with a markedly increased risk of asthma.[32] Several potential risk factors are being investigated, such as race and poverty, adherence to asthma treatment,[33] and factors related to the disproportionate exposures associated with socioeconomic disadvantage such as indoor and outdoor exposure to pollution and cockroach infestation.[34] At least, early in life, cockroach exposure has been associated with the development of sensitization to cockroach allergen[35] and wheeze[36] in infants living in inner-city areas of the USA. Problems related to inner city asthma will be discussed in more detail in a subsequent chapter of this book.

Time Trends in the Prevalence of Allergic Diseases

Numerous studies have investigated the trends in the occurrence of allergic disorders.[37] Data collected over the last 40 years in industrialized countries indicate a significant increase in the prevalence of asthma, hay fever and atopic dermatitis. The investigators all used identical questionnaires in similar population samples at different times. Therefore, these studies are reliable indicators of changes in prevalence over time. Most studies lack objective measurements such as airway responsiveness and atopic sensitization. However, the consistent and strong increase in the prevalence of allergic conditions indicates that a true increase in the prevalence has occurred.

Despite the use of different methods and definitions of asthma, most studies from industrialized countries suggest an overall increase in the prevalence of asthma and wheezing between 1960 and 1990. Most studies have been performed among children and little is known about time trends among adults. Twenty-year trends of the prevalence of treated asthma among pediatric and adult members of a large US health maintenance organization were reported recently.[38] During the period 1967–1987, the treated prevalence of asthma increased significantly in all age-sex categories except males aged 65 and older. In the USA, the greatest increase was detected among children and young adults living in inner cities.[39]

Recent studies suggest that in some areas this trend continues unabated. Kuehni and colleagues from the UK reported that among preschool children the prevalence of all types of wheezing increased from 1990 up to 1998.[40] In contrast, studies for Italy showed that among school children surveyed in 1974, 1992 and 1998 the prevalence of asthma had increased significantly during the 1974–1992 period, whereas it remained stable over the last 4 years.[41] Similar findings have been reported from Germany and Switzerland where prevalence rates may have reached a plateau since the 1990s.[42,43] On a global scale, time trends in the prevalence of asthma and allergic rhinoconjunctivitis have been assessed in ISAAC Phase III.[44] The findings indicate that international differences in symptom prevalence have reduced with decreases in prevalence in English-speaking countries and western Europe and increases in prevalence in regions where prevalence was previously low, i.e. in low- to mid-income countries.

Environmental Risk Factors for Allergic Diseases

Air Pollution

The geographical variation in the prevalence of asthma in children does not coincide with variations in air pollution levels. The increase in the prevalence of asthma and allergies seen over the last decades was paralleled by a decrease in emissions of SO_2 and particles from coal combustion, and an increase of emissions from motor vehicle traffic. There is a growing number of studies suggesting that increased exposure to traffic exhausts, particularly diesel exhausts, may be a risk factor for the new onset of asthma.[45] Since most studies so far have used cross-sectional designs with all the limitations discussed above, there is a need for prospective studies which on a personal level e.g. using geographical information systems link pollution data to the incidence of various wheezing phenotypes.

In panel and time-series studies, air pollutants, such as fine particles and ozone, reduce lung function among children already affected by asthma and increase symptoms and medication use. Likewise, emergency room visits, general practitioner activities and hospital admissions for asthma and wheeze are positively associated with ambient air pollution levels. There is, thus, ample evidence to suggest that increasing pollutant concentrations and exposure to traffic emissions can trigger and exacerbate preexisting disease,[46] even when taking pollen and mold counts as well as influenza epidemics into account.

Besides pollution, other environmental factors such as domestic water supply may be relevant for the inception of atopic dermatitis. An ecological study of the relation between domestic water hardness and the prevalence of atopic eczema among British schoolchildren was performed.[47] Geographical information systems were used to link the geographical distribution of eczema in the study area to four categories of domestic water-hardness data. Among the primary school children aged 4 to 16 years, a significant relation between the prevalence of atopic eczema and water hardness, both before and after adjustment for potential confounding factors, was found. The 1-year period prevalence was 17.3% in the highest water-hardness category and 12.0% in the lowest category (adjusted odds ratio = 1.54; 95% confidence interval = 1.19–1.99). The effect on recent eczema symptoms was stronger than on lifetime prevalence, which may indicate that water hardness acts more on existing dermatitis by exacerbating the disorder or prolonging its duration rather than as a cause of new cases.

Environmental Tobacco Smoke

The effects of exposure to environmental tobacco smoke (ETS) on children have been extensively studied and numerous surveys have consistently reported an association between ETS exposure and respiratory diseases. Strong evidence exists that passive smoking increases the risk of lower respiratory tract illnesses such as bronchitis, wheezy bronchitis and pneumonia in infants and young children. Maternal smoking during pregnancy and early childhood has been shown to be strongly associated with impaired lung growth and diminished lung function[3,4] which in turn may predispose infants to develop transient early wheezing. In children with asthma, parental smoking increases symptoms and the frequency of asthma attacks. A series of epidemiological studies has also been performed to determine the effect of ETS exposure on the inception, prevalence and severity of asthma. In most cross-sectional and longitudinal studies, ETS exposure appears to be an important risk factor for the development of childhood asthma. Conversely, no unequivocal association between ETS exposure, atopic sensitization and atopic dermatitis was seen.

Nutrition

There is increasing evidence relating body mass index to the prevalence and incidence of asthma in children and adults, males, and more consistently, in adolescent females.[48] It is unlikely that the association is attributable to reverse causation, i.e. that asthma precedes obesity because of exercise-induced symptoms. Rather, weight gain can antedate the development of asthma. Weight reduction among asthmatic patients can also result in improvements of lung function.[48] Potential explanations are that both are programmed to occur in early life, or that mechanical factors promote asthma symptoms, or that gastro-esophageal reflux as a result of obesity induces asthma. Furthermore, physical inactivity may promote both obesity and asthma.

Fruit, vegetable, cereal and starch consumption, intake of various fatty acids, vitamins A, C, D, E, minerals and antioxidants have all been studied.[37] However, diet is complex and difficult to measure, and standardized tools are still lacking. All methods pertaining to food frequency, individual food items, food patterns and serum nutrients can introduce substantial misclassification, and the close correlation of many nutrients presents problems when trying to identify independent effects. In cross-sectional surveys a wide range of nutrients appear to have an effect on asthma outcomes. The evidence from prospective studies and randomized clinical trials is, however, far less consistent or conclusive.[49] Maternal nutrition during pregnancy may play a role but data are scarce. Intervention studies promoting avoidance of cow's milk and eggs during pregnancy have failed to achieve protection from asthma[50] and breast-feeding does, likewise, not prevent asthma. Recent studies showing a positive association between breast-feeding and asthma may reflect adherence to recommendations rather than being a causal factor for asthma.

Allergen Exposure

There is much controversy as to the role of allergen exposure for the development of atopic sensitization towards this allergen. While in some studies, a clear, almost linear dose-response relation between allergen exposure and sensitization has been found,[51] others described a bell-shaped association with higher levels of exposures relating to lower rates of atopic sensitization.[52] Part of the discrepancy may relate to the type of allergen, since mostly cat but not house dust mite allergen exposure has been shown, in some studies, to exert protective effects at higher levels of exposure.

The relationship between allergen, particularly house dust mite exposure, and asthma has been studied for many years. Overall, there is little evidence suggesting a positive association between allergen exposure and the development of childhood asthma. Intervention studies have failed to show convincing evidence of a reduction in asthma risk after the implementation of avoidance strategies.[53] Furthermore, in a prospective birth cohort the overall incidence of asthma up to the age of 7 years was not related to indoor allergen levels early in life.[54] However, after refining the analysis for different wheezing phenotypes, a role for indoor allergen exposure among children developing atopic sensitization in the first 3 years of life for the progression of allergic asthma into school age, became apparent.[5] Thus, for certain asthma phenotypes, but not for others, allergen exposure may play a role. Other co-factors of exposure should, however, also be taken into account, such as exposure to microbial compounds. For example, levels of endotoxin have been shown to modify the effect of allergen exposure,[55] Also, keeping cats and dogs does, in most studies, not increase the risk of allergic diseases. In contrast, protective effects on the development of allergic illnesses have been reported when pets, in particular dogs, have been kept in the first year of life of the index child.[56]

Family Size, Infections and Hygiene

Strachan first reported that sibship size is inversely related to the prevalence of childhood atopic diseases.[57] This observation has since been confirmed by numerous studies, all showing that atopy, hay fever and atopic eczema were inversely related to increasing numbers of siblings. In contrast, the relation between family size and childhood asthma and airway hyperresponsiveness is less clear. However, underlying causes of this consistent protective effect remain unknown.

Viral infections of the respiratory tract are the major precipitants of acute exacerbations of wheezing illness at any age. Yet, viral respiratory infections are very common during infancy and early childhood and most children do not suffer from any aftermath relating to these infections, including infections with respiratory syncitial virus and rhinovirus.[58] Thus, host factors in children susceptible to the development of wheezing illnesses and asthma are likely to play a major role. Deficiencies in innate immune responses have been shown to contribute to a subject's susceptibility to rhinovirus infections, the most prevalent cause of lower respiratory tract viral infections in infants associated with asthma development.[59]

An inverse relation between asthma and the overall burden of respiratory infections may, however, also exist. Evidence for this assumption derives from a number of sources. First, it had been observed that in developing countries such as in Papua New Guinea and the Fiji Islands, as well as in east European countries, asthma is inversely related to the overall burden of respiratory infections. Several studies investigating children in daycare have rather consistently shown that exposure to a daycare environment in the first months of life is associated with a significantly reduced risk of wheezing, hay fever and atopic sensitization at school age and adolescence.[60,61] It remains, however, unclear whether the burden of infections or other exposures in daycare early in life account for this protective effect. Several reports have shown that sero-positivity for hepatitis A, *Toxoplasma gondii* or *Helicobacter pylori* are related to a significantly lower prevalence of atopic sensitization, allergic rhinitis and allergic asthma as compared to their sero-negative peers.[62] The use of antibiotics has been proposed as a risk factor for asthma and allergic diseases. In most cross-sectional studies a positive relation between antibiotics and asthma has been found which is, however, most likely to be attributable to reverse causation. Early in life, when it is difficult to diagnose asthma, antibiotics are often prescribed for respiratory symptoms in wheezy children and thus are positively associated with asthma later in life. Most studies using a prospective design have, however, failed to identify antibiotics as a risk factor antedating the new onset of asthma.[63] Similar problems arise when interpreting the positive relation between paracetamol use and asthma seen in cross-sectional studies.[64] Intervention trials are needed to come to firm conclusions.

Active and chronic helminthic infections were reported to be protective from atopy, but findings are less consistent for wheeze and asthma.[65] Part of the discrepancies in the literature reporting associations between helminths and allergic diseases may be the load of parasitic infestation and the type of helminths in a particular area. Microbial stimulation, both from normal commensals and pathogens through the gut, may be another route of exposure which may have altered the normal intestinal colonization pattern in infancy. Thereby, the induction and maintenance of oral tolerance of innocuous antigens, such as food proteins and inhaled allergens may substantially be hampered. These hypotheses, though intriguing, have to date not been supported by epidemiological evidence since significant methodological difficulties arise when attempting to measure the microbial pattern of the intestinal flora.

Exposure to microbes does, however, not only occur through invasive infection of human tissues. Viable germs and nonviable parts of microbial organisms are ubiquitous in nature and can be found in varying concentrations in our daily indoor and outdoor environments, and also in urban areas. These microbial products are recognized by the innate immune system as danger signals, even in the absence of overt infection, and induce a potent inflammatory response. Therefore, environmental exposure to microbial products may play a crucial role for the maturation of a child's immune response, enabling tolerance of other components of its natural environment such as pollen and animal dander.

A number of studies have in fact shown that environmental exposure to endotoxin, a component of the cell wall of Gram negative bacteria, is inversely related to the development of atopic sensitization and atopic dermatitis.[66] Yet, endotoxin exposure is a risk factor for wheezing and asthma as shown in a number of studies.[67] Muramic acid, a component of the cell wall of all bacteria, but more abundantly in Gram positive bacteria, has been inversely related to asthma and wheeze, but not atopy.[68] Compounds related to fungal exposures, such as extracellular polysaccharides derived from *Penicillium* spp. and *Aspergillus* spp. have also been inversely associated with asthma.[69] These microbial compounds are found in higher abundance in farming rather than nonfarming environments, and may, in part, contribute to the protective 'farm effect'.

Gene–Environment Interactions

The genetics of asthma will be discussed in a later chapter and are touched on here only in the context of environmental exposures. In general, the identification of novel genes for asthma suggests that many genes with small effects, rather than a few genes with strong effects, contribute to the development of asthma.[70] These genetic effects may, in part, differ with respect to a subject's environmental exposures, although some genes may also exert their effect independently of the environment.

A number of gene–environment interactions have been found which are discussed in detail by von Mutius[70] and Le Souef.[71] These interactions confer additional biologic plausibility for the identified environmental exposures in the inception of asthma and allergic diseases. For example, the interaction of polymorphisms in the *TLR2* gene with a farming environment or daycare settings is highly suggestive of microbial exposures underlying this observation. The consideration of environmental factors into genetic analyses may further help to reveal some genetic effects that are masked by stronger environmental exposures. Finally, the analysis of gene–environment interactions may result in the identification of individuals who are particularly vulnerable to certain environmental exposures.

Conclusions

Large variations in the prevalence of childhood and adult asthma and allergies have been reported. In affluent, urbanized centers, prevalences are generally higher than in poorer centers. Lower levels are seen, especially in some rural areas in Africa, Asia and among farmers' children in Europe. Numerous environmental factors have been scrutinized, but no conclusive explanation for the rising trends has been found. Future challenges are to tackle the complex interplay between environmental factors and genetic determinants.

References

1. Emanuel MB. Hay fever, a post industrial revolution epidemic: a history of its growth during the 19th century. Clin Allergy 1988;18:295–304.
2. Morgan WJ, Stern DA, Sherrill DL, et al. Outcome of asthma and wheezing in the first 6 years of life: follow-up through adolescence. Am J Respir Crit Care Med 2005;172:1253–8.
3. Dezateux C, Stocks J, Dundas I, et al. Impaired airway function and wheezing in infancy: the influence of maternal smoking and a genetic predisposition to asthma. Am J Respir Crit Care Med 1999;159:403–10.
4. Tager IB, Ngo L, Hanrahan JP. Maternal smoking during pregnancy: effects on lung function during the first 18 months of life. Am J Respir Crit Care Med 1995;152:977–83.
5. Illi S, von Mutius E, Lau S, et al. Perennial allergen sensitisation early in life and chronic asthma in children: a birth cohort study. Lancet 2006;368:763–70.
6. von Mutius E. Paediatric origins of adult lung disease. Thorax 2001;56:153–7.
7. von Mutius E. Risk factors for atopic dermatitis. In: Bieber TLD, editor. Atopic dermatitis. New York, Basel: Marcel Dekker; 2002. p. 111–22.
8. ISAAC. Worldwide variation in prevalence of symptoms of asthma, allergic rhinoconjunctivitis, and atopic eczema: ISAAC. The International Study of Asthma and Allergies in Childhood (ISAAC) Steering Committee. Lancet 1998;351:1225–32.
9. Burney PG, Luczynska C, Chinn S, et al. The European Community Respiratory Health Survey. Eur Respir J 1994;7:954–60.
10. Janson C, Anto J, Burney P, et al. The European Community Respiratory Health Survey: what are the main results so far? European Community Respiratory Health Survey II. Eur Respir J 2001;18:598–611.
11. Pearce N, Sunyer J, Cheng S, et al. Comparison of asthma prevalence in the ISAAC and the ECRHS. ISAAC Steering Committee and the European Community Respiratory Health Survey. International Study of Asthma and Allergies in Childhood. Eur Respir J 2000;16:420–6.
12. Zhao T, Wang HJ, Chen Y, et al. Prevalence of childhood asthma, allergic rhinitis and eczema in Urumqi and Beijing. J Paediatr Child Health 2000;36:128–33.
13. Faniran AO, Peat JK, Woolcock AJ. Prevalence of atopy, asthma symptoms and diagnosis, and the management of asthma: comparison of an affluent and a non-affluent country. Thorax 1999;54:606–10.
14. Scrivener S, Yemaneberhan H, Zebenigus M, et al. Independent effects of intestinal parasite infection and domestic allergen exposure on risk of wheeze in Ethiopia: a nested case-control study. Lancet 2001;358:1493–9.
15. Pearce N, Pekkanen J, Beasley R. How much asthma is really attributable to atopy? Thorax 1999;54:268–72.
16. Weinmayr G, Weiland SK, Bjorksten B, et al. Atopic sensitization and the international variation of asthma symptom prevalence in children. Am J Respir Crit Care Med 2007;176:565–74.
17. Powell CV, Nolan TM, Carlin JB, et al. Respiratory symptoms and duration of residence in immigrant teenagers living in Melbourne, Australia. Arch Dis Child 1999;81:159–62.
18. Waite DA, Eyles EF, Tonkin SL, et al. Asthma prevalence in Tokelauan children in two environments. Clin Allergy 1980;10:71–5.
19. Leung R. Asthma, allergy and atopy in South-east Asian immigrants in Australia. Aust N Z J Med 1994;24:255–7.
20. von Mutius E, Martinez FD, Fritzsch C, et al. Prevalence of asthma and atopy in two areas of West and East Germany. Am J Respir Crit Care Med 1994;149:358–64.
21. Bjorksten B, Dumitrascu D, Foucard T, et al. Prevalence of childhood asthma, rhinitis and eczema in Scandinavia and Eastern Europe. Eur Respir J 1998;12:432–7.
22. Braback L, Breborowicz A, Julge K, et al. Risk factors for respiratory symptoms and atopic sensitisation in the Baltic area. Arch Dis Child 1995;72:487–93.
23. Nowak D, Heinrich J, Jorres R, et al. Prevalence of respiratory symptoms, bronchial hyperresponsiveness and atopy among adults: West and East Germany. Eur Respir J 1996;9:2541–52.
24. Schafer T, Ring J. Epidemiology of allergic diseases. Allergy 1997;52:14–22; discussion 35–6.
25. Wong GW, Hui DS, Chan HH, et al. Prevalence of respiratory and atopic disorders in Chinese schoolchildren. Clin Exp Allergy 2001;31:1225–31.
26. Viinanen A, Munhbayarlah S, Zevgee T, et al. The protective effect of rural living against atopy in Mongolia. Allergy 2007;62:272–80.
27. von Mutius E, Radon K. Living on a farm: impact on asthma induction and clinical course. Immunol Allergy Clin North Am 2008;28:631–47, ix–x.
28. Leynaert B, Guilloud-Bataille M, Soussan D, et al. Association between farm exposure and atopy, according to the CD14 C-159T polymorphism. J Allergy Clin Immunol 2006;118:658–65.
29. Portengen L, Sigsgaard T, Omland O, et al. Low prevalence of atopy in young Danish farmers and farming students born and raised on a farm. Clin Exp Allergy 2002;32:247–53.
30. Smit LA, Zuurbier M, Doekes G, et al. Hay fever and asthma symptoms in conventional and organic farmers in The Netherlands. Occup Environ Med 2007;64:101–7.
31. Riedler J, Braun-Fahrlander C, Eder W, et al. Early life exposure to farming environment is essential for protection against the development of asthma and allergy: a cross-sectional survey. Lancet 2001;358:1129–33.
32. Webber MP, Carpiniello KE, Oruwariye T, et al. Prevalence of asthma and asthma-like symptoms in inner-city elementary schoolchildren. Pediatr Pulmonol 2002;34:105–11.
33. Bauman LJ, Wright E, Leickly FE, et al. Relationship of adherence to pediatric asthma morbidity among inner-city children. Pediatrics 2002;110:e6.
34. Rauh VA, Chew GR, Garfinkel RS. Deteriorated housing contributes to high cockroach allergen levels in inner-city households. Environ Health Perspect 2002;110(Suppl 2):323–7.
35. Alp H, Yu BH, Grant EN, et al. Cockroach allergy appears early in life in inner-city children with recurrent wheezing. Ann Allergy Asthma Immunol 2001;86:51–4.
36. Litonjua AA, Carey VJ, Burge HA, et al. Exposure to cockroach allergen in the home is associated with incident doctor-diagnosed asthma and recurrent wheezing. J Allergy Clin Immunol 2001;107:41–7.
37. Eder W, Ege MJ, von Mutius E. The asthma epidemic. N Engl J Med 2006;355:2226–35.
38. Vollmer WM, Osborne ML, Buist AS. 20-year trends in the prevalence of asthma and chronic airflow obstruction in an HMO. Am J Respir Crit Care Med 1998;157:1079–84.
39. Eggleston PA, Buckley TJ, Breysse PN, et al. The environment and asthma in U.S. inner cities. Environ Health Perspect 1999;107(Suppl 3):439–50.
40. Kuehni CE, Davis A, Brooke AM, et al. Are all wheezing disorders in very young (preschool) children increasing in prevalence? Lancet 2001;357:1821–5.
41. Ronchetti R, Villa MP, Barreto M, et al. Is the increase in childhood asthma coming to an end? Findings from three surveys of schoolchildren in Rome, Italy. Eur Respir J 2001;17:881–6.
42. Zollner IK, Weiland SK, Piechotowski I, et al. No increase in the prevalence of asthma, allergies, and atopic sensitisation among children in Germany: 1992–2001. Thorax 2005;60:545–8.
43. Grize L, Gassner M, Wuthrich B, et al. Trends in prevalence of asthma, allergic rhinitis and atopic dermatitis in 5–7-year old Swiss children from 1992 to 2001. Allergy 2006;61:556–62.
44. Asher MI, Montefort S, Bjorksten B, et al. Worldwide time trends in the prevalence of symptoms of asthma, allergic rhinoconjunctivitis, and eczema in childhood: ISAAC Phases One and Three repeat multicountry cross-sectional surveys. Lancet 2006;368:733–43.
45. Gilliland FD. Outdoor air pollution, genetic susceptibility, and asthma management: opportunities for intervention to reduce the burden of asthma. Pediatrics 2009;123(Suppl 3):S168–73.
46. O'Connor GT, Neas L, Vaughn B, et al. Acute respiratory health effects of air pollution on children with asthma in US inner cities. J Allergy Clin Immunol 2008;121:1133–9 e1.
47. McNally NJ, Williams HC, Phillips DR, et al. Atopic eczema and domestic water hardness. Lancet 1998;352:527–31.
48. Schaub B, von Mutius E. Obesity and asthma, what are the links? Curr Opin Allergy Clin Immunol 2005;5:185–93.
49. McKeever TM, Britton J. Diet and asthma. Am J Respir Crit Care Med 2004;170:725–9.
50. Falth-Magnusson K, Kjellman NI. Allergy prevention by maternal elimination diet during late pregnancy – a 5-year follow-up of a randomized study. J Allergy Clin Immunol 1992;89:709–13.

51. Lau S, Nickel R, Niggemann B, et al. The development of childhood asthma: lessons from the German Multicentre Allergy Study (MAS). Paediatr Respir Rev 2002;3:265–72.

52. Platts-Mills T, Vaughan J, Squillace S, et al. Sensitisation, asthma, and a modified Th2 response in children exposed to cat allergen: a population-based cross-sectional study. Lancet 2001;357:752–6.

53. Simpson A, Custovic A. Allergen avoidance in the primary prevention of asthma. Curr Opin Allergy Clin Immunol 2004;4:45–51.

54. Lau S, Illi S, Sommerfeld C, et al. Early exposure to house-dust mite and cat allergens and development of childhood asthma: a cohort study. Multicentre Allergy Study Group. Lancet 2000;356: 1392–7.

55. Litonjua AA, Milton DK, Celedon JC, et al. A longitudinal analysis of wheezing in young children: the independent effects of early life exposure to house dust endotoxin, allergens, and pets. J Allergy Clin Immunol 2002;110:736–42.

56. Campo P, Kalra HK, Levin L, et al. Influence of dog ownership and high endotoxin on wheezing and atopy during infancy. J Allergy Clin Immunol 2006;118:1271–8.

57. Strachan DP. Hay fever, hygiene, and household size. Br Med J 1989;299:1259–60.

58. Long CE, McBride JT, Hall CB. Sequelae of respiratory syncytial virus infections. A role for intervention studies. Am J Respir Crit Care Med 1995;151:1678–80; discussion 80–1.

59. Johnston SL. Overview of virus-induced airway disease. Proc Am Thorac Soc 2005;2:150–6.

60. Ball TM, Castro-Rodriguez JA, Griffith KA, et al. Siblings, day-care attendance, and the risk of asthma and wheezing during childhood. N Engl J Med 2000;343:538–43.

61. Celedon JC, Wright RJ, Litonjua AA, et al. Day care attendance in early life, maternal history of asthma, and asthma at the age of 6 years. Am J Respir Crit Care Med 2003;167:1239–43.

62. Matricardi PM. The role of early infections, hygiene and intestinal micro-flora. Pediatr Pulmonol Suppl 2004;26:211–2.

63. Bremner SA, Carey IM, DeWilde S, et al. Early-life exposure to antibac-terials and the subsequent development of hayfever in childhood in the UK: case-control studies using the General Practice Research Database and the Doctors' Independent Network. Clin Exp Allergy 2003;33:1518–25.

64. Beasley R, Clayton T, Crane J, et al. Association between paracetamol use in infancy and childhood, and risk of asthma, rhinoconjunctivitis, and eczema in children aged 6–7 years: analysis from Phase Three of the ISAAC programme. Lancet 2008;372:1039–48.

65. Yazdanbakhsh M, Matricardi PM. Parasites and the hygiene hypothesis: regulating the immune system? Clin Rev Allergy Immunol 2004;26:15–24.

66. Gehring U, Bolte G, Borte M, et al. Exposure to endotoxin decreases the risk of atopic eczema in infancy: a cohort study. J Allergy Clin Immunol 2001;108:847–54.

67. Braun-Fahrlander C, Riedler J, Herz U, et al. Environmental exposure to endotoxin and its relation to asthma in school-age children. N Engl J Med 2002;347:869–77.

68. van Strien RT, Engel R, Holst O, et al. Microbial exposure of rural school children, as assessed by levels of N-acetyl-muramic acid in mattress dust, and its association with respiratory health. J Allergy Clin Immunol 2004;113:860–7.

69. Ege MJ, Frei R, Bieli C, et al. Not all farming environments protect against the development of asthma and wheeze in children. J Allergy Clin Immunol 2007;119:1140–7.

70. von Mutius E. Gene-environment interactions in asthma. J Allergy Clin Immunol 2009;123:3–11; quiz 2–3.

71. Le Souef PN. Gene-environmental interaction in the development of atopic asthma: new developments. Curr Opin Allergy Clin Immunol 2009;9:123–7.

Natural History of Allergic Diseases and Asthma

Andrew H. Liu • Fernando D. Martinez • Lynn M. Taussig

Natural history studies of allergic diseases and asthma are fundamental for predicting disease onset and prognosis. Such studies reveal a developmental 'allergic march' in childhood, from the early onset of atopic dermatitis (AD) and food allergies in infancy, to asthma, allergic rhinitis (AR), and inhalant allergen sensitization in later childhood. Allergy and asthma of earlier onset and greater severity are generally associated with disease persistence. Therefore, allergy and asthma commonly develop during the early childhood years, the period of greatest immune maturation and lung growth. This highlights the importance of growth and development in a conceptual framework for allergy and asthma pathogenesis.

This chapter reviews the allergic march of childhood and its different clinical manifestations: food allergies, AD, inhalant allergies, AR, and asthma. The natural history of anaphylaxis, an allergic condition not currently implicated in the allergic march, is also covered. Interventions that reduce the prevalence of allergy and asthma are reviewed toward the end of the chapter. The findings and conclusions presented in this chapter are largely based on long-term prospective (i.e., 'natural history') studies. Complementary reviews of the epidemiology of allergic diseases in childhood can be found in Chapter 1, and the prevention and natural history of food allergy in Chapter 47.

It is important to acknowledge current investigational deficits in our understanding of natural history. So far, childhood natural history studies have largely investigated modern metropolitan cohorts and may, therefore, be relevant only for people living in modernized locales. Epidemiologic findings that (1) AR, asthma, and aeroallergen sensitization are less common in children raised in rural areas of developing countries and in farming communities and (2) increased asthma severity occurs in asthmatic children of low-income families in US inner-city communities suggest that the natural history of allergic diseases and asthma is strongly influenced by environmental, lifestyle, and disease management factors.

Allergic March of Childhood

Natural history studies with the following design features provide a firm epidemiologic foundation for risk factor assessments and etiologic hypotheses: (1) long-term cohort studies of a prospective design minimize biases resulting from poor parental recall; (2) multiple evaluations over time provide important checkpoints during the dynamic period of childhood growth and development; and (3) the inclusion of objective disease measurements strengthens these studies by validating subjective disease assessments (i.e. questionnaire data).

Three prospective, longitudinal, birth cohort studies exemplify optimized natural history studies that are rich resources for our current understanding of the development and outcome of allergy and asthma in childhood: (1) the Tucson Children's Respiratory Study (CRS) in Tucson, Arizona (begun in 1980); (2) a Kaiser-based study in San Diego, California (begun in 1981); and the German Multicentre Allergy Study (MAS) in Germany (begun in 1990). The major findings of these studies have been consistent and reveal a common pattern of allergy and asthma development that begins in infancy.

1. The highest incidence of AD and food allergies is in the first 2 years of life (Figure 2-1). It is generally believed that infants rarely manifest allergic symptoms in the first month of life. By 3 months of age, however, AD, food allergies, and wheezing problems are common.
2. This is paralleled by a high prevalence of food allergen sensitization in the first 2 years of life.[1] Early food allergen sensitization is an important risk factor for food allergies, AD, and asthma.
3. Allergic airways diseases generally begin slightly later in childhood (see Figure 2-1). Most persistent asthma begins before 12 years of age. Childhood asthma often initially manifests with a lower respiratory tract infection or bronchiolitis episodes in the first few years of life.
4. AR commonly begins in childhood, although there is also good evidence that AR often develops in early adulthood.[2,3]
5. The development of AR and persistent asthma is paralleled by a rise in inhalant allergen sensitization. Perennial inhalant allergen sensitization (i.e. cat dander, dust mites) emerges between 2 to 5 years of age, and seasonal inhalant allergen sensitization becomes apparent slightly later in life (ages 3 to 5 years).

Early Immune Development Underlying Allergies

A paradigm of immune development underlies allergy development and progression in early childhood and is the subject of Chapter 6. Briefly, the immune system of the fetus is maintained in a tolerogenic state, preventing adverse immune responses and rejection between the mother and fetus. Placental interleukin-10 (IL-10) suppresses the production of immune-potentiating inter-

©2010 Elsevier Ltd, Inc, BV
DOI: 10.1016/B978-1-4377-0271-2.00002-X

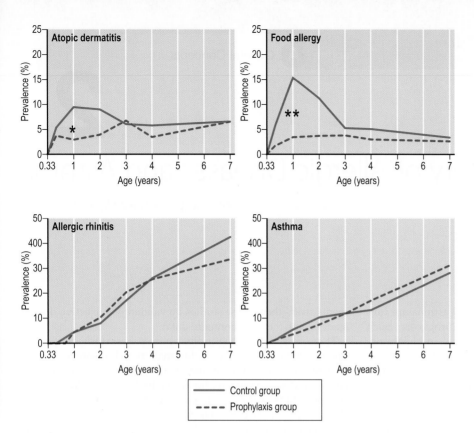

Figure 2-1 Allergic march of early childhood. Period prevalence of atopic dermatitis, food allergy, allergic rhinitis, and asthma from birth to 7 years in prophylactic-treated (allergenic food avoidance) and untreated (control) groups (Kaiser Permanente; San Diego). * $P \leq 0.05$; **$P < 0.01$. (Data from Zeiger RS, Heller S J. Allergy Clin Immunol 1995;95:1179–1190; and Zeiger RS, Heller S, Mellon MH, et al. J Allergy Clin Immunol 1989;84:72–89.)

feron gamma (IFN-γ) by fetal immune cells. IFN-γ downregulates the production of pro-allergic cytokines, such as IL-4 and IL-13. The reciprocal relationship between these cytokines and the immune cells that produce them defines 'T-helper 2' (Th2), pro-allergic immune responses (i.e., IL-4, IL-13), and antiallergic 'T-helper 1' (Th1) immune development (i.e. IFN-γ). Thus the conditions that favor immune tolerance in utero may also foster allergic immune responses. Current studies suggest that newborn immune responses to ubiquitous ingested and inhaled proteins are Th2-biased.[4] Postnatally, encounters with these common allergenic proteins lead to the development of mature immune responses to them. The underlying immune characteristics of allergic diseases – allergen-specific memory Th2 cells and immunoglobulin (IgE) – can be viewed as aberrant manifestations of immune maturation that typically develop during these early years, and might have its roots in the inadequate or delayed development of regulatory T lymphocytes that can inhibit them. Longitudinal prospective studies in young children have provided evidence for this pro-allergic immune developmental process.

Total Serum IgE Levels

At birth, cord blood IgE levels are almost undetectable, but these levels increase during the first 6 years of life. Elevated serum IgE levels in infancy have been associated with persistent asthma in later childhood.[5] High serum IgE levels in later childhood (i.e. after 11 years of age) have also been well correlated with bronchial hyperresponsiveness (BHR) and asthma.[6,7]

Allergen-Specific IgE

In two birth cohort (up to 5 years old) studies of immunoglobulin G and E (IgG and IgE) antibody development to common food

and inhalant allergens, IgG antibodies to milk and egg proteins were detectable in nearly all subjects in the first 12 months of life, implying that the infant immune system sees and responds to commonly ingested proteins.[8,9] In comparison, food allergen-specific IgE (especially to egg) was measurable in approximately 30% of subjects at 1 year of age. Low-level IgE responses to food allergens in infancy were common and transient, and sometimes occurred before introduction of the foods into the diet. In children who developed clinical allergic conditions, higher levels and persistence of food allergen-specific IgE were typical.

Of seasonal inhalant allergens, ragweed and grass allergen-specific IgGs were detectable in approximately 25% of subjects at 3 to 6 months of age, and steadily increased to 40% to 50% by 5 years of age.[10,11] In comparison, allergen-specific IgE was detected in <5% of subjects from 3 to 12 months of age, and increased in prevalence to approximately 20% by 5 years of age. Therefore, allergen-specific IgE production emerges in the preschool years and persists in those who develop clinical allergies.

Allergen-Specific Th2 Lymphocytes

The development of allergen-specific antibody production is indicative of allergen-specific T lymphocytes that are guiding the development and differentiation of B lymphocytes to produce IgE through secreted Th2-type cytokines (i.e., IL-4, IL-13) and cell surface molecular interactions (i.e., CD40/CD40 ligand). T cell-derived IL-4, IL-5, and GM-CSF also support eosinophil and mast cell development and differentiation in allergic inflammation. A current paradigm for allergic disease suggests that pro-allergic Th2 cells are (1) differentiated to produce cytokines that direct allergic responses and inflammation and (2) opposed by Th1 cells that produce counter-regulatory cytokines (e.g., IFN-γ) that inhibit Th2 differentiation. As an example of this Th2/Th1 paradigm, peripheral blood mononuclear cells from infants who ultimately manifest allergic disease at 2 years of age produce more pro-allergic Th2 cytokines (i.e. IL-4) to allergen-specific stimulation in vitro.[10] In comparison, infants who continue to be nonallergic (i.e. no allergic disease and/or no allergen sensitization in later childhood) produce more counter-regulatory IFN-γ to nonspecific[5,11] and allergen-specific[10] stimuli.

Infants with diminished Th1 responses may be more susceptible to developing asthma for additional reasons. Bronchiolitic infants who continued to have persistent wheezing and airflow obstruction also produce less IFN-γ.[12] This suggests that infants who produce less IFN-γ to ubiquitous allergens and to airway viral infections are susceptible to chronic allergic diseases and asthma because (1) they are less able to impede the development of allergen-specific T cells and IgE and (2) they are more likely to manifest persistent airways abnormalities following respiratory viral infections.

Childhood Asthma

Approximately 80% of asthmatic patients report disease onset before 6 years of age.[13] However, of all young children who experience recurrent wheezing, only a minority will go on to have persistent asthma in later life. The most common form of recurrent wheezing in preschool children occurs primarily with viral infections (Box 2-1). These 'transient wheezers' or 'wheezy bronchitics' are not at an increased risk of having asthma in later life. Transient wheezing is associated with airways viral infections, smaller airways and lung size, male gender, low birth weight, and prenatal environmental tobacco smoke (ETS) exposure.

Persistent asthma commonly begins and coexists with the large population of transient wheezers (see Box 2-1). Persistent asthma is strongly associated with allergy, which is evident in the early childhood years as clinical conditions (i.e. AD, AR, food allergies) or by testing for allergen sensitization to inhalant and food allergens (e.g. IgE, allergy skin testing). Severity of childhood asthma, determined clinically or by lung function impairment, also predicts asthma persistence into adulthood.

Early Childhood: Transient vs Persistent Asthma

In the Tucson CRS study, ≈50% of young children experienced a period of recurrent wheezing and/or coughing in the first 6 years of life.[14] These early-childhood wheezers were further subdivided into (1) 'transient early wheezers,' with wheezing only <3 years; (2) 'persistent wheezers,' with manifestations through the first 6 years; and (3) 'late-onset wheezers,' with manifestations only after 3 years. Transient wheezers comprised the largest proportion of the group at 20%; persistent and late-onset wheezers made up slightly smaller proportions (14% and 15%, respectively). Of these three groups, persistent wheezers had the greatest likelihood of persistent asthma in later childhood (Figure 2-2). By age 16 years, ≈50% of those with persistent or late-onset wheezing in early life continued to have recurrent wheezing/coughing episodes.[15] In contrast, the prevalence of persistent asthma in the transient wheezer group was ≈20% and not different from nonwheezers.

Lung function in the Tucson CRS was measured in the first year of life (before the occurrence of lower respiratory tract infections) and at 6 years of age. Interestingly, transient wheezers had the lowest airflow measures in infancy, suggesting that they had the narrowest airways and/or the smallest lungs at birth.[14] Their reduced lung function improved significantly by age 6 years, but continued to be lower than normal at age 16 years.[15] In comparison, persistent wheezers demonstrated normal lung function in the first few months of life but a significant decline in airflow measures by 6 years of age that persisted as lower than normal at age 16 years.[15] Therefore, lung function in transient early and persistent wheezers remained lower than normal nonwheezers through age 16 years, indicating two different clinical patterns of recurrent wheezing in early childhood that are associated with persistently low lung function established early in life.

Some children with BHR in early life are also more likely to have persistent asthma. Investigators of a birth cohort in Perth, Australia, found that BHR at 1 month of age was associated with lower lung function (i.e. FEV_1 and FVC) and a higher likelihood of asthma at 6 years of age.[16] Interestingly, congenital BHR was not associated with total serum IgE, eosinophilia, allergen sensitization, or BHR at 6 years of age and was independent of gender,

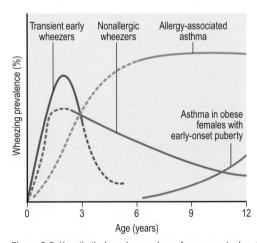

Figure 2-2 Hypothetical yearly prevalence for recurrent wheezing phenotypes in childhood (Tucson Children's Respiratory Study, Tucson, Arizona). This classification does not imply that the groups are exclusive. Dashed lines suggest that wheezing can be represented by different curve shapes resulting from many different factors, including overlap of groups. (Modified from Stein RT, Holberg CJ, Morgan WJ, et al. Thorax 1997;52:946–952.)

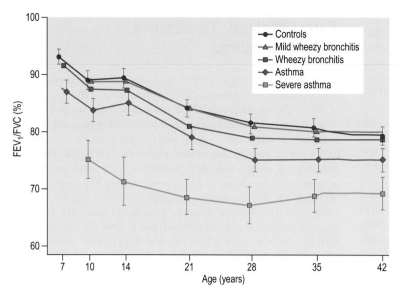

Figure 2-3 Natural history of lung function from childhood to adulthood (Melbourne Longitudinal Study of Asthma, Melbourne, Australia). Subjects were classified according to their diagnosis at time of enrollment: no-wheezing control; mild wheezy bronchitis; wheezy bronchitis; asthma; and severe asthma. Lung function is represented as FEV_1 corrected for lung volume (FEV_1/FVC ratio). Mean values and standard error bars are shown. (Adapted from Oswald H, Phelan PD, Lanigan A, et al. Pediatr Pulmonol 1997;23:14–20; with data for age 42 years from Horak E, Lanigan A, Roberts M, et al. BMJ 2003; 326(7386):422–423.)

family history of asthma, and maternal smoking. In the Tucson CRS study, BHR, measured at age 6 years, predicted chronic and newly diagnosed asthma at age 22 years.[17]

Asthma from Childhood to Adulthood

A cohort of 7-year-old children with asthma living in Melbourne, Australia, was restudied for persistence and severity of asthma at 10, 14, 21, 28, 35, and 42 years of age. At 42 years of age, 71% of the asthmatics and 89% of the severe asthmatics continued to have asthma symptoms; 76% of the severe asthmatics reported frequent or persistent asthma.[18] In comparison, 15% of 'mild wheezy bronchitics' (i.e. wheezing only with colds at 7 years of age) and 28% of 'wheezy bronchitics' (i.e., at least 5 episodes of wheezing with colds) reported frequent or persistent asthma. These observations – that many children with asthma experience disease remission or improvement in early adulthood but that severe asthma persists with age – are remarkably similar to those of several other natural history studies of childhood asthma into adulthood.[19-22]

Spirometric measures of lung function of the Melbourne study children initially revealed that asthmatics (especially severe asthmatics) had lung function impairment, whereas wheezy bronchitics (i.e., 'transient' wheezers) had lung function that was not different from that of nonasthmatics. Over the ensuing years these differences in lung function impairment between groups persisted in parallel, without a greater rate of decline in lung function in any group (Figure 2-3).[18,23] Beginning from birth, in the Tucson CRS, low lung function in infancy also persisted through ages 11, 16, and 22 years.[24] However, some children with persistent asthma demonstrated progressive decline in lung function. In the longitudinal CAMP study, ≈25% of elementary school-age children with persistent asthma manifested progressive decline in lung function annually for 4 years.[25] Risk factors for progressive decline in lung function included male gender, younger age, and hyperinflation. These findings support the importance of the early childhood years in lung and asthma development. The establishment of chronic disease and lung function impairment in early life appears to predict persistent asthma and lung dysfunction well into adulthood; however, progressive decline in lung function can occur in some children during school-age years.

BOX 2-2 Key concepts

Risk Factors for Persistent Asthma

Allergy

Atopic dermatitis

Allergic rhinitis

Elevated total serum IgE levels (first year of life)

Peripheral blood eosinophilia >4% (2 to 3 years of age)

Inhalant and food allergen sensitization

Gender

Males

- Transient wheezing
- Persistent allergy-associated asthma

Females

- Asthma associated with obesity and early-onset puberty
- 'Triad' asthma (adulthood)

Parental Asthma

Lower Respiratory Tract Infections

Rhinovirus, respiratory syncytial virus

Severe bronchiolitis (i.e. requiring hospitalization)

Pneumonia

Environmental Tobacco Smoke Exposure (Including Prenatal)

Risk Factors for Persistent Asthma

Natural history studies of asthma have identified biologic, genetic, and environmental risk factors for persistent asthma (Box 2-2). From the Tucson CRS, a statistical optimization of the major risk factors for persistent childhood asthma provided 97% specificity and 77% positive predictive value for persistent asthma in later childhood (Figure 2-4).[26]

Allergy

Essentially all of the current natural history studies have found that allergic disease and evidence of pro-allergic immune devel-

At least 4 wheezing episodes, plus:	
1 Major criterion	**or 2 Minor criteria**
Parental asthma	Allergic rhinitis
Eczema	Wheezing apart from colds
Inhalant allergen sensitization	Eosinophils ≥ 4%
	Food allergen sensitization

Figure 2-4 Modified Asthma Predictive Index for children (Tucson Children's Respiratory Study, Tucson, Arizona). Through a statistically optimized model for 2- to 3-year-old children with frequent wheezing in the past year, one major criterion or two minor criteria provided 77% positive predictive value and 97% specificity for persistent asthma in later childhood. (Adapted from from Castro-Rodriguez JA, Holberg CH, Wright AL, et al. Am J Respir Crit Care 2000;162:1403–1406; and Guilbert TW, Morgan WJ, Zeiger RS, et al. J Allergy Clin Immunol 2004;114:1282–1287.)

opment are significant risk factors for persistent asthma. For example, in the Tucson CRS, early AD, AR, elevated serum IgE levels in the first year of life, and peripheral blood eosinophilia were all significant risk factors for persistent asthma.[14,26] In the Berlin MAS study, additional risk factors for asthma and BHR at age 7 years included persistent sensitization to foods (i.e. hen's egg, cow's milk, wheat and/or soy) and perennial inhalant allergens (i.e. dust mite, cat dander), especially in early life.[27,28] The combination of allergic sensitization to major indoor allergens (dog, cat and/or mite) by age 3 years with higher levels of allergen exposure in the home was associated with persistent wheezing and lower lung function into adolescence.[29] In the Kaiser San Diego study, milk or peanut allergen sensitization was a risk factor for asthma.[30] Natural history studies of asthma that have extended into adulthood continue to find allergy to be a risk factor for persistent asthma.[20,21] Since the eight-center Childhood Asthma Management Program (CAMP) study of 1041 asthmatic children ages 5 to 12 years found that 88% were sensitized to at least one inhalant allergen at study enrollment, allergy-associated asthma appears to be the most common form of asthma in elementary school-age children in the USA.[31] Furthermore, in the International Study of Asthma and Allergies in Childhood (ISAAC), strong correlations between high asthma prevalence and both high allergic rhinoconjunctivitis and high AD prevalence in different sites throughout the world suggest that allergy-associated asthma is also the most common form of childhood asthma worldwide.[32] In children with recurrent cough or wheeze in early life, early manifestations of atopy are well-regarded predictive risk factors for persistent lung dysfunction and clinical disease (Figure 2-4).[33,34]

Gender

Male gender is a risk factor for both transient wheezing and persistent asthma in childhood.[14,30] This is generally believed to be caused by the smaller airways of young boys when compared with girls.[35,36] Later in childhood, BHR and inhalant allergen sensitization are more prevalent in boys than in girls.[37,38] For asthma persistence from childhood to adulthood, female gender is a risk factor for greater asthma severity[20] and BHR.[19] Female children who become overweight are also more likely to develop asthma in adolescence, an association not appreciated in males.[39] These observations are consistent with the higher prevalence of asthma in males in childhood and in females in adulthood.[13]

Parental History of Asthma

Infants whose parents report a history of childhood asthma have lower lung function and are more likely to wheeze in early life,[40,41] in later childhood,[14,30] and in adulthood.[20] However, in a two-generation, longitudinal study in Aberdeen, Scotland, the children of well-characterized subjects without atopy or asthma were found to have a surprisingly high prevalence of allergen sensitization (56%) and wheezing (33%).[42] Similarly, in the MAS study, the majority of children with AD and/or asthma in early childhood were born to nonallergic parents.[43] For example, of the study's asthmatic children at 5 years of age, 57% were born to parents without an atopic history. Therefore allergen sensitization and asthma seem to be occurring at high rates, even in persons considered to be at low genetic risk for allergy and asthma.

Lower Respiratory Tract Infections

Certain respiratory viruses have been associated with persistent wheezing problems in children. It is not known if persistent airways abnormalities are primarily the result of virus-induced damage, vulnerable individuals revealing their airway susceptibility to virus-induced airflow obstruction, or airways injury with aberrant repair. In long-term studies, infants hospitalized with respiratory syncytial virus (RSV) bronchiolitis (most occurred by 4 months of age) were significantly more likely to have asthma and lung dysfunction through age 13 years.[44] In the Tucson CRS birth cohort, 91% of lower respiratory tract infections (LRTIs) in the first 3 years of life were cultured for common pathogens: 44% were RSV-positive, 14% were parainfluenza-positive, 14% were culture-positive for other respiratory pathogens, and 27% were culture-negative.[45] Followed prospectively, infants with RSV LRTI were more likely to have wheezing symptoms at 6 years of age but not at later ages (i.e. 11 and 13 years old). However, young children who had radiographic evidence of pneumonia or croup symptoms accompanying wheezing were more likely to have persistent asthma symptoms and lung function impairment at 6 and 11 years of age.[46,47]

Improved PCR-based detection methods have affirmed a strong association between rhinovirus infection and asthma exacerbations, such that ≈40–70% of wheezing illnesses and asthma exacerbations in children can be attributed to rhinovirus.[48–50] People with asthma do not appear to be more susceptible to rhinovirus infection; but they are more likely to develop an LRTI with symptoms that are more severe and longer lasting.[51] In the Childhood Origins of Asthma (COAST) birth cohort study, 90% of children with rhinovirus-associated wheezing episodes at age 3 years had asthma at age 6 years, such that a rhinovirus-associated wheezing episode at age 3 years was a stronger predictor of subsequent asthma than aeroallergen sensitization (odds ratios 25.6 versus 3.4).[52] This supports the premise that individuals with lower airway vulnerability to common respiratory viruses are at risk for wheezing episodes and persistent asthma.

Environmental Tobacco Smoke Exposure

ETS exposure is a risk factor for wheezing problems at all ages. Prenatal ETS exposure is associated, in a dose-dependent manner, with wheezing manifestations and decreased lung function in infancy and early childhood.[53,54] Postnatal ETS exposure is associated with a greater likelihood of wheezing in infancy,[41] transient wheezing, and persistent asthma in childhood.[14] Cigarette smoking has also been strongly associated with persistent asthma and asthma relapses in adulthood.[21]

ETS exposure is also associated with food allergen sensitization,[55] AR, hospitalization for LRTIs, BHR, and elevated serum IgE levels.[56,57] In a 7-year prospective study, ETS exposure was associated with greater inhalant allergen sensitization and reduced lung function.[30]

Asthma- and Allergy-Protective Influences

Some lifestyle differences may impart asthma- and/or allergy-protective effects. Natural history studies have started to contribute some epidemiologic evidence in support of these hypotheses.

Breast-Feeding

Numerous studies have investigated the potential of early breast-feeding as a protective influence against the development of allergy and asthma. Meta-analyses of prospective studies of exclusive breast-feeding for 4 or more months from birth have been associated with less AD and asthma (summary odds ratios of 0.68 and 0.70, respectively).[58,59] In the Tucson CRS, breast-feeding generally reduced the risk of recurrent wheezing up to 2 years of age (odds ratio 0.45); however, in a subgroup of atopic children who were exclusively breast-fed for 4 months by asthmatic mothers, the risk of persistent asthma between 6 and 13 years of age was increased (odds ratio 8.7),[60] and their lung function through age 16 years was lower.[61] This surprising finding was corroborated by findings that infants breast-fed by mothers with higher IgE levels also had higher IgE levels at ages 6 and 11 years.[62] Nevertheless, when considered with many other health and developmental attributes of breast-feeding, prolonged breast-feeding should still be recommended.

Microbial Exposures

Numerous epidemiologic studies have found that a variety of microbial exposures are associated with a lower likelihood of allergen sensitization, allergic disease, and asthma. This has led to a 'hygiene' hypothesis, which proposes that the reduction of microbial exposures in childhood in modernized locales has led to the rise in allergy and asthma.[63] This hypothesis is actually based on immune development. Microbes and their molecular components are potent inducers of Th1-type and regulatory immune development and immune memory. Theoretically, microbial exposures in early life, by promoting Th1-type immune memory and appropriate immune regulation, might prevent the development of allergen sensitization and diseases, while strengthening the immune response and controlling inflammation to common respiratory viral infections.

To address this hypothesis, natural history studies have begun to explore the relationships between microbes and their components (e.g. home environmental bacterial endotoxin) to the development of allergies and asthma:

1. In the Tucson CRS, children raised in larger families or in daycare from an early age (believed to be surrogate measures for more respiratory infections and microbial exposures) were less likely to have asthma symptoms in later childhood.[64] In the German MAS study, more runny nose colds in the first 3 years of life were associated with a lower likelihood

of allergen sensitization, asthma, and BHR at 7 years of age.[65] A dose-dependent effect was observed, such that children who experienced at least 8 colds by age 3 years had an adjusted odds ratio of 0.16 for asthma at age 7 years.

2. In infants and children, higher house-dust endotoxin levels were associated with less AD,[66-68] inhalant allergen sensitization,[69,70-72] AR, and asthma.[73,74] The strength of this evidence is apparent in these studies, which are prospective or demonstrate dose-response relationships. Complementary immunological studies reveal that higher house-dust endotoxin levels were associated with increased proportions of Th1-type cells,[69] higher levels of IFN-γ from stimulated peripheral blood samples,[75,76] and immune down-regulation of endotoxin-stimulated blood samples.[73] In contrast to these atopy-protective influences, higher endotoxin levels were associated with more wheezing, often in the same studies where a protective effect on atopy in early life was concurrently observed.[66,68,70,73,77]

3. Since gastrointestinal (GI) microbiota stimulate and shape early immune development, some investigators identified differences in the bacteria in stool samples from newborns and infants who ultimately go on to develop allergic disease. The stools of infants who develop allergy had more clostridia and *Staphylococcus aureus*, while nonallergic infants had more enterococci, bifidobacteria, lactobacilli, and *Bacteroides*,[78-81] However, in another study, bacteroides colonization in infants' stools was associated with a higher prevalence of early-onset asthma.[82] Using culture-independent methods of microbiota diversity, the stool of 1-week-old infants who subsequently developed AD was significantly less diverse than their noneczema counterparts.[83] Alterations in the gut flora of infants from dietary and environmental differences (i.e. breast versus formula feeding, semi-sterile food, antibiotic use, siblings and/or pets) may have an allergy-protective effect on the developing immune system.

Pet Ownership

Multiple longitudinal birth cohort studies have observed dog and/or cat ownership to be associated with a lower likelihood of AD, allergen sensitization, and asthma.[84-86] Similarly, in farming and rural locales, a lower likelihood of allergy and asthma has been associated with animal contact or the keeping of domestic animals in the home.[87] Two meta-analyses of numerous studies of domestic animal exposure and allergy and asthma outcomes generally found a protective effect.[88,89] Although the mechanism(s) for this protective association is unclear, one possibility is that greater bacterial exposure occurs with animal contact and/or animal/petkeeping in the home. Indoor pets are a major factor associated with higher indoor endotoxin levels in metropolitan homes.[87]

Vitamin D

There is current conjecture that vitamin D supplementation can prevent allergy and asthma. It has been hypothesized that modern lifestyles with greater time spent indoors have fostered a propensity for vitamin D deficiency, resulting in more asthma and allergy.[90,91] The scientific rationale is appealing: vitamin D has been recently shown to bolster innate antimicrobial and regulatory T lymphocyte responses, and improve immune responses to corticosteroids and allergen immunotherapy in the lab.[90] Complementing this mechanistic science, three birth cohorts studies have observed that high maternal vitamin D intake during pregnancy was associated with a lower risk of recurrent/persistent wheeze or asthma in preschool childhood.[92-94] In children with asthma, vitamin D insufficiency has been associated with a greater likelihood of severe exacerbations, and higher serum total IgE levels and eosinophil counts.[95] The potential preventive and thereapeutic benefits of vitamin D supplementation on allergy and asthma are prime targets for clinical trials to reconcile these important questions.

Other Types of Childhood Asthma

Although males are more likely to experience childhood asthma, the incidence of new-onset cases of asthma becomes more common in females in early adolescence. One contributor to this gender shift in asthma onset was described in the Tucson CRS. Female children who became overweight between 6 and 11 years of age (defined as body mass index ≥85th percentile) were more likely to develop new-onset asthma between 11 and 13 years of age (see Figure 2-2).[39] This effect was strongest in females with early-onset puberty (i.e. before age 11 years) and was not observed in males.

Asthma mediated by occupational-type exposures is often not considered in children, and yet some children are raised in settings where occupational-type exposures can mediate asthma in adults (e.g. children raised on farms or with farm animals in the home). Children with hypersensitivity and exposure to other common airways irritants or air pollutants such as ETS, endotoxin, ozone, sulphur dioxide, or cold air may also contribute to the pool of nonatopic children with persistent asthma. 'Triad' asthma, characteristically associated with hyperplastic sinusitis/nasal polyposis and/or hypersensitivity to nonsteroidal antiinflammatory medications (e.g. aspirin, ibuprofen), rarely occurs in childhood.

Atopic Dermatitis

AD usually begins during the preschool years and persists throughout childhood. Two prospective birth cohort studies have found the peak incidence of AD to be in the first 2 years of life (see Figure 2-1).[30,96] Although 66% to 90% of patients with AD have clinical manifestations before 7 years of age,[97,98] eczematous lesions in the first 2 months of life are rare. Natural history studies of AD have reported a wide variation (35% to 82%) in disease persistence throughout childhood.[98,99] The greatest remission in AD seems to occur between 8 and 11 years of age and, to a lesser extent, between 12 and 16 years.[98] Natural history studies of AD may have underestimated the persistent nature of the disease for reasons that include (1) AD definition – some studies have included other forms of dermatitis that have a better prognosis over time (i.e. seborrheic dermatitis),[100] (2) AD recurrence – a recent 23-year birth cohort study found that many patients who went into disease remission in childhood had an AD recurrence in early adulthood,[98] and (3) AD manifestation – it is generally believed that patients with childhood AD will often evolve to manifest hand and/or foot dermatitis as adults.

Parental history of AD is an important risk factor for childhood AD. This apparent heritability complements studies revealing a high concordance rate of AD among monozygotic versus dizygotic twins (0.72 vs 0.23, respectively).[101] In a risk factor assessment for AD in the first 2 years of life, higher levels of maternal education and living in less crowded homes were risk factors for early-onset AD.[102] The environmental/lifestyle risk factors

AD severity	Initial examination		4 years later		
	Inhalant ± food	Food only	Inhalant ± food	Food only	Asthma and/or AR
Mild	15%	20%	31%	6%	15%
Moderate	18%	26%	52%	6%	32%
Severe	20%	45%	100%	0%	75%

Figure 2-5 Atopic dermatitis (AD) in young children (2 months to 3 years of age) and allergen sensitization (to food and inhalant allergens), asthma, and allergic rhinoconjunctivitis (AR) 4 years later. At enrollment, AD severity was determined, and no subjects had AR or asthma. Four years later, 88% of subjects had a marked improvement or complete resolution of AD. However, all children with severe AD at enrollment were sensitized to inhalant allergens, and 75% had asthma and/or AR. (From Patrizi A, Guerrini V, Ricci G, et al. Pediatr Dermatol 2000; 17:261–265.)

reported for AR and asthma are similar. A meta-analysis of prospective breast-feeding studies concluded that exclusive breast-feeding of infants with a family history of atopy for at least the first 3 months of life is associated with a lower likelihood of childhood AD (odds ratio 0.58). This protective effect was not observed, however, in children without a family history of atopy.[58]

Initial AD disease severity seems predictive of later disease severity and persistence. Of adolescents with moderate to severe AD, 77% to 91% continued to have persistent disease in adulthood.[103] In comparison, of adolescents with mild AD, 50% had AD in adulthood. Food allergen sensitization and exposure in early childhood also contribute to AD development and disease severity. Food allergen sensitization is associated with greater AD severity[30,104] Furthermore, elimination of common allergenic foods in infancy (i.e. soy, milk, egg, peanuts) is associated with a lower prevalence of allergic skin conditions up to age 2 years (see Figure 2-1).[30]

Natural history studies have found early childhood AD to be a major risk factor for food allergen sensitization in infancy,[105] inhalant allergen sensitization,[105,106] and persistent asthma in later childhood.[14,26] In particular, severe AD in early childhood is associated with a high prevalence of allergen sensitization and airways allergic disease in later childhood (i.e. 4 years later; Figure 2-5). Indeed, in young patients with severe AD, 100% developed inhalant allergen sensitization and 75% developed an allergic respiratory disease (mostly asthma) over 4 years. In contrast to severe AD, patients with mild to moderate AD were not as likely to develop allergen sensitization (36%) or an allergic respiratory disease (26%). More information on current concepts of barrier and immune dysfunction in AD, and the role of food hypersensitivity, can be found in Chapters 53 and 51, respectively.

Allergic Rhinitis

Many people develop AR during childhood. Two prospective birth cohort studies reported a steady rise in total (i.e. seasonal and perennial) AR prevalence, reaching 35% to 40% by age 7 years.[30,107] Seasonal AR emerged after 2 years of age and increased steadily to 15% by age 7 years.[107]

AR also commonly begins in early adulthood. In a 23-year cohort study of Brown University students beginning in their freshman year, perennial AR developed in 4.8% at 7 years and 14% at 23 years of follow-up.[2,3] The incidence increase for seasonal AR was substantially greater: 13% at 7 years and 41% at 23

15

years of follow-up.[2,3] Allergen skin test sensitization and asthma were prognostic risk factors for the development of AR.

AR persistence has been evaluated in adult patients. Three follow-up studies of adult AR patients have found a disease remission rate of 5% to 10% by 4 years[108] and 23% by 23 years.[2] In the 23-year follow-up study, 55% of the follow-up subjects reported improvement in rhinitis. Onset of disease in early childhood was associated with greater improvement.[2]

Food Allergy

Food-adverse reactions in childhood include food hypersensitivity that is IgE-mediated and manifests as classic allergic symptoms of immediate onset. Other food-allergic reactions, such as eosinophilic gastroenteropathy and delayed-onset reactions, have variable associations with foods and lack natural history studies.

Natural history studies reveal that the prevalence of food hypersensitivity is greatest in the first few years of life, affecting 5% to 15% of children in their first year of life.[109,110] Most children become tolerant of or seem to 'outgrow' their food allergies to milk, soy, and egg within a few years. In a prospective study of young children with milk allergy, most became nonallergic within a few years: 50% by 1 year of age, 70% by 2 years, and 85% by 3 years.[111] Older children and adults with food allergies are less likely to become tolerant (26% to 33%).[112,113] Long-term follow-up studies of peanut-allergic children found that loss of clinical hypersensitivity was uncommon, especially in children with anaphylactic symptoms in addition to urticaria and/or AD.[114,115] Allergies to other nuts, fish, and shellfish are also believed to be more persistent. It is purported that allergen avoidance diets in food-allergic children increase their likelihood of losing clinical hypersensitivity, but this has not been well studied.[113]

Hypersensitivity to milk at 1 year of age was a risk factor for additional food allergies in later childhood.[116,117] Furthermore, food hypersensitivity in early life (i.e. to milk, egg, peanut) was found to be a risk factor for AD[118,119] and, later, asthma.[27,30] More information on the natural history and prevention of food allergy can be found in Chapter 47.

Anaphylaxis

Anaphylaxis in children can result from numerous possible exposures (e.g. foods, antibiotics, insulin, insect venoms, latex) and is sometimes anaphylactoid (clinically similar but non-IgE-mediated reaction, such as occurs with radio-contrast media and aspirin/nonsteroidal antiinflammatory drugs) or idiopathic. A history of AR or asthma is a risk factor for anaphylaxis to foods and latex.[120] A history of asthma, pollenosis, or food and/or drug allergy is a surprising risk factor for anaphylactoid reactions to radio-contrast media, with a higher prevalence of adverse reactions to ionic versus nonionic contrast media observed.[121] In contrast, atopy is not a risk factor for anaphylaxis to insulin,[122] penicillin,[123] or insect stings.[124] The natural history of anaphylactic reactions in children has been studied prospectively only for food-induced anaphylaxis (described previously) and bee sting anaphylaxis.

In a Johns Hopkins study examining the natural history of bee venom allergy in children, venom-allergic children with a history of mild generalized reactions were randomly assigned to venom immunotherapy or no treatment and then subjected to a repeat sting in a medical setting 4 years later.[125] Systemic allergic reac-

tions occurred in 1.2% of the treated group and 9.2% of the untreated group. Moreover, no systemic reactions that occurred were more severe than the original incidents. In a smaller study of children and adults with venom hypersensitivity, repeat sting challenges, at least 5 years after the original incidents, induced no systemic reactions in those who originally presented with only urticaria/angioedema but did induce systemic reactions in 21% of those who originally had respiratory and/or cardiovascular complications.[126]

These studies suggest that insect sting anaphylaxis is often self-limited in children, with spontaneous remission usually occurring within 4 years. Those at greatest risk of persistent hypersensitivity include those with previous severe anaphylactic episodes. Conversely, those children with mild systemic reactions to bee stings are less likely to have an allergic reaction on re-sting, and any future anaphylactic episodes from bee stings are not likely to be severe. Finally, in a re-challenge study of subjects with no clinical response to a first sting challenge, 21% experienced anaphylaxis to the second challenge, and, of those, one half developed symptomatic hypotension requiring epinephrine.[127]

Gene-Environment Interactions

Gene-environment interactions validate the central paradigm that allergy and asthma development results from common environmental exposures affecting the inherently susceptible host. There are several notable examples related to childhood asthma and AD:

1. *CD14, endotoxin and dogs:* Polymorphisms in genes encoding proteins that mediate endotoxin recognition can modify endotoxin responsiveness. A common polymorphism in the promoter region (-260C-to-T) of the CD14 gene (endotoxin promoter/enhancer protein) has been one of the most studied polymorphisms with regard to asthma and allergies. Functionally, the -260CT CD14 promoter polymorphism alters the transcriptional regulation of CD14; the T allele increases CD14 transcription by reducing the binding of proteins that inhibit gene transcription.[128] Some studies have found that the C allele of the -260 CD14 promoter polymorphism increases the risk for allergic sensitization,[129,130] while others have not.[131,132] Furthermore, some studies show this allele to have either protective or risk effects, depending on the type of environment in which the individuals live. These discrepancies are likely to be owing to different levels of exposure to endotoxin or similar microbial components. For example, in a birth cohort study, only the low-responder, 'CC' homozygous, group demonstrated strong dose-response relationships between higher house dust endotoxin levels and less subsequent allergic sensitization to inhalant allergens, less AD and more nonatopic wheeze.[133] Similarly, the C allele was found to be protective in children living in a subset of homes where measured endotoxin levels were high.[134] In another birth cohort study, the protective effect of dog ownership on AD in infancy occurred only in those who were of the CD14 'TT' genotype.[86]

2. *Glutathione S-transferases (GSTs), environmental tobacco smoke (ETS), and diesel exhaust:* Genetic susceptibility to common air pollutant exposures increases the risk of childhood asthma. For example, polymorphisms in the endogenous antioxidant GST genes (e.g. GSTM1 null) were associated with less asthma in children; these associations were strengthened when genetic GST susceptibility was combined with maternal smoking.[135-137] In a longitudinal birth cohort study, diesel

exhaust particulate exposure was associated with persistent wheezing only in those children carrying a specific genotypic variant in GST-P1 (valine at position 105).[138] Similar to the GST polymorphisms, genetic variants in chromosome 17q21 increased the risk of early-onset asthma; this risk was further increased by early ETS exposure.[139]

3. *Filaggrin and cat exposure*: Loss-of-function mutations in the gene encoding filaggrin (important to skin physical barrier) have been associated with the development of AD. In two independent birth cohorts, cat ownership further increased the risk of developing AD in infants with filaggrin mutations.[140] The effect of cat exposure was independent of allergic sensitization, and not observed with either dog ownership or mite allergen levels.

These findings demonstrate how ordinary environmental exposures conspire with genetic susceptibilities to exert stronger effects on the development of asthma and allergy than either genes or environmental exposures alone.

Prevention Studies

Early-intervention studies to prevent the development of allergic disease and asthma have had limited success so far. Nevertheless, because of their prospective design, such studies can add valuable insights to the natural history of allergic diseases.

Avoidance of Allergenic Foods

Perhaps the best-studied intervention so far has been a 7-year follow-up of a randomized, controlled intervention study performed at Kaiser Permanente in San Diego, California, in which the common allergenic foods (cow's milk, peanut, egg, fish) were eliminated from the diets of at-risk infants (i.e. with one parent with an atopic disorder and allergen sensitization) from the third trimester of pregnancy to 24 months of life[110] (see Figure 2-1). Although this intervention significantly reduced the prevalence of food allergen sensitization, AD, and urticarial rash in the first year of life,[110] a lower prevalence of allergic disease did not persist at either age 4 or 7 years[30] (see Figure 2-1). Furthermore, no effect was observed on inhalant allergen sensitization or allergic airways conditions.

Inhalant Allergen Elimination/Reduction

Randomized clinical trials of home inhalant allergen reduction beginning prebirth have had mixed results. An intensive indoor allergen reduction intervention did not affect the risk of respiratory symptoms, wheeze, rhinitis, or AD at age 3 years; although intervention was associated with a higher prevalence of allergic sensitization, it was conversely associated with better lung function, i.e. lower airways resistance.[141] Addition of thorough dust mite reduction measures to food allergen avoidance for 1 year reduced the likelihood of AD from 1 to 4 years of age and reduced the incidence of allergen sensitization at age 4 years.[142-144] Decreased asthma was observed in the first year of life but not at age 2 or 4 years. An intervention including house dust, pets, and ETS avoidance, breast-feeding, and delayed introduction of solid foods was associated with a lower risk of asthma at age 7 years; BHR, allergic sensitization, AR, and AD were not affected.[145] A systematic review and meta-analysis of three multi-faceted and 6 mono-faceted allergen reduction trials suggested that exposure reduction to multiple indoor allergens, but not mono-allergen interventions, modestly reduced the likelihood of asthma in children.[146] The modest effect of these allergen reduction interventions may be attributable to the partial effectiveness of these specific interventions in lowering home allergen levels, allergen exposure that occurs outside of the home, and the potential unintended effect of the interventions on other environmental disease modifiers (e.g. endotoxin). Improving allergen reduction/elimination (i.e dehumidification[147]) could potentially be more effective. Dust mite-sensitive children with asthma who have been moved to high-altitude locales without dust mite allergen,[148,149] or whose bedrooms have undergone extensive mite reduction measures,[58,59,150] experience significant asthma improvement, sometimes dramatically.

Breast-Feeding

This has been best addressed in prospective studies, discussed earlier in this chapter.

Environmental Tobacco Smoke Elimination/Reduction

The acquisition of definitive proof of the preventive value of reducing or eliminating ETS exposure in infancy and childhood has been hindered by the difficulties in achieving long-term smoking cessation in randomized, controlled studies. ETS exposure at all ages, from prenatal exposure of mothers to smoking in asthmatic adults, is associated with more wheezing problems and more severe disease and is discussed earlier in this chapter. When considered with other health benefits of ETS exposure avoidance, this is strongly recommended.

Pharmacologic Intervention

Several studies have attempted to determine if conventional therapy for allergy and asthma may be able to alter the natural course of the allergic march or to prevent persistent allergic disease and chronic asthma.

Antihistamines

In the Early Treatment of the Atopic Child (ETAC) study, the antihistamine cetirizine was administered for 18 months to young children at high risk for asthma. Of subjects receiving cetirizine, only young children with early allergen sensitization to mites or grass pollen were less likely to develop asthma symptoms during the treatment period.[151] Eighteen months after cetirizine discontinuation, a slightly lower incidence of asthma symptoms continued for the cetirizine-treated, grass-allergic subjects only.[152]

Conventional 'Controller' Pharmacotherapy for Asthma

In the CAMP study, 5- to 12-year-old children were treated with daily inhaled corticosteroid (ICS, budesonide), daily inhaled nonsteroidal antiinflammatory medication (nedocromil), or placebo for more than 4 years.[27] Study medication was then discontinued. During treatment, the ICS-treated subjects demonstrated significant improvement in most of the clinical outcomes and lung function measures of asthma, including BHR to methacholine. After ICS discontinuation, however, the mean BHR of the ICS-treated group regressed to that of the placebo group.

Nedocromil-treated subjects did not improve BHR when compared with placebo. This suggests that, although long-term ICS administration in school-age children with asthma significantly improves asthma severity, it does not increase the likelihood of asthma remission in later childhood or adulthood.

Similarly, randomized controlled trials with ICS administered earlier in life have not demonstrated a preventive effect on the development of persistent asthma. Intermittent 2-week ICS courses administered to infants for episodic wheezing in the first 3 years of life neither improved their wheezing episodes nor their likelihood of developing persistent wheezing.[153] Daily ICS administered to infants with 1–2 prior confirmed wheezing episodes did not improve asthma, wheeze, or lung function outcomes at age 5 years.[154] Daily ICS administered for 2 years to toddler-age children meeting modified asthma predictive index criteria for persistent asthma (Figure 2-4) improved clinical asthma while on treatment, but did not alter the likelihood of asthma persistence during a third treatment-free year.[155] Although, as a meta-analysis of 29 studies of infants and preschoolers with recurrent wheezing or asthma concluded, daily ICS improves respiratory symptoms, exacerbations, and lung function,[156] it does not appear to improve the natural course of asthma.

Allergen-Specific Immunotherapy

Allergen-specific immunotherapy (AIT) has been studied to determine if it can reduce the likelihood of asthma development in children with AR. A recently published randomized, controlled study found that a 3-year AIT course administered to children with birch and/or grass pollen AR reduced rhinoconjunctivitis severity, conjunctival sensitivity to allergen, and the likelihood of developing asthma at 2 and 7 years after AIT discontinuation.[157,158] AIT also prevents the development of new sensitization to inhalant allergens.[159,160] These studies suggest that AIT may alter the allergic march of inhalant allergen sensitization and asthma, but the difficulties and risks of conventional AIT in children warrant careful consideration.

Probiotics

Some studies suggest that oral probiotic supplementation in infancy may prevent atopy by promoting Th1-type and/or regulatory T lymphocyte immune development. In breast-feeding mothers who received lactobacillus supplementation, their breast milk had higher concentrations of the antiinflammatory cytokine TGF-β, and their infants had a reduced risk of AD of 0.32.[161] Lactobacillus ingestion has also been associated with increased infant peripheral blood IL-10 production and serum IL-10 levels.[162] A meta-analysis of 6 randomized controlled trials to prevent AD in children, usually beginning with maternal intake before birth, reported less AD in the probiotic-treated group.[163] Other clinical trials with lactobacillus or combined pro-/prebiotics demonstrated reduced respiratory infection illnesses in young children.[164–166] A large RCT (n = 1018) of pre-/probiotic supplementation to prevent allergies found no significant differences in allergic sensitization, AD, AR, or asthma at 5 years of age; however, it significantly reduced the odds ratio (0.47) of IgE-associated allergic disease in cesarean-delivered children.[167] Differences in the specific probiotic strains used in the different clinical trials may contribute to the differences in findings between studies.

To summarize, allergic diseases and asthma commonly develop in the early childhood years. Current paradigms of immune development and lung growth shape the understanding of disease pathogenesis. The systemic nature of these conditions is such that manifestations of one allergic condition are often risk factors for others (e.g. AD and allergen sensitization are risk factors for persistent asthma). Although many allergy and asthma sufferers improve and can even become disease-free as adults, those with severe disease and some particular conditions (e.g. peanut allergy) are likely to have lifelong disease.

References

1. Kulig M, Bergmann R, Klettke U, et al. Natural course of sensitization to food and inhalant allergens during the first 6 years of life. J Allergy Clin Immunol 1999;103:1173–9.
2. Greisner WA, Settipane RJ, Settipane GA. Co-existence of asthma and allergic rhinitis: a 23-year follow-up study of college students. Allergy Asthma Proc 1998;19:185–8.
3. Hagy GW, Settipane GA. Risk factors for developing asthma and allergic rhinitis: a 7-year follow-up study of college students. J Allergy Clin Immunol 1976;58:330–6.
4. Prescott SL, Macaubas C, Holt BJ, et al. Transplacental priming of the human immune system to environmental allergens: universal skewing of initial T cell responses toward the Th2 cytokine profile. J Immunol 1998;160:4730–7.
5. Martinez FD, Stern DA, Wright AL, et al. Association of interleukin-2 and interferon-g production by blood mononuclear cells in infancy with parental allergy skin tests and with subsequent development of atopy. J Allergy Clin Immunol 1995;96:652–60.
6. Burrows B, Sears MR, Flannery EM, et al. Relation of the course of bronchial responsiveness from age 9 to age 15 to allergy. Am J Respir Crit Care Med 1995;152:1302–8.
7. Sears MR, Burrows B, Flannery EM, et al. Relation between airway responsiveness and serum IgE in children with asthma and in apparently normal children. N Engl J Med 1991;325:1067–71.
8. Hattevig G, Kjellman B, Johansson SG, et al. Clinical symptoms and IgE responses to common food proteins in atopic and healthy children. Clin Allergy 1984;14:551–9.
9. Rowntree S, Cogswell JJ, Platts-Mills TAE, et al. Development of IgE and IgG antibodies to food and inhalant allergens in children at risk of allergic disease. Arch Dis Child 1985;60:727–35.
10. Prescott SL, Macaubas C, Smallacombe TB, et al. Development of allergen-specific T cell memory in atopic and normal children. Lancet 1999;353:196–200.
11. Tang ML, Kemp AS, Thorburn J, et al. Reduced interferon-gamma secretion in neonates and subsequent atopy. Lancet 1994;344:983–5.
12. Renzi PM, Turgeon JP, Marcotte JE, et al. Reduced interferon-g production in infants with bronchiolitis and asthma. Am J Resp Cut Care Med 1999;159:1417–22.
13. Yunginger JW, Reed CE, O'Connell, EJ, et al. A community-based study of the epidemiology of asthma: incidence rates, 1964–1983. Am Rev Respir Dis 1992;146:888–94.
14. Martinez FD, Wright AL, Taussig LM, et al. Asthma and wheezing in the first six years of life. N Engl J Med 1995;332:133–8.
15. Morgan WJ, Stern DA, Sherrill DL, et al. Outcome of asthma and wheezing in the first 6 years of life: follow-up through adolescence. Am J Respir Crit Care Med 2005;72:1253–8.
16. Palmer LJ, Rye PJ, Gibson NA, et al. Airway responsiveness in early infancy predicts asthma, lung function, and respiratory symptoms by school age. Am J Respir Crit Care Med 2001;163:37–42.
17. Stern DA, Morgan WJ, Halonen M, et al. Wheezing and bronchial hyperresponsiveness in early childhood as predictors of newly diagnosed asthma in early adulthood: a longitudinal birth-cohort study. Lancet 2008;372:1058–64.
18. Horak E, Lanigan A, Roberts M, et al. Longitudinal study of childhood wheezy bronchitis and asthma: outcome at age 42. Br Med J 2003;326:422–3.
19. Godden DJ, Ross S, Abdalla M, et al. Outcome of wheeze in childhood. Am J Respir Crit Care Med 1994;149:106–12.
20. Jenkins MA, Hopper JL, Bowes G, et al. Factors in childhood as predictors of asthma in adult life. Br Med J 1994;309:90–3.
21. Strachan DP, Butland BK, Anderson HR. Incidence and prognosis of asthma and wheezing illness from early childhood to age 33 in a national British cohort. Br Med J 1996;312:1195–9.
22. Sears MR, Greene JM, Willan AR, et al. A longitudinal, population-based, cohort study of childhood asthma followed to adulthood. N Engl J Med 2003;349:1414–22.
23. Oswald H, Phelan PD, Lanigan A, et al. Childhood asthma and lung function in mid-adult life. Pediatr Pulmonol 1997;23:14–20.
24. Stern DA, Morgan WJ, Wright AL, et al. Poor airway function in early infancy and lung function by age 22 years: a non-selective longitudinal cohort study. Lancet 2007;370:758–64.

25. Covar RA, Spahn JD, Murphy JR, et al. Childhood Asthma Management Program Research Group. Progression of asthma measured by lung function in the childhood asthma management program. Am J Respir Crit Care Med 2004;170:234–41.

26. Castro-Rodriguez JA, Holberg CJ, Wright AL, et al. A clinical index to define risk of asthma in young children with recurrent wheezing. Am J Respir Crit Care Med 2000;162:1403–6.

27. Kulig M, Bergmann R, Tacke U, et al. Long-lasting sensitization to food during the first two years precedes allergic airway disease: the MAS Study Group, Germany. Pediatr Allergy Immunol 1998;9:61–7.

28. Lau S, Illi S, Sommerfeld C, et al. Early exposure to house-dust mite and cat allergens and development of childhood asthma: a cohort study – Multicentre Allergy Study Group. Lancet 2000;356:1392–7.

29. Illi S, von Mutius E, Lau S, et al. Multicentre Allergy Study (MAS) group. Perennial allergen sensitisation early in life and chronic asthma in children: a birth cohort study. Lancet 2006;368:763–70.

30. Zeiger RS, Heller S. The development and prediction of atopy in high-risk children: follow-up at age seven years in a prospective randomized study of combined maternal and infant food allergen avoidance. Allergy Clin Immunol 1995;95:1179–90.

31. The Childhood Asthma Management Program Research Group. Long-term effects of budesonide or nedocromil in children with asthma. N Engl J Med 2000;343:1054–63.

32. ISAAC Steering Committee. Worldwide variation in prevalence of symptoms of asthma, allergic rhinoconjunctivitis, and atopic eczema: ISAAC. Lancet 1998;351:1225–32.

33. Guilbert TW, Morgan WJ, Zeiger RS, et al. Atopic characteristics of children with recurrent wheezing at high risk for the development of childhood asthma. J Allergy Clin Immunol 2004;114:1282–7.

34. National Institutes of Health, National Heart, Lung, and Blood Institute. National Asthma Education and Prevention Program, Expert Panel Report 3: Guidelines for the Diagnosis and Management of Asthma 2007;(NIH Publication No. 07-4051), pp. 1–417.

35. Taussig LM. Maximal expiratory flows at functional residual capacity: a test of lung function for young children. Am Rev Respir Dis 1977;116:1031–7.

36. Tepper RS, Morgan WJ, Cota K, et al. Physiologic growth and development of the lung during the first year of life. Am Rev Respir Dis 1986;134:513–9.

37. Peat JK, Salome CM, Xuan W. On adjusting measurements of airway responsiveness for lung size and airway caliber. Am J Respir Crit Care Med 1996;154:870–5.

38. Sears MR, Burrows B, Flannery EM, et al. Atopy in childhood. I. Gender and allergen-related risks for development of hay fever and asthma. Clin Exp Allergy 1993;23:941–8.

39. Castro-Rodriguez JA, Holberg CJ, Morgan WJ, et al. Increased incidence of asthma-like symptoms in girls who become overweight or obese during the school years. Am J Respir Cut Care Med 2001;163:1344–9.

40. Camilli AE, Holberg CJ, Wright AL, et al. Parental childhood respiratory illness and respiratory illness in their infants: Group Health Medical Associates. Pediatr Pulmonol 1993;16:275–80.

41. Dezateux C, Stocks J, Dundas I, et al. Impaired airway function and wheezing in infancy. Am J Respir Crit Care Med 1999;159:403–10.

42. Christie GL, Helms PJ, Godden DJ, et al. Asthma, wheezy bronchitis, and atopy across two generations. Am J Respir Crit Care Med 1999;159:125–9.

43. Wahn U. Review Series VI: The immunology of fetuses and infants: what drives the allergic march? Allergy 2000;55:591–9.

44. Sigurs N, Gustafsson PM, Bjarnason R, et al. Severe respiratory syncytial virus bronchiolitis in infancy and asthma and allergy at age 13. Am J Respir Crit Care Med 2005;171:137–41.

45. Stein RT, Sherrill D, Morgan WJ, et al. Respiratory syncytial virus in early life and risk of wheeze and allergy by age 13 years. Lancet 1999;354:541–5.

46. Castro-Rodriguez JA, Holberg CJ, Wright AL, et al. Association of radiologically ascertained pneumonia before age 3 yr with asthma-like symptoms and pulmonary function during childhood: a prospective study. Am J Respir Crit Care Med 1999;159:1891–7.

47. Castro-Rodriguez JA, Holberg CJ, Morgan WJ, et al. Relation of two different subtypes of croup before age three to wheezing atopy, and pulmonary function during childhood: a prospective study. Pediatrics 2001;107:512–8.

48. Rakes GP, Arruda E, Ingram JM, et al. Rhinovirus and respiratory syncytial virus in wheezing children requiring emergency care: IgE and eosinophil analyses. Am J Respir Crit Care Med 1999;159:785–90.

49. Johnston NW, Johnston SL, Duncan JM, et al. The September epidemic of asthma exacerbations in children: a search for etiology. J Allergy Clin Immunol 2005;115:132–8.

50. Lemanske RF Jr, Jackson DJ, Gangnon RE, et al. Rhinovirus illnesses during infancy predict subsequent childhood wheezing. J Allergy Clin Immunol 2005;116:571–7.

51. Corne JM, Marshall C, Smith S, et al. Frequency, severity, and duration of rhinovirus infections in asthmatic and non-asthmatic individuals: a longitudinal cohort study. Lancet 2002;359:831–4.

52. Jackson DJ, Gangnon RE, Evans MD, et al. Wheezing rhinovirus illnesses in early life predict asthma development in high-risk children. Am J Respir Crit Care Med 2008;178:667–72.

53. Stein RT, Holberg CJ, Sherrill D, et al. Influence of parental smoking on respiratory symptoms during the first decade of life: the Tucson Children's Respiratory Study. Am J Epidemiol 1999;149:1030–7.

54. Hanrahan JP, Tager IB, Segal MR, et al. The effect of maternal smoking during pregnancy on early infant lung function. Am Rev Respir Dis 1992;145:1129–35.

55. Kulig M, Luck W, Lau S, et al. Effect of pre- and postnatal tobacco smoke exposure on specific sensitization to food and inhalant allergens during the first 3 years of life. Multicenter Allergy Study Group, Germany. Allergy 1999;54:220–8.

56. Barbee RA, Halonen M, Kaltenborn W, et al. A longitudinal study of serum IgE in a community cohort: correlations with age, sex, smoking, and atopic status. J Allergy Clin Immunol 1987;79:919–27.

57. Sherrill DL, Halonen M, Burrows B. Relationships between total serum IgE, atopy, and smoking: a twenty-year follow-up analysis. J Allergy Clin Immunol 1994;94:954–62.

58. Gdalevich M, Mimouni D, David M, et al. Breast-feeding and the onset of atopic dermatitis in childhood: a systematic review and meta-analysis of prospective studies. J Am Acad Dermatol 2001;45:520–7.

59. Gdalevich M, Mimouni D, Mimouni M. Breast-feeding and the risk of bronchial asthma in childhood: a systematic review with meta-analysis of prospective studies. J Pediatr 2001;139:261–6.

60. Wright AL, Holberg CJ, Taussig LM, et al. Factors influencing the relation of infant feeding to asthma and recurrent wheeze in childhood. Thorax 2001;56:192–7.

61. Guilbert TW, Stern DA, Morgan WJ, et al. Effect of breastfeeding on lung function in childhood and modulation by maternal asthma and atopy. Am J Respir Crit Care Med 2007;176:843–8.

62. Wright AL, Sherrill D, Holberg CJ, et al. Breast-feeding, maternal IgE, and total serum IgE in childhood. J Allergy Clin Immunol 1999;104:589–94.

63. Liu AH. Hygiene hypothesis for allergy and asthma. In: Martin RJ, Sutherland ER, editors. Lung biology in health and disease Series. New York: Informa Healthcare USA Inc; p. 32–59.

64. Ball TM, Castro-Rodriguez JA, Griffith KA, et al. Siblings, day-care attendance, and the risk of asthma and wheezing during childhood. N Engl J Med 2000;343:538–43.

65. Illi S, von Mutius E, Lau S, et al. Early childhood infectious diseases and the development of asthma up to school age: a birth cohort study. Br Med 2001;322:390–5.

66. Gehring U, Bolte G, Borte M, et al. Exposure to endotoxin decreases the risk of atopic eczema in infancy: a cohort study. J Allergy Clin Immunol 2001;108:847–54.

67. Phipatanakul W, Celedon JC, Raby BA, et al. Endotoxin exposure and eczema in the first year of life. Pediatrics 2004;114:13–8.

68. Perzanowski MS, Miller RL, Thorne PS, et al. Endotoxin in inner-city homes: associations with wheeze and eczema in early childhood. J Allergy Clin Immunol 2006;117:1082–9.

69. Gereda JE, Leung DYM, Thatayatikom A, et al. Relation between house-dust endotoxin exposure, type 1 T cell development, and allergen sensitization in infants at high risk of asthma. Lancet 2000;355:1680–3.

70. Celedon JC, Milton DK, Ramsey CD, et al. Exposure to dust mite allergen and endotoxin in early life and asthma and atopy in childhood. J Allergy Clin Immunol 2007;120:144–9.

71. Gehring U, Bischof W, Fahlbusch B, et al. House dust endotoxin and allergic sensitization in children. Am J Resp Crit Care Med 2002;166:939–44.

72. Gehring U, Heinrich J, Hoek G, et al. Bacteria and mould components in house dust and children's allergic sensitisation. Eur Respir J 2007;29:1144–53.

73. Braun-Fahrlander C, Riedler J, Herz U, et al. Environmental exposure to endotoxin and its relation to asthma in school-age children. N Engl J Med 2002;347:869–77.

74. Douwes J, Siebers R, Wouters I, et al. Endotoxin, (1 -> 3)-beta-D-glucans and fungal extra-cellular polysaccharides in New Zealand homes: a pilot study. Ann Agric Environ Med 2006;13:361–5.

75. Roponen M, Hyvarinen A, Hirvonen M-R, et al. Change in IFN-g-producing capacity in early life and exposure of environmental microbes. J Allergy Clin Immunol 2005;116:1048–52.

76. Bufford JD, Reardon CL, Li Z, et al. Effects of dog ownership in early childhood on immune development and atopic diseases. Clin Exp Allergy 2008;38:1635–43.

77. Park JH, Gold DR, Spiegelman DL, et al. House dust endotoxin and wheeze in the first year of life. Am J Respir Crit Care Med 2001;163:322–8.

78. Bjorksten B, Sepp E, Julge K, et al. Allergy development and the intestinal microflora during the first year of life. J Allergy Clin Immunol 2001;108:516–20.

79. Kalliomaki M, Kirjavainen P, Eerola E, et al. Distinct patterns of neonatal gut microflora in infants in whom atopy was and was not developing. J Allergy Clin Immunol 2001;107:129–34.

80. Bjorksten B, Naaber P, Sepp E, et al. The intestinal microflora in allergic Estonian and Swedish 2-year old children. Clin Exp Allergy 1999;29(342–6).

81. Sjogren YM, Jenmalm MC, Bottcher MF, et al. Altered early infant gut microbiota in children developing allergy up to 5 years of age. Clin Exp Allergy 2009;39:518–26.

82. Vael C, Nelen V, Verhulst SL, et al. Early intestinal Bacteroides fragilis colonisation and development of asthma. BMC Pulm Med 2008;8:19.

83. Wang M, Karlsson C, Olsson C, et al. Reduced diversity in the early fecal microbiota of infants with atopic eczema. J Allergy Clin Immunol 2008;121:129–34.

84. Remes ST, Castro-Rodriguez JA, Holberg CJ, et al. Dog exposure in infancy decreases the subsequent risk of frequent wheeze but not of atopy. J Allergy Clin Immunol 2001;108:509–15.

85. Ownby DR, Johnson CC, Peterson EL. Exposure to dogs and cats in the first year of life and risk of allergic sensitization at 6 to 7 years of age. JAMA 2002;288:963–72.

86. Gern JE, Reardon CL, Hoffjan S, et al. Effects of dog ownership and genotype on immune development and atopy in infancy. J Allergy Clin Immunol 2004;113:307–14.

87. Liu AH. Endotoxin exposure in allergy and asthma: reconciling a paradox. J Allergy Clin Immunol 2002;109:379–92.

88. Tse K, Horner AA. Defining a role for ambient TLR ligand exposures in the genesis and prevention of allergic disease. Semin Immunopathol 2008;30:53–62.

89. Takkouche B, Gonzáles-Barcala F-J, Etminan M, et al. Exposure to furry pets and the risk of asthma and allergic rhinitis: a meta-analysis. Allergy 2008;63:857–64.

90. Litonjua AA. Childhood asthma may be a consequence of vitamin D deficiency. Curr Opin Allergy Clin Immunol 2009;9:202–7.

91. Litonjua AA, Weiss ST. Is vitamin D deficiency to blame for the asthma epidemic? J Allergy Clin Immunol 2007;120:1031–5.

92. Camargo CA Jr, Rifas-Shiman SL, Litonjua AA, et al. Maternal intake of vitamin D during pregnancy and risk of recurrent wheeze in children at 3 y of age. Am J Clin Nutr 2007;85:788–95.

93. Devereux G, Litonjua AA, Turner SW, et al. Maternal vitamin D intake during pregnancy and early childhood wheezing. Am J Clin Nutr 2007;85:853–9.

94. Erkkola M, Kaila M, Nwaru BI, et al. Maternal vitamin D intake during pregnancy is inversely associated with asthma and allergic rhinitis in 5-year-old children. Clin Exp Allergy 2009;39:875–82.

95. Brehm JM, Celedón JC, Soto-Quiros ME, et al. Serum vitamin D levels and markers of severity of childhood asthma in Costa Rica. Am J Respir Crit Care Med 2009;179:765–71.

96. Bergmann RL, Bergmann KE, Lau-Schadensdorf S, et al. Atopic diseases in infancy: the German multicenter atopy study (MAS-90). Pediatr Allergy Immunol 1994;5:19–25.

97. Hanifin JM, Rajka G. Diagnostic features of atopic dermatitis. Ada Dermatol Venereol (suppl) 1980;92:44–7.

98. Williams HC, Strachan DP. The natural history of childhood eczema: observations from the British 1958 cohort study. Br J Dermatol 1998;139:834–9.

99. Linna O. Ten-year prognosis for generalized infantile eczema. Acta Pediatr 1992;81:1013.

100. Vickers CFH. The natural history of atopic eczema. Acta Dermatol Venereal 1980;92:113–5.

101. Schultz Larsen F. Atopic dermatitis: a genetic-epidemiologic study in a population-based twin sample. J Am Acad Dermatol 1993;28:719–23.

102. Harris JM, Cullinan P, Williams HC, et al. Environmental associations with eczema in early life. Br J Dermatol 2001;144:795–802.

103. Lammintausta K. Prognosis of atopic dermatitis: a prospective study in early adulthood. Int J Dermatol 1991;30:563–8.

104. Guillet G, Guillet MH. Natural history of sensitizations in atopic dermatitis. Arch Dermatol 1992;128:187–92.

105. Patrizi A, Guerrini V, Ricci G, et al. The natural history of sensitizations to food and aeroallergens in atopic dermatitis: a 4-year follow-up. Pediatr Dermatol 2000;17:261–5.

106. Bergmann RL, Edenharter G, Bergmann KE, et al. Atopic dermatitis in early infancy predicts allergic airway disease at 5 years. Clin Exp Allergy 1998;28:965–70.

107. Kulig M, Klettke U, Wahn V, et al. Development of seasonal allergic rhinitis during the first 7 years of life. J Allergy Clin Immunol 2000;106:832–9.

108. Broder I. Epidemiology of asthma and allergic rhinitis in a total community, Tecumseh, Michigan. IV. Natural history. J Allergy Clin Immunol 1974;54:100.

109. Bock SA. Prospective appraisal of complaints of adverse reactions to foods in children during the first 3 years of life. Pediatrics 1987;79:683–8.

110. Zeiger RS, Heller S, Mellon MH, et al. Effect of combined maternal and infant food-allergen avoidance on development of atopy in early infancy: a randomized study. J Allergy Clin Immunol 1989;84:72–89.

111. Host A. Cow's milk protein allergy and intolerance in infancy: some clinical, epidemiological and immunological aspects. Pediatr Allergy Immunol 1994;5:1–36.

112. Bock SA. The natural history of food sensitivity. J Allergy Clin Immunol 1982;69:173–7.

113. Sampson HA, Scanlon SM. Natural history of food hypersensitivity in children with atopic dermatitis. J Pediatr 1989;115:23–7.

114. Spergel JM, Beausoleil JL, Pawlowski NA. Resolution of childhood peanut allergy. Ann Allergy Asthma Immunol 2000;85:435–7.

115. Vander Leek TK, Liu AH, Stefanski K, et al. The natural history of peanut allergy in young children and its association with serum peanut-specific IgE. J Pediatr 2000;137:749–55.

116. Hill DJ, Bannister DG, Hosking CS, et al. Cow milk allergy within the spectrum of atopic disorders. Clin Exp Allergy 1994;24:1137–43.

117. Host A, Halken S. A prospective study of cow milk allergy in Danish infants during the first 3 years of life: clinical course in relation to clinical and immunological type of hypersensitivity reaction. Allergy 1990;45:587–96.

118. Cogswell JJ, Halliday DF, Alexander JR. Respiratory infections in the first year of life in children at risk of developing atopy. Br Med J 1982;284:1011–3.

119. Van Asperen PP, Kemp AS, Mellis CM. Skin test reactivity and clinical allergen sensitivity in infancy. J Allergy Clin Immunol 1984;73:381–6.

120. Fernandez de Corres L, Moneo I, Munoz D, et al. Sensitization from chestnuts and bananas in patients with urticaria and anaphylaxis from contact with latex. Ann Allergy 1993;70:35–9.

121. Katayama H, Yamaguchi K, Kozuka T, et al. Adverse reactions to ionic and nonionic contrast media: a report from the Japanese Committee on the Safety of Contrast Media. Radiology 1990;175:621–8.

122. Lieberman P, Patterson R, Metz R, et al. Allergic reactions to insulin. JAMA 1971;215:1106–12.

123. Green GR, Rosenblum A. Report of the Penicillin Study Group – American Academy of Allergy. J Allergy Clin Immunol 1971;48:331–43.

124. Settipane GA, Klein DE, Boyd GK. Relationship of atopy and anaphylactic sensitization: a bee sting allergy model. Clin Allergy 1978;8:259–65.

125. Valentine MD, Schuberth KC, Kagey-Sobotka A, et al. The value of immunotherapy with venom in children with allergy to insect stings. N Engl J Med 1990;323:1601–3.

126. Savliwala MN, Reisman RE. Studies of the natural history of stinging-insect allergy: long-term follow-up of patients without immunotherapy. J Allergy Clin Immunol 1987;80:741–5.

127. Franken HH, Dubois AE, Minkema HJ, et al. Lack of reproducibility of a single negative sting challenge response in the assessment of anaphylactic risk in patients with suspected yellow jacket hypersensitivity. J Allergy Clin Immunol 1994;93:431–6.

128. LeVan TD, Bloom JW, Bailey TJ, et al. A common single nucleotide polymorphism in the CD14 promoter decreases the affinity of Sp protein binding and enhances transcriptional activity. J Immunol 2001;167:5838–44.

129. Baldini M, Lohman IC, Halonen M, et al. A Polymorphism* in the 5′ flanking region of the CD14 gene is associated with circulating soluble CD14 levels and with total serum immunoglobulin E. Am J Respir Cell Mol Biol 1999;20:976–83.

130. Koppelman GH, Reijmerink NE, Colin Stine O, et al. Association of a promoter polymorphism of the CD14 gene and atopy. Am J Respir Crit Care Med 2001;163:965–9.

131. Litonjua AA, Belanger K, Celedon JC, et al. Polymorphisms in the 5′ region of the CD14 gene are associated with eczema in young children. J Allergy Clin Immunol 2005;115:1056–62.

132. Ober C, Tsalenko A, Parry R, et al. A second-generation genomewide screen for asthma-susceptibility alleles in a founder population. Am J Hum Genet 2000;67:1154–62.

133. Simpson A, John SL, Jury F, et al. Endotoxin exposure, CD14, and allergic disease: an interaction between genes and the environment. Am J Respir Crit Care Med 2006;174:386–92.

134. Eder W, Klimecki W, Yu L, et al. Opposite effects of CD 14/-260 on serum IgE levels in children raised in different environments. J Allergy Clin Immunol 2005;116:601–7.

135. Gilliland FD, Li YF, Dubeau L, et al. Effects of glutathione S-transferase M1, maternal smoking during pregnancy, and environmental tobacco smoke on asthma and wheezing in children. Am J Respir Crit Care Med 2002 Aug 15;166:457–63.

136. Kabesch M, Hoefler C, Carr D, et al. Glutathione S transferase deficiency and passive smoking increase childhood asthma. Thorax 2004;59:569–73.

137. Breton CV, Vora H, Salam MT, et al. Variation in the GST mu locus and tobacco smoke exposure as determinants of childhood lung function. Am J Respir Crit Care Med 2009;179:601–7.

138. Schroer KT, Biagini Myers JM, Ryan PH, et al. Associations between multiple environmental exposures and glutathione S-Transferase P1 on persistent wheezing in a birth cohort. J Pediatr 2009;154:401–8

139. Bouzigon E, Corda E, Aschard H, et al. Effect of 17q21 variants and smoking exposure in early-onset asthma. N Engl J Med 2008;359:1985–94.

140. Bisgaard H, Simpson A, Palmer CN, et al. Gene-environment interaction in the onset of eczema in infancy: filaggrin loss-of-function mutations enhanced by neonatal cat exposure. PLoS Med 2008;5:e131.

141. Woodcock A, Lowe LA, Murray CS, et al. NAC Manchester Asthma and Allergy Study Group. Early life environmental control: effect on symptoms, sensitization, and lung function at age 3 years. Am J Respir Crit Care Med 2004;170:433–9.

142. Arshad SH, Matthews S, Gant C, et al. Effect of allergen avoidance on development of allergic disorders in infancy. Lancet 1992;339:1493–7.

143. Hide DW, Matthews S, Matthews L, et al. Effect of allergen avoidance in infancy on allergic manifestations at age two years. J Allergy Clin Immunol 1994;93:842–6.

144. Hide DW, Matthews S, Tariq S, et al. Allergen avoidance in infancy and allergy at 4 years of age. Allergy 1996;51:89–93.

145. Chan-Yeung M, Ferguson A, Watson W, et al. The Canadian Childhood Asthma Primary Prevention Study: outcomes at 7 years of age. J Allergy Clin Immunol 2005;116:49–55.

146. Maas T, Kaper J, Sheikh A, et al. Mono and multifaceted inhalant and/or food allergen reduction interventions for preventing asthma in children at high risk of developing asthma. Cochrane Database Syst Rev 2009;(3):CD006480.

147. Arlian LG, Neal JS, Morgan MS, et al. Reducing relative humidity is a practical way to control dust mites and their allergens in homes in temperate climates. J Allergy Clin Immunol 2001;107:99–104.

148. Boner AL, Niero E, Antolini I, et al. Pulmonary function and bronchial hyperreactivity in asthmatic children with house dust mite allergy during prolonged stay in the Italian Alps (Misurina, 1756 m). Ann Allergy 1985;54:42–5.

149. Grootendorst DC, Dahlen SE, Van Den Bos JW, et al. Benefits of high-altitude allergen avoidance in atopic adolescents with moderate to severe asthma, over and above treatment with high-dose inhaled steroids. Clin Exp Allergy 2001;31:400–8.

150. Murray AB, Ferguson AC. Dust-free bedrooms in the treatment of asthmatic children with house dust or house dust mite allergy: a controlled trial. Pediatrics 1983;71:418–22.

151. ETAC Study Group: Allergic factors associated with the development of asthma and the influence of cetirizine in a double-blind, randomized, placebo-controlled trial: first results of ETAC. Early treatment of the atopic child. Pediatr Allergy Immunol 1998;9:116–24.

152. Warner JO. A double-blinded, randomized, placebo-controlled trial of cetirizine in preventing the onset of asthma in children with atopic dermatitis: 18 months' treatment and 18 months' posttreatment follow-up. J Allergy Clin Immunol 2001;108:929–37.

153. Bisgaard H, Hermansen MN, Loland L, et al. Intermittent inhaled corticosteroids in infants with episodic wheezing. N Engl J Med 2006;354:1998–2005.

154. Murray CS, Woodcock A, Langley SJ, et al. IFWIN study team. Secondary prevention of asthma by the use of Inhaled Fluticasone propionate in Wheezy Infants (IFWIN): double-blind, randomised, controlled study. Lancet 2006;368:754–62.

155. Guilbert TW, Morgan WJ, Zeiger RS, et al. Long-term inhaled corticosteroids in preschool children at high risk for asthma. N Engl J Med 2006;354:1985–97.

156. Castro-Rodriguez JA, Rodrigo GJ. Efficacy of inhaled corticosteroids in infants and preschoolers with recurrent wheezing and asthma: a systematic review with meta-analysis. Pediatrics 2009;123:e519–25.

157. Moller C, Dreborg S, Ferdousi HA, et al. Pollen immunotherapy reduces the development of asthma in children with seasonal rhinoconjunctivitis (the PAT-study). J Allergy Clin Immunol 2002;109:251–6.

158. Jacobsen L, Niggemann B, Dreborg S, et al. (The PAT investigator group). Specific immunotherapy has long-term preventive effect of seasonal and perennial asthma: 10-year follow-up on the PAT study. Allergy 2007;62:943–8.

159. Purello-D'Ambrosio F, Gangemi S, Merendino RA, et al. Prevention of new sensitizations in monosensitized subjects submitted to specific immunotherapy or not: a retrospective study. Clin Exp Allergy 2001;31:1295–302.

160. Des Roches A, Paradis L, Menardo JL, et al. Immunotherapy with a standardized *Dermatophagoides pteronyssinus* extract. VI. Specific immunotherapy prevents the onset of new sensitizations in children. J Allergy Clin Immunol 1997;99:450–3.

161. Rautava S, Kalliomaki M, Isolauri E. Probiotics during pregnancy and breast-feeding might confer immunomodulatory protection against atopic disease in the infant. J Allergy Clin Immunol 2002;109:119–21.

162. Pessi T, Sutas Y, Hurme M, et al. Interleukin-10 generation in atopic children following oral *Lactobacillus rhamnosus* GG. Clin Exp Allergy 2000;30:1804–8.

163. Lee J, Seto D, Bielory L. Meta-analysis of clinical trials of probiotics for prevention and treatment of pediatric atopic dermatitis. J Allergy Clin Immunol 2008;121:116–21 e11.

164. Hatakka K, Savilahti E, Ponka A, et al. Effect of long term consumption of probiotic milk on infections in children attending day care centers: double blind, randomized trial. Br Med J 2001;322:1–5.

165. Kukkonen K, Savilahti E, Haahtela T, et al. Long-term safety and impact on infection rates of postnatal probiotic and prebiotic (synbiotic) treatment: randomized, double-blind, placebo-controlled trial. Pediatrics 2008;122:8–12.

166. Rautava S, Salminen S, Isolauri E. Specific probiotics in reducing the risk of acute infections in infancy: a randomised, double-blind, placebo-controlled study. Br J Nutr 2009;101:1722–6.

167. Kuitunen M, Kukkonen K, Juntunen-Backman K, et al. Probiotics prevent IgE-associated allergy until age 5 years in cesarean-delivered children but not in the total cohort. J Allergy Clin Immunol 2009;123:335–41.

CHAPTER 3

The Genetics of Allergic Disease and Asthma

Matthew J. Rose-Zerilli • Shelley A. Davis • Stephen T. Holgate • John W. Holloway

Since the first report of linkage of a region of the human genome with allergic disease,[1] considerable effort has been made to identify the genetic factors that modify susceptibility to allergic diseases, severity of disease in affected individuals, and the response to treatment. Since the first report of linkage between chromosome 11q13 and atopy in 1989, there have been thousands of published studies of the genetics of asthma and other allergic diseases. Our knowledge of how genetic variation between individuals determines susceptibility, severity and response to treatment has expanded considerably, providing intriguing insights into the pathophysiology of these complex disorders. In this chapter we outline the approaches used to undertake genetic studies of common diseases such as atopic dermatitis and asthma and provide examples of how these approaches are beginning to reveal new insights into the pathophysiology of allergic diseases.

Why Undertake Genetic Studies of Allergic Disease?

Susceptibility to allergic disease is likely to result from the inheritance of many mutant genes. Unfortunately, as in many other complex disorders, in allergic diseases any specific biochemical defect(s) at the cellular level that cause the disease are unknown, even though considerable knowledge has accrued on molecular pathways involved in pathogenesis. By undertaking research into the genetic basis of these conditions, these mutant genes and their abnormal gene products can be identified solely by the anomalous phenotypes they produce. Identifying the genes that produce these disease phenotypes will provide a greater understanding of the fundamental mechanisms of these disorders, stimulating the development of specific new drugs or biologics to both relieve and prevent symptoms. In addition, genetic variants may also influence the response to therapy and the identification of individuals with altered response to current drug therapies will allow optimization of current therapeutic measures (i.e. disease stratification and pharmacogenetics). The study of genetic factors in large longitudinal cohorts with extensive phenotype and environmental information will allow the identification of external factors that initiate and sustain allergic diseases in susceptible individuals and the periods of life in which this occurs, with a view to identifying those environmental factors that could be modified for disease prevention or for changing the natural history of the disorder. For example, early identification of vulnerable children would allow targeting of preventative therapy or environmental intervention, such as avoidance of allergen exposure. Genetic screening in early life may eventually become a practical and cost-effective option for allergic disease prevention.

Approaches to Genetic Studies of Complex Genetic Diseases

What is a Complex Genetic Disease?

The use of genetic analysis to identify genes responsible for simple mendelian traits such as cystic fibrosis[2] has become almost routine in the 30 years since it was recognized that genetic inheritance can be traced with naturally occurring DNA sequence variation.[3] However, many of the most common medical conditions known to have a genetic component to their etiology, including diabetes, hypertension, heart disease, schizophrenia, and asthma, have much more complex inheritance patterns.

Complex disorders show a clear hereditary component, however the mode of inheritance does not follow any simple mendelian pattern. Furthermore, unlike single-gene disorders, they tend to have an extremely high prevalence. Asthma occurs in at least 10% of children in the UK, and atopy is as high as 40% in some population groups.[4] This compares with a frequency of one of the most common mendelian disorders, cystic fibrosis, of 1 in 2000 live white births. Characteristic features of mendelian diseases are that they are rare and involve mutations in a single gene which are severe and result in large phenotypic effects that may be independent of environmental influences. In contrast, complex disease traits are common and involve many genes, with 'mild' mutations leading to small phenotypic effects with strong environmental interactions.

How to Identify Genes Underlying Complex Disease

Before any genetic study of a complex disease can be initiated, there are a number of different factors that need to be considered. These include: (1) assessing the heritability of a disease of interest to establish whether there is indeed a genetic component to the disease in question; (2) defining the phenotype (or physical characteristics) to be measured in a population; (3) the size and nature of the population to be studied; (4) determining which genetic markers are going to be typed in the DNA samples obtained from the population; (5) how the relationships between the genetic data and the phenotype measures in individuals are to be

©2010 Elsevier Ltd, Inc, BV
DOI: 10.1016/B978-1-4377-0271-2.00003-1

analyzed and (6) how this data can be used to identify the genes underlying the disease.

One of the most important considerations in genetic studies of complex disease susceptibility is the choice of the methods of genetic analysis to be used. This choice will both reflect and be reflected in the design of the study. Will the study be a population study or a family-based study? What numbers of subjects will be needed?

Inheritance

The first step in any genetic analysis of a complex disease is to determine whether genetic factors contribute at all to an individual's susceptibility to disease. The fact that a disease has been observed to 'run in families' is insufficient evidence to begin molecular genetic studies as this can occur for a number of reasons, including common environmental exposure and biased ascertainment, as well as having a true genetic component. There are a number of approaches that can be taken to determine if genetics contributes to a disease or disease phenotype of interest including family studies, segregation analysis, twin and adoption studies, heritability studies, and population-based relative risk to relatives of probands.

There are three main steps involved in the identification of genetic mechanisms for a disease.[5,6]

1. Determine whether there is familial aggregation of the disease – does the disease occur more frequently in relatives of cases than of controls?
2. If there is evidence for familial aggregation, is this because of genetic effects or other factors such as environmental or cultural effects?
3. If there are genetic factors, which specific genetic mechanisms are operating?

The exact methods used in this process will vary depending on a number of disease-specific factors. For example, is the disease of early or late onset, and is the phenotype in question discrete or continuous (e.g. insulin resistance or blood pressure)?

Family studies involve the estimation of the frequency of the disease in relatives of affected, compared with unaffected, individuals. The strength of the genetic effect can be measured as λ_R, where λ_R is the ratio of risk to relatives of type R (e.g. sibs, parents, offspring, etc.) compared with the population risk ($\lambda_R = \kappa_R/\kappa$, where κ_R is the risk to relatives of type R and κ is the population risk). The stronger the genetic effect, the higher the value of λ. For example, for a recessive single gene mendelian disorder such as cystic fibrosis, the value of λ is about 500; for a dominant disorder such as Huntington's disease, it is about 5000. For complex disorders the values of λ are much lower, e.g. 20–30 for multiple sclerosis, 15 for insulin-dependent diabetes mellitus (IDDM), and 4 to 5 for Alzheimer's disease. It is important to note, though, that λ is a function of both the strength of the genetic effect and the frequency of the disease in the population. Therefore a disease with a λ of 3 to 4 does not mean that genes are less important in that trait than in a trait with a λ of 30 to 40. A strong effect in a very common disease will have a smaller λ than the same strength of effect in a rare disease.

Determining the relative contribution of common genes versus common environment to clustering of disease within families can be undertaken using twin studies where the concordance of a trait in monozygotic and dizygotic twins is assessed. Monozygotic twins have identical genotypes, whereas dizygotic twins share, on average, only one half of their genes. In both cases, they share the same childhood environment. Therefore, a disease that has a genetic component is expected to show a higher rate of concordance in monozygotic than in dizygotic twins.

Another approach used to disentangle the effects of nature versus nurture in a disease is in adoption studies, where, if the disease has a genetic basis, the frequency of the disease should be higher in biologic relatives of probands than in their adopted family.

Once familial aggregation with a probable genetic etiology for a disease has been established, the mode of inheritance can be determined by observing the pattern of inheritance of a disease or trait by observing how it is distributed within families. For example, is there evidence of a single major gene and is it dominantly or recessively inherited? Segregation analysis is the most established method for this purpose. The observed frequency of a trait in offspring and siblings is compared with the distribution expected with various modes of inheritance. If the distribution is significantly different than predicted, that model is rejected. The model that cannot be rejected is therefore considered the most likely. However, for complex disease, it is often difficult to undertake segregation analysis because of the multiple genetic and environmental effects making any one model hard to determine. This has implication for the methods of analysis of genetic data in studies, because some methods, such as the parametric lod score approach, require a model to be defined to obtain estimates of parameters such as gene frequency and penetrance (see later).

Phenotype

Studies of a genetic disorder require that a phenotype be defined, to which genetic data are compared. Phenotypes can be classified in two ways. They may be complex, such as asthma or atopy, and are likely to involve the interaction of a number of genes. Alternatively, intermediate phenotypes may be used, such as bronchial hyperresponsiveness (BHR) and eosinophilia for asthma and serum immunoglobulin E (IgE) levels and specific IgE responsiveness or positive skin prick tests to particular allergens for atopy. Together, these phenotypes contribute to an individual's expression of the overall complex disease phenotype but are likely to involve the interaction of fewer genetic influences, thus increasing the chances of identifying specific genetic factors predisposing toward the disease. Phenotypes may also be discrete or qualitative, such as the presence or absence of wheeze, atopy and asthma, or quantitative. Quantitative phenotypes, such as blood pressure (mm Hg), lung function measures (e.g. FEV_1) and serum IgE levels, are phenotypes that can be measured as a continuous variable. With quantitative traits, no arbitrary cut-off point has to be assigned (making quantitative trait analysis important) because clinical criteria used to define an affected or an unaffected phenotype may not reflect whether an individual is a gene carrier or not. In addition, the use of quantitative phenotypes allows the use of alternative methods of genetic analysis that, in some situations, can be more powerful. Most recently, cluster analysis has been used to identify individual phenotypic expressions of asthma in a population sample.[7,8]

Population

Having established that the disease or phenotype of interest does have a genetic component to its etiology, the next step is to recruit a study population in which to undertake genetic analyses to identify the gene(s) responsible. The type and size of study population recruited depend heavily on a number of interrelated factors, including the epidemiology of the disease, the method of genetic epidemiologic analysis being used, and the class of genetic markers genotyped. For example, the recruitment of families is necessary to undertake linkage analysis, whereas association studies are better suited to either a randomly selected or case-control cohort. In family-based linkage studies, the age of onset of a disease will determine whether it is practical to collect multigenerational families or affected sibpairs for analysis. Equally, if a disease is rare, then actively recruiting cases and matched controls will be a more practical approach than recruiting a random population that would need to be very large to have sufficient power.

Genetic Markers

Genetic markers used can be any identifiable site within the genome (locus) where the DNA sequence is variable (polymorphic between individuals). The most common genetic markers used for linkage analysis are microsatellite markers comprising short lengths of DNA consisting of repeats of a specific sequence (e.g. CA_n). The number of repeats varies between individuals, thus providing polymorphic markers that can be used in genetic analysis to follow the transmission of a chromosomal region from one generation to the next. Single-nucleotide polymorphisms (SNPs) are the simplest class of polymorphism in the genome resulting from a single base substitution: e.g. cytosine substituted for thymidine. SNPs are much more frequent than microsatellites in the human genome, occurring in introns, exons, promoters, and intergenic regions, with several million SNPs now having been identified and mapped.[9] Another source of variation in the human genome that has recently been recognized to be present to a much greater extent than was previously thought are copy number variations (CNVs). CNVs are either a deletion or insertion of a large piece of DNA sequence; CNVs can contain whole genes and therefore are correlated with gene expression in a dose-dependent manner.[10] Recent sequencing of an individual human genome revealed that non-SNP variation (which includes CNVs) made up 22% of all variation in that individual but involved 74% of all variant DNA bases in that genome.[11]

Approaches to Analysis

The method chosen to analyze the molecular genetic data obtained by the typing of genetic markers within a study cohort, like the cohort recruited and the selection of genetic markers, is interdependent on the other parameters of the study. There are two main approaches. Linkage analysis involves proposing a model to explain the inheritance pattern of phenotypes and genotypes observed in a pedigree.[12] Linkage is evident when a gene that produces a phenotypic trait and its surrounding markers are co-inherited. In contrast, those markers not associated with the anomalous phenotype of interest will be randomly distributed among affected family members as a result of the independent assortment of chromosomes and crossing over during meiosis. The evidence for linkage of a genomic region to a phenotype of interest is usually expressed in terms of the ratio of their odds of the two hypotheses (linkage or non linkage), the likelihood ratio (LR), or more equivalently by the lod score, $Z = \log_{10}(LR)$.[13] In complex disease, non-parametric linkage approaches, such as allele sharing, are usually used. Allele-sharing methods test whether the inheritance pattern of a particular chromosomal region is not consistent with random mendelian segregation by showing that pairs of affected relatives inherit identical copies of the region more often than would be expected by chance.[14] Because allele-sharing methods are non-parametric, it is not necessary to define a model for the inheritance of the trait, making allele-sharing methods more robust than linkage analysis: affected relatives should show excess sharing even in the presence of incomplete penetrance, phenocopy, genetic heterogeneity, and high-frequency disease alleles. Affected sib-pair analysis is the simplest form of allele-sharing analysis. Because both sib-

lings are affected, the disease genes are assumed to have acted, and therefore, non-penetrant individuals are excluded from the analysis. Two sibs can show identical-by-descent (IBD) sharing for no, one, or two copies of any locus (with a 1:2:1 distribution expected under random segregation). Excess allele sharing can be measured with a simple χ^2 test.

Association studies do not examine inheritance patterns of alleles; rather, they are case-control studies based on a comparison of allele frequencies between groups of affected and unaffected individuals from a population. A particular allele is said to be associated with the trait if it occurs at a significantly higher frequency among affected individuals as compared with those in the control group. The odds ratio of the trait in individuals is then assessed as the ratio of the frequency of the allele in the affected population compared with the unaffected population. The greatest problem in association studies is the selection of a suitable control group to compare with the affected population group. Although association studies can be performed with any random DNA polymorphism, they have the most significance when applied to polymorphisms that have functional consequences in genes relevant to the trait (candidate genes).

It is important to remember with association studies that there are a number of reasons leading to an association between a phenotype and a particular allele:

- A positive association between the phenotype and the allele will occur if the allele is the cause of, or contributes to, the phenotype. This association would be expected to be replicated in other populations with the same phenotype, unless there are several different alleles at the same locus contributing to the same phenotype, in which case association would be difficult to detect, or if the trait was predominantly the result of different genes in the other population (genetic heterogeneity).
- Positive associations may also occur between an allele and a phenotype if that particular allele is in linkage disequilibrium with the phenotype-causing allele. That is, the allele tends to occur on the same parental chromosome that also carries the trait-causing mutation more often than would be expected by chance. Linkage disequilibrium will occur when most causes of the trait are the result of relatively few ancestral mutations at a trait-causing locus and the allele is present on one of those ancestral chromosomes and lies close enough to the trait-causing locus that the association between them has not been eroded away through recombination between chromosomes during meiosis.
- Positive association between an allele and a trait can also be artefactual as a result of recent population admixture. In a mixed population, any trait present in a higher frequency in a subgroup of the population (e.g. an ethnic group) will show positive association with an allele that also happens to be more common in that population subgroup.[15] Thus, to avoid spurious association arising through admixture, studies should be performed in large, relatively homogeneous populations. An alternative method to test for association in the presence of linkage is the 'transmission test for linkage disequilibrium'. (transmission/disequilibrium test [TDT]).[16,17] The TDT uses families with at least one affected child, and the transmission of the associated marker allele from a heterozygous parent to an affected offspring is evaluated. If a parent is heterozygous for an associated allele *A1* and a non-associated allele *A2*, then *A1* should be passed on to the affected child more often than *A2*.

Historically, association studies were not well suited to whole genome searches in large mixed populations. Because linkage disequilibrium extends over very short genetic distances in an old population, many more markers would need to be typed to 'cover' the whole genome. Therefore genome-wide searches for association were more favorable in young, genetically isolated populations because linkage disequilibrium extends over greater distances and the number of disease-causing alleles is likely to be fewer.

However, recent advances in array-based SNP genotyping technologies and haplotype mapping of the human genome[18] have presented the possibility of simultaneously determining millions of SNPs throughout the genome of an individual. This breakthrough has made genome-wide association studies of disease a reality and identification of casual genes less challenging than positional cloning of genes by linkage analysis. Genome-wide association studies (GWAS) have revolutionized the study of genetic factors in complex common disease over the last few years.[19,20] For more than 150 phenotypes – from common diseases to physiological measurements such as height and BMI and biological measurements such as circulating lipid levels and blood eosinophil levels, GWAS have provided compelling statistical associations for over hundreds of different loci in the human genome.[21]

Identify Gene

If, as in most complex disorders, the exact biochemical or physiologic basis of the disease is unknown, there are three main approaches to finding the disease gene(s). One method is to test markers randomly spaced throughout the entire genome for linkage with the disease phenotype. If linkage is found between a particular marker and the phenotype, then further typing of genetic markers including SNPs and association analysis will enable the critical region to be further narrowed; the genes positioned in this region can be examined for possible involvement in the disease process and the presence of disease-causing mutations in affected individuals. This approach is often termed *positional cloning,* or *genome scanning* if the whole genome is examined in this manner. Although this approach requires no assumptions to be made as to the particular gene involved in genetic susceptibility to the disease in question, it does require considerable molecular genetic analysis to be undertaken in large family cohorts, involving considerable time, resource and expense.

This approach has now largely been superceded by genome-wide association studies using SNPs evenly spaced throughout the genome as an assumption-free approach to locate disease-associated genes involved in disease pathogenesis. As GWAS utilize large data sets, up to one million SNPs to test for association, stringent genotype calling, quality control, population stratification (genomic controls) and statistical techniques have been developed to handle the analysis of such data.[22] Studies start by reporting single marker analyses of primary outcome; SNPs are considered to be strongly associated if the P-values are below the 1% false discovery rate (FDR) or showing weak association above 1% but below the 5% FDR. A cluster of P-values below the 1% FDR from SNPs in one chromosomal location is defined as the region of, 'maximal association' and is the first candidate gene region to examine further, with analysis of secondary outcome measures, gene database searches, fine mapping to find the causal locus and replication in other cohorts/populations. It is unlikely that the SNP showing the strongest association will be the causal locus, as SNPs are chosen to provide maximal coverage of variation in that region of the genome and not on biological function. Therefore, GWAS will often include fine mapping/haplotype analysis of the region with the aim of identifying the causal locus. If linkage disequilibrium prevents the identification

of a specific gene in a haplotype block then it may be necessary to utilize different racial and ethnic populations to hone in on the causative candidate gene that accounts for the genetic signal in GWAS.[23]

Finally, in the candidate gene approach, variation in individual genes is directly assessed for association with the disease phenotype of interest. In general, candidate genes are selected for analysis because of a known role for the encoded product of the gene in the disease process. The gene is then screened for polymorphism, which is tested for association with the disease or phenotype in question. A hybrid approach is the selection of candidate genes based not only on their function but also on their position within a genetic region previously linked to the disease (positional candidate). This approach may help to reduce the considerable work required to narrow a large genetic region of several megabases of DNA identified through linkage containing tens to hundreds of genes to one single gene to test for association with the disease.

Once a gene has been identified, further work is required to understand its role in the disease pathogenesis. Further molecular genetic studies may help to identify the precise genetic polymorphism that is having functional consequences for the gene's expression or function as opposed to those that are merely in linkage disequilibrium with the causal SNP. Often the gene identified may be completely novel and cell and molecular biology studies will be needed to understand the gene product's role in the disease and to define genotype/phenotype correlations. Furthermore, by using cohorts with information available on environmental exposures, it may be possible to define how the gene product may interact with the environment to cause disease. Ultimately, knowledge of the gene's role in disease pathogenesis may lead to the development of novel therapeutics.

Allergy and Asthma as Complex Genetic Diseases

From studies of the epidemiology and heritability of allergic diseases, it is clear that these are complex diseases in which the interaction between genetic and environmental factors plays a fundamental role in the development of IgE-mediated sensitivity and the subsequent development of clinical symptoms. The development of IgE responses by an individual, and therefore allergies, is the function of several genetic factors. These include the regulation of basal serum immunoglobulin production, the regulation of the switching of Ig-producing B cells to IgE, and the control of the specificity of responses to antigens. Furthermore, the genetic influences on allergic diseases such as asthma are more complex than those on atopy alone, involving not only genes controlling the induction and level of an IgE-mediated response to allergen but also 'lung-' or 'asthma'-specific genetic factors that result in the development of asthma. This also applies equally to other clinical manifestations of atopy such as rhinitis and atopic dermatitis.

Phenotypes for Allergy and Allergic Disease: What Should We Measure?

The term *atopy* (from the Greek word for 'strangeness') was originally used by Coca and Cooke[24] in 1923 to describe a particular predisposition to develop hypersensitivity to common allergens associated with an increase of circulating reaginic antibody, now defined as IgE, and with clinical manifestations such as whealing-type reactions, asthma, and hay fever. Today, even if the definition of *atopy* is not yet precise, the term is commonly used to define a disorder that involves IgE antibody responses to ubiquitous allergens that is associated with a number of clinical disorders such as asthma, allergic dermatitis, allergic conjunctivitis, and allergic rhinitis.

Atopy can be defined in several ways including: raised total serum IgE levels, the presence of antigen-specific IgE antibodies, and/or a positive skin test to common allergens. Furthermore, because of their complex clinical phenotype, atopic diseases can be studied using intermediate or surrogate disease-specific measurements, such as BHR or lung function for asthma. As discussed earlier, phenotypes can be defined in several ways, ranging from subjective measures (e.g. symptoms), objective measures (e.g. BHR, blood eosinophils or serum IgE levels), or both. In addition, some studies have used quantitative scores that are derived from both physical measures such as serum IgE and BHR and questionnaire data.[25,26] It is a lack of a clear definition of atopic phenotypes that presents the greatest problem when reviewing studies of the genetic basis of atopy, with multiple definitions of the same intermediate phenotype often being used in different studies.

The Heritability of Atopic Disease: Are Atopy and Atopic Disease Heritable Conditions?

In 1916, the first comprehensive study of the heritability of atopy was undertaken by Robert Cooke and Albert Vander Veer[27] at the Department of Medicine of the Postgraduate Hospital and Medical School of New York. Although the atopic conditions they included, as well as those excluded (e.g. eczema), may be open for debate today, the conclusions nonetheless remain the same. That there is a high heritable component to the development of atopy and atopic disease, and as is now more clearly understood biologically, this is owing to the inheritance of a tendency to generate specific IgE responses to common proteins.

Subsequent to the work of Cooke and Vander Veer, the results of many studies have established that atopy and atopic disease such as asthma, rhinitis, and eczema have strong genetic components. Family studies have shown an increased prevalence of atopy, and phenotypes associated with atopy, among the relatives of atopic compared with non-atopic subjects.[28-30] In a study of 176 normal families, Gerrard and colleagues[31] found a striking association between asthma in the parent and asthma in the child, between hay fever in the parent and hay fever in the child, and between eczema in the parent and eczema in the child. These studies suggest that 'end-organ sensitivity', or which allergic disease an allergic individual will develop, is controlled by specific genetic factors, differing from those that determine susceptibility to atopy per se. This hypothesis is borne out by a questionnaire study involving 6665 families in southern Bavaria. Children with atopic diseases had a positive family history in 55% of cases compared with 35% in children without atopic disease (*P* < 0.001).[32] Subsequent researchers used the same population to investigate familial influences unique to the expression of asthma and found that the prevalence of asthma alone (i.e. without hay fever or eczema) increased significantly if the nearest of kin had asthma alone (11.7% vs 4.7%, *P* < 0.0001). A family history of eczema or hay fever (without asthma) was unrelated to asthma in the offspring.[33]

Numerous twin studies[34-40] have shown a significant increase in concordance among monozygotic twins compared with dizygotic twins, providing further evidence for a genetic component to atopy. Atopic asthma has also been widely studied, and both

twin and family studies have shown a strong heritable component to this phenotype.[38,39,41-43] Using a twin-family model, Laitinen and colleagues[44] reported that in families with asthma in successive generations, genetic factors alone accounted for as much as 87% of the development of asthma in offspring, and the incidence of the disease in twins with affected parents is 4-fold compared with the incidence in twins without affected parents. This indicates that asthma is recurring in families as a result of shared genes rather than shared environmental risk factors. This has been further substantiated in a study of 11 688 Danish twin pairs. Using additive genetic and non-shared environmental modeling, it was suggested that 73% of susceptibility to asthma was the result of the genetic component. However, a substantial part of the variation in liability of asthma was the result of environmental factors; there also was no evidence for genetic dominance or shared environmental effects.[45]

Molecular Regulation of Atopy and Atopic Disease, I: Susceptibility Genes

Positional Cloning by Genome-Wide Screens

Many genome-wide screens for atopy and atopic disorder susceptibility genes have now been completed.[46,47] The results of these studies reflect the genetic and environmental heterogeneity seen in allergic disorders. Multiple regions of the genome have been observed to be linked to varying phenotypes with differences between cohorts recruited from both similar and different populations. This illustrates the difficulty of identifying susceptibility genes for complex genetic diseases. Different genetic loci will show linkage in populations of different ethnicities and different environmental exposures. Therefore, the identification of a gene(s) underlying the linkage observed poses a major challenge. As mentioned earlier, in studies of complex disease, the real challenge has not been identification of regions of linkage but rather identification of the precise gene and genetic variant underlying the observed linkage. To date, several genes have been identified as the result of positional cloning using a genome-wide scan for allergic disease phenotypes including for example *ADAM33, GPRA, DPP10, PHF11* and *UPAR* for asthma and *COL29A1* for atopic dermatitis (See Table 3-1).

Genes Identified by Genome-Wide Association Studies

To date several genome-wide association studies have been performed with great success in allergic diseases, such as asthma, eczema and allergic sensitization; Table 3-2 describes some of the associated genes. The first novel asthma susceptibility locus to be identified by a GWAS approach contains the *ORMDL3* and *GSDML* genes on Chromosome 17q12-21.1.[48] 317 000 SNPs (in genes or surrounding sequences) were characterized in 994 subjects with childhood onset asthmatics and 1243 non-asthmatics. After adjusting markers for quality control and population stratification, 7 SNPs remained above the 1% False Discovery Rate (FDR) threshold and mapped to a 112 kb region at 17q21. The authors performed internal replication of association by genotyping nine of the associated SNPs in the 17q21 locus in 2320 subjects (200 asthmatic cases and 2120 controls) and found 5 SNPs to be significantly associated with disease (P < 0.01). Global gene expression levels were measured in Epstein-Barr virus transformed lymphoblastoid (B cell) derived cell lines and tran-

Table 3-1 Summary of Positionally Cloned Genes for Atopy and Allergic Disease Phenotypes

Gene Name (Gene ID)	Chr	Associated Phenotypes	Gene Product: Possible Functional Role in Asthma or Allergic Disease	Associated Variation	Size of Study	Population	Reference of Initial Study	Replication of Association
OPN3+CML (23596+1122)	1q43	Asthma Atopic asthma BHR	Opsin 3 & choroideremia-like (Rab escort protein 2): Likely role of OPN3 in the regulation of peripheral circadian rhythms and TH1 and TH2 cells polarization	Multiple SNPs (linkage signal from rs614251)	294 families (1151 subjects) 442 families	Danish UK* Norway	White et al[150]	YES[150]
DPP10 (57628)	2q14.1	Asthma Atopy (SPT) Asthma severity	Dipeptidyl peptidase: Potassium channel regulator with no detectable protease activity. Involved in Cytokine processing (especially in T cells)	D2S308*3/*5 Multiple SNPs Haplotypes	244 families	Australian UK German	Allen et al[151]	YES[151]
COL29A1 (256076)	3q22.1	Atopic dermatitis	Collagen, type XXIX alpha 1: Novel epidermal ECM collagen. Expressed in the skin, lung, small intestine and colon. Distinct lack of COL29A1 in outer viable layers of the epidermis in AD patients	M3CS075 M3CS233 Multiple SNPs (rs4688761 had strongest association) Haplotypes	199 families (427 children) for discovery 292 families (481 children) for replication	European	Soderhall et al[152]	YES[152]
CYFIP2 (26999)	5q33.3	Atopic asthma Childhood asthma	Cytoplasmic fragile X mental retardation (FMRP) interaction protein 2: May be involved in differentiation of T cells	Multiple SNPs Haplotypes	155 families	Korean	Noguchi et al[153]	NO
HLA-G (3135)	6p21.3	Asthma BHR Atopy	Class I, Histo-compatibility antigen-G: Inhibits Th1-mediated inflammation and only the soluble form (HLA-G5) is expressed in asthmatic bronchial epithelial cells	D6S1281 MOGc Multiple SNPs	129 families	Caucasian Hutterite Dutch	Nicolae et al[154]	YES[154]
GPRA (387129)	7q14.3	Asthma Total IgE BHR Specific IgE Childhood asthma	G-Protein coupled receptor: Bronchial epithelial and smooth muscle surface receptor. May modulate asthma by increasing expression levels in tissues and potential inhibitory effect of GPRA-A on cell growth[155]	Haplotypes	86 families & 103 trios	Finnish Canadian German Italian Chinese	Laitinen et al[156]	YES[156-160]
IRAK-M (11213)	12q14.3	Early onset persistent asthma	Interleukin-1 receptor associated kinase 3: Negative regulator of TOLL-like receptor/IL-1R pathways. Master regulator of NF-Kappaβ and inflammation	Haplotypes	100 families	Sardinian Italian	Balaci et al[161]	YES[161]
PHF11 (51131)	13q14.3	Total IgE Asthma Asthma severity	Zinc Finger transcription factor: Possibly involved in Chromatin mediated transcription regulation. B cell clonal expansion and regulation of immunoglobulin expression may operate through shared mechanisms at this locus	Multiple SNPs Haplotypes	230 families	Australian UK European	Zhang et al[162]	YES[162,163]
UPAR (5329)	19q13	Asthma Lung function decline (FEV₁) BHR	Plasminogen activator, urokinase receptor: Key role in formation of serine protease plasmin. Implicated in many physiologic processes including; cell differentiation, proliferation, migration and fibrinolysis. May contribute to the pathogenesis of asthma via airway remodeling	Multiple SNPs Haplotypes	46 & 341 families 200 families	UK Dutch	Barton et al[164]	YES[164]
ADAM33 (80332)	20p13	Asthma+BHR	Metalloproteinase: Involved in airway remodelling by fibroblasts and smooth muscle hyperactivity	D20S482 Multiple SNPs Haplotypes	460 families	Caucasian (UK & US)	Van Eerdewegh et al[165]	YES[166-174]

Table 3-2 Summary of Genome-Wide Association Studies for Atopy and Allergic Disease Phenotypes

Identification Method	Gene Name (Gene ID)	Chr	Associated Phenotype	Gene Product: Possible Functional Role in Asthma or Allergic Disease	Associated Variation	Size of Study	Population	Reference of Initial Study	Replication of Association
Whole Genome Association	FCERIA (2205)	1q23	IgE levels Allergic sensitization	*Fc fragment of IgE, high affinity I-receptor for; alpha polypeptide:* Alpha unit of the IgE receptor. Initiates the inflammation and hypersensitivity responses to allergens	SNP (rs2251746 rs2427837)	1530 individuals. Replication in 4 independent samples (n = 9769)	European	Weidinger et al[59]	YES[59]
	IL1RL1 (9173)	2q12	Blood eosinophil counts Asthma Non-atopic asthma	*Interleukin1 receptor-like 1:* Studies of the mouse gene suggest that this receptor can be induced by pro-inflammatory stimuli, and may be involved in the function of helper T cells	SNP (rs1420101)	9392 12118 5212 7996 cases & 44890 controls	Icelandic European East Asians 10 different populations	Gudbjartsson et al[57]	YES[57]
	WDR36 (134430)	5q22	Blood eosinophil counts Atopic asthma	*WD repeat domain 36:* May facilitate formation of heterotrimeric or multiprotein complexes. Members of this family are involved in a variety of cellular processes, including cell cycle progression, signal transduction, apoptosis, and gene regulation	SNP (rs2416257)	9392 12118 5212 7996 cases & 44890 controls	Icelandic European East Asians 10 different populations	Gudbjartsson et al[57]	YES[57]
	RAD50 (10111)	5q23	IgE levels Atopic eczema & asthma	*RAD50 homolog (S. cerevisiae):* This protein is important for DNA double-strand break repair, cell cycle checkpoint activation, telomere maintenance, and meiotic recombination	SNP (rs2706347, rs3798135, rs2040704, rs7737470)	1530 individuals. Replication in 4 independent samples (n = 9769)	European	Weidinger et al[59]	YES[59]
	MYB (4602)	6q23	Blood eosinophil counts Atopic asthma	*v-myb myeloblastosis viral oncogene homolog:* nuclear transcription factor implicated in proliferation, survival and differentiation of hematopoietic stem and progenitor cells	SNP (rs9494145)	9392 12118 5212 7996 cases & 44890 controls	Icelandic European East Asians 10 different populations	Gudbjartsson et al[57]	YES[57]

	Gene	Locus	Phenotype	Function	Marker	Population	Samples	Reference	Replicated
	IL33 (90865)	9q24	Blood eosinophil counts Atopic asthma	Interleukin-33: An IL-1-like cytokine ligand for the IL-1 receptor-related protein ST2, activating mast cells and Th2 lymphocytes	SNP (rs3939286)	Icelandic European East Asians 10 different populations	9392 12118 5,212 7996 cases & 44890 controls	Gudbjartsson et al[57]	YES[57]
	CTNNA3 (29119)	10q22.2	Toluene diisocyanate-induced asthma	Catenin (cadherin-associated protein), alpha 3: Key molecule in the E-cadherin-mediated cell-cell adhesion complex. a-Catenin is an invasion suppressor and tumour-growth suppressor that inhibits Ras-MAPK activation. Genetic polymorphisms might disturb the defence systems of the airway epithelium, increasing airway hyperresponsiveness to environmental toxins such as TDI	SNP (rs1076205, rs7088181, rs4378283)	Korean	84 TDI asthma cases & 263 unexposed healthy controls	Kim et al[58]	NO
	ORMDL3 (94103)	17q12-17q21.1	Childhood onset asthma	ORMDL3: Trans-membrane protein anchored in the endoplasmic reticulum. Unknown function	SNP (rs7216389) & ORMDL3 mRNA expression	Caucasian *German †UK	994 asthmatics and 1243 controls. Replicated in 2320* and 3301† individuals	Moffatt et al[48]	YES[48]
Genome-Wide Gene Expression	PENDRIN (5172)	7q31	Mucus production in bronchial asthma	Solute carrier family 26, member 4: Transmembrane protein that acts as an anion transporter and can be induced by IL13. Critical mediator of mucus production in airway epithelial cells		Pendrin-expressing NCI-H292 cells in vitro and mouse lungs	NA	Nakao et al[175]	NO
Combination Approach	TNC (3371)	9p33	Asthma	Tenacin C: Extracellular matrix glycoprotein. Sub-epithelial marker for asthma severity and response to therapy. May affect the integrity and stiffness of asthma airways	SNP 44513A/T (in exon 17)	Japanese	446 adult asthmatics 658 non-asthmatic controls[176]	Linkage: Wjst et al[177] Association: Matsuda et al[176] Expression: Yuyama et al[178]	NO

script levels from one gene, *ORMDL3*, were strongly associated with disease-associated markers (P < 10^{-22} for rs7216389) identified by the GWAS.

Importantly, subsequent studies have replicated the association between variation in the Chr 17q21 region (mainly rs7216389) and childhood asthma in ethnically diverse populations.[49–52] Further information on the role of this locus in asthmatic susceptibility has been provided by Bouzignon and colleagues[53] who showed that SNPs on 17q21 and located in the *IKZF3-ZPBP2-GSDML-ORMDL3* gene cluster were found to be associated particularly with early-onset asthma (≤ 4 yrs of age), whereas no association was found for late-onset asthma. Furthermore, adjusting for early life smoke exposure revealed a 2.9-fold increase in risk compared to unexposed early-onset asthmatics.

However, a recent study of association between SNPs and gene expression levels found that a distant SNP rs1051740 (greater than 4 megabases away and on a different chromosome) in the *EPHX1* gene associates with *ORMDL3* gene expression at a more significant level than rs7216389.[54] Therefore, it is important to remember that considerable work is still required to fully characterize this region of the genome before accepting *ORMDL3* as the causal gene through 'guilt by association'.[55,56] The identification of the 17q21 locus as a novel susceptibilty gene for asthma illustrates the power of the GWAS approach. It is likely that further such studies will reveal considerable insight in to the pathogenesis of allergic disease in the near future. Indeed, GWAS studies have already resulted in the identification of novel genes underlying blood eosinophil levels (and also associated with asthma),[57] occupational asthma,[58] total serum IgE levels[59] and eczema.[60]

These studies show the power of the GWAS approach for identifying complex disease susceptibility variants and the number is likely to rapidly increase in the near future. However, as for other complex diseases such as Crohn's disease and diabetes (which have been extensively studied using GWAS approaches), the results from studies performed to date do not fully explain the heritability of common complex disease. However, geneticists remain optimistic, as it is believed that this 'missing heritability' can be accounted for.[61] It is thought that this inability to find genes could be explained by limitations of GWAS, such as other variants not screened for, analyses not adjusted for gene-environment and gene-gene interactions or epigenetic changes in gene expression. One explanation for missing heritability, after assessing common genetic variation in the genome, is that rare variants (below the frequency of SNPs included in GWAS studies) of high genetic effect, or common copy number variants may be responsible for some of the genetic heritability of common complex diseases.[9] The discovery of rare, high penetrance loss-of-function mutations in the filaggrin gene predisposing individuals to ichthyosis vulgaris, atopic dermatitis and asthma in the presence of atopic dermatitis (discussed later on in this chapter) is supporting evidence for the rare variant hypothesis.

Candidate Gene/Gene Region Studies

A large number of candidate regions have been studied for both linkage to and association with a range of atopy-related phenotypes. In addition, SNPs in the promoter and coding regions of a wide range of candidate genes have been examined. Candidate genes are selected for analysis based on a wide range of evidence, for example: biological function, differential expression in disease, involvement in other diseases with phenotypic overlap, affected tissues, cell type(s) involved and findings from animal

models. There are now more than 500 studies that have examined polymorphism in more than 200 genes for association with asthma and allergy phenotypes.[47,62] When assessing the significance of association studies, it is important to consider several things. For example, was the size of the study adequately powered if negative results are reported? Were the cases and controls appropriately matched? Could population stratification account for the associations observed? In the definitions of the phenotypes, which phenotypes have been measured (and which have not)? How were they measured? Regarding correction for multiple testing, have the authors taken multiple testing into account when assessing the significance of association? Publications by Weiss,[63] Hall,[64] and Tabor and colleagues[65] review these issues in depth.

It is also important to remember that statistical association is only that, i.e. a statistic; it does not necessarily imply that the genetic variant in question has a direct effect on gene expression or protein function. Genetic variants showing association with a disease are not necessary causal because of the phenomenon of linkage disequilibrium (LD). LD is the non-random association of adjacent polymorphisms on a single strand of DNA in a population; the allele of one polymorphism in an LD block (haplotype) can predict the allele of adjacent polymorphisms (one of which could be the causal variant). Consequently, an association seen between polymorphism A and a disease phenotype may not indicate that polymorphism A is affecting gene function but rather that it is merely in LD with polymorphism B that is exerting an effect on gene function or expression in the same or an adjacent gene.

Positive association may also represent a Type I error; candidate gene studies have suffered from non-replication of findings between studies, which may be due to poor study design, population stratification, different LD patterns between individuals of different ethnicity and differing environmental exposures between study cohorts. The genetic association approach can also be limited by under-powered studies and loose phenotype definitions.[66] The inherent complexities in the accurate assessment of the role of polymorphisms in a candidate gene involved in disease susceptibility are clearly illustrated by the examples provided from studies of the gene *IL13*.

Interleukin-13: An Example of a Candidate Gene

Given the importance of Th-2 mediated inflammation in allergic disease, and the biological roles of *IL13*, including, switching B cells to produce IgE, wide-ranging effects on epithelial cells, fibroblasts, and smooth muscle promoting airway remodeling and mucus production, *IL13* is a strong biological candidate gene. Furthermore, *IL13* is also a strong positional candidate. The gene encoding *IL13*, like *IL4*, is located in the Th2 cytokine gene cluster on chromosome 5q31 within 12 kb of *IL4*,[67] with which it shares 40% homology. This genomic location has been extensively linked with a number of phenotypes relevant to allergic disease including asthma, atopy, specific and total IgE responses, blood eosinophils and BHR.[68]

Which IL13 Polymorphism is Important (And What Phenotype)?

A number of polymorphisms have now been identified in the *IL13* gene. Van der Pouw-Kraan and colleagues[69] identified a single-base pair substitution in the promoter of *IL13* adjacent to a consensus nuclear factor of activated T cell binding sites. Using a sample of 101 asthmatics and 107 controls, they observed an increased frequency of homozygotes in the asthmatic group (13 of 107 vs 2 of 107, $P = 0.002$, odds ratio = 8.3). Additional in vitro experiments demonstrated that the polymorphism was associated with reduced inhibition of *IL13* production by cyclosporin and increased transcription factor binding. In addition to promoter polymorphisms of *IL13*, an amino acid polymorphism of *IL13* has been described: R110Q (rs20541).[70–72] Hypotheses proposed to explain the association of this *IL13* polymorphism and development of atopic disease include: decreased affinity for the decoy receptor IL13Rα2, increased functional activity through IL13Rα1 and enhanced stability of the molecule in plasma (Reviewed in Kasaian et al[73]).

In 2005, Vladich and colleagues[74] showed that the 110Q variant enhances the effector mechanisms of allergic inflammation compared to the wildtype 110R IL13 molecule. The *IL13* 110Q was found to be more active than *IL13* 110R in inducing STAT6 phosphorylation and CD23 expression in monocytes and hydrocortisone-dependent IgE switching in B cells. Subsequently, *IL13* 110Q was demonstrated to have a lower affinity for the IL-13Rα2 decoy receptor and produced a more sustained eotaxin response in primary human fibroblasts expressing low levels of IL-13Rα2 than was observed for 110R *IL13*.[75] In cells expressing high levels of IL-13Rα2 the response was similar between 110Q and 110R *IL13*; the authors concluded that the ability of R110Q to contribute to an allergic response was dependant on its reduced affinity and naturally occurring levels of IL-13Rα2.

The work of Graves and colleagues[70] and Liu and colleagues[76] show strong associations between this *IL13* polymorphism and atopy in children. However, neither study examined associations with asthma. In contrast, the study of Heinzmann and colleagues[71] shows that in adults, polymorphisms in *IL13* are associated with asthma and not with atopy. Howard and colleagues[77] also showed that the −1112 C/T variant of *IL13* contributes significantly to BHR susceptibility ($P = 0.003$) but not to total serum IgE levels. Thus it is possible that polymorphisms in *IL13* may confer susceptibility to airway remodelling in persistent asthma, as well as to allergic inflammation in early life.

Is It Really IL13?

As discussed previously, positive association observed between a SNP and phenotype, does not imply that the SNP is casual. The SNP tested may be acting as a proxy marker for an adjacent untyped polymorphism in LD in the gene, or even adjacent genes. *IL13* lies adjacent to *IL4*, an equally strong biological candidate in which SNPs have shown association with relevant phenotypes,[78] therefore association observed with *IL13* SNPs may simply represent a proxy measure of the effect of polymorphisms in *IL4*. As both *IL13* and *IL4* are good functional candidates for atopy and asthma, polymorphism in either or both of them may be affecting disease susceptibility, or even potentially neither of them. For example, a recent genome-wide association study of total IgE levels reported significant associations between polymorphisms in an adjacent gene *RAD50* and total serum IgE levels,[59] in a region containing a number of evolutionary conserved non-coding sequences that may play a role in regulating *IL4* and *IL13* transcription.[79] However, given the extensive biologic evidence for functionality and recent studies examining polymorphisms across the gene region showing independent effects of the *IL13* R110Q SNP; it is likely that the reported *IL13* associations are real.

What About the Environment?

In addition to rigorous study design (adequate power, relevant genes in a pathway, haplotypes of polymorphisms within each gene and relevant phenotypes), genetic studies should consider

environmental exposure of individuals in the cohort. Many studies have observed positive associations of specific genetic polymorphisms with differential response to environmental factors in asthma and other respiratory phenotypes.[80,81] *IL13* levels have been shown to be increased in children whose parents smoke[82] and interaction between *IL13* -1112 C/T and smoking with childhood asthma as an outcome has been reported,[83] as well as evidence for this same SNP modulating the adverse affect of smoking on lung function in adults.[84] Thus differences in smoking exposure between studies may account for some of the differences in findings between studies.

What About Gene-Gene Interaction?

Any observed association of *IL13* polymorphism should have its effect reported in context by considering other variation in other relevant genes whose products may modulate its effects. For example, there are a number of other functional polymorphisms in genes encoding other components of the *IL4/IL13* signaling pathway (*IL4, IL13, IL4RA, IL13Rα1, IL13Rα2* and *STAT6*), and there is evidence that there may be a synergistic effect on disease risk in inheriting more than one of these variants.[85]

The *IL13* polymorphism studies illustrate many of the difficulties of genetic analysis in complex disease. Replication is often not found between studies and this may be accounted for by the lack of power to detect the small increases in disease risk that are typical for susceptibility variants in complex disease. Differences in genetic make up;[86,87] in environmental exposure between study populations; and failure to 'strictly replicate'[66] in either phenotype (IgE and atopy vs asthma and BHR) or genotype (different polymorphisms in the same gene) can all contribute to the lack of replication between studies. Furthermore, studies of a single polymorphism, or even a single gene in isolation, are likely to underestimate the contribution of a particular variant or gene to disease by not considering interactions with other genetic factors. Interaction with environmental exposure provides an additional layer of complexity.

Analysis of Clinically Defined Subgroups

One approach to the genetic analysis of complex disease that has proved successful in other complex genetic disorders, such as Type 2 diabetes, is to identify genes in a rare, severely affected subgroup of patients, in whom disease appears to follow a pattern of inheritance that indicates the effect of a single major gene. The assumption is that mutations (polymorphisms) of milder functional effect in the same gene in the general population may play a role in susceptibility to the complex genetic disorder. One example of this has been the identification of the gene encoding the protein filaggrin as a susceptibility gene for atopic dermatitis.

Filaggrin

Filaggrin (filament-aggregating protein) has a key role in epidermal barrier function. The protein is a major component of the protein-lipid cornified envelope of the epidermis important for water permeability and blocking the entry of microbes and allergens.[88] In 2002, the condition ichthyosis vulgaris, a severe skin disorder characterized by dry flaky skin and a predisposition to atopic dermatitis and associated asthma, was mapped to the epidermal differentiation complex on chromosome 1q21; this gene complex includes the filaggrin gene (FLG).[89] In 2006, Smith and colleagues[90] reported that loss of function mutations in the filaggrin gene caused ichthyosis vulgaris.

Noting the common occurrence of atopic dermatitis in individuals with ichthyosis vulgaris, these researchers subsequently showed that common loss of function variants (combined carrier frequencies of 9% in the European population[91]) were associated with atopic dermatitis in the general population.[92] Subsequent studies have association confirmed with atopic dermatitis,[93-95] and also with asthma[96] and allergy[97] but only in the presence of atopic dermatitis. Atopic dermatitis in children is often the first sign of atopic disease and these studies of filaggrin mutation have provided a molecular mechanism for the co-existence of asthma and dermatitis. It is thought that deficits in epidermal barrier function could initiate systemic allergy by allergen exposure through the skin and start the 'atopic march' in susceptible individuals.[98,99]

Molecular Regulation of Atopy and Atopic Disease, II: Disease-Modifying Genes

The concept of genes interacting to alter the effects of mutations in susceptibility genes is not unknown. A proportion of interfamilial variability can be explained by differences in environmental factors and differences in the effect of different mutations in the same gene. Intrafamilial variability, especially in siblings, cannot be so readily accredited to these types of mechanisms. Many genetic disorders are influenced by 'modifier' genes that are distinct from the disease susceptibility loci.

Genetic Influences on Disease Severity

Very few studies of the heritability of IgE-mediated disease have examined phenotypes relating to severity. Sarafino and Goldfedder[100] studied 39 monozygotic twin pairs and 55 same-sex dizygotic twin pairs for the heritability of asthma and asthma severity. Asthma severity (as measured by frequency and intensity of asthmatic episodes) was examined in twin pairs concordant for asthma. Severity was significantly correlated for monozygotic pairs but not for dizygotic pairs, suggesting the there are distinct genetic factors that determine asthma severity as opposed to susceptibility.

A number of studies have examined associations between asthma severity and polymorphisms in candidate genes but the conclusive identification of genetic factors contributing to asthma severity has been hampered by the lack of clear, easily applied, accurate phenotype definitions for asthma severity that distinguish between the underlying severity and level of therapeutic control. For example, it has been suggested that β_2-adrenergic receptor polymorphisms could influence asthma severity, and the Arg16Gly polymorphism has been associated with measures of asthma severity.[101] However, it is not clear whether this reflects β_2-adrenergic receptor polymorphism affecting patients' responses to β_2 agonists and hence leading to poor therapeutic control or whether, regardless of their effects on treatment, polymorphism of the β_2-adrenergic receptor leads to more severe chronic asthma.[102] The development of such phenotypes in conjunction with more extensive studies of the genetics of asthma severity may allow identification of at-risk individuals and targeting of prophylactic therapy. For example, a recent retrospective study of the Childhood Asthma Management Program (CAMP) cohort showed that variation in the gene encoding the low affinity IgE receptor, FCER2, is associated with high IgE levels and increased frequency of severe exacerbations despite inhaled corticosteroid treatment.[103]

Genetic Regulation of Response to Therapy: Pharmacogenetics

Genetic variability may not only play a role in influencing susceptibility to allergy but may also modify its severity or influence the effectiveness of therapy.[104] In asthma, patient response to drugs, such as bronchodilators, corticosteroids and antileukotrienes is heterogeneous.[105,106] In the future, identification of such pharmacogenetic factors has the potential to allow individualized treatment plans based on an individual's genetic background.[107] One of the most investigated pharmacogenetic effects has been the effect of polymorphisms at the gene encoding the β_2-adrenergic receptor, ADRB2, on the bronchodilator response to inhaled short- and long-acting β agonists.

Clinical studies have shown that β_2-adrenergic receptor polymorphisms may influence the response to bronchodilator treatment. The two most common polymorphisms of the receptor are at amino acid 16 (Arg16Gly) and at amino acid 27 (Gln27Glu).[108] Asthmatic patients carrying the Gly16 polymorphism have been shown to be more prone to develop bronchodilator desensitization,[109] whereas children who are homozygous or heterozygous for Arg16 are more likely to show positive responses to bronchodilators.[110] Studies in vitro have shown that the Gly16 increases down-regulation of the β_2-adrenergic receptor after exposure to a β_2 agonist. In contrast, the Glu27 polymorphism appears to protect against agonist-induced down-regulation and desensitization of the β_2-adrenergic receptor.[111,112]

However, a study of 190 asthmatics examined whether β_2-adrenergic receptor genotype affects the response to regular versus as-needed albuterol use.[113] During a 16-week treatment period, there was a small but significant decline in morning peak flow in patients homozygous for the Arg16 polymorphism who used albuterol regularly. The effect was magnified during the 4-week run-out period when all patients returned to albuterol as needed. However, other studies have suggested that response to bronchodilator treatment is genotype independent.[114,115]

In contrast to the possible effects on short-acting bronchodilators, pharmacogenetic analysis of β_2-adrenergic receptor polymorphisms have found no effect on response to long-acting β_2 agonist therapy in combination with corticosteroids.[116,117] These findings are difficult to explain in the light of the studies discussed linking the Gly16 allele with BHR, β_2 agonist effectiveness, and asthma severity but may indicate that the co-administration of corticosteroids abrogates the effect of variation of ADRB2. The complexity of the genotype by response effects observed for variation in ADRB2 makes clinical application limited at this time, and may require the use of detailed haplotypic variation to fully understand the role that variation at this locus plays in regulating β_2 agonist response.[118]

While glucocorticoid therapy is a potent antiinflammatory treatment for asthma, there is a subset of asthmatics who are poor responders and clinical studies have shown that those with severe disease are more likely to have glucocorticoid resistance.[119] Numerous mutations in the glucocorticoid receptor gene that alter expression, ligand binding and signal trans-activation have been identified; however, these are rare and studies in asthma have not revealed an obvious correlation between any specific polymorphism in the glucocorticoid receptor gene and a response to corticosteroid treatment. However, a number of studies have examined variations in components of the downstream signaling pathways or other related genes. For example, Tantisira and colleagues[120] have shown that variation in Adenyl cylase 9 gene predicts improved bronchodilator response following corticosteroid treatment, and also identified variation in the *CRHR1* locus[121,122] and the gene encoding *TBX21*[123] as potential markers for steroid responsiveness.

Genetic polymorphism may also play a role in regulating responses to anti-leukotrienes.[105] In part, this is mediated by polymorphism in both *ALOX5* and other components of the leukotriene biosynthetic pathway.[124-126] There is also a substantial overlap in the genetic modulation of response to the two classes of leukotriene modifier drugs (5-LO inhibitor and Cysteinyl LT1 receptor antagonists).[127] Genetic variation in the leukotriene biosynthetic pathway has also been shown to be associated with increased susceptibility to several chronic disease phenotypes including myocardial infarction,[128,129] stroke,[129,130] atherosclerosis,[131] and asthma,[132] suggesting variation in leukotriene production increases risk and severity of inflammation in many conditions.

The aim of pharmacogenetic approaches is to maximize the therapeutic response and minimize any side-effects. To date there is no direct pharmacogenetic test for asthma treatment. However, there is a growing body of research suggesting that development of these tests would be of great benefit to develop new drugs, tailor treatment and provide better control of asthma in individuals who are predisposed to poor response, than using current prescription methodology based on clinical trials that do not account for inter-individual variability in drug response that is genetically determined.

Epigenetics and Allergic Disease

The role of epigenetics is being increasingly recognized as playing an important role as a mechanism by which the environment can alter disease risk in an individual. The term *epigenetics* refers to biological processes that regulate gene activity but which do not alter the DNA sequence. Epigenetic factors include modification of histones by acetylation and methylation, and DNA methylation. Modification of histones, around which the DNA is coiled, alters the rate of transcription, altering protein expression. DNA methylation involves the addition of a methyl group to specific cytosine bases, suppressing gene expression. DNA methylation patterns can be heritable. Importantly, both changes to histones and DNA methylation can be induced in response to environmental exposures such as tobacco smoke and alterations in early life environment, e.g. maternal nutrition.[133]

There is evidence that epigenetic factors are important in allergic disease. For example, a number of studies have linked altered birth weight and/or head circumference at birth (proxy markers for maternal nutrition), with an increase in adult IgE levels and risk of allergic disease.[134-136] A recent study has also shown that increased environmental particulate exposure from traffic pollution results in a dose-dependant increase in peripheral blood DNA methylation.[137]

The effect of epigenetics has been observed over more than just a single generation. For example, in humans, trans-generational effects have been observed where the initial environmental exposure occurred in F_0 generation and changes in disease suceptibilty were still evident in F_2 (grandchildren). Pembery and colleagues[138] showed that exposures, such as poor nutrition or smoking during the slow growth period of the F_0 generation, resulted in effects on life expectancy and growth through the

male line and female line in the F_2 generation, although there had been no further exposure. Observations such as grandmaternal smoking increasing the risk of childhood asthma in their grandchildren,[139] supports the concept that trans-generational epigenetic effects (mediated by DNA methylation) may be operating in allergic disease. Other support comes from the study of animal models, for example in one model where mice were exposed to in utero supplementation with methyl donors and exhibited enhanced airway inflammation following allergen challenge.[140] It is probable in the near future that the study of large prospective birth cohorts with information on maternal environmental exposures during pregnancy are likely to provide important insights into the role of epigenetic factors in the heritability of allergic disease.[141]

Conclusions

The varying and sometimes conflicting results of studies to identify allergic disease susceptibility genes reflect the genetic and environmental heterogeneity seen in allergic disorders and illustrate the difficulty of identifying susceptibility genes for complex genetic diseases. This is the result of a number of factors, including difficulties in defining phenotypes and population heterogeneity with different genetic loci showing association in populations of differing ethnicity and differing environmental exposure. However, despite this, there is now a rapidly expanding list of genes robustly associated with a wide range of allergic disease phenotypes.

This leads to the question, is it possible to predict the likelihood that an individual will develop allergic disease? To an extent, clinicians already make some predictions of the risk of developing allergic disease through the use of family history and this has been shown to have some validity.[142] However, at present, we are not in a position to utilize the rapidly accumulating knowledge of genetic variants that influence allergic disease progression in clinical practice. This simply reflects the complex interactions between different genetic and environmental factors required, both to initiate disease and determine progression to a more severe phenotype in an individual, meaning that the predictive value of variation in any one gene is low, with a typical genotype relative risk of 1.1–1.5.[143]

However, it is possible that, as our knowledge of the genetic factors underlying disease increases, the predictive power of genetic testing will increase sufficiently to enable its use in clinical decision making (Box 3-1). For example, simulation studies based on the use of 50 genes relevant for disease development demonstrated that an area under a curve (AUC) of 0.8 can be reached if the genotype relative risk is 1.5 and the risk allele frequency is 10%.[143,144] Whether this is likely to improve on diagnostics using traditional risk factor assessment is a separate issue. Recent analyses of the power of genetic testing to predict risk of Type 2 diabetes (for which many more genetic risk factors have been identified through genome-wide approaches than for allergic disease at this stage) demonstrate that, currently, the inclusion of common genetic variants has only a small effect on the ability to predict the future development of the condition.[145,146] This has led to some questioning the 'disproportionate attention and resources' given to genetic studies in the prevention of common disease.[147] However, the identification of further risk factors and the development of better methods for incorporating genetic factors into risk models are likely to substantially increase the value of genotypic risk factors and may also provide a means for predicting progression to severe disease and targeting of preventative treatment in the future.[148]

Whatever the future value of genetic studies of allergic disease in predicting risk, it is unlikely that this will be the area of largest impact of genetics studies on the treatment and prevention of these conditions. Rather, it is the insight the genetic studies have provided, and undoubtedly will continue to provide, into disease pathogenesis. It is clear from genetic studies of allergic disease that the propensity to develop atopy is influenced by factors different than those that influence atopic disease. However, these disease factors require interaction with atopy (or something else)

to trigger disease. For example, in asthma, bronchoconstriction is triggered mostly by an allergic response to inhaled allergen accompanied by eosinophilic inflammation in the lungs, but in some people who may have 'asthma susceptibility genes' but not atopy, asthma is triggered by other exposures, such as toluene diiso-cyanate. It is possible to group the genes indentified into four broad groups (Figure 3-1). Firstly, there is a group of genes that are involved in directly modulating response to environmental exposures. These include genes encoding components of the innate immune system that interact with levels of microbial exposure to alter risk of developing allergic immune

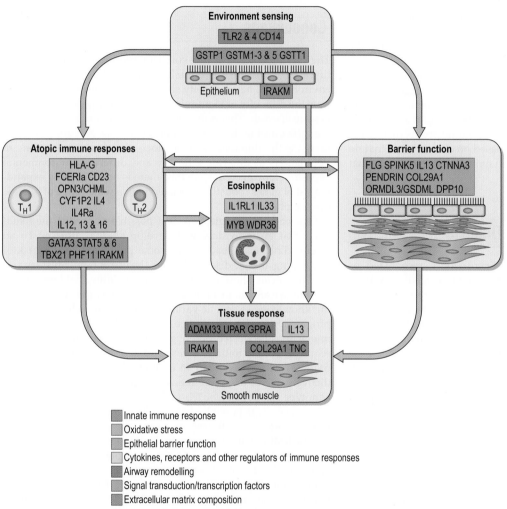

Figure 3-1 Susceptibility genes for allergic disease: a large number of robustly associated genes have been identified that predispose to allergic disease. These can be broadly divided into four main groups. **Group 1 – sensing the environment.** This group of genes encodes molecules that directly modulate the effect of environmental risk factors for allergic disease. For example, genes such as *TLR2*, *TLR4* and *CD14* encoding components of the innate immune system interact with levels of microbial exposure to alter risk of developing allergic immune responses. Polymorphism of Glutathione-S-transferase genes (*GSTM1*, *-2*, *-3*, and *-5*, *GSTT1*, and *GSTP1*) has been shown to modulate the effect of exposures involving oxidant stress such as tobacco smoke and air pollution on asthma susceptibility. **Group 2 – barrier function.** The body is also protected from environmental exposure through the direct action of the epithelial barrier both in the airways and in the dermal barrier of the skin. A high proportion of the novel genes identified for susceptibility to allergic disease through genome-wide linkage and association approaches has been shown to be expressed in the epithelium. This includes genes, such as *FLG*, that directly affect dermal barrier function and are associated, not only with increased risk of atopic dermatitis, but also with increased atopic sensitization and inflammatory products produced directly by the epithelium such as chemokines and defensins. Other novel genes such as *ORMDL3/GSDML* are also expressed in the epithelium and may have a role in possibly regulating epithelial barrier function. **Group 3 – regulation of (atopic) inflammation.** This group of genes includes genes that regulate Th1/Th2 differentiation and effector function such as *IL13*, *IL4RA*, *STAT6*, *TBX21* (encoding T-bet) and *GATA3*, as well as genes such as *IRAKM* and *PHF11* that potentially regulate both atopic sensitization and the level inflammation that occurs at the end organ location for allergic disease (airway, skin, nose, etc.). This also includes the genes recently identified as regulating the level of blood eosinophilia using a GWAS approach (*IL1RL1*, *IL33*, *MYB* and *WDR36*). **Group 4 – tissue response genes.** This group of genes appears to modulate the consequences of chronic inflammation such as airway remodeling. They include genes such as *ADAM33* expressed in fibroblasts and smooth muscle and *COL29A1*, encoding a novel collagen expressed in the skin and linked to atopic dermatitis. It is important to recognize that some genes may affect more than one component, for example *IL13* may regulate atopic sensitization through switching B cells to produce IgE but also has direct effects on the airway epithelium and mesenchyme promoting goblet cell metaplasia and fibroblast proliferation.

BOX 3-1 Key concepts

What Can Genetics Studies of Allergic Disease Tell Us?

Greater Understanding of Disease Pathogenesis

- Identification of novel genes and pathways leading to new pharmacologic targets for developing therapeutics

Identification of Environmental Factors that Interact with an Individual's Genetic Make-up to Initiate Disease

- Prevention of disease by environmental modification

Identification of Susceptible Individuals

- Early-in-life screening and targeting of preventative therapies to at-risk individuals to prevent disease

Targeting of Therapies

- Subclassification of disease on the basis of genetics and targeting of specific therapies based on this classification
- Determination of the likelihood of an individual responding to a particular therapy (pharmacogenetics) and individualized treatment plans

---

BOX 3-2 Key concepts

Genetic Effects on Allergy and Allergic Disease

Determine Susceptibility Atopy

- *'Th2' or 'IgE switch' genes*
  Determine specific target-organ disease in atopic individuals
- *Asthma susceptibility genes*
  'Lung-specific factors' that regulate susceptibility of lung epithelium/fibroblasts to remodeling in response to allergic inflammation, such as *ADAM33*
- *Atopic dermatitis susceptibility genes*
  Genes that regulate dermal barrier function, such as FLG

Influence the Interaction of Environmental Factors with Atopy and Allergic Disease

- Determining immune responses to factors that drive Th1/Th2 skewing of the immune response, such as *CD14* and *TLR4* polymorphism and early childhood infection
- Modulating the effect of exposures involving oxidant stress such as tobacco smoke and air pollution on asthma susceptibility
- Altering interaction between environmental factors and established disease, such as genetic polymorphism regulating responses to respiratory syncytial virus infection and asthma symptoms

Modify Severity of Disease

- Examples are tumor necrosis factor α polymorphisms and asthma severity

Regulate Response to Therapy

- Pharmacogenetics
- Examples are β₂-adrenergic receptor polymorphism and response to β₂ agonists

---

responses as well as detoxifying enzymes such as the Glutathione S-transferase genes that modulate the effect of exposures involving oxidant stress, such as tobacco smoke and air pollution. The second major group that includes many of the genes identified through hypothesis independent genome-wide approaches is a group of genes involved in maintaining the integrity of the epithelial barrier at the mucosal surface and signaling of the epithelium to the immune system following environmental exposure. For example, polymorphisms in FLG that directly affect dermal barrier function are associated, not only with increased risk of atopic dermatitis, but also with increased atopic sensitization. The third group of genes are those that regulate the immune response, including those such as *IL13, IL4RA, STAT6, TBX21* (encoding Tbet), *HLAG* and *GATA3* that regulate Th1/Th2 differentiation and effector function, but also others such as *IRAKM* and *PHF11* that may regulate the level of inflammation that occurs at the end organ for allergic disease (i.e. airway, skin, nose, etc.). Finally, but not least, a number of genes appear to be involved in determining the tissue response to chronic inflammation, such as airway remodelling. They include genes such as *ADAM33* expressed in fibroblasts and smooth muscle and *COL29A1* encoding a novel collagen expressed in the skin and linked to atopic dermatitis.

Thus, the insights provided by the realization that genetic variation in genes regulating atopic immune responses are not the only, or even the major, factor in determining susceptibility to allergic disease, has highlighted the importance of local tissue response factors and epithelial susceptibility factors in the pathogenesis of allergic disease.[149] This is possibly the greatest contribution that genetic studies have made to the study of allergic disease and where the most impact in the form of new therapeutics targeting novel pathways of disease pathogenesis is likely to occur.

In conclusion, over the past 15 years, there have been many linkage and association studies examining genetic susceptibility to atopy and allergic disease resulting in the unequivocal identification of a number of loci that alter the susceptibility of an individual to allergic disease. While further research is needed to confirm previous studies and to understand how these genetic variants alter gene expression and/or protein function, and therefore contribute to the pathogenesis of disease, genetic studies have already helped to change our understanding of these conditions. In the future, the study of larger cohorts and the pooling of data across studies will be needed to allow the determination of the contribution of identified polymorphisms to susceptibility and how these polymorphisms interact with each other and the environment to initiate allergic disease. Furthermore it is now apparent that the added complexity of epigenetic influences on allergic disease needs to be considered. Despite these challenges for the future, genetic approaches to the study of allergic disease have clearly shown that they can lead to identification of new biologic pathways involved in the pathogenesis of allergic disease, the development of new therapeutic approaches, and the identification of at-risk individuals (Box 3-2).

References

1. Cookson WO, Sharp PA, Faux JA, et al. Linkage between immunoglobulin E responses underlying asthma and rhinitis and chromosome 11q. Lancet 1989;1:1292–5.
2. Kerem B, Rommens JM, Buchanan JA, et al. Identification of the cystic fibrosis gene: genetic analysis. Science 1989;245:1073–80.
3. Botstein D, White RL, Skolnick M, et al. Construction of a genetic linkage map in man using restriction fragment length polymorphisms. Am J Hum Genet 1980;32:314–31.

4. Pearce N, Weiland S, Keil U, et al. Self-reported prevalence of asthma symptoms in children in Australia, England, Germany and New Zealand: an international comparison using the ISAAC protocol. Eur Respir J 1993;6:1455–61.

5. King MC, Lee GM, Spinner NB, et al. Genetic epidemiology. Annu Rev Public Health 1984;5:1–52.

6. Farrer LA, Cupples LA. Determining the genetic component of a disease. In: Haines JL, Pericak-Vance MA, eds. Approaches to gene mapping in complex human diseases. New York, USA: Wiley-Liss, Inc., 1998.

7. Haldar P, Pavord ID, Shaw DE, et al. Cluster analysis and clinical asthma phenotypes. Am J Respir Crit Care Med 2008;178:218–24.

8. Weatherall M, Travers J, Shirtcliffe PM, et al. Distinct clinical phenotypes of airways disease defined by cluster analysis. Eur Respir J 2009;34:812–8.

9. Frazer KA, Murray SS, Schork NJ, et al. Human genetic variation and its contribution to complex traits. Nat Rev Genet 2009;10:241–51.

10. Feuk L, Marshall CR, Wintle RF, et al. Structural variants: changing the landscape of chromosomes and design of disease studies. Hum Mol Genet 2006;15(Spec No 1):R57–66.

11. Levy S, Sutton G, Ng PC, et al. The diploid genome sequence of an individual human. PLoS Biol 2007;5:e254.

12. Peddle L, Rahman P. Genetic epidemiology of complex phenotypes. Methods Mol Biol 2009;473:187–201.

13. Morton N. Major loci for atopy? Clin Exp Allergy 1992;22:1041–3.

14. Almasy L, Blangero J. Contemporary model-free methods for linkage analysis. Adv Genet 2008;60:175–93.

15. Cooper RS, Tayo B, Zhu X. Genome-wide association studies: implications for multiethnic samples. Hum Mol Genet 2008;17:R151–5.

16. Spielman RS, McGinnis RE, Ewens WJ. Transmission test for linkage disequilibrium: the insulin gene region and insulin-dependent diabetes mellitus (IDDM). Am J Hum Genet 1993;52:506–16.

17. Spielman RS, Ewens WJ. The TDT and other family-based tests for linkage disequilibrium and association. Am J Hum Genet 1996;59:983–9.

18. A haplotype map of the human genome. Nature 2005;437:1299–320.

19. Altshuler D, Daly MJ, Lander ES. Genetic mapping in human disease. Science 2008;322:881–8.

20. McCarthy MI, Abecasis GR, Cardon LR, et al. Genome-wide association studies for complex traits: consensus, uncertainty and challenges. Nat Rev Genet 2008;9:356–69.

21. Hindorff LA, Junkins HA, Mehta JP, et al. A catalog of published genome-wide association studies. Available at: wwwgenomegov/ 26525384; Accessed 24 March 2009.

22. Amos CI. Successful design and conduct of genome-wide association studies. Hum Mol Genet 2007;16(Spec No. 2):R220–5.

23. Lam AC, Powell J, Wei WH, et al. A combined strategy for quantitative trait loci detection by genome-wide association. BMC Proc 2009;3(Suppl 1):S6.

24. Coca A, Cooke R. On the classification of the phenomena of hypersensitiveness. J Immunol 1923;8:163–80.

25. Lawrence S, Beasley R, Doull I, et al. Genetic analysis of atopy and asthma as quantitative traits and ordered polychotomies. Ann Human Genet 1994;58:359–68.

26. Wilkinson J, Grimley S, Collins A, et al. Linkage of asthma to markers on chromosome 12 in a sample of 240 families using quantitative phenotype scores. Genomics 1998;53:251–9.

27. Cooke RA, Vander Veer A. Human sensitisation. J Immunol 1916;16:201–305.

28. Hayashi T, Kawakami N, Kondo N, et al. Prevalence of and risk factors for allergic diseases: comparison of two cities in Japan. Ann Allergy Asthma Immunol 1995;75:525

29. Jenkins MA, Hopper JL, Giles GG. Regressive logistic modeling of familial aggregation for asthma in 7,394 population-based nuclear families. Genet Epidemiol 1997;14:317–32.

30. Bazaral M, Orgel HA, Hamburger RN. IgE levels in normal infants and mothers and an inheritance hypothesis. J Immunol 1971;107:794–801.

31. Gerrard JW, Vickers P, Gerrard CD. The familial incidence of allergic disease. Ann Allergy 1976;36:10–5.

32. Dold S, Wjst M, von Mutius E, et al. Genetic risk for asthma, allergic rhinitis, and atopic dermatitis. Arch Dis Child 1992;67:1018–22.

33. von Mutius E, Nicolai T. Familial aggregation of asthma in a South Bavarian population. Am J Respir Crit Care Med 1996;153:1266–72.

34. Duffy DL, Martin NG, Battistutta D, et al. Genetics of asthma and hay fever in Australian twins. Am Rev Respir Dis 1990;142:1351–8.

35. Wuthrich B, Baumann E, Fries RA, et al. Total and specific IgE (RAST) in atopic twins. Clin Allergy 1981;11:147–54.

36. Sarafino EP, Goldfedder J. Genetic factors in the presence, severity, and triggers of asthma. Arch Dis Child 1995;73:112–6.

37. Husby S, Holm NV, Christensen K, et al. Cord blood immunoglobulin E in like-sexed monozygotic and dizygotic twins. Clin Genet 1996;50:332–8.

38. Hopp RJ, Bewtra AK, Watt GD, et al. Genetic analysis of allergic disease in twins. J Allergy Clin Immunol 1984;73:265–70.

39. Harris JR, Magnus P, Samuelsen SO, et al. No evidence for effects of family environment on asthma: a retrospective study of Norwegian twins. Am J Respir Crit Care Med 1997;156:43–9.

40. Hanson B, McGue M, Roitman-Johnson B, et al. Atopic disease and immunoglobulin E in twins reared apart and together. Am J Hum Genet 1991;48:873–9.

41. Sibbald B, Horn ME, Gregg I. A family study of the genetic basis of asthma and wheezy bronchitis. Arch Dis Child 1980;55:354–7.

42. Sibbald B, Turner-Warwick M. Factors influencing the prevalence of asthma among first degree relatives of extrinsic and intrinsic asthmatics. Thorax 1979;34:332–7.

43. Longo G, Strinati R, Poli F, et al. Genetic factors in nonspecific bronchial hyperreactivity: an epidemiologic study. Am J Dis Child 1987;141:331–4.

44. Laitinen T, Rasanen M, Kaprio J, et al. Importance of genetic factors in adolescent asthma: a population-based twin-family study. Am J Respir Crit Care Med 1998;157:1073–8.

45. Skadhauge LR, Christensen K, Kyvik KO, et al. Genetic and environmental influence on asthma: a population-based study of 11,688 Danish twin pairs. Eur Respir J 1999;13:8–14.

46. Ober C. Susceptibility genes in asthma and allergy. Curr Allergy Asthma Rep 2001;1:174–9.

47. Ober C, Hoffjan S. Asthma genetics 2006: the long and winding road to gene discovery. Genes Immun 2006;7:95–100.

48. Moffatt MF, Kabesch M, Liang L, et al. Genetic variants regulating ORMDL3 expression contribute to the risk of childhood asthma. Nature 2007;448:470–3.

49. Galanter J, Choudhry S, Eng C, et al. ORMDL3 gene is associated with asthma in three ethnically diverse populations. Am J Respir Crit Care Med 2008;177:1194–200.

50. Leung TF, Sy HY, Ng MC, et al. Asthma and atopy are associated with chromosome 17q21 markers in Chinese children. Allergy 2009;64:621–8.

51. Tavendale R, Macgregor DF, Mukhopadhyay S, et al. A polymorphism controlling ORMDL3 expression is associated with asthma that is poorly controlled by current medications. J Allergy Clin Immunol 2008;121:860–3.

52. Wu H, Romieu I, Sienra-Monge JJ, et al. Genetic variation in ORM1-like 3 (ORMDL3) and gasdermin-like (GSDML) and childhood asthma. Allergy 2009;64:629–35.

53. Bouzigon E, Corda E, Aschard H, et al. Effect of 17q21 variants and smoking exposure in early-onset asthma. N Engl J Med 2008;359:1985–94.

54. Duan S, Huang RS, Zhang W, et al. Genetic architecture of transcript-level variation in humans. Am J Hum Genet 2008;82:1101–13.

55. Holloway JW, Koppelman GH. 17q21 variants and asthma - questions and answers. N Engl J Med 2008;359:2043–5.

56. Wjst M. ORMDL3–guilt by association? Clin Exp Allergy 2008;38:1579–81.

57. Gudbjartsson DF, Bjornsdottir US, Halapi E, et al. Sequence variants affecting eosinophil numbers associate with asthma and myocardial infarction. Nat Genet 2009;41:342–7.

58. Kim SH, Cho BY, Park CS, et al. Alpha-T-catenin (CTNNA3) gene was identified as a risk variant for toluene diisocyanate-induced asthma by genome-wide association analysis. Clin Exp Allergy 2009;39:203–12.

59. Weidinger S, Gieger C, Rodriguez E, et al. Genome-wide scan on total serum IgE levels identifies FCER1A as novel susceptibility locus. PLoS Genet 2008;4:e1000166.

60. Esparza-Gordillo J, Weidinger S, Folster-Holst R, et al. A common variant on chromosome 11q13 is associated with atopic dermatitis. Nat Genet 2009;41:596–601.

61. Maher B. Personal genomes: the case of the missing heritability. Nature 2008;456:18–21.

62. Vercelli D. Discovering susceptibility genes for asthma and allergy. Nat Rev Immunol 2008;8:169–82.

63. Weiss ST. Association studies in asthma genetics. Am J Respir Crit Care Med 2001;164:2014–5.

64. Hall I. Candidate gene studies in respiratory disease: avoiding the pitfalls. Thorax 2002;57:377–8.

65. Tabor HK, Risch NJ, Myers RM. Candidate gene approaches for studying complex genetic traits: practical considerations. Nat Rev Genet 2002;3:391–7.

66. Holloway JW, Koppelman GH. Identifying novel genes contributing to asthma pathogenesis. Curr Opin Allergy Clin Immunol 2007;7:69–74.

67. Frazer KA, Ueda Y, Zhu Y, et al. Computational and biological analysis of 680 kb of DNA sequence from the human 5q31 cytokine gene cluster region. Genome Res 1997;7:495–512.

68. Hoffjan S, Nicolae D, Ober C. Association studies for asthma and atopic diseases: a comprehensive review of the literature. Respir Res 2003;4:14.

69. van der Pouw Kraan T, van Veen A, Boeije L, et al. An IL-13 promoter polymorphism associated with increased risk of allergic asthma. Genes Immun 1999;1:61–5.

70. Graves PE, Kabesch M, Halonen M, et al. A cluster of seven tightly linked polymorphisms in the IL-13 gene is associated with total serum IgE levels in three populations of white children. J Allergy Clin Immunol 2000;105:506–13.

71. Heinzmann A, Mao XQ, Akaiwa M, et al. Genetic variants of IL-13 signalling and human asthma and atopy. Hum Mol Genet 2000;9:549–59.

72. Pantelidis P, Jones MG, Welsh KI, et al. Identification of four novel interleukin-13 gene polymorphisms. Genes Immun 2000;1:341–5.

73. Kasaian MT, Miller DK. IL-13 as a therapeutic target for respiratory disease. Biochem Pharmacol 2008;76:147–55.

74. Vladich FD, Brazille SM, Stern D, et al. IL-13 R130Q, a common variant associated with allergy and asthma, enhances effector mechanisms essential for human allergic inflammation. J Clin Invest 2005;115:747–54.

75. Andrews AL, Bucchieri F, Arima K, et al. Effect of IL-13 receptor alpha2 levels on the biological activity of IL-13 variant R110Q. J Allergy Clin Immunol 2007;120:91–7.

76. Liu X, Nickel R, Beyer K, et al. An IL13 coding region variant is associated with a high total serum IgE level and atopic dermatitis in the German multicenter atopy study (MAS- 90). J Allergy Clin Immunol 2000;106:167–70.

77. Howard TD, Whittaker PA, Zaiman AL, et al. Identification and association of polymorphisms in the interleukin-13 gene with asthma and atopy in a Dutch population. Am J Respir Cell Mol Biol 2001;25:377–84.

78. Li Y, Guo B, Zhang L, et al. Association between C-589T polymorphisms of interleukin-4 gene promoter and asthma: a meta-analysis. Respir Med 2008;102:984–92.

79. Loots GG, Locksley RM, Blankespoor CM, et al. Identification of a coordinate regulator of interleukins 4, 13, and 5 by cross-species sequence comparisons. Science 2000;288:136–40.

80. Le Souef PN. Gene-environmental interaction in the development of atopic asthma: new developments. Curr Opin Allergy Clin Immunol 2009;9:123–7.

81. von Mutius E. Gene-environment interactions in asthma. J Allergy Clin Immunol 2009;123:3–11; quiz 2–3.

82. Feleszko W, Zawadzka-Krajewska A, Matysiak K, et al. Parental tobacco smoking is associated with augmented IL-13 secretion in children with allergic asthma. J Allergy Clin Immunol 2006;117:97–102.

83. Sadeghnejad A, Karmaus W, Arshad SH, et al. IL13 gene polymorphisms modify the effect of exposure to tobacco smoke on persistent wheeze and asthma in childhood: a longitudinal study. Respir Res 2008;9:2.

84. Sadeghnejad A, Meyers DA, Bottai M, et al. IL13 promoter polymorphism 1112C/T modulates the adverse effect of tobacco smoking on lung function. Am J Respir Crit Care Med 2007;176:748–52.

85. Kabesch M, Schedel M, Carr D, et al. IL-4/IL-13 pathway genetics strongly influence serum IgE levels and childhood asthma. J Allergy Clin Immunol 2006;117:269–74.

86. Battle NC, Choudhry S, Tsai HJ, et al. Ethnicity-specific gene-gene interaction between IL-13 and IL-4Ralpha among African Americans with asthma. Am J Respir Crit Care Med 2007;175:881–7.

87. Hunninghake GM, Soto-Quiros ME, Avila L, et al. Polymorphisms in IL13, total IgE, eosinophilia, and asthma exacerbations in childhood. J Allergy Clin Immunol 2007;120:84–90.

88. Presland RB, Coulombe PA, Eckert RL, et al. Barrier function in transgenic mice overexpressing K16, involucrin, and filaggrin in the suprabasal epidermis. J Invest Dermatol 2004;123:603–6.

89. Compton JG, DiGiovanna JJ, Johnston KA, et al. Mapping of the associated phenotype of an absent granular layer in ichthyosis vulgaris to the epidermal differentiation complex on chromosome 1. Exp Dermatol 2002;11:518–26.

90. Smith FJ, Irvine AD, Terron-Kwiatkowski A, et al. Loss-of-function mutations in the gene encoding filaggrin cause ichthyosis vulgaris. Nat Genet 2006;38:337–42.

91. Brown SJ, McLean WH. Eczema genetics: current state of knowledge and future goals. J Invest Dermatol 2009;129:543–52.

92. Palmer CN, Irvine AD, Terron-Kwiatkowski A, et al. Common loss-of-function variants of the epidermal barrier protein filaggrin are a major predisposing factor for atopic dermatitis. Nat Genet 2006;38:441–6.

93. Sandilands A, O'Regan GM, Liao H, et al. Prevalent and rare mutations in the gene encoding filaggrin cause ichthyosis vulgaris and predispose individuals to atopic dermatitis. J Invest Dermatol 2006;126:1770–5.

94. Barker JN, Palmer CN, Zhao Y, et al. Null mutations in the filaggrin gene (FLG) determine major susceptibility to early-onset atopic dermatitis that persists into adulthood. J Invest Dermatol 2007;127:564–7.

95. Weidinger S, Illig T, Baurecht H, et al. Loss-of-function variations within the filaggrin gene predispose for atopic dermatitis with allergic sensitizations. J Allergy Clin Immunol 2006;118:214–9.

96. Palmer CN, Ismail T, Lee SP, et al. Filaggrin null mutations are associated with increased asthma severity in children and young adults. J Allergy Clin Immunol 2007;120:64–8.

97. Marenholz I, Nickel R, Ruschendorf F, et al. Filaggrin loss-of-function mutations predispose to phenotypes involved in the atopic march. J Allergy Clin Immunol 2006;118:866–71.

98. Vercelli D. Of flaky tails and itchy skin. Nat Genet 2009;41:512–3.

99. Fallon PG, Sasaki T, Sandilands A, et al. A homozygous frameshift mutation in the mouse Flg gene facilitates enhanced percutaneous allergen priming. Nat Genet 2009;41:602–8.

100. Sarafino EP, Goldfedder J. Genetic-factors in the presence, severity, and triggers of asthma. Arch Dis Child 1995;73:112–6.

101. Contopoulos-Ioannidis DG, Manoli EN, Ioannidis JP. Meta-analysis of the association of beta2-adrenergic receptor polymorphisms with asthma phenotypes. J Allergy Clin Immunol 2005;115:963–72.

102. Holloway JW, Yang IA. Beta2-Adrenergic receptor polymorphism and asthma: true or false? J Allergy Clin Immunol 2005;115:960–2.

103. Tantisira KG, Silverman ES, Mariani TJ, et al. FCER2: a pharmacogenetic basis for severe exacerbations in children with asthma. J Allergy Clin Immunol 2007;120:1285–91.

104. Palmer LJ, Silverman ES, Weiss ST, et al. Pharmacogenetics of Asthma. Am J Respir Crit Care Med 2002;165:861–6.

105. Malmstrom K, Rodriguez-Gomez G, Guerra J, et al. Oral montelukast, inhaled beclomethasone, and placebo for chronic asthma: a randomized, controlled trial. Montelukast/Beclomethasone Study Group. Ann Intern Med 1999;130:487–95.

106. Szefler SJ, Phillips BR, Martinez FD, et al. Characterization of within-subject responses to fluticasone and montelukast in childhood asthma. J Allergy Clin Immunol 2005;115:233–42.

107. Hall IP, Sayers I. Pharmacogenetics and asthma: false hope or new dawn? Eur Respir J 2007;29:1239–45.

108. Reihsaus E, Innis M, MacIntyre N, et al. Mutations in the gene encoding for the b_2-adrenergic receptor in normal and asthmatic subjects. Am J Respir Cell Mol Biol 1993;8:334–9.

109. Tan S, Hall IP, Dewar J, et al. Association between b_2-adrenoceptor polymorphism and susceptibility to bronchodilator desensitisation in moderately severe stable asthmatics. Lancet 1997;350:995–9.

110. Martinez FD, Graves PE, Baldini M, et al. Association between genetic polymorphisms of the b_2-adrenoceptor and response to albuterol in children with and without a history of wheezing. J Clin Invest 1997;100:3184–8.

111. Green SA, Turki J, Innis M, et al. Amino-terminal polymorphisms of the human b_2-adrenergic receptor impart distinct agonist-promoted regulatory properties. Biochemistry 1994;33:9414–9.

112. Green SA, Turki J, Bejarano P, et al. Influence of b_2-adrenergic receptor genotypes on signal transduction in human airway smooth muscle cells. Am J Respir Cell Mol Biol 1995;13:25–33.

113. Israel E, Drazen JM, Liggett SB, et al. The effect of polymorphisms of the b_2-adrenergic receptor on the response to regular use of albuterol in asthma. Am J Respir Crit Care Med 2000;162:75–80.

114. Lipworth BJ, Hall IP, Tan S, et al. Effects of genetic polymorphism on ex vivo and in vivo function of beta2-adrenoceptors in asthmatic patients. Chest 1999;115:324–8.

115. Hancox RJ, Sears MR, Taylor DR. Polymorphism of the b2-adrenoceptor and the response to long-term b2-agonist therapy in asthma. Eur Respir J 1998;11:589–93.

116. Bleecker ER, Postma DS, Lawrance RM, et al. Effect of ADRB2 polymorphisms on response to longacting beta2-agonist therapy: a pharmacogenetic analysis of two randomised studies. Lancet 2007;370:2118–25.

117. Bleecker ER, Yancey SW, Baitinger LA, et al. Salmeterol response is not affected by beta2-adrenergic receptor genotype in subjects with persistent asthma. J Allergy Clin Immunol 2006;118:809–16.

118. Hawkins GA, Weiss ST, Bleecker ER. Clinical consequences of ADRbeta2 polymorphisms. Pharmacogenomics 2008;9:349–58.

119. Chan MT, Leung DY, Szefler SJ, et al. Difficult-to-control asthma: clinical characteristics of steroid-insensitive asthma. J Allergy Clin Immunol 1998;101:594–601.

120. Tantisira KG, Small KM, Litonjua AA, et al. Molecular properties and pharmacogenetics of a polymorphism of adenylyl cyclase type 9 in

The Genetics of Allergic Disease and Asthma

asthma: interaction between beta-agonist and corticosteroid pathways. Hum Mol Genet 2005;14:1671–7.

121. Tantisira KG, Lake S, Silverman ES, et al. Corticosteroid pharmacogenetics: association of sequence variants in CRHR1 with improved lung function in asthmatics treated with inhaled corticosteroids. Hum Mol Genet 2004;13:1353–9.

122. Tantisira KG, Lazarus R, Litonjua AA, et al. Chromosome 17: association of a large inversion polymorphism with corticosteroid response in asthma. Pharmacogenet Genomics 2008;18:733–7.

123. Tantisira KG, Hwang ES, Raby BA, et al. TBX21: a functional variant predicts improvement in asthma with the use of inhaled corticosteroids. Proc Natl Acad Sci U S A 2004;101:18099–104.

124. Fowler SJ, Hall IP, Wilson AM, et al. 5-Lipoxygenase polymorphism and in-vivo response to leukotriene receptor antagonists. Eur J Clin Pharmacol 2002;58:187–90.

125. Klotsman M, York TP, Pillai SG, et al. Pharmacogenetics of the 5-lipoxygenase biosynthetic pathway and variable clinical response to montelukast. Pharmacogenet Genomics 2007;17:189–96.

126. Lima JJ, Zhang S, Grant A, et al. Influence of leukotriene pathway polymorphisms on response to montelukast in asthma. Am J Respir Crit Care Med 2006;173:379–85.

127. Tantisira KG, Lima J, Sylvia J, et al. 5-Lipoxygenase pharmacogenetics in asthma: overlap with Cys-leukotriene receptor antagonist loci. Pharmacogenet Genomics 2009.

128. Helgadottir A, Manolescu A, Helgason A, et al. A variant of the gene encoding leukotriene A4 hydrolase confers ethnicity-specific risk of myocardial infarction. Nat Genet 2006;38:68–74.

129. Helgadottir A, Manolescu A, Thorleifsson G, et al. The gene encoding 5-lipoxygenase activating protein confers risk of myocardial infarction and stroke. Nat Genet 2004;36:233–9.

130. Helgadottir A, Gretarsdottir S, St Clair D, et al. Association between the gene encoding 5-lipoxygenase-activating protein and stroke replicated in a Scottish population. Am J Hum Genet 2005;76:505–9.

131. Dwyer JH, Allayee H, Dwyer KM, et al. Arachidonate 5-lipoxygenase promoter genotype, dietary arachidonic acid, and atherosclerosis. N Engl J Med 2004;350:29–37.

132. Holloway JW, Barton SJ, Holgate ST, et al. The role of LTA4H and ALOX5AP polymorphism in asthma and allergy susceptibility. Allergy 2008;63:1046–53.

133. Jirtle RL, Skinner MK. Environmental epigenomics and disease susceptibility. Nat Rev Genet 2007;8:253–62.

134. Benn CS, Jeppesen DL, Hasselbalch H, et al. Thymus size and head circumference at birth and the development of allergic disease. Clin Exp Allergy 2001;31:1862–6.

135. Fergusson DM, Crane J, Beasley R, et al. Perinatal factors and atopic disease in childhood. Clin Exp Allergy 2006;27:1394–401.

136. Godfrey KM, Barker DJ, Osmond C. Disproportionate fetal growth and raised IgE concentration in adult life. Clin Exp Allergy 2006;24:641–8.

137. Baccarelli A, Wright RO, Bollati V, et al. Rapid DNA methylation changes after exposure to traffic particles. Am J Respir Crit Care Med 2009;179:572–8.

138. Pembery ME, Bygren LO, Kaati G, et al. The ALSPAC study team. Sex-specific, male-line transgenerational responses inhumans. Eur J Hum Genet 2006;14:159–66.

139. Li Y, Langholx B, Salam MT, et al. Maternal and grandmaternal smoking patterns are associated with early childhood asthma. Chest 2005;127:1232–41.

140. Hollingsworth JW, Maruoka S, Boon K, et al. In utero supplementation with methyl donors enhances allergic airway disease in mice. J Clin Invest 2008;118:3462–9.

141. Miller RL, Ho SM. Environmental epigenetics and asthma: current concepts and call for studies. Am J Respir Crit Care Med 2008;177:567–73.

142. Burke W, Fesinmeyer M, Reed K, et al. Family history as a predictor of asthma risk. Am J Prev Med 2003;24:160–9.

143. Koppelman GH, te Meerman GJ, Postma DS. Genetic testing for asthma. Eur Respir J 2008;32:775–82.

144. Janssens AC, Aulchenko YS, Elefante S, et al. Predictive testing for complex diseases using multiple genes: fact or fiction? Genet Med 2006;8:395–400.

145. Lyssenko V, Jonsson A, Almgren P, et al. Clinical risk factors, DNA variants, and the development of type 2 diabetes. N Engl J Med 2008;359:2220–32.

146. Meigs JB, Shrader P, Sullivan LM, et al. Genotype score in addition to common risk factors for prediction of type 2 diabetes. N Engl J Med 2008;359:2208–19.

147. Narayan KM, Weber MB. Clinical risk factors, DNA variants, and the development of type 2 diabetes. N Engl J Med 2009;360:1360; author reply 1.

148. Holloway JW, Yang IA, Holgate ST. Interpatient variability in rates of asthma progression: can genetics provide an answer? J Allergy Clin Immunol 2008;121:573–9.

149. Holgate ST, Davies DE, Powell RM, et al. Local genetic and environmental factors in asthma disease pathogenesis: chronicity and persistence mechanisms. Eur Respir J 2007;29:793–803.

150. White JH, Chiano M, Wigglesworth M, et al. Identification of a novel asthma susceptibility gene on chromosome 1qter and its functional evaluation. Hum Mol Genet 2008;17:1890–903.

151. Allen M, Heinzmann A, Noguchi E, et al. Positional cloning of a novel gene influencing asthma from chromosome 2q14. Nat Genet 2003;35:258–63.

152. Soderhall C, Marenholz I, Kerscher T, et al. Variants in a novel epidermal collagen gene (COL29A1) are associated with atopic dermatitis. PLoS Biol 2007;5:e242.

153. Noguchi E, Yokouchi Y, Zhang J, et al. Positional identification of an asthma susceptibility gene on human chromosome 5q33. Am J Respir Crit Care Med 2005;172:183–8.

154. Nicolae D, Cox NJ, Lester LA, et al. Fine mapping and positional candidate studies identify HLA-G as an asthma susceptibility gene on chromosome 6p21. Am J Hum Genet 2005;76:349–57.

155. Vendelin J, Pulkkinen V, Rehn M, et al. Characterization of GPRA, a novel G protein-coupled receptor related to asthma. Am J Respir Cell Mol Biol 2005;33:262–70.

156. Laitinen T, Polvi A, Rydman P, et al. Characterization of a common susceptibility locus for asthma-related traits. Science 2004;304:300–4.

157. Feng Y, Hong X, Wang L, et al. G protein-coupled receptor 154 gene polymorphism is associated with airway hyperresponsiveness to methacholine in a Chinese population. J Allergy Clin Immunol 2006;117:612–7.

158. Kormann MS, Carr D, Klopp N, et al. G-Protein-coupled receptor polymorphisms are associated with asthma in a large German population. Am J Respir Crit Care Med 2005;171:1358–62.

159. Malerba G, Lindgren CM, Xumerle L, et al. Chromosome 7p linkage and GPR154 gene association in Italian families with allergic asthma. Clin Exp Allergy 2007;37:83–9.

160. Melen E, Bruce S, Doekes G, et al. Haplotypes of G protein-coupled receptor 154 are associated with childhood allergy and asthma. Am J Respir Crit Care Med 2005;171:1089–95.

161. Balaci L, Spada MC, Olla N, et al. IRAK-M is involved in the pathogenesis of early-onset persistent asthma. Am J Hum Genet 2007;80:1103–14.

162. Zhang Y, Leaves NI, Anderson GG, et al. Positional cloning of a quantitative trait locus on chromosome 13q14 that influences immunoglobulin E levels and asthma. Nat Genet 2003;34:181–6.

163. Jang N, Stewart G, Jones G. Polymorphisms within the PHF11 gene at chromosome 13q14 are associated with childhood atopic dermatitis. Genes Immun 2005;6:262–4.

164. Barton S, Koppelman G, Vonk J, et al. UPAR polymorphisms are associated with asthma, uPAR expression and lung function decline. J Allergy Clin Immunol 2009;[In press].

165. Van Eerdewegh P, Little RD, Dupuis J, et al. Association of the ADAM33 gene with asthma and bronchial hyperresponsiveness. Nature 2002;(In press).

166. Hirota T, Hasegawa K, Obara K, et al. Association between ADAM33 polymorphisms and adult asthma in the Japanese population. Clin Exp Allergy 2006;36:884–91.

167. Howard TD, Postma DS, Jongepier H, et al. Association of a disintegrin and metalloprotease 33 (ADAM33) gene with asthma in ethnically diverse populations. J Allergy Clin Immunol 2003;112:717–22.

168. Kedda MA, Duffy DL, Bradley B, et al. ADAM33 haplotypes are associated with asthma in a large Australian population. Eur J Hum Genet 2006;14:1027–36.

169. Lee JH, Park HS, Park SW, et al. ADAM33 polymorphism: association with bronchial hyper-responsiveness in Korean asthmatics. Clin Exp Allergy 2004;34:860–5.

170. Noguchi E, Ohtsuki Y, Tokunaga K, et al. ADAM33 polymorphisms are associated with asthma susceptibility in a Japanese population. Clin Exp Allergy 2006;36:602–8.

171. Qiu YM, Luo YL, Lai WY, et al. [Association between ADAM33 gene polymorphism and bronchial asthma in South China Han population]. Nan Fang Yi Ke Da Xue Xue Bao 2007;27:485–7.

172. Sakagami T, Jinnai N, Nakajima T, et al. ADAM33 polymorphisms are associated with aspirin-intolerant asthma in the Japanese population. J Hum Genet 2007;52:66–72.

173. Schedel M, Depner M, Schoen C, et al. The role of polymorphisms in ADAM33, a disintegrin and metalloprotease 33, in childhood asthma and lung function in two German populations. Respir Res 2006;7:91.

174. Werner M, Herbon N, Gohlke H, et al. Asthma is associated with single-nucleotide polymorphisms in ADAM33. Clin Exp Allergy 2004;34: 26–31.

175. Nakao I, Kanaji S, Ohta S, et al. Identification of pendrin as a common mediator for mucus production in bronchial asthma and chronic obstructive pulmonary disease. J Immunol 2008;180:6262–9.

176. Matsuda A, Hirota T, Akahoshi M, et al. Coding SNP in tenascin-C Fn-III-D domain associates with adult asthma. Hum Mol Genet 2005;14: 2779–86.

177. Wjst M, Fischer G, Immervoll T, et al. A genome-wide search for linkage to asthma. German Asthma Genetics Group. Genomics 1999;58: 1–8.

178. Yuyama N, Davies DE, Akaiwa M, et al. Analysis of novel disease-related genes in bronchial asthma. Cytokine 2002;19:287–96.

CHAPTER

4

Regulation and Biology of Immunoglobulin E

Hans C. Oettgen

Normally present at very low levels in plasma, antibodies of the immunoglobulin E (IgE) isotype were first discovered in 1967, decades after the description of IgG, IgA, and IgM. IgE antibodies are produced primarily by plasma cells in mucosal-associated lymphoid tissue and their levels are uniformly elevated in patients suffering from atopic conditions like asthma, allergic rhinitis, and atopic dermatitis. Production of allergen-specific IgE in atopic individuals is driven both by a genetic predisposition to the synthesis of this isotype as well as by environmental factors, including chronic allergen exposure. The lineage commitment by B cells to produce IgE involves irreversible genetic changes at the immunoglobulin heavy chain gene locus and is very tightly regulated. It requires both cytokine signals (interleukin [IL]-4 and IL-13) and interaction of TNF receptor family members on the B cell surface with their ligands.

IgE antibodies exert their biologic functions via the high-affinity IgE receptor, FcεRI, and the low-affinity receptor, CD23. In the classic immediate hypersensitivity reaction, the interaction of polyvalent allergens with IgE bound to mast cells via FcεRε triggers receptor aggregation, which initiates a series of signals that result in the release of vasoactive and chemotactic mediators of acute tissue inflammation. Clinical manifestations of IgE-induced immediate hypersensitivity include systemic anaphylaxis (triggered by foods, drugs, and insect stings), bronchial edema with smooth muscle constriction and acute airflow obstruction in asthmatic patients (following allergen inhalation), angioedema and urticaria.

Although best known for their critical function in mediating antigen-specific immediate hypersensitivity reactions, IgE antibodies also exert potent immunoregulatory effects including regulation of IgE receptor expression and mast cell survival. IgE antibodies directly up-regulate the surface expression of their receptors FcεRI and CD23 on mast cells and B cells, respectively, in a positive feedback loop that may augment ongoing allergic responses. IgE signaling via FcεRI provides an anti-apoptotic signal for mast cells. CD23-bound IgE facilitates allergen uptake by B cells that can present captured antigen to specific T cells resulting in augmented secondary immune responses. Occupancy of CD23 by its ligand also inhibits proteolytic shedding of sCD23, a soluble fragment with immunomodulatory properties. This chapter will describe in detail the regulation of IgE synthesis and provide an overview of the biologic actions of IgE antibodies and their role in allergic pathogenesis.

Components of the Immune Response

Immunoglobulin E Protein Structure and Gene Organization

Immunoglobulin E (IgE) antibodies are tetramers consisting of two light chains (κ or λ) and two ε-heavy chains (Figure 4-1 and Box 4-1). The heavy chains each contain a variable (V_H) region and four constant region domains. The V_H domain, together with the V-regions of the light chains (V_L), confers antibody specificity and the Cε domains confer isotype-specific functions, including interaction with FcεRI and CD23. IgE antibodies are heavily glycosylated and contain numerous intrachain and interchain disulfide bonds. The exons encoding the ε-heavy chain domains are located in the Cε locus near the 3' end of the immunoglobulin heavy chain locus (IgH) (Figure 4-2).[1] Additional exons, M1 and M2, encode hydrophobic sequences present in the ε-heavy chain mRNA splice isoforms encoding transmembrane IgE in IgE+ B cells. In contrast to IgG antibodies, which have a half-life of about 3 weeks, IgE antibodies are very short-lived in plasma ($T_{1/2}$ less than 1 day) but they can remain fixed to mast cells in tissues for weeks or months.

The assembly of a functional IgE gene requires two sequential processes of DNA excision and ligation.[2,3] In the first, which occurs in pre-B cells, individual V_H, D, and J_H exons randomly combine to generate a $V_H DJ_H$ cassette encoding an antigen-specific V_H domain. In B cells that have undergone 'productive' $V_H DJ_H$ rearrangements (e.g. no stop codons have been introduced during assembly), this $V_H DJ_H$ cassette is situated just upstream of the Cμ and Cδ exons so that functional μ- and δ-heavy chain transcripts can be produced. A similar process then occurs at the κ or λ light chain loci to produce functional light chains. The assembled heavy (μ or δ) and light (κ or λ) chains are then expressed at the cell surface, marking the transition from pre-B cell to immature B cell. B cells at this point in their maturation have a fixed antigenic specificity dictated by the V-D-J sequences of their heavy and light chains.

A second DNA excision and ligation process, called *class switch recombination* (CSR), must occur before B cells can produce antibodies of other isotypes, including IgE. These antibodies retain their original $V_H DJ_H$ cassette and antigenic specificity but

©2010 Elsevier Ltd, Inc, BV
DOI: 10.1016/B978-1-4377-0271-2.00004-3

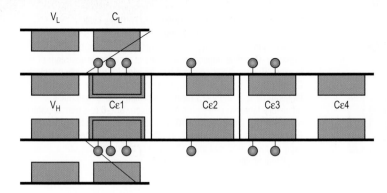

Figure 4-1 IgE antibody structure. IgE antibodies are tetramers containing two immunoglobulin light chains and two immunoglobulin ε-heavy chains connected by interchain disulfide bonds as indicated. Each light chain contains one V_L and one C_L immunoglobulin domain and each ε-heavy chain contains an N-terminal V_H domain and four Cε domains. Intrachain disulfide bonds are contained within each of these immunoglobulin domains. The Cε domains contain IgE isotype-specific sequences important for interactions with IgE receptors FcεRI and CD23. IgE antibodies are relatively heavily glycosylated; glycosylation sites are indicated with circles.

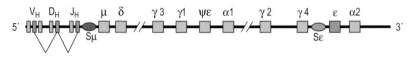

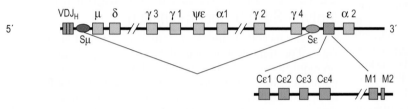

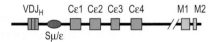

Figure 4-2 The human immunoglobulin heavy chain gene locus; deletional class switch recombination. **(A)** The human immunoglobulin heavy chain locus contains clusters of V_H, D_H and J_H cassettes that are stochastically rearranged during B cell ontogeny. This process, which involves DNA excision and repair, results in the assembly of a complete VDJ exon encoding an antigen-binding V_H domain. Pre-B cells that have completed this rearrangement are capable of producing intact μ-heavy chains and, following an analogous process of light chain rearrangements, can produce intact IgM antibodies. **(B)** Production of other antibody isotypes, bearing the original antigenic specificity, requires an additional excision and repair process, deletional 'class switch recombination' (CSR). For IgE isotype switching, this process involves the excision of a large piece of genomic DNA spanning from Sμ switch sequences just upstream of the μ-heavy chain exons to the Sε sequence 5′ of the Cε exons. **(C)** Ligation of the VDJ sequences to the Cε locus then gives rise to an intact ε-heavy chain gene containing a V_H-encoding VDJ exon and exons Cε1-4 encoding the constant region domains of ε-heavy chain. The M1 and M2 exons encode trans-membrane sequences that are present in RNA splice isoforms encoding the membrane IgE of IgE+ B cells.

BOX 4-1 Key concepts

Components of the Immune Response

IgE Antibodies, Genes, and Receptors

• IgE structure	IgE protein
	IgE gene arrangement
• IgE class switch	Germline transcription
recombination	Structure of the Iε promoter
	Cytokine regulation of germline transcription
	CD40/CD154 signaling
	TACI/BAFF signaling
	Activation-induced cytidine deaminase
	DNA double strand breaks and repair
• IgE receptors	FcεRI
	CD23

exchange C_H cassettes of various isotypes to construct different heavy chains and effect distinct biologic functions. In this tightly regulated and irreversible process, sometimes referred to as deletional switch recombination, a long stretch of genomic DNA spanning from the Sε region between V_HDJ_H and Cμ to Sε upstream of the Cε locus is excised (see Figure 4-2). The DNA products of this reaction include an extrachromosomal circle of

intervening DNA and the contiguous V_HDJ_H and Cε sequences, joined by Sμ-Sε ligation, to generate a functional IgE gene. A complex series of cytokine signals and cell surface interactions collaborate to trigger deletional switch recombination in B cells destined for IgE production.

Regulation of IgE Isotype Switching

ε-Germline Transcription Precedes Isotype Switch Recombination

Before deletional isotype switch recombination is initiated, cytokine signals provided by IL-4 and/or IL-13 induce RNA transcription in the IgH locus of B cells. This occurs at the unrearranged or 'germline' ε-heavy chain locus driven from a promoter 5′ of the Iε exon, located just upstream of the Sε switch recombination region and the four Cε exons (Figure 4-3). This is referred to as ε-germline RNA and the transcripts include a 140-bp Iε exon as well as exons Cε1-Cε4.[4,5] As Iε contains several stop codons, germline transcripts do not encode functional proteins and have been referred to as 'sterile.'[6] B cells in which the I exon or its promoter have been mutated are unable to undergo isotype switching, indicating that germline transcription is a prerequisite of deletional switch recombination.[7–9] Conversely,

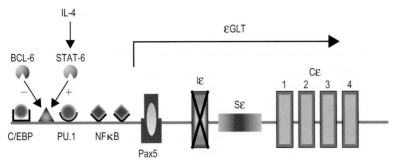

Figure 4-3 ε-Germline transcription (*εGLT*). Class switch recombination is invariably preceded by a process of RNA transcription at the C_H locus being targeted by specific cytokine signals. ε-Germline transcripts originate at a promoter upstream of the Iε exon. This promoter contains binding sites for transcription factors C/EBP, PU.1, STAT-6, NFκB (2 sites), and Pax5. STAT-6 activation is triggered by IL-4 and IL-13 receptor signaling and is the critical regulatory factor in ε-germline transcription. BCL-6 is a transcriptional repressor that binds to the STAT-6 target site and inhibits εGLT. Germline transcripts contain Iε and Cε1-4 exons but, because the Iε exon contains stop codons ('X'), these RNAs do not encode a functional protein.

introduction of an active promoter upstream of the I exon not only promotes germline transcription but also promotes isotype switching.[10]

Regulation of Germline Transcription, The Iε Promoter

Initiation of germline transcription is regulated by the Iε promoter that contains binding sites for several known transcription factors including STAT-6, NFκB, BSAP (Pax5), C/EBP, and PU.1 (see Figure 4-3). Accessibility of the promoter is regulated by the non-histone chromosomal protein, HMG-I(Y).[11] This repression is released upon IL-4-driven phosphorylation of the protein.[12,13] Translocation of activated STAT-6 to the nucleus is triggered by IL-4 and IL-13 signaling. STAT-6 activation appears to be the key regulator of ε-germline transcription. Although neither BSAP nor NFκB nuclear-binding activities have been shown to be altered by cytokine signaling, these promoter elements must be present for normal Iε promoter function.[14,15] The requirement for NFκB may be related to a physical interaction and resultant synergism in promoter activation between NFκB and STAT-6.[16] CD40 signaling also stimulates NFκB activation and may enhance cytokine-driven germline transcription by activating the NFκB promoter elements. Isotype switching is impaired in NFκB p50[-/-] mice[17] and enhanced in mice lacking the NFκB inhibitor IkB-α.[18] BSAP overexpression can drive Iε transcription and promote IgE isotype switching.[19] PU.1, like NFκB, may synergize with STAT-6 in activating the promoter.[20]

BCL-6, a POZ/zinc-finger transcription factor expressed in B cells, is an important negative regulator of the Iε promoter. BCL-6 binds to STAT-6 sites and can repress the induction of ε-germline transcripts by IL-4.[21,22] BCL-6 is induced by the cytokine, IL-21, which is known to suppress IgE production in B cells and which has been reported to induce apoptosis of IgE[+] B cells.[23] IL-21 is important in germinal center formation and germinal centers have relatively low levels of IgE production.[23,24] Consistent with this model, BCL-6[-/-] mice have enhanced IgE isotype switching, whereas BCL-6[-/-] STAT-6[-/-] animals do not produce IgE. As IL-4- and IL-13–induced STAT-6 activation supports not only IgE germline transcription but also Th2 differentiation, expression of CD23, and up-regulation of VCAM, alterations in the regulation or function of BCL-6 are likely to have a great impact on allergy pathogenesis.

Cytokines IL-4 and IL-13 Activate STAT-6

The cytokines IL-4 and IL-13 are potent inducers of ε-germline transcription in B cells.[5,25,26] The multimeric receptors for these two cytokines share the IL-4R-αchain. The type I IL-4 receptor, which binds IL-4, is composed of the ligand-binding IL-4Rα and the signal-transducing common cytokine receptor γ-chain γc. The type II receptor, which can bind either IL-4 or IL-13, contains

the IL-4R-α chain along with an IL-13 binding chain, IL-13Rα1. IL-4 receptor signaling triggers the activation of Janus family tyrosine kinases Jak-1 (via IL-4Rα), Jak-3 (via γc) and TYK2 (via IL-13Rα).[27-30] These activated Jaks then phosphorylate tyrosine residues in the intracellular domains of the receptor chain. These phosphotyrosines serve as binding sites for STAT-6, which is, in turn, phosphorylated and then dimerizes and translocates to the nucleus.[31,32]

CD40/CD154 Provides Second Signal for Isotype Switch Recombination

The cytokines IL-4 and IL-13 are very efficient inducers of ε-germline transcription, and this transcription is an absolute prerequisite for isotype switching. However, cytokine-induced germline transcription alone is not sufficient to drive B cells to complete the genomic deletional switch recombination reaction that gives rise to a functional IgE gene. A second signal, provided by the interaction of the TNF receptor family member CD40 on B cells with its ligand, CD154, on activated T cells, is required to bring the process to completion.

CD154 is transiently expressed on antigen/MCH-stimulated T cells.[33] T cell CD154 induces CD40 aggregation on B cells, triggering signal transduction via four intracellular proteins belonging to the TRAF family of TNF-receptor associated factors.[34,35] TRAF-2, -5, and -6 promote the dissociation of NFκB from its inhibitor, IκB, allowing NFκB to translocate to the nucleus and synergize with STAT-6 to activate the Iε promoter as described above.[36,37] In addition to inducing TRAF association and signaling, aggregation of CD40 activates protein tyrosine kinases (PTKs) including Jak-3, which play an important role in immunoglobulin class switching.[38,39] CD154 is encoded on the X chromosome. Boys with X-linked immunodeficiency with hyper-IgM (XHIM) are deficient in CD154. Consequently, their B cells are unable to produce IgG, IgA, or IgE.[40-44] Mice with a targeted disruption of the CD154 or CD40 genes have the same defect in antibody production.[45-47]

Alternative Second Signals for Isotype Switch Recombination

Recently, alternative switching pathways have been defined in which the second 'switch' signal is provided not by CD40/CD154 ligation but rather by interaction of other TNF-like molecules with their receptors. One such TNF family member, BAFF, binds to its receptor TACI on cytokine-stimulated B cells, inducing isotype switching even in the absence of CD40.[48,49] BAFF/TACI-driven switching may be of particular importance at mucosal sites, especially IgA production in the gastrointestinal tract. Defects in this pathway underlie some cases of IgA deficiency.[50,51] Although BAFF can drive IgE switching, its physio-

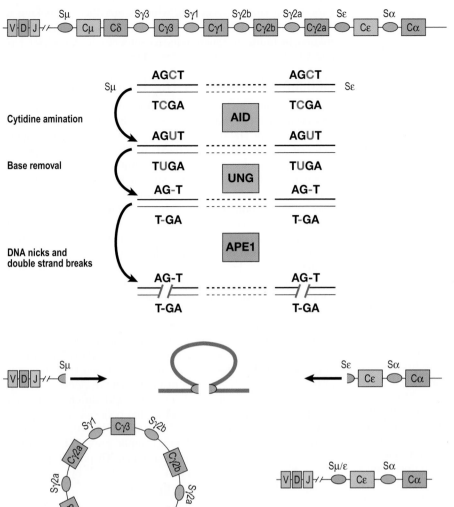

Figure 4-4 Activation-induced cytidine deaminase (*AID*) is recruited to sites of cytokine-driven germline transcription (Sμ and Sε) in the IgH locus where it catalyzes cytidine deamination to uracil. Uracil glyosylase (*UNG*) introduces abasic sites which are then converted to nicks by apurinic/apyridinimic endonuclease 1 (*APE1*). Subsequent double-strand DNA breaks followed by end joining of the Sμ and Sε sequences leads to the generation of an intact VDJ-Cε$_{1-4}$ ε-heavy chain gene along with an excised episomal DNA circle containing the intervening sequences.

logic relevance in IgE regulation remains to be clarified. It has been reported that respiratory epithelium produces BAFF, with elevations of the factor in BAL of segmental allergen-challenged subjects.[52,53] In addition, it has been demonstrated that IgE class switch recombination occurs, not only in central lymphoid organs, but also in the respiratory mucosa of patients with allergic rhinitis and asthma.[54]

Cytokine-Stimulated Germline Transcripts and CD40-Induced AID Collaborate to Execute Switch Recombination

It has been known for some time that deletional class switch recombination stimulated by cytokines and CD40/CD154 requires the synthesis of new proteins and it has been inferred that these proteins might constitute the enzymatic apparatus required for the excision of intervening genomic DNA and ligation of V$_H$DJ$_H$ cassette to the Cε locus in CSR. In 1999 a subtractive approach was used to identify one of these proteins as activation-induced cytidine deaminase (AID), which is expressed in activated splenic B cells and in the germinal centers of lymph nodes.[55,56] AID-deficient mice have elevated IgM levels and a major defect in isotype switching with absent IgG, IgE, and IgA. A rare autosomal form of hyper-IgM syndrome (HIGM2), which

is associated with striking lymphoid hypertrophy, has now been attributed to mutations in the AID gene.[57] An unanticipated phenotype of both mice and humans with AID mutations is a decrease in somatic V region hypermutation during active antibody responses.

Transfection of AID, which has homology to APOBEC, an RNA editing enzyme into fibroblasts is adequate to confer switch recombination in an artificial switch construct.[58] AID is recruited to sites of active germline transcription where it deaminates deoxy-cytidine residues within the C-rich Sε and Sμ sequences, generating uracils and consequent U:G mismatches (see Figure 4-4).[59,60] Subsquent removal of these uracils by the enzyme, uracil glycocylase (UNG) results in the introduction of abasic sites. The enzyme apurinic/apyrimidinic endonuclease 1, APE1, generates nicks at these sites which ultimately lead to double-stranded DNA breaks. In subsequent steps of the process, analogous breaks, located at Sμ between V$_H$DJ$_H$ and the Cμ exons are annealed to generate a functional IgE gene. The heterogeneous nature of the Sμ-Sε junctions suggests a nonhomologous end-joining mechanism such as would be generated by the DNA repair enzymes, Ku70, Ku80, and DNA-PKcs. Consistent with this possibility, B cells lacking Ku70, Ku80, and DNA-PKcs, all of which are involved in nonhomologous end joining, cannot execute isotype switching normally.[61,62]

Regulation of Allergen-Specific T Cell Responses

The execution of IgE isotype switch recombination in B cells, as detailed previously, requires that cytokine (IL-4 and IL-13) signals and the CD40 ligand, CD154 signal, be delivered in a coordinated fashion. Both these stimuli are provided by Th2-type allergen-specific T-helper cells. Thus, the mechanisms that regulate expansion and survival of Th2 cells are crucial in regulating IgE responses.

Th2 Helper T Cell Development

Naïve CD4⁺ Th cells have the capacity to differentiate into a number of distinct types of effector helper, each with distinct capacities for induction of cellular immune responses (Th1), antibody production and allergic responses (Th2), inflammatory responses (Th17) and regulation (Treg, see Figure 4-5). These Th types are further characterized by the expression of specific transcription factors which maintain their specific lineage commitments and direct their respective cytokine transcription profiles. Some of the Th lineages can be identified by specific cell surface markers. Th1 cells, which arise under the direction of IL-12 or IL-18, express abundant IFN-γ and IL-2 and are important in immunity to intracellular pathogens. Th1 cells are further characterized by the presence of the transcription factor, T-bet. The relatively recently identified Th subset, Th17, is induced in the presence of TGF-β and IL-6 and produces IL-17, TNF-α and IL-1. Th17 cells harbor the transcription factors RORγt and STAT3 and are important in driving neutrophil recruitment and inflammatory responses. As their name implies, Treg, which are generated in the presence of TGF-β and IL-2 (absent IL-6) are important in controlling immune responses via immunsuppresive cytokines including TGF-β and IL-10. The transcription factor associated with this lineage is FoxP3.

The critical Th cells promoting IgE production are Th2 which are induced by IL-4, express the transcription factor GATA-3 and produce IL-4, IL-5, IL-6, IL-9, IL-10, IL-13, and GM-CSF. Th2 cells express cell surface receptors, which target their trafficking to allergic sites and trigger activation in settings of allergic inflammation, including the chemokine receptors CCR3, CCR4, CRTh2, and CCR8 and the IL-33 receptor, T1/ST2.[63–66]

Genetic Influences on Th2 Development

Both host and environmental factors promote the Th2 shift observed in allergic individuals. Some inbred mouse strains have a propensity for Th2-dominated responses to particular antigens, whereas others are characterized by Th1-dominant responses indicating a significant genetic contribution to T-helper cell differentiation. It is possible that specific evolutionary pressures exerted by particular pathogen exposures might account for this; mice with a dominant Th1 response mount effective attacks against intracellular pathogens such as *Leishmania*.[67,68] In contrast, those with enhanced Th2 responsiveness may be at an advantage in the elimination of parasites.[69] In humans it is clear that the tendency to develop allergic responses to antigens also varies greatly among individuals raised within nearly identical environments and that this allergic tendency is familial.

Genetic predispositions toward Th1 or Th2 are partly accounted for by T cell autonomous tendencies to transcribe Th1 versus Th2 cytokines, but are also the result of a wide range of influences external to T cells.[70] Perhaps the most potent Th1/Th2-polarizing effect is exerted by the cytokine milieu, particularly tissue levels of IL-4, IL-12, and IFN-γ. IL-4 promotes Th2 responses and suppresses Th1 development. IL-12 drives Th1 differentiation (an effect that is greatly potentiated by the presence of IFN-γ) and can inhibit and even reverse Th2 development. In ongoing immune responses these cytokines can be provided by existing T cells already committed to a particular Th phenotype. In de novo allergen encounters, cytokines produced by cells of the 'innate' immune response may tip the balance.

Antigen-Presenting Cell Function in Th Differentiation

Naïve T cells initially encounter antigens as MHC-bound processed peptides on the surface of antigen-presenting cells (APCs). The most potent APCs are dendritic cells (DCs), which reside in tissues as immature sentinels and sample antigens in their milieu. Upon activation, these cells acquire mature APC function and migrate to regional lymphoid tissues where they efficiently activate antigen-specific T helper cells via MHC-peptide complexes. Dendritic cells obtained from various lymphoid tissues in vivo or cultured ex vivo under a range of conditions all express MHC II and, following activation, express costimulatory molecules, including CD80/86. However, there is some functional heterogeneity among DCs, especially with respect to the ability to induce Th1 versus Th2 T helper responses.[71] DC-derived IL-12 drives Th1 responses; IL-23, TGFβ and IL-6 support Th17 induction and IL-10 drives both Treg and Th2.[72]

Microbial Products and Dendritic Cell Phenotype

The recent understanding that Th polarity may be determined by DC polarity obviously begs the following question: what determines DC polarity? IFN-γ favors DC1 development, whereas histamine and PGE₂ promote the development of DC2.[73–75] IL-10 may negatively regulate DC production of IL-12.[76] Conserved microbial structures, which signal via the Toll-like receptor (TLR) family of receptors, can shift DC polarity. Dendritic cells express a range of TLR and the specific effects of ligand binding by each of these receptors on DC phenotype remain to be fully eluci-

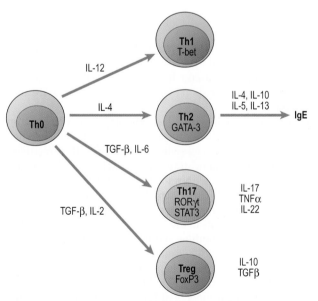

Figure 4-5 CD4⁺ T-helper cell differentiation. CD4⁺ T-helper cells undergo a process of differentiation to Th1 (producing IL-2, IFN-γ, and TNF-α), Th2 (producing IL-4, IL-5, IL-6, IL-9, IL-10, IL-13, and GM-CSF), Th17 (producing IL-17, TNFα and IL-22) and Treg (producing IL-10 and TGF-β) phenotypes. Each lineage is further characterized by the presence of specific transcription factors (as indicated in the nuclei). The critical regulator of IgE production is the Th2 lineage which uniquely produces IL-4.

dated. The default state of mucosal DC appears to be skewed towards Th2 induction with relatively low basal IL-12 and constitutive production of IL-10.[77]

Non-T Cell Sources of IL-4: Mast Cells, Basophils, NKT Cells, and NK Cells

Although allergen-specific T-helper cells committed to the Th2 lineage are a major source of IL-4 in allergic tissues and may predominate during chronic or memory responses to allergen, several other cell types can provide IL-4 and IL-13 and may be more important in initial allergen encounters. Mast cells, which are abundant in the respiratory and gastrointestinal mucosa, are excellent producers of both IL-4 and IL-13 following activation via IgE/FcεRI.[78,79] Basophils are rapidly induced in response to allergens or parasites and consitutively produce large quantities of IL-4. They have been implicated as the critical initial IL-4 source in some murine model systems of Th2 induction in vivo.[80-87] NK1.1+ CD4+ T (NKT) cells are another source of IL-4. These cells express a very restricted repertoire of αβ T cell receptors and interact with the non-classical MHC class I molecule, CD1.[88] The intravenous injection of anti-CD3 in mice induces large amounts of IL-4, derived primarily from these NKT cells. Mice with abundant NKT cells have enhanced IL-4 production

and IgE synthesis, whereas those depleted of the same population show suppressed Th2 responses.[89] NK cells may also provide IL-4 early in immune responses to allergens. Both cultured and freshly isolated human NK cells have been shown to be differentiated to produce either IL-10 and IFN-γ (NK1) or IL-5 and IL-13 (NK2), a polarity analogous to that observed in Th1 versus Th2 T-helper cells.[90,91] In light of the strong association between asthma flares and viral respiratory infections, particularly in the first 2 to 3 years of life, the NK contribution to tissue cytokine levels may be important.

IgE Receptors

FcεRI Structure

The high-affinity IgE receptor FcεRI is a multimeric complex expressed in two isoforms, a tetrameric αβγ2 receptor present on mast cells and basophils and a trimeric αγ2 receptor expressed, albeit at levels 10-fold to 100-fold lower, by several cell lineages including eosinophils, platelets, mono-cytes, dendritic cells, and cutaneous Langerhans cells[92] (Figure 4-6). The α chain contains two extracellular immunoglobulin-related domains and is responsible for binding IgE. The β-subunit of the receptor con-

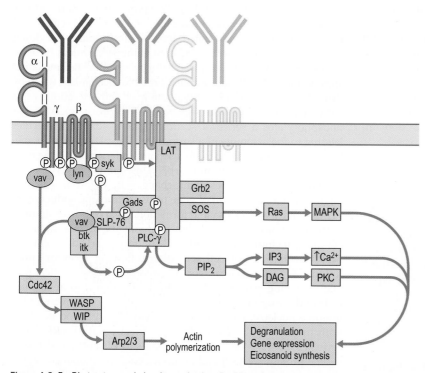

Figure 4-6 FcεRI structure and signal transduction. FcεRI is a tetramer containing an IgE-binding α-chain (with two extracellular immunoglobulin-type domains), a disulfide-linked, signal-transducing dimer of γ-chains, each of which contains an intracellular immunoreceptor tyrosine-based activation motif (ITAM) and a tetramembrane spanner β-chain that also contains a cytosolic ITAM and serves to augment FcεRI surface expression and signal transduction intensity. Trimeric forms of the receptor, lacking the β-chain, can be expressed on some cell types.

Aggregation of the receptor by the interaction of its ligand, IgE, with polymeric antigens induces signal transduction. The β-chain–associated protein tyrosine kinase, lyn, in aggregated receptor complexes phosphorylates (P) the β- and γ-chain ITAMs, generating docking sites for the SH2-domain containing kinase, syk. Activated syk phosphorylates the membrane-associated scaffolding protein LAT as well as the adapter, SLP-76 (which is also bound to LAT via the Grb-2 homolog, Gads). These proteins have no inherent enzymatic activity but serve to assemble a membrane-associated supramolecular complex of proteins that brings together a number of signaling molecules. LAT and SLP-76 both recruit PLC-γ, whose activity is enhanced by the SLP-76–associated kinases btk and itk. PLC-γ activation results in the conversion of PIP2 (phosphatidylinositol 4,5-bisphosphate) into inositol trisphosphate (IP3) and diacyl glycerol (DAG) with resultant increases in intracellular Ca2+ and activation of protein kinase C (PKC).

Alongside this protein tyrosine kinase pathway, FcεRI aggregation triggers a vav/cytoskeletal signaling cascade. The guanine nucleotide exchange factor, vav, which is directly associated with FcεRI-"γ as well as with SLP-76, activates the GTPase Cdc42 which, in turn, induces a conformational change in a complex of proteins, WASP and WIP, associated with the cytoskeleton. This exposes binding sites for Arp2/3, a complex of proteins that mediates actin polymerization. Vav activation also drives the stress-activated protein kinase (SAPK) pathway. Vav and Sos, another guanine nucleotide exchange factor, also result in the ativation of the Ras/MAPK pathway. The combined effects of elevated Ca2+, PKC activation, actin polymerization, and SAPK activation drive mast cell degranulation, eicosanoid formation and induction of gene expression.

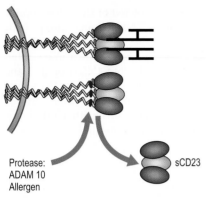

Figure 4-7 CD23 structure. CD23 is a type II transmembrane protein (with intracellular N-terminus) that contains α-helical coiled stalks and oligomerizes at the cell surface. Occupancy of the receptor by IgE stabilizes the receptor. In the absence of the IgE ligand, protease-sensitive sites appear *(ovals)* and endogenous proteases (ADAM10) as well as proteases present in allergens such as Der p 1 cleave CD23, shedding soluble sCD23 into the milieu.

tains four transmembrane-spanning domains with both N- and C-terminal ends on the cytosolic side of the plasma membrane. FcεRI-β appears to have two functions that result in enhanced receptor activity. β-chain expression both enhances cell surface density of FcεRI and amplifies the signal transduced following activation of the receptor by IgE aggregation.[92-95] The γ-chains (which have homology to the ζ and η chains important in T cell receptor signaling) exist as disulfide-linked dimers with transmembrane domains and cytoplasmic tails. The β and γ chains perform critical signal transduction functions and their intracellular domains contain immunoreceptor tyrosine-based activation motifs (ITAMs), 18 amino acid long tyrosine-containing sequences that constitute docking sites for SH2 domain-containing signaling proteins.

CD23 Expression and Structure

Although its common designation as the 'low-affinity' IgE receptor implies differently, CD23 actually has a fairly high affinity for IgE with a K_A of about 10^8.[96,97] A wide variety of cell types express CD23 in humans, including B cells, Langerhans cells, follicular dendritic cells, T cells, and eosinophils.[98] It is a type II transmembrane protein with a C-type lectin domain, making it the only immunoglobulin receptor that is not in the Ig superfamily.[99-101] Adjacent to its lectin domain, CD23 has sequences that are predicted to give rise to α-helical coiled-coil stalks (Figure 4-7). As a result, CD23 is known to have a tendency to multimerize and only oligomeric CD23 will bind IgE.[102] CD23 has homology to the asialo glycoprotein receptor, suggesting a role for CD23 in endocytosis. In addition to binding IgE, CD23 binds to a second ligand, the B cell surface molecule, CD21.[103,104]

Principles of Disease Mechanism

Once produced, allergen-specific IgE antibodies engage their receptors and trigger a wide variety of tissue-specific responses. The cellular and molecular mechanisms of pathogenesis giving rise to specific allergic disorders are presented in great detail later in this textbook. This section will provide a general overview of the consequences of IgE interaction with its receptors, including immediate hypersensitivity, late-phase reactions, regulation of IgE receptor expression, and immune modulation (Box 4-2).

BOX 4-2 Key concepts

Principles of Disease Mechanism

Effector Functions of IgE

• Mast cell activation/FcεRI	FcεRI signaling – antigen dependent
	Immediate hypersensitivity reactions
	Late-phase reactions
	FcεRI signaling – antigen independent
• IgE regulation of IgE receptors	FcεRI
	CD23
• IgE regulation of mast cell homeostasis	Enhanced mast cell survival
• CD23 functions	IgE antigen capture
	Regulation of IgE synthesis by CD23 and by CD23

Mast Cell Activation and Homeostasis

FcεRI Signaling

FcεRI has high affinity for IgE (Kd 10^{-8} M) and under physiologic conditions mast cell and basophil FcεRI is fully occupied by IgE antibodies. Aggregation of this receptor-bound IgE by an encounter with polyvalent allergen triggers a cascade of signaling events[105,106] (see Figure 4-6). Receptor aggregation induces transphosphorylation of intracellular ITAMs on FcεRI-β and FcεRI-γ by receptor-associated lyn tyrosine kinase, providing docking sites to recruit the SH2-containing syk protein tyrosine kinase. Syk levels are decreased during chronic IgE-mediatied stimulation of FcεRI, suggesting a possible mechanism whereby drug desensitization might attenuate mast cell activation at this early step in the signaling cascade.[107] Receptor-associated syk phosphorylates a series of scaffolding and adapter molecules leading to the assembly of a supramolecular plasma membrane-localized signaling complex, focused around the scaffolding molecules LAT1/2, SLP-76 and Grb2. This complex recruits and activates PLCγ with resultant changes in cytosolic calcium, degranulation, activation of gene transcription and induction of PLA2 activity with eicosanoid formation. Mast cells from animals with mutations in several key components of this signaling complex, including LAT and SLP-76, have markedly inhibited FcεRI-mediated mast cell activation following receptor cross-linking.[108,109] Cytoskeletal reorganization provides a critical parallel signaling pathway driven by FcεRI aggregation in mast cells and basophils. This cytoskeletal signaling is driven by the guanine nucleoside exchange factor vav.[110] Vav associates both with the SLP-76/LAT complex and directly with FcεRI.[111] Vav activates Cdc42, a GTPase, which binds to Wiskott-Aldrich syndrome protein (WASP) and induces a conformational change in the cytoskeletal WASP/WASP-interacting protein (WIP) protein complex, allowing interaction with the actin-polymerizing Arp2/3 complex.[108,112] Vav (as well as Sos, another GTP exchanger) also activates the Ras pathway with resultant transcriptional activation.

In the classic immediate hypersensitivity reaction, cross-linking of IgE induces the complex signaling cascade just described, resulting in the release of preformed mediators including histamine, proteoglycans, and proteases; transcription of cytokines (IL-4, TNF, IL-6); and de novo synthesis of prostaglandins (PGD_2) and leukotrienes (LTD_4). In the airways of asthmatic patients, these mediators rapidly elicit bronchial mucosal edema, mucus production, and smooth muscle constriction and, eventually, recruit an inflammatory infiltrate. In asthmatic patients subjected to allergen inhalation, these cellular and molecular events result in an acute obstruction of airflow with a drop in FEV_1, an effect which can be blocked by inhibition of IgE with a monoclonal anti-IgE antibody.[113,114]

In many subjects exposed to allergens by inhalation, ingestion, cutaneous exposure, or injection, immediate responses are followed 8 to 24 hours later by a second, delayed-phase reaction, designated the late-phase response (LPR). LPR can manifest as delayed or repeated onset of airflow obstruction, gastrointestinal symptoms, skin inflammation, or anaphylaxis hours after initial allergen exposure and after the acute response has completely subsided. In animal models, IgE antibodies can transfer both acute and LPR sensitivity to allergen challenge.[115] Interference with mast cell activation or inhibition of the mast cell mediators blocks the onset of both acute-phase and late-phase responses.[116] It has been proposed that chronic obstructive symptoms in asthma patients subjected to recurrent environmental allergen exposure result from persistent late-phase responses.[117,118]

Antigen-Independent IgE Signaling Via FcεRI and IgE Effects on Mast Cell Homeostasis

Although IgE-mediated signaling via FcεRI has long been believed to be dependent on antigen-mediated receptor aggregation, some recent evidence suggests that the binding of IgE per se, in the absence of antigen, provides a signal to mast cells and basophils. Experiments using cultured bone marrow mast cells have revealed that monomeric IgE has a survival-enhancing effect, protecting these cells from apoptosis following the withdrawal of growth factor.[119,120] This effect is mediated via FcεRI; no antiapoptotic effect is observed in FcεRI-deficient mast cells exposed to IgE. A number of other mast cell functions have been reported to be induced by IgE alone, in the absence of antigen-including cytokine production, histamine release, leukotriene synthesis and calcium flux.[121-124]

Parasitic infestation and allergic inflammation, which are both associated with elevated IgE levels, trigger mast cell expansion in affected tissues. The observation that IgE antibodies promote the viability of cultured mast cells suggests that IgE might similarly regulate mast cell survival in vivo. Indeed, there is evidence that mast cell induction in parasitized mice or animals exposed to allergens depends upon the presence of IgE antibodies.[125,126] Thus, in addition to their role in allergen-triggered mast cell activation, IgE antibodies are key regulators of mast cell homeostasis.

IgE Regulation of Receptors

The expression of both FcεRI and CD23 is positively regulated by their mutual ligand, IgE. FcεRI expression is markedly diminished on peritoneal mast cells from IgE-deficient mice and this defect can be reversed in vivo by injection of IgE antibodies.[127-129] Low FcεRI expression in IgE$^{-/-}$ mice is associated with diminished mast cell activation following IgE sensitization and allergen exposure. Treatment of allergic subjects with anti-IgE has been shown to induce a decrease in IgE receptor expression on mast cells, basophils and dendritic cells.[130-132]

CD23 expression on cultured B cells is enhanced in the presence of IgE, which, by occupancy of its receptor, prevents proteolytic degradation of CD23 and shedding into the medium.[96,133] This shedding is mediated by the endogenous protease, ADAM10 but can also be triggered by allergens.[134,135] This regulatory interaction between IgE and CD23 is operative in vivo as well; B cells from IgE$^{-/-}$ animals have markedly diminished CD23 levels and

intravenous injection of IgE induces normal CD23 expression.[136] Restoration of CD23 expression can be induced using monomeric IgE and is antigen independent. Exposure to IgE does not alter transcription of mRNA encoding CD23 or the FcεRI subunits but rather modulates receptor turnover and proteolytic shedding.[137] The positive feedback interaction between IgE and its receptors may have implications in terms of augmenting allergic responses in atopic individuals with high IgE levels.

CD23 Function: Antigen Capture

Several investigators have now shown that the binding of allergen by specific IgE facilitates allergen uptake by CD23-bearing cells for processing and presentation to T cells.[138-140] Mice immunized intravenously with antigen produce stronger IgG responses when antigen-specific IgE is provided at the time of immunization.[141,142] As expected, CD23$^{-/-}$ mice cannot display augmentation of immune responses by IgE but acquire responsiveness to IgE following reconstitution with cells from CD23$^+$ donors.[143,144] These findings suggest a scenario in which preformed allergen-specific IgE present in the bronchial and gut mucosa of patients with recurrent allergen exposure would enhance immune responses upon repeated allergen inhalation or ingestion.

CD23 Function: IgE Regulation

In addition to its role in allergen uptake, CD23 appears to have regulatory influences on IgE synthesis and allergic inflammation. Although the data in this area have seemed to be conflicting at times, the emerging consensus from human and animal studies is that ligation of membrane-bound CD23 on B cells suppresses IgE production. Ligation of CD23 on human B cells by activating antibodies inhibits IgE synthesis[145] and transgenic mice overexpressing CD23 have suppressed IgE responses.[146,147] Conversely, mice rendered CD23-deficient by targeted gene disruption have increased and sustained specific IgE titers following immunization, also consistent with a suppressive effect of membrane-bound CD23.[148] This enhanced tendency toward IgE synthesis in CD23$^{-/-}$ mice is also observed following allergen inhalation and is accompanied by increased eosinophilic inflammation of the airways.[149-152]

In contrast, there have been reports that soluble CD23 (sCD23) fragments, which are generated by proteolytic cleavage, may enhance IgE production, either by direct interaction with B cells (via CD21) or by binding to IgE, thereby blocking its interaction with membrane-bound CD23.[153] The IgE-enhancing effects of crude sCD23 have not yet been reproduced with recombinant sCD23[154] and it is unclear whether this discrepancy arises from IgE-inducing activity attributable to other components of sCD23-containing culture supernatants or whether the lack of activity of recombinant sCD23 is the consequence of a nonphysiologic structure. Recent data implicate a role for allergens, some of which are proteases, as effectors of CD23 cleavage and for IgE itself as a stabilizer of membrane CD23 and inhibitor of proteolytic shedding.[155] Two possible consequences of such allergen-mediated cleavage would be decreased suppressive signaling to the B cell via CD23, along with increased production of activating sCD23 fragments, both promoting IgE production. Inhibition of proteolytic activity of Der p 1 blocks its ability to induce IgE responses in vivo both in normal and humanized scid mice.[156,157] Similar effects are observed in culture systems. Metalloproteinase inhibitors block sCD23 shedding in cultures of tonsillar B cells or peripheral blood mononuclear cells and this is accompanied by decreased IgE production following stimulation with IL-4.[158]

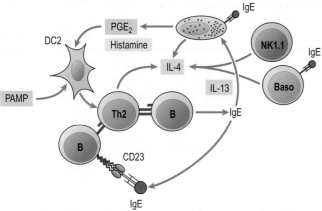

Figure 4-8 The IgE network: cellular and cytokine control of IgE production in allergic tissues and amplification of allergic responses by preformed IgE. A confluence of cellular and molecular stimuli supports IgE synthesis in the tissues of asthmatic patients. Tissue DCs are driven toward a Th2-promoting DC2 phenotype by a variety of environmental influences, including exposure to microbial 'pathogen-associated molecular patterns' *(PAMPs)* and histamine and PGE$_2$ (both of which can be provided by mast cells). Activated DC2s translocate to mucosal- or skin-associated lymphoid tissues where they attain competence as antigen-presenting cells (APCs) and drive the generation of Th2 cells. B cells also serve as APCs, a function that is augmented when preformed IgE (generated during previous allergen encounter) is present and can facilitate B cell antigen uptake via CD23.

IL-4 and IL-13 are derived from numerous cellular sources. In the setting of recurrent allergen challenge, pre-existing, allergen-specific Th2 T cells are likely to provide a major source of IL-4. Additional producers of IL-4 include NKT cells and mast cells. Mast cell IL-4 synthesis can be triggered via FcεRI in the presence of preformed IgE. IL-4 and IL-13 along with cognate T-B interactions involving antigen presentation and CD40 signaling then support IgE isotype switching in B cells.

Conclusions

To summarize, IgE antibodies are invariably elevated in individuals affected by the atopic conditions of asthma, allergic rhinitis, and atopic dermatitis. The production of IgE follows a series of complex genomic rearrangements in B cells, called deletional class switch recombination, a process that is tightly regulated by the cytokines IL-4 and IL-13 along with T-B cell interaction and CD40/CD154 signaling. IgE antibodies exert their biologic effects via receptors FcεRI and CD23. It is now clear that, in addition to mediating the classic immediate hypersensitivity reactions by inducing acute mediator release by mast cells, IgE antibodies have a number of immunomodulatory functions (Figure 4-8). These include up-regulation of IgE receptors, promotion of mast cell survival, enhancement of allergen uptake by B cells for antigen presentation, and induction of Th2 cytokine expression by mast cells and may all collaborate to amplify and perpetuate allergic responses in susceptible individuals. Thus blockade of IgE effects, using novel anti-IgE therapies, may ultimately prove to have a broad benefit.

References

1. Liu FT. Gene expression and structure of immunoglobulin epsilon chains. Crit Rev Immunol 1986;6:47–69.
2. Chaudhuri J, Alt FW. Class-switch recombination: interplay of transcription, DNA deamination and DNA repair. Nat Rev Immunol 2004;4: 541–52.
3. Oettgen HC. Regulation of the IgE isotype switch: new insights on cytokine signals and the functions of varepsilon germline transcripts [In Process Citation]. Curr Opin Immunol 2000;12:618–23.
4. Del Prete G, Maggi E, Parronchi P, et al. IL-4 is an essential factor for the IgE synthesis induced in vitro by human T cells clones and their supernatants. J Immunol 1988;140:4193–8.
5. Vercelli D, Jabara H, Arai K-I, et al. Induction of human IgE synthesis requires interleukin 4 and T/B interactions involving the T cell receptor/CD3 complex and MHC class II antigens. J Exp Med 1989;169: 1295–307.
6. Gauchat J-F, Lebman D, Coffman R, et al. Structure and expression of germline ε transcripts in human B cells induced by interleukin 4 to switch to IgE production. J Exp Med 1990;172:463–73.
7. Jung S, Rajewsky K, Radbruch A. Shutdown of class switch recombination by deletion of a switch region control element. Science 1993;259: 984–87.
8. Lorenz M, Jung S, Radbruch A. Switch transcripts in immunoglobulin class switching. Science 1995;267:1825–8.
9. Zhang J, Bottaro A, Li S, et al. A selective defect in IgG2b switching as a result of targeted mutation of the I gamma 2b promoter and exon. EMBO J 1993;12:3529–37.
10. Bottaro A, Lansford R, Xu L, et al. S region transcription per se promotes basal IgE class switch recombination but additional factors regulate the efficiency of the process. EMBO J 1994;13:665–74.
11. Kim J, Reeves R, Rothman P, et al. The non-histone chromosomal protein HMG-I(Y) contributes to repression of the immunoglobulin heavy chain germ-line epsilon RNA promoter. Eur J Immunol 1995;25:798–808.
12. Wang DZ, Ray P, Boothby M. Interleukin 4-inducible phosphorylation of HMG-I(Y) is inhibited by rapamycin. J Biol Chem 1995;270:22924–32.
13. Wang DZ, Cherrington A, Famakin-Mosuro B, et al. Independent pathways for de-repression of the mouse Ig heavy chain germ-line epsilon promoter: an IL-4 NAF/NF-IL-4 site as a context-dependent negative element. Int Immunol 1996;8:977–89.
14. Monticelli S, De Monte L, Vercelli D. Molecular regulation of IgE switching: let's walk hand in hand. Allergy 1998;53:6–8.
15. Thienes CP, De Monte L, Monticelli S, et al. The transcription factor B cell-specific activator protein (BSAP) enhances both IL-4- and CD40-mediated activation of the human epsilon germline promoter. J Immunol 1997;158:5874–82.
16. Shen CH, Stavnezer J. Interaction of stat6 and NF-kappaB: direct association and synergistic activation of interleukin-4-induced transcription. Mol Cell Biol 1998;18:3395–404.
17. Sha WC, Liou HC, Tuomanen EI, et al. Targeted disruption of the p50 subunit of NF-kappa B leads to multifocal defects in immune responses. Cell 1995;80:321–30.
18. Chen CL, Singh N, Yull FE, et al. Lymphocytes lacking IkappaB-alpha develop normally, but have selective defects in proliferation and function [In Process Citation]. J Immunol 2000;165:5418–27.
19. Qiu G, Stavnezer J. Overexpression of BSAP/Pax-5 inhibits switching to IgA and enhances switching to IgE in the I.29 mu B cell line. J Immunol 1998;161:2906–18.
20. Stutz AM, Woisetschlager M. Functional synergism of STAT6 with either NF-kappa B or PU.1 to mediate IL-4-induced activation of IgE germline gene transcription. J Immunol 1999;163:4383–91.
21. Harris MB, Chang CC, Berton MT, et al. Transcriptional repression of Stat6-dependent interleukin-4-induced genes by BCL-6: specific regulation of iepsilon transcription and immunoglobulin E switching. Mol Cell Biol 1999;19:7264–75.
22. Kitayama D, Sakamoto A, Arima M, et al. A role for Bcl6 in sequential class switch recombination to IgE in B cells stimulated with IL-4 and IL-21. Mol Immunol 2008;45:1337–45.
23. Harada M, Magara-Koyanagi K, Watarai H, et al. IL-21-induced Bepsilon cell apoptosis mediated by natural killer T cells suppresses IgE responses. J Exp Med 2006;203:2929–37.
24. Suto A, Nakajima H, Hirose K, et al. Interleukin 21 prevents antigen-induced IgE production by inhibiting germ line C(epsilon) transcription of IL-4-stimulated B cells. Blood 2002;100:4565–73.
25. Defrance T, Carayon P, Billian G, et al. Interleukin 13 is a B cell stimulating factor. J Exp Med 1994;179:135–43.
26. Punnonen J, Aversa G, Cocks B, et al. Interleukin 13 induces interleukin 4-independent IgG4 and IgE synthesis and CD23 expression by human B cells. Proc Natl Acad Sci, USA 1993;90:3730–4.
27. Palmer-Crocker P, Hughes C, Pober J. IL-4 and IL-13 activate the JAK2 tyrosine kinase and STAT6 in cultured human vascular endothelial cells through a common pathway that does not involve the gc chain. J Clin Invest 1996;98:604–9.
28. Rolling C, Treton D, Beckmann P, et al. JAK3 associates with the human interleukin 4 receptor and is tyrosine phosphorylated following receptor triggering. Oncogene 1995;10:1757–61.
29. Welham M, Learmonth L, Bone H, et al. Interleukin-13 signal transduction in lymphohemopoietic cells. J Biol Chem 1995;270:12286–96.
30. Witthuhn B, Silvennoinen O, Miura O, et al. Involvement of the Jak-3 Janus kinase in signalling by interleukins 2 and 4 in lymphoid and myeloid cells. Nature 1994;370:153–7.
31. Ivashkiv L. Cytokines and STATs: how can signals achieve specificity? Immunity 1995;3:1–4.
32. Schindler C, Kashleva H, Pernis A, et al. STF-IL-4: a novel IL-4-induced signal transducing factor. EMBO J 1994;13:1350–6.

33. Grewal I, Flavell R. A central role of CD40 ligand in the regulation of CD4+ T cell responses. Immunol Today 1996;17:410–4.

34. Cheng G, Cleary AM, Ye Z, et al. Involvement of CRAF1, a relative of TRAF, in CD40 signaling. Science 1995;267:1494–8.

35. Ishida T, Mizushima S, Azuma S, et al. Identification of TRAF6, a novel tumor necrosis factor receptor-associated protein that mediates signaling from an amino-terminal domain of the CD40 cytoplasmic region. J Biol Chem 1996;271:28745–8.

36. Iciek LA, Delphin SA, Stavnezer J. CD40 cross-linking induces Ig epsilon germline transcripts in B cells via activation of NF-kappaB: synergy with IL-4 induction. J Immunol 1997;158:4769–79.

37. Messner B, Stutz A, Albrecht B, et al. Cooperation of binding sites for STAT6 and NFkB/rel in the IL-4-induced up-regulation of the human IgE germline promoter. J Immunol 1997;159:3330–7.

38. Faris M, Gaskin F, Geha R, et al. Tyrosine phosphorylation defines a unique transduction pathway in human B cells mediated via CD40. Trans Assoc Amer Phys 1993;106:187–95.

39. Ren C, Morio T, Fu S, et al. Signal transduction via CD40 involves activation of lyn kinase and phosphatidylinositol-3-kinase, and phosphorylation of phospholipase C gamma 2. J Exp Med 1994;179:673–80.

40. Allen RC, Armitage RJ, Conley ME, et al. CD40 ligand gene defects responsible for X-linked hyper-IgM syndrome [see comments]. Science 1993;259:990–3.

41. Aruffo A, Farrington M, Hollenbaugh D, et al. The CD40 ligand, gp39, is defective in activated T cells from patients with X-linked hyper-IgM syndrome. Cell 1993;72:291–300.

42. DiSanto JP, Bonnefoy JY, Gauchat JF, et al. CD40 ligand mutations in x-linked immunodeficiency with hyper-IgM [see comments]. Nature 1993;361:541–3.

43. Fuleihan R, Ramesh N, Loh R, et al. Defective expression of the CD40 ligand in X chromosome-linked immunoglobulin deficiency with normal or elevated IgM. Proc Natl Acad Sci U S A 1993;90:2170–3.

44. Korthauer U, Graf D, Mages HW, et al. Defective expression of T cell CD40 ligand causes X-linked immunodeficiency with hyper-IgM [see comments]. Nature 1993;361:539–41.

45. Castigli E, Alt FW, Davidson L, et al. CD40-deficient mice generated by recombination-activating gene-2-deficient blastocyst complementation. Proc Natl Acad Sci U S A 1994;91:12135–9.

46. Kawabe T, Naka T, Yoshida K, et al. The immune responses in CD40-deficient mice: impaired immunoglobulin class switching and germinal center formation. Immunity 1994;1:167–78.

47. Xu J, Foy T, Laman J, et al. Mice deficient for CD40 ligand. Immunity 1994;1:423–31.

48. Castigli E, Geha RS. TACI, isotype switching, CVID and IgAD. Immunol Res 2007;38:102–11.

49. Castigli E, Wilson SA, Scott S, et al. TACI and BAFF-R mediate isotype switching in B cells. J Exp Med 2005;201:35–9.

50. Castigli E, Wilson SA, Garibyan L, et al. TACI is mutant in common variable immunodeficiency and IgA deficiency. Nat Genet 2005;37:829–34.

51. Castigli E, Wilson S, Garibyan L, et al. Reexamining the role of TACI coding variants in common variable immunodeficiency and selective IgA deficiency. Nat Genet 2007;39:430–1.

52. Kato A, Truong-Tran AQ, Scott AL, et al. Airway epithelial cells produce B cell-activating factor of TNF family by an IFN-beta-dependent mechanism. J Immunol 2006;177:7164–72.

53. Kato A, Xiao H, Chustz RT, et al. Local release of B cell-activating factor of the TNF family after segmental allergen challenge of allergic subjects. J Allergy Clin Immunol 2009.

54. Cameron L, Gounni AS, Frenkiel S, et al. S epsilon S mu and S epsilon S gamma switch circles in human nasal mucosa following ex vivo allergen challenge: evidence for direct as well as sequential class switch recombination. J Immunol 2003;171:3816–22.

55. Muramatsu M, Kinoshita K, Fagarasan S, et al. Class switch recombination and hypermutation require activation-induced cytidine deaminase (AID), a potential RNA editing enzyme [see comments]. Cell 2000;102:553–63.

56. Muramatsu M, Sankaranand VS, Anant S, et al. Specific expression of activation-induced cytidine deaminase (AID), a novel member of the RNA-editing deaminase family in germinal center B cells. J Biol Chem 1999;274:18470–6.

57. Revy P, Muto T, Levy Y, et al. Activation-induced cytidine deaminase (AID) deficiency causes the autosomal recessive form of the Hyper-IgM syndrome (HIGM2) [see comments]. Cell 2000;102:565–75.

58. Okazaki IM, Kinoshita K, Muramatsu M, et al. The AID enzyme induces class switch recombination in fibroblasts. Nature 2002;416:340–5.

59. Longerich S, Basu U, Alt F, et al. AID in somatic hypermutation and class switch recombination. Curr Opin Immunol 2006;18:164–74.

60. Soulas-Sprauel P, Rivera-Munoz P, Malivert L, et al. V(D)J and immunoglobulin class switch recombinations: a paradigm to study the regulation of DNA end-joining. Oncogene 2007;26:7780–91.

61. Manis JP, Dudley D, Kaylor L, et al. IgH class switch recombination to IgG1 in DNA-PKcs-deficient B cells. Immunity 2002;16:607–17.

62. Manis JP, Gu Y, Lansford R, et al. Ku70 is required for late B cell development and immunoglobulin heavy chain class switching. J Exp Med 1998;187:2081–9.

63. Annunziato F, Galli G, Cosmi L, et al. Molecules associated with human Th1 or Th2 cells. Eur Cytokine Netw 1998;9:12–6.

64. Coyle AJ, Lloyd C, Tian J, et al. Crucial role of the interleukin 1 receptor family member T1/ST2 in T helper cell type 2-mediated lung mucosal immune responses. J Exp Med 1999;190:895–902.

65. Sallusto F, Mackay CR, Lanzavecchia A. Selective expression of the eotaxin receptor CCR3 by human T helper 2 cells. Science 1997;277:2005–7.

66. Sallusto F, Mackay CR, Lanzavecchia A. The role of chemokine receptors in primary, effector, and memory immune responses. Annu Rev Immunol 2000;18:593–620.

67. Sadick MD, Heinzel FP, Shigekane VM, et al. Cellular and humoral immunity to Leishmania major in genetically susceptible mice after in vivo depletion of L3T4+ T cells. J Immunol 1987;139:1303–9.

68. Sadick MD, Locksley RM, Tubbs C, et al. Murine cutaneous leishmaniasis: resistance correlates with the capacity to generate interferon-gamma in response to Leishmania antigens in vitro. J Immunol 1986;136:655–61.

69. Pritchard DI, Hewitt C, Moqbel R. The relationship between immunological responsiveness controlled by T- helper 2 lymphocytes and infections with parasitic helminths. Parasitology 1997;115:S33–44.

70. Murphy KM, Ouyang W, Szabo SJ, et al. T helper differentiation proceeds through Stat1-dependent, Stat4- dependent and Stat4-independent phases. Curr Top Microbiol Immunol 1999;238:13–26.

71. Kalinski P, Hilkens CM, Wierenga EA, et al. T cell priming by type-1 and type-2 polarized dendritic cells: the concept of a third signal. Immunol Today 1999;20:561–7.

72. Pasare C, Medzhitov R. Toll pathway-dependent blockade of CD4+CD25+ T cell-mediated suppression by dendritic cells. Science 2003;299:1033–6.

73. Kalinski P, Schuitemaker JH, Hilkens CM, et al. Prostaglandin E2 induces the final maturation of IL-12-deficient CD1a+CD83+ dendritic cells: the levels of IL-12 are determined during the final dendritic cell maturation and are resistant to further modulation. J Immunol 1998;161:2804–9.

74. Mazzoni A, Young HA, Spitzer JH, et al. Histamine regulates cytokine production in maturing dendritic cells, resulting in altered T cell polarization. J Clin Invest 2001;108:1865–73.

75. Vieira PL, de Jong EC, Wierenga EA, et al. Development of Th1-inducing capacity in myeloid dendritic cells requires environmental instruction. J Immunol 2000;164:4507–12.

76. Kalinski P, Hilkens CM, Snijders A, et al. IL-12-deficient dendritic cells, generated in the presence of prostaglandin E2, promote type 2 cytokine production in maturing human naive T helper cells. J Immunol 1997;159:28–35.

77. Stumbles PA, Thomas JA, Pimm CL, et al. Resting respiratory tract dendritic cells preferentially stimulate T helper cell type 2 (Th2) responses and require obligatory cytokine signals for induction of Th1 immunity. J Exp Med 1998;188:2019–31.

78. Galli SJ. Complexity and redundancy in the pathogenesis of asthma: reassessing the roles of mast cells and T cells. J Exp Med 1997;186:343–7.

79. Toru H, Pawankar R, Ra C, et al. Human mast cells produce IL-13 by high-affinity IgE receptor cross-linking: enhanced IL-13 production by IL-4-primed human mast cells. J Allergy Clin Immunol 1998;102:491–502.

80. Denzel A, Maus UA, Rodriguez Gomez M, et al. Basophils enhance immunological memory responses. Nat Immunol 2008;9:733–42.

81. Gauchat JF, Henchoz S, Mazzei G, et al. Induction of human IgE synthesis in B cells by mast cells and basophils. Nature 1993;365:340–3.

82. Yanagihara Y, Kajiwara K, Basaki Y, et al. Induction of human IgE synthesis in B cells by a basophilic cell line, KU812. Clin Exp Immunol 1997;108:295–301.

83. Yanagihara Y, Kajiwara K, Basaki Y, et al. Cultured basophils but not cultured mast cells induce human IgE synthesis in B cells after immunologic stimulation. Clin Exp Immunol 1998;111:136–43.

84. Aoki I, Kinzer C, Shirai A, et al. IgE receptor-positive non-B/non-T cells dominate the production of interleukin 4 and interleukin 6 in immunized mice. Proc Natl Acad Sci U S A 1995;92:2534–8.

85. Khodoun MV, Orekhova T, Potter C, et al. Basophils initiate IL-4 production during a memory T-dependent response. J Exp Med 2004;200:857–70.

86. Sokol CL, Barton GM, Farr AG, et al. A mechanism for the initiation of allergen-induced T helper type 2 responses. Nat Immunol 2008;9:310–8.

87. Mukai K, Matsuoka K, Taya C, et al. Basophils play a critical role in the development of IgE-mediated chronic allergic inflammation independently of T cells and mast cells. Immunity 2005;23:191–202.

88. Yoshimoto T, Bendelac A, Hu-Li J, et al. Defective IgE production by SJL mice is linked to the absence of CD4+, NK1.1+ T cells that promptly produce interleukin 4. Proc Natl Acad Sci U S A 1995;92:11931–4.

89. Bendelac A, Hunziker RD, Lantz O. Increased interleukin 4 and immunoglobulin E production in transgenic mice overexpressing NK1 T cells. J Exp Med 1996;184:1285–93.

90. Deniz G, Akdis M, Aktas E, et al. Human NK1 and NK2 subsets determined by purification of IFN-gamma-secreting and IFN-gamma-nonsecreting NK cells. Eur J Immunol 2002;32:879–84.

91. Hoshino T, Winkler-Pickett RT, Mason AT, et al. IL-13 production by NK cells: IL-13-producing NK and T cells are present in vivo in the absence of IFN-gamma. J Immunol 1999;162:51–9.

92. Kinet JP. The high-affinity IgE receptor (Fc epsilon RI): from physiology to pathology. Annu Rev Immunol 1999;17:931–72.

93. Dombrowicz D, Lin S, Flamand V, et al. Allergy-associated FcRbeta is a molecular amplifier of IgE- and IgG-mediated in vivo responses. Immunity 1998;8:517–29.

94. Donnadieu E, Jouvin MH, Kinet JP. A second amplifier function for the allergy-associated Fc(epsilon)RI- beta subunit. Immunity 2000;12:515–23.

95. Lin S, Cicala C, Scharenberg AM, et al. The Fc(epsilon)RIbeta subunit functions as an amplifier of Fc(epsilon)RIgamma-mediated cell activation signals. Cell 1996;85:985–95.

96. Lee WT, Conrad DH. Murine B cell hybridomas bearing ligand-inducible Fc receptors for IgE. J Immunol 1986;136:4573–80.

97. Vander-Mallie R, Ishizaka T, Ishizaka K. Lymphocyte bearing Fc receptors for IgE. VIII. Affinity of mouse IgE for FceR on mouse B lymphocytes. J Immunol 1982;128:2306–12.

98. Delespesse G, Sarfati M, Hofstetter H, et al. Structure, function and clinical relevance of the low affinity receptor for IgE. Immunol Invest 1988;17:363–87.

99. Bettler B, Hofstetter H, Rao M, et al. Molecular structure and expression of the murine lymphocyte low-affinity receptor for IgE (Fc epsilon RII). Proc Natl Acad Sci U S A 1989;86:7566–70.

100. Gould HJ, Sutton BJ. IgE in allergy and asthma today. Nat Rev Immunol 2008;8:205–17.

101. Kikutani H, Inui S, Sato R, et al. Molecular structure of human lymphocyte receptor for immunoglobulin E. Cell 1986;47:657–65.

102. Dierks SE, Bartlett WC, Edmeades RL, et al. The oligomeric nature of the murine Fc epsilon RII/CD23: implications for function. J Immunol 1993;150:2372–82.

103. Aubry J-P, Pochon S, Graber P, et al. CD21 is a ligand for CD23 and regulates IgE production. Nature 1992;358:505–7.

104. Aubry JP, Pochon S, Gauchat JF, et al. CD23 interacts with a new functional extracytoplasmic domain involving N-linked oligosaccharides on CD21. J Immunol 1994;152:5806–13.

105. Gilfillan AM, Rivera J. The tyrosine kinase network regulating mast cell activation. Immunol Rev 2009;228:149–69.

106. Rivera J, Gonzalez-Espinosa C, Kovarova M, et al. The architecture of IgE-dependent mast cell signalling. ACI International 2002;14:25–36.

107. Macglashan D, Miura K. Loss of syk kinase during IgE-mediated stimulation of human basophils. J Allergy Clin Immunol 2004;114:1317–24.

108. Pivniouk VI, Martin TR, Lu-Kuo JM, et al. SLP-76 deficiency impairs signaling via the high-affinity IgE receptor in mast cells. J Clin Invest 1999;103:1737–43.

109. Saitoh S, Arudchandran R, Manetz TS, et al. LAT is essential for Fc(epsilon)RI-mediated mast cell activation. Immunity 2000;12:525–35.

110. Manetz TS, Gonzalez-Espinosa C, Arudchandran R, et al. Vav1 regulates phospholipase cgamma activation and calcium responses in mast cells. Mol Cell Biol 2001;21:3763–74.

111. Song JS, Gomez J, Stancato LF, et al. Association of a p95 Vav-containing signaling complex with the FcepsilonRI gamma chain in the RBL-2H3 mast cell line. Evidence for a constitutive in vivo association of Vav with Grb2, Raf-1, and ERK2 in an active complex. J Biol Chem 1996;271:26962–70.

112. Pivniouk VI, Snapper SB, Kettner A, et al. Impaired signaling via the high-affinity IgE receptor in Wiskott-Aldrich syndrome protein-deficient mast cells. Int Immunol 2003;15:1431–40.

113. Fahy JV, Fleming HE, Wong HH, et al. The effect of an anti-IgE monoclonal antibody on the early- and late-phase responses to allergen inhalation in asthmatic subjects [see comments]. Am J Respir Crit Care Med 1997;155:1828–34.

114. Howarth PH, Durham SR, Kay AB, et al. The relationship between mast cell-mediator release and bronchial reactivity in allergic asthma. J Allergy Clin Immunol 1987;80:703–11.

115. Shampain MP, Behrens BL, Larsen GL, et al. An animal model of late pulmonary responses to Alternaria challenge. Am Rev Respir Dis 1982;126:493–8.

116. Cockcroft DW, Murdock KY. Comparative effects of inhaled salbutamol, sodium cromoglycate and beclomethasone dipropionate on allergen-induced early astmatic responses, late asthmatic responses and increased bronchial responsiveness to histamine. J Allergy Clin Immunol 1987;79:734–40.

117. Cartier A, Thomson NC, Frith PA, et al. Allergen-induced increase in bronchial responsiveness to histamine: relationship to the late asthmatic response and change in airway caliber. J Allergy Clin Immunol 1982;70:170–7.

118. McFadden ER, Gilbert IA. Asthma. N Engl J Med 1992;327:1928–37.

119. Asai K, Kitaura J, Kawakami Y, et al. Regulation of mast cell survival by IgE. Immunity 2001;14:791–800.

120. Kalesnikoff J, Huber M, Lam V, et al. Monomeric IgE stimulates signaling pathways in mast cells that lead to cytokine production and cell survival. Immunity 2001;14:801–11.

121. Kitaura J, Song J, Tsai M, et al. Evidence that IgE molecules mediate a spectrum of effects on mast cell survival and activation via aggregation of the FcepsilonRI. Proc Natl Acad Sci U S A 2003;100:12911–6.

122. Pandey V, Mihara S, Fensome-Green A, et al. Monomeric IgE stimulates NFAT translocation into the nucleus, a rise in cytosol Ca2+, degranulation, and membrane ruffling in the cultured rat basophilic leukemia-2H3 mast cell line. J Immunol 2004;172:4048–58.

123. Tanaka S, Takasu Y, Mikura S, et al. Antigen-independent induction of histamine synthesis by immunoglobulin E in mouse bone marrow-derived mast cells. J Exp Med 2002;196:229–35.

124. Kawakami T, Kitaura J. Mast cell survival and activation by IgE in the absence of antigen: a consideration of the biologic mechanisms and relevance. J Immunol 2005;175:4167–73.

125. Mathias CB, Freyschmidt EJ, Caplan B, et al. IgE influences the number and function of mature mast cells, but not progenitor recruitment in allergic pulmonary inflammation. J Immunol 2009;182:2416–24.

126. Gurish MF, Bryce PJ, Tao H, et al. IgE enhances parasite clearance and regulates mast cell responses in mice infected with Trichinella spiralis. J Immunol 2004;172:1139–45.

127. Lantz CS, Yamaguchi M, Oettgen HC, et al. IgE regulates mouse basophil FceRI expression in vivo. J Immunol 1997;158:2517–21.

128. Yamaguchi M, Lantz CS, Oettgen HC, et al. IgE enhances mouse mast cell FceRI expression in vitro and in vivo: evidence for a novel amplification mechanism for IgE-dependent reactions. J Exp Med 1997;185:663–72.

129. Yamaguchi M, Lantz CS, Oettgen HC, et al. IgE enhances mouse mast cell Fc(epsilon)RI expression in vitro and in vivo: evidence for a novel amplification mechanism in IgE-dependent reactions. J Exp Med 1997;185:663–72.

130. Beck LA, Marcotte GV, MacGlashan D, et al. Omalizumab-induced reductions in mast cell Fce psilon RI expression and function. J Allergy Clin Immunol 2004;114:527–30.

131. Prussin C, Griffith DT, Boesel KM, et al. Omalizumab treatment down-regulates dendritic cell FcepsilonRI expression. J Allergy Clin Immunol 2003;112:1147–54.

132. Saini SS, MacGlashan DW Jr, Sterbinsky SA, et al. Down-regulation of human basophil IgE and FC epsilon RI alpha surface densities and mediator release by anti-IgE-infusions is reversible in vitro and in vivo. J Immunol 1999;162:5624–30.

133. Lee WT, Rao M, Conrad DH. The murine lymphocyte receptor for IgE. IV. The mechanism of ligand-specific receptor upregulation on B cells. J Immunol 1987;139:1191–8.

134. Weskamp G, Ford JW, Sturgill J, et al. ADAM10 is a principal 'sheddase' of the low-affinity immunoglobulin E receptor CD23. Nat Immunol 2006;7:1293–8.

135. Lemieux GA, Blumenkron F, Yeung N, et al. The low affinity IgE receptor (CD23) is cleaved by the metalloproteinase ADAM10. J Biol Chem 2007;282:14836–44.

136. Kisselgof AB, Oettgen HC. The expression of murine B cell CD23, in vivo, is regulated by its ligand, IgE. Int Immunol 1998;10:1377–84.

137. Borkowski TA, Jouvin MH, Lin SY, et al. Minimal requirements for IgE-mediated regulation of surface Fc epsilon RI. J Immunol 2001;167:1290–6.

138. Kehry MR, Hudak SA. Characterization of B cell populations bearing Fce receptor II. Cell Immunol 1989;118:504–15.

139. Pirron U, Schlunck T, Prinz JC, et al. IgE-dependent antigen focusing by human B lymphocytes is mediated by the low-affinity receptor for IgE. Eur J Immunol 1990;20:1547–51.

140. Van der Heijden FL, Joost van Neerven RJ, van Katwijk M, et al. Serum-IgE-facilitated allergen presentation in atopic disease. J Immunol 1993;150:643–50.

141. Gustavsson S, Hjulstrom S, Liu T, et al. CD23/IgE-mediated regulation of the specific antibody response in vivo. J Immunol 1994;152:4793–800.

142. Heyman B, Liu T, Gustavsson S. In vivo enhancement of the specific antibody response via the low-affinity receptor for IgE. Eur J Immunol 1993;23:1739–42.

143. Fujiwara H, Kikutani H, Suematsu S, et al. The absence of IgE antibody-mediated augmentation of immune responses in CD23-deficient mice. Proc Natl Acad Sci U S A 1994;91:6835–39.

144. Gustavsson S, Wernersson S, Heyman B. Restoration of the antibody response to IgE/antigen complexes in CD23- deficient mice by CD23+ spleen or bone marrow cells. J Immunol 2000;164:3990–5.

145. Sherr E, Macy E, Kimata H, et al. Binding the low affinity Fc epsilon R on B cells suppresses ongoing human IgE synthesis. J Immunol 1989;142:481–9.

146. Payet ME, Woodward EC, Conrad DH. Humoral response suppression observed with CD23 transgenics. J Immunol 1999;163:217–23.

147. Payet-Jamroz M, Helm SL, Wu J, et al. Suppression of IgE responses in CD23-transgenic animals is due to expression of CD23 on nonlymphoid cells. J Immunol 2001;166:4863–9.

148. Yu P, Kosco-Vilbois M, Richards M, et al. Negative feedback regulation of IgE synthesis by murine CD23. Nature 1994;369:753–6.

149. Cernadas M, De Sanctis GT, Krinzman SJ, et al. CD23 and allergic pulmonary inflammation: potential role as an inhibitor. Am J Respir Cell Mol Biol 1999;20:1–8.

150. Haczku A, Takeda K, Hamelmann E, et al. CD23 exhibits negative regulatory effects on allergic sensitization and airway hyperresponsiveness. Am J Respir Crit Care Med 2000;161:952–60.

151. Haczku A, Takeda K, Hamelmann E, et al. CD23 deficient mice develop allergic airway hyperresponsiveness following sensitization with ovalbumin. Am J Respir Crit Care Med 1997;156:1945–55.

152. Riffo-Vasquez Y, Spina D, Thomas M, et al. The role of CD23 on allergen-induced IgE levels, pulmonary eosinophilia and bronchial hyperresponsiveness in mice. Clin Exp Allergy 2000;30:728–38.

153. Saxon A, Ke Z, Bahati L, et al. Soluble CD23 containing B cell supernatants induce IgE from peripheral blood B lymphocytes and costimulate with interleukin-4 in induction of IgE. J Allergy Clin Immunol 1990;86:333–44.

154. Uchibayashi N, Kikutani H, Barsumian EL, et al. Recombinant soluble Fc epsilon receptor II (Fc epsilon RII/CD23) has IgE binding activity but no B cell growth promoting activity. J Immunol 1989;142:3901–8.

155. Schulz O, Laing P, Sewell HF, et al. Der p I, a major allergen of the house dust mite, proteolytically cleaves the low-affinity receptor for human IgE (CD23). Eur J Immunol 1995;25:3191–4.

156. Gough L, Schulz O, Sewell HF, et al. The cysteine protease activity of the major dust mite allergen Der p 1 selectively enhances the immunoglobulin E antibody response. J Exp Med 1999;190:1897–902.

157. Mayer RJ, Bolognese BJ, Al-Mahdi N, et al. Inhibition of CD23 processing correlates with inhibition of IL-4- stimulated IgE production in human PBL and hu-PBL-reconstituted SCID mice [see comments]. Clin Exp Allergy 2000;30:719–27.

158. Christie G, Barton A, Bolognese B, et al. IgE secretion is attenuated by an inhibitor of proteolytic processing of CD23 (Fc epsilonRII). Eur J Immunol 1997;27:3228–35.

CHAPTER

5

Inflammatory Effector Cells/Cell Migration

Charles W. DeBrosse • Marc E. Rothenberg

One of the hallmarks of allergic disorders is the accumulation of an abnormally large number of leukocytes, including eosinophils, neutrophils, lymphocytes, basophils, and macrophages, in the inflammatory tissue. There is substantial evidence that inflammatory cells are major effector cells in the pathogenesis of allergic disorders. Therefore understanding the mechanisms by which leukocytes accumulate and are activated in tissues is very relevant to allergic diseases. Substantial progress has been made in understanding the specific molecules involved in leukocyte migration and the specific mechanisms by which effector cells participate in disease pathogenesis. In particular, cellular adhesion proteins, integrins, and chemoattractant cytokines (chemokines) have emerged as critical molecules in these processes. Chemokines are potent leukocyte chemoattractants, cellular activating factors, and histamine-releasing factors, making them attractive new therapeutic targets for the treatment of allergic disease. This chapter focuses on recently emerging data on the mechanisms by which specific leukocyte subsets are recruited into allergic tissues and the mechanisms by which they participate in disease pathogenesis.

Allergic Inflammation

Experimentation in the allergy field has largely focused on analysis of the cellular and molecular events induced by allergen exposure in sensitized animals and humans.[1-3] In patient studies, naturally sensitized individuals are challenged by exposure to allergen.[4] In the animal models, mice are typically subjected to sensitization with antigen (e.g., ovalbumin [OVA]) in the presence of adjuvant (e.g. alum) via intraperitoneal injection.[5] Subsequently, mice are challenged by exposure to mucosal allergen and pathologic responses are monitored. In other animal models, nonsensitized mice are repeatedly exposed to mucosal allergens and the development of experimental allergy is monitored.[6] Though no animal model precisely mimics human disease, experimentation in animals has provided a framework to identify the critical effector cells, and inflammatory mediators involved in allergic responses.

The animal and human experimental systems have demonstrated that allergic inflammatory responses are often biphasic. For example, asthma is characterized by a biphasic bronchospasm response, consisting of an early-phase asthmatic response (EAR) and a late-phase asthmatic response (LAR)[7] (Figure 5-1). The EAR phase is characterized by immediate bronchoconstriction in the absence of pronounced airway inflammation or morphologic changes in the airway tissue.[7,8] The EAR phase has been shown to directly involve IgE mast cell mediated release of histamine, prostaglandin D_2, and cysteinyl-peptide leukotrienes, which are potent mediators of bronchoconstriction. After the immediate response, individuals with asthma often experience an LAR, which is characterized by persistent bronchoconstriction associated with extensive airway inflammation and morphologic changes to the airways.[7,9-11] Clinical investigations have demonstrated that the LAR is associated with increased levels of inflammatory cells, in particular activated T lymphocytes and eosinophils (see Figure 5-1). The elevated levels of T lymphocytes and eosinophils correlate with increased levels of eosinophilic constituents in the bronchoalveolar lavage fluid (BALF), the degree of airway epithelial cell damage, enhanced bronchial responsiveness to inhaled spasmogens, and disease severity[7,10-15] Analysis of tissue biopsy samples from patients with allergic disorders has revealed that chronic inflammation is associated with a variety of processes, including tissue remodeling. Asthmatic tissue is characterized by the accumulation of a large number of inflammatory cells, increased mucus production, epithelial shedding and hypertrophy, mucus and smooth muscle cell hyperplasia/metaplasia, hyperplasia and metaplasia of submucosal mucus glands, and fibrosis.[2,16-20]

In summary, allergic responses involve a complex interplay of diverse cells including infiltrating leukocytes and residential cells including endothelial, epithelial, and smooth muscle cells.[2,16,18] This interface results in elevated production of IgE, mucus, eosinophils, complement proteins, and enhanced tissue reactivity to allergens or other stimulants.[19,20]

Effector Cells

T Cells

T cells are specialized leukocytes distinguished by their expression of antigen-specific receptors that arise from somatic gene rearrangement. Two major subpopulations were originally defined based on the expression of the CD4 and CD8 antigens and their associated function. CD4$^+$ T cells recognize antigen in association with MHC class II molecules and are primarily involved in orchestrating immune responses, whereas CD8$^+$ cells recognize antigen in association with MHC class I molecules and are primarily involved in cytotoxicity. More recently, populations of regulatory T cells have been characterized. Regulatory T cells include a subpopulation of natural killer (NK) T cells, as well as CD4$^+$ CD25$^+$ Fox p 3$^+$ T cells; both populations appear to be chief sources of regulatory cytokines, including interleukin (IL)-4 and IL-10.[21] The absence or decrease in function of

DOI: 10.1016/B978-1-4377-0271-2.00005-5

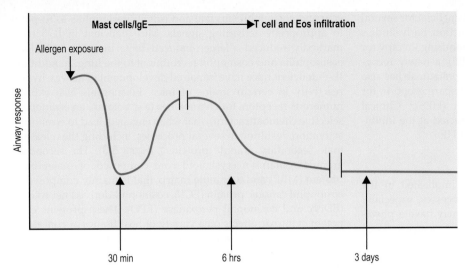

Mast cells/IgE ──────────────▶ T cell and Eos infiltration

Airway response

Allergen exposure

30 min   6 hrs   3 days

Figure 5-1 Early- and late-phase allergic responses. The airway response (e.g. forced expiratory volume in the first second [FEV$_1$]) is illustrated when an allergen-sensitized individual is experimentally exposed to an allergen; a biphasic bronchospasm response, consisting of an early-phase asthmatic response (EAR) and a late-phase asthmatic response (LAR), is shown. The EAR phase is characterized by immediate bronchoconstriction in the absence of pronounced airway inflammation or morphologic changes in the airways tissue. The EAR phase has been shown to directly involve IgE mast cell-mediated release histamine, prostaglandin D$_2$, and cysteinyl-peptide leukotrienes, which are potent mediators of bronchoconstriction. After the immediate response, the airway recovers but later undergoes marked decline in function, which is characterized by more persistent bronchoconstriction associated with extensive airway inflammation (involving T cells and eosinophils).

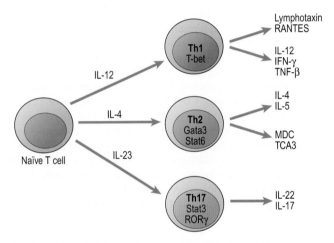

Lymphotaxin
RANTES

Th1
T-bet

IL-12
IFN-γ
TNF-β

IL-12

IL-4
IL-5

Naïve T cell

IL-4

Th2
Gata3
Stat6

MDC
TCA3

IL-23

Th17
Stat3
RORγ

IL-22
IL-17

Figure 5-2 Chemokine and chemokine receptor expression by Th1 and Th2 cells. Th0 cells differentiate into Th1 or Th2 cells following their activation by antigen-presenting cells (APCs). IL-12 promotes the development of Th1 cells that preferentially express CCR5 and CXCR3. IL-4 promotes the development of Th2 cells that preferentially express CCR3, CCR4, and CCR8. IL-23 and TGF-β are responsible for driving Th17 development. In addition to expressing distinct cytokines (IL-2, IL-4, IL-5, IL-13, and IFN-γ), murine T cells have recently been shown to express a unique panel of chemokines, as indicated. The unique transcription factors responsible for driving cytokine development are identified.

T regulatory cells leads to an increase in activity of both Th1 and Th2 lymphocytes and is associated with the development of autoimmunity.[22] Impairment of T regulatory function has also been implicated in the development of the predominantly CD4$^+$ Th2 response seen in allergic disease, though this hypothesis is controversial.[23]

CD4$^+$ T lymphocytes have central roles in allergic responses by regulating the production of IgE and the effector function of mast cells and eosinophils.[24] CD4$^+$ T lymphocytes can be divided into two distinct subsets, which are primarily based on their restricted cytokine profiles and different immune functions (Figure 5-2). CD4$^+$ Th1-type T lymphocytes produce IL-2, tumor necrosis factor (TNF)-β (lymphotoxin), and interferon (IFN)-γ and are involved in delayed-type hypersensitivity responses. Th2 lymphocytes (Th2 cells) secrete IL-4, IL-5, IL-9, IL-10, and IL-13 and promote antibody responses and allergic inflammation (see Figure 5-2).

Clinical investigations indicate that CD4$^+$ T lymphocytes are activated and are predominantly of the Th2-type subclass in allergic disorders. Notably, there is a strong correlation between the presence of CD4$^+$ Th2 lymphocytes and disease severity, suggesting an integral role for these cells in the pathophysiology of allergic diseases.[25,26] Th2 cells are thought to induce asthma through the secretion of cytokines that activate inflammatory and residential effector pathways both directly and indirectly.[27] In particular, IL-4 and IL-13 are produced at elevated levels in the allergic tissue and are thought to be central regulators of many of the hallmark features of the disease.[28] However, in addition to Th2 cells, inflammatory cells within the allergic tissue also produce IL-4, IL-13, and a variety of other cytokines.[29,30] IL-4 promotes Th2 cell differentiation, IgE production, tissue eosinophilia, and, in the case of asthma, morphologic changes to the respiratory epithelium and airway hyperreactivity.[31,32] IL-13 induces IgE production, mucus hypersecretion, eosinophil recruitment and survival, airway hyperreactivity, the expression of CD23, adhesion systems, and chemokines.[28,33,34] IL-4 and IL-13 share similar signaling requirements such as utilization of the IL-4 receptor (R) α chain and the induction of Janus kinase 1 and signal transducer and activator of transcription (STAT)-6.[35-37] A critical role for IL-13 in orchestration of experimental asthma has been suggested by the finding that a soluble IL-13 receptor homolog blocks many of the essential features of experimental asthma.[38,39] Furthermore, mice deficient in the IL-4Rα chain have impaired eosinophil recruitment and mucus production, but still develop airway hyperreactivity.[40] Mice with the targeted deletion of STAT-6 have impaired development of asthma including inflammatory cell infiltrates, IL-13 production, and airway hyperreactivity.[41-44] Collectively, these studies have provided the rationale for the development of multiple therapeutic agents that interfere with specific inflammatory pathways. (Box 5-1). Monoclonal antibodies developed to block the function of IgE and IL-5 have been evaluated in clinical trials. Anti-IgE has shown to be beneficial in the treatment of patients with allergen-induced asthma that is refractory to traditional therapy.[45] Initial studies on the treatment of moderate atopic asthma with the anti-IL-5 antibody mepolizumab, demonstrated mixed results.[46] However, recent studies in refractory eosinophilic, steroid-dependent asthma demonstrated that mepolizumab was effective in reducing asthma exacerbations, increasing quality of life, and reducing the maximum dose of prednisone required for asthma control.[47,48] The use of mepolizumab among a well-defined subset of patients with severe, eosinophil-mediated asthma may be helpful in the future.

Mepolizumab has also been proven to be beneficial for several disorders associated with elevated IL-5 production. Early studies have demonstrated that mepolizumab is a promising therapy for the treatment of eosinophilic esophagitis (EE), a newly recognized allergic disorder of the esophagus.[49] Mepolizumab has also been shown to be an efficacious and steroid-sparing option for the treatment of hypereosinophilic syndrome (HES).[50] Clinical trials investigating the role of antibodies directed at the inhibition of IL-5 are still ongoing for both EE and HES.

Eosinophils

Eosinophils are multifunctional leukocytes implicated in the pathogenesis of numerous inflammatory processes, especially allergic disorders.[51] In addition, eosinophils may have a physiologic role in organ morphogenesis (e.g. postgestational mammary gland development).[52] Eosinophils selectively express the receptor for IL-5, a cytokine that regulates eosinophil expansion and eosinophil survival and primes eosinophils to respond to appropriate activating signals. Mice deficient in IL-5 have markedly reduced allergen-induced bone marrow and blood eosinophilia and eosinophil recruitment to the lung. In addition, IL-5-deficient mice have impaired development of airway hyperreactivity in certain strains of mice. Eosinophils also express numerous receptors for chemokines (e.g. eotaxin, an eosinophil-selective chemoattractant), that when engaged, lead to eosinophil activation, resulting in several processes, including the release of toxic secondary granule proteins[30] (Figure 5-3). The secondary granule contains a crystalloid core composed of major basic protein (MBP) and a granule matrix that is mainly composed of eosinophil cationic protein (ECP), eosinophil-derived neurotoxin (EDN), and eosinophil peroxidase (EPO). These proteins elicit potent cytotoxic effects on a variety of host tissues at concentrations similar to those found in biologic fluid from patients with eosinophilia. The cytotoxic effects of eosinophils may be elicited through multiple mechanisms including degrading cellular ribonucleic acid because ECP and EDN have substantial functional and structural homology to a large family of ribonuclease genes.[53,54] Notably, ECP and EDN are the most divergent family of coding sequences in the human genome (compared with other species), even though their homologs have conserved RNase activity. The strong positive evolutionary pressure to modulate this family of proteins suggests a critical role for these enzymes and eosinophils in host survival, perhaps related to the antiviral activity of these molecules. EDN is a potent activator of TLR2, capable of activating dendritic cells to polarize Th2 responses.[55] ECP also inserts ion-nonselective pores into the membranes of target cells, which may allow the entry of the cytotoxic proteins.[56] Further proinflammatory damage is caused by the generation of unstable oxygen radicals formed by the respiratory burst oxidase apparatus and EPO. Furthermore, direct degranulation of mast cells and basophils is triggered by MBP. In addition to being

---

BOX 5-1 Key concepts

T Cells

- Mature T cells are primarily divided into CD4+ and CD8+ cells.
- T cells express antigen-specific T cell receptors (TCR) that recognize antigen in the context of major histocompatibility molecules (MHC).
- CD4+ T cells are engaged by antigen in the context of class II molecules.
- CD4+ T cells are divided into Th1 and Th2 cells.
- Th1 cells are major producers of Th1 cytokines (e.g. interferon-gamma) and Th2 cells are major producers of Th2 cytokines (e.g. IL-4, IL-5, IL-13).

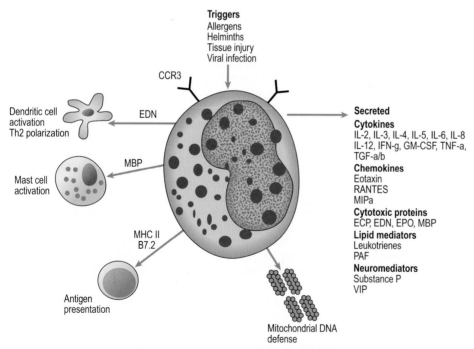

Triggers
Allergens
Helminths
Tissue injury
Viral infection

CCR3

EDN

Dendritic cell activation
Th2 polarization

MBP

Mast cell activation

MHC II
B7.2

Antigen presentation

Mitochondrial DNA defense

Secreted
Cytokines
IL-2, IL-3, IL-4, IL-5, IL-6, IL-8
IL-12, IFN-g, GM-CSF, TNF-a,
TGF-a/b
Chemokines
Eotaxin
RANTES
MIPa
Cytotoxic proteins
ECP, EDN, EPO, MBP
Lipid mediators
Leukotrienes
PAF
Neuromediators
Substance P
VIP

Figure 5-3 Schematic diagram of an eosinophil and its diverse properties. Eosinophils are bilobed granulocytes that respond to diverse stimuli including allergens, helminths, viral infections, allografts, and nonspecific tissue injury. Eosinophils express the receptor for IL-5, a critical eosinophil growth and differentiation factor, as well as the receptor for eotaxin and related chemokines (CCR3). The secondary granules contain four primary cationic proteins designated eosinophil peroxidase (EPO), major basic protein (MBP), eosinophil cationic protein (ECP), and eosinophil-derived neurotoxin (EDN). All four proteins are cytotoxic molecules; also, ECP and EDN are ribonucleases. In addition to releasing their preformed cationic proteins, eosinophils can release a variety of cytokines, chemokines and neuromediators and generate large amounts of LTC$_4$. Last, eosinophils can be induced to express MHC class II and costimulatory molecules and may be involved in propagating immune responses by presenting antigen to T cells.

cytotoxic, MBP directly increases smooth muscle reactivity by causing dysfunction of vagal muscarinic M2 receptors.[57] By acting as a competitive inhibitor of M2 receptors, MBP increases acetylcholine release that is likely to be at least one mechanism for induction of airway hyperresponsiveness.[58] Vagal dysfunction induced by eosinophil MBP may be an important pathway involved in asthma where eosinophils frequently cluster around airway nerves, and the release of MBP is seen in fatal asthma.[58] Recent data suggest that Alternaria can also directly activate eosinophils through its interaction with the cell surface receptor CD11b.[59] This finding demonstrates that eosinophils can be directly activated by environmental allergens and suggests that eosinophils may have a role in innate immune responses. Activation of eosinophils also leads to the generation of large amounts of LTC_4, which induces increased vascular permeability, mucus secretion, and smooth muscle constriction.[60] Also, activated eosinophils generate a wide range of cytokines including IL-1, -3, -4, -5, and -13; GM-CSF; transforming growth factor (TGF)-α/β; TNF-α; RANTES (regulated on activation, normal T cells expressed and secreted); macrophage inflammatory protein (MIP)-1α; and eotaxin, indicating that they have the potential to sustain or augment multiple aspects of the immune response, inflammatory reaction, and tissue repair process.[29] Interestingly, specimens from patients with eosinophilic disorders often display eosinophils undergoing marked degranulation near nerves, suggesting that they may indeed be involved in promoting inflammatory changes to neurons.[61,62] The gastric dysmotility during experimental oral antigen-induced gastrointestinal inflammation is associated with eosinophils in the proximity of damaged nerves, suggesting a causal role for eosinophils in nerve dysfunction.[63] Experimental eosinophil accumulation in the gastrointestinal tract is associated with the development of weight loss, which is attenuated in eotaxin-deficient mice that have a deficiency in gastrointestinal eosinophils.[64] Eosinophils also have the capacity to initiate antigen-specific immune responses by acting as antigen-presenting cells. Consistent with this, eosinophils express relevant costimulatory molecules (CD40, CD28, CD86, B7),[65,66] secrete cytokines capable of inducing T cell proliferation and maturation (IL-2, IL-4, IL-6, IL-10, IL-12),[29,67,68] and can be induced to express MHC class II molecules.[67] Interestingly, experimental adoptive transfer of antigen-pulsed eosinophils induces antigen-specific T cell responses in vivo[69] (Box 5-2). Finally, it has been shown that the gastrointestinal eosinophils have a unique and fascinating innate effector response. It appears that eosinophils may eliminate invading bacteria by ejecting their mitochondrial DNA, which is encased in highly cationic proteins.[70] Evidence continues to emerge suggesting that eosinophils have an important role in innate immune responses, in addition to their well-established role in allergic disease.

Mast Cells

Mast cells are major effector cells involved in allergic responses; in addition, they are important cytokine-producing cells that are involved in nonallergic processes such as the innate immune responses (Figure 5-4). In contrast to other hematopoietic cells that complete their differentiation in the bone marrow, mast cell progenitors leave the bone marrow and complete their differentiation in tissues. Elegant studies in mice have demonstrated that mast cell development from bone marrow cells is dependent on IL-3, and their tissue differentiation is primarily dependent on stem cell factor (SCF). These studies have been primarily conducted in two mast cell-deficient strains of mice: one strain has a homozygous deficiency in the white spotting locus (W), whereas the other strain has deficiencies at the steel locus (Sl).[71] Mice deficient in the W locus can be cured by adoptive transfer of normal bone marrow because they are deficient in the SCF receptor (c-kit), whereas mice deficient in the Sl locus cannot be cured with adaptive transfer of bone marrow because they are deficient in SCF itself.[72,73] Mast cell-deficient mice have been instrumental in defining the critical role of mast cells in experimental anaphylaxis.[74] In addition, mast cells have been shown to contribute to the chronic inflammation associated with the LAR in experimental asthma.[74] In contrast to the mast cell culture conditions in the murine system (which depend on IL-3), mature human mast cells are obtained by culturing progenitor cells with SCF, IL-6, and IL-10. Furthermore, treatment of mature human mast cells with IL-4 induces further maturation, including enhancing their capacity for IgE-dependent activation and their enzymatic machinery for synthesizing PGD_2 and cysteinyl leukotrienes.[75]

Mast cells exist as heterogeneous populations depending on the tissue microenvironment in which they reside and on the immunologic status of the individual. In work with rodents, the terms *mucosal mast cell* (MMC) and *connective tissue mast cell* (CTMC) have emerged, but designating these two populations of mast cells by tissue location alone is an oversimplification. In general, MMCs express less sulfated proteoglycans (chondroitin sulfate) in their granules than CTMCs and hence have different staining characteristics with metachromatic stains. In addition, mast cell populations express distinct granule proteases; in humans, the mast cell nomenclature is based on neutral protease expression. Human cells that express only tryptase (MC_T) are distinguished from mast cells that express tryptase, chymase, carboxypeptidase, and cathepsin G (MC_{TC}). In normal tissues,

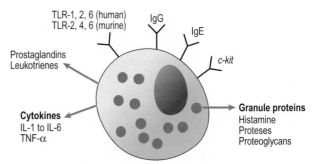

Figure 5-4 Schematic diagram of a mast cell and its products. Mast cells are mononuclear cells that express high-affinity IgE receptors and contain a large number of metachromatic granules. Mast cells express *c-kit*, the receptor for stem cell factor (SCF), a critical mast cell growth and differentiation factor. The secondary granule of a mast cell also contains abundant levels of proteases, proteoglycans, and histamine. In addition to releasing their preformed proteins, mast cells can also release a variety of cytokines and generate large amounts of prostaglandins (PGD_2) and leukotrienes (LTC_4). Mast cells also express Toll-like receptors (*TLR*) indicating that mast cells participate during innate immune responses.

MC_T cells are the predominant cells in the lung and small intestine mucosa, whereas MC_{TC} cells are the predominant types found in the skin and gastrointestinal submucosa.

Mast cell activation occurs through several pathways; classically, a multivalent allergen cross-links IgE molecules bound to the high-affinity IgE receptor (FcεRI) exclusively expressed by mast cells and basophils. In addition, mast cells directly respond to a variety of other agents including calcium ionophore A23187, basic polypeptides (polylysine, polyargi-nine), eosinophil granule proteins, morphine sulfate, chemokines, formyl-methionyl-leucyl-phenylalanine (fMLP) peptides, complement degradation products (e.g. C5a), and substance P. Mast cells undergo regulated exocytosis of their granules resulting in the release of preformed mediators; in addition, activated mast cells undergo de novo synthesis and release of a variety of potent mediators (such as prostaglandin D_2 and LTC_4). Preformed mediators in mast cells include biogenic amines such as histamine (a vasodilator), various neutral proteases, a variety of cytokines, acid hydrolases (e.g. β-hexosaminidase), and proteoglycans. Notably, nearly 20% of the protein of human mast cells is composed of tryptase, a proinflammatory protease with a wide range of activities (e.g. cleavage of complement proteins).[76] Mast cells store a variety of cytokines in their granules (e.g. TNF-α, IL-1, IL-4, IL-5, and IL-6 and chemokines including IL-8) and, after activation with allergens or cytokines, mast cells can increase their synthesis and secretion of these cytokines.[77] It is well established that mast cell products contribute to the early phase of allergic responses, but the contribution of mast cell products such as cytokines has been less clear. Although the exact contribution of mast cell-derived cytokines compared with lymphocyte-derived cytokines has been debated, mast cells appear to be a chief source of TNF-α in asthmatic lung (Box 5-3).

Basophils

Basophils are hematopoietic cells that arise from a granulocyte-monocyte progenitor (GMP) that shares its lineage with mast cells and eosinophils.[78] Basophils complete their development in the bone marrow and circulate as mature cells, representing less than 2% of blood leukocytes. Similar to mast cells, basophils express substantial levels of FcεRI and store histamine in their granules. They are distinguished from mast cells by their segmented nuclei, ultrastructural features, growth factor requirements, granule constituents, and surface marker expression (*c-kit*–, FcεRI+).[79] Basophils are more readily distinguished from eosinophils microscopically due to differences in the their nuclei, cytoplasmic granules and appearance on hematoxylin and eosin stained tissues. In the human system, they develop largely in response to IL-3 in a process augmented by TGF-β. Mature basophils maintain expression of the IL-3 receptor, and IL-3 is a potent basophil priming and activating cytokine.[80]

Several processes activate basophils; notably, on cross-linking of their surface-bound IgE, basophils release preformed mediators including histamine and proteases and synthesize LTC_4. In addition, they secrete cytokines such as IL-4 and IL-13; notably, the amount of IL-4 secreted by basophils appears to be substantial compared with Th2 cells.[81] Similar to eosinophils, basophils are also activated by IgA (by expressing FcαR) and by CCR3 ligands. Basophils also express several other chemokine receptors, including CCR2, whose ligands are potent histamine-releasing factors. The development of monoclonal antibodies that specifically recognize basophils (the respective antigens recognized are 2D7 and basogranin), as well as advancements in FACS analysis and microaray technology,[82–84] have lead to the reliable detection of basophils in allergic tissue. Through the utilization of this technology, basophils have been demonstrated to be recruited in allergen-induced, late-phase skin reactions and are present in increased numbers in asthma models as well[85,86] (Box 5-4).

Basophils have also been implicated in a unique IgG-mediated mechanism of anphaylaxis. It appears as though this mechanism of anaphylaxis is dependent upon IgG, macrophages and platelet activating factor (PAF). Elegant mouse studies have demonstrated that mice deficient in IgE, FcεRI and mast cells still experience anaphylaxis via an IgG-mediated process.[87] However, IgG-mediated anaphylaxis is abolished in basophil-deficient mice.[88] Further investigations are needed to define the role of basophils in this newly described anaphylactic pathway.

Macrophages

Macrophages are tissue-dwelling cells that originate from hematopoietic stem cells in the bone marrow and are subsequently derived from circulating blood monocytes.[89] Under healthy conditions, bone marrow colony-forming cells rapidly progress through monoblast and promonocyte stages to monocytes, which subsequently enter the bloodstream for about 3 days, where they account for about 5% of circulating leukocytes in most species. On entering various tissues, monocytes terminally differentiate into morphologically, histochemically, and functionally distinct tissue macrophage populations that have the capacity to survive for several months.[90] Tissue-specific populations of macrophages include dendritic cells (skin, gut), Kupfer cells (liver), and alveolar macrophages (lung).

Macrophage colony-stimulating factor (M-CSF) 1 promotes monocyte differentiation into macrophages, and mice with a genetic mutation in CSF1 have a deficiency of tissue macrophages.[91] In addition, GM-CSF promotes the survival, differentiation, proliferation, and function of myeloid progenitors as well as the proliferation and function of macrophages.[92] An unexpected but critical role for GM-CSF in lung homeostasis was revealed by ablation of murine loci for GM-CSF[93] which results in pulmonary alveolar proteinosis (PAP) and abnormalities of alveolar macrophage function. Interestingly, the ability of GM-CSF to regulate macrophage differentiation is dependent on PU.1, an ETS-family transcription factor that also regulates myeloid and B cell lineage development.[94]

Tissue macrophages contribute to innate immunity by virtue of their ability to migrate, phagocytose, and kill microorganisms and to recruit and activate other inflammatory cells. By expressing Toll-like receptor-mediated pathogen recognition molecules that induce the release of cytokines capable of programming adaptive immune responses, macrophages provide important links between innate and adaptive immunity.[95] Macrophages also express high- and low-affinity receptors for IgG (Fcr/RI/II) and complement receptors (CR1) that promote their activation. Activated macrophages produce a variety of pleiotropic proinflammatory cytokines such as IL-1, TNF-α, and IL-8, as well as lipid mediators (e.g. leukotrienes and prostaglandins). Notably, macrophages express costimulatory molecules (e.g. CD86) and are potent antigen-presenting cells capable of efficiently activating antigen-specific T cells. In addition, macrophages actively metabolize arginine via two competing pathways, depending on their cytokine polarization.[96] For example; IFN-γ and lipopolysaccharide (LPS) augment the expression of inducible nitric oxide synthase (iNOS), which results in the production of NO, a potent smooth muscle and endothelial cell regulator. Alternatively, the treatment of macrophages with IL-4 or IL-13 induces the expression of arginase, which preferentially shunts arginine away from NOS (thus promoting bronchoconstriction). Arginase metabolizes arginine into ornithine, a precursor for polyamines and proline, critical regulators of cell growth and collagen deposition, respectively. A substantial body of evidence has revealed that macrophages are critical effector cells in allergic responses. For example, peripheral blood monocytes from asthmatic individuals secrete elevated levels of superoxide anion and GM-CSF.[97] In addition, the lung tissue and BALF from asthmatic individuals have elevated levels of macrophages.[98] Consistent with this, the asthmatic lung has overexpression of macrophage-active chemokines (e.g., MCP-1).[99]

We now recognize that there are at least two distinct subsets of macrophages, classically and alternatively activated macrophages. Classically activated macrophages are associated with a proinflammatory response and are activated by Th1 cytokines, whereas alternatively activated macrophages, so named because they are activated in the presence of Th2 cytokines, are associated with resolution of inflammation and tissue repair. Alternatively activated macrophages may serve as a link between the innate and adaptive immune system and further investigation into their function in allergic disorders is needed.

Dendritic Cells

Dendritic cells are unique antigen-presenting cells that have a pivotal role in innate and acquired immune responses. These cells originate in the bone marrow and subsequently migrate into the circulation before they assume tissue locations as immature dendritic cells, incidentally at locations where maximum allergen encounter occurs (e.g. skin, gastrointestinal tract, and airways). Immature dendritic cells are potent in antigen uptake, efficient in capturing pathogens, and producers of potent cytokines (e.g. IFN-α and IL-12). By expressing pattern recognition receptors, dendritic cells directly recognize a variety of pathogens. Immature dendritic cells express the CC chemokine receptor (CCR) 6 that binds to MIP-3a and β-defensin, which are produced locally in tissues such as those in the lung.[100] After antigen uptake, dendritic cells rapidly cross into the lymphatic vessels and migrate into draining secondary lymphoid tissue. During this migration, the dendritic cells undergo maturation, which is characterized by down-regulation in their capacity to capture antigen, up-regulation of antigen processing and presentation capabilities, and up-regulation of CCR7, which likely promotes dendritic cell recruitment to secondary lymphoid organs (which express CCR7 ligands).[101] After presentation of antigen to antigen-specific T cells in the T cell-rich areas of secondary lymphoid organs, dendritic cells mainly undergo apoptosis.

Dendritic cells are composed of heterogeneous populations based on ultrastructural features, surface molecule expression, and function. In human blood, dendritic cells are divided into three types including two myeloid-derived subpopulations and another lymphoid-derived population (plasmacytoid dendritic cells).[102] The myeloid populations are divided into CD1+ and CD1-. CD1 is a molecule involved in the presentation of glycolipids to T cells. CD1c+ myeloid dendritic cells also express high levels of CD11c (complement receptor-4 [iC3b receptor]), whereas the CD1c- population expresses lower levels of CD11c. The plasmacytoid dendritic cell population is CD1c-, CD11c-, but is distinguished by its high levels of IL-3 receptor expression. This population of dendritic cells appears to be a primary source of IFN-α. Dendritic cells can be cultured from freshly isolated human cord or peripheral blood; myeloid dendritic cells are primarily derived in response to stimulation with GM-CSF, TNF-α, and IL-4, whereas plasmacytoid dendritic cells develop in culture with IL-3.

Dendritic cells can differentially influence Th cell differentiation preferentially by induction of Th1 or Th2 cell responses (see Figure 5-2). There is evidence that the same population of dendritic cells can influence Th1 and Th2 differentiation depending on several factors. For example, the ratio between dendritic cells and T cells has profound effects on influencing Th1 and Th2 differentiation.[103] In addition, Th1 polarized effector dendritic cells induce Th1 responses, whereas Th2 polarized dendritic cells induce Th2 responses.[102] Also, plasmacytoid dendritic cells stimulated first with the IL-3 and then with CD40 ligand (before adding naïve T cells) induce strong Th1 responses but no Th2 cytokine production. Finally, dendritic cells that express specific costimulatory molecules may promote distinct Th differentiation; for example, expression of B7-related protein (ICOS ligand) promotes Th2 development.[104] As such, dendritic cells are likely to have critical roles in the development of allergic responses. Recent studies indicate that dendritic cells are required for the development of eosinophilic airway inflammation in response to inhaled antigen.[105] Importantly, adoptive transfer of antigen-pulsed dendritic cells has been shown to be sufficient for the induction of Th2 responses and eosinophilic airway inflammation to inhaled antigen.[101,106] Finally, elevated levels of CD1a+, MHC class II+ dendritic cells, are found in the lung of atopic asthmatics compared with nonasthmatics[101] (Box 5-5).

Neutrophils

Neutrophils are bone marrow-derived granulocytes that account for the largest proportion of cells in most inflammatory sites. Neutrophils develop in the bone marrow by the sequential differentiation of progenitor cells into myeloblasts, promyelocytes, and then myelocytes, an ordered process regulated by growth factors such as GM-CSF. Granulocyte-CSF promotes the terminal differentiation of neutrophils, which normally reside in the bloodstream for only 6 to 8 hours. A significant pool of

Dendritic Cells

- Dendritic cells normally exist as tissue surveillance cells.
- On contact with antigen (e.g. invading pathogen), dendritic cells migrate via lymphatics to secondary lymphoid organs.
- Immature dendritic cells are chief sources of innate cytokines (e.g. interferon-α).
- Mature dendritic cells are potent antigen-presenting cells.
- Dendritic cells can preferentially activate Th1 or Th2 responses.

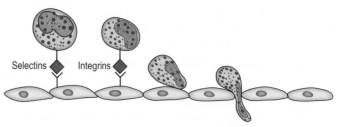

Selectins   Integrins

Figure 5-5 Overview of leukocyte migration. The trafficking of leukocytes into various tissues is regulated by a complex network of signaling events between leukocytes in the circulation and endothelial cells lining blood vessels. These interactions involve a multistep process including (1) leukocyte rolling (mediated by endothelial selectin and specific leukocyte ligands), (2) rapid activation of leukocyte integrins, (3) firm adhesion between endothelial molecules and counterligands on leukocytes, and (4) transmigration of leukocytes through the endothelial layer.

marginated neutrophils exists in select tissues,[107] allowing rapid mobilization of neutrophils in response to a variety of triggers (e.g. IL-8, LTB₄ PAF).

Activated neutrophils have the capacity to release a variety of products at inflammatory sites, which may induce tissue damage. These products include those of primary (azurophilic), secondary (or specific), and tertiary granules, including proteolytic enzymes, oxygen radicals, and lipid mediators (LTB₄, PAF, and thromboxane A2). Neutrophil granules contain more than 20 enzymes; of these, elastase, collagenase, and gelatinase have the greatest potential for inducing tissue damage. Neutrophil-derived defensins, lysozyme, and cathepsin G have well-defined roles in antibacterial defense. In fact, recent studies have suggested that the major function of superoxide release into the phagocytic vesicle is increasing the concentration of intravesicle H^+ and K^+, permitting conditions for optimal protease-mediated bacterial killing.[108] Although neutrophils are not the predominant cell type associated with allergic disorders, there are several studies that have demonstrated a correlation and possible role for neutrophils in the pathogenesis of allergic disease.[109] Individuals who die within 1 hour of the onset of an acute asthma attack have neutrophil-dominant airway inflammation,[110] suggesting that neutrophils may have a pathogenic role in some clinical situations. Collectively, these data suggest an important role for neutrophils in the acute and chronic manifestations of allergen-induced asthma.

Leukocyte Recruitment

The trafficking of leukocytes into various tissues is regulated by a complex network of signaling events between leukocytes in the circulation and endothelial cells lining blood vessels. These interactions involve a multistep process including (1) leukocyte rolling (mediated by endothelial selectin and specific leukocyte ligands), (2) rapid activation of leukocyte integrins, (3) firm adhesion between endothelial molecules and counterligands on leukocytes, and (4) transmigration of leukocytes through the endothelial layer (Figure 5-5). Chemokines are thought to have a central role in modulating this multistep process by (1) activating both the leukocytes and the endothelium and (2) increasing leukocyte integrin and adhesion molecule interaction affinity. The multistep signaling cascade must occur rapidly to allow for the leukocytes to reduce rolling velocity, mediate adherence, and extravasate into tissues in response to a chemokine gradient (see Figure 5-5). In addition to mediating leukocyte movement from the bloodstream into tissues, chemokines use similar steps to mediate leukocyte-directed motion across other tissue barriers such as respiratory epithelium. The ultimate distribution of leukocytes in particular tissue locations represents a balance between cell recruitment and cell death (Box 5-6).

Leukocyte Trafficking

- Leukocytes bind to the endothelium via low-affinity reversible interactions mediated by selectins.
- Tight adhesion of leukocytes to endothelium is mediated by specific adhesion molecules such as integrins (e.g., β2-integrins).
- Leukocyte migration into tissues is regulated by chemoattractants.
- The level of a particular leukocyte in an inflammatory site is a result of the net balance between cell recruitment and cell death (e.g. apoptosis).

Leukocyte Chemoattraction

Chemokine and Chemokine Receptor Families

Chemokines represent a large family of chemotactic cytokines that have been divided into four groups, designated CXC, CC, C, and CX3C, depending on the spacing of conserved cysteines (Figure 5-6). These four families of chemokines are grouped into distinct chromosomal loci (see Figure 5-6). The CXC and CC groups, in contrast to the C and CX3C chemokines, contain many members and have been studied in greatest detail. The CXC chemokines mainly target neutrophils, whereas the CC chemokines target a variety of cell types including macrophages, eosinophils, and basophils. The current chemokine receptor nomenclature uses CC, CXC, XC, or CX3C (to designate chemokine group) followed by R (for receptor) and then a number. The new chemokine nomenclature substitutes the R for L (for ligand) and the number is derived from the one already assigned to the gene encoding the chemokine from the SCY (small secreted cytokine) nomenclature. Thus a given gene has the same number as its protein ligand (e.g. the gene encoding eotaxin-1 is *SCYA11*, and the chemokine is referred to as CCL11). Table 5-1 summarizes the chemokine family using this nomenclature.

Chemokines induce leukocyte migration and activation by binding to specific G protein-coupled, seven-transmembrane-spanning cell surface receptors (GPCRs).[111] Although chemokine receptors are similar to many GPCRs, they have unique structural motifs such as the amino acid sequence DRYLAIV in the second intracellular domain.[111,112] There have been five CXCR receptors identified, which are referred to as CXCR1 through CXCR5, and 10 human CC chemokine receptor genes cloned, which are known as CCR1 through CCR10 (Figure 5-7). The

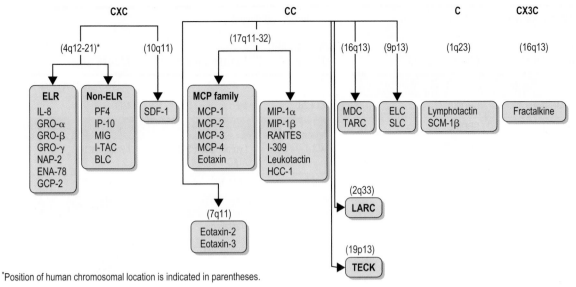

Figure 5-6 Human chemokine family.

CCR1	CCR2	CCR3	CCR4	CCR5	CCR6	CCR7	CCR8	CCR9	CCR10
CCL3		CCL5							
CCL5		CCL7							
CCL7	CCL2	CCL8							
CCL14	CCL7	CCL11		CCL3					
CCL15	CCL8	CCL13	CCL17	CCL4		CCL19			CCL27
CCL23	CCL13	CCL15	CCL22	CCL5	CCL20	CCL21	CCL1	CCL25	CCL28
		CCL24							
		CCL26							
		CCL28							

(A)

CXCR1	CXCR2	CXCR3	CXCR4	CXCR5
	CXCL1			
	CXCL2			
	CXCL3			
	CXCL5			
	CXCL6	CXCL9		
CXCL6	CXCL7	CXCL10		
CXCL8	CXCL8	CXCL11	CXCL12	CXCL13

(B)

Figure 5-7 Ligands for CC **(A)** and CXC **(B)** receptor families.

chemokine and leukocyte selectivities of chemokine receptors overlap extensively; a given leukocyte often expresses multiple chemokine receptors, and more than one chemokine typically binds to the same receptor (see Figure 5-7).

Chemokine Receptor Signal Transduction

Chemokine receptors are, for the most part, inhibited by pertussis toxin, indicating that they are primarily coupled to G proteins.[111] Receptor activation leads to a cascade of intracellular signaling events that in turn lead to activation of phosphatidylinositol-specific phospholipase C, protein kinase C, small GTPases, Src-related tyrosine kinases, phophatidyl-inositol-3-OH kinases, and protein kinase B. Phospholipase C delivers two secondary messengers, inositol-1,4,5 triphosphate, which releases intracellular calcium, and diacylglycerol, which activates protein kinase C. Multiple phosphorylation events are triggered by chemokines. Phosphatidylinositol-3-OH kinase can be activated by the βγ subunit of G proteins, small GTP-ases or Src-related tyrosine kinases. Phosphorylation of the tyrosine kinase, RAFTK, a member of the focal adhesion kinase family, has been shown to be induced by signaling through CCR5.[113] Mitogen-activated

protein kinases have also been shown to be phosphorylated and activated within 1 minute after exposure of leukocytes to chemokines.[114] In addition to triggering intracellular events, engagement with ligand induces rapid chemokine receptor internalization. Ligand-induced internalization of most chemokine receptors occurs independent of calcium transients, G protein coupling, and protein kinase C, indicating a mechanism different from that with the induction of chemotaxis. Thus chemokine receptor internalization may provide a mechanism for chemokines to also halt leukocyte trafficking in vivo.

Regulation of Chemokine and Chemokine Receptor Expression

The main stimuli for the secretion of chemokines are the early proinflammatory cytokines, such as IL-1 and TNF-α, bacterial products such as LPS, and viral infection[115-117] (Figure 5-8). In addition, products of the adaptive arm of the immune system, including both Th1 and Th2 cells, IFN-γ and IL-4, respectively, also induce the production of chemokines independently and in synergy with IL-1 and TNF-α. Although there are many

Table 5-1 Systematic Names for Human and Mouse Ligands

Systematic Name	Human Ligand	Mouse Ligand
CXC Family		
CXCL1	GRO-α/MGSA-α	GRO/KC?*
CXCL2	GRO-β/MGSA-β	GRO/KC?
CXCL3	GRO-γ/MGSA-γ	GRO/KC?
CXCL4	PF4	PF4
CXCL5	EN A-78	LIX?
CXCL6	GCP-2	Ckα-3
CXCL7	NAP-2	?
CXCL8	IL-8	?
CXCL9	Mig	Mig
CXCL10	IP-10	IP-10
CXCL11	I-TAC	?
CXCL12	SDF-1α/β	SDF-1
CXCL13	BLC/BCA-1	BLC/BCA-1
CXCL14	BRAK/bolekine	BRAK
CXCL15	?	Lungkine
CC Family		
CCL1	I-309	TCA-3, P500
CCL2	MCP-1/MCAF	JE ?
CCL3	MIP-1α/LD78α	MIP-1α
CCL4	MIP-1β	MIP-1β
CCL5	RANTES	RANTES
CCL6	?	C10, MRP-1
CCL7	MCP-3	MARC?
CCL8	MCP-2	MCP-2?
CCL9/10	?	MRP-2, CCF18, MIP-1γ
CCL11	Eotaxin	Eotaxin
CCL12	?	MCP-5
CCL13	MCP-4	?
CCL14	HCC-1	?
CCL15	HCC-2/Lkn-1/MIP-1δ	?
CCL16	HCC-4/LEC	LCC-1
CCL17	TARC	TARC
CCL18	DC-CK1/PARC/AMAC-1	?
CCL19	MIP-3β/ELC/exodus-3	MIP-3β/ELC/exodus-3
CCL20	MIP-3α/LARC/exodus-1	MIP-3α/LARC/exodus-1
CCL21	6Ckine/SLC/exodus-2	6Ckine/SLC/exodus-2/TCA-4
CCL22	MDC/STCP-1	ABCD-1
CCL23	MPIF-1	?
CCL24	MPIF-2/Eotaxin-2	Eotaxin-2
CCL25	TECK	TECK
CCL26	Eotaxin-3	?

Table 5-1 Continued

Systematic Name	Human Ligand	Mouse Ligand
CCL27	CTACK/ILC	ALP/CTACK/ILC/ESkine
CCL28	MEC	MEC
C Family		
XCL1	Lymphotactin/SCM-1α/ATAC	Lymphotactin
XCL2	SCM-1β	?
CX3C Family		
CX3CL1	Fractalkine	Neurotactin

*A question mark indicates that the mouse and human homologs are ambiguous.

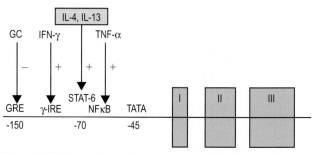

Figure 5-8 Regulatory elements in chemokine promoter. Depicted are the positions of the transcription factor motifs and the regulatory cytokines of the eotaxin-1 promoter. The three exons of the gene are depicted with rectangles. Positive signals are indicated with (+), whereas inhibitory signals are indicated with (−). Notably, IL-4/IL-13 via STAT-6 induces transcription; IFN-γ induces transcription through an IFN response element (γ-IRE), and TNF-α induces transcription through NFκB. Glucocorticoids (GC) inhibit transcription via the glucocorticoid response element (GRE).

similarities in the regulation of chemokines, important differences that may have implications for asthma are beginning to be appreciated. For example, in the healthy lung, epithelial cells are the primary source of chemokines; however, in the inflamed lung, infiltrating cells within the submucosa are a major cellular source of chemokines.[118] Furthermore, the induced expression of chemokines by TNF-α or IL-1 treatment of epithelial cells is suppressed by the steroid dexamethasone.[119] This may be relevant to the clinical effectiveness of inhaled glucocorticoids at decreasing the eosinophil-rich inflammatory exudate characteristically seen in the respiratory tract of individuals with asthma.

Analysis of the 5' flanking regions of most chemokines reveals several conserved regulatory elements that may explain the observed regulation of the chemokine genes by cytokines and glucocorticoids[120,121] (see Figure 5-8). Of note, nuclear factor kappa B (NFκB), glucocorticoid response element (GRE), gamma interferon response element (γIRE), Sp1, and E2A binding site motifs are well conserved in both human and mouse chemokine promoters. For example, the eotaxin promoter in mice and humans has NFκB and STAT-6 sequences; mutation of the NFκB and STAT-6 sites impairs eotaxin promoter activity in response to TNF-α and IL-4, respectively.[122] NFκB is a nuclear factor that is activated after the stimulation of cells with various immunologic agents, such as LPS, IL-1, and TNF-α. NFκB has been shown to be important for the transcriptional activation of selected chemokines. For example, a single NFκB binding site is essential for TNF-α and IL-1 induced expression of the MCP-1[123] and growth-regulated oncogene-α (GRO-α)[124] genes and LPS-induced expression of the MIP-2 gene.[125] GRE mediates glucocorticoid regulation of transcription.[126] Deletion analysis of the GRE from the IL-8 promoter revealed that this element participated in dexamethasone suppression of IL-8 expression.[127] In vitro, the glucocorticoid budesonide inhibits eotaxin promoter-driven reporter gene activity and accelerates the decay of eotaxin mRNA.[128] These studies indicate that glucocorticoids inhibit chemokine expression through multiple mechanisms of action.

Chemokine receptors are constitutively expressed on some cells, whereas they are inducible on others. For example, CCR1 and CCR2 are constitutively expressed on monocytes but are expressed on lymphocytes only after IL-2 stimulation.[129,130] Activated lymphocytes are then responsive to multiple CC chemokines that use these receptors, including the MCPs. In addition, some constitutive receptors can be down-modulated by biologic response modifiers. For example, IL-10 was shown to modify the activity of CCR1, CCR2, and CCR5 on dendritic cells and monocytes.[131] Normally, dendritic cells mature in response to inflammatory stimuli, and shift from expressing CCR1, CCR2, CCR5, and CCR6 to CCR7 expression. However, IL-10 blocks the chemokine receptor switch. Importantly, although CCR1, CCR2, and CCR5 remain detectable on the cell surface and bind appropriate ligands, they do not signal in calcium mobilization and chemotaxis assays. Thus IL-10 converts chemokine receptors to functional decoy receptors, thereby serving a down-regulatory function (Box 5-7).

Chemokine Regulation of Leukocyte Effector Function

Chemoattraction

Structural motifs in the primary amino acid sequence of chemokines have an important impact on their chemoattractive ability. For example, CXC chemokines are mainly chemoattractants for neutrophils and lymphocytes. Furthermore, ELR (Glu-Leu-Arg)-containing CXC chemokines (e.g. IL-8) are mainly chemoattractive on neutrophils, whereas non-ELR CXC chemokines (e.g. IP-10) chemoattract selected populations of lymphocytes. In contrast to cellular specificity of CXC chemokines, CC chemokines are active on a variety of leukocytes, including dendritic cells, monocytes, basophils, lymphocytes, and eosinophils. For example, as their names imply, all MCPs have strong chemoat-

tractive activity for monocytes. However, they display partially overlapping chemoattractant activity on basophils and eosinophils. In particular, MCP-2, MCP-3, and MCP-4 have basophil and eosinophil chemoattractive activity, but MCP-1 is only active on basophils. In distinction to the MCPs, the eotaxin subfamily of chemokines (e.g. eotaxin-1, -2, and -3) has limited activity on macrophages but are potent eosinophil and basophil chemoattractants.[132,133] Chemokines also work in concert with other cytokines to promote leukocyte trafficking. IL-5 collaborates with eotaxin in promoting tissue eosinophilia by (1) increasing the pool of circulating eosinophils (by stimulating eosinophilopoiesis and bone marrow release) and (2) priming eosinophils to have enhanced responsiveness to eotaxin. The ability of two cytokines (IL-5 and eotaxin) that are relatively eosinophil selective to cooperate in promoting tissue eosinophilia offers a molecular explanation for the occurrence of selective tissue eosinophilia in human allergic diseases.

Cellular Activation

In addition to promoting leukocyte accumulation, chemokines are potent cell activators. After binding to the appropriate G protein-linked, seven-transmembrane-spanning receptor, chemokines elicit transient intracellular calcium flux, actin polymerization, oxidative burst with release of superoxide free radicals, the exocytosis of secondary granule constituents, and increased avidity of integrins for their adhesion molecules. For example, in basophils, chemokine-induced cellular activation results in degranulation with the release of histamine and the de novo generation of LTC$_4$.[115,134,135] Basophil activation by chemokines requires cellular priming with IL-3, IL-5, or GM-CSF for the maximal effect of each chemokine, highlighting the cooperativity between cytokines and chemokines.

Hematopoiesis

In addition to being involved in leukocyte accumulation, chemokines also have a role in regulating hematopoiesis. These functions include (1) chemotaxis of hematopoietic progenitor cells (HPC), (2) suppression and enhancement activity on HPC proliferation and differentiation, and (3) mobilization of HPCs to the peripheral blood[136]. For example, stromal cell-derived factor (SDF)-1, a CXC chemokine, is critical for B cell lymphopoiesis and bone marrow myelopoiesis as demonstrated by gene targeting.[137] Furthermore, eotaxin has been shown to directly stimulate the release of eosinophilic progenitor cells and mature eosinophils from the bone marrow.[138] Eotaxin synergizes with stem cell factor in stimulating yolk sac development into mast cells in vitro[139] and has been shown to function as a GM-CSF after allergic challenge in the lungs.[140]

Regulation of Dendritic Cells

A central question in allergy research is to understand the mechanism for initial allergen recognition in mucosal surfaces. Tissue resident dendritic cells are believed to have a fundamental role in this process because they are able to efficiently take up, process, and deliver antigens to lymphoid tissues. The migration pattern of dendritic cells is complex and is thought to involve a coordinated chemokine-signaling network. Dendritic cell progenitors from the bone marrow migrate into nonlymphoid tissues where they develop into immature dendritic cells that have an active role in antigen uptake and processing. Antigen stimulation and the production of inflammatory cytokines promote the differentiation of immature dendritic cells into mature presenting dendritic cells. This promotes dendritic cell

Inflammatory Effector Cells/Cell Migration

trafficking from the periphery to regional lymph nodes via afferent lymphatics. On reaching the lymph nodes, dendritic cells home in on T cell-rich regions where they present the processed antigen to naïve T cells and generate an antigen-specific primary T cell response. As part of the maturation program, immature dendritic cells up-regulate the expression of CCR7 and become responsive to ELC and SLC, chemokines responsible for their trafficking to lymph nodes. At the same time, they decrease the expression of CCR1, CCR2, and CCR5, the receptors for inflammatory chemokines.[141-143]

Modulation of T Cell Immune Responses

T lymphocytes have been shown to express a majority of chemokine receptors, thus making them potentially responsive to a large number of different chemokines. Characterization of chemokine receptor expression has shown that T lymphocytes display a dynamic expression pattern of chemokine receptors, and it is the differential expression of receptors during T lymphocyte maturation and differentiation that is thought to allow for individual chemokine-specific functionality on T lymphocytes.[144] As mentioned previously, CCR7 plays an important role in trafficking of naïve T cells into lymph nodes.[145] On activation, T cells may express an array of chemokine receptors. They thus become sensitive to inflammatory chemokines, including MIP-1α, MIP-1β, MCP-3, and RANTES, which are thought to mediate T cell trafficking to sites of inflammation.[146] Also, specific subsets of memory T cells can be distinguished based on their expression of CCR7 and the propensity to migrate into lymph nodes.[147] Chemokines have an important role in the induction of inflammatory responses and are central in selecting the type of immune response (Th1 vs Th2). During bacterial or viral infections IP-10, Mig, IL-8, and I-TAC production correlates with the presence of CD4+ Th1-type T cells. In contrast, during allergic inflammatory responses, eotaxin, RANTES, MCP-2, MCP-3, and MCP-4 are induced, and the majority of the CD4+ T lymphocytes are of the Th2-type phenotype. The characterization of chemokine receptor expression on T lymphocytes suggests that this may be explained by the expression of CXCR3 and CCR5 predominantly on Th1-type T cells, whereas CCR3, CCR4, and CCR8 have been associated with Th2-type T cells (see Figure 5-2). In addition, Th1 and Th2 cells secrete distinct chemokines[148] (see Figure 5-2). In mice, Th1 cells preferentially secrete RANTES and lymphotactin, whereas Th2 cells secrete MDC and TCA3. Interestingly, supernatants from Th2 cells preferentially attract Th2 cells. These data suggest that the presence of specific patterns of chemokine receptors on T cell subsets predicts which subset will be preferentially accumulated at sites of inflammation. Alternatively, chemokines may directly influence the differentiation of naïve T cells to the Th1 or Th2 phenotype. MIP-1α and MCP-1 have been described as capable of inducing the differentiation of Th1 and Th2 cells,[149] and MCP-1-deficient mice have defective Th2 responses.[150] Consistent with this, Bcl-6-deficient animals express high levels of chemokines, including MCP-1, and have systemic Th2-type inflammation.[151]

Chemokines and Chemokine Receptors Strongly Implicated in Allergic Disorders

Eotaxin/CCR3

Because eosinophilia is a hallmark feature of allergic inflammation, a large body of research has focused on the analysis of chemokine receptors and signaling pathways on eosinophils. Eosinophils from most healthy donors express CCR3 at the

BOX 5-8 Key concepts

Chemokines in Allergic Responses

- Chemokines regulate leukocyte recruitment.
- Chemokines are potent cellular activating factors.
- Chemokines are potent histamine-releasing factors.
- Th2 cytokines (e.g. IL-4 and IL-13) are potent inducers of allergy-associated chemokines (e.g., eotaxin).
- In allergic tissue, chemokines are frequently produced by epithelial cells.

highest level[133,152,153] and have significantly lower levels of CCR1. Consistent with the expression of CCR1 and CCR3, eosinophils respond to MIP-1α, RANTES, MCP-2, MCP-3, MCP-4, eotaxin-1, eotaxin-2, and eotaxin-3. CCR3 appears to function as the predominant eosinophil chemokine receptor because CCR3 ligands are generally more potent eosinophil chemoattractants. Furthermore, an inhibitory monoclonal antibody specific for CCR3 blocks the activity of RANTES, a chemokine that could signal through CCR1 or CCR3 in eosinophils.[154] The importance of eotaxin and CCR3 in orchestrating eosinophil recruitment into allergic tissue is highlighted from results with eotaxin- and CCR3-deficient mice. Eotaxin-deficient mice have a major impairment in the baseline level of tissue eosinophils and a reduction in early eosinophil recruitment into the asthmatic lung.[155] In addition, CCR3-deficient mice have impaired eosinophil recruitment into the skin and lung in a model of allergy induced via cutaneous allergen sensitization.[156] The eotaxin/CCR3 pathway is not the only signaling system important for eosinophil tissue recruitment; eosinophils have recently been shown to express or respond to ligands of CCR6, CXCR3, and CXCR4.[157-159] For instance, eosinophils isolated from allergic donors responded to MIP-3α in chemotaxis and calcium mobilization assays. Importantly, eosinophils isolated from non-allergic donors failed to respond to MIP-3α.[157] In contrast, in this study, 50% of eosinophils from nonallergic donors express CXCR3 by FACS analysis and these cells respond in functional assays. The significance of these chemokine receptors in eosinophil accumulation in healthy and diseased states remains to be elucidated (Box 5-8).

Genetic Polymorphisms Affecting Cellular Migration in Allergic Responses

Polymorphisms in individual chemokines and chemokine receptor genes are likely to influence the course of allergic disorders. For example, CCR5Δ32 is a 32-bp deletion in the CCR5 gene that is associated with protection against HIV strains that are tropic for this receptor. Notably, this genetic polymorphism also appears to protect against asthma.[160] Also, a polymorphism in the RANTES promoter (G→A at position bp401) appears to increase the susceptibility to atopic dermatitis in children.[161] The polymorphism confers higher transcriptional activity and a new GATA transcription binding site. A similar mutation (G→A at position bp403 of the RANTES promoter) is associated with increased susceptibility to both asthma and atopy because the proportion of individuals carrying the mutant allele is higher in atopic and nonatopic asthma patients.[162] In addition, the polymorphism is associated with increased aeroallergen skin test positivity, and homozygosity is associated with increased risk of airway obstruction.

Therapeutic Approach to Interfering with Chemokines

One of the actions of glucocorticoids is to inhibit the transcription and/or stability of chemokine mRNA (see Figure 5-8). However, the ideal pharmaceutical agent would interfere with the selective function of critical chemokines and/or their receptors in the pathophysiology of disease but not in protective immune responses. CCR3 represents such a potential target because preliminary studies indicate that it is likely to be critically involved in allergic inflammation and antagonizing CCR3 would selectively target eosinophils, basophils, and Th2 cells. Also, CCR4 and CCR8 may be potential targets because both are reported to be Th2 specific and involved in recruitment of Th2 cells in allergic inflammation.[163,164] CCR8 represents a potentially attractive target as CCR8-deficient mice have shown impaired antigen-driven Th2 responses and pulmonary eosinophilia.[164]

Chemokine and/or chemokine receptor inhibition has thus been an active area of research. Studies have also been fueled by the finding that natural chemokine receptor mutations block the HIV coreceptor function of selected chemokine receptors (e.g. CCR2 and CCR5), suggesting that pharmaceutical targeting of chemokine receptors is a promising strategy for treatment of HIV infection.[165,166] There are several potential approaches for blockade of chemokines and their receptors. One approach is to develop humanized monoclonal antibodies against chemokines and/or their receptors.[167] Specifically, an antibody directed against a chemokine receptor (e.g. CCR3) would offer an advantage over antibodies against chemokines because actions of multiple chemokines through a single receptor would be affected. Another approach involves developing receptor antagonists based on chemokine protein modifications. One such agent has been derived by the addition of a single methionine to the amino terminus of RANTES (designated Met-RANTES).[168,169] This agent acts as a strong competitive inhibitor of CCR1, CCR3, and CCR5. In vivo studies have demonstrated significant reduction in eosinophil numbers after Met-RANTES administration in a murine model of allergic airway inflammation.[170] The success of protein antagonists has already been recognized by viruses, some of which have developed their own chemokine antagonists. For example, the human herpes simplex virus-8 genome encodes for two chemokine-related proteins, and one of these, vMIP-II, is a potent broad-spectrum antagonist against both CXC and CC chemokine receptors.[171,172] Also, small molecule inhibitors of chemokine receptors have recently been described and display potent inhibition at nanomolar concentrations in vitro.[173,174] Three companies have reported the development of small-molecule CCR3 antagonists[175,176] these compounds share the presence of a hydrophobic group some distance from a basic nitrogen group. It has been postulated that the basic nitrogen group interacts with a key anionic residue in or near the seven-transmembrane region of the receptor, as found with antagonists of the monoamine receptors, which are seven-transmembrane-spanning receptors. However, no in vivo data are yet available (Box 5-9).

An additional approach to inhibiting chemokines can be induction of prolonged desensitization to chemokine stimulation.[177] It may be possible to induce cellular desensitization by promoting chemokine receptor internalization.[178] Alternatively, the transcription or translation of specific chemokines or chemokine receptors could be blocked. For example, antisense oligonucleotides and transcription factor inhibitors specifically designed to interact with regulatory regions in chemokine receptors may have clinical use. A more detailed understanding of the regulation of chemokine and chemokine receptor genes is necessary for the development of these approaches.

> **BOX 5-9** Key concepts
>
> **Chemokine Blockade**
>
> - Experimental models (e.g. knockouts and neutralizing antibodies) have demonstrated an essential role for chemokines in allergic responses.
> - Chemokine receptors can be blocked with small-molecule inhibitors (e.g. receptor antagonists).
> - Chemokine inhibition can be accomplished with humanized neutralizing antibodies.
> - The treatment of allergic diseases with chemokine inhibitors is not likely to be accomplished unless several receptors and/or ligand groups are simultaneously blocked.

Conclusions

Allergic disorders involve the complex interplay of a large number of leukocytes (especially mast cells, eosinophils, neutrophils, lymphocytes, basophils, and dendritic cells) and structural tissue cells (especially epithelial and smooth muscle cells). A combination of mouse and human studies has been used to define the specific mechanisms involved in leukocyte activation, migration, and effector function. In particular, cellular adhesion proteins, integrins, and chemokines have emerged as critical molecules involved in leukocyte accumulation and activation. Also, a combination of innate activation pathways (involving mast cells, dendritic cells, and eosinophils) that induce proinflammatory pathways and adaptive immune pathways have been elucidated. Although we are in the early phases of analysis of disease pathogenesis, we have already identified critical pathways that are currently being therapeutically targeted in patients. It is the author's hope that this chapter has provided the appropriate framework for the reader to understand (and contribute to) the next generation of clinical intervention strategies for the treatment of allergic disorders.

Acknowledgments

This work was supported in part by National Institutes of Health grants R01-AI42242, R01-AI45898, HL-076383, A1070235, and DK076893.

References

1. Leong KP, Huston DP. Understanding the pathogenesis of allergic asthma using mouse models. Ann Allergy Asthma Immunol 2001;87:96–109.
2. Wills-Karp M. Immunologic basis of antigen-induced airway hyperresponsiveness. Annu Rev Immunol 1999;17:255–81.
3. O'Byrne PM, Inman MD, Parameswaran K. The trials and tribulations of IL-5, eosinophils, and allergic asthma. J Allergy Clin Immunol 2001;108:503–8.
4. Makker HK, Montefort S, Holgate S. Investigative use of fibreoptic bronchoscopy for local airway challenge in asthma. Eur Respir J 1993;6:1402–8.
5. Lloyd CM, Gonzalo JA, Coyle AJ, et al. Mouse models of allergic airway disease. Adv Immunol 2001;77:263–95.
6. Kurup VP, Mauze S, Choi H, et al. A murine model of allergic bronchopulmonary aspergillosis with elevated eosinophils and IgE. J Immunol 1992;148:3783–8.
7. Wardlaw AJ, Dunnette S, Gleich GJ, et al. Eosinophils and mast cells in bronchoalveolar lavage in subjects with mild asthma. Relationship to bronchial hyperreactivity. Am Rev Respir Dis 1988;137:62–9.

8. Broide DH, Firestein GS. Endobronchial allergen challenge in asthma. J Clin Invest 1991;88:1048–53.

9. Lam S, LeRiche J, Phillips D, et al. Cellular and protein changes in bronchial lavage fluid after late asthmatic reaction in patients with red cedar asthma. J Allergy Clin Immunol 1987;80:44–50.

10. Beasley R, Roche WR, Roberts JA, et al. Cellular events in the bronchi in mild asthma and after bronchial provocation. Am Rev Respir Dis 1989;139:806–17.

11. De Monchy JG, Kauffman HF, Venge P, et al. Bronchoalveolar eosinophilia during allergen-induced late asthmatic reactions. Am Rev Respir Dis 1985;131:373–6.

12. Fukuda T, Dunnette SL, Reed CE, et al. Increased numbers of hypodense eosinophils in the blood of patients with bronchial asthma. Am Rev Respir Dis 1985;132:981–5.

13. Gleich GJ, Flavahan NA, Fujisawa T, et al. The eosinophil as a mediator of damage to respiratory epithelium: a model for bronchial hyperreactivity. J Allergy Clin Immunol 1988;81:637–48.

14. Walker C, Kaegi MK, Braun P, et al. Activated T cells and eosinophilia in bronchoalveolar lavages from subjects with asthma correlated with disease severity. J Allergy Clin Immunol 1991;88:935–42.

15. Broide DH, Gleich GJ, Cuomo AJ, et al. Evidence of ongoing mast cell and eosinophil degranulation in symptomatic asthma airway. J Allergy Clin Immunol 1991;88:637–48.

16. Bochner BS, Undem BJ, Lichtenstein LM. Immunological aspects of allergic asthma. Annu Rev Immunol 1994;12:295–335.

17. Wilson JW, Li X. The measurement of reticular basement membrane and submucosal collagen in the asthmatic airway. Clin Exp Allergy 1997;27:363–71.

18. Barnes PJ. New directions in allergic diseases: mechanism-based antiinflammatory therapies. J Allergy Clin Immunol 2000;106:5–16.

19. Broide DH. Molecular and cellular mechanisms of allergic disease. J Allergy Clin Immunol 2001;108:S65–71.

20. Humbles AA, Lu B, Nilsson CA, et al. A role for the C3a anaphylatoxin receptor in the effector phase of asthma. Nature 2000;406:998–1001.

21. Annacker O, Pimenta-Araujo R, Burlen-Defranoux O, et al. On the ontogeny and physiology of regulatory T cells. Immunol Rev 2001;182: 5–17.

22. Viglietta V, Baecher-Alan C, Weiner HL. Loss of functional suppression by CD4+CD25+ regulatory Tcells in patients with multiple sclerosis. J Exp Med 2004;199:971–9.

23. Umetsu DT, DeKruyff RH. The regulation of allergy and asthma. Immunol Rev 2006;212:238–55.

24. Hogan SP, Foster PS. Cytokines as targets for the inhibition of eosinophilic inflammation. Pharmacol Ther 1997;74:259–83.

25. Robinson DS, Hamid Q, Ying S, et al. Predominant TH2-like bronchoalveolar T lymphocyte population in atopic asthma. N Engl J Med 1992;326:298–304.

26. Hogan SP, Koskinen A, Mattaei KI, et al. Interleukin-5-producing CD4+ T cells play a pivotal role in aeroallergen-induced eosinophilia, bronchial hyperreactivity, and lung damage in mice. Am J Respir Crit Care Med 1998;157:210–8.

27. Ray A, Cohn L. Th2 cells and GATA-3 in asthma: new insights into the regulation of airway inflammation. J Clin Invest 1999;104: 985–93.

28. Wills-Karp M. IL-12/IL-13 axis in allergic asthma. J Allergy Clin Immunol 2001;107:9–18.

29. Kita H. The eosinophil: a cytokine-producing cell? J Allergy Clin Immunol 1996;97:889–92.

30. Rothenberg ME. Eosinophilia. N Engl J Med 1998;338:1592–600.

31. Brusselle GG, Kips JC, Tavernier JH, et al. Attenuation of allergic airway inflammation in IL-4 deficient mice. Clin Exp Allergy 1994;24: 73–80.

32. Rankin JA, Picarella DE, Geba GP, et al. Phenotypic and physiologic characterization of transgenic mice expressing interleukin 4 in the lung: lymphocytic and eosinophilic inflammation without airway hyperreactivity. Proc Natl Acad Sci U S A 1996;93:7821–5.

33. Bochner BS, Klunk DA, Sterbinsky SA, et al. IL-13 selectively induces vascular cell adhesion molecule-1 expression in human endothelial cells. J Immunol 1995;154:799–803.

34. Zhu Z, Homer RJ, Wang Z, et al. Pulmonary expression of interleukin-13 causes inflammation, mucus hypersecretion, subepithelial fibrosis, physiologic abnormalities, and eotaxin production. J Clin Invest 1999;103: 779–88.

35. Murata T, Noguchi PD, Puri RK. IL-13 induces phosphorylation and activation of JAK2 Janus kinase in human colon carcinoma cell lines: similarities between IL-4 and IL-13 signaling. J Immunol 1996;156: 2972–8.

36. Takeda K, Tanaka T, Shi W, et al. Essential role of Stat6 in IL-4 signalling. Nature 1996;380:627–30.

37. Takeda K, Kamanaka M, Tanaka T, et al. Impaired IL-13-mediated functions of macrophages in STAT6-deficient mice. J Immunol 1996;157: 3220–2.

38. Grunig G, Warnock M, Wakil AE, et al. Requirement for IL-13 independently of IL-4 in experimental asthma. Science 1998;282:2261–3.

39. Wills-Karp M, Luyimbazi J, Xu X, et al. Interleukin-13: central mediator of allergic asthma. Science 1998;282:2258–61.

40. Mattes J, Yang M, Siqueira A, et al. IL-13 induces airways hyperreactivity independently of the IL-4R alpha chain in the allergic lung. J Immunol 2001;167:1683–92.

41. Mathew A, MacLean JA, DeHaan E, et al. Signal transducer and activator of transcription 6 controls chemokine production and T helper cell type 2 cell trafficking in allergic pulmonary inflammation. J Exp Med 2001;193:1087–96.

42. Akimoto T, Numata F, Tamura M, et al. Abrogation of bronchial eosinophilic inflammation and airway hyperreactivity in signal transducers and activators of transcription (STAT)6-deficient mice. J Exp Med 1998;187:1537–42.

43. Kuperman D, Schofield B, Wills-Karp M, et al. Signal transducer and activator of transcription factor 6 (Stat6)-deficient mice are protected from antigen-induced airway hyperresponsiveness and mucus production. J Exp Med 1998;187:939–48.

44. Yang M, Hogan SP, Henry PJ, et al. Interleukin-13 mediates airways hyperreactivity through the IL-4 receptor-alpha chain and STAT-6 independently of IL-5 and eotaxin. Am J Respir Cell Mol Biol 2001;25:522–30.

45. Busse W, Corren J, Lanier BQ, et al. Omalizumab, anti-Ige recombinant humanized monoclonal antibody for the threatment of severe allergic asthma. J Allergy Clin Immunol 2001;108:184–90.

46. Flood-Page P, Swenson C, Faiferman I, et al. A study to evaluate the safety and efficacy of mepolizumab in patients with moderate persistent asthma. Am J Respir Crit Care Med 2007;176:1062–71.

47. Haldar P, Brightling CE, Hargadon B, et al. Mepolizumab and exacerbations of refractory eosinophilic asthma. N Engl J Med 2009;360:973–84.

48. Nair P, Pizzichini MM, Kjarsgaard M, et al. Mepolizumab for prednisone-dependent asthma with sputum eosinophilia. N Engl J Med 2009;360:985–93.

49. Stein ML, Collins MH, Villanueva JM, et al. Antil-IL-5 (mepolizumab) therapy for eosinophilic esophagitis. J Allergy Clin Immunol 2006;118:1312–9.

50. Rothenberg ME, Klion AD, Roufosse FE, et al. Treatment of patients with the hypereosinophilic syndrome with mepolizumab. N Engl J Med 2008;358:1215–28.

51. Weller PF. The immunobiology of eosinophils. N Engl J Med 1991;324:1110–8.

52. Gouon-Evans V, Rothenberg ME, Pollard JW. Postnatal mammary gland development requires macrophages and eosinophils. Development 2000;127:2269–82.

53. Slifman NR, Loegering DA, McKean DJ, et al. Ribonuclease activity associated with human eosinophil-derived neurotoxin and eosinophil cationic protein. J Immunol 1986;137:2913–7.

54. Rosenberg HF, Dyer KD, Tiffany HL, et al. Rapid evolution of a unique family of primate ribonuclease genes. Nat Genet 1995;10:219–23.

55. Yang D, Chen Q, Su SB, et al. Eosinophil-derived neurotoxin acts as an alrmin to activate the TLR2-MyD88 signal pathway in dendritic cells and enhances Th2 immune responses. J Exp Med 2008;205:79–90.

56. Young JD, Peterson CG, Venge P, et al. Mechanism of membrane damage mediated by human eosinophil cationic protein. Nature 1986; 321:613–6.

57. Jacoby DB, Gleich GJ, Fryer AD. Human eosinophil major basic protein is an endogenous allosteric antagonist at the inhibitory muscarinic M2 receptor. J Clin Invest 1993;91:1314–8.

58. Jacoby DB, Costello RM, Fryer AD. Eosinophil recruitment to the airway nerves. J Allergy Clin Immunol 2001;107:211–8.

59. Yoon J, Ponikau JU, Lawrence CB, et al. Innate antifungal immunity of human eosinophils mediated by a beta 2 integrin, CD11b. J Immunol 2008;181:2907–15.

60. Lewis RA, Austen KF, Soberman RJ. Leukotrienes and other products of the 5-lipoxygenase pathway Biochemistry and relation to pathobiology in human diseases. N Engl J Med 1990;323:645–55.

61. Stead RH. Innervation of mucosal immune cells in the gastrointestinal tract. Reg Immunol 1992;4:91–9.

62. Dvorak AM, Onderdonk AB, McLeod RS, et al. Ultrastructural identification of exocytosis of granules from human gut eosinophils in vivo. Int Arch Allergy Immunol 1993;102:33–45.

63. Hogan SP, Mishra A, Brandt EB, et al. A pathological function for eotaxin and eosinophils in eosinophilic gastrointestinal inflammation. Nat Immunol 2001;2:353–60.

64. Hogan SP, Mishra A, Brandt EB, et al. The chemokine eotaxin is a central mediator of experimental eosinophilic gastrointestinal allergy. J Allergy Clin Immunol 1999;105:S379.

65. Ohkawara Y, Lim KG, Xing Z, et al. CD40 expression by human peripheral blood eosinophils. J Clin Invest 1996;97:1761–6.

66. Woerly G, Roger N, Loiseau S, et al. Expression of CD28 and CD86 by human eosinophils and role in the secretion of type 1 cytokines (inter-

leukin 2 and interferon gamma). Inhibition by immunoglobulin a complexes. J Exp Med 1999;190:487–96.

67. Lucey DR, Nicholson WA, Weller PF. Mature human eosinophils have the capacity to express HLA-DR. Proc Natl Acad Set U S A 1989;86:1348–51.

68. Lacy P, Levi-Schaffer F, Mahmudi Azer S, et al. Intracellular localization of interleukin-6 in eosinophils from atopic asthmatics and effects of interferon gamma. Blood 1998;91:2508–16.

69. Shi HZ, Humbles A, Gerard C, et al. Lymph node trafficking and antigen presentation by endobronchial eosinophils. J Clin Invest 2000;105:945–53.

70. Yousefi S, Gold JA, Andina N, et al. Catapul-like release of mitochondrial DNA by eosinophils contributes to antibacterial defense. Nat Med 2008;14:949–53.

71. Kitamura Y, Go S, Hatanaka K. Decrease of mast cells in W/Wv mice and their increase by bone marrow transplantation. Blood 1978;52:447–52.

72. Geissler EN, Ryan MA, Housman DE. The dominant-white spotting (W) locus of the mouse encodes the c-kit proto-oncogene. Cell 1988;55:185–92.

73. Flanagan JG, Leder P. The kit ligand: a cell surface molecule altered in steel mutant fibroblasts. Cell 1990;63:185–94.

74. Williams CM, Galli SJ. The diverse potential effector and immunoregulatory roles of mast cells in allergic disease. J Allergy Clin Immunol 2000;105:847–59.

75. Hsieh FH, Lam BK, Penrose JF, et al. T helper cell type 2 cytokines coordinately regulate immunoglobulin E-dependent cysteinyl leukotriene production by human cord blood-derived mast cells: profound induction of leukotriene C(4) synthase expression by interleukin 4. J Exp Med 2001;193:123–33.

76. Oh SW, Pae CI, Lee DK, et al. Tryptase inhibition blocks airway inflammation in a mouse asthma model. J Immunol 2002;168:1992–2000.

77. Bradding P, Roberts JA, Britten KM, et al. Interleukin-4, -5, and -6 and tumor necrosis factor-alpha in normal and asthmatic airways: evidence for the human mast cell as a source of these cytokines. Am J Respir Cell Mol Biol 1994;10:471–80.

78. Boyce JA, Friend D, Matsumoto R, et al. Differentiation in vitro of hybrid eosinophil/basophil granulocytes: autocrine function of an eosinophil developmental intermediate. J Exp Med 1995;182:49–57.

79. Schwartz LB. Mast cells and basophils. Clin Allergy Immunol 2002;16:3–42.

80. Miura K, Saini SS, Gauvreau G, et al. Differences in functional consequences and signal transduction induced by IL-3, IL-5, and nerve growth factor in human basophils. J Immunol 2001;167:2282–91.

81. Devouassoux G, Foster B, Scott LM, et al. Frequency and characterization of antigen-specific IL-4- and IL-13-producing basophils and T cells in peripheral blood of healthy and asthmatic subjects. J Allergy Clin Immunol 1999;104:811–9.

82. Kepley CL, Craig SS, Schwartz LB. Identification and partial characterization of a unique marker for human basophils. J Immunol 1995;154:6548–55.

83. McEuen AR, Buckley MG, Compton SJ, et al. Development and characterization of a monoclonal antibody specific for human basophils and the identification of a unique secretory product of basophil activation. Lab Invest 1999;79:27–38.

84. Grützkau A, Kögel H, et al. Detection of intracellular interleukin-8 in human mast cells: flow cytometry as a guide for immunoelectron microscopy. J Histochem Cytochem 1997;45:935–45.

85. Irani AM, Huang C, Xia HZ, et al. Immunohistochemical detection of human basophils in late-phase skin reactions. J Allergy Clin Immunol 1998;101:354–62.

86. Ying S, Robinson DS, Meng Q, et al. C-C chemokines in allergen-induced late-phase cutaneous responses in atopic subjects: association of eotaxin with early 6-hour eosinophils, and of eotaxin-2 and monocyte chemoattractant protein-4 with the later 24-hour tissue eosinophilia, and relationship to basophils and other C-C chemokines (monocyte chemoat-tractant protein-3 and RANTES). J Immunol 1999;163:3976–84.

87. Khodoun M, Strait R, Orekov T, et al. Peanuts can contribute to anaphylactic shock by activating complement. J Allergy Clin Immunol 2009;123:342–51.

88. Tsujimura Y, Obata K, Mukai K, et al. Basophils play a pivotal role in innunoglobulin-G-mediated but not immunoglobulin-E- mediated systemic anaphylaxis. Immunity 2008;28:581–9.

89. Thomas ED, Ramberg RE, Sale GE, et al. Direct evidence for a bone marrow origin of the alveolar macrophage in man. Science 1976;192:1016–8.

90. Hume DA, Robinson AP, MacPherson GG, et al. The mononuclear phagocyte system of the mouse defined by immunohistochemical localization of antigen F4/80. Relationship between macrophages, Langerhans cells, reticular cells, and dendritic cells in lymphoid and hematopoietic organs. J Exp Med 1983;158:1522–36.

91. Begg SK, Radley JM, Pollard JW, et al. Delayed hematopoietic development in osteopetrotic (op/op) mice. J Exp Med 1993;177:237–42.

92. Trapnell BC, Whitsett JA. GM-CSF regulates pulmonary surfactant homeostasis and alveolar macrophage-mediated innate host defense. Annu Rev Physiol 2002;64:775–802.

93. Dranoff G, Crawford AD, Sadelain M, et al. Involvement of granulocyte-macrophage colony-stimulating factor in pulmonary homeostasis. Science 1994;264:713–6.

94. Shibata Y, Berclas PY, Chroneos ZC, et al. GM-CSF regulates alveolar macrophage differentiation and innate immunity in the lung through PU.1. Immunity 2001;15:557–67.

95. Aderem A, Ulevitch RJ. Toll-like receptors in the induction of the innate immune response. Nature 2000;406:782–7.

96. Mills CD. Macrophage arginine metabolism to ornithine/urea or nitric oxide/citrulline: a life or death issue. Cut Rev Immunol 2001;21:399–425.

97. Rivier A, Pene J, Rabesandratana H, et al. Blood monocytes of untreated asthmatics exhibit some features of tissue macrophages. Clin Exp Immunol 1995;100:314–8.

98. Poston RN, Chanez P, Lacoste JY, et al. Immunohistochemical characterization of the cellular infiltration in asthmatic bronchi. Am Rev Respir Dis 1992;145:918–21.

99. Sousa AR, Lane SJ, Nakhosteen JA, et al. Increased expression of the monocyte chemoattractant protein-1 in bronchial tissue from asthmatic subjects. Am J Respir Cell Mol Biol 1994;10:142–7.

100. Randolph GJ. Dendritic cell migration to lymph nodes: cytokines, chemokines, and lipid mediators. Semin Immunol 2001;13:267–74.

101. Lambrecht BN. The dendritic cell in allergic airway diseases: a new player to the game. Clin Exp Allergy 2001;31:206–18.

102. Keller R. Dendritic cells: their significance in health and disease. Immunol Lett 2001;78:113–22.

103. Tanaka H, Demeure CE, Rubio M, et al. Human monocyte-derived dendritic cells induce naive T cell differentiation into T helper cell type 2 (Th2) or Th1/Th2 effectors: role of stimulator/responder ratio. J Exp Med 2000;192:405–12.

104. Hutloff A, Dittrich AM, Beier KC, et al. ICOS is an inducible T cell co-stimulator structurally and functionally related to CD28. Nature 1999;397:263–6.

105. Lambrecht BN, Salomon B, Klatzmann D, et al. Dendritic cells are required for the development of chronic eosinophilic airway inflammation in response to inhaled antigen in sensitized mice. J Immunol 1998;160:4090–7.

106. Lambrecht BN, De Veerman M, Coyle AJ, et al. Myeloid dendritic cells induce Th2 responses to inhaled antigen, leading to eosinophilic airway inflammation. J Clin Invest 2000;106:551–9.

107. Cartwright GE, Athens JW, Winthrobe MM. The kinetics of granulopoiesis in normal man. Blood 1964;24:780–803.

108. Reeves EP, Lu H, Jacobs HL, et al. Killing activity of neutrophils is mediated through activation of proteases by K+ flux. Nature 2002;416:291–7.

109. Kelly C, Ward C, Stenton CS, et al. Number and activity of inflammatory cells in bronchoalveolar lavage fluid in asthma and their relation to airway responsiveness. Thorax 1988;43:684–92.

110. Sur S, Crotty TB, Kephart GM, et al. Sudden-onset fatal asthma: a distinct entity with few eosinophils and relatively more neutrophils in the airway submucosa? Am Rev Respir Dis 1993;148:713–9.

111. Murphy PM. The molecular biology of leukoctye chemoattractant receptors. Annu Rev Immunol 1994;12:593–633.

112. Gerard C, Gerard NP. The proinflammatory seven-transmembrane segment receptors of the leukocyte. Curr Opin Immunol 1994;6:140–5.

113. Ganju RK, Dutt P, Wu L, et al. Beta-chemokine receptor CCR5 signals via the novel tyrosine kinase RAFTK. Blood 1998;91:791–7.

114. Boehme SA, Sullivan SK, Crowe PD, et al. Activation of mitogen-activated protein kinase regulates eotaxin-induced eosinophil migration. J Immunol 1999;163:1611–8.

115. Proost P, Wuyts A, Van Damme J. Human monocyte chemotactic proteins-2 and -3: structural and functional comparison with MCP-1. J Leukoc Biol 1996;59:67–74.

116. Garcia-Zepeda EA, Rothenberg ME, Ownbey RT, et al. Human eotaxin is a specific chemoattractant for eosinophil cells and provides a new mechanism to explain tissue eosinophilia. Nat Med 1996;2:449–56.

117. Stellato C, Collins P, Ponath PD, et al. Production of the novel C-C chemokine MCP-4 by airway cells and comparison of its biological activity to other C-C chemokines. J Clin Invest 1997;99:926–36.

118. Minshall EM, Cameron L, Lavigne F, et al. Eotaxin mRNA and protein expression in chronic sinusitis and allergen-induced nasal responses in seasonal allergic rhinitis. Am J Respir Cell Mol Biol 1997;17:683–90.

119. Lilly CM, Nakamura H, Kesselman H, et al. Expression of eotaxin by human lung epithelial cells: induction by cytokines and inhibition by glucocorticoids. J Clin Invest 1997;99:1767–73.

120. Nelson PJ, Kim HT, Manning WC, et al. Genomic organization and transcriptional regulation of the RANTES chemokine gene. J Immunol 1993;151:2601–12.

121. Garcia-Zepeda EA, Rothenberg ME, Weremowicz S, et al. Genomic organization, complete sequence, and chromosomal location of the gene for human eotaxin (SCYA11), an eosinophil-specific CC chemokine. Genomics 1997;41:471–6.

122. Matsukura S, Stellato C, Plitt JR, et al. Activation of eotaxin gene transcription by NF-kappaB and STAT6 in human airway epithelial cells. J Immunol 1999;163:6876–83.

123. Ueda A, Okuda K, Ohno S, et al. NF-kappa B and Sp1 regulate transcription of the human monocyte chemoattractant protein-1 gene. J Immunol 1994;153:2052–63.

124. Anisowicz A, Messineo M, Lee SW, et al. An NF-kappa B-like transcription factor mediates IL-1/TNF-alpha induction of gro in human fibroblasts. J Immunol 1991;147:520–7.

125. Widmer U, Manogue KR, Cerami A, et al. Genomic cloning and promoter analysis of macrophage inflammatory protein (MIP)-2, MIP-1 alpha, and MIP-1 beta, members of the chemokine superfamily of proinflammatory cytokines. J Immunol 1993;150:4996–5012.

126. Beato M. Gene regulation by steroid hormones. Cell 1989;56:335–44.

127. Mukaida N, Gussella GL, Kasahara T, et al. Molecular analysis of the inhibition of interleukin-8 production by dexamethasone in a human fi-brosarcoma cell line. Immunology 1992;75:674–9.

128. Stellato C, Matsukura S, Fal A, et al. Differential regulation of epithelial-derived C-C chemokine expression by IL-4 and the glucocorticoid budesonide. J Immunol 1999;163:5624–32.

129. Loetscher P, Seitz M, Baggiolini M, et al. Interleukin-2 regulates CC chemokine receptor expression and chemotactic responsiveness in T lymphocytes. J Exp Med 1996;184:569–77.

130. Loetscher M, Gerber B, Loetscher P, et al. Chemokine receptor specific for IP10 and mig: structure, function, and expression in activated T lymphocytes. J Exp Med 1996;184:963–9.

131. D'Amico G, Frascaroli G, Bianchi G, et al. Uncoupling of inflammatory chemokine receptors by IL-10: generation of functional decoys. Nat Immunol 2000;1:387–91.

132. Yamada H, Hirai K, Miyamasu M, et al. Eotaxin is a potent chemotaxin for human basophils. Biochem Biophys Res Commun 1997;231:365–8.

133. Luster AD, Rothenberg ME. Role of monocyte chemoattractant protein and eotaxin subfamily of chemokines in allergic inflammation. J Leukoc Biol 1997;62:620–33.

134. Alam R, Lett-Brown MA, Forsythe PA, et al. Monocyte chemotactic and activating factor is a potent histamine-releasing factor for basophils. J Clin Invest 1992;89:723–8.

135. Alam R, Forsythe P, Stafford S, et al. Monocyte chemotactic protein-2, monocyte chemotactic protein-3, and fibroblast-induced cytokine: three new chemokines induce chemotaxis and activation of basophils. J Immunol 1994;153:3155–9.

136. Kim CH, Broxmeyer HE. Chemokines for immature blood cells: effects on migration, proliferation, and differentiation. In: Rothenberg ME, editor. Chemokines in allergic disease. New York: Marcel Dekker; 2000.

137. Nagasawa T, Hirota S, Tachibana K, et al. Defects of B cell lymphopoiesis and bone-marrow myelopoiesis in mice lacking the CXC chemokine PBSF/SDF-1. Nature 1996;382:635–8.

138. Palframan RT, Collins PD, Williams TJ, et al. Eotaxin induces a rapid release of eosinophils and their progenitors from the bone marrow. Blood 1998;91:2240–8.

139. Quackenbush EJ, Aguirre V, Wershil BK, et al. Eotaxin influences the development of embryonic hematopoietic progenitors in the mouse. J Leukoc Biol 1997;62:661–6.

140. Peled A, Gonzalo JA, Lloyd C, et al. The chemotactic cytokine eotaxin acts as a granulocyte-macrophage colony-stimulating factor during lung inflammation. Blood 1998;91:1909–16.

141. Sallusto F, Schaerli P, Loetscher P, et al. Rapid and coordinated switch in chemokine receptor expression during dendritic cell maturation. Eur J Immunol 1998;28:2760–9.

142. Sozzani S, Luini W, Borsatti A, et al. Receptor expression and responsiveness of human dendritic cells to a defined set of CC and CXC chemokines. J Immunol 1997;159:1993–2000.

143. Dieu-Nosjean MC, Vicari A, Lebecque S, et al. Regulation of dendritic cell trafficking: a process that involves the participation of selective chemokines. J Leukoc Biol 1999;66:252–62.

144. Rollins BJ. Chemokines. Blood 1997;90:909–28.

145. Gunn MD, Tangemann K, Tam C, et al. A chemokine expressed in lymphoid high endothelial venules promotes the adhesion and chemotaxis of naive T lymphocytes. Proc Natl Acad Sci U S A 1998;95:258–63.

146. Ward SG, Bacon K, Westwick J. Chemokines and T lymphocytes: more than an attraction. Immunity 1998;9:1–11.

147. Sallusto F, Lenig D, Forster R, et al. Two subsets of memory T lymphocytes with distinct homing potentials and effector functions. Nature 1999;401:708–12.

148. Zhang S, Lukacs NW, Lawless VA, et al. Cutting edge: differential expression of chemokines in Th1 and Th2 cells is dependent on Stat6 but not Stat4. J Immunol 2000;165:10–4.

149. Karpus WJ, Kennedy KJ. MIP-1alpha and MCP-1 differentially regulate acute and relapsing autoimmune encephalomyelitis as well as Th1/Th2 lymphocyte differentiation. J Leukoc Biol 1997;62:681–7.

150. Gu L, Tseng S, Horner RM, et al. Control of TH2 polarization by the chemokine monocyte chemoattractant protein-1. Nature 2000;404:407–11.

151. Toney LM, Cattoretti G, Graf JA, et al. BCL-6 regulates chemokine gene transcription in macrophages. Nat Immunol 2000;1:214–20.

152. Ponath PD, Qin S, Post TW, et al. Molecular cloning and characterization of a human eotaxin receptor expressed selectively on eosinophils. J Exp Med 1996;183:2437–48.

153. Daugherty BL, Siciliano SJ, DeMartino JA, et al. Cloning, expression, and characterization of the human eosinophil eotaxin receptor. J Exp Med 1996;183:2349–54.

154. Heath H, Qin SX, Rao P, et al. Chemokine receptor usage by human eosinophils: the importance of CCR3 demonstrated using an antagonistic monoclonal antibody. J Clin Invest 1997;99:178–84.

155. Rothenberg ME. Eotaxin: an essential mediator of eosinophil trafficking into mucosal tissues. Am J Respir Cell Mol Biol 1999;21:291–5.

156. Ma W, Bryce PJ, Humbles AA, et al. CCR3 is essential for skin eosinophilia and airway hyperresponsiveness in a murine model of allergic skin inflammation. J Clin Invest 2002;109:621–8.

157. Sullivan SK, McGrath DA, Liao F, et al. MIP-3alpha induces human eosinophil migration and activation of the mitogen-activated protein kinases (p42/p44 $MAPK$). J Leukoc Biol 1999;66:674–82.

158. Nagase H, Miyamasu M, Yamaguchi M, et al. Expression of CXCR4 in eosinophils: functional analyses and cytokine-mediated regulation. J Immunol 2000;164:5935–43.

159. Jinquan T, Jing C, Jacobi HH, et al. CXCR3 expression and activation of eosinophils: role of IFN-gamma-inducible protein-10 and monokine induced by IFN-gamma. J Immunol 2000;165:1548–56.

160. Gerard C, Rollins BJ. Chemokines and disease. Nat Immunol 2001;2:108–15.

161. Nickel RG, Casolaro V, Wahn U, et al. Atopic dermatitis is associated with a functional mutation in the promoter of the C-C chemokine RANTES. J Immunol 2000;164:1612–6.

162. Fryer AA, Spiteri MA, Bianco A, et al. The −403 G→A promoter polymorphism in the RANTES gene is associated with atopy and asthma. Genes Immun 2000;1:509–14.

163. Lloyd CM, Delaney T, Nguyen T, et al. CC chemokine receptor (CCR)3/eotaxin is followed by CCR4/monocyte-derived chemokine in mediating pulmonary T helper lymphocyte type 2 recruitment after serial antigen challenge in vivo. J Exp Med 2000;191:265–74.

164. Chensue SW, Lukacs NW, Yang TY, et al. Aberrant in vivo T helper type 2 cell response and impaired eosinophil recruitment in CC chemokine receptor 8 knockout mice. J Exp Med 2001;193:573–84.

165. Dean M, Carrington M, Winkler C, et al. Genetic restriction of HIV-1 infection and progression to AIDS by a deletion allele of the CKR5 structural gene. Hemophilia Growth and Development Study, Multicen-ter AIDS Cohort Study, Multicenter Hemophilia Cohort Study, San Francisco City Cohort, ALIVE Study. Science 1996;273:1856–62.

166. Smith MW, Dean M, Carrington M, et al. Contrasting genetic influence of CCR2 and CCR5 variants on HIV-1 infection and disease progression. Hemophilia Growth and Development Study (HGDS), Multicenter AIDS Cohort Study (MACS), Multicenter Hemophilia Cohort Study (MHCS), San Francisco City Cohort (SFCC), ALIVE Study. Science 1997;277:959–65.

167. Sabroe I, Conroy DM, Gerard NP, et al. Cloning and characterization of the guinea pig eosinophil eotaxin receptor, C-C chemokine receptor-3: blockade using a monoclonal antibody in vivo. J Immunol 1998;161:6139–47.

168. Proudfoot AE, Power CA, Hoogewerf AJ, et al. Extension of recombinant human RANTES by the retention of the initiating methionine produces a potent antagonist. J Biol Chem 1996;271:2599–603.

169. Elsner J, Petering H, Hochstetter R, et al. The CC chemokine antagonist Met-RANTES inhibits eosinophil effector functions through the chemokine receptors CCR1 and CCR3. Eur J Immunol 1997;27:2892–8.

170. Gangur V, Oppenheim JJ. Are chemokines essential or secondary participants in allergic responses? Ann Allergy Asthma Immunol 2000;84:569–79.

171. Moore PS, Boshoff C, Weiss RA, et al. Molecular mimicry of human cytokine and cytokine response pathway genes by KSHV. Science 1996;274:1739–44.

172. Kledal TN, Rosenkilde MM, Coulin F, et al. A broad-spectrum chemokine antagonist encoded by Kaposi's sarcoma-associated her-pesvirus. Science 1997;277:1656–9.

173. White JR, Lee JM, Young PR, et al. Identification of a potent, selective non-peptide CXCR2 antagonist that inhibits interleukin-8-induced neutrophil migration. J Biol Chem 1998;273:10095–8.

174. Hesselgesser J, Ng HP, Liang M, et al. Identification and characterization of small molecule functional antagonists of the CCR1 chemokine receptor. J Biol Chem 1998;273:15687–92.

175. Bertrand CP, Ponath PD. CCR3 blockade as a new therapy for asthma. Expert Opin Invest Drugs 2000;9:43–52.

176. Sabroe I, Peck MJ, Van Keulen BJ, et al. A small molecule antagonist of chemokine receptors CCR1 and CCR3: potent inhibition of eosinophil function and CCR3-mediated HIV-1 entry. J Biol Chem 2000;275: 25985–92.

177. Rutledge BJ, Rayburn H, Rosenberg R, et al. High level monocyte chemoattractant protein-1 expression in transgenic mice increases their susceptibility to intracellular pathogens. J Immunol 1995;155: 4838–43.

178. Zimmermann N, Conkright JJ, Rothenberg ME. CC chemokine receptor-3 undergoes prolonged ligand-induced internalization. J Biol Chem 1999;274:12611–8.

6

The Developing Immune System and Allergy

Elysia M. Hollams • Julie Rowe • Patrick G. Holt

The prevalence of allergic diseases has risen markedly since the 1960s, particularly in the developed countries of the western world. The diseases manifest initially during childhood, and have become more prevalent and persistent in successive birth cohorts, although there is evidence that prevalence may have peaked in several countries. The ultimate expression of allergic disease results from complex interactions between genetic and environmental factors, neither of which have yet been comprehensively characterized. There is increasing evidence that the level of complexity inherent in the pathogenesis of allergic diseases may be even greater than is currently contemplated, as an additional set of crucial factors appear to be involved. Notably, it appears likely that the ultimate effect(s) of these 'gene x environment' interactions within individuals may also be related to the developmental status of the relevant target tissues at the time the interactions occur.

The following discussion is presented in two major subsections. First, our current understanding of the maturation of the immune system is broadly summarized. Second, recent findings relating to the etiology of allergic disease in general (and atopic asthma in particular) are presented, with a particular focus upon the role of immune developmental factors during infancy and early childhood.

Immune Function During Fetal Life

The initial stage of hematopoiesis in the human fetus occurs in extraembryonic mesenchymal tissue and in the mesoderm of the yolk sac, and pluripotent erythroid and granulo-macrophage progenitors are detectable in the latter at around the fourth week of gestation (Box 6-1). These cells appear subsequently in the fetal circulation and by weeks 5 to 6 in the liver, which at that stage of development is the major site of hematopoiesis. Within the liver, the interactions between stromal cells and haematopoietic cells play an important role in regulation. Specifically, the expression of fibronectin by stromal cells is increased during the second trimester and is believed to result in enhanced proliferation and differentiation of haematopoietic cells.[1] The spleen and thymus are seeded from the liver, and by the eighth week of development CD7[+] precursor cells are found in the thymus;[2-4] stem cells do not appear in bone marrow until around the 12th week of gestation.[5] T cells recognizable by expression of characteristic T cell receptor (TcR)/CD3 are found in peripheral lymphoid organs from weeks 13 to 15 of gestation onwards,[6-8] despite the lack of well-defined thymic cortical and medullary regions and

mature epithelial components.[2] These early T cells also express CD2 and CD5.[4] The maturation of nonlymphoid components within peripheral lymphoid tissues progresses even more slowly and takes up to 20 weeks.[8-11]

The fetal gastrointestinal tract may be an additional site for extrathymic T cell differentiation in the human fetus, as has been reported in the mouse.[12] T cells are detectable in the intestinal mucosa by 12 weeks of gestation,[13] and many of these express the CD8αα phenotype, in particular within Peyer's patches.[14] In the mouse, CD8αα cells appear to be thymus independent and are believed to develop in the gut. Although there is no direct evidence for this in humans, it is noteworthy, initially, that fetal gut lamina propria lymphocytes are an actively proliferating population as indicated by constitutive expression of Ki67, and there is little or no overlap between gut-derived and blood-derived TcRβ transcripts.[15]

The gut mucosa may also be a major site for differentiation of TcRγ/δ cells during fetal life. Rearranged TcRδ genes are first detectable in the gut at 6 to 9 weeks of gestation,[16] which is earlier than is observed in the thymus. The liver is another significant extrathymic site for TcRγ/δ differentiation in humans, including a unique subset expressing CD4.[17]

The capacity to respond to polyclonal stimuli such as phytohemagglutinin (PHA) is first seen at 15 to 16 weeks of gestation.[18] The degree to which the fetal immune system can respond to foreign antigens has not been clearly established. On the one hand, the offspring of mothers infected during pregnancy with a range of pathogens including mumps,[19] ascaris,[20] malaria,[21] schistosomes,[22] and helminths[23] display evidence of pathogen-specific T cell reactivity at birth, whereas infection with other organisms such as toxoplasma[24] may induce tolerance. Additionally, vaccination of pregnant women with tetanus toxoid results in the appearance of IgM in the fetal circulation that is indicative of fetal T cell sensitization.[25] Similarly, vaccination of pregnant women against influenza results in the presence of influenza-specific IgM in cord blood, and virus-specific CD8[+] T cells detected by the use of major histocompatability complex (MHC) tetramers.[26] There is also a variety of evidence based on in vitro lymphoproliferation of cord blood mononuclear cells (CBMCs)[27] and recently the presence of low levels of immunoglobulin E (IgE) in cord blood[28] which suggests that environmental antigens to which pregnant women are exposed may in some circumstances prime T cell responses transplacentally. However, these conclusions have been challenged on the basis of a variety of evidence of low specificity of cord blood responses to allergen and on the kinetics of postnatal development of allergen specific Th-memory,[29] and the issue remains contentious.[30]

DOI: 10.1016/B978-1-4377-0271-2.00006-7

Maturation of the Immune System

- Weeks 5–6 of gestation: pluripotent erythroid and granulomacrophage progenitors are detected in the liver
- Week 8 of gestation: CD7$^+$ precursor cells found in the thymus
- Week 12 of gestation: stem cells appear in bone marrow
- Weeks 13–15 of gestation: T cells found in peripheral lymphoid organs
- Weeks 15–16 of gestation: fetal T cells respond to mitogen
- IgM responses develop in fetus following maternal vaccination
- Infant T cells express CD1, PNA, and CD38, indicative of mature thymocytes
- Proportion of CD45RO$^+$ CD4$^+$ T cells increase from < 10% at birth to > 65% in adulthood, reflecting progressive antigenic exposure
- Adult peripheral blood T cells express CCR-1, -2, -5, and -6 and CXCR-3 and CXCR-4, whereas cord blood expresses only CXCR-4, reflecting decreased capacity to respond to proinflammatory signals at birth
- At infancy, cytotoxic effector functions and capacity to drive B cell immunoglobulin production are attenuated

Studies examining lymphocyte subsets in cord blood from babies born at gestational ages between 20 and 42 weeks found that the proportion of cord NK cells increased with gestational age, while the proportion of CD4$^+$ cells and the ratio of CD4$^+$:CD8$^+$ cells decreased.[31,32] It is noteworthy that, despite the lack of significant numbers of CD4$^+$ and CD8$^+$ CD45RO$^+$ T cells in cord blood, fetal spleen and cord blood samples from premature infants contain these cells in relatively high frequency.[33] These 'postactivated or memory' T cells were unresponsive to recombinant IL-2, suggesting they may have been anergized by earlier contact with self- or environmental antigens.[33] CD4$^+$ CD25$^+$ T regulatory cells are detected in fetal lymphoid tissue, and they have been shown to have a suppressive effect on fetal CD4$^+$ and CD8$^+$ T cells expressing the activation antigen CD69.[34] Fetal thymic exposure to high-avidity TcR ligand has been shown to promote development of T regulatory cells in mice, while exposure to low-affinity TcR ligand did not; it appears that T regulatory cells require a higher ligand avidity for positive selection than conventional T cells.[35] Interestingly, expression and function of T regulatory cells has been found to be impaired at birth in the offspring of atopic mothers.[36]

These findings collectively suggest that the fetal immune system develops at least partial functional competence before birth but lacks the full capacity to generate sustained immune responses; although IgM responses develop in the fetus following maternal tetanus vaccination, there is no evidence of class-switching in the offspring until they are actively vaccinated.[25] Given the fact that the fetal immune system can generate at least primary immune responses against external stimuli, the question arises as to how immune responses within or in close contact with the fetal compartment are regulated. The necessity for tight control of these responses becomes obvious in light of findings that a variety of T cell cytokines are exquisitely toxic to the placenta.[37] Part of this control may be at the level of transcription factor expression.

It is also pertinent to question how potential immunostimulatory interactions between cells derived from fetal and maternal bone marrow are regulated at the fetomaternal interface. In par-

ticular, it has been clearly demonstrated that fetal cells readily traffic into the maternal circulation,[38–42] potentially sensitizing the maternal immune system against paternal HLA antigens present on the fetal cells. However, it is clear from recent studies[43] that the maternal immune system, in the vast majority of circumstances, successfully eradicates fetal cells from the peripheral circulation while remaining functionally tolerant of the fetus. This suggests that tolerance of the fetal allograft is a regionally controlled process that is localized to the fetomaternal interface.

The mechanisms that regulate the induction and expression of immune responses in this milieu are complex and multilayered. The first line of defense appears to be a local immunosuppressive 'blanket' maintained via the local production within the placenta by trophoblasts and macrophages of metabolites of tryptophan generated via indolamine 2,3-dioxygenase, which are markedly inhibitory against T cell activation and proliferation.[44] Constitutive production of high levels of IL-10 by placental trophoblasts provides a second broad-spectrum immunosuppressive signal to dampen local T cell responses,[45] as well as the homeostatic function of alternatively activated macrophages.[46]

A second line of defense operates to protect against T cell activation events that evade suppression via these pathways. Two such mechanisms involve the expression of FasL on cells within the placenta, providing a potential avenue for apoptosis-mediated elimination of locally activated T cells,[47,48] and the presence of maternally derived CD4$^+$ CD25$^+$ T regulatory cells, which are recruited to the fetomaternal interface where they act to dampen fetus-specific responses.[49] These mechanisms are complemented by a series of pathways that operate to selectively dampen production at the fetomaternal interface of Th1 cytokines, in particular, of interferon-gamma (IFN-γ). This cytokine plays an important role in implantation,[50] but if produced in suprathreshold levels at later stages of pregnancy, triggered, for example, by local immune responses against microbial or alloantigens, IFN-γ (and other Th1 cytokines) can potentially cause placental detachment and fetal resorption.[51,52] These Th2-trophic mechanisms involve local production of a range of immunomodulators including IL-10,[45] which programs antigen-presenting cells (APCs) for Th2 switching;[53] progesterone, which directly inhibits IFN-γ gene transcription;[54–56] and PGE2, which promotes Th2 switching via effects upon APCs, dendritic cells in particular.[53]

Resistance to Infection During Pregnancy

It is well established that infancy represents a period of high susceptibility to infection with a range of pathogens including bacteria and fungi[57] and, in particular, viruses.[58–60] The expression of cell-mediated immunity during active viral infection is attenuated in infants in comparison to older age groups,[61–63] and the subsequent generation of virus-specific immunologic memory is also inefficient.[64] These findings suggest that a range of developmentally related deficiencies in innate and adaptive immunologic mechanisms are operative in the immediate postnatal period, and the nature and clinical significance of the latter are the subject of increasingly intensive research.

Surface Phenotype of T Cells in Early Life

Total lymphocyte counts in peripheral blood are higher in infancy than in adulthood,[65] and at birth T cell levels are twice those of adults. Longitudinal studies on individual infants indicate a further rapid doubling in T cell numbers in the circulation during the first 6 weeks of life, which is maintained throughout infancy.[66] Surface marker expression on infant T cells differs markedly from that observed in adults. The most noteworthy characteristics are frequent expression of CD1[67] and PNA[68] antigens and CD38.[66,69,70] These three antigens are considered to mark mature thymocytes as opposed to circulating 'mature' naïve T cells.

Analyses performed on CD38+ cord blood cells have reinforced this view. In particular, animal model studies on thymic output have led to the development of an accurate technique for phenotypic identification of recent thymic emigrants (RTE), which are newly produced peripheral naïve T cells that retain a distinct phenotypic signature of recent thymic maturation that distinguishes them from long-lived naïve T cells produced at remote sites. This approach involves the measurement of T cell receptor excision circles (TRECs), which are stable extrachromosomal products generated during the process of variable/diverse/ joining (VDJ) TcR gene rearrangement. These excision DNA circles are not replicated during mitosis and as a consequence become diluted with each round of cell division. Employing this procedure, Hassan and Reen[70] have demonstrated that the majority of circulating CD4+ CD45R+ human T cells at birth are RTE as reflected by their high level of expression of TRECs. Analogous to thymocytes, the RTE were highly susceptible to apoptosis,[70] and unlike mature adult-derived CD4+ CD45RA+ naïve T cells they were uniquely responsive to common 7-chain cytokines, particularly IL-7.[70,71] Whereas IL-7 promotes their proliferation and survival, IL-7-exposed RTE could not reexpress recombination-activating gene-2 gene expression in vitro. These findings suggest that postthymic naïve peripheral T cells in early infancy are at a unique stage in ontogeny as RTEs, during which they can undergo homeostatic regulation including survival and antigen-independent expansion while maintaining their preselected TcR repertoire.[70]

The patterns of postnatal change in T cell surface marker expression have been analyzed in several recent studies. Of relevance to the preceding conclusions are observations noting the presence of relatively high numbers of T cells coexpressing both CD4 and CD8 during infancy, which is also a hallmark of immaturity.[66,72,73] In contrast, expression of CD57 on T cells, which marks non-MHC-restricted cytotoxic cells, is infrequent, as are T cells coexpressing IL-2 and HLA-DR, which is indicative of recent activation.[72] The expression of other activation markers such as CD25, CD69, and CD154, is also low.[66]

Of particular interest in relation to the understanding of overall immune competence during postnatal life are changing patterns of surface CD45RA and CD45RO on T cells. T cells exported from the thymus express the CD45RA isoform of the leukocyte common antigen CD45, and after activation switch to CD45RO expression. Most postactivated neonatal CD4+ CD45RO+ T cells are short-lived and die within a matter of days, but a subset of these is believed to be programmed to enter the long-lived recirculating T cell compartment as T memory cells.[74] The proportion of CD45RO+ cells within the CD4+ T cell compartment progressively increases from a baseline of less than 10% at birth up to 65% in adulthood, reflecting age-dependent accumulation of antigenic exposure.[66,72,74-79] The rate of increase within the TcRα/β and TcRγ/δ populations is approximately equivalent and is slightly more rapid for CD4+ T cells relative to CD8+ T cells.[79] The relative proportion of CD45RO+ putative memory T cells attain adult-equivalent levels within the teen years,[72,79] but it is noteworthy that the population spread during the years of childhood is very wide.[79] This suggests substantial heterogeneity within the pediatric population in the efficiency of mechanisms regulating

the generation of T helper memory, an issue that is discussed next in more detail.

Functional Phenotype of T Cells During Infancy and Early Childhood

T cell function during infancy exhibits a variety of qualitative and quantitative differences relative to that observed in adults. Employing a limiting dilution analytic system, it has been demonstrated that at least 90% of peripheral blood CD4+ T cells from adults can give rise to stable T cell clones, whereas the corresponding (mean) figure for immunocompetent T cell precursors in infants was less than 35%.[80] It was also observed that cloning frequencies within the infant population were bimodally distributed, with a significant subset of ostensibly normal healthy subjects displaying particularly low cloning frequencies of no more than 20%.[80]

In apparent contrast to these findings, the magnitude of initial T cell proliferation induced by polyclonal T cell mitogens such as PHA in short-term cultures is higher at birth than subsequently during infancy and adulthood.[81,82] However, proliferation is not sustained, which may reflect the greater susceptibility of neonatal T cells to apoptosis postactivation[70] and/or decreased production of IL-2.[83,84] In contrast, activation induced by TcR stimulation[85] and cross-linking CD2[83,86] or CD28[87] is reduced.

In addition to these deficiencies, neonatal T cells are hyperresponsive to IL-4[88] and hyporesponsive to IL-12[89] relative to adults, the latter being associated with reduced receptor expression.[90] Neonates also have reduced capacity to produce IL-12 which can last into childhood; our work has suggested that slow maturation of IL-12 synthetic capacity can be attributed to deficiencies in the number and/or function of dendritic cells.[91]

Neonatal T cells exhibit heightened susceptibility to anergy induction poststimulation with bacterial superantigen, employing protocols that do not tolerize adult T cells.[92,93] The latter has been ascribed to deficient IL-2 production,[92] but may alternatively be related to developmentally related deficiencies in the Ras signaling pathway, which have been associated with secondary unresponsiveness to alloantigen stimulation by T cells from neonates.[94] Additional aberrations in intracellular signaling pathways reported in neonatal T cells include phospholipase C and associated Lck expression,[95] protein kinase C,[96] and CD28, which is associated with dysfunction in FasL-mediated cytotoxicity[97] and reduced NFκB production.[87]

Profiles of chemokine receptor expression and responsiveness in neonatal T cells have been observed to differ distinctly from those in adults. In particular, adult peripheral blood T cells expressed CCR-1, -2, -5, -6 and CXCR-3 and CXCR-4, whereas those from cord blood expressed only CXCR-4, reflecting markedly attenuated capacity to respond to signals from inflammatory foci.[98]

Evidence from a range of studies indicates that both cytotoxic effector functions[99,100] and capacity to provide help for B cell immunoglobulin production[99-103] are attenuated during infancy. These functional deficiencies are likely to be the result of a combination of factors that include decreased expression of CD40L,[99,101,102] reduced expression of cytokine receptors,[90,104] and decreased production of a wide range of cytokines following stimulation.[80,84,105-111] The mechanism(s) underlying these reduced cytokine responses are unclear, but factors intrinsic to the T cells themselves,[80,112] as well as those involving accessory cell functions,[112-114] appear to be involved.

The IFN-γ gene is under tight regulation during fetal development, presumably to prevent rejection of the fetus by the mother's immune system that may result from excessive IFN-γ in the uterine environment.[115] Expression of IFN-γ is modulated in part at the epigenetic level via gene methylation, with transcriptional activity inhibited by hypermethylation of DNA. This laboratory has demonstrated hypermethylation at multiple CpG sites in the proximal promoter region of the IFN-γ gene in CD4[+] CD45RA[+] T cells in cord blood relative to their adult counterparts.[116] We subsequently demonstrated that in vitro differentiation of CD4([+]) T cells down the Th1 but not Th2 pathway is accompanied by progressive demethylation of CpG sites in the IFN-γ promoter, which is most marked in neonatal cells.[117] While atopy development by age 2 was not associated with variations in methylation patterns in cord blood T cells, IFN-γ promoter methylation was reduced in CD8([+]) T cells from atopic children in the age range in which hyperproduction of IFN-γ has recently been identified as a common feature of the atopic phenotype.

It has been proposed that many naïve neonatal T cells may have low-affinity TcRs, reduced affinity for T cell activation, and that expansion may take place without production of conventional memory T cells. If this is the case, cytokine responses to antigens in cord blood might have little relevance to immune responses to the same antigens later in childhood. It is possible that the relevance of cord-blood responses to those in later life vary according to antigen. Indeed, the allergen reactivity of neonatal T cells appears to consist predominantly of a default response by recent thymic emigrants which provides an initial burst of short-lived cellular immunity in the absence of conventional T cell memory; this response is limited in duration and intensity by parallel activation of regulatory T cells.[118] Our studies in a longitudinal birth cohort comprised of children at high risk (i.e. one or both parents allergic) examined how the immune function in early childhood relates to infection and development of allergy. We found that priming of Th2 responses associated with persistent HDM-IgE production in a high-risk cohort occurred entirely postnatally, as HDM-reactivity in cord blood appeared to be nonspecific and was unrelated to subsequent development of allergen-specific Th2 memory or IgE.[29] However, a different story emerged when polyclonal responses to mitogen were assessed in this cohort by measuring PHA-induced cytokines from cultured CBMCs, and correlated with rate of respiratory infections up to age 5.[119] The ratio of PHA-induced IL-10/IL-5 was highly predictive of subsequent severe infection, with high IL-5 responses increasing infection risk and high IL-10 responses reducing it. We suggest that the relevant underlying mechanisms may involve IL-10-mediated feedback inhibition of IL-5-dependent eosinophil-induced inflammation, which is a common feature of antiviral responses in early childhood.[119] Additionally, the same immunophenotype appears associated with reduced capacity to produce IL-21,[119] and it is significant to note that a series of recent studies point to a crucial role for this cytokine in resistance to persistent viral infection.[120-122] The relevance of cord blood responses to immune function in later life may depend upon environmental factors and associated exposures to infection during pregnancy. A study performed in a malaria endemic region of Kenya, examining mononuclear cell responses to malaria antigen, found that the fine specificity of lymphocyte proliferation and cytokine secretion was similar in cord and adult blood mononuclear cells.[123] Stimulation with overlapping peptides to identify dominant malaria T cell epitopes also showed that cord blood cells from neonates whose mothers who had been malaria-infected during pregnancy were 4-fold more likely to acquire a peptide-specific immune response. It was therefore proposed that the fetal malaria response functions in a competent adaptive manner which may help to protect neonates from severe malaria during infancy.[123]

Research in recent years has identified a new subset of T helper cells which produce IL-17, named Th17 cells. Th17 cells appear to mediate tissue inflammation by supporting neutrophil recruitment and survival, proinflammatory cytokine production by structural cells and matrix degradation (reviewed in Schmidt-Weber et al[124]). Recent studies have shown that all IL-17-producing cells originate exclusively from CD161[+] naïve CD4[+] T cells of umbilical cord blood and the postnatal thymus in response to a combination of IL-1 beta and IL-23.[125] Human naïve CD4[+] T cells can give rise to either Th1 or Th17 cells in the presence of IL-1 beta and IL-23, with IL-12 presence determining Th1 development. Additionally, a subset of IL-17-producing cells possessed the ability to produce IFN-γ even after their development from CD4[+] T cells, perhaps representing an intermediate Th1/Th17 phenotype.[125]

Innate Immunity in Neonates

Research in recent years has shown that the innate and adaptive arms of the immune system are interconnected. Competent adaptive immune function is important for switching off innate immune responses, and defects in innate immunity are believed to play a role in the development of allergy. Toll-like receptors (TLRs) are central to the function of the innate immune system, and there are at least 10 known human TLRs that recognize pattern motifs present in bacteria, viruses or other prokaryotes.

Premature newborns are particularly susceptible to severe bacterial infections. A study investigating mechanisms behind this phenomenon demonstrated that TLR4 expression is dependent on gestational aging; pre-term infants show decreased expression of TLR4 on monocytes compared to full-term newborns, both of which were lower than in adults.[126] Similarly, cytokine production following bacterial lipopolysaccharide (LPS) stimulation was significantly lower in whole blood cultures from pre-term compared to full-term infants, both of which were significantly lower than those from adults. Subsequent studies examining TLR2 expression found that although TLR2 levels did not differ between pre-term and full-term neonates, levels of the proximal downstream adaptor molecule myeloid differentiation factor MyD88 were significantly reduced in pre-term newborns, along with cytokine responses to TLR2 ligand.[127]

Studies examining the effect of breast-feeding on neonatal innate immune response have found that breast milk from days 1–5 postpartum negatively modulated TLR2 and TLR3 ligand responses, while enhancing those of TLR4 and 5.[128] Breast milk has been found to contain sCD14 and sTLR2 in addition to unidentified TLR-modulatory factors.[129,130] It has been suggested that the differential modulation of TLR function by breast milk may serve to promote efficient response to potentially harmful LPS-producing Gram-negative bacteria via TLR4 while allowing the establishment of Gram-positive bifidobacteria as the predominant intestinal microflora.[128]

Neonatal immune responses to microbial stimuli appear to be affected by maternal allergy. CBMCs from children with atopic mothers have been observed to have significantly lower expression of TLR2 and TLR4 than their mothers, both before and after microbial stimulation, a disparity that was not seen between nonatopic mothers and their children.[131] In addition, CBMC from children with atopic mothers produced less IL-6 in response to peptidoglycan stimulation than those from children with nonatopic mothers.[131] In another study, CBMC stimulation with the TLR2 ligand peptidoglycan led to secretion of IL-10 and induction of FOXP3 which varied according to maternal atopy; CBMCs from newborns with maternal atopy showed reduced induction of these factors compared to those without maternal atopy.[132]

A recent study from our laboratory focused on the ontogeny of the innate immune system and examined the cytokine secretory capacity of mononuclear cells from subjects at various ages between birth and adulthood.[133] Cells were primed with IFN-γ then stimulated with LPS; production of IL-6, IL-10, IL-12, IL-18, IL-23, TNF-α and myxovirus resistance protein A (MXA: a cytokine induced by type I interferon in response to virus infection) was measured and compared. The developmental pattern between 1 year and 13 years showed that levels of all cytokines increased with age, with levels of some cytokines further increasing in adulthood. However, a subset of cytokines showed hyperexpression in CBMCs. There appeared to be major differences in developmental regulation between the MyD88-dependent (TNF-α, IFN-γ, IL-6 and IL-10), cytokines, which were hyperexpressed by CBMCs relative to infant peripheral blood mononuclear cells (PBMCs), compared to the MyD88-independent cytokines (IL-12, IL-18, IL-23 and MXA) which were expressed at lower levels in both CBMCs and PBMCs from infants than in PBMCs from older age groups.[133]

There appears to be a gradual maturation of phagocytic capacity by innate immune cells over time. The phagocytic activity of fetal neutrophils and monocytes has been observed to be significantly lower than that of healthy neonates and adults, and a direct relationship between gestational age and number of phagocytozing granulocytes has been demonstrated.[134] Similarly, the activity of natural killer cells in infants is significantly correlated with gestational age and significantly impaired compared to children and adults.[31]

B Cell Function in Early Life

Certain aspects of B cell function in neonates appear unique in relation to adults. In particular, large numbers of neonatal B cells express CD5,[135,136] together with activation markers such as IL-2R and CD23.[135] It has been postulated that these CD5− B cells act as a 'first line of defense' in primary antibody responses in neonates utilizing a preimmune repertoire, in contrast to CD5− B cells in which response patterns are acquired following antigen contact.[137] Unlike adult B cells, these neonatal B cells proliferate readily in the presence of IL-2 or IL-4 without requirement of further signals.[135,138-140] An additional (albeit less frequent) neonatal B cell subset that expresses IgD, IgM, CD23, and CD11b and is CD5 variable spontaneously secretes IgM antibodies against a range of autoantigens.[135]

Conventional B cell function, that is, antibody production following infection or vaccination, is reduced in infants relative to adults,[64] and some in vitro studies suggest that this may be related to a defect in isotype switching.[141] The relative contributions of the T cell and B cell compartments to this deficiency in immunoglobulin production are widely debated, but the consensus is that both cell types play a role.

As noted previously, T cells in infants do not readily express high levels of CD40L[99-103] unless provided with particularly potent activating stimuli.[142] CD40L represents a critical signal for T helper cell-induced class switching[143] and the generally low expression on neonatal T cells may thus be a limiting factor in the process. Reduced T cell cytokine production[80,84,105-111] may further exacerbate the problem. However, although immunoglobulin production by neonatal B cells is low in the presence of neonatal T helper cells, production levels can be markedly improved if mature T helper cells or adequate soluble signals are provided.[103,138,144] However, the neonatal B cells still fail to reach adult-equivalent levels of production, suggesting that an intrinsic defect also exists.

Antigen-Presenting Cell Populations

The key 'professional' antigen-presenting cell (APC) populations in this context are the mononuclear phagocytes (MPCs), dendritic cells (DCs), and B cells. The precise role of each cell type in different types of immune response is not completely clear, although it is evident that DCs represent the most potent APC for priming the naïve T cell system against antigens encountered at low concentrations (e.g. virus and environmental allergens).

Ontogenic studies on human MPCs have been essentially limited to blood monocytes. Neonatal populations appear comparable to the adult in number and phagocytic activity[145,146] and display reduced chemotactic responses[147] and reduced capacity for secretion of inflammatory cytokines such as tumor necrosis factor-α.[148] Their capacity to present alloantigen to T cells is reportedly normal,[149] but they display reduced levels of MHC class II expression.[150] Several studies have implicated poor accessory cell function of infant blood monocytes as cofactors in the reduced IFN-γ responses of infant T cells to polyclonal mitogens such as PHA,[112-114] possibly as a result of diminished elaboration of costimulator signals. Macrophage populations at mucosal sites such as the lung and airways have important immunoregulatory roles in adults,[151] but it is not clear whether these mechanisms are operative in early life. A murine study from our group indicates lower levels of expression of immunomodulatory molecules including IL-10 and NO by lung macrophages during the neonatal period.[152]

B cells are also recognized as important APCs, in particular for secondary immune responses.[153,154] In murine systems it has been demonstrated that neonatal B cells function poorly as APCs relative to their adult counterparts and do not reach adult-equivalent levels of activity until after weaning.[145,155]

As noted previously, DCs are the most potent APC population in adult experimental animals for initiation of primary immunity and, in this regard, have been designated as the 'gatekeepers' of the immune response.[156] The distribution and phenotypes of these cells appear comparable in murine and human tissues, and it is accordingly reasonable to speculate that the proposed role of murine DCs as the link between the innate and adaptive arms of the immune system[156-159] is also applicable to man. Importantly, in the context of allergic disease comparative studies on DCs from mucosal sites in humans and experimental animals suggest very similar functional characteristics.[160]

DCs commence seeding into peripheral tissues relatively early in gestation,[161] and at birth recognizable networks of these cells can be detected in a variety of tissues including epidermis,[161-163] intestinal mucosa,[164,165] and the upper and lower respiratory tract.[166,167] The cells within these DC networks in perinatal tissues are typically present at lower densities and express lower levels of surface MHC class II relative to adults,[162,163,167] hinting at developmentally related variations in function phenotype. Recent murine studies have emphasized these differences. Notably, the phenomenon of neonatal tolerance in mice has recently been ascribed to the relative inability of neonatal DCs from central lymphoid organs to present Th1-inducing signals to T cells, leading to the preferential generation of Th2-biased immune responses.[168] Of particular relevance to studies on susceptibility to infectious and allergic diseases in infancy, our group has demonstrated that in the rat, the airway mucosal DC compartment develops postnatally very slowly, and does not obtain adult-equivalent levels of tissue density, MHC class II expression, and capacity to respond to local inflammatory stimuli until after biologic weaning.[167,169]

Data based on immunohistochemical studies of autopsy tissues suggest that the kinetics of postnatal maturation of airway DC networks in humans may be comparably slow.[170,171] Recent reports suggest that the numbers of circulating HLA-DR$^+$ DCs are reduced at birth relative to adults[172] and these cells display diminished APC activity.[173] Additionally, analysis of cord blood monocyte-derived DC functions indicates diminished expression of HLA-DR, CD80, and CD40 and attenuated production of IL-12p35 in response to stimuli such as LPS, poly (I:C), and CD40 ligation.[174] However, studies using human CD8$^+$ T cell clones to compare the ability of neonatal and adults DCs to present and process antigen using the MHC class I pathway found that neonatal DCs were not defective in their ability to perform these functions.[175] Recent studies have shown that synergistic stimulation of neonatal DCs by ligands for multiple TLRs is required for efficient differentiation, signaling and T cell priming; membrane associated TLR4 and intracellular TLR3 were found to act in synergy with endosomal TLR4 to induce functional maturation of neonatal DCs.[176] Interestingly, cord blood monocyte-derived DC have also been shown to express higher levels of IL-27 following TLR stimulation, which may compensate for the diminished ability of neonatal DCs to produce IL-12.[177]

Eosinophils and Mast Cells

Eosinophils and mast cells play key roles in the pathogenesis of allergic disease, and perform important functions in relation to host resistance to certain pathogens. Eosinophilia at 3 months of age has been linked to enhanced risk for later development of atopic disease,[178] but little additional data on disease association are available. Several earlier observations are suggestive of developmentally related problems in eosinophil trafficking in early life. In particular, inflammatory exudates in neonates frequently contain elevated numbers of eosinophils,[179–181] and eosinophilia is common in premature infants.[182,183] The mechanism(s) underlying these developmental variations in eosinophil function are unclear, but some evidence suggests a role for integrin expression including Mac-1[184] and L-selectin.[185]

Adult mucosal tissues contain discrete populations of mucosal mast cells (MMCs) and connective tissue mast cells (CTMCs), respectively, within epithelia and underlying lamina propria. No direct information is available on the ontogeny of these MCs in human tissues, but indirect evidence suggests that they seed into gut tissues during infancy in response to local inflammatory stimulation.[186] Our group has examined the kinetics of postnatal development of MCs in the rat respiratory tract, and has reported that both MMC and CTMC populations develop slowly between birth and weaning.[187] MC-derived proteases appear transiently in serum around the time of weaning in the rat, suggesting that the immature MC populations may be unstable or are undergoing local stimulation at this time,[188] and a similar transient peak of MC-tryptase is observed in human serum during infancy.[189]

Direct functional studies on MCs from immature subjects are lacking. However, a 2001 report employed oligonucleotide microarray technology to examine IL-4-induced gene expression in cultured MCs derived from cord blood versus adult peripheral blood, and the results indicate that expression of FcɛR1α is 10-fold higher in adult-derived MCs.[190] This suggests that during infancy the capacity to express IgE-mediated immunity may be restricted.

Vaccine Immunity in Early Life

Significant aspects of immune function are immature at birth, not reaching adult capacity for several years. For example, the in utero generation of vaccine-specific IgM following maternal immunization against either influenzae or tetanus demonstrates the ability of the fetus to generate an active, albeit immature, immune response because no switch from IgM to IgG is evident until later during infancy, following boosting.[191,26] After birth, there is a progressive maturation of the capacity to generate adult-like responses, both quantitatively and qualitatively. After measles-mumps-rubella vaccination, the seroconversion rate against measles is age-dependent, with those vaccinated between 9 and 11 months having significantly lower antibody titers than those vaccinated between 15 and 17 months.[192] In another study, Gans and colleagues[193] observed that, while antibody responses were lower in infants receiving the measles vaccine at 6 months than those vaccinated at 9 or 12 months, there was no significant difference in in vitro antigen-specific IFN-γ or IL-12 production. However, when these responses were compared to those of adults, the infants produced significantly lower levels of IL-12 after in vitro stimulation with measles antigen.[193] These deficient responses in infants were increased to approximate adult responses by the addition of exogenous IL-12 and IL-15, which suggests that lower APC function may play a role in the response of infants.[194] In mice, significant B and T cell vaccine responses were obtained as early as the first year of life. However, neonatal responses differed qualitatively from those in adults, with neonates having a decreased ratio of IgG2a/IgG1 and higher in vitro vaccine-specific IL-5 and decreased IFN-γ.[195]

In a prospective cohort of 132 infants, we have examined the response to the tetanus component of the diphtheria/tetanus/ acellular pertussis (DTaP) vaccine and compared these responses to age-related changes in systemic Th1 and Th2 cytokine function. Our results indicate early Th1 and Th2 cytokine responses to the vaccine antigen. Although Th2 vaccine-specific responses persisted throughout the study period, Th1 responses were transient.[196,197] These results are similar to those observed in mice, with balanced Th1/Th2 vaccine responses generated in neonatal animals. However, Th2 secondary responses predominated in mice first vaccinated as neonates, suggesting that Th1 cells may not be well maintained early in life.[198]

Interestingly, in our study, although vaccine-specific IFN-γ production declined after the final priming DTaP dose at 6 months, between 12 and 18 months in the absence of further vaccination there was a marked resurgence in these responses, coinciding with a parallel increase in overall IFN-γ production capacity.[197] Ausiello and colleagues[199] reported a similar finding in relation to increased pertussis-specific IFN-γ responses in the absence of further vaccination, which was attributed to boosting by covert infection with *Bordetella pertussis*. With regard to our findings, we hypothesize that the vaccine-independent upswing of Th1 responses may reflect boosting by environmental antigens that cross-react with tetanus toxoid. However, given the parallel increase in polyclonal IFN-γ-secreting capacity over the same period, a more likely explanation is that changes in accessory cell function permit more efficient in vitro expression of IFN-γ memory responses by previously primed tetanus toxoid-specific Th1 cells. In this context, it is pertinent to note that it has been demonstrated that given a mature source of accessory cells, peripheral blood T cell IFN-γ production in response to polyclonal mitogen stimulation can be boosted to approximate that of adults.[112,113] Moreover, vaccine-specific Th2 memory responses in PBMCs from previously vaccinated 1-year-old children are markedly enhanced if responding cultures are supplemented with homologous 'in vitro matured' accessory cells.[200] Similarly, vaccination with the use of powerful stimuli such as BCG[201,202] or selective Th1-driving agents such as IL-12,[203] plasmid DNA,[204] and CpG-containing oligonucleotides[205] can all induce adult-like Th1 responses in early life, presumably through activation of accessory cell function.

Slow postnatal maturation of IFN-γ production capacity is linked to genetic risk for atopy. There is some evidence to suggest that delayed Th1 maturation may reduce the capacity of children at high risk of atopy to respond to vaccination efficiently in infancy. In response to BCG vaccination in infancy, failure to develop long-lasting delayed-type hypersensitivity responses to tuberculin was associated with increased risk of atopy at 12 years.[206] In addition, children who develop atopic dermatitis had a reduced ability to respond to pneumococcal vaccination.[207] With regard to the DTP vaccine, we also have observed that infants at high risk of atopy had specific responses to tetanus toxoid that were consistently more Th2 skewed, displaying higher Th2/Th1 ratios.[197] This difference was no longer evident in these subjects at 18 months.[197] Furthermore, in another study we have shown that in vitro proliferative responses to tetanus toxoid during infancy were inversely related to the atopic phenotype.[208] It is important to stress that, in our experience, these differences appear transient, and after the completion of the standard priming/boosting vaccine schedule at age 6 years, there was no significant difference in vaccine response when comparing atopic patients to their nonatopic counterparts.[209] However, the possibility remains that transient hyporesponsiveness to vaccines during infancy in subjects genetically at high risk of developing atopy may confer significant risk for infection from the organisms targeted by the vaccines, and further work needs to be done to clarify this issue.

Postnatal Maturation of Immune Functions and Allergic Sensitization

Studies from a number of groups have highlighted the importance of the early postnatal period in relation to the development of long-lasting response patterns to environmental allergens. In particular, it is becoming clear that initial priming of the naïve immune system typically occurs before weaning and may consolidate into stable immunologic memory before the end of the preschool years. Given that the underlying immunologic processes involve the coordinate operations of the full gamut of innate and adaptive immune mechanisms, issues relating to developmentally determined functional competence during this life phase may be predicted to be of major importance.

In relation to initial priming of the T cell system against allergens, reports from numerous groups indicate the presence of T cells responsive to food and inhalant allergens in cord blood.[210-214] Cloning of these cells and subsequent DNA genotyping indicated fetal as opposed to maternal origin,[215] and the array of cytokines produced in vitro in their responses are dominated by Th2 cytokines, although IFN-γ is also observed, suggestive of a Th0-like pattern.[215] The issue of how initial priming of these cells occurs remains to be resolved. It is possible that transplacental transport of allergen, perhaps conjugated with maternal IgG, may be responsible, and some indirect supporting evidence based on in vitro perfusion studies has been published recently to support this notion.[216] Alternatively, initial T cell priming may be against cross-reacting antigens as opposed to native allergen, and the uncertain relationship between maternal allergen

exposure and newborn T cell reactivity is consistent with this view.[217,218] The mucosal T cell epitope map of the typical cord blood T cell response to ovalbumin (OVA), involving multiple regions of the OVA molecule,[219] suggests major qualitative differences relative to conventional adult T cell responses.

Regardless of how initial T cell responses are primed, it is clear that direct exposure to environmental allergens during infancy drives the early responses down one of two alternate pathways. In the majority of (nonatopic) subjects, the Th2 cytokine component of these early responses progressively diminishes, and by the age of 5 years, in vitro T cell responses to allergens comprise a combination of low-level IFN-γ and IL-10 production.[219-221] In contrast, a subset of children develop positive skin prick test (SPT) reactivity to one or more allergens, and in vitro stimulation of PBMCs with the latter elicits a mixed or Th0-like response pattern comprising IL-4, IL-5, IL-9, IL-10, IL-13, and IFN-γ.[221] This latter pattern closely resembles that seen in the majority of adult atopic patients, and much more commonly develops in atopic family history-positive (AFH+) children than in their AFH- counterparts.

It is increasingly debated whether it remains useful to describe these differing responses in human atopic and nonatopic patients within the framework of the murine Th1/Th2 paradigm, which was based upon the concept of reciprocal and/or antagonistic patterns of Th-memory expression. In this context, recent studies from our group[222,223] indicate that reciprocal patterns of expression of the transcription factor GATA-3, analogous to those that distinguish Th1 from Th2 polarized cell lines (with regard to down-regulation versus up-regulation, respectively, poststimulation), are reiterated during the allergen-specific recall responses of CD4+ T cells from nonatopic versus atopic subjects. This suggests that the Th1/Th2 model still provides a potentially useful framework for the study of allergic responses, despite the strong likelihood of significant interspecies differences.

The central issue in relation to understanding the initial phase of allergic sensitization in childhood concerns the molecular basis for genetic susceptibility to development of Th2-polarized memory against inhalant allergens, and the key to the resolution of this puzzle may lie in a more comprehensive understanding of the mechanisms that drive postnatal maturation of adaptive immune function. In this regard we have reported earlier that genetic risk for atopy was associated with delayed postnatal maturation of Th-cell function, in particular Th1 function, and that this may increase risk for consolidating Th2-polarized memory against allergens during childhood. The evidence originally presented was based on decreased peripheral blood T cell cloning frequency and diminished IFN-γ production by T cell clones in AFH+ infants relative to their counterparts,[80] and these findings have been substantiated in several independent laboratories employing bulk culture studies with neonatal PBMCs.[224-229] We have proposed that this phenomenon may derive from inappropriate postnatal persistence of one or more of the mechanisms responsible for selective damping of Th1 immunity during fetal life.[230] Alternatively, given that the postnatal maturation of adaptive immunity is essentially driven by microbial signals from the outside environment,[230-232] one or more deficiencies in relevant receptors or downstream signaling pathways may retard this process. Genetic variations described in CD14 may be an archetypal example,[233,234] and similar variants in one or more of the Toll receptor genes constitute additional likely candidates. These possibilities are of particular interest in light of reports that environmental exposure to airborne bacterial lipopolysaccharide in childhood may be protective against Th2-mediated sensitization to inhalant allergens.[235,236] Environmental exposures to a farming environment, endotoxin in house dust and exposure to cats and dogs in the first three months of life have been found to enhance IFN-γ-producing capacity.[237]

Although low IFN-γ response capacity in neonates has been identified as a risk factor for allergy by our group and others, longitudinal studies have suggested that this Th1 deficiency may be transient and reversible, such that by 18 months of age, Th1 function in children with atopic family history is equivalent to or greater than that in children without atopic family history.[197] We found in studies focusing on CBMC from AFH+ children that early development of sensitization amongst this low-IFN-γ-producing group is maximal amongst those with the highest IFN-γ responses, suggesting a potentially dualistic role for IFN-γ in atopy pathogenesis.[238] This conclusion is reinforced by the results of other studies in older (school age) children which suggest a positive role for IFN-γ in airway symptomatology in atopics.[239,240]

Further research is required to elucidate the complex regulatory mechanisms that govern generation of different patterns of allergen-specific Th memory during childhood. However, it is also becoming clear that an additional, and related, set of complexities needs to be considered. It is now evident that only a subset of atopic patients progress to development of severe persistent allergic diseases, in particular atopic asthma,[241] and it is likely that these subjects suffer additional and/or particularly intense inflammatory insults to target tissues. In this context, epidemiologic evidence suggests that risk for development of persistent asthma is most marked in children who display early allergic sensitization to inhalants[242,243] and who develop severe wheezing and lower respiratory tract infections during infancy.[243-245] This has given rise to the suggestion that susceptibility to development of the airways remodeling characteristic of chronic asthma[246] may, in many circumstances, be the long-term result of inflammation-induced changes in lung and airway differentiation during critical stages of early growth during childhood. It is additionally noteworthy that resistance to respiratory infections is also mediated by the same Th1 mechanisms just identified as attenuated in children at risk of atopy,[247] suggesting that the same set of genetic mechanisms may be responsible for airways inflammation induced via the viral infection and atopic pathways in children at high risk of asthma (Box 6-2).

An additional variable that merits more detailed research in this context is the role of airway DC populations. In the adult, these cells regulate the Th1/Th2 balance in immune responses to airborne antigens[248] and also mediate primary and secondary immunity to viral pathogens.[156] However, airway DC networks develop very slowly postnatally, apparently 'driven' by exposure to inhaled airborne irritants,[134] in particular bacterial LPS.[249,250] Hence the rate at which this key cell population gains competence to respond to maturation-inducing stimuli, and then to orchestrate appropriately balanced T cell responses against viral pathogens and allergens, may be a key determinant of overall susceptibility to allergic disease. Variations in the genes that govern the functions of these cells in early life are thus likely to be of major importance in the etiology of a variety of disease processes, in particular atopic asthma and related syndromes.

As only a subset of patients with atopy develop more severe allergic diseases, the ability to identify these patients early, and to choose treatment strategies accordingly, could potentially improve patient outcome. A variety of independent studies suggest that prospective evaluation of blood IgE levels, particularly in early childhood, may significantly aid in early identification of at-risk subjects.[251]

References

1. Lambropoulou M, Tamiolakis D, Venizelos I, et al. Induction of hepatic haematopoiesis with fibronectin expression by EMT stromal cells during the second trimester of development. Clin Exp Med 2007;7:115–21.
2. Haynes BF, Martin ME, Kay HH, et al. Early events in human T cell ontogeny: phenotypic characterization and immunohistologic localization of T cell precursors in early human fetal tissues. J Exp Med 1988;168:1061–80.
3. Compana D, Janossy G, Coustan-Smith E, et al. The expression of T cell receptor-associated proteins during T cell ontogeny in man. J Immunol 1989;142:57–66.
4. Haynes BF, Singer KH, Denning SM, et al. Analysis of expression of CD2, CD3, and T cell antigen receptor molecules during early human fetal thymic development. J Immunol 1988;141:3776–84.
5. Migliaccio G, Migliaccio AR, Petti S, et al. Human embryonic hemopoiesis: kinetics of progenitors and precursors underlying the yolk sac to liver transition. J Clin Invest 1986;78:51–60.
6. Asma GEM, Van Den Bergh RL, Vossen JM. Use of monoclonal antibodies in a study of the development of T lymphocytes in the human fetus. Clin Exp Immunol 1983;53:429–36.
7. Royo C, Touraine J-L, De Bouteiller O. Ontogeny of T lymphocyte differentiation in the human fetus: acquisition of phenotype and functions. Thymus 1987;10:57–73.
8. Timens W, Rozeboom T, Poppema S. Fetal and neonatal development of human spleen: an immunohistological study. Immunology 1987;60:603–9.
9. Markgraf R, von Gaudecker B, Muller-Hermelink H-K. The development of the human lymph node. Cell Tissue Res 1982;225:387–413.
10. Vellguth S, von Gaudecker B, Muller-Hermelink H-K. The development of the human spleen: ultrastructural studies in fetuses from the 14th to 24th week of gestation. Cell Tissue Res 1985;242:579–92.
11. Namikawa R, Mizuno T, Matsuoka H, et al. Ontogenic development of T and B cells and non-lymphoid cells in the white pulp of human spleen. Immunology 1986;57:61–9.
12. Fichtelius KE. The gut epithelium: a first level lymphoid organ? Exp Cell Res 1968;49:87–104.
13. Spencer J, MacDonald TT, Finn T, et al. The development of gut-associated lymphoid tissue in the terminal ileum of fetal human intestine. Clin Exp Immunol 1986;64:536–43.
14. Latthe M, Terry L, MacDonald TT. High frequency of CD8 alpha alpha homodimer-bearing T cells in human fetal intestine. Eur J Immunol 1994;24:1703–5.
15. Howie D, Spencer J, DeLord D, et al. Extrathymic T cell differentiation in the human intestine early in life. J Immunol 1998;161:5862–72.
16. McVay LD, Jaswal SS, Kennedy C, et al. The generation of human gamma delta T cell repertoires during fetal development. J Immunol 1998;160:5851–60.
17. Wucherpfennig KW, Liao YJ, Prendergast M, et al. Human fetal liver gamma/delta T cells predominantly use unusual rearrangements of the T cell receptor delta and gamma loci expressed on both CD4+ CD8- and CD4- CD8- gamma/delta T cells. J Exp Med 1993;177:425–32.
18. Stites DP, Carr MC, Fudenberg HH. Ontogeny of cellular immunity in the human fetus: development of responses to phytohaemagglutinin and to allogeneic cells. Cell Immunol 1974;11:257–71.
19. Aase JM, Noren GR, Reddy DV, et al. Mumps-virus infection in pregnant women and the immunologic response of their offspring. N Engl J Med 1972;286:1379–82.

BOX 6-2 Key concepts

Role of Immune Developmental Factors on Allergic Response

- Dendritic cells (DCs) are the most potent antigen-presenting cells for priming naïve T cells against antigens encountered at low concentrations.
- Neonatal DCs present weak Th1-inducing signals to T cells, leading to preferential generation of Th2 immune responses.
- Slow postnatal maturation of interferon-gamma production capacity is linked to genetic risk for atopy.
- Postnatal maturation of adaptive immunity is driven by microbial signals.
- A deficiency in microbial receptors (e.g. CD14, Toll receptors) or downstream signaling pathways may prevent the development of polarized Th1 responses.

20. Sanjeevi CB, Vivekanandan S, Narayanan PR. Fetal response to maternal ascariasis as evidenced by anti-*Ascaris lumbricoides* IgM antibodies in the cord blood. Acta Pediatr Scand 1991;80:1134–8.

21. Fievet N, Ringwald P, Bickii J. Malaria cellular immune responses in neonates from Cameroon. Parasite Immunol 1996;18:483–90.

22. Novato-Silva E, Gazzinelli G, Colley DG. Immune responses during human schistosomiasis mansoni. XVIII. Immunologic status of pregnant women and their neonates. Scand J Immunol 1992;35:429–47.

23. King CL, Malhotra I, Mungai P, et al. B cell sensitization to helminthic infection develops in utero in humans. J Immunol 1998;160:3578–84.

24. McLeod R, Mack DG, Boyer K, et al. Phenotypes and functions of lymphocytes in congenital toxoplasmosis. J Lab Clin Med 1990;116:623–35.

25. Gill TJ, Repetti CF, Metlay LA. Transplacental immunisation of the human fetus to tetanus by immunisation of the mother. J Clin Invest 1983;72:987–96.

26. Rastogi D, Wang C, Mao X, et al. Antigen-specific immune responses to influenza vaccine in utero. J Clin Invest 2007;117:1637–46.

27. Holt PG. Primary allergic sensitization to environmental antigens: perinatal T cell priming as a determinant of responder phenotype in adulthood. J Exp Med 1996;183:1297–1301.

28. Pfefferle PI, Sel S, Ege MJ, et al. Cord blood allergen-specific IgE is associated with reduced IFN-gamma production by cord blood cells: the Protection against Allergy-Study in Rural Environments (PASTURE) Study. J Allergy Clin Immunol 2008;122:711–6.

29. Rowe J, Kusel M, Holt BJ, et al. Prenatal versus postnatal sensitization to environmental allergens in a high-risk birth cohort. J Allergy Clin Immunol 2007;119:1164–73.

30. Holt PG. Prenatal versus postnatal priming of allergen specific immunologic memory: the debate continues. J Allergy Clin Immunol 2008;122:717–8.

31. Gasparoni A, Ciardelli L, Avanzini A, et al. Age-related changes in intracellular TH1/TH2 cytokine production, immunoproliferative T lymphocyte response and natural killer cell activity in newborns, children and adults. Biol Neonate 2003;84:297–303.

32. Perez A, Gurbindo MD, Resino S, et al. NK cell increase in neonates from the preterm to the full-term period of gestation. Neonatology 2007;92:158–63.

33. Byrne JA, Stankovic AK, Cooper MD. A novel subpopulation of primed T cells in the human fetus. J Immunol 1994;152:3098–106.

34. Michaelsson J, Mold JE, McCune JM, et al. Regulation of T cell responses in the developing human fetus. J Immunol 2006;176:5741–8.

35. Yu P, Haymaker CL, Divekar RD, et al. Fetal exposure to high-avidity TCR ligand enhances expansion of peripheral T regulatory cells. J Immunol 2008;181:73–80.

36. Schaub B, Liu J, Hoppler S, et al. Impairment of T-regulatory cells in cord blood of atopic mothers. J Allergy Clin Immunol 2008;121:1491–9, 1499 e1–13.

37. Wegmann TG, Lin H, Guilbert L, et al. Bidirectional cytokine interactions in the maternal-fetal relationship: is successful pregnancy a Th2 phenomenon? Immunol Today 1993;14:353–6.

38. Herzenberg LA, Bianchi DW, Schroder J, et al. Fetal cells in the blood of pregnant women: detection and enrichment by fluorescence-activated cell sorting. Proc Natl Acad Sci U S A 1979;76:1453–5.

39. Lo Y-MD, Wainscoat JS, Gillmer MDG, et al. Prenatal sex determination by DNA amplification from maternal peripheral blood. Lancet 1989;9:1363–5.

40. Bianchi DW, Zickwolf GK, Yih MC, et al. Erythroid-specific antibodies enhance detection of fetal nucleated erythrocytes in maternal blood. Prenat Diagn 1993;13:293–300.

41. Wachtel S, Elias S, Price J, et al. Fetal cells in the maternal circulation: isolation by multiparameter flow cytometry and confirmation by polymerase chain reaction. Hum Reprod 1991;6:1466–9.

42. Price JO, Elias S, Wachtel SS, et al. Prenatal diagnosis with fetal cells isolated from maternal blood by multiparameter flow cytometry. Am J Obstet Gynecol 1994;165:1731–7.

43. Bonney EA, Matzinger P. The maternal immune system's interaction with circulating fetal cells. J Immunol 1997;158:40–7.

44. Munn DH, Zhou M, Attwood JT, et al. Prevention of allogeneic fetal rejection by tryptophan catabolism. Science 1998;281:1191–3.

45. Roth I, Corry DB, Locksley RM, et al. Human placental cytotrophoblasts produce the immunosuppressive cytokine interleukin 10. J Exp Med 1996;184:539–48.

46. Kzhyshkowska J, Gratchev A, Schmuttermaier C, et al. Alternatively activated macrophages regulate extracellular levels of the hormone placental lactogen via receptor-mediated uptake and transcytosis. J Immunol 2008;180:3028–37.

47. Guller S, LaChapelle L. The role of placental Fas ligand in maintaining immune privilege at maternalfetal interface. Semin Reprod Endocrinol 1999;17:39–44.

48. Hammer A, Blaschitz A, Daxbock C, et al. Gas and Fasligand are expressed in the uteroplacental unit of first-trimester pregnancy. Am J Reprod Immunol 1999;41:41–51.

49. Tilburgs T, Roelen DL, van der Mast BJ, et al. Evidence for a selective migration of fetus-specific CD4+CD25bright regulatory T cells from the peripheral blood to the decidua in human pregnancy. J Immunol 2008;180:5737–45.

50. Ashkar AA, Di Santo JP, Croy BA. Interferon gamma contributes to initiation of uterine vascular modification, decidual integrity, and uterine natural killer cell maturation during normal murine pregnancy. J Exp Med 2000;192:259–69.

51. Krishnan L, Guilbert LJ, Wegmann TG, et al. T helper 1 response against *Leishmania major* in pregnant C57BL/6 mice increases implantation failure and fetal resorptions. J Immunol 1996;156:653–62.

52. Krishnan L, Guilbert LJ, Russell AS, et al. Pregnancy impairs resistance of C57BL/6 mice to *Leishmania major* infection and causes decreased antigen-specific IFN-g responses and increased production of T helper 2 cytokines. J Immunol 1996;156:644–52.

53. Hilkens CM, Vermeulen H, Joost van Neerven RJ, et al. Differential modulation of T helper type 1 (Th1) and T helper type 2 (Th2) cytokine secretion by prostaglandin E$_2$ critically depends on interleukin-2. Eur J Immunol 1995;25:59–63.

54. Piccinni M-P, Giudizi M-G, Biagiotti R, et al. Progesterone favours the development of human T helper cells producing Th2-type cytokines and promotes both IL-4 production and membrane CD30 expression in established Th1 cell clones. J Immunol 1995;155:128–33.

55. Szekeres-Bartho J, Faust Z, Varga P, et al. The immunological pregnancy-protective effect of progesterone is manifested via controlling cytokine production. Am J Reprod Immunol 1996;35:348–51.

56. Szekeres-Bartho J, Wegmann TG. A progesterone-dependent immunomodulatory protein alters the Th1/Th2 balance. J Reprod Immunol 1996;31:81–95.

57. Miller ME. Phagocyte function in the neonate: selected aspects. Pediatrics 1979;64:709–12.

58. Wilson CB. Immunologic basis for increased susceptibility of the neonate to infection. J Pediatr 1986;108:1–12.

59. Burchett SK, Corey L, Mohan KM, et al. Diminished interferon-g and lymphocyte proliferation in neonatal and postpartum primary herpes simplex virus infection. J Infect Dis 1992;165:813–8.

60. Siegrist CA. Vaccination in the neonatal period and early infancy. Int Rev Immunol 2000;19:195–219.

61. Friedmann PS. Cell-mediated immunological reactivity in neonates and infants with congenital syphilis. Clin Exp Immunol 1977;30:271–6.

62. Starr SE, Tolpin MD, Friedman HM, et al. Impaired cellular immunity to cytomegalovirus in congenitally infected children and their mothers. J Infect Dis 1979;140:500–5.

63. Hayward AR, Herberger M, Saunders D. Herpes simplex virus-stimulated gamma-interferon production by newborn mononuclear cells. Pediatr Res 1986;20:398–400.

64. Hayward AR, Groothuis J. Development of T cells with memory phenotype in infancy. Adv Exp Med Biol 1991;310:71–6.

65. Comans-Bitter WM, de Groot R, van den Beemd R, et al. Immunophenotyping of blood lymphocytes in childhood: reference values for lymphocyte subpopulations. J Pediatr 1997;130:388–93.

66. de Vries E, de Bruin-Versteeg S, Comans-Bitter WM, et al. Longitudinal survey of lymphocyte subpopulations in the first year of life, Pediatr Res 2000; 47:528–37.

67. Griffiths-Chu S, Patterson JAK, Berger CL, et al. Characterization of immature T cell subpopulations in neonatal blood. Blood 1984;64:296–300.

68. Maccario R, Nespoli L, Mingrat G, et al. Lymphocyte subpopulations in the neonate: identification of an immature subset of OKT8-positive, OKT3-negative cells. J Immunol 1983;130:1129–31.

69. Clement LT, Vink PE, Bradley GE. Novel immunoregulatory functions of phenotypically distinct subpopulations of CD4+ cells in the human neonate. J Immunol 1990;145:102–8.

70. Hassan J, Reen DJ. Human recent thymic emigrants: identification, expansion and survival characteristics. J Immunol 2001;167:1970–6.

71. Hassan J, Reen DJ. IL-7 promotes the survival and maturation but not differentiation of human postthymic CD4 + T cells. Eur J Immunol 1998;28:3057–65.

72. Hannet I, Erkeller-Yuksel F, Lydyard P, et al. Developmental and maturational changes in human blood lymphocyte subpopulations. Immunol Today 1992;13:215–8.

73. Calado RT, Garcia AB, Falcao RP. Age-related changes of immunophenotypically immature lymphocytes in normal human peripheral blood. Cytometry 1999;38:133–7.

74. Hassan J, Reen DJ. Neonatal CD4+ CD45RA+ T cells: precursors of adult CD4+ CD45RA+ T cells? Res Immunol 1993;144:87–92.

75. Sanders ME, Makgoba MW, Shaw S. Human naive and memory T cells: reinterpretation of helper-inducer and suppressor-inducer subsets. Immunol Today 1988;9:195–9.

76. Gerli R, Bertotto A, Spinozzi F, et al. Phenotypic dissection of cord blood immunoregulatory T cell subsets by using a two-color immunofluorescence study. Clin Immunol Immunopathol 1986;40:429–35.

77. Kingsley G, Pitzalis C, Waugh A, et al. Correlation of immunoregulatory function with cell phenotype in cord blood lymphocytes. Clin Exp Immunol 1988;73:40–5.

78. Bradley L, Bradley J, Ching D, et al. Predominance of T cells that express CD45R in the CD4 + helper/inducer lymphocyte subset of neonates. Clin Immunol Immunopathol 1989;51:426–35.

79. Hayward A, Lee J, Beverley PCL. Ontogeny of expression of UCHL1 antigen on TcR-1 + (CD4/8) and TcR delta + T cells. *Euro* J Immunol 1989;19:771–3.

80. Holt PG, Clough JB, Holt BJ, et al. Genetic 'risk' for atopy is associated with delayed postnatal maturation of T cell competence. Clin Exp Allergy 1992;22:1093–9.

81. Pirenne H, Aujard Y, Eljaafari A, et al. Comparison of T cell functional changes during childhood with the ontogeny of CDw29 and CD45RA expression on CD4+ T cells. Pediatr Res 1992;32:81–6.

82. Stern DA, Hicks MJ, Martinez FD, et al. Lymphocyte subpopulation number and function in infancy. Dev Immunol 1992;2:175–9.

83. Hassan J, Reen DJ. Cord blood CD4 + CD45RA + T cells achieve a lower magnitude of activation when compared with their adult counterparts, Immunology 1997;90:397–401.

84. Hassan J, Reen DJ. Reduced primary antigen-specific T cell precursor frequencies in neonates is associated with deficient interleukin-2 production. Immunology 1996;87:604–8.

85. Bertotto A, Gerli R, Lanfrancone L, et al. Activation of cord T lymphocytes. II. Cellular and molecular analysis of the defective response induced by anti-CD3 monoclonal antibody. Cell Immunol 1990;127:247–59.

86. Gerli R, Agea E, Muscat C, et al. Activation of cord T lymphocytes. III. Role of LFA-1/ICAM-1 and CD2/LFA-3 adhesion molecules in CD3-induced proliferative response. Cell Immunol 1993;148:32–47.

87. Hassan J, O'Neill S, O'Neill LAJ, et al. Signaling via DC28 of human naive neonatal T lymphocytes. Clin Exp Immunol 1995;102:192–8.

88. Early EM, Reen DJ. Antigen-independent responsiveness to interleukin-4 demonstrates differential regulation of newborn human T cells. Eur J Immunol 1996;26:2885–9.

89. Shu U, Demeure CE, Byun D-G, et al. Interleukin 12 exerts a differential effect on the maturation of neonatal and adult human CD45RO – CD4 T cells. J Clin Invest 1994;94:1352–8.

90. Zola H, Fusco M, Weedon H, et al. Reduced expression of the interleukin-2-receptor g chain on cord blood lymphocytes: relationship to functional immaturity of the neonatal immune response. Immunology 1996;87:86–91.

91. Upham JW, Lee PT, Holt BJ, et al. Development of interleukin-12-producing capacity throughout childhood. Infect Immun 2002;70:6583–8.

92. Takahashi N, Imanishi K, Nishida H, et al. Evidence for immunologic immaturity of cord blood T cells. J Immunol 1995;155:5213–9.

93. Macardle PJ, Wheatland L, Zola H. Analysis of the cord blood T lymphocyte response to superantigen. Hum Immunol 1999;60:127–39.

94. Porcu P, Gaddy J, Broxmeyer HE. Alloantigen-induced unresponsiveness in cord blood T lymphocytes is associated with defective activation of Ras. Proc Natl Acad Sci U S A 1998;95:4538–43.

95. Miscia S, Du Baldassarre A, Sabatino G, et al. Inefficient phospholipase C activation and reduced Lck expression characterize the signaling defect of umbilical cord T lymphocytes. J Immunol 1999;163:2416–24.

96. Whisler RL, Newhouse YG, Grants IS, et al. Differential expression of the a- and b-isoforms of protein kinase C in peripheral blood T and B cells from young and elderly adults. Mech Ageing Dev 1995;77:197–211.

97. Sato K, Nagayama H, Takahasji TA. Aberrant CD3- and CD28-mediated signaling events in cord blood T cells are associated with dysfunctional regulation of Fas ligand-mediated cytotoxicity. J Immunol 1999;162:4464–71.

98. Sato K, Kawasaki H, Nagayama H, et al. Chemokine receptor expressions and responsiveness of cord blood T cells. J Immunol 2001;166:1659–66.

99. Andersson U, Bird AG, Britten S, et al. Human and cellular immunity in humans studied at the cellular level from birth to two years. Immunol Rev 1981;57:5–19.

100. Hayward AR. Development of lymphocyte responses in humans, the fetus and newborn. Immunol Rev 1981;57:43–61.

101. Durandy A, De Saint Basile G, Lisowska-Grospierre B, et al. Undetectable CD40 ligand expression on T cells and low B cell responses to CD40 binding antagonists in human newborns. J Immunol 1995;154:1560–8.

102. Fuleihan R, Ahern D, Geha RS. Decreased expression of the ligand for CD40 in newborn lymphocytes. Eur J Immunol 1994;24:1925–8.

103. Splawski JB, Lipsky PE. Cytokine regulation of immunoglobulin secretion by neonatal lymphocytes. J Clin Invest 1991;88:967–77.

104. Zola H, Fusco M, MacArdle PJ, et al. Expression of cytokine receptors by human cord blood lymphocytes: comparison with adult blood lymphocytes. Pediatr Res 1995;38:397–403.

105. Lee SM, Suen Y, Chang L, et al. Decreased interleukin-12 (IL-12) from activated cord versus adult peripheral blood mononuclear cells and up-regulation of interferon-g, natural killer, and lymphokine-activated killer activity by IL-12 in cord blood mononuclear cells. Blood 1996;88:945–54.

106. Chheda S, Palkowetz KH, Garofalo R, et al. Decreased interleukin-10 production by neonatal monocytes and T cells: relationship to decreased production and expression of tumor necrosis factor-a and its receptors. Pediatr Res 1996;40:475–83.

107. Qian JX, Lee SM, Suen Y, et al. Decreased interleukin-15 from activated cord versus adult peripheral blood mononuclear cells and the effect of interleukin-15 in upregulating antitumor immune activity and cytokine production in cord blood. Blood 1997;90:3106–17.

108. Scott ME, Kubin M, Kohl S. High level interleukin-12 production, but diminished interferon-g production, by cord blood mononuclear cells. Pediatr Res 1997;41:547–53.

109. Kotiranta-Ainamo A, Rautonen J, Rautonen N. Interleukin-10 production by cord blood mononuclear cells. Pediatr Res 1997;41:110–3.

110. Chalmers IMH, Janossy G, Contreras M, et al. Intracellular cytokine profile of cord and adult blood lymphocytes. Blood 1998;92:11–8.

111. Adkins B. T cell function in newborn mice and humans. Immunol Today 1999;20:330–5.

112. Wilson CB, Westall J, Johnston L, et al. Decreased production of interferon gamma by human neonatal cells: intrinsic and regulatory deficiencies. J Clin Invest 1986;77:860–7.

113. Taylor S, Bryson YJ. Impaired production of gamma-interferon by newborn cells *in vitro* is due to a functionally immature macrophage. J Immunol 1985;134:1493–8.

114. Lewis DB, Yu CC, Meyer J, et al. Cellular and molecular mechanisms for reduced interleukin 4 and interferon-gamma production by neonatal T cells. J Clin Invest 1991;87:194–202.

115. Murphy SP, Tayade C, Ashkar AA, et al. Interferon gamma in successful pregnancies. Biol Reprod 2009;80:848–59.

116. White GP, Watt PM, Holt BJ, et al. Differential patterns of methylation of the IFN-(γ promoter at CpG and non-CpG sites underlie differences in IFN-(γ gene expression between human neonatal and adult CD45RO- T cells. J Immunol 2002;168:2820–7.

117. White GP, Hollams EM, Yerkovich ST, et al. CpG methylation patterns in the IFNgamma promoter in naive T cells: variations during Th1 and Th2 differentiation and between atopics and non-atopics. Pediatr Allergy Immunol 2006;17:557–64.

118. Thornton CA, Upham JW, Wikstrom ME, et al. Functional maturation of CD4+CD25+CTLA4+CD45RA+ T regulatory cells in human neonatal T cell responses to environmental antigens/allergens. J Immunol 2004;173:3084–92.

119. Zhang G, Rowe J, Kusel M, et al. Interleukin-10/interleukin-5 responses at birth predict risk for respiratory infections in children with atopic family history. Am J Respir Crit Care Med 2009;179:205–11.

120. Frohlich A, Kisielow J, Schmitz I, et al. IL-21R on T cells is critical for sustained functionality and control of chronic viral infection. Science 2009;324:1576–80.

121. Elsaesser H, Sauer K, Brooks DG. IL-21 is required to control chronic viral infection. Science 2009;324:1569–72.

122. Yi JS, Du M, Zajac AJ. A vital role for interleukin-21 in the control of a chronic viral infection. Science 2009;324:1572–6.

123. Malhotra I, Wamachi AN, Mungai PL, et al. Fine specificity of neonatal lymphocytes to an abundant malaria blood-stage antigen: epitope mapping of *Plasmodium falciparum* MSP1(33). J Immunol 2008;180:3383–90.

124. Schmidt-Weber CB, Akdis Mb, Akdis CA. TH17 cells in the big picture of immunology. J Allergy Clin Immunol 2007;120:247–54.

125. Cosmi L, De Palma R, Santarlasci V, et al. Human interleukin 17-producing cells originate from a CD161+CD4+ T cell precursor. J Exp Med 2008;205:1903–16.

126. Forster-Waldl E, Sadeghi K, Tamandl D, et al. Monocyte toll-like receptor 4 expression and LPS-induced cytokine production increase during gestational aging. Pediatr Res 2005;58:121–4.

127. Sadeghi K, Berger A, Langgartner M, et al. Immaturity of infection control in preterm and term newborns is associated with impaired toll-like receptor signaling. J Infect Dis 2007;195:296–302.

128. LeBouder E, Rey-Nores JE, Raby AC, et al. Modulation of neonatal microbial recognition: TLR-mediated innate immune responses are specifically and differentially modulated by human milk. J Immunol 2006;176:3742–52.

129. Labeta MO, Vidal K, Nores JE, et al. Innate recognition of bacteria in human milk is mediated by a milk-derived highly expressed pattern recognition receptor, soluble CD14. J Exp Med 2000;191:1807–12.

130. LeBouder E, Rey-Nores JE, Rushmere NK, et al. Soluble forms of Toll-like receptor (TLR)2 capable of modulating TLR2 signaling are present in human plasma and breast milk. J Immunol 2003;171:6680–9.

131. Amoudruz P, Holmlund U, Malmstrom V, et al. Neonatal immune responses to microbial stimuli: is there an influence of maternal allergy? J Allergy Clin Immunol 2005;115:1304–10.

132. Schaub B, Campo M, He H, et al. Neonatal immune responses to TLR2 stimulation: influence of maternal atopy on Foxp3 and IL-10 expression. Respir Res 2006;7:40.

133. Yerkovich ST, Wikstrom ME, Suriyaarachchi D, et al. Postnatal development of monocyte cytokine responses to bacterial lipopolysaccharide. Pediatr Res 2007;62:547-52.

134. Strunk T, Temming P, Gembruch U, et al. Differential maturation of the innate immune response in human fetuses. Pediatr Res 2004;56:219-26.

135. Barbouche R, Forveille M, Fischer A, et al. Spontaneous IgM autoantibody production in vitro by B lymphocytes of normal human neonates. Scand J Immunol 1992;35:659-67.

136. Durandy A, Thuillier L, Forveille M, et al. Phenotypic and functional characteristics of human newborns' B lymphocytes. J Immunol 1990;144:60-5.

137. Casali P, Notkins AL. CD5 + B lymphocytes polyreactive antibodies and the human B cell repertoire. Immunol Today 1989;10:364-7.

138. Watson W, Oen K, Ramdahin R, et al. Immunoglobulin and cytokine production by neonatal lymphocytes. Clin Exp Immunol 1991;83:169-74.

139. Caligaris-Cappio F, Riva M, Tesio L, et al. Human normal CD5 + B lymphocytes can be induced to differentiate to CD5 – B lymphocytes with germinal center cell features. Blood 1989;73:1259-64.

140. Punnonen J. The role of interleukin-2 in the regulation of proliferation and IgM synthesis of human newborn mononuclear cells. Clin Exp Immunol 1989;75:421-5.

141. Lewis DB, Wilson CB. Developmental immunology and role of host defenses in fetal and neonatal susceptibility to infection. In: Remington JS, Klein JO, eds: Infectious diseases of the fetus and newborn infant. Philadelphia: WB Saunders; 2001.

142. Splawski JB, Nishioka J, Nishioka Y, et al. CD40 ligand is expressed and functional on activated T cells. J Immunol 1996;156:119-27.

143. Stavnezer J. Antibody class switching. Adv Immunol 1996;61:79-146.

144. Gauchat JF, Gauchat D, De Weck AL, et al. Cytokine mRNA levels in antigen-stimulated peripheral blood mononuclear cells. Eur J Immunol 1989;7:804-10.

145. Morris JF, Hoyer JT, Pierce SK. Antigen presentation for T cell interleukin-2 secretion is a late acquisition of neonatal B cells. Eur J Immunol 1992;22:2923-8.

146. Van Tol MJD, Ziljstra J, Thomas CMG, et al. Distinct role of neonatal and adult monocytes in the regulation of the in vitro antigen-induced plaque-forming cell response in man. J Immunol 1984;134:1902-8.

147. Serushago B, Issekutz AC, Lee SH, et al. Deficient tumour necrosis factor secretion by cord blood mononuclear cells upon in vitro stimulation with Listeria monocytogenes. J Interferon Cytokine Res 1996;16:381-7.

148. Weston WL, Carson BS, Barkin RM, et al. Monocyte-macrophage function in the newborn. Am J Dis Child 1977;131:1241-2.

149. Clerici M, DePalma L, Roilides E, et al. Analysis of T helper and antigen-presenting cell functions in cord blood and peripheral blood leukocytes from healthy children of different ages. J Clin Invest 1993;91:2829-36.

150. Stiehm ER, Sztein MB, Oppenheim JJ. Deficient DR antigen expression on human cord blood monocytes: reversal with lymphokines. Clin Immunol Immunopathol 1984;30:430-6.

151. Holt PG. Regulation of antigen-presenting cell function(s) in lung and airway tissues. Eur Respir J 1993;6:120-9.

152. Lee PT, Holt PG, McWilliam AS. Ontogeny of rat pulmonary alveolar function: evidence for a selective deficiency in IL-10 and nitric oxide production by newborn alveolar macrophages. Cytokine 2001;15:53-7.

153. Chesnut RW, Grey HM. Antigen presentation by B cells and its significance in T-B interactions. Adv Immunol 1986;39:51-82.

154. Pierce SK, Morris JF, Grusby MJ, et al. Antigen-presenting function of B lymphocytes. Immunol Rev 1988;106:149-56.

155. Muthukkumar S, Goldstein J, Stein KE. The ability of B cells and dendritic cells to present antigen increases ontogeny. J Immunol 2000;165:4803-13.

156. Steinman RM. The dendritic cell system and its role in immunogenicity. Annu Rev Immunol 1991;9:271-96.

157. Janeway CA. The immune response evolved to discriminate infectious nonself from noninfectious self. Immunol Today 1992;13:11-16.

158. McWilliam AS, Napoli S, Marsh AM, et al. Dendritic cells are recruited into the airway epithelium during the inflammatory response to a broad spectrum of stimuli. J Exp Med 1996;184:2429-32.

159. Matzinger P. Tolerance, danger, and the extended family. Annu Rev Immunol 1994;12:991-1045.

160. Holt PG, Stumbles PA. Regulation of immunologic homeostasis in peripheral tissues by dendritic cells: the respiratory tract as a paradigm. J Allergy Clin Immunol 2000;105:421-9.

161. Foster CA, Holbrook KA. Ontogeny of Langerhans cells in human embryonic and fetal skin: cell densities and phenotypic expression relative to epidermal growth. Am J Anat 1989;184:157-64.

162. Mizoguchi S, Takahashi K, Takeya M, et al. Development, differentiation and proliferation of epidermal Langerhans cells in rat ontogeny studied by a novel monoclonal antibody against epidermal Langerhans cells, RED-1. J Leukoc Biol 1992;52:52-61.

163. Romani N, Schuler G, Fritsch P. Ontogeny of Ia-positive and Thy-1-positive leukocytes of murine epidermis. J Invest Dermatol 1986;86:129-33.

164. Mayrhofer G, Pugh CW, Barclay AN. The distribution, ontogeny and origin in the rat of Ia-positive cells with dendritic morphology and of Ia antigen in epithelia, with special reference to the intestine. Eur J Immunol 1983;13:112-22.

165. Brandtzaeg P, Halstensen TS, Huitfeldt HS, et al. Epithelial expression of HLA, secretory component (poly-Ig receptor), and adhesion molecules in the human alimentary tract. Ann N Y Acad Sci 1992;664:157-79.

166. McCarthy KM, Gong JL, Telford JR, et al. Ontogeny of Ia+ accessory cells in fetal and newborn rat lung. Am J Respir Cell Mol Biol 1992;6:349-56.

167. Nelson DJ, McMenamin C, McWilliam AS, et al. Development of the airway intraepithelial dendritic cell network in the rat from class II MHC (Ia) negative precursors: differential regulation of Ia expression at different levels of the respiratory tract. J Exp Med 1994;179:203-12.

168. Ridge JP, Fuchs EJ, Matzinger P. Neonatal tolerance revisited: turning on newborn T cells with dendritic cells. Science 1996;271:1723-6.

169. Nelson DJ, Holt PG. Defective regional immunity in the respiratory tract of neonates is attributable to hyporesponsiveness of local dendritic cells to activation signals. J Immunol 1995;155:3517-24.

170. Stoltenberg L, Thrane PS, Rognum TO. Development of immune response markers in the trachea in the fetal period and the first year of life. Pediatr Allergy Immunol 1993;4:13-9.

171. Holt PG. Dendritic cell ontogeny as an aetiological factor in respiratory tract diseases in early life. Thorax 2001;56:419-20.

172. Sorg RV, Kogler G, Wernet P. Identification of cord blood dendritic cells as an immature CD11c- population. Blood 1999;93:2302-7.

173. Hunt DW, Huppertz HI, Jiang HJ, et al. Studies of human cord blood dendritic cells: evidence for functional immaturity. Blood 1994;84:4333-43.

174. Goriely S, Vincart B, Stordeur P, et al. Deficient IL-12(p35) gene expression by dendritic cells derived from neonatal monocytes. J Immunol 2001;166:2141-6.

175. Gold MC, Robinson TL, Cook MS, et al. Human neonatal dendritic cells are competent in MHC class I antigen processing and presentation. PLoS ONE 2007;2:e957.

176. Krumbiegel D, Zepp F, Meyer CU. Combined Toll-like receptor agonists synergistically increase production of inflammatory cytokines in human neonatal dendritic cells. Hum Immunol 2007;68:813-22.

177. Krumbiegel D, Anthogalidis-Voss C, Markus H, et al. Enhanced expression of IL-27 mRNA in human newborns. Pediatr Allergy Immunol 2008;19:513-6.

178. Borrese MP, Odelram H, Irander K, et al. Peripheral blood eosinophilia in infants at three months of age is associated with subsequent development of atopic disease in early childhood. J Allergy Clin Immunol 1995;95:694-8.

179. Bullock JD, Robertson AF, Bodenbender JG, et al. Inflammatory response in the neonate re-examined. Pediatrics 1969;44:58-61.

180. Eitzman DV, Smith RT. The nonspecific inflammatory cycle in the neonatal infant. Am J Dis Child 1959;97:326-34.

181. Roberts RL, Ank BJ, Salusky IB, et al. Purification and properties of peritoneal eosinophils from pediatric dialysis patients. J Immunol Methods 1990;126:205-11.

182. Bhat AM, Scanlon JW. The pattern of eosinophilia in premature infants. J Pediatr 1981;98:612-6.

183. Gibson EL, Vaucher Y, Corrigan JJ. Eosinophilia in premature infants: relationship to weight gain. J Pediatr 1979;95:99-101.

184. Smith JB, Kunjummen RD, Raghavender BH. Eosinophils and neutrophils of human neonates have similar impairments of quantitative up-regulation of Mac-1 (CD11b/CD18) expression in vitro. Pediatr Res 1991;30:355-61.

185. Smith JB, Kunjummen RD, Kishimoto TK, et al. Expression and regulation of L-selectin on eosinophils from human adults and neonates. Pediatr Res 1992;32:465-71.

186. Spencer J, Isaacson PG, Walker-Smith JA, et al. Heterogeneity in intraepithelial lymphocyte subpopulations in fetal and postnatal human small intestine. J Pediatr Gastroenterol Nutr 1989;9:173-7.

187. Wilkes LK, McMenamin C, Holt PG. Postnatal maturation of mast cell subpopulations in the rat respiratory tract. Immunology 1992;75:535-41.

188. Cummins AG, Munro GH, Miller HRP, et al. Association of maturation of the small intestine at weaning with mucosal mast cell activation in the rat. J Cell Biol 1988;66:417-23.

189. Cummins AG, Eglinton BA, Gonzalez A, et al. Immune activation during infancy in healthy humans. J Clin Immunol 1994;14:107-15.

190. Iida M, Matsumoto K, Tomita H, et al. Selective down-regulation of high-affinity IgE receptor (Fc εRI) α-chain messenger RNA among tran-

scriptome in cord blood-derived versus adult peripheral blood-derived cultured human mast cells. Blood 2001;97:1016–22.

191. Dastur FD, Shastry P, Iyer E, et al. The foetal immune response to maternal tetanus toxoid immunization. J Assoc Physicians India 1993;41:94–6.

192. Klinge J, Lugauer S, Korn K, et al. Comparison of immunogenicity and reactogenicity of a measles, mumps and rubella (MMR) vaccine in German children vaccinated at 9–11, 12–14 or 15–17 months of age. Vaccine 2000;18:3134–40.

193. Gans HA, Maldonado Y, Yasukawa LL, et al. IL-12, IFN-g, and T cell proliferation to measles in immunized infants. J Immunol 1999;162:5569–75.

194. Gans HA, Yasukawa LL, Zhang CZ, et al. Effects of interleukin-12 and interleukin-15 on measles-specific T cell responses in vaccinated infants. Viral Immunol 2008;21:163–72.

195. Barrios C, Brawand P, Berney M, et al. Neonatal and early life immune responses to various forms of vaccine antigens qualitatively differ from adult responses: predominance of a Th2-biased pattern which persists after adult boosting. Eur J Immunol 1996;26:1489–96.

196. Rowe J, Macaubas C, Monger T, et al. Antigen-specific responses to diphtheria-tetanus-acellular pertussis vaccine in human infants are initially Th2 polarized. Infect Immun 2000;68:3873–7.

197. Rowe J, Macaubas C, Monger T, et al. Heterogeneity in diphtheria-tetanus-acellular pertussis vaccine-specific cellular immunity during infancy: relationship to variations in the kinetics of postnatal maturation of systemic Th1 function. J Infect Dis 2001;184:80–8.

198. Adkins B, Du R-Q. Newborn mice develop balanced Th1/Th2 primary effector responses in vivo but are biased to Th2 secondary responses. J Immunol 1998;160:4217–24.

199. Ausiello CM, Lande R, Urbani F, et al. Cell-mediated immune responses in four-year-old children after primary immunization with acellular pertussis vaccines. Infect Immunol 1999;67:4064–71.

200. Upham JW, Rate A, Rowe J, et al. Dendritic cell immaturity during infancy restricts the capacity to express vaccine-specific T cell memory. Infect Immun 2006;74:1106–12.

201. Marchant A, Goetghebuer T, Ota M, et al. Newborns develop a Th1-type immune response to Mycobacterium bovis bacillus Calmette-Guérin vaccination. J Immunol 1999;163:2249–55.

202. Vekemans J, Amedei A, Ota MO, et al. Neonatal bacillus Calmette-Guérin vaccination induced adult-like IFN-γ production by CD4+ T lymphocytes. Eur J Immunol 2001;31:1531–35.

203. Arulanandam BP, Van Cleave VH, Metzger DW. IL-12 is a potent neonatal vaccine adjuvant. Eur J Immunol 1999;29:256–64.

204. Martinez X, Brandt C, Saddallah F, et al. DNA immunization circumvents deficient induction of T helper type 1 and cytotoxic T lymphocyte responses in neonates and during early life. Proc Natl Acad Sci U S A 1997;94:8726–31.

205. Kovarik J, Bozzotti P, Love-Homan L, et al. CpG oligodeoxynucleotides can circumvent the Th2 polarization of neonatal responses to vaccines but may fail to fully direct Th2 responses established by neonatal priming. J Immunol 1999;162:1611–7.

206. Shirakawa T, Enomoto T, Shimazu S, et al. Inverse association between tuberculin responses and atopic disorder. Science 1997;275:77–9.

207. Arkwright PD, Patel L, Moran A, et al. Atopic eczema is associated with delayed maturation of the antibody response to pneumococcal vaccine. Clin Exp Immunol 2000;122:16–9.

208. Prescott SL, Sly PD, Holt PG. Raised serum IgE associated with reduced responsiveness to DPT vaccination during infancy. Lancet 1998;351:1489.

209. Holt PG, Rudin A, Macaubas C, et al. Development of immunologic memory against tetanus toxoid and pertactin antigens from the diphtheria-tetanus-pertussis vaccine in atopic versus nonatopic children. J Allergy Clin Immunol 2000;105:1117–22.

210. Kondo N, Kobayashi Y, Shinoda S, et al. Cord blood lymphocyte responses to food antigens for the prediction of allergic disorders. Arch Dis Child 1992;67:1003–7.

211. Piccinni M-P, Mecacci F, Sampognaro S, et al. Aeroallergen sensitization can occur during fetal life. Int Arch Allergy Immunol 1993;102:301–3.

212. Piastra M, Stabile A, Fioravanti G, et al. Cord blood mononuclear cell responsiveness to beta-lactoglobulin: T cell activity in 'atopy-prone; and 'non-atopy-prone' newborns. Int Arch Allergy Immunol 1994;104:358–65.

213. Miles EA, Warner JA, Jones AC, et al. Peripheral blood mononuclear cell proliferative responses in the first year of life in babies born to allergic parents. Clin Exp Allergy 1996;26:780–8.

214. Holt PG, O'Keeffe PO, Holt BJ, et al. T cell 'priming' against environmental allergens in human neonates: sequential deletion of food antigen specificities during infancy with concomitant expansion of responses to ubiquitous inhalant allergens. Ped Allergy Immunol 1995;6:85–90.

215. Prescott SL, Macaubas C, Holt BJ, et al. Transplacental priming of the human immune system to environmental allergens: universal skewing of initial T cell responses towards the Th-2 cytokine profile. J Immunol 1998;160:4730–7.

216. Szepfalusi Z, Loibichler C, Pichler J, et al. Direct evidence for transplacental allergen transfer. Pediatr Res 2000;48:404–7.

217. Bjorksten B, Holt BJ, Baron-Hay MJ, et al. Low-level exposure to house dust mites stimulates T cell responses during early childhood independent of atopy. Clin Exp Allergy 1996;26:775–9.

218. Smillie FI, Elderfield AJ, Patel F, et al. Lymphoproliferative responses in cord blood and at one year: no evidence for the effect of in utero exposure to dust mite allergens. Clin Exp Allergy 2001;31:1194–1204.

219. Yabuhara A, Macaubas C, Prescott SL, et al. Th-2-polarised immunological memory to inhalant allergens in atopics is established during infancy and early childhood. Clin Exp Allergy 1997;27:1261–9.

220. Prescott SL, Macaubas C, Smallacombe T, et al. Development of allergen-specific T cell memory in atopic and normal children. Lancet 1999;353:196–200.

221. Macaubas C, Sly PD, Burton P, et al. Regulation of Th-cell responses to inhalant allergen during early childhood. Clin Exp Allergy 1999;29:1223–31.

222. Macaubas C, Holt PG. Regulation of cytokine production in T cell responses to inhalant allergen: GATA-3 expression distinguishes between Th1- and Th2-polarized immunity. Int Arch Allergy Immunol 2001;124:176–9.

223. Macaubas C, Lee PT, Smallacombe TB, et al. Reciprocal patterns of allergen-induced GATA-3 expression in peripheral blood mononuclear cells from atopics vs. non-atopics. Clin Exp Allergy 2002;32:97–106.

224. Rinas U, Horneff G, Wahn V. Interferon-gamma production by cord-blood mononuclear cells is reduced in newborns with a family history of atopic disease and is independent from cord blood IgE-levels, Pediatr Allergy Immunol 1993;4:60–4.

225. Tang MLK, Kemp AS, Thorburn J, et al. Reduced interferon-g secretion in neonates and subsequent atopy. Lancet 1994;344:983–6.

226. Liao SY, Liao TN, Chiang BL, et al. Decreased production of IFNg and increased production of IL-6 by cord blood mononuclear cells of newborns with a high risk of allergy. Clin Exp Allergy 1996;26:397–405.

227. Martinez FD, Stern DA, Wright AL, et al. Association of interleukin-2 and interferon-g production by blood mononuclear cells in infancy with parental allergy skin tests and with subsequent development of atopy. J Allergy Clin Immunol 1995;96:652–60.

228. Warner JA, Miles EA, Jones AC, et al. Is deficiency of interferon gamma production by allergen-triggered cord blood cells a predictor of atopic eczema? Clin Exp Allergy 1994;24:423–30.

229. Williams TJ, Jones CA, Miles EA, et al. Fetal and neonatal IL-13 production during pregnancy and at birth and subsequent development of atopic symptoms. J Allergy Clin Immunol 2000;105:951–9.

230. Holt PG, Macaubas C. Development of long-term tolerance versus sensitisation to environmental allergens during the perinatal period. Curr Opin Immunol 1997;9:782–7.

231. Holt PG. Environmental factors and primary T cell sensitisation to inhalant allergens in infancy: reappraisal of the role of infections and air pollution. Pediatr Allergy Immunol 1995;6:1–10.

232. Martinez FD, Holt PG. The role of microbial burden in the aetiology of allergy and asthma. Lancet 1999;354:12–5.

233. Baldini M, Lohman IC, Halonen M, et al. A polymorphism in the 5′ flanking region of the CD14 gene is associated with circulating soluble CD14 levels with total serum IgE. Am J Resp Cell Mol Biol 1999;20:976–83.

234. Hartel C, Rupp J, Hoegemann A, et al. 159C>T CD14 genotype–functional effects on innate immune responses in term neonates. Hum Immunol 2008;69:338–43.

235. Von Ehrenstein OS, Von Mutius E, Illi S, et al. Reduced risk of hay fever and asthma amongst children of farmers. Clin Exp Allergy 2000;30:187–93.

236. Gereda JE, Leung DYM, Thatayatikom A, et al. Relation between house-dust endotoxin exposure, type 1 T cell development, and allergen sensitisation in infants at high risk of asthma. Lancet 2000;355:1680–3.

237. Roponen M, Hyvarinen A, Hirvonen MR, et al. Change in IFN-gamma-producing capacity in early life and exposure to environmental microbes. J Allergy Clin Immunol 2005;116:1048–52.

238. Rowe J, Heaton T, Kusel M, et al. High IFN-gamma production by CD8+ T cells and early sensitization among infants at high risk of atopy. J Allergy Clin Immunol 2004;113:710–6.

239. Heaton T, Rowe J, Turner S, et al. An immunoepidemiological approach to asthma: identification of in-vitro T cell response patterns associated with different wheezing phenotypes in children. Lancet 2005;365:142–9.

240. Hollams EM, Deverell M, Serralha M, et al. Elucidation of asthma phenotypes in atopic teenagers via parallel immunophenotypic and clinical profiling. J Allergy Clin Immunol 2009;124:463–70, 70e1–26.

241. Woolcock AJ, Peat JK, Trevillion LM. Is the increase in asthma prevalence linked to increase in allergen load? Allergy 1995;50:935–40.

242. Peat JK, Salome CM, Woolcock AJ. Longitudinal changes in atopy during a 4-year period: relation to bronchial hyperresponsiveness and respiratory symptoms in a population sample of Australian schoolchildren. J Allergy Clin Immunol 1990;85:65–74.

243. Martinez FD, Wright AL, Taussig LM, et al. Asthma and wheezing in the first six years of life. N Engl J Med 1995;332:133–8.

244. Welliver RC, Duffy L. The relationship of RSV-specific immunoglobulin E antibody responses in infancy, recurrent wheezing, and pulmonary function at age 7–8 years. Pediatr Pulmonol 1993;15:19–27.

245. Oddy WH, de Klerk N, Sly PD, et al. The effects of respiratory infections, atopy, and breastfeeding on childhood asthma. Eur Respir J 2002;19: 899–905.

246. Holgate ST. The inflammation-repair cycle in asthma: the pivotal role of the airway epithelium. Clin Exp Allergy 1998;28 (suppl 5):97–103.

247. Holt PG, Sly PD. Interactions between respiratory tract infections and atopy in aetiology of asthma. Eur Respir J 2002;19:1–8.

248. Stumbles PA, Thomas JA, Pimm CL, et al. Resting respiratory tract dendritic cells preferentially stimulate Th2 responses and require obligatory cytokine signals for induction of Th1 immunity. J Exp Med 1998;188:2019–31.

249. Schon-Hegrad MA, Oliver J, McMenamin PG, et al. Studies on the density, distribution, and surface phenotype of intraepithelial class II major histocompatibility complex antigen (Ia)-bearing dendritic cells (DC) in the conducting airways. J Exp Med 1991;173:1345–56.

250. McWilliam AS, Nelson D, Thomas JA, et al. Rapid dendritic cell recruitment is a hallmark of the acute inflammatory response at mucosal surfaces. J Exp Med 1994;179:1331–6.

251. Sly PD, Boner AL, Bjorksten B, et al. Early identification of atopy in the prediction of persistent asthma in children. Lancet 2008;372:1100–6.

CHAPTER

7

Approach to the Child with Recurrent Infections

Howard M. Lederman • Erwin W. Gelfand

Many children who present for allergy evaluation have chronic/recurrent infections of the upper and lower respiratory tracts. Allergy may predispose the patient to such symptoms because swelling of the nasal mucosa causes obstruction of the sinus ostia and the eustachian tubes. However, one must be alert to the possibility of other underlying problems, including primary immunodeficiency diseases, secondary immunodeficiency caused by human immunodeficiency virus (HIV) or Epstein-Barr virus (EBV) infection, cystic fibrosis, disorders of ciliary structure and function, swallowing dysfunction and pulmonary aspiration caused by anatomic or physiologic abnormalities, and aspirated foreign body. Environmental factors such as exposure to cigarette smoke, daycare, and the number of household members must also be considered. This chapter provides an approach to evaluating children for these disorders.

Definition of Recurrent Infections

It is difficult to assign a precise frequency of infections that defines increased susceptibility to infection (Box 7-1).[1] For example, chronic/recurrent otitis media is very common in the first 2 years of life but thereafter decreases in frequency. Rather than defining an arbitrary number of ear infections that is too many, the nature and pattern of those infections provide a more reliable guide to identify the child who deserves further evaluation. Ear infections that increase in frequency after the age of 2 years, ear infections associated with mastoiditis, ear infections associated with infections at other sites, and ear infections occurring in the context of failure to thrive should raise the suspicion of an underlying disorder. Similarly, it is unusual for a child to have more than one episode of pneumonia per decade of life, chronic sinusitis, or chronic bronchitis.

Other clues to an abnormal susceptibility to infection include a history of infections at multiple anatomic locations or relatively unusual infections such as sepsis, mastoiditis, septic arthritis, osteomyelitis, and meningitis. In some instances, patients may present with one or more infections that are unusually severe, lead to an unexpected complication (e.g. empyema or fistula formation), or are caused by an organism of relatively low virulence (e.g. *Aspergillus* or *Pneumocystis jirovecii*).

Sometimes, the most challenging aspect of evaluating the past medical history is assessing the reliability of the data. It may be difficult to distinguish pneumonia from atelectasis with fever in children with reactive airway disease. Sinusitis is easily mistaken for purulent rhinitis, unless a computed tomography scan documents sinus involvement. Diarrhea may be the result of infection or an adverse effect of antibiotic therapy. Finally, with the often rapid institution of antibiotic therapy, the infections in a patient with an immune deficiency may not be severe or progressive. Indeed, many patients ultimately diagnosed with a primary immune deficiency present with an infection history that is not distinguishable from normal children.

It is also important to account for environmental exposure. There may be an obvious explanation for frequent infections in an infant attending a large daycare center during the winter months, whereas the same number of infections might raise concern if an only child were cared for in his or her home. Similarly, exposure to cigarette smoke and drinking from a bottle in a supine position are known risk factors for respiratory tract symptoms. A sometimes useful clue is whether the child has had distinctly more infections than his/her siblings by a comparable age.

Early diagnosis of an underlying disorder is critical because it may lead to more effective approaches to therapy and appropriate anticipatory guidance. Furthermore, because some underlying disorders are inherited in mendelian fashion, early diagnosis is essential for making genetic information available to the families of affected individuals.

The Clinical Presentation of Underlying Disorders

Allergy

Patients with allergic disease, rhinitis, and/or asthma often have symptoms of both acute and chronic sinusitis.[2] There is little to distinguish the symptoms or mucopurulent discharge in patients with immunodeficiency compared with those with allergic disease. Similarly, radiographic studies do not discriminate between the two. History is important because flare-ups of sinusitis often accompany exacerbations of the underlying allergic symptoms, and patients may report more symptomatic improvement when treated with corticosteroids than when treated with antibiotics. In general, a history of atopy makes a diagnosis of antibody deficiency less likely because the ability to produce specific immunoglobulin E (IgE) antibodies usually indicates normal B and T cell function.

Recurrent sinopulmonary infection is the most frequent illness associated with selective IgA deficiency. IgA deficiency and allergy may also be associated. Even in blood bank donors in whom IgA deficiency was accidentally discovered, allergy may

DOI: 10.1016/B978-1-4377-0271-2.00007-9

Guidelines for Identifying Children with Increased Susceptibility to Infection

Frequency

More than one episode of pneumonia per decade of life

Increasing frequency of otitis media in children older than 2 years

Persistent otitis media and drainage despite patent tympanostomy tubes

Persistent sinusitis despite medical and, when appropriate, surgical treatment

Severity

Pneumonia with empyema

Bacterial meningitis, arthritis, or osteomyelitis

Sepsis

Mastoiditis

Infection with Opportunistic Pathogens

Pneumocystis jirovecii pneumonia

Mucocutaneous candidiasis

Invasive fungal infection

Vaccine-acquired poliomyelitis

Bacille Calmette-Guérin infection after vaccination

Infections at Multiple Anatomic Locations

Lack of Other Epidemiologic Explanations (e.g. daycare center, exposure to cigarette smoke, environmental allergies)

Anatomic or Physiologic Features Suggestive of a Syndrome Complex

Failure to Thrive

Clinical Features of Immmunodeficiency

Increased Susceptibility to Infection

Chronic/recurrent infections without other explanations

Infection with organism of low virulence

Infection of unusual severity

Autoimmune or Inflammatory Disease

Target cells (e.g. hemolytic anemia, immune thrombocytopenia, thyroiditis)

Target tissues (e.g. rheumatoid arthritis, vasculitis, systemic lupus erythematosus)

Syndrome Complexes

Other immunodeficiency diseases may be diagnosed because of their known association with syndrome complexes.

Infection

An increased susceptibility to infection is the hallmark of the primary immunodeficiency diseases. In most patients, the striking clinical feature is the chronic or recurring nature of the infections rather than the fact that individual infections are unusually severe.[1] However, not all immunodeficient patients are diagnosed after recurrent infections. In some, the first infection may be sufficiently unusual to raise the question of immunodeficiency. For example, an infant who presents with infection caused by *P. jerovicii* or another opportunistic pathogen is likely to be immunodeficient even if it is his or her first recognized infection.

Autoimmune/Chronic Inflammatory Disease

Immunodeficient patients can present with autoimmune or chronic inflammatory diseases. It is thought that the basic abnormality leading to immunodeficiency may also lead to faulty discrimination between self and nonself and thus susceptibility for developing an autoimmune disease. The manifestations of these disorders may be limited to a single target cell or organ (e.g. autoimmune hemolytic anemia, immune thrombocytopenia, autoimmune thyroiditis) or may involve a number of different target organs (e.g. vasculitis, systemic lupus erythematosus, or rheumatoid arthritis). The autoimmune and inflammatory diseases are more commonly seen in particular primary immunodeficiency diseases, most notably common variable immunodeficiency,[8] selective IgA deficiency, chronic mucocutaneous candidiasis,[9] and deficiencies of early components (C1 through C4) of the classic complement pathway.[10]

Occasionally, a disorder that appears to be autoimmune in nature may in fact be due to an infectious agent. For example, the dermatomyositis that is sometimes seen in patients with X-linked agammaglobulinemia is actually a manifestation of chronic enterovirus infection and not an autoimmune disease.

Syndrome Complexes

Immunodeficiency can be seen as one part of a constellation of signs and symptoms in a syndrome complex.[11] In fact, the

be twice as common as in healthy donors.[3] The most common allergic disorders in IgA-deficient individuals are rhinosinusitis, eczema, conjunctivitis, and asthma.[4]

Because of the association between allergy and sinusitis, a careful history may often be sufficient, obviating the need for extensive testing for immunodeficiency. Screening for IgA deficiency may be of some help in understanding the association between the two in IgA-deficient individuals. Management of sinusitis should be medical with avoidance of surgery, unless all else fails. Improvement in asthma symptoms after sinus surgery is questionable and only transient at best.

Immunodeficiency

The primary immunodeficiency diseases were originally viewed as rare disorders, characterized by severe clinical expression early in life. However, it has become clear that these diseases are not as uncommon as originally suspected, that their clinical expression can sometimes be relatively mild, and that they are seen nearly as often in adolescents and adults as they are in infants and children.[5–7] In fact, the presentation of immunodeficiency may be so subtle that the diagnosis will be made only if the physician is alert to that possibility.

Patients with primary immunodeficiency diseases most often are recognized because of their increased susceptibility to infection, but these patients may also present with a variety of other clinical manifestations (Box 7-2). In fact, noninfectious manifestations, such as autoimmune disease, may be the first or the predominant clinical symptom of the underlying immunodeficiency.

Table 7-1 Examples of Immunodeficiency Syndromes that May Increase Susceptibility to Sinopulmonary Infections

Syndrome	Clinical Presentation	Immunologic Abnormality	Other Contributing Factors
Ataxia telangiectasia	Ataxia, telangiectasia	Variable B and T lymphocyte dysfunction	Dysfunctional swallow with pulmonary aspiration
DiGeorge syndrome	Congenital heart disease, hypoparathyroidism, abnormal facies	Thymic hypoplasia or aplasia	Craniofacial anomalies including cleft palate; physiologic abnormalities including dysfunction of soft palate
Dysmotile cilia syndromes	Situs inversus, male infertility, ectopic pregnancy, upper and lower respiratory tract infections	None	
Hyper-IgE syndrome	Coarse facies, eczematoid rash, retained primary teeth, bone fractures, pneumonia	Elevated serum IgE, eosinophilia	
Wiskott-Aldrich syndrome	Thrombocytopenia, eczema	Variable B and T lymphocyte dysfunction	

recognition that a patient has a syndrome in which immunodeficiency occurs may allow a diagnosis of immunodeficiency to be made before there are any clinical manifestations of that deficiency (Table 7-1). For example, children with the DiGeorge syndrome are usually identified initially because of the neonatal presentation of congenital heart disease, hypocalcemic tetany, or both. This should lead to T lymphocyte evaluation before the onset of opportunistic infections. Similarly, a diagnosis of Wiskott-Aldrich syndrome can often be made in young boys with eczema and thrombocytopenia even before the onset of infections.

Cystic Fibrosis

Cystic fibrosis (CF) is one of the most common autosomal recessive disorders among white populations, occurring with an incidence of almost 1:3000 live newborns.[12] The classic presentation of CF with chronic/recurrent sinopulmonary infections caused by *Pseudomonas* and *Staphylococcus,* diarrhea with malabsorption, and failure to thrive, is easy to recognize. New methods for diagnosis have led to the recognition of a broader clinical phenotype, including patients whose first or only manifestation is chronic/recurrent sinusitis.[13,14] The diagnosis of CF should be considered in any patient with chronic/recurrent sinopulmonary infections, especially if *Pseudomonas, Staphylococcus,* nontypeable *Hemophilus influenzae,* or *Burkholderia cepacia* are identified as pathogens.

Abnormalities of Airway Anatomy and Physiology

A variety of anatomic abnormalities may increase a child's susceptibility to upper and lower respiratory tract infections. Some anatomic abnormalities, such as craniofacial anomalies involving the palate and the nose, may be readily apparent on physical examination. Others, such as bronchogenic cysts and extra lobar pulmonary sequestrations, may be suspected when recurrent infections occur at a single anatomic site.[15] Unilateral otitis media and sinusitis in a young child should prompt an investigation for a nasal foreign body.

Abnormalities of airway muscle function may cause similar symptoms. Swallowing dysfunction with aspiration may be obvious in a child with cerebral palsy who coughs and gags when eating. More subtle clues are a history of drooling or the presence of dysarthria.

Disorders of Ciliary Structure and Function

Primary ciliary dyskinesia (PCD) is a rare problem, estimated to occur with an incidence of less than 1:10000 in the general population.[16] In most cases, it is inherited as an autosomal recessive trait, but PCD is genetically and clinically heterogeneous. Affected individuals have chronic/recurrent rhinitis, otitis media, sinusitis, pneumonia, and bronchiectasis that begin at an early age. In approximately half of the cases, there are accompanying abnormalities of laterality such as situs in-versus or heterotaxy, and complex congenital heart disease has been reported in approximately 10% of individuals with PCD. Abnormal ciliary function of spermatozoa can cause infertility in males, and abnormal ciliary function in the fallopian tubes can result in ectopic pregnancy.

Cilia are complex structures formed from a set of nine peripheral microtubular doublets surrounding two single central microtubules. PCD can be caused by abnormalities of any of the structural proteins: inner or outer dynein arms, radial spokes, or microtubules. PCD can also be caused by disordered orientation of cilia on mucosal surfaces, preventing them from beating in a synchronized wave that clears mucus from the airways. Advances in identification of specific mutations in functional genes has revealed the possibility of ciliary dysfunction despite normal ultrastructural findings.[17]

Secondary Immunodeficiency

Immunodeficiency may occur secondary to other illnesses or medications.[18] A variety of infections, particularly viruses, may cause either temporary or long-lived abnormalities of humoral and/or cell-mediated immunity. Such viruses include HIV, measles, and EBV, among others. Malnutrition or malabsorption can cause hypogammaglobulinemia and impaired cell-mediated immunity. A number of medications, most notably corticosteroids and chemotherapeutic agents, are immunosuppressive; phenytoin therapy has been associated with secondary IgA deficiency and even panhypogammaglobulinemia. Posttraumatic splenectomy, or the 'autosplenectomy' that occurs at an early age in sickle cell anemia, leads to an increased risk of sepsis. Susceptibility to infection is dependent on the secondary immunodeficiency that is caused by these or other agents; that is, patients with acquired deficiency of humoral immunity are at highest risk for infections with encapsulated bacteria and enteroviruses, whereas patients with acquired deficiency of cell-mediated

Table 7-2 Patterns of Illness Associated with Primary Immunodeficiency

Disorder	Illnesses	
	Infection	Other
Antibody	Sinopulmonary (pyogenic, encapsulated bacteria) Gastrointestinal (enteroviruses, *Giardia lamblia*)	Autoimmune disease (autoantibodies, inflammatory bowel disease)
Cell-mediated immunity	Pneumonia (pyogenic bacteria, *Pneumocystis jerovicii*, viruses) Gastrointestinal (viruses) Skin, mucous membranes (fungi)	
Phagocytosis	Skin, reticuloendothelial system, abscesses (*Staphylococcus*, enteric bacteria, fungi, mycobacteria)	
Complement	Sepsis and other blood-borne encapsulated bacteria (*Streptococcus*, *Pneumococcus*, *Neisseria*)	Autoimmune disease (systemic lupus erythematosus, glomerulonephritis)

immunity are at risk for infection by a wide variety of bacterial, fungal, and viral pathogens.

Laboratory Tests for Underlying Disorders

Immunodeficiency

Although the clinician can suspect immune system dysfunction after a careful review of the history and physical examination, specific diagnoses are rarely evident without use of the laboratory. However, the types of infections and other symptoms should help to focus the laboratory work-up on specific parts of the immune system (Table 7-2). For example, patients with antibody deficiency typically have sinopulmonary infections as a prominent presenting feature.[19] Deficiency of cell-mediated immunity predisposes individuals to develop infections caused by *P. jirovecii*, other fungi, and a variety of viruses.[20] Abnormalities of phagocytic function should be suspected when patients have recurrent skin infections or visceral abscesses.[21] Patients with complement deficiency most often present with bacterial sepsis or immune complex-mediated diseases.[22] Although still controversial, patients who are deficient in mannose-binding lectin may present with recurrent respiratory tract infections for the first several years of life.[23]

Screening tests that should be performed in almost all patients include a complete blood count with differential and quantitative measurement of serum immunoglobulins. Other tests should be guided by the clinical features of the patient (Table 7-3). Finally, whenever primary immunodeficiency is suspected, consideration must also be given to secondary causes of immunodeficiency, including HIV infection, therapy with antiinflammatory medications (e.g. corticosteroids), and other underlying illnesses (e.g. lymphoreticular neoplasms and viral infections such as infectious mononucleosis).

Examination of the Peripheral Blood Smear

The complete blood count with examination of the blood smear is an inexpensive and readily available test that provides important diagnostic information relating to a number of immunodeficiency diseases. Neutropenia most often occurs secondary to immunosuppressive drugs, infection, malnutrition, or autoimmunity but may be a primary problem (congenital or cyclic neutropenia). In contrast, persistent neutrophilia is characteristic of leukocyte adhesion molecule deficiency,[24] and abnormal cyto-

Table 7-3 Screening Tests for Underlying Disorders

Suspected Abnormality	Diagnostic Tests
Antibody	Quantitative immunoglobulins (IgG, IgA, IgM) Antibody response to immunization
Cell-mediated immunity	Lymphocyte count T lymphocyte enumeration (CD3, CD4, CD8) T cell function in vitro: proliferation to mitogens and antigens Delayed-type hypersensitivity tests Human immunodeficiency virus serology
Complement	Total hemolytic complement (CH_{50})
Phagocytosis	Neutrophil count

plasmic granules may be seen in the peripheral blood smear of patients with Chediak-Higashi syndrome.[25]

The blood is predominantly a 'T cell organ'; that is, the majority (50% to 70%) of peripheral blood lymphocytes are T cells, whereas only 5% to 15% are B cells. Therefore lymphopenia is usually a presenting feature of T cell or combined immunodeficiency disorders such as severe combined immunodeficiency disease or DiGeorge syndrome.

Thrombocytopenia may occur as a secondary manifestation of immunodeficiency but is often a presenting manifestation of the Wiskott-Aldrich syndrome. A unique finding in the latter group of patients is an abnormally small platelet (and lymphocyte) volume,[26] a measurement that is easily made with automated blood counters.

Examination of red blood cell morphology can yield clues about splenic function. Howell-Jolly bodies may be visible in peripheral blood in cases of splenic dysfunction or asplenia.[27] However, the converse is not always true, and the absence of Howell-Jolly bodies does not ensure that splenic function is normal.

Evaluation of Humoral Immunity

Measurement of serum immunoglobulin levels is an important screening test to detect immunodeficiency for three reasons: (1) more than 80% of patients diagnosed with a primary disorder of immunity will have abnormalities of serum immunoglobulin levels; (2) immunoglobulin measurements yield indirect information about several disparate aspects of the immune system because immunoglobulin synthesis requires the coordinated function of B lymphocytes, T lymphocytes, and monocytes; and (3) the measurement of serum immunoglobulin levels is readily available, highly reliable, and relatively inexpensive. The initial screening test for humoral immune function is the quantitative measurement of serum immunoglobulins. Neither serum protein electrophoresis nor immunoelectrophoresis is sufficiently sensitive or quantitative to be useful for this purpose. Quantitative measurements of serum IgG, IgA, and IgM levels will identify patients with panhypogammaglobulinemia as well as those with deficiencies of an individual immunoglobulin class, such as selective IgA deficiency. Interpretation of results must be made in view of the marked variations in normal immunoglobulin levels with age;[28] therefore age-related normal values must always be used for comparison. Different reference ranges are necessary in the first year of life for very low birth-weight, premature infants.[29]

A clue to immunodeficiency may be a low-normal IgG level in an individual with recurrent infections. One would expect a high normal IgG level if the cause of the recurrent infections does not involve the immune system. In such cases, it is critical to assess antibody function in addition to immunoglobulin levels. Antibody levels generated in response to childhood immunization with tetanus toxoid, pneumococcal or *H. influenzae* polysaccharide/protein conjugate vaccines are usually the most convenient to measure. In children over the age of 18 to 24 months, it is also important to assess antibody responses to polysaccharide antigens because these responses may be deficient in some patients who can respond normally to protein and polysaccharide/protein conjugate antigens.[30] Antibody can be measured in response to immunization with the 23 valent pneumococcal capsular polysaccharide vaccine. Alternatively, because the ABO blood group antigens are polysaccharides, quantifying isoagglutinin titers (usually of the IgM class) can assess antipolysaccharide antibody. However, the value of this test in the young child is limited because many normal children do not have significant isoagglutinin titers.[31] Live viral (e.g. oral polio, measles, mumps, rubella, varicella) and live bacterial (e.g. bacille Calmette-Guérin) vaccines should never be used for the evaluation of suspected immunodeficiency because they may cause disseminated infection in an immunocompromised host.

The role for IgG subclass measurements is controversial.[32] There are four subclasses of IgG, and selective deficiencies of each of these have been described. However, the significance of an IgG subclass deficiency in the presence of normal antibody responses to protein and polysaccharide antigens is not known. Most specialists therefore rely on antibody measurements and find that information about IgG subclass levels adds to the expense but not to the diagnosis.

Evaluation of Cell-Mediated Immunity

Testing for defects of cell-mediated immunity is relatively difficult because of the lack of good screening tests. Lymphopenia is suggestive of T lymphocyte deficiency because T lymphocytes constitute the majority (50% to 70%) of peripheral blood mononuclear cells. However, lymphopenia is not always present in patients with T lymphocyte functional defects. Similarly, the lack of a thymus silhouette on chest radiography is rarely helpful in the evaluation of T lymphocyte disorders because the thymus of normal children may rapidly involute after stress and provide the appearance of thymic hypoplasia.

Indirect information about the T cell compartment may be obtained by subset analysis of peripheral blood T lymphocytes with appropriate monoclonal antibodies, such as anti-CD3 for total T cells, anti-CD4, and anti-CD8.[33] Patients with severe combined immunodeficiency and DiGeorge syndrome generally have decreased numbers of CD3, CD4, and CD8 T lymphocytes. In contrast, patients infected with HIV have decreased T lymphocyte levels because there is a selective loss of CD4 lymphocytes. Further analysis of T cell numbers can evaluate expression of the α/β or γ/δ T cell receptor, and the distribution of CD45RA (naïve) and CD45RO (memory) subsets. With increasing availability of antibodies specific to cell surface proteins, subtle defects associated with deficiencies of specific subsets of T cells are being described, such as deficiencies of regulatory T cells.

As enumeration does not indicate function, assessment of the proliferative response of T cells to nonspecific mitogens (phytohemagglutinin, concanavalin A, pokeweed mitogen) or specific antigens (tetanus, candida) can be performed.[34] This involves culturing of peripheral blood mononuclear cells with these stimuli and assessing de novo DNA synthesis by tritiated thymidine incorporation into newly synthesized DNA. The response to any other antigen can be evaluated in a similar manner.

Delayed-type hypersensitivity (DTH) skin testing with a panel of antigens can be used to screen for cell-mediated immune function, but there are significant limitations to its use:[35-39] (1) it is difficult to find standardized antigens prepared for DTH testing; (2) prior exposure to antigen is a prerequisite; (3) normal patients may have transient depression of DTH with acute viral infections such as infectious mononucleosis; (4) a positive skin test to some antigens does not ensure that the patient has normal cell-mediated immunity to all antigens (e.g. patients with chronic mucocutaneous candidiasis have a limited defect in which cell-mediated immunity is generally intact except for their response to *Candida*); (5) normal children under the age of 12 months frequently are unresponsive to all of the antigens in the panel. When negative, DTH skin tests are therefore generally not helpful for the evaluation of suspected T lymphocyte abnormalities that present early in life (e.g. severe combined immunodeficiency or DiGeorge syndrome).

Evaluation of the Complement System

Most of the genetically determined deficiencies of complement can be detected with the total serum hemolytic complement (CH_{50}) assay.[40] Because this assay depends on the functional integrity of all of the components of the classic complement pathway (C1 through C9), a genetic deficiency of any of these components leads to a marked reduction or absence of total hemolytic complement activity. Utilization of any of these components, for example in an autoimmune disease, generally reduces but does not eliminate total hemolytic complement activity. Mannose-binding lectin can be measured by ELISA. Alternative pathway deficiencies (e.g. factor H, factor I, and properdin) are extremely rare; they may be suspected if the CH_{50} is in the low range of normal and the serum C3 level is low. AH_{50} is an assay of alternative pathway activity that is helpful. The final identification of the specific complement component that is deficient usually rests on both functional and immunochemical tests, and highly specific assays have been developed for each of the individual components.

Evaluation of Phagocytic Cells

Evaluation of phagocytic cells usually entails assessment of both their number and function. Disorders such as congenital agranulocytosis or cyclic neutropenia that are characterized by a deficiency in phagocytic cell number can be easily detected by evaluating a white blood cell count and differential. Beyond that, assessment of phagocytic cell function is relatively specialized because it depends on a variety of in vitro assays, including measurement of directed cell motility (chemotaxis), ingestion (phagocytosis), and intracellular killing (bactericidal activity).[41] The most common of the phagocyte function disorders, chronic granulomatous disease, can be diagnosed by the nitroblue tetrazolium (NBT) dye test[42] or by using the flow cytometric dihydrorhodamine (DHR)[43] test, both of which measure the oxidative metabolic response of neutrophils and monocytes.

Evaluation of Cilia

For suspected ciliary dyskinesia, ciliary structure and function must be assessed. Structure is assessed by electron microscopy of tissue obtained from the nasal mucosa, tonsils, adenoids, or bronchial mucosa. Because tobacco smoke, other pollutants, and infection may cause secondary abnormalities of cilia, it is sometimes difficult to find an appropriate tissue to sample. The microscopic examination should look for the presence of an anatomic defect that is consistent from cilia to cilia, such as the absence of dynein arms, and assess the orientation of cilia on the epithelium. With secondary causes, the structural abnormalities vary from cilia to cilia.[44] At the same time that tissue is obtained for electron microscopy, epithelial cell brushings from the nasal turbinates or bronchi can be examined for ciliary waveform and beat frequency. Assessments of mucociliary clearance are usually made by placing a small particle of saccharin on the anterior portion of the middle turbinate and then measuring the time until the patient tastes the saccharin.[45] For this test, the subject must sit quietly without sniffing or sneezing, and it is therefore difficult to perform in young children. A sweet taste should be evident within 1 hour in normal subjects, but the test has a very high rate of false-positive results. In individuals with a high suspicion for one of the ciliary defects, genetic screening for one of the mutations may be necessary.

Cystic Fibrosis

In most cases, the diagnosis of CF can be made by measuring the chloride concentration in sweat after iontophoresis of pilocarpine.[46] A minimum acceptable volume or weight of sweat must be collected to ensure an average sweat rate of greater than $1 \text{ g/m}^2/\text{min}$, and the diagnosis can be made with certainty if the sweat chloride concentration is greater than 60 mmol/L. However, this test may be falsely negative, especially among those patients who have an atypical clinical presentation. If the clinical suspicion of CF is high, especially in the absence of some of the features of the more common CF mutations, other useful diagnostic tests include mutation analysis of the CF transmembrane conductance regulator (CFTR) gene and/or measurement of potential differences across the nasal epithelium (nasal PD). The genetic testing is commercially available; the measurement of nasal PD is not widely available and should still be considered a research tool.

Evaluation for Human Immunodeficiency Virus and Other Immunosuppressive Virus Infections

Many techniques for the diagnosis of viral infection focus on the serologic detection of antibodies to viral proteins. There are, however, several problems with the sole reliance on antibody detection techniques. First, antibody tests will not detect infection in patients during the 'window period' between the time

---

of infection and seroconversion. For HIV infections, 95% of infected individuals will seroconvert within 6 months of infection, although 'window periods' of as long as 35 months have been reported.[47,48] Second, if the virus induces immunodeficiency, it may inhibit the production of antiviral antibodies.[49] Thus in a patient with known or suspected immunodeficiency, viral cultures as well as tests to detect viral antigens and nucleic acids should be performed in addition to serologic tests.[50]

Conclusions

The majority of children with recurrent respiratory tract infections will have environmental risk factors such as exposure to daycare or cigarette smoke, or are atopic with associated problems with allergies. It is the task of the allergist to identify the individuals who are most likely to have an underlying deficiency of host defense and to perform appropriate screening tests for such disorders. Early identification is critical for optimal clinical management and genetic counseling (Box 7-3).

Helpful Website

Immune Deficiency Foundation website (www.primaryimmune.org)

References

1. Stiehm ER, Ochs HD, Winkelstein JA. Immunodeficiency disorders: general considerations. In: Stiehm ER, Ochs HD, Winkelstein JA, editors. Immunologic disorders in infants and children. ed 5. Philadelphia: Elsevier/Saunders; 2004.
2. Rachelefsky GS, Katz RM, Siegel SC. Chronic sinus disease with associated reactive airway disease in children. Pediatrics 1984;73:526–9.
3. Kaufman HS, Hobbs JR. Immunologic deficiencies in an atopic population. Lancet 1970;2:1061–3.
4. Plebani A, Monafo V, Ugazio AG, et al. Comparison of the frequency of atopic diseases in children with severe and partial IgA deficiency. Int Arch Allergy Appl Immunol 1987;82:485–6.
5. Geha RS, Notarangelo LD, Casanova JL, et al. International Union of Immunological Societies Primary Immunodeficiency Diseases Classification Committee. Primary immunodeficiency diseases: an update from the International Union of Immunological Societies Primary Immunodeficiency Diseases Classification Committee. J Allergy Clin Immunol 2007;120:776–94.

6. Bonilla FA, Geha RS. Update on primary immunodeficiency diseases. J Allergy Clin Immunol 2006;117(2 Suppl):S435–41.

7. Bonilla FA, Bernstein IL, Khan DA, et al. American Academy of Allergy, Asthma and Immunology; American College of Allergy, Asthma and Immunology; Joint Council of Allergy, Asthma and Immunology. Practice parameter for the diagnosis and management of primary immunodeficiency. Ann Allergy Asthma Immunol 2005;94(5 Suppl 1):S1–63.

8. Chapel H, Cunningham-Rundles C. Update in understanding common variable immunodeficiency disorders (CVIDs) and the management of patients with these conditions, Br J Haematol. 2009 Mar 27 (Epub ahead of print).

9. Herrod HG. Chronic mucocutaneous candidiasis and complications of non-*Candida* infection: a report of the Pediatric Immunodeficiency Collaborative Study Group. J Pediatr 1990;116:377–82.

10. Barilla-LaBarca ML, Atkinson JP. Rheumatic syndromes associated with complement deficiency. Curr Opin Rheumatol 2003;15:55–60.

11. Ming JE, Stiehm ER, Graham JM Jr. Syndromic immunodeficiencies: genetic syndromes associated with immune abnormalities. Crit Rev Clin Lab Sci 2003;40:587–642.

12. Davies JC, Alton EW, Bush A. Cystic fibrosis. Br Med J 2007;335:1255–9.

13. Wiatrak BJ, Meyer CM III, Cottin RT. Cystic fibrosis presenting with sinus disease in children. Am J Dis Child 1993;147:258–60.

14. Wang X-J, Maylan B, Leopold DA, et al. Mutation in the gene responsible for cystic fibrosis and predisposition to chronic rhinosinusitis in the general population. JAMA 2000;284:1814–9.

15. Winters WD, Effmann EL. Congenital masses of the lung: prenatal and postnatal imaging evaluation. J Thorac Imaging 2001;16:196–206.

16. Bush A, Chodhari R, Collins N, et al. Primary ciliary dyskinesia: current state of the art. Arch Dis Child 2007;92:1136–40.

17. Leigh MW, Zariwala MA, Knowles MR. Primary ciliary dyskinesia: improving the diagnostic approach. Curr Opin Pediatr 2009;21:320–5.

18. Bonilla FA. Secondary immune deficiency due to medications and infections (other than HIV) In: Stiehm ER, editor. UpToDate. Waltham, MA; 2008.

19. Ochs HD, Smith CIE. X-linked agammaglobulinemia: a clinical and molecular analysis. Medicine 1996;75:287–99.

20. Buckley RH. Primary cellular immunodeficiencies. J Allergy Clin Immunol 2002;109:747–57.

21. Rosenzweig SD, Holland S. Phagocyte immunodeficiencies and their infections. J Allergy Clin Immunol 2004;113:620–6.

22. Walport MJ. Complement. N Engl J Med 2001;344:1058–66, 1140–4.

23. Koch A, Melbye M, Sorensen P, et al. Acute respiratory tract infections and mannose-binding lectin insufficiency during early childhood. JAMA 2001;285:1316–21.

24. Anderson DC, Springer TA. Leukocyte adhesion deficiency: an inherited defect in the Mac-1, LFA-1, and p150, 95 glycoproteins. Annu Rev Med 1987;38:175–94.

25. Introne W, Boissy RE, Gahl WA. Clinical, molecular, and cell biological aspects of Chediak-Higashi syndrome. Mol Genet Metab 1999;68:283–303.

26. Corash L, Shafer B, Blaese RM. Platelet-associated immunoglobulin, platelet size, and the effect of splenectomy in the Wiskott-Aldrich syndrome. Blood 1985;65:1439–43.

27. Pearson HA, Gallagher D, Chilcote R, et al. Developmental pattern of splenic dysfunction in sickle cell disorders. Pediatrics 1985;76:392–7.

28. Jolliff CR, Cost KM, Stivrins PC, et al. Reference intervals for serum IgG, IgA, IgM, C3 and C4 as determined by rate nephelometry. Clin Chem 1982;28:126–8.

29. Ballow M, Cates KL, Rowe JC, et al. Development of the immune system in very low birth weight (less than 1500 g) premature infants: concentrations of plasma immunoglobulins and patterns of infections. Pediatr Res 1986;20:899–904.

30. Boyle RJ, Le C, Balloch A, et al. The clinical syndrome of specific antibody deficiency in children. Clin Exp Immunol 2006;146:486–92.

31. Auf de Maur C, Hodel M, Nydegger UE, et al. Age dependency of ABO histo-blood group antibodies: reexamination of an old transfusion dogma. Transfusion 1993;33:915–8.

32. Buckley RH. Immunoglobulin G subclass deficiency: fact or fancy? Curr Allergy Asthma Rep 2002;2:356–60.

33. Shearer WT, Rosenblatt HM, Gelman RS, et al. Pediatric AIDS Clinical Trials Group. Lymphocyte subsets in healthy children from birth through 18 years of age: the Pediatric AIDS Clinical Trials Group P1009 study. J Allergy Clin Immunol 2003;112:973–80.

34. Folds JD, Schmitz JL. Clinical and laboratory assessment of immunity. J Allergy Clin Immunol. 2003;111(2 Suppl):S702–11.

35. Centers for Disease Control and Prevention. Anergy skin testing and preventive therapy for HIV-infected persons: revised recommendations. MMWR Morb Mortal Wkly Rep 1997;46(RR-15):1–19.

36. Gordon EH, Krouse HA, Kinney JL, et al. Delayed cutaneous hypersensitivity in normals: choice of antigens and comparison to in vitro assays of cell-mediated immunity. J Allergy Clin Immunol 1983;72:487–94.

37. Palmer DL, Reed WP. Delayed hypersensitivity skin testing. II. Clinical correlates and anergy. J Infect Dis 1974;130:138–43.

38. Kniker WT, Anderson CT, McBryde JL, et al. Multitest CMI for standardized measurement of delayed cutaneous hypersensitivity and cell-mediated immunity: normal values and proposed scoring system for healthy adults in the USA. Ann Allergy 1984;52:75–82.

39. Kniker WT, Lesourd BM, McBryde JL, et al. Cell-mediated immunity assessed by multitest CMI skin testing in infants and preschool children. Am J Dis Child 1985;139:840–5.

40. Wen L, Atkinson JP, Giclas PC. Clinical and laboratory evaluation of complement deficiency. J Allergy Clin Immunol 2004;113:585–93.

41. Elloumi HZ, Holland SM. Diagnostic assays for chronic granulomatous disease and other neutrophil disorders. Methods Mol Biol 2007;412:505–23.

42. Baehner RL, Nathan DG. Quantitative nitroblue tetrazolium test in chronic granulomatous disease. N Engl J Med 1968;278:971–976.

43. Roesler J, Emmendorffer A. Diagnosis of chronic granulomatous disease. Blood 1991;78:1387–9.

44. Carson JL, Collier AM, Hu S-CS. Acquired ciliary defects in nasal epithelium of children with acute viral upper respiratory infections. N Engl J Med 1985;312:463–8.

45. Stanley P, MacWilliam L, Greenstone M, et al. Efficacy of a saccharin test for screening to detect abnormal mucociliary clearance. Br J Dis Chest 1984;78:62–5.

46. Rosenstein BJ, Cutting GR, for the Cystic Fibrosis Foundation Consensus Panel. The diagnosis of cystic fibrosis: a consensus statement. J Pediatr 1998;132:589–95.

47. Horsburgh CH Jr, Jason J, Longini IM Jr, et al. Duration of human immunodeficiency virus infection before detection of antibody. Lancet 1989;2:637–40.

48. Imagawa DT, Lee MH, Wolinsky SM, et al. Human immunodeficiency virus type 1 infection in homosexual men who remain seronegative for prolonged periods. N Engl J Med 1989;320:1458–62.

49. Saulsbury FT, Wykoff RF, Boyle RJ. Transfusion-acquired human immunodeficiency virus infection in twelve neonates: epidemiologic, clinical and immunologic features. Pediatr Infect Dis J 1987;6:544–9.

50. Centers for Disease Control and Prevention. Revised guidelines for HIV counseling, testing, and referral and revised recommendations for HIV screening of pregnant women. MMWR Morb Mortal Wkly Rep 2001;50(RR-19):1–110.

CHAPTER 8

Antibody Deficiency

Francisco A. Bonilla

Primary immunodeficiencies result from inherited or spontaneous genetic lesions affecting immune system function. These are subdivided into defects of adaptive and innate immunity. Defects of adaptive immunity are further subdivided into humoral, cellular, and combined immunodeficiencies arising as a result of T and/or B lymphocyte dysfunction. The disorders of innate immunity result from defects of some lymphocyte subsets such as natural killer cells, phagocytes, the complement system, or signaling systems such as the Toll-like receptors.[1,2] Humoral immunodeficiencies, also called antibody deficiencies, are characterized by low serum levels of one or more immunoglobulin classes and/or relative impairment of antibody responses to antigen challenge. This arises as the result of a defect intrinsic to the antibody-producing cells (B cells) or of a failure of communication between T cells and B cells (T cell help for antibody production). Cell-mediated immunity is intact.

The most common complications of humoral immunodeficiency are recurrent bacterial infections of the upper and lower respiratory tract.[3] Other organ systems frequently infected include the gastrointestinal tract, skin, and the central nervous and musculoskeletal systems. These infections are generally caused by the same organisms virulent in immunocompetent hosts, predominantly encapsulated bacteria such as *Streptococcus pneumoniae*, *Haemophilus influenzae*, *Staphylococcus aureus*, and *Neisseria meningitidis*. Viral infections are usually cleared normally by these patients, although some enteric viruses (particularly echoviruses) may cause severe disease. Antibody deficient individuals will have a higher frequency of recurrence with the same agents, since they often do not produce neutralizing antibodies or B cell memory. Additional infectious diseases may be associated with particular syndromes.[1]

The most severely affected patients have frequent episodes of pneumonia and other invasive bacterial infections, and frequent severe viral infections. However, presentation with milder infections such as treatment-resistant recurrent otitis media and sinusitis are also frequently seen. Unfortunately, there are no clinically based criteria that have been well validated for predicting which children with recurrent otitis media or sinusitis or one or two episodes of pneumonia will have an identifiable immunologic defect. A high index of suspicion for antibody deficiency should be maintained in these cases.[3]

Table 8-1 contains a classification of humoral immunodeficiencies according to known gene defects, as well as clinically defined entities.

Epidemiology and Etiology

Estimates of the incidence and prevalence of immunodeficiency based on survey or registry data both range from about 1:10 000–1:2000.[4] One recent retrospective study of a single county (Olmsted County, Minnesota, USA) reported an incidence of 10.3 cases of primary immunodeficiency per 100 000 person-years during the period 2001–2006.[5] A recent estimate of the prevalence of primary immunodeficiency used a random telephone dialing strategy to identify cases of diagnosed primary immunodeficiency overall in US households (10 005 households comprising 26 657 individuals were surveyed).[6] These authors concluded that the prevalence of primary immunodeficiency is 1:1200 individuals with a 95% confidence interval of 1:1956–1:824. Based on survey and registry data worldwide, antibody deficiencies account for 57% of all diagnosed primary immunodeficiencies.[4]

X-linked Agammaglobulinemia

Ogden Bruton published the classic description of this disorder in 1952. This condition is, therefore, often called 'Bruton's agammaglobulinemia.'[7] It is caused by a defect in a signal-transducing protein known as Bruton's tyrosine kinase (BTK).[8] BTK is expressed in B cells at all stages of development, as well as in monocytes, macrophages, mast cells, erythroid cells, and platelets. BTK transduces signals from the B cell immunoglobulin receptor, as well as other signaling pathways. In its absence, B cell development is impeded at an early stage (the pro-B cell to pre-B cell transition).

Only males are affected, and they are often asymptomatic during infancy. During this period, they are protected by maternal antibodies acquired through placental transfer during gestation. Maternal IgG gradually disappears, and infectious complications usually begin by the age of 9 to 18 months. The absence of visible tonsils or palpable lymph nodes is notable on examination. Laboratory investigation reveals absent or very low serum levels of immunoglobulins and B cells. Neutropenia is not uncommon and may occur in up to 25% of patients. This often resolves when the load of bacterial infection is reduced by antibiotic therapy.

Despite normal cellular immunity, patients with X-linked agammaglobulinemia (XLA) are prone to certain viral infections, including chronic enteroviral meningoencephalitis and vaccine-

©2010 Elsevier Ltd, Inc, BV
DOI: 10.1016/B978-1-4377-0271-2.00008-0

Table 8-1 Classification of Humoral Immunodeficiencies

Disease	Gene
Known Genetic Basis	
X-linked (Bruton's) agammaglobulinemia (XLA), Bruton's tyrosine kinase	BTK
Autosomal recessive agammaglobulinemia (AR AGAM):	
Immunoglobulin M constant region (Cµ)	IGHM
Signal transducing molecule Ig-α	CD79A
Surrogate light chain	CD179B
B cell linker protein	BLNK
Translocation of LRRC8	LRRC8
Hyper-IgM syndrome (HIM)	
X-linked (XHIM, HIM1), tumor necrosis factor superfamily member 5 (CD154, CD40 ligand)	TNFSF5
Autosomal recessive:	
Activation-induced cytidine deaminase (HIM2)	AICDA
Tumor necrosis factor receptor superfamily member 5 (CD40) (HIM3)	TNFRSF5
Uracil nucleoside glycosylase (HIM5)	UNG
Common variable immunodeficiency	
Inducible costimulator	ICOS
CD19	CD19
Transmembrane activator and calcium mobilizing ligand interactor (TACI, also tumor necrosis factor receptor superfamily 13B)	TNFRSF13B
Unknown Genetic Basis	
Common variable immunodeficiency	
IgA deficiency	
IgG subclass deficiency	
Specific antibody deficiency with normal immunoglobulins	
Transient hypogammaglobulinemia of infancy	
Hypogammaglobulinemia, unspecified	

associated poliomyelitis. These susceptibilities indicate the importance of specific antibody for control of these agents. Additional infections described in these patients include mycoplasma or ureaplasma arthritis.[9] Opportunistic infections such as *Pneumocystis jiroveci* pneumonia are seen only very rarely.[10]

About half of XLA patients have a family history of affected male relatives on the maternal side.[8] Autosomal recessive forms of agammaglobulinemia with a virtually identical phenotype (see later) must be distinguished among those without a family history. BTK is expressed in platelets and monocytes and may be detected by flow cytometry, which may be used as a screening test.[11,12] This method is also useful for detecting carrier females who have random X-chromosome inactivation in monocytes or megakaryocytes and two populations: BTK+ and BTK−.

Some patients with BTK mutations have an 'atypical' phenotype with low numbers of B cells and low-level antibody production.[13] Some of these atypical XLA cases were misdiagnosed as having common variable immunodeficiency (see later) before the recognition of the BTK kinase defect.[1] There is no consistent genotype-phenotype correlation in XLA.[1] Even siblings with identical mutations may show divergent clinical features. Female carriers of XLA show nonrandom X chromosome inactivation in their B cells, and this can be used for carrier detection.

Autosomal Recessive Agammaglobulinemia

Agammaglobulinemia with autosomal recessive inheritance is relatively rare, accounting for about 15% of agammaglobulinemia, overall.[8] Mutations of the immunoglobulin (Ig)-µ heavy-chain locus, the λ5 surrogate light chain, or the signal transducing molecules Igα (CD79a) and Igβ (CD79b), all prevent formation of Ig receptors on pre-B cells and mature B cells.[8,14] Mutations in the gene encoding the signal transduction protein BLNK (B cell linker protein) have also been described.[8] Finally, a single female patient has been described with a translocation interrupting the gene encoding a protein with unknown function called leucine rich repeat containing 8 (LRRC8).[15] All of these autosomal recessive defects arrest B cell development at early stages of development within the bone marrow. The clinical presentation is very similar to XLA.

Common Variable Immunodeficiency

Common variable immunodeficiency (CVID) encompasses several distinct conditions having in common a (relatively) late-onset humoral immunodeficiency.[16-19] CVID patients have recurrent sinopulmonary bacterial infections characteristic of antibody deficiency. Additional manifestations of CVID may include asthma, chronic rhinitis, chronic giardiasis, and recurrent or chronic arthropathy. Acute and chronic enteroviral infections, including meningoencephalitis, may also be seen in CVID. The apparent 'atopic' symptoms found in about 10% of patients occur in the absence of allergen-specific immunoglobulin E (IgE). Malabsorption, inflammatory bowel disease, and autoimmune syndromes such as pernicious anemia and autoimmune cytopenias (thrombocytopenia, anemia, and neutropenia) also occur with increased frequency. Other diseases such as autoimmune polyglandular syndrome type 2 have also been described.[20,21] In addition, noncaseating granulomatous disease resembling sarcoidosis may be encountered in the skin or viscera, even in children. In one study, 6 of 9 individuals with granulomatous lung disease had evidence of infection with human herpesvirus 8.[22]

Lymphoproliferation may cause splenomegaly, adenopathy, and intestinal lymphonodular hyperplasia, and patients with CVID also have a higher incidence of gastrointestinal and lymphoid malignancy. The relative risk of lymphoma has been estimated to be 10- to 20-fold greater than in the general population.[23] Most are B cell non-Hodgkin's lymphomas; some arise in mucosal associated lymphoid tissue (MALT). While EBV is prominent in lymphomas in several primary immunodeficiencies, it is uncommon in CVID.[24] Thymoma with CVID with low B cell numbers has been designated Good's syndrome.[25] It is not clear if this represents a distinct diagnostic entity. Opportunistic infections (such as *P. jiroveci* pneumonia) occur more frequently in Good's syndrome, and the prognosis may be worse than that for the typical CVID patient.

Immunologic findings in CVID are variable, possibly reflecting heterogeneity in the pathophysiology. Hypogammaglobulinemia and impaired specific antibody production are universal, by definition. In addition, patients often have low IgA and/or IgM. The levels of particular Ig isotypes in a patient with CVID are often static over time, but fluctuations may occur. Patients have variable numbers of B cells and T cells.

Upon activation, B cells frequently 'switch' isotype production from IgM and IgD to IgG, IgA, or IgE (see the section on 'Hyper-IgM Syndromes'). Memory B cells express the surface marker CD27. The levels of peripheral blood 'switched' (IgM−IgD−) memory (CD27+) B cells correlate with disease phenotype in CVID. Levels below 1–2% of peripheral B cells are associated with a higher rate of severe infection, autoimmune disease, lymphoproliferation and lymphoma.[26-28] The T cell phenotype in CVID is also variable. Low levels of naïve (CD45RA[+]) CD4 T cells correlate with elements of the disease spectrum similar to those just listed.[29]

X-linked lymphoproliferative disease (XLP) results from mutations in the signaling lymphocyte associated molecule (SLAM)-associated protein (SAP) signal transducing molecule encoded by the SH2D1A gene. Some of these patients have dysgammaglobulinemias of various types, and a few had been classified as having CVID before the discovery of the genetic basis of XLP.[30] It is important to rule out XLP in males with a CVID phenotype because prognosis and therapy are distinct for these disorders. XLP patients have virtually absent natural killer T (NKT) cells and this test can be used as a screen. Rarely, male patients with BTK mutations may be misdiagnosed as having CVID.[31]

Causative genetic lesions have been identified in approximately 1% of patients with CVID. Deficiency of inducible co-stimulator (ICOS) expressed on activated T cells leads to a form of CVID with panhypogammaglobulinemia, low B cells (including low switched memory B cells) and recurrent infections.[32] Autoimmune and lymphoproliferative complications do not occur. A very similar phenotype has been found in a small number of CVID patients with defects of the B cell membrane glycoprotein CD19.[33]

Functionally important polymorphisms of the transmembrane activator and calcium mobilizing ligand interactor (TACI, TNFRSF13B) are found in a higher proportion of CVID patients (in the order of 5–10%) in comparison to the general population (1%).[34,35] Patients with CVID may be homozygous or heterozygous for mutations in TACI. However, these alterations in TACI are likely not to be entirely disease-causing, since some healthy individuals harboring the same genetic changes have been identified.[36,37] Similarly, mutations of the *E. coli* mutS human homologue 5 (MSH5) have been found in some individuals with CVID or IgA deficiency (see below).[38] As is the case with TACI, these changes in MSH5 are also observed in some asymptomatic individuals, indicating a role for additional disease-associated genes.

IgA Deficiency

Human IgA is divided into two subclasses: IgA1 and IgA2. These are encoded by separate genes in the heavy-chain C region locus on chromosome 14. IgA1 constitutes 80% to 90% of serum IgA; both contribute equally to secretory IgA. Both IgA1 and IgA2 subclasses are affected in IgA deficiency (IGAD). Very low levels of total IgA (<7 mg/dL) are found in about 1:500–700 whites.[39] This is called selective IGAD. Clinical associations with levels of IgA that are above this threshold, but still below the lower limit of the normal range ('low' IgA) are not well established. Most individuals with IGAD are asymptomatic. In a population of patients with chronic bacterial sinusitis, IGAD is more prevalent than in healthy individuals.[40] Furthermore, 20 years of prospective follow-up of IgA-deficient blood donors showed an increased incidence of respiratory infections and autoimmune disease.[41] Atopic disease is found frequently among IgA-deficient patients.[42] In addition, autoimmune syndromes and malignancies very similar to those associated with CVID occur with greater frequency in IGAD. Rare cases of IGAD may evolve into CVID or improve over time.[43] About one third of IGAD patients have a concomitant IgG subclass deficiency (see later). This association is more frequently accompanied by deficits in specific antibody production and significant infectious complications.[44,45]

No disease-causing genetic defects underlying IGAD have been defined. IgA deficiency and CVID have been associated with human leukocyte antigen (HLA) haplotypes A1-B8-DR3, B14-DR1, and B44.[38] As many as 13% of patients homozygous for A1-B8-DR3 may be IgA deficient. The polymorphisms of MSH5 described above are associated with the A1-B8-DR3 extended haplotype and have also been found in individuals with IGAD. IGAD has been reported in patients after chemotherapy[46] or treatment with anticonvulsants such as phenytoin.[47] In the latter case, the effect was reversible with drug discontinuation.

IgG Subclass Deficiency

Human IgG is divided into four subclasses designated IgG1, 2, 3, and 4, each encoded by different Ig constant region genes. Each represents approximately 67%, 23%, 7%, and 3% of the total IgG, respectively. IgG subclasses are produced in different relative amounts depending on the antigenic stimulus.[48] For example, IgG1 predominates in responses to soluble protein antigens, and responses to pneumococcal capsular polysaccharides consist almost entirely of the IgG2 subclass.

A disproportionately low level of one or more of the four IgG subclasses with normal total serum IgG constitutes an IgG subclass deficiency (IGGSD). Individuals with IGGSD may present with recurrent sinopulmonary infections caused by common respiratory bacterial pathogens.[49,50] Frequent viral infections and recurrent diarrhea (infectious or allergic in nature) are also seen. Additional clinical manifestations may include atopic diseases and rheumatologic disorders as is the case in IGAD and CVID. IGGSD has been reported in patients with HIV infection/AIDS,[51] combined immunodeficiencies such as ataxia-telangiectasia,[52] and after bone marrow transplantation.[53] Patients with IGGSDs in childhood often improve with time, although the IgG subclass abnormality may never normalize completely. When IGGSD is diagnosed in adulthood, resolution is much less likely. As is true of IGAD, IGGSD is not commonly the result of genetic lesions in the human Ig heavy-chain locus.[49] Mutations preventing expression of cell surface IgG2 have been found in a few reported cases of IgG2 deficiency.

Considerable diagnostic controversy arises due to variations in immunoglobulin subclass determinations depending on laboratory methods, as well as significant differences in normal ranges depending on age and ethnicity. Furthermore, most individuals with isolated low IgG subclass levels are asymptomatic, rendering its significance questionable in patients with recurrent infections. However, some studies show a higher prevalence of subclass deficiency in groups of patients with chronic or recurrent sinopulmonary bacterial infection.[50] Not all of these patients have demonstrably impaired specific antibody responses to vaccines or infectious challenge. Thus the connection between IgG subclass deficiency and susceptibility to infection or other disease may be difficult to demonstrate.

Specific Antibody Deficiency with Normal Immunoglobulins

There exists a population of patients with recurrent infections and poor antibody responses (mainly to polysaccharide antigens) who have normal levels of antibody classes and subclasses. This has been called 'specific antibody deficiency with normal immunoglobulins' (SADNI), or 'functional antibody deficiency.'[54] In a retrospective study of 90 patients evaluated for immunodeficiency in one tertiary care center, SADNI was the most frequent diagnosis (23% of patients).[55] The relationship of SADNI to other humoral immunodeficiencies is unclear, although these patients are clinically very similar to those with IGGSD and recurrent infections.

Transient Hypogammaglobulinemia of Infancy

In humans, IgG is actively transported from the maternal to the fetal circulation during gestation, mainly during the third trimester. Maternal antibody has a half-life in the infant's circulation between 20 and 30 days. A physiologic nadir of serum IgG occurs at 3 to 9 months of age as maternal Ig is cleared and newborn IgG production gradually begins. Transient hypogammaglobulinemia of infancy (THI) is an IgG deficiency of unknown cause that begins in infancy and resolves spontaneously by 36 to 48 months of age.[56] Thus, the diagnosis can be confirmed only after IgG levels normalize. By definition, the serum IgG is lower than is normal for age. As is the case in IGAD and IGGSD, many of these children are asymptomatic. Beginning at about 6 months of age, some of these IgG-deficient children manifest the types of recurrent infections associated with hypogammaglobulinemia. Some cases may also be associated with food allergy. Severe infections are not often seen, but vaccine strain polio meningoencephalitis has been reported in one case of THI.[57]

Lymphocyte populations in THI are usually normal, as are various measures of lymphocyte function in vitro. B cell numbers may be elevated in some patients.[56] Most children with THI have normal antibody responses to immunization and other antigen challenges well before their serum antibody levels enter the normal range. Inadequate antibody responses do not exclude the diagnosis of THI but should prompt further investigation for other forms of immunodeficiency.

Hyper-IgM Syndromes

The eponym 'hyper-IgM syndrome' (HIM) has been applied to a pattern of immunodeficiency with a prominent defect in Ig class switching, whereby a B cell changes from production of IgM and IgD to other isotypes such as IgG, IgA, or IgE. If this process is impaired, IgM production predominates in antibody responses with very few, if any, other isotypes being produced (hence the term 'hyper-IgM syndrome'). The X-linked hyper-IgM syndrome (sometimes abbreviated XHIM or HIM1) is a combined immunodeficiency resulting from mutation of the tumor necrosis factor superfamily member 5 (TNFSF5) gene.[58,59] This molecule is also called CD154 or CD40 ligand. Many would consider this to be most appropriately classified as a combined immunodeficiency, because the interactions of T cells with antigen-presenting cells and effector mononuclear cells are significantly impaired. However, HIM1 is often classified with antibody deficiencies because hypogammaglobulinemia is such a prominent feature.

Usually within the first 2 years of life, patients with HIM1 develop the types of recurrent bacterial infections generally seen in hypogammaglobulinemia.[58-60] They are also prone to opportunistic infections from fungal pathogens such as *Pneumocystis* or *Histoplasma*. Additional infections noted most frequently include anemia due to parvovirus and sclerosing cholangitis due to *Cryptosporidium*. Noninfectious complications include neutropenia and liver and certain hematologic malignancies.

B cell numbers are normal; IgG is usually low and IgM high; more than half of patients lack IgA. Specific antibody formation is often impaired. Patients make IgM in response to immunization or infection but little, if any, IgG is produced. Antibody levels wane rapidly, and there are no memory responses. Secondary lymphoid tissues are poorly developed and do not contain germinal centers. The diagnosis may be established by demonstrating a failure of T cells to express CD40 ligand on mitogenic stimulation.

Various forms of hyper-IgM syndrome with autosomal recessive inheritance have also been described. One of these results from mutations in the gene encoding tumor necrosis factor receptor superfamily member 5 (TNFRSF5), also known as CD40.[61] Because this is the ligand for TNFSF5, the molecule affected in XHIM, all of the same cellular interactions are affected, and the pathophysiology is identical.

Two additional forms of autosomal recessive hyper-IgM syndrome are due to mutations of the genes encoding the enzymes activation-induced cytidine deaminase (AID) and uracil nucleoside glycosylase (UNG).[62] Bacterial sinopulmonary infections occur in the majority of patients. Less frequent complications include diarrhea with failure to thrive and massive lymphadenopathy.

Differential Diagnosis

Clinical entities that mimic (or even coexist with) antibody deficiency are listed in Box 8-1. The most frequent presentation of antibody deficiency includes recurrent, frequent, and severe upper and lower respiratory tract infections with encapsulated bacteria, and viruses.[3] Of course, antibody deficiency may accompany cellular immunodeficiency (i.e. combined immunodeficiency). If the cellular immune defect is not profound, the manifestations related to the antibody deficiency component may predominate in the clinical presentation. Normal cellular immune function should be confirmed in all cases of significant abnormalities of humoral immunity (see next section and Figure 8-1).

BOX 8-1

Differential Diagnosis of Antibody Deficiency

Primary humoral immunodeficiency

Secondary or acquired humoral immunodeficiency (immunosuppression, cancer)

Primary combined immunodeficiency

    Severe combined immunodeficiency

    Wiskott-Aldrich syndrome

    DiGeorge syndrome

    Ataxia-telangiectasia

    Other

Secondary or acquired combined immunodeficiency (HIV/AIDS)

Complement deficiency

Phagocytic cell defect

    Chronic granulomatous disease

    Leukocyte adhesion defect

    Chédiak-Higashi syndrome

    Neutropenia

Allergic rhinosinusitis

Anatomic obstruction of Eustachian tube or sinus ostia (tumor, foreign body, lymphoid hyperplasia)

Cystic fibrosis

Ciliary dysfunction

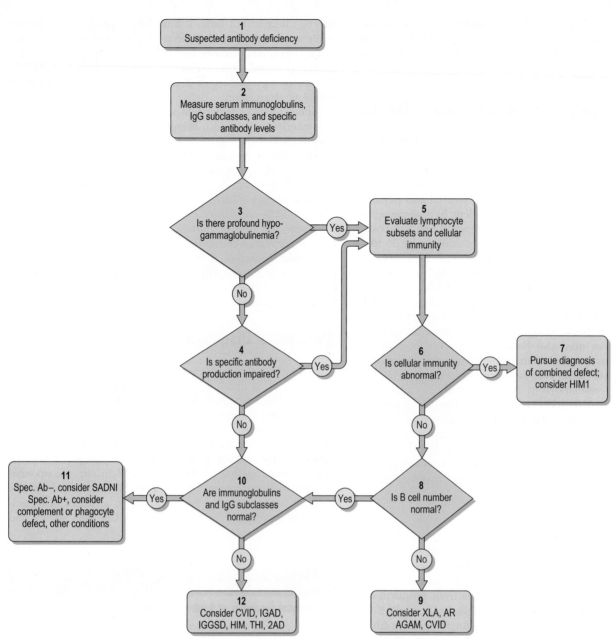

Figure 8-1 Algorithm for evaluation of the patient with suspected antibody deficiency (see text for annotations and abbreviations).

Complement deficiency may present with the infectious complications characteristic of antibody deficiency. Patients with phagocyte defects frequently present with distinct infectious complications, such as deep-seated abscesses or cellulitis, which are not as often seen in antibody deficiencies although they do occur occasionally.

Some 'nonimmune' disorders of host defense may mimic antibody deficiencies, such as cystic fibrosis. Ciliary dysmotility syndromes may have a presentation identical to that of antibody deficiency. Nasopharyngeal anatomic defects or hyperplasia of lymphoid tissue may lead to Eustachian tube or ostiomeatal obstruction and lead to recurrent or chronic otitis media and/or sinusitis. Allergic rhinosinusitis may also lead to sinus and nasopharyngeal mucosal inflammation, promoting mucus stasis and infection. As mentioned, atopic disease (or clinically similar pathology in the absence of IgE) may accompany antibody deficiencies such as CVID, IGAD, and IGGSD. Based on other clinical features of the case in question, some or all of these disorders should be investigated in patients with normal humoral

immunity in the setting of infections characteristic of antibody deficiency.

Evaluation

Figure 8-1 shows an algorithm that may be applied to patients suspected of having humoral immunodeficiency. Some combined immunodeficiencies have characteristic clinical features that should prompt investigation of cellular immune function, even if the history of infections at the time of evaluation is more suggestive of antibody deficiency. Examples include the eczema and thrombocytopenia of Wiskott-Aldrich syndrome, ataxic gait in ataxia-telangiectasia, etc. This algorithm assumes that there are no such features because evaluation of cellular immunity would be undertaken immediately in such cases. The following annotations correspond to the numbered elements in Figure 8-1.

1. The descriptions of the various diseases mentioned point out the characteristic elements of a medical history that

should arouse suspicion of impaired antibody production, with the main element being recurrent upper and lower respiratory tract bacterial infections. Physical examination is generally not specific, often showing only the presence or sequelae of microbial infections. Visible or palpable lymphoid tissue may be scarce or absent in some cases, especially in areas rich in B cells (e.g. tonsils). This is most often the case in the agammaglobulinemias. Specific diagnosis rests entirely on the laboratory evaluation.[1]

2. The initial laboratory examination of humoral immunity consists of measuring the levels of various Ig isotypes (IgG, IgA, IgM, and possibly IgG subclasses) in serum, as well as a measure of function or specific antibody production (Table 8-2).[63] Specific antibody titers both to protein and polysaccharide antigens should be measured. These substances differ in how they stimulate antibody production, and clinically significant disease may result from a selective inability to respond to polysaccharide antigens (see earlier). Antibody levels for protein vaccine antigens such as tetanus and diphtheria are often determined. Antibodies against the capsular polysaccharide (polyribose phosphate [PRP]) of *H. influenzae* type B (HIB) may also be measured. It is important to note that current HIB vaccines couple the PRP to a protein carrier, and PRP titers in immunized children, although specific for a polysaccharide, are indicative of immune response to a protein.

Similar considerations apply to measurement of antibodies against pneumococcal capsular polysaccharides. Antibody levels measured after natural exposure or immunization with unconjugated pneumococcal vaccines are indicative of polysaccharide responses. Newer pneumococcal vaccines also couple the polysaccharide to a protein carrier, and responses to these vaccines are indicative of protein antigen response. The interpretation of pneumococcal polysaccharide responses is complex.1,[64,65] It is often helpful to assess responses to as large a number of serotypes as possible, to include types present in the conjugate vaccine, as well as those contained only in the unconjugated vaccines. The 4-fold rise in antibody level is still generally regarded as the accepted criterion of response to a single type. However, the likelihood of a 4-fold rise decreases as the pre-immunization level increases.[64,65] In addition, a level of 1.3 μg/mL is considered a criterion of protection with respect to a single type in the setting of a standardized ELISA method.[65] Note that this precise standard method is not used in all clinical laboratories. Although many children less than 2 years of age may respond well to some pneumococcal types, many normal children respond poorly. In general, children of 2 to 5 years of age have protective antibody or a 4-fold rise in level for 50% of pneumococcal types. Individuals who are 6 years old or more will normally respond to at least 70% of serotypes.[65]

If initial measurements of specific antibodies are low, response to booster immunization should be assessed. Postvaccination levels may be determined after 4 to 6 weeks. One must bear in mind that polysaccharide antibody responses are less reliable in normal children under the age of 2 years, and negative responses to these antigens in these patients should be interpreted with caution.[66] Serum isohemagglutinins are naturally occurring antibodies against ABO blood group antigens. They are produced in response to polysaccharide antigens of gut flora, and measurement is sometimes a useful indicator of polysaccharide immunity.[65]

3. Profound hypogammaglobulinemia with serum IgG of less than 100 mg/dL in an infant or less than 200 to 300 mg/dL

Table 8-2 Reference Ranges for Serum Immunoglobulins and Specific Antibody Levels*

Age	IgG (mg/dL)	IgA (mg/dL)	IgM (mg/dL)
0–1 mo	700–1300	0–11	5–30
1–4 mo	280–750	6–50	15–70
4–7 mo	200–1200	8–90	10–90
7–13 mo	300–1500	16–100	25–115
13 mo–3 yr	400–1300	20–230	30–120
3–6 yr	600–1500	50–150	22–100
6-yr adult	639–1344	70–312	56–352

Age	IgG1 (mg/dL)	IgG2 (mg/dL)	IgG3 (mg/dL)	IgG4 (mg/dL)
Cord	435–1084	143–453	27–146	1–47
0–3 mo	218–496	40–167	4–23	1–120
3–6 mo	143–394	23–147	4–100	1–120
6–9 mo	190–388	37–60	12–62	1–120
9 mo–2 yr	286–680	30–327	13–82	1–120
2–4 yr	381–884	70–443	17–90	1–120
4–6 yr	292–816	83–513	8–111	2–112
6–8 yr	422–802	113–480	15–133	1–138
8–10 yr	456–938	163–513	26–113	1–95
10–12 yr	456–952	147–493	12–179	1–153
12–14 yr	347–993	140–440	23–117	1–143
Adult	422–1292	117–747	41–129	10–67

	Tetanus Toxoid (IU/mL)	PRP (HIB) (ng/mL)	Pneumococcus
Protective level	0.15	1000	1000
Adequate response	4-fold rise	4-fold rise	4-fold rise

	Isohemagglutinin Titer	
Age	Anti-A	Anti-B
0–6 mo	Unpredictable	Unpredictable
6 mo–2 yr	≥1:4–8	≥1:4–8
2–10 yr	1:4–256	1:16–256
10-yr adult	≥1:4–8	≥1:4–8

*These are normal ranges from the laboratories of Children's Hospital, Boston, MA (except isohemagglutinins, see Fong SW, Qaqundah BY, Taylor WF. Transfusion 1974;14:551). Normal ranges are method-dependent and should be validated for each laboratory. These reference ranges are intended for educational purposes only.

in an older child or adult should prompt additional evaluation of lymphocyte populations and cellular immune function to investigate combined immunodeficiency and B cell number.[1,63]

4. Specific antibody responses may be impaired as a result of the failure of T cell help for antibody production, even if

serum Ig levels are normal or near normal. This situation should also prompt an evaluation of cellular immunity.[1]

5. Cellular immunity is evaluated because of either severe hypogammaglobulinemia or impaired specific antibody production.

6. **and 7.** If cellular immunity is abnormal, then the eventual diagnosis will be a form of combined immunodeficiency. Recall that HIM1 is often classified as a combined immunodeficiency.

8. Cellular immunity is normal; it is important to determine whether there appears to be a significant impairment of B cell development.

9. B cells are usually absent or severely reduced in X-linked or autosomal recessive agammaglobulinemia (XLA or AR AGAM). A positive family history of affected male relatives on the mother's side establishes the diagnosis of XLA.[67] Demonstration of maternal carrier status (nonrandom inactivation of X chromosomes in maternal B cells) is presumptive evidence; the diagnosis should be confirmed by molecular analysis. B cells may also be low in some cases of CVID.

10. At this point, either there is no severe hypogammaglobulinemia and specific antibody formation is not significantly impaired or specific antibody is reduced, a cellular immunologic evaluation is normal, and the B cell number is normal. Most of the remaining diagnoses are clinically defined, in part by the serum Ig profile.

11. If specific antibody formation is impaired (Spec.Ab−) and serum immunoglobulins are normal, then the diagnosis is SADNI. Otherwise, all measurements are normal (Spec. Ab+), and alternative explanations for recurrent infections should be sought. See the discussion on 'Differential Diagnosis'.

12. There is an immunoglobulin abnormality, with or without demonstrable impairment of specific antibody production. Possible diagnoses include CVID, a form of HIM, IGAD, IGGSD, THI, and possibly secondary antibody deficiency.

Treatment

There are two principal modalities used to treat patients with antibody deficiencies: antimicrobial therapy (and prophylaxis) and immunoglobulin replacement (Box 8-2). Agammaglobulinemia, CVID, and HIM are clear indications for immediate replacement therapy with immunoglobulin.[1] Antibiotics are used as necessary to treat infectious complications before or during IgG replacement. The choice of antibiotic depends on the site of infection, severity, past history of infections and antibiotic use, and microbiologic data, where available. Doses do not need to be adjusted for immunodeficiency; however, resolution may be slower in comparison with immunocompetent patients, and treatment may need to be prolonged.

The role of IgG in the therapy of IGAD, IGGSD, and specific antibody deficiency is not as clear. These patients are probably best managed initially with therapeutic and prophylactic antibiotics and thorough evaluation to rule out other potential predisposing factors (e.g. anatomic defects, environmental allergies). If standard preventive regimens[68] are not effective, prophylaxis may be attempted by using half of the therapeutic daily dose of the antibiotic of choice. If infections continue to occur with unacceptable frequency or severity, and especially if antibody responses to immunization are poor, gamma globulin replacement is indicated.

BOX 8-2 Therapeutic principles

Care of Patients with Antibody Deficiency

Therapy for Existing Infections

Antimicrobial chemotherapy, standard-dose regimens are appropriate

Intravenous immunoglobulin, doses range from 300–800 mg/kg q2–4 weeks (see text)

Subcutaneous immunoglobulin, doses range from 50–300 mg/kg semiweekly–q2 weeks

Prevention of Further Infections

Immunoglobulin replacement

Antimicrobial chemoprophylaxis	Children	Adults
Amoxicillin	20 mg/kg qd or ÷ bid	500 mg qd/bid
Trimethoprim (TMP)/ sulfamethoxazole (dosing for TMP)	5 mg/kg qd	160 mg qd
Azithromycin	10 mg/kg qwk	250–500 mg qwk

Supportive Care

Fluid and nutritional support, enteral, parenteral

Cardiopulmonary support

IgG replacement therapy may provide some antibody deficient patients with an almost normal lifestyle. Studies in patients with agammaglobulinemia (serum IgG of less than 100 mg/mL) have clearly shown that relatively high-dose regimens of monthly IgG replacement (600 mg/kg) versus a low-dose (200 mg/kg) regimen are superior, as determined by subjective criteria such as chest radiographs, pulmonary function, and rates of major or minor infections.[69] Maintaining a trough serum IgG level of greater than 500 to 600 mg/dL is beneficial. Most patients do well with about 300 to 500 mg/kg, usually at 2- to 4-week intervals. Adjustment of both the dose and the infusion interval is empirical. One randomized crossover study in 41 hypogammaglobulinemic patients compared low-dose (300 mg/kg in adults, 400 mg/kg in children) with high-dose (double the low dose) monthly IVIG therapy.[70] High-dose therapy was associated with significant reduction in both number (3.5 vs 2.5 per patient over 9 months) and duration (median, 33 days vs 21 days) of infections. Note that IgG replacement is also available by subcutaneous infusion.[71] Similar cumulative dose regimens are achieved by administering smaller doses at more frequent intervals (usually weekly). Thus, even when peripheral access is problematic, placement of a central catheter is not required.

Patients with XLA and CVID should be treated with IgG replacement therapy.[71] A retrospective study of bacterial infections in XLA patients showed a reduction in incidence from 0.4 to 0.06 episodes per patient per year with IVIG therapy.[72] Some viral infections, including enteroviral meningoencephalitis, may occur (although rarely) in patients, even while receiving IVIG. IgG replacement leads to prompt and dramatic reduction in the incidence of pneumonia in patients with CVID.[73] Most patients with XLA and CVID do well with IgG replacement therapy (see later). Occasionally, antibiotic prophylaxis is also required.

Anaphylactoid reactions to IgA containing blood products (including IVIG) occur rarely in IgA-deficient CVID patients with circulating anti-IgA antibodies.[74] These reactions occur in a subset of individuals having undetectable IgA and high titer IgG anti-IgA antibodies. Note that anti-IgA antibodies are not found in individuals with any measurable level of serum IgA. The threshold antibody level for reaction is unknown. If anti-IgA antibodies are present, IgG replacement therapy is best administered via the subcutaneous route, as it has been demonstrated to be safe in this situation.[75,76]

There are no randomized trials of IgG replacement therapy in IGAD, IGGSD, specific antibody deficiency, or THI. One open trial of IVIG in 12 patients with IgG3 subclass deficiency for whom antibiotic prophylaxis failed found significant reductions in the frequency of acute sinusitis and otitis media.[77] Another retrospective study indicated that IVIG was of benefit for a substantial fraction of patients with IGGSD.[50] Patients with IGGSD and SADNI have also been included in some clinical trials of IVIG products. One such study compared IVIG with equivalent cumulative monthly doses administered by subcutaneous infusion on a weekly basis.[78] There were no differences in efficacy or rate of adverse events. Symptomatic IGGSD or THI should be managed initially with antibiotic prophylaxis. Failure of preventive antibiotic treatment may justify a period of gamma globulin replacement. After 6 to 12 months, infusions should be stopped and antibody production reevaluated. Children with recurrent infections, regardless of immunoglobulin class or subclass levels, and normal responses to immunization may be difficult to manage. The benefit of gamma globulin replacement is less predictable, although an attempt is probably warranted in patients with significant infectious complications in the absence of other predisposing factors and for whom antibiotic prophylaxis fails.

HIM1 is usually treated with IgG replacement and trimethoprim/sulfamethoxazole prophylaxis of *P. jiroveci* pneumonia.[58–60] Neutropenia in this disorder sometimes responds to granulocyte colony-stimulating factor (G-CSF, or filgrastim). HIM1 is curable with bone marrow transplantation. Successful sequential liver and bone marrow transplantation has also been reported. IgG therapy alone with or without the use of antibiotic prophylaxis is generally adequate therapy for otherwise uncomplicated autosomal recessive hyper-IgM syndrome.

Conclusions

There are no prospective studies that define the 'true' incidence of clinically significant antibody deficiency. Some diagnostic controversy still exists with respect to what constitutes 'clinically significant' rates or severity of infection, and there are no criteria regarding such histories that have proven sensitivity or specificity leading toward diagnosis of antibody deficiency. Thus it is important to maintain an index of suspicion in cases where an infectious predisposition appears to exist (see Box 8-3).

One prospective analysis of patients presenting with hypogammaglobulinemia under the age of 4 years showed three distinct patterns over time.[79] In group 1, composed of 29 patients (83%), IgG and its subclass levels and antibody responses all became normal and infections ceased; in group 2 (3 patients, or 9%) IgG levels remained low, and antibody production was poor; and in the remaining 3 patients (group 3), IgG levels became normal, but antibody production remained poor. Group 1 would be classified as THI and group 3 as SADNI. Group 2 consists of uncharacterized, persistent hypogammaglobulinemia. This could include atypical XLA, CVID, HIM, or undefined conditions. Invasive infections and low tetanus antibody level at presentation were the most significant predictors of persistent hypogammaglobulinemia. A more recent study arrived at similar conclusions.[80]

Although it may be reassuring that a large proportion of these patients appear to improve with time, this will certainly not be the case for all. Even for patients who are destined to recover

---

BOX 8-3 Key concepts

Antibody Deficiencies

- A clinician must maintain an index of suspicion for immunodeficiency when confronted with patients with infections considered unusual with respect to frequency, severity, response to treatment, or organism.
- The possibility of antibody deficiency in particular should be considered when the history includes pyogenic upper and lower respiratory tract infections.
- Early diagnosis is critical for reducing morbidity and mortality rates for immunodeficiency diseases.
- To provide the most efficient and complete approach to diagnosis and management, referral to a clinical immunology specialist is indicated where there is clear evidence for, or suspicion of, antibody or other immunodeficiency syndrome.
- Intravenous or subcutaneous immunoglobulin replacement therapy and antibiotic prophylaxis are the main modalities for management of antibody deficiency disorders.
- With IVIG and antibiotics, many patients with agammaglobulinemia or hypogammaglobulinemia may lead normal or near-normal lives.

---

completely, early diagnosis is critical for preventing significant morbidity and mortality (Box 8-3).

Helpful Websites

The American Academy of Allergy, Asthma and Immunology website (www.aaaai.org)

The Clinical Immunology Society website (www.clinimmsoc.org/)

The Immune Deficiency Foundation website (www.primaryimmune.org)

The Immunodeficiency Resource website (www.uta.fi/imt/bioinfo/idr)

The Primary Immunodeficiency Resource Center (www.info4pi.org)

References

1. Bonilla FA, Bernstein IL, Khan DA, et al. Practice parameter for the diagnosis and management of primary immunodeficiency. Ann Allergy Asthma Immunol 2005;94:S1.
2. Geha RS, Notarangelo LD, Casanova JL, et al. Primary immunodeficiency diseases: an update from the International Union of Immunological Societies Primary Immunodeficiency Diseases Classification Committee. J Allergy Clin Immunol 2007;120:776.
3. Wood P, Stanworth S, Burton J, et al. Recognition, clinical diagnosis and management of patients with primary antibody deficiencies: a systematic review. Clin Exp Immunol 2007;149:410.
4. Rezaei N, Bonilla FA, Sullivan KE, et al. An introduction to primary immunodeficiency diseases. In: Rezaei N, Aghamohammadi A, Notarangelo L, editors. Primary immunodeficiency diseases: definition, diagnosis, management. Berlin: Springer-Verlag; 2008, p. 1.
5. Joshi AY, Iyer VN, Hagan JB, et al. Incidence and temporal trends of primary immunodeficiency: a population-based cohort study. Mayo Clin Proc 2009;84:16.
6. Boyle JM, Buckley RH. Population prevalence of diagnosed primary immunodeficiency diseases in the United States. J Clin Immunol 2007;27:497.
7. Bruton OC. Agammaglobulinemia. Pediatrics 1952;9:722.
8. Conley ME, Broides A, Hernandez-Trujillo V, et al. Genetic analysis of patients with defects in early B cell development. Immunol Rev 2005;203:216.
9. Bloom KA, Chung D, Cunningham-Rundles C. Osteoarticular infectious complications in patients with primary immunodeficiencies. Curr Opin Rheumatol 2008;20:480.

10. Alibrahim A, Lepore M, Lierl M, et al. Pneumocystis carinii pneumonia in an infant with X-linked agammaglobulinemia. J Allergy Clin Immunol 1998;101:552.

11. Futatani T, Watanabe C, Baba Y, et al. Bruton's tyrosine kinase is present in normal platelets and its absence identifies patients with X-linked agammaglobulinaemia and carrier females. Br J Haematol 2001;114:141.

12. Kanegane H, Futatani T, Wang Y, et al. Clinical and mutational characteristics of X-linked agammaglobulinemia and its carrier identified by flow cytometric assessment combined with genetic analysis. J Allergy Clin Immunol 2001;108:1012.

13. Mueller OT, Hitchcock R. Gene symbol: BTK. Disease: agammaglobulinaemia. Hum Genet 2008;124:299.

14. Ferrari S, Lougaris V, Caraffi S, et al. Mutations of the Igbeta gene cause agammaglobulinemia in man. J Exp Med 2007;204:2047.

15. Sawada A, Takihara Y, Kim JY, et al. A congenital mutation of the novel gene LRRC8 causes agammaglobulinemia in humans. J Clin Invest 2003;112:1707.

16. Chapel H, Lucas M, Lee M, et al. Common variable immunodeficiency disorders: division into distinct clinical phenotypes. Blood 2008;112:277.

17. Oksenhendler E, Gerard L, Fieschi C, et al. Infections in 252 patients with common variable immunodeficiency. Clin Infect Dis 2008;46:1547.

18. Quinti I, Soresina A, Spadaro G, et al. Long-term follow-up and outcome of a large cohort of patients with common variable immunodeficiency. J Clin Immunol 2007;27:308.

19. Wehr C, Kivioja T, Schmitt C, et al. The EUROclass trial: defining subgroups in common variable immunodeficiency. Blood 2008;111:77.

20. Cunningham-Rundles C. Autoimmune manifestations in common variable immunodeficiency. J Clin Immunol 2008;28(Suppl 1):S42.

21. Lopes-da-Silva S, Rizzo LV. Autoimmunity in common variable immunodeficiency. J Clin Immunol 2008;28(Suppl 1):S46.

22. Wheat WH, Cool CD, Morimoto Y, et al. Possible role of human herpesvirus 8 in the lymphoproliferative disorders in common variable immunodeficiency. J Exp Med 2005;202:479.

23. Chua I, Quinti I, Grimbacher B. Lymphoma in common variable immunodeficiency: interplay between immune dysregulation, infection and genetics. Curr Opin Hematol 2008;15:368.

24. Gompels MM, Hodges E, Lock RJ, et al. Lymphoproliferative disease in antibody deficiency: a multi-centre study. Clin Exp Immunol 2003;134:314.

25. Agarwal S, Cunningham-Rundles C. Thymoma and immunodeficiency (Good syndrome): a report of 2 unusual cases and review of the literature. Ann Allergy Asthma Immunol 2007;98:185.

26. Ko J, Radigan L, Cunningham-Rundles C. Immune competence and switched memory B cells in common variable immunodeficiency. Clin Immunol 2005;116:37.

27. Piqueras B, Lavenu-Bombled C, Galicier L, et al. Common variable immunodeficiency patient classification based on impaired B cell memory differentiation correlates with clinical aspects. J Clin Immunol 2003;23:385.

28. Warnatz K, Denz A, Drager R, et al. Severe deficiency of switched memory B cells (CD27(+)IgM(–)IgD(–)) in subgroups of patients with common variable immunodeficiency: a new approach to classify a heterogenous disease. Blood 2002;99:1544.

29. Giovannetti A, Pierdominici M, Mazzetta F, et al. Unravelling the complexity of T cell abnormalities in common variable immunodeficiency. J Immunol 2007;178:3932.

30. Morra M, Silander O, Calpe S, et al. Alterations of the X-linked lymphoproliferative disease gene SH2D1A in common variable immunodeficiency syndrome. Blood 2001;98:1321.

31. Weston SA, Prasad ML, Mulligan CG, et al. Assessment of male CVID patients for mutations in the Btk gene: how many have been misdiagnosed? Clin Exp Immunol 2001;124:465.

32. Salzer U, Maul-Pavicic A, Cunningham-Rundles C, et al. ICOS deficiency in patients with common variable immunodeficiency. Clin Immunol 2004;113:234.

33. van Zelm MC, Reisli I, van der Burg M, et al. An antibody-deficiency syndrome due to mutations in the CD19 gene. N Engl J Med 2006;354:1901.

34. Castigli E, Wilson SA, Garibyan L, et al. TACI is mutant in common variable immunodeficiency and IgA deficiency. Nat Genet 2005;37:829.

35. Salzer U, Chapel HM, Webster AD, et al. Mutations in TNFRSF13B encoding TACI are associated with common variable immunodeficiency in humans. Nat Genet 2005;37:820.

36. Pan-Hammarstrom Q, Salzer U, Du L, et al. Reexamining the role of TACI coding variants in common variable immunodeficiency and selective IgA deficiency. Nat Genet 2007;39:429.

37. Zhang L, Radigan L, Salzer U, et al. Transmembrane activator and calcium-modulating cyclophilin ligand interactor mutations in common variable immunodeficiency: clinical and immunologic outcomes in heterozygotes. J Allergy Clin Immunol 2007;120:1178.

38. Sekine H, Ferreira RC, Pan-Hammarstrom Q, et al. Role for Msh5 in the regulation of Ig class switch recombination. Proc Natl Acad Sci U S A 2007;104:7193.

39. Weber-Mzell D, Kotanko P, Hauer AC, et al. Gender, age and seasonal effects on IgA deficiency: a study of 7293 Caucasians. Eur J Clin Invest 2004;34:224.

40. Tahkokallio O, Seppala IJ, Sarvas H, et al. Concentrations of serum immunoglobulins and antibodies to pneumococcal capsular polysaccharides in patients with recurrent or chronic sinusitis. Ann Otol Rhinol Laryngol 2001;110:675.

41. Koskinen S, Tolo H, Hirvonen M, et al. Long-term follow-up of anti-IgA antibodies in healthy IgA-deficient adults. J Clin Immunol 1995;15:194.

42. Cunningham-Rundles C. Physiology of IgA and IgA deficiency. J Clin Immunol 2001;21:303.

43. Aghamohammadi A, Mohammadi J, Parvaneh N, et al. Progression of selective IgA deficiency to common variable immunodeficiency. Int Arch Allergy Immunol 2008;147:87.

44. Edwards E, Razvi S, Cunningham-Rundles C. IgA deficiency: clinical correlates and responses to pneumococcal vaccine. Clin Immunol 2004;111:93.

45. Kutukculer N, Karaca NE, Demircioglu O, et al. Increases in serum immunoglobulins to age-related normal levels in children with IgA and/or IgG subclass deficiency. Pediatr Allergy Immunol 2007;18:167.

46. Uram R, Rosoff PM. Isolated IgA deficiency after chemotherapy for acute myelogenous leukemia in an infant. Pediatr Hematol Oncol 2003;20:487.

47. Braconier JH. Reversible total IgA deficiency associated with phenytoin treatment. Scand J Infect Dis 1999;31:515.

48. Ferrante A, Beard LJ, Feldman RG. IgG subclass distribution of antibodies to bacterial and viral antigens. Pediatr Inf Dis J 1990;9:S16.

49. Pan Q, Hammarstrom L. Molecular basis of IgG subclass deficiency. Immunol Rev 2000;178:99.

50. Olinder-Nielsen AM, Granert C, Forsberg P, et al. Immunoglobulin prophylaxis in 350 adults with IgG subclass deficiency and recurrent respiratory tract infections: a long-term follow-up. Scand J Infect Dis 2007;39:44.

51. Bartmann P, Grosch-Worner I, Wahn V, et al. IgG2 deficiency in children with human immunodeficiency virus infection. Eur J Pediatr 1991;150:234.

52. Aucouturier P, Bremard-Oury C, Griscelli C, et al. Serum IgG subclass deficiency in ataxia telangiectasia. Clin Exp Immunol 1987;68:392.

53. Kristinsson VH, Kristinsson JR, Jonmundsson GK, et al. Immunoglobulin class and subclass concentrations after treatment of childhood leukemia. Pediatr Hematol Oncol 2001;18:167.

54. Boyle RJ, Le C, Balloch A, et al. The clinical syndrome of specific antibody deficiency in children. Clin Exp Immunol 2006;146:486.

55. Javier FC 3rd, Moore CM, Sorensen RU. Distribution of primary immunodeficiency diseases diagnosed in a pediatric tertiary hospital. Ann Allergy Asthma Immunol 2000;84:25.

56. Dorsey MJ, Orange JS. Impaired specific antibody response and increased B cell population in transient hypogammaglobulinemia of infancy. Ann Allergy Asthma Immunol 2006;97:590.

57. Inaba H, Hori H, Ito M, et al. Polio vaccine virus-associated meningoencephalitis in an infant with transient hypogammaglobulinemia. Scand J Infect Dis 2001;33:630.

58. Lougaris V, Badolato R, Ferrari S, et al. Hyper immunoglobulin M syndrome due to CD40 deficiency: clinical, molecular, and immunological features. Immunol Rev 2005;203:48.

59. Winkelstein JA, Marino MC, Ochs H, et al. The X-linked hyper-IgM syndrome: clinical and immunologic features of 79 patients. Medicine (Baltimore) 2003;82:373.

60. Bonilla FA, Geha RS. CD154 deficiency and related syndromes. Immunol Allergy Clin North Am 2001;21:65.

61. Ferrari S, Giliani S, Insalaco A, et al. Mutations of CD40 gene cause an autosomal recessive form of immunodeficiency with hyper IgM. Proc Natl Acad Sci U S A 2001;98:12614.

62. Durandy A, Taubenheim N, Peron S, et al. Pathophysiology of B cell intrinsic immunoglobulin class switch recombination deficiencies. Adv Immunol 2007;94:275.

63. Agarwal S, Cunningham-Rundles C. Assessment and clinical interpretation of reduced IgG values. Ann Allergy Asthma Immunol 2007;99:281.

64. Hare ND, Smith BJ, Ballas ZK. Antibody response to pneumococcal vaccination as a function of preimmunization titer. J Allergy Clin Immunol 2009;123:195.

65. Paris K, Sorensen RU. Assessment and clinical interpretation of polysaccharide antibody responses. Ann Allergy Asthma Immunol 2007;99:462.

66. Leinonen M, Sakkinen A, Kalliokoski R, et al. Antibody response to 14-valent pneumococcal capsular polysaccharide vaccine in pre-school age children. Pediatr Infect Dis 1986;5:39.

67. Conley ME, Rohrer J, Minegishi Y. X-linked agammaglobulinemia. Clin Rev Allergy Immunol 2000;19:183.

68. De Diego JI, Prim MP, Alfonso C, et al. Comparison of amoxicillin and azithromycin in the prevention of recurrent acute otitis media. Int J Pediatr Otorhinolaryngol 2001;58:47.

69. Orange JS, Hossny EM, Weiler CR, et al. Use of intravenous immunoglobulin in human disease: a review of evidence by members of the

Primary Immunodeficiency Committee of the American Academy of Allergy, Asthma and Immunology. J Allergy Clin Immunol 2006;117:S525.

70. Eijkhout HW, van Der Meer JW, Kallenberg CG, et al. The effect of two different dosages of intravenous immunoglobulin on the incidence of recurrent infections in patients with primary hypogammaglobulinemia: a randomized, double-blind, multicenter crossover trial. Ann Intern Med 2001;135:165.

71. Berger M. Subcutaneous administration of IgG. Immunol Allergy Clin North Am 2008;28:779.

72. Quartier P, Debre M, De Blic J, et al. Early and prolonged intravenous immunoglobulin replacement therapy in childhood agammaglobuline-mia: a retrospective survey of 31 patients. J Pediatr 1999;134:589.

73. Busse PJ, Razvi S, Cunningham-Rundles C. Efficacy of intravenous immunoglobulin in the prevention of pneumonia in patients with common variable immunodeficiency. J Allergy Clin Immunol 2002; 109:1001.

74. Horn J, Thon V, Bartonkova D, et al. Anti-IgA antibodies in common variable immunodeficiency (CVID): diagnostic workup and therapeutic strategy. Clin Immunol 2007;122:156.

75. Sundin U, Nava S, Hammarstrom L. Induction of unresponsiveness against IgA in IgA-deficient patients on subcutaneous immunoglobulin infusion therapy. Clin Exp Immunol 1998;112:341.

76. Ahrens N, Hoflich C, Bombard S, et al. Immune tolerance induction in patients with IgA anaphylactoid reactions following long-term intrave-nous IgG treatment. Clin Exp Immunol 2008;151:455.

77. Barlan IB, Geha RS, Schneider LC. Therapy for patients with recurrent infections and low serum IgG3 levels. J Allergy Clin Immunol 1993; 92:353.

78. Chapel HM, Spickett GP, Ericson D, et al. The comparison of the efficacy and safety of intravenous versus subcutaneous immunoglobulin replace-ment therapy. J Clin Immunol 2000;20:94.

79. Dalal I, Reid B, Nisbet-Brown E, et al. The outcome of patients with hypogammaglobulinemia in infancy and early childhood. J Pediatr 1998;133:144.

80. Moschese V, Graziani S, Avanzini MA, et al. A prospective study on children with initial diagnosis of transient hypogammaglobulinemia of infancy: results from the Italian Primary Immunodeficiency Network. Int J Immunopathol Pharmacol 2008;21:343.

9

T Cell Immunodeficiencies

Luigi D. Notarangelo

T lymphocytes are an essential component of adaptive immunity. Through cytolytic activity and release of Th1 cytokines (such as interferon [IFN]-γ) they mediate resistance to intracellular pathogens. In addition, interaction of T cells with B lymphocytes and antigen-presenting cells on the one hand, and release of soluble mediators such as interleukin (IL)-4 and IL-10 on the other, is essential in order to mount T-dependent antibody responses to soluble and particulate antigens, thus contributing to defense against extracellular pathogens. Consequently, severe defects in T cell development and/or function result in severe combined immunodeficiency (SCID), a heterogeneous group of disorders characterized by increased susceptibility to severe infections since early in life.[1] The overall frequency of these disorders is estimated to be 1 in 50 000 to 100 000 live births.

In addition, T lymphocytes play a crucial role in maintaining peripheral immune homeostasis. In keeping with this, it has been demonstrated that impaired development and/or function of regulatory T lymphocytes are associated with immune dysregulation and autoimmunity. Because of the differences in clinical presentation, this chapter will discuss SCID and other congenital T cell disorders separately. For a more detailed discussion of genetically determined T cell mediated autoimmune diseases, bone marrow transplantation, and gene therapy the reader is referred to Chapters 15, 18 and 20.

Severe Combined Immunodeficiency

Etiology

SCID includes a heterogeneous group of disorders that present with a distinct immunologic phenotype, and are caused by mutations of different genes (Table 9-1). These defects affect various steps in T cell development, and can be grouped as follows:

- *Defects of lymphocyte survival*: adenosine deaminase (ADA) deficiency, reticular dysgenesis
- *Signaling defects*: X-linked SCID, JAK3 deficiency, IL-7R deficiency, CD45 deficiency
- *Defects of expression and signaling through the pre-T cell receptor (pre-TCR) and the TCR*: defects of RAG1, RAG2, Artemis, Cernunnos, DNA ligase IV (LIG4), DNA protein kinase catalytic subunit (DNA-PKcs), defects of CD3 chains (CD3δ, CD3ε, CD3ζ), CD45 deficiency.

Occasionally, hypomorphic mutations in these genes may allow for residual T cell development, with or without significant clinical notes of immune dysreactivity and immunopathology. These conditions, and other defects at later stages in T cell development, will be discussed separately in this chapter (see 'Other Combined Immunodeficiencies').

SCID Caused by Adenosine Deaminase Deficiency

Adenosine deaminase (ADA) is a ubiquitously expressed enzyme that mediates conversion of adenosine into inosine, and of deoxyadenosine into deoxyinosine. Deficiency of ADA, inherited as an autosomal recessive trait, accounts for 5–10% of all cases of SCID. Lack of ADA results in intracellular accumulation of deoxyadenosine and of its phosphorylated metabolites, among which dATP is particularly toxic to lymphoid precursors.[2-4] Consequently, complete ADA deficiency is characterized by extreme lymphopenia (T⁻ B⁻ NK⁻ SCID) and extra-immune manifestations (reflecting the housekeeping nature of the *ADA* gene) since early in life. However, partial defects of the enzyme may result in less severe clinical presentation (delayed or late-onset forms) that may even present in adulthood.[5]

Reticular Dysgenesis

This rare form of SCID is characterized by a combined defect in lymphoid and myeloid differentiation, associated with sensorineural deafness.[6] The disease is inherited as an autosomal recessive trait and is due to mutations of the *AK2* gene, encoding for adenylate kinase 2, that controls intramitochondrial levels of ADP. AK2 deficiency results in lack of energetic substrates and increased cell death in lymphoid progenitors and in myeloid precursors committed to neutrophil differentiation.[7,8]

X-Linked Severe Combined Immunodeficiency (SCIDX1, γc Deficiency)

SCIDX1 is the most common form of SCID in humans, with an estimated incidence of 1:100 000–1:150 000 live births. Inherited as an X-linked trait, it is characterized by complete absence of both T and NK lymphocytes, with a preserved development of B lymphocytes (T⁻ B⁺ NK⁻ SCID). The disease is caused by mutations in the *IL2RG* gene, that encodes for the IL2 receptor common gamma chain (IL-2Rγc, γc).[9] The γc-chain is constitutively expressed by T, B, and NK cells, as well as myeloid cells and other cell types, including keratinocytes. The γc protein is an integral component of various cytokine receptors, namely IL-2R, IL-4R, IL-7R, IL-9R, IL-15R and IL-21R. In all of these receptors, the γc is coupled with the intracellular tyrosine kinase Janus-associated

©2010 Elsevier Ltd, Inc, BV
DOI: 10.1016/B978-1-4377-0271-2.00009-2

Table 9-1 Genetic and Immunologic Features of Combined Immune Deficiency

Disease	Gene	Inheritance	Circulating Lymphocytes		
			T	B	NK
B⁻SCID					
Reticular dysgenesis	AK2	AR	↓↓	↓	↓↓
RAG deficiency, T⁻ B⁻SCID	RAG1, RAG2	AR	↓↓	↓↓	N
Radiation-sensitive T⁻ B⁻SCID	DCLRE1C (Artemis)	AR	↓↓	↓↓	N
	PRKDC (DNA-PKcs)	AR	↓↓	↓↓	N
	LIG4	AR	↓↓	↓↓	N
	NHEJ1 (Cernunnos/XLF)	AR	↓↓	↓	N
T⁻ B⁺ SCID					
X-linked SCID	IL2RG	XL	↓↓	N/↑	↓↓
Jak-3 deficiency	Jak-3	AR	↓↓	N/↑	↓↓
IL-7R deficiency	IL7RA	AR	↓↓	N/↑	N
CD45 deficiency	CD45	AR	↓↓	↓	↓
Purine metabolism deficiency					
Adenosine deaminase deficiency	ADA	AR	↓↓	↓	↓
Nucleoside phosphorylase deficiency	PNP	AR	↓↓	↓/N	↓/N
Omenn syndrome	RAG1, RAG2, DCLRE1C, LIG4, ADA	AR	↓/N	↓↓	N
	IL7R, RMRP	AR	↓/N	N	N
	IL2RG	XL	↓/N	N	↓↓
ZAP-70 deficiency	ZAP70	AR	↓ (↓↓ CD8)	N	N
CD25 deficiency	IL2RA	AR	↓	N	N
CD3 deficiency					
CD3δ deficiency	CD3D	AR	↓	N	N
CD3ε deficiency	CD3E	AR	↓	N	N
CD3ζ deficiency	CD3Z	AR	↓	N	N
Calcium flux defects					
Stim1 deficiency	STIM1	AR	N	N	N
Orai1 deficiency	ORAI1	AR	N	N	N
Coronin1-A deficiency	CORO1A	AR	↓	N	N
STAT5b deficiency	STAT5B	AR	↓	N	N
Human nude phenotype	FOXN1	AR	↓↓	N	N
MHC class I deficiency	TAP1, TAP2, TAPBP	AR	↓ (↓↓CD8)	N	N
MHC class II deficiency	CIITA, RFXANK, RFX5, RFXAP	AR	↓ (↓↓CD4)	N	N
X-linked hyper-IgM syndrome	CD40LG (TNFS5)	XL	N	N	N
ID with multiple intestinal atresia	?	AR (?)	↓	↓	N
Cartilage hair hypoplasia	RMRP	AR	↓/N	N	N
Schimke syndrome	SMARCAL1	AR	↓	N	N

T, T lymphocytes; *B*, B lymphocytes; *NK*, natural killer lymphocytes; *AR*, autosomal recessive; *XL*, X-linked; *N*, normal.

kinase (JAK)-3, that mediates signal transduction.[10] The SCID-X1 phenotype reflects impaired signaling through multiple cytokine receptors. In particular, lack of circulating T and NK cells in SCIDX1 males reflects defective signaling through IL-7R and IL-15R, respectively. Altogether, a variety of genetic defects in the *IL2RG* gene have been identified in SCIDX1.[11] Whereas in most cases. defects in the *IL2RG* gene result in T⁻ B⁺ NK⁻ SCID, some mutations may impair, but do not completely abolish, cytokine-mediated signaling, possibly resulting in atypical presentations.

Jak-3 Deficiency

Jak-3 is a cytoplasmic tyrosine kinase that is physically and functionally associated with the γc in all of the γc-containing cytokine receptors, namely IL-2R, IL-4R, IL-7R, IL-9R, IL-15R, and IL-21R.[12]

Mutations of the *JAK3* gene result in a clinical and immunologic phenotype (i.e. T⁻ B⁺ NK⁻ SCID) that is undistinguishable from SCIDX1,[13,14] but with an autosomal pattern of inheritance.

IL-7Rα Deficiency

IL-7Rα deficiency results in an autosomal recessive form of SCID characterized by selective absence of circulating T lymphocytes, with preserved development of B and NK cells (T⁻ B⁺ NK⁺ SCID).[15,16] IL-7 is produced by stromal cells in bone marrow and in the thymus. The IL-7R consists of two subunits, the γc chain and the IL-7R α chain. IL-7 provides survival and proliferative signals to IL-7R⁺ lymphoid progenitor cells. In humans, mutations that impair expression or function of IL-7R result in an early block in T cell development, but do not compromise B cell development. This is at variance with what is observed in *il7r⁻/⁻* (and in *il7*$^{-/-}$) mice, in which both T and B cell development are abrogated.[17]

T⁻ B⁻ SCID Caused by Defective VDJ Recombination

B and T lymphocytes recognize foreign antigen through specialized receptors: the immuno-globulin (Ig) and the T cell receptor (TCR), respectively. The highly polymorphic antigen recognition regions of these receptors are composed of variable/diversity/joining (VDJ) gene segments that undergo somatic rearrangement prior to their expression by a mechanism known as VDJ recombination.[18] The process of VDJ recombination is initiated when the lymphoid-specific recombinase activating gene 1 (RAG1) and RAG2 proteins recognize specific recombination signal sequences (RSS) that flank each of the V, D, and J gene elements, and introduce a DNA double-strand break in this region.[19,20] Subsequently, a variety of ubiquitously expressed proteins (including Ku70, Ku80, DNA-PKcs, XRCC4, DNA ligase IV, Artemis and Cernunnos/XLF) involved in recognition and repair of DNA damage mediate the final steps of the VDJ recombination process.

Accordingly, defects of V(D)J recombination cause complete absence of both T and B lymphocytes, with preserved presence of NK cells (T⁻ B⁻ NK⁺ SCID). This represents the second most common immunologic phenotype of SCID in humans.[21] These patients can be further divided into two subgroups according to their cellular response in vitro to ionizing radiations. Patients with *RAG1* and *RAG2* mutations are not impaired in the mechanisms of DNA double-strand break (dsb) repair, and hence do not exhibit increased cellular radiosensitivity.[22] In contrast, patients with defects of Artemis, LIG4, Cernunnos/XLF or DNA-PKcs show increased radiosensitivity, reflecting impaired dsb repair.[23–27] Among these forms, Artemis deficiency is particularly common among Athabascan-speaking Native Americans, with an estimated incidence of approximately 1 in 2000 live births.

CD3 Deficiencies

The CD3 complex consists of CD3γ, δ, ε and ζ chains, and is required to mediate signaling through the pre-TCR and the TCR.[28–31] In humans, defects of the CD3 δ, ε or ζ chains cause autosomal recessive T⁻ B⁺ NK⁺ SCID. In contrast, CD3γ deficiency is associated with a partial T cell lymphopenia, and a variable clinical phenotype.[32,33]

CD45 Deficiency

Two unrelated patients have been reported in whom SCID was caused by the complete absence of the CD45 protein, a phosphatase that modulates signaling through the TCR/CD3 complex.[34,35] The immunologic phenotype is characterized by complete lack of T cells, with normal to increased B cell counts.

Other Combined Immunodeficiencies

Omenn Syndrome

Omenn syndrome (OS) is a combined immunodeficiency that affects infants of both sexes who present with generalized exudative erythrodermia, enlarged lymph nodes, hepatosplenomegaly, severe respiratory infections, diarrhea, failure to thrive, hypoproteinemia with edema, and eosinophilia[36] (Figure 9-1). This clinical phenotype may mimic graft-versus-host disease, and may in fact occasionally be seen in SCID infants with transplacental passage of alloreactive maternal T cells. Although the

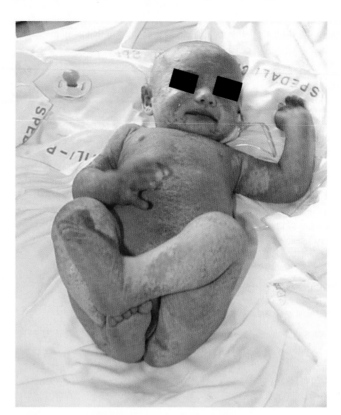

Figure 9-1 Typical clinical features in an infant with Omenn's syndrome. Note generalized erythrodermia with scaly skin, alopecia, and oedema.

latter condition is also referred to as *Omenn-like syndrome,* the term *Omenn syndrome* is reserved for cases in which presence of allogeneic T cells has been ruled out.

The molecular pathogenesis of OS has long remained obscure. However, the demonstration of oligoclonal, activated T cells in OS infants and the simultaneous occurrence of OS and of T⁻ B⁺ SCID in two siblings[37] suggest that OS may be genetically related to T⁻ B⁺ SCID and may reflect defective T and B lymphocyte differentiation. This hypothesis was proved when hypomorphic mutations in *RAG1* and *RAG2* genes were demonstrated in OS patients.[38,39] More recently, it has been recognized that OS may be caused also by hypomorphic defects in other genes, including *Artemis,*[40] *IL7R,*[41] *LIG4,*[42] *RMRP,*[43] *IL2RG,*[44] *ADA,*[45] and *ZAP70.*[46] These defects permit some intrathymic T cell differentiation, with generation of oligoclonal T cells that undergo peripheral expansion, possibly in response to autoantigens. Impaired thymic expression of aire, a transcription factor involved in expression and presentation of self-antigens, has been reported in patients with OS, and may favor survival of autoreactive T cell clones.[47]

Nucleoside Phosphorylase Deficiency

Purine nucleoside phosphorylase (PNP) converts guanosine into guanine and deoxyguanosine to deoxyguanine. PNP deficiency is inherited as an autosomal recessive trait and results in accumulation of phosphorylated deoxyguanosine metabolites (and of dGTP in particular) that inhibit ribonucleotide reductase, whose activity is essential to DNA synthesis. Although PNP is widely expressed, its deficiency is particularly deleterious to lymphoid development, and especially to T cell generation, and to the central nervous system. Consequently, patients with PNP deficiency experience progressive and severe T cell lymphopenia, associated with neurological deterioration.[48]

ZAP-70 Deficiency

Zeta-associated protein of 70 kDa (ZAP-70) is an intracellular tyrosine kinase that is required for T cell activation following engagement of the CD3/TCR complex. Stimulation of T cells through TCR results in activation of the p56lck kinase, which mediates tyrosine phosphorylation of immunoreceptor tyrosine-based activation motifs (ITAMs) in the CD3- γ, -δ, -ε and -ζ chains. ZAP-70 is then recruited into the CD3/TCR complex through binding of its SH2 domains to phosphorylated ITAM motifs of the ζ chain.[49] ZAP-70 itself then becomes phosphorylated by Src-family protein tyrosine kinases, and this phosphorylation triggers ZAP-70 activation, allowing activation of downstream signaling molecules such as linker for activation of T cells (LATs) and SLP-76.[50]

ZAP-70 deficiency is inherited as an autosomal recessive trait, and results in impaired T cell development and function.[51-53] ZAP-70-deficient patients have a profound deficiency of peripheral CD8+ T cells; however, the function of CD4+ T lymphocytes is also affected.

p56lck Deficiency

p56lck is a src-tyrosine kinase that is critically involved in TCR-mediated signaling, contributing to phosphorylation of the ITAM motifs of the proteins of the CD3/TCR complex. Defective expression of p56lck has been found in a SCID infant, whose immunologic phenotype consisted of panhypogammaglobulinemia, lymphopenia with a reduced proportion of CD4+ T cells, and reduced in vitro proliferative responses to CD3 cross-linking.[54]

Major Histocompatibility Complex (MHC) Class II Deficiency

The primary basis for this immunodeficiency resides in the inability of T cells to recognize antigens in the context of self-MHC class II molecules expressed by antigen-presenting cells. In particular, lack of MHC class II molecules expression on the surface of thymic epithelial cells results in an inability to positively select CD4+ thymocytes, and hence, in the very low number of circulating CD4+ lymphocytes. In addition, the ability to mount antibody responses is also impaired.

MHC class II deficiency has an autosomal recessive pattern of inheritance and is more common in northern Africa. The pathophysiology of the disease resides in abnormalities of transcription factors that govern MHC class II antigen expression by binding to MHC class II genes proximal promoter. Four different genetic variants are known, owing to mutations of the *CIITA*, *RFXANK*, *RFX5*, and *RFXAP* genes.[55-58] Of these, CIITA acts as a master regulator for MHC class II antigens expression.

MHC Class I Deficiency

Human leukocyte antigen (HLA) class I molecules are polymorphic cell surface glycoproteins that play an essential role in presenting antigenic peptides to cytotoxic T lymphocytes, and in modulating the activity of natural killer (NK) cells that bear HLA class I–binding receptors. HLA class I molecules are composed of a polymorphic heavy chain, associated with β2-microglobulin (β2M). The assembly of HLA class I molecules occurs in the lumen of the endoplasmic reticulum (ER), where they are loaded with peptides derived from the degradation of intracellular organisms. These peptides are transported into the ER via transporter associated with antigen presentation (TAP) proteins.[59] TAP consists of two structurally related subunits (TAP1 and

TAP2), which interact to form a functional peptide transporter system. In addition, the tapasin protein plays an important role in the loading process. Defects in TAP1, TAP2 or Tapasin result in impaired peptide-HLA class I/β2M complex formation and eventually lead to reduced surface expression of HLA class I molecules.[60-62]

A reduced number of circulating CD8+ T cells can be observed, because positive selection of CD8+ lymphocytes in the thymus depends on MHC class I molecules recognition. However, this defect is usually incomplete, reflecting residual MHC class I expression.

Human 'Nude' Phenotype (FOXN1 Defect)

In two siblings, a severe T cell immunodeficiency with complete lack of CD8+ T cells was found in association with alopecia.[63] The disease is caused by the mutation of the *FOXN1* gene, whose abnormality accounts for the SCID nude phenotype in mice. *FOXN1* encodes for a transcription factor that is critical for maturation of the thymic microenvironment.

Coronin-1A Deficiency

Coronin 1A is an actin regulator that plays a key role in the egress of thymocytes and trafficking of naïve T lymphocytes to secondary lymphoid organs. Mutations of the *CORO1A* gene have been reported in a single patient with combined immunodeficiency characterized by T cell lymphopenia and poor antibody responses.[64]

Deficiency of Calcium-Release Activated Channels (CRAC)

Lymphocyte activation depends on calcium mobilization. In particular, TCR-induced activation results in release of Ca^{2+} from the endoplasmic reticulum (ER) stores, and this favors Ca^{2+} entry through the Ca^{2+}-release activated channels (CRAC) located in the cell membrane. The Orai1 protein constitutes the pore-forming subunits of the CRAC channel. Mutations of the *ORAI1* gene in humans account for an autosomal recessive immunodeficiency.[65] In contrast to typical cases of SCID, T cell development is unaffected; however. in vitro proliferation of peripheral T cells to mitogens is drastically reduced, and there is no Ca^{2+} influx following T cell activation. In spite of hypergammaglobulinemia, specific antibody responses are typically absent.

STAT5b Deficiency

STAT5b is a transcription factor that is activated in response to growth hormone (GH) and cytokines, including IL-2. STAT5b deficiency is a rare autosomal recessive condition that is characterized by the association of short stature with GH insensitivity and a variable degree of immune deficiency and immune dysregulation.[66,67]

Combined Immunodeficiency with Multiple Intestinal Atresias

The association of combined immune deficiency with multiple gastrointestinal atresia has been observed in a few families.[68,69] The molecular cause of this disease, with a presumed autosomal recessive inheritance, remains unknown.

IL-2R α (CD25) Deficiency

IL-2-mediated signaling is essential to maintain peripheral immune homeostasis. Deficiency of the α chain of the IL-2 receptor (IL-2Rα, CD25) results in immune dysregulation and lymphoproliferation with clinical features that may mimic immune dysregulation-polyendocrinopathy-enteropathy-X-linked (IPEX) syndrome.[70] However, the disease can also present with early-onset severe and recurrent viral and bacterial infections, oral thrush, and chronic diarrhea, associated with lymphadenopathy and hepatosplenomegaly, reduced CD4+ T cell counts, and low in vitro proliferative response to mitogens.[71]

Differential Diagnosis of Combined Immunodeficiencies

All forms of SCID are characterized by typical clinical signs (Box 9-1), consisting of early-onset severe infections (interstitial pneumonia, chronic diarrhea, persistent candidiasis), that lead to growth failure[21,72] (Figure 9-2). Infections are sustained by bacteria, viruses, and fungi. Demonstration that the infection is sustained by an opportunistic pathogen (such as *Pneumocystis jiroveci*, cytomegalovirus) should immediately raise the suspicion of SCID. Skin manifestations are also common (rash, generalized erythroderma, alopecia). These may reflect the presence of auto-reactive T cell clones (such as in OS), or may represent manifestations of a true graft-versus-host disease (GvHD) caused by transplacental passage of alloreactive maternal T lymphocytes. Maternal T cell engraftment is a common finding in SCID, but is only observed in patients with complete lack of T cell immunity.[73] Most often asymptomatic, transplacental passage of maternal T lymphocytes may occasionally result in clinical signs of GvHD: skin rash, liver dysfunction, cytopenia (as a result of bone marrow aggression), and eosinophilia.[73]

Some forms of combined immunodeficiency may present with typical clinical and laboratory features. Adenosine deaminase deficiency is often characterized by cupping and flaring of the ribs and by liver dysfunction that in most cases is caused by accumulation of toxic metabolites in the liver, and not by infections.[74] In addition, the clinical onset of PNP deficiency is often marked by autoimmune hemolytic anemia; furthermore, progressive and severe neurodegeneration, with regression of psychomotor skills, is typically observed in this disease.[75] Sensorineural deafness is part of the phenotype of reticular dysgenesis,[6] whereas microcephaly and growth abnormalities are seen in patients with immunodeficiency due to impairment of DNA repair.[23,25,26] Alopecia is seen in patients with FOXN1 deficiency.[63] The phenotype of MHC class I deficiency is distinct, and consists of recurrent sinopulmonary infections and deep skin ulcers.

Because infections mark the clinical onset of SCID, the differential diagnosis should be focused to consider alternative causes of severe infections. Congenital heart disease, pulmonary defects, cystic fibrosis, and secondary immune deficiencies (such as perinatal HIV infection) should be included in the differential diagnosis. However, it is important to remember that SCID is a medical emergency. Because of this, all infants with a possible diagnosis of SCID need to be carefully and rapidly evaluated by means of appropriate laboratory assays (see Box 9-1 and below).

Infants with SCID may also present as 'red babies,' with generalized erythroderma (caused by transplacental passage of maternal T cells or by OS). The differential diagnosis in this case includes severe allergy, various forms of ichthyosis, IPEX (immune dysregulation, polyendocrinopathy, enteropathy, X-linked),[76] and Netherton's syndrome. In the latter, hair shaft anomalies are frequently observed.

Because SCID and other combined immunodeficiencies are inherited disorders, a thorough family history (aiming at ascertaining the possibility of parental consanguinity or of other affected individuals in the family) should be part of the general approach to infants with possible SCID.

BOX 9-1   Key concepts

Clinical and Laboratory Elements in the Diagnosis of SCID

Clinical Features

- Positive family history (X-linked, other siblings affected, parental consanguinity)
- Presentation early in life (within the first 4 to 6 months of age)
- Severe respiratory infections (interstitial pneumonia)
- Protracted diarrhea
- Failure to thrive
- Persistent candidiasis
- Skin rash, erythrodermia

Laboratory Elements

- Lymphopenia (ALC:<2000/μL)
- Reduced number (<1500/μL) of circulating CD3+ T cells
- Very low to undetectable levels of serum immunoglobulins*
- Very low to absent in vitro proliferative response to mitogens

SCID, Severe combined immunodeficiency.
*IgG serum levels may initially be normal because of transplacental passage of maternal IgG.

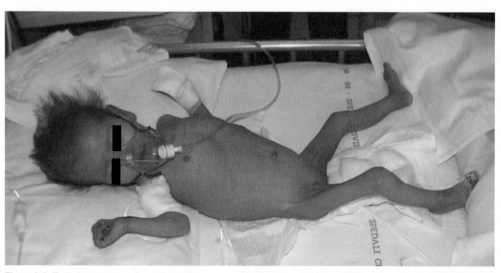

Figure 9-2 Typical appearance of an infant with severe combined immunodeficiency (SCID). Note severe growth failure and respiratory distress.

Evaluation and Management

A correct diagnosis of SCID should be established as soon as possible in order to offer an optimal perspective on treatment. The most rapid tool to consolidate the diagnosis of SCID is represented by analysis of the absolute lymphocyte count; lymphopenia is observed in most SCID infants.[77] Importantly, in normal infants the lymphocyte count tends to be high (>2000 and to 10 000 cells/μL) as compared to later periods in life; thus, values below 2000 lymphocytes/μL have been proposed to identify infants at risk of SCID at birth.[77] However, a proportion of SCID infants are not lymphopenic. This may reflect the presence of a reasonable number of autologous lymphocytes (as observed in OS, MHC class II deficiency, ZAP-70 deficiency) or the transplacental passage of maternal T cells. Consequently, and regardless of the total lymphocyte count, all infants with clinical features suggestive of SCID should be evaluated for the distribution of lymphocyte subsets by flow cytometry and functional assays (see Box 9-1). Immunophenotypic evaluation should include characterization and enumeration of total (CD3$^+$) T lymphocytes, CD4$^+$ and CD8$^+$ T cell subsets, B (CD19$^+$) lymphocytes, and NK (CD16$^+$) cells. In most cases, such a panel of immunophenotyping will reveal the diagnosis of SCID, and also orient towards specific gene defects. More subtle analysis may then be applied to selected cases. For instance, differential diagnosis between a γ_c or a Jak-3 defect in a male infant with T$^-$ B$^+$ NK$^-$ SCID may often be resolved by analyzing γ_c expression on the surface of lymphocytes by flow cytometry.[78] The immunologic work-up of patients with possible maternal T cell engraftment or with OS should also include analysis of the expression of CD45RA and CD45R0 markers on the surface of CD4$^+$ and of CD8$^+$ lymphocytes. In fact, early in life the vast majority of T lymphocytes normally carry the CD45RA antigen (a marker of naïve T cells). In contrast, circulating T lymphocytes from patients with SCID and maternal T cell engraftment or with OS have an activated/memory profile, and hence express the CD45R0 antigen. In any case, in vitro proliferative responses to mitogens are drastically reduced in all patients with SCID. Low or undetectable levels of IgA and IgG may support the diagnosis of SCID; however, IgG serum levels may initially be normal because of transplacental passage of maternally derived antibodies.

The selective deficiency of CD4$^+$ lymphocytes may suggest MHC class II deficiency. In such cases, analysis of MHC class II antigens on the surface of B lymphocytes and monocytes prompts the diagnosis.

Extreme lymphopenia is often observed in ADA deficiency. Measurement of enzymatic ADA and PNP activity, and of dATP and dGTP levels in red blood cells, is important to reach a final diagnosis of ADA or PNP deficiency. Importantly, whenever ADA or PNP deficiencies are suspected, use of red cell transfusions should be delayed, if possible, until determination of enzymatic activity has been performed.

T cell receptor excision circles (TRECs) are a by-product of V(D)J recombination and are present as episomal DNA fragments in newly generated T lymphocytes. Levels of TRECs in circulating lymphocytes are particularly high in newborns and infants, and progressively decline with age. No TRECs are detected in infants with SCID. Assessment of TREC levels by polymerase chain reaction has been proposed for newborn screening of SCID,[79] and has recently entered a pilot phase in Wisconsin and Massachusetts in the USA.

Ultimately, now that the genes responsible for most forms of SCID have been identified, mutation analysis represents an important diagnostic tool.[80] All infants with a probable diagnosis of SCID should be evaluated for specific gene defects (see Table 9-1), as this may not only allow definitive diagnosis but may also provide important information for accurate genetic counseling and possible future prenatal diagnosis in the family. However, it is important to emphasize that the diagnosis of SCID should not be based strictly on demonstration of a specific gene defect, as this would often require too much time. In contrast, careful evaluation of clinical and laboratory data is sufficient to pose a diagnosis of SCID, so that the procedures to achieve definitive treatment may be immediately initiated.

Treatment

The main therapeutic strategies for SCID are illustrated in Box 9-2. Optimal treatment of SCID is based on hematopoietic cell transplantation (HCT). Transplantation from an HLA-identical family donor can cure > 90% of infants with SCID, and excellent results have been obtained with transplantation from haploidentical family donors or matched unrelated donors.[77,81,82] Survival after transplantation from HLA-mismatched related donors is optimal (> 90%) if performed early in life (< 3.5 months of age),[77,83] but is only 50–70% if performed at > 3.5 months. Lung infection prior to HCT and a B$^-$ immunologic SCID phenotype are associated with less favorable outcome.[84] Recent data of long-term follow-up after HCT for SCID indicate that the majority of the transplanted infants enjoy a good quality of life; however, autoimmune manifestations, infections, and growth and nutritional problems are observed in a proportion of them, and are more common among those who fail to attain robust and persistent T and B cell immune reconstitution.[85,86] Furthermore, ADA deficiency, PNP deficiency and SCID with increased cellular radiosensitivity are associated with progressive neurological deterioration and developmental problems, even after successful engraftment.[87-89]

Prior to HCT, SCID infants need to be protected from infections. Prophylactic trimethoprim-sulfamethoxazole is effective in preventing *P. jiroveci* pneumonia (PJP). Intravenous immunoglobulins should be administered regularly, regardless of

---

BOX 9-2 Therapeutic principles

Treatment of Infants with SCID

- Always consider an infant with putative SCID as a medical emergency.
- Treat any infections promptly and aggressively.
- Take into account the high frequency of *Pneumocystis jiroveci* pneumonia (PJP). Take appropriate measures to evaluate this possibility (chest X-ray, bronchoalveolar lavage). If PJP is suspected or proven, use trimethoprim-sulfamethoxazole (20 mg/kg/d IV).
- If growth failure is present, start parenteral nutrition.
- Start prophylaxis of PJP with trimethoprim-sulfamethoxazole (5 mg/kg/d).
- Start prophylaxis of fungal infections with fluconazole (5 mg/kg/d).
- Give intravenous immunoglobulins regularly (400 mg/kg/21 days).
- Isolate the infant in a protected environment (laminar-flow unit).
- Always irradiate blood products, if transfusions are necessary.
- Avoid administration of live-attenuated vaccines.
- Immediately plan for a hematopoietic cell transplantation once the diagnosis of SCID has been established.

SCID, Severe combined immunodeficiency.

serum IgG levels. Isolation in a protected environment and supportive treatment with parenteral nutrition and transfusions may also improve the health status of SCID infants while waiting for HCT. Importantly, blood products need to be irradiated because alloreactive T cells contained in the transfusion would invariably cause rapidly fatal GVHD.[21]

Alternative therapeutic approaches are available in selected cases. Patients affected with ADA deficiency who do not have an HLA-identical donor may be treated with weekly intramuscular injections of polyethylene glycole-conjugated ADA (PEG-ADA). This treatment usually results in immune reconstitution and clinical improvement, although T lymphocyte counts tend to remain lower than normal.[3,90]

Successful immune reconstitution has been achieved after gene therapy in 17/20 infants with X-linked SCID,[91,92] however, 5 of these 20 patients have developed leukemic proliferation due to insertional mutagenesis.[93,94] In contrast, gene therapy with the use of a nonmyeloablative conditioning regimen has been successfully used in a series of patients with ADA deficicency.[95,96]

DiGeorge Anomaly

Etiology

Originally described in 1965, DiGeorge anomaly (DGA) is a developmental anomaly characterized by thymic hypoplasia, hypoparathyroidism with consequent hypocalcemia, congenital heart disease, and facial dysmorphisms.[97] The majority of patients have a partial monosomy of the 22q11 region of chromosome 22. This deletion may also associate with overlapping clinical phenotypes, such as velo-cardio-facial syndrome and CHARGE syndrome.[97] The vast majority have residual thymus and have a milder immunodeficiency (partial DGA),[97] whereas approximately 1% of the patients show complete absence of the thymus and extreme T cell lymphopenia (complete DGA).[98] In some cases, patients with complete DGA may develop a variable number of oligoclonal, activated and functionally anergic T lymphocytes. This phenotype is also referred to as 'complete atypical DGA' and may clinically manifest with skin erythrodermia and lymphadenopathy, resembling OS.[98]

Diagnosis

Typical cases of DGA should be suspected early after birth because of the association of heart defect (especially interrupted aortic arch type B or truncus arteriosus) with hypocalcemic seizures. Micrognathia, hypertelorism, antimongoloid slant of the eyes, and ear malformation are also common (Figure 9-3). Feeding problems, microcephaly, speech delay, and neurobehavioral problems (including bipolar disorders, autistic spectrum disorders and schizophrenia) are frequently observed.[97] While DGA patients rarely suffer from severe immunodeficiency, persistent candidiasis, chronic diarrhea, and P. jiroveci pneumonia are indicators of a severe thymic defect and require prompt investigation of the immune system, with enumeration of lymphocyte subsets and assessment of in vitro proliferative response to mitogens. Patients with partial DGA tend to show variable T cell lymphopenia, but in vitro proliferative responses to mitogens and antibody responses are normal.[97]In patients with possible DGA, monosomy of the 22q11 region should be investigated by fluorescent in situ hybridization (FISH). However, DGA may also occur in the absence of 22q11 deletion.

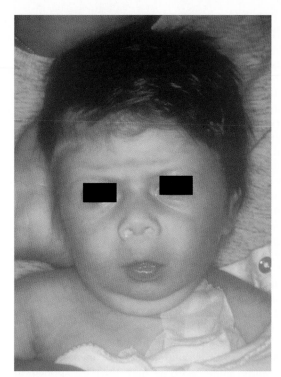

Figure 9-3 Facial dysmorphic features in an infant with DiGeorge syndrome. Note hypertelorism, enlarged nasal root, anteroverted nostrils, low-set ears, and micrognathia.

Management and Treatment

Heart defects are the most severe manifestation of the disease, and should be treated aggressively if necessary. Hypocalcemia requires supplementation with calcium and vitamin D; however, in most cases seizures do not recur beyond the neonatal period. If a significant immune defect is present, prophylaxis of P. jiroveci pneumonia with trimethoprim-sulfamethoxazole is indicated. Live-attenuated vaccines can be safely administered to patients with partial DGA who have good cellular immunity; however, these vaccines are contraindicated in patients with complete DGA. Thymic transplantation is the treatment of choice for patients with complete (typical or atypical) DGA, and results in good (75%) long-term survival and immune reconstitution, although T lymphocyte counts tend to remain lower than normal.[98] Unmanipulated bone marrow transplantation from HLA-identical donors can also lead to immune reconstitution in patients with complete DGA, through a mechanism that involves peripheral expansion of T lymphocytes contained in the graft.[99]

Syndromes with Significant T Cell Deficiency

Immuno-Osseous Syndromes

Cartilage Hair Hypoplasia

Cartilage hair hypoplasia (CHH) is an autosomal recessive disease, characterized by short-limbed dwarfism, light-colored hypoplastic hair and a variable degree of immunodeficiency, associated with an increased occurrence of bone marrow dysplasia, malignancies and Hirschsprung's disease. The disease is more common among the Amish and the Finns, and is due to mutations of the gene encoding for the untranslated RNA component of the ribonuclease mitochondrial RNA processing

(*RMRP*) complex, that is involved in cleavage of ribosomal RNA, processing of mitochondrial RNA, and cell cycle control.[100] The majority of patients have a limited susceptibility to bacterial and viral infections; however, some may present with severe infections early in life and show an immunological phenotype of SCID. Furthermore, both Omenn syndrome and selective CD8+ lymphocytopenia have been reported in CHH.[101,102] Various degrees of T cell lymphopenia, and reduced in vitro function of T lymphocytes, have been frequently observed. Hematopoietic cell transplantation may be required in patients with CHH and a SCID or OS phenotype.

Schimke Syndrome

Schimke syndrome is characterized by dwarfism with short neck and trunk due to spondyloepiphyseal dysplasia, progressive renal impairment evolving to renal failure, facial dysmorphisms, lentigines, immunodeficiency, and increased occurrence of bone marrow failure and of early-onset atherosclerosis.[103] The disease is inherited as an autosomal recessive trait and is due to mutations of the *SMARCAL1* gene, that encodes for a chromatin remodeling protein.[103] T cell lymphopenia is common, and may occasionally be severe enough to cause SCID. Recurrent bacterial, viral or fungal infections are seen in almost half of the patients.

Immunodeficiency Syndromes with Defective DNA Repair

Ataxia-telangiectasia (AT) is an autosomal recessive disorder characterized by telangiectasia, progressive ataxia, recurrent respiratory tract infections, and an increased susceptibility to tumors (leukemia, lymphoma, dysgerminoma, and gonadoblastoma).[104] Cells derived from AT patients show an increased sensitivity to ionizing radiation. The disease is caused by mutations of the *ATM* gene, which maps at 11q22-23. This gene encodes for a large protein that participates in the repair of DNA breakage and controls cell cycle and cellular apoptosis.[105]

Nijmegen breakage syndrome (NBS) is characterized by microcephaly, growth retardation, bird-like facies, increased susceptibility to infections, and higher occurrence of tumors. Inherited as an autosomal recessive trait, the disease is caused by mutations of the *NBS1* gene, which encodes for nibrin, another protein involved in DNA repair.[106]

A subgroup of patients with an *AT-like disorder* have been identified in whom the defect was in the *hMRE11* gene, which encodes for another component of the DNA repair machinery that associates with nibrin.[107]

DNA ligase IV (LIG4) is an enzyme involved in nonhomologous DNA end-joining and V(D)J recombination. Deficiency of this enzyme is inherited as an autosomal recessive trait and results in *LIG4 syndrome*, characterized by microcephaly, growth abnormalities, increased susceptibility to malignancies, and pancytopenia.[108] The immunodeficiency of LIG4 syndrome can be variable, but occasionally may be severe and cause T− B− SCID or OS.[26,42]

Differential Diagnosis

Although these disorders share similar findings (increased susceptibility to infections, higher risk of tumors), they also present typical features that permit differential diagnosis. Ocular telangiectasias and progressive ataxia are early signs of AT, and usually occur within the first few years of life. Confirmation of the diagnosis is provided by the demonstration of increased serum levels of alpha-fetoprotein (AFP). Development of reciprocal chromosomal translocations (mostly involving chromosomes 7 and 14) in a fraction of T lymphocytes is common. In contrast, patients affected with NBS do not develop telangiectasias or ataxia, and show normal AFP levels; however, they also present somatic chromosomal translocations.[104]

Laboratory investigations in patients with AT, AT-like disease, or NBS show progressive reduction of the T cell number (particularly the CD4+ subset), with impaired in vitro proliferative response to mitogens. IgA deficiency is common and is often associated with low/undetectable IgG2 and IgG4. These defects are more severe in AT than in NBS.[104]

Management and Treatment

At present, there is no definitive cure for AT and NBS. Use of prophylactic antibiotics, chest physiotherapy, and administration of intravenous immunoglobulins may decrease the risk of infections. Careful monitoring of the clinical conditions may allow early recognition of tumors. However, in spite of these measures, the prognosis remains poor, particularly in AT patients, and infections and tumors are the main causes of death.[104] Exposure to ionizing radiations should be avoided, if possible. Hematopoeitic cell transplantation has been performed in a few patients with LIG4 syndrome, with variable results.

Wiskott-Aldrich Syndrome

Etiology

Wiskott-Aldrich syndrome (WAS) is an X-linked disorder characterized by eczema, congenital thrombocytopenia with small-sized platelets, and immune deficiency. The responsible gene, named *WASP*, maps at Xp11.2 and encodes for a protein involved in cytoskeleton reorganization in hematopoietic cells.[109] Most patients with typical WAS have mutations that impair expression and/or function of the WASP protein. However, some missense mutations are associated with a milder phenotype (isolated X-linked thrombocytopenia, XLT) (Figure 9-4).[110]

Differential Diagnosis

The diagnosis of WAS is relatively simple, if all elements of the triad (eczema, thrombocytopenia, and immune deficiency) are present; however, this happens only in one third of the cases.

The immune deficiency of WAS may manifest as recurrent bacterial and viral infections, autoimmune manifestations, and increased occurrence of tumors (leukemia, lymphoma). Immunologic laboratory abnormalities include lymphopenia (particularly among CD8+ lymphocytes), impaired in vitro proliferation to immobilized anti-CD3, reduced serum IgM with increased levels of IgA and IgE, and inability to mount effective antibody responses, especially to T-independent antigens.[109] Analysis of intracellular WASP protein expression by flow cytometry may assist in the diagnosis; absence of the protein is most often associated with a severe clinical phenotype, whereas XLT patients tend to show residual protein expression that is usually associated with missense mutations in exons 1 and 2 of the gene.[110] Somatic reversion, leading to WASP protein expression in a proportion of cells (mostly in T lymphocytes) has been observed in several patients, but its implications on the evolution of the clinical phenotype are unclear.[111]

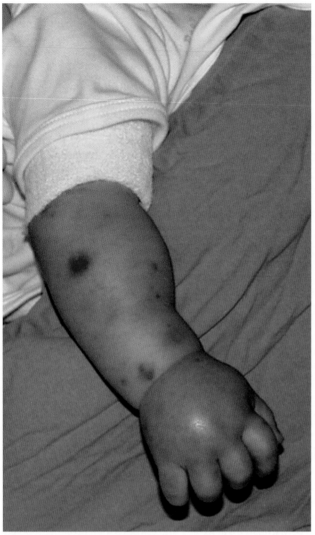

Figure 9-4 Severe vasculitis and petechiae in a child with Wiskott-Aldrich syndrome.

Management and Treatment

The only curative approach to WAS is represented by hematopoietic cell transplantation (HCT), that gives optimal results when performed from HLA-identical family donors or early in life from matched unrelated donors.[81,112] Mixed chimerism after HCT has been associated with increased risk of autoimmunity.[113] Administration of intravenous immunoglobulins, regular antibiotic prophylaxis, topical steroids to control eczema, and use of vigorous immune suppression for autoimmunity are the hallmarks of conservative treatment. Splenectomy may be indicated in case of severe and refractory thrombocytopenia; however, it carries the risk of overwhelming sepsis.

Hyper-IgM Syndromes due to CD40 Ligand (CD40L) or to CD40 Deficiency

Etiology

CD40 ligand (CD40L, CD154) is a cell-surface molecule predominantly expressed by activated CD4⁺ T lymphocytes. Interaction of CD40L with its counter-receptor CD40 (expressed by B and dendritic cells, macrophages, endothelial cells, and some epithe-lial cells) is essential for germinal center formation, terminal differential of B lymphocytes, and effective defense against intracellular pathogens. Mutations in the *CD40LG (TNFSF5)* gene, mapping at Xq26, result in X-linked hyper-IgM syndrome (HIGM1), characterized by an increased occurrence of bacterial and opportunistic infections, chronic diarrhea (often sustained by *Cryptosporidium*), liver/biliary tract disease, and susceptibility to liver and gut tumors.[114,115]

Differential Diagnosis

Presentation early in life with opportunistic infections (PJP) requires differential diagnosis with SCID and other forms of severe T cell defects. The typical immunoglobulin profile (undetectable or very low serum IgG and IgA, with normal to increased IgM) may also be observed in common variable immunodeficiency or in autosomal recessive hyper-IgM caused by defects in the *AID, UNG* or in the *CD40* genes. Neutropenia is a common finding. The diagnosis of HIGM1 is made based on the demonstration of defective expression of CD40L (but not of other activation markers) on the surface of T cells following in vitro activation, and is eventually confirmed by mutation analysis.[114]

Management and Treatment

Treatment is based on regular use of intravenous immunoglobulins, prophylactic trimethoprim-sulfamethoxazole, and use of sterile/filtered water to prevent *Cryptosporidium* infection. Monitoring of liver/biliary tract morphology and function by ultrasound scanning, measurement of appropriate laboratory parameters of liver and biliary tract function, and, when indicated, liver biopsy is also advised. Severe neutropenia may be treated with recombinant granulocyte colony-stimulating factor (G-CSF). In spite of these measures, the long-term prognosis is poor because of severe infections and liver disease. The only curative approach is represented by HCT, and better results are achieved when transplantation is performed prior to development of lung problems or of *Cryptosporidium* infection.[116]

Conclusions

Irrespective of the specific definitive diagnosis, all forms of T cell immunodeficiencies are characterized by significant morbidity and some of them also by high early-onset mortality rates, thus emphasizing the critical role played by T lymphocytes in ensuring effective immune defense mechanisms and in maintaining homeostasis. Consequently, it is a primary physician's responsibility to perform accurate clinical and laboratory evaluation of patients with a putative T cell immunodeficiency. Whereas clinical history and physical examination may disclose the diagnosis in some forms of T cell immunodeficiency (e.g. Wiskott-Aldrich syndrome, ataxia-telangiectasia, and cartilage hair hypoplasia), laboratory evaluation is most often required to provide a definitive diagnosis. In spite of the heterogeneity of this group of disorders, simple laboratory assays (total lymphocyte count and subsets distribution, in vitro proliferative responses are usually sufficient to confirm the suspicion. It is noteworthy that some forms of T cell immunodeficiencies (SCID in particular) represent true medical emergencies, and warrant prompt and accurate evaluation, and treatment by HCT. Based on recent experience, it is likely that gene therapy may be successfully applied in a broader group of disorders in the near future.

References

1. Fischer A. Severe combined immunodeficiencies (SCID). Clin Exp Immunol 2000;122:143–9.

2. Apasov SG, Blackburn MR, Kellems RE, et al. Adenosine deaminase deficiency increases thymic apoptosis and causes defective T cell receptor signaling. J Clin Invest 2001;108:131–41.

3. Malacarne F, Benicchi T, Notarangelo LD, et al. Reduced thymic output, increased spontaneous apoptosis and oligoclonal B cells in polyethylene glycol-adenosine deaminase-treated patients. Eur J Immunol 2005;35: 3376–86.

4. Cassani B, Mirolo M, Cattaneo F, et al. Altered intracellular and extracellular signaling leads to impaired T cell functions in ADA-SCID patients. Blood 2008;111:4209–19.

5. Ozsahin H, Arredondo-Vega FX, Santisteban I, et al. Adenosine deaminase deficiency in adults. Blood 1997;89:2849–55.

6. de Vaal OM, Seynhaeve V. Reticular dysgenesia. Lancet 1959;ii: 1123–4.

7. Pannicke U, Honig M, Hess I, et al. Reticular dysgenesis (aleukocytosis) is caused by mutations in the gene encoding mitochondrial adenylate kinase 2. Nat Genet 2009;41:101–5.

8. Lagresle-Peyrou C, Six EM, Picard C, et al. Human adenylate kinase 2 deficiency causes a profound hematopoietic defect associated with sensorineural deafness. Nat Genet 2009;41:106–11.

9. Noguchi M, Yi H, Rosenblatt HM, et al. Interleukin-2 receptor gamma chain mutation results in X-linked severe combined immunodeficiency in humans. Cell 1993;73:147–57.

10. Leonard WJ, Noguchi M, Russell SM, et al. The molecular basis of X-linked severe combined immunodeficiency: the role of the interleukin-2 receptor gamma chain as a common gamma chain, gamma c. Immunol Rev 1994;138:61–86.

11. Puck JM. IL2RGbase: a database of γc-chain defects causing human XSCID. Immunol Today 1996;17:507–11.

12. O'Shea JJ, Notarangelo LD, Johnston JA, et al. Advances in the understanding of cytokine signal transduction: the role of Jaks and STATs in immunoregulation and the pathogenesis of immunodeficiency. J Clin Immunol 1997;17:431–47.

13. Macchi P, Villa A, Giliani S, et al. Mutations of Jak-3 gene in patients with autosomal severe combined immune deficiency (SCID). Nature 1995;377:65–8.

14. Russell SM, Tayebi N, Nakajima H, et al. Mutation of Jak3 in a patient with SCID: essential role of Jak3 in lymphoid development. Science 1995;270:797–800.

15. Puel A, Leonard WJ. Mutations in the gene for the IL-7 receptor result in T-B+ NK+ severe combined immunodeficiency disease. Curr Opin Immunol 2000;12:468–73.

16. Puel A, Ziegler S, Buckley RH, et al. Defective IL7R expression in TB+ NK+ severe combined immunodeficiency. Nat Genet 1998;20:394–7.

17. Peschon JJ, Morrissey PJ, Grabstein KH, et al. Early lymphocyte expansion is severely impaired in interleukin 7 receptor-deficient mice. J Exp Med 1994;180:1955–60.

18. Sekiguchi J, Frank K. V(D)J recombination. Curr Biol 1999;22:835.

19. Schatz DG, Oettinger MA, Baltimore D. The V(D)J recombination activating gene. RAG-1, Cell 1989;59:1035–48.

20. Oettinger MA, Schatz DG, Gorka C, et al. RAG-1 and RAG-2, adjacent genes that synergistically activate V(D)J recombination. Science 1990; 248:1517–23.

21. Stephan JL, Vlekova V, Le Deist F, et al. Severe combined immunodeficiency: a retrospective single-center study of clinical presentation and outcome in 117 patients. J Pediatr 1993;123:564–72.

22. Schwarz K, Gauss GH, Ludwig L, et al. RAG mutations in human B cell-negative SCID. Science 1996;274:97–9.

23. Moshous D, Callebaut I, de Chasseval R, et al. Artemis, a novel DNA double-strand break repair/V(D)J recombination protein, is mutated in human severe combined immune deficiency. Cell 2001;105:177–86.

24. van der Burg M, Ijspeert H, Verkaik NS, et al. A DNA-PKcs mutation in a radiosensitive T-B- SCID patient inhibits Artemis activation and nonhomologous end-joining. J Clin Invest 2009;119:91–8.

25. Buck D, Moshous D, de Chasseval R, et al. Severe combined immunodeficiency and microcephaly in siblings with hypomorphic mutations in DNA ligase IV. Eur J Immunol 2006;36:224–35.

26. van der Burg M, van Veelen LR, Verkaik NS, et al. A new type of radiosensitive T-B-NK+ severe combined immunodeficiency caused by a LIG4 mutation. J Clin Invest 2006;116:137–45.

27. Buck D, Malivert L, de Chasseval R, et al. Cernunnos, a novel nonhomologous end-joining factor, is mutated in human immunodeficiency with microcephaly. Cell 2006;124:287–99.

28. Dadi HK, Simon AJ, Roifman CM. Effect of CD3delta deficiency on maturation of alpha/beta and gamma/delta T cell lineages in severe combined immunodeficiency. N Engl J Med 2003;349:1821–8.

29. de Saint Basile G, Geissmann F, Flori E, et al. Severe combined immunodeficiency caused by deficiency in either the delta or the epsilon subunit of CD3. J Clin Invest 2004;114:1512–7.

30. Rieux-Laucat F, Hivroz C, Lim A, et al. Inherited and somatic CD3zeta mutations in a patient with T cell deficiency. N Engl J Med 2006;354:1913–21.

31. Roberts JL, Lauritsen JP, Cooney M, et al. T-B+NK+ severe combined immunodeficiency caused by complete deficiency of the CD3zeta subunit of the T cell antigen receptor complex. Blood 2007;109:3198–206.

32. Arnaiz-Villena A, Timon M, Corell A, et al. Primary immunodeficiency caused by mutations in the gene encoding the CD3-gamma subunit of the T lymphocyte receptor. N Engl J Med 1992;327:529–33.

33. Recio MJ, Moreno-Pelayo MA, Kilic SS, et al. Differential biological role of CD3 chains revealed by human immunodeficiencies. J Immunol 2007;178:2556–64.

34. Kung C, Pingel JT, Heikinheimo M, et al. Mutations in the tyrosine phosphatase CD45 gene in a child with severe combined immunodeficiency disease. Nat Med 2000;6:343–5.

35. Tchilian EZ, Wallace DL, Wells RS, et al. A deletion in the gene encoding the CD45 antigen in a patient with SCID. J Immunol 2001;166: 1308–13.

36. Omenn GS. Familial reticuloendotheliosis with eosinophilia. N Engl J Med 1965;273:427–32.

37. De Saint-Basile G, Le Deist F, de Villartay JP, et al. Restricted heterogeneity of T lymphocytes in combined immunodeficiency with hypereosinophilia (Omenn's syndrome). J Clin Invest 1991;87:1352–9.

38. Villa A, Santagata S, Bozzi F, et al. Partial V(D)J recombination activity leads to Omenn syndrome. Cell 1998;93:885–96.

39. Villa A, Sobacchi C, Notarangelo LD, et al. V(D)J recombination defects in lymphocytes due to Rag mutations: a severe immunodeficiency with a spectrum of clinical presentation. Blood 2001;97:81–8.

40. Ege M, Ma Y, Manfras B, et al. Omenn syndrome due to ARTEMIS mutations. Blood 2005;105:4179–86.

41. Giliani S, Bonfim C, de Saint Basile G, et al. Omenn syndrome in an infant with IL7RA gene mutation. J Pediatr 2006;148:272–4.

42. Grunebaum E, Bates A, Roifman CM. Omenn syndrome is associated with mutations in DNA ligase IV. J Allergy Clin Immunol 2008; 122:1219–20.

43. Roifman CM, Gu Y, Cohen A. Mutations in the RNA component of RNase mitochondrial RNA processing might cause Omenn syndrome. J Allergy Clin Immunol 2006;117:897–903.

44. Wada T, Yasui M, Toma T, et al. Detection of T lymphocytes with a second-site mutation in skin lesions of atypical X-linked severe combined immunodeficiency mimicking Omenn syndrome. Blood 2008;112:1872–5.

45. Roifman CM, Zhang J, Atkinson A, et al. Adenosine deaminase deficiency can present with features of Omenn syndrome. J Allergy Clin Immunol 2008;121:1056–8.

46. Turul T, Tezcan I, Artac H, et al. Clinical heterogeneity can hamper the diagnosis of patients with ZAP70 deficiency. Eur J Pediatr 2009;168: 87–93.

47. Cavadini P, Vermi W, Facchetti F, et al. AIRE deficiency in thymus of 2 patients with Omenn sindrome. J Clin Invest 2005;115:728–32.

48. Markert ML, Finkel BD, McLaughlin TM, et al. Mutations in purine nucleoside phosphorylase deficiency. Hum Mutat 1997;9:118–21.

49. Chan AC, van Oers NSC, Tran A, et al. Differential expression of ZAP-70 and Syk protein tyrosine kinases, and the role of this family of protein tyrosine kinases in TCR signaling. J Immunol 1994;152: 4758–64.

50. van Leeuwen JEM, Samelson LE. T cell antigen-receptor signal transduction. Curr Opin Immunol 1999;11:242–8.

51. Chan AC, Kadlecek TA, Elder ME, et al. ZAP-70 deficiency in an autosomal recessive form of severe combined immunodeficiency. Science 1994;264:1599–601.

52. Arpaia E, Shahar M, Dadi H, et al. Defective T cell receptor signaling and CD8+ thymic selection in humans lacking Zap-70 kinase. Cell 1994;76: 947–58.

53. Elder ME, Lin D, Clever J, et al. Human severe combined immunodeficiency due to a defect in ZAP-70, a T cell tyrosine kinase. Science 1994;264:1596–9.

54. Goldman FD, Ballas ZK, Schutte BC, et al. Defective expression of p56lck in an infant with severe combined immunodeficiency. J Clin Invest 1998;102:421–9.

55. Steimle V, Otten LA, Zufferey M, et al. Complementation cloning of an MHC class II transactivator mutated in hereditary MHC class II deficiency (or bare lymphocyte syndrome). Cell 1993;75:135–46.

56. Masternak K, Barras E, Zufferey M, et al. A gene encoding a novel RFX-associated transactivator is mutated in the majority of MHC class II deficiency patients. Nat Genet 1998;20:273–7.

57. Steimle V, Durand B, Barras E, et al. A novel DNA-binding regulatory factor is mutated in primary MHC class II deficiency (bare lymphocyte syndrome). Genes Dev 1995;9:1021–32.

58. Durand B, Sperisen P, Emery P, et al. RFXAP, a novel subunit of the RFX DNA binding complex is mutated in MHC class II deficiency. EMBO J 1997;16:1045–55.

59. Gadola SD, Moins-Teisserenc HT, Trowsdale J, et al. TAP deficiency syndrome. Clin Exp Immunol 2000;121:173–8.

60. de la Salle H, Zimmer J, Fricker D, et al. HLA class I deficiencies due to mutations in subunit 1 of the peptide transporter TAP1. J Clin Invest 1999;103:9–13.

61. de la Salle H, Hanau D, Fricker D, et al. Homozygous human TAP peptide transporter mutation in HLA class I deficiency. Science 1994;265:237–41.

62. Yabe T, Kawamura S, Sato M, et al. A subject with a novel type I bare lymphocyte syndrome has tapasin deficiency due to deletion of 4 exons by Alu-mediated recombination. Blood 2002;100:1496–8.

63. Frank J, Pignata C, Panteleyev AA, et al. Exposing the human nude phenotype. Nature 1999;398:473–4.

64. Shiow LR, Roadcap DW, Paris K, et al. The actin regulator coronin 1A is mutant in a thymic egress-deficient mouse strain and in a patient with severe combined immunodeficiency. Nat Immunol 2008;9:1307–15.

65. Feske S, Gwack Y, Prakriya M, et al. A mutation in Orai1 causes immune deficiency by abrogating CRAC channel function. Nature 2006;441:179–85.

66. Kofoed EM, Hwa V, Little B, et al. Growth hormone insensitivity associated with a STAT5b mutation. N Engl J Med 2003;349:1139–47.

67. Bernasconi A, Marino R, Ribas A, et al. Characterization of immunodeficiency in a patient with growth hormone insensitivity secondary to a novel STAT5b gene mutation. Pediatrics 2006;118:e1584–1592.

68. Moreno LA, Gottrand F, Turck D, et al. Severe combined immunodeficiency syndrome associated with autosomal recessive familial multiple gastrointestinal atresias. Am J Med Genet 1990;37:143–6.

69. Walker MW, Lovell MA, Thaddeus EK, et al. Multiple areas of intestinal atresia associated with immunodeficiency and posttransfusion graftversus-host disease. J Pediatr 1993;123:93–5.

70. Caudy AA, Reddy ST, Chatila T, et al. CD25 deficiency causes an immune dysregulation, polyendocrinopathy, enteropathy, X-linked-like syndrome, and defective IL-10 expression from CD4 lymphocytes. J Allergy Clin Immunol 2007;19:482–7.

71. Sharfe N, Dadi HK, Shahar M, et al. Human immune disorder arising from mutation of the a chain of the interleukin-2 receptor. Proc Natl Acad Sci U S A 1997;94:3168–71.

72. Buckley RH, Schiff RI, Schiff SE, et al. Human severe combined immunodeficiency: genetic, phenotypic, and functional diversity in one hundred eight infants. J Pediatr 1997;130:378–87.

73. Muller SM, Ege M, Pottharst A, et al. Transplacentally acquired maternal T lymphocytes in severe combined immunodeficiency: a study of 121 patients. Blood 2001;98:1847–51.

74. Bollinger ME, Arredondo-Vega FX, Santisteban I, et al. Hepatic dysfunction as a complication of adenosine deaminase deficiency. N Engl J Med 1996;334:1367–71.

75. Carson DA, Carrera CJ. Immunodeficiency secondary to adenosine deaminase deficiency and purine nucleoside phosphorylation deficiency. Semin Hematol 1990;27:260–9.

76. Bennett CL, Ochs HD. IPEX is a unique X-linked syndrome characterized by immune dysfunction, polyendocrinopathy, enteropathy, and a variety of autoimmune phenomena. Curr Opin Pediatr 2001;13:533–8.

77. Buckley RH. Molecular defects in human severe combined immunodeficiency and approaches to immune reconstitution. Annu Rev Immunol 2004;22:625–55.

78. Notarangelo LD, Giliani S, Mazza C, et al. Of genes and phenotypes: the immunological and molecular spectrum of combined immune deficiency. Defects of the γc-JAK3 signaling pathway as a model. Immunol Rev 2000;178:39–48.

79. Puck JM; SCID Newborn Screening Working Group. Population-based newborn screening for severe combined immunodeficiency: steps toward implementation. J Allergy Clin Immunol 2007;120:760–8.

80. Fischer A. Primary immunodeficiency diseases: an experimental model for molecular medicine. Lancet 2001;357:1863–9.

81. Antoine C, Muller S, Cant A, et al. Long-term survival and transplantation of haemopoietic stem cells for immunodeficiencies: report of the European experience 1968–99. Lancet 2003;361:553–60.

82. Grunebaum E, Mazzolari E, Porta F, et al. Bone marrow transplantation for severe combined immune deficiency. JAMA 2006;295:508–18.

83. Myers LA, Patel DD, Puck JM, et al. Hematopoietic stem cell transplantation for severe combined immunodeficiency in the neonatal period leads to superior thymic output and improved survival. Blood 2002;99:872–8.

84. Bertrand Y, Landais P, Friedrich W, et al. Influence of severe combined immunodeficiency phenotype on the outcome of HLA non-identical, T cell-depleted bone marrow transplantation: a retrospective European survey from the European group for bone marrow transplantation and the European Society for Immunodeficiency. J Pediatr 1999;134:740–8.

85. Mazzolari E, Forino C, Guerci S, et al. Long-term immune reconstitution and clinical outcome after stem cell transplantation for severe T cell immunodeficiency. J Allergy Clin Immunol 2007;120:892–9.

86. Neven B, Leroy S, Decaluwe H, et al. Long-term outcome after haematopoietic stem cell transplantation of a single-centre cohort of 90 patients with severe combined immunodeficiency: long-term outcome of HSCT in SCID. Blood 2009;113:4114–24.

87. Honig M, Albert MH, Schulz A, et al. Patients with adenosine deaminase deficiency surviving after hematopoietic stem cell transplantation are at high risk of CNS complications. Blood 2007;109:3595–602.

88. Baguette C, Vermylen C, Brichard B, et al. Persistent developmental delay despite successful bone marrow transplantation for purine nucleoside phosphorylase deficiency. J Pediatr Hematol Oncol 2002;24:69–71.

89. Titman P, Pink E, Skucek E, et al. Cognitive and behavioral abnormalities in children after hematopoietic stem cell transplantation for severe congenital immunodeficiencies. Blood 2008;12:3907–13.

90. Booth C, Hershfield M, Notarangelo L, et al. Management options for adenosine deaminase deficiency; proceedings of the EBMT satellite workshop (Hamburg, March 2006). Clin Immunol 2007;123:139–47.

91. Hacein-Bey-Abina S, Le Deist F, Carlier F, et al. Sustained correction of X-linked severe combined immunodeficiency by ex vivo gene therapy. N Engl J Med 2002;346:1185–93.

92. Gaspar HB, Parsley KL, Howe S, et al. Gene therapy of X-linked severe combined immunodeficiency by use of a pseudotyped gammaretroviral vector. Lancet 2004;364:2181–7.

93. Hacein-Bey-Abina S, Garrigue A, Wang GP, et al. Insertional oncogenesis in 4 patients after retrovirus-mediated gene therapy of SCID-X1. J Clin Invest 2008;118:3132–42.

94. Howe SJ, Mansour MR, Schwarzwaelder K, et al. Insertional mutagenesis combined with acquired somatic mutations causes leukemogenesis following gene therapy of SCID-X1 patients. J Clin Invest 2008;118:3143–50.

95. Aiuti A, Slavin S, Aker M, et al. Correction of ADA-SCID by stem cell gene therapy combined with nonmyeloablative conditioning. Science 2002;296:2410–3.

96. Aiuti A, Cattaneo F, Galimberti S, et al. Gene therapy for immunodeficiency due to adenosine deaminase deficiency. N Engl J Med 2009;360:447–58.

97. Kobrynski LJ, Sullivan KE. Velocardiofacial syndrome, DiGeorge syndrome: the chromosome 22q11.2 deletion syndromes. Lancet 2007;370:1443–52.

98. Markert ML, Devlin BH, Alexieff MJ, et al. Review of 54 patients with complete DiGeorge anomaly enrolled in protocols for thymus transplantation: outcome of 44 consecutive transplants. Blood 2007;109:4539–47.

99. Land MH, Garcia-Lloret MI, Borzy MS, et al. Long-term results of bone marrow transplantation in complete DiGeorge syndrome. J Allergy Clin Immunol 2007;120:908–15.

100. Ridanpaa M, van Eenennaam H, Pelin K, et al. Mutations in the RNA component of RNase MRP cause a pleiotropic human disease, cartilagehair hypoplasia. Cell 2001;104:195–203.

101. Roifman CM, Gu Y, Cohen A. Mutations in the RNA component of RNase mitochondrial RNA processing might cause Omenn syndrome. J Allergy Clin Immunol 2006;117:897–903.

102. Kavadas FD, Giliani S, Gu Y, et al. Variability of clinical and laboratory features among patients with ribonuclease mitochondrial RNA processing endoribonuclease gene mutations. J Allergy Clin Immunol 2008;122:1178–84.

103. Boerkoel CF, O'Neill S, Andre JL, et al. Manifestations and treatment of Schimke immuno-osseous dysplasia: 14 new cases and a review of the literature. Eur J Pediatr 2000;159:1–7.

104. Gennery AR, Cant AC, Jeggo PA. Immunodeficiency associated with DNA repair defect. Clin Exp Immunol 2000;121:1–7.

105. Savitsky K, Bar-Shira A, Gilad S, et al. A single ataxia-telangiectasia gene with a product similar to PI-3 kinase. Science 1995;268:1749–53.

106. Varon R, Vissinga C, Platzer M, et al. Nibrin, a novel DNA double-strand break repair protein, is mutated in Nijmegen breakage syndrome. Cell 1998;93:467–76.

107. Stewart GS, Maser RS, Stankovic T, et al. The DNA double-strand break repair gene hMRE11 is mutated in individuals with an ataxia-telangiectasia-like disorder. Cell 1999;99:577–87.

108. O'Driscoll M, Cerosaletti KM, Girard PM, et al. DNA ligase IV mutations identified in patients exhibiting developmental delay and immunodeficiency. Mol Cell 2001;8:1175–85.

109. Ochs HD, Thrasher AJ. The Wiskott-Aldrich syndrome. J Allergy Clin Immunol 2006;117:725–38.

110. Jin Y, Mazza C, Christie JR, et al. Mutations of the Wiskott-Aldrich Syndrome Protein (WASP): hotspots, effect on transcription, and translation and phenotype/genotype correlation. Blood 2004;104:4010–9.

111. Davis BR, Candotti F. Revertant somatic mosaicism in the Wiskott-Aldrich syndrome. Immunol Res 2009;44:127–31.

112. Pai SY, DeMartiis D, Forino C, et al. Stem cell transplantation for the Wiskott-Aldrich syndrome: a single-center experience confirms efficacy of matched unrelated donor transplantation. Bone Marrow Transplant 2006;38:671–9.

113. Ozsahin H, Cavazzana-Calvo M, Notarangelo LD, et al. Long-term outcome following hematopoietic stem-cell transplantation in Wiskott-Aldrich syndrome: collaborative study of the European Society for Immunodeficiencies and European Group for Blood and Marrow Transplantation. Blood 2008;111:439–45.

114. Notarangelo LD, Hayward AR. X-linked immunodeficiency with hyper IgM (X-HIM). Clin Exp Immunol 2000;120:349–405.

115. Winkelstein JA, Marino MC, Ochs H, et al. The X-linked hyper-IgM syndrome: clinical and immunologic features of 79 patients. Medicine (Baltimore) 2003;82:373–84.

116. Gennery AR, Khawaja K, Veys P, et al. Treatment of CD40 ligand deficiency by hematopoietic stem cell transplantation: a survey of the European experience 1993–2002. Blood 2004;103:1152–7.

10

Pediatric Human Immunodeficiency Virus Infection

Filiz O. Seeborg • Mary E. Paul • William T. Shearer

Human immunodeficiency virus (HIV) infection in pediatrics is a deadly disease of infants who are infected at the time of birth, through breast-feeding, or through adult-type high-risk behaviors in adolescence. Prior to the mid 1990s, pediatric HIV infection had been marked by more rapid disease progression than was seen in HIV-infected adults. Since that time, better clinical, immunologic, and virologic outcomes of pediatric HIV infection have been achieved with the implementation of highly active antiretroviral therapy (HAART). The key to success with therapy involves meeting the patient's psychosocial needs, providing the understanding and tools necessary for compliance, addressing and correcting formulation and dosing problems when possible, and having the patient or guardian committed to achieving adherence approaching 100% for antiretroviral therapy (ART) doses.

Epidemiology and Etiology

Twenty-five years after the first clinical evidence of HIV was recognized, HIV infection remains the fourth leading cause of death worldwide. The Joint United Nations Programme on HIV/AIDS (UNAIDS) estimated that globally, 33 million people were living with HIV in 2007.[1] Sub-Saharan Africa remains most heavily affected by HIV, accounting for 67% of all people infected with HIV. An estimated 370 000 children under 15 years of age became infected with HIV during the year 2007. Globally, the number of children younger than 15 years of age living with HIV increased from 1.6 million in 2001 to 2.0 million in 2007.[1] Young people aged 15 to 24 years of age account for 45% of all new infections in adults worldwide.[2] An estimated 56 300 adolescents and adults were newly infected with HIV in 2006 in the United States.[2] The Centers for Disease Control and Prevention (CDC) reported that the number of newly diagnosed HIV/AIDS cases decreased among children less than 13 years of age while this rate increased among persons aged 15 to 29 years from 2004 through 2007.[3] The number of adults and adolescents living with HIV infection in the USA at the end of 2006 was approximately 1.1 million including those not yet diagnosed and those who had already progressed to AIDS.[4] Seventy percent of those were between 25 and 49 years of age, and 5% were between the ages of 13 and 24 years. HIV infection was diagnosed in 159 children in 2007, all but 20 of whom became infected through mother-to-child transmission (MTCT).[3] The CDC estimated that there were 7181 children living with HIV/AIDS in the USA at the end of 2007, of whom 91% had been exposed perinatally.[3]

Prevention of MTCT of HIV in the USA and Europe has been a tremendous success, such that transmission rates of less than 2% have been achieved.[5] Mother-to-infant transmission can occur during gestation, at the time of delivery or in the intrapartum period, or postpartum as a result of breast-feeding. The majority of perinatal transmission occurs during late pregnancy, close to the time of delivery.[6] Maternal factors associated with an increased risk for transmission include low $CD4^+$ T lymphocyte counts,[7] high HIV viral load,[5] presence of HIV in the genital tract,[8] advanced HIV disease, the presence of p24 antigen in serum,[9] placental inflammation,[8] maternal-fetal microtransfusions,[10] premature rupture of membranes, and premature delivery. HIV-infected women are counseled to forgo breast-feeding as postnatal HIV transmission risk is around 1% per month of breast-feeding.[11] A randomized trial from Nairobi, Kenya found that breast-fed infants had a significantly higher incidence of HIV infection compared to those fed formula (36.7 vs 20.5%); feeding infant formula was estimated to prevent 44% of HIV-1 infections in these infants.[12] However, there is continuing debate over the importance of breast-feeding of infants in developing countries because of the threat of chronic diarrhea and death due to the use of contaminated water used to prepare artificial formulas.[13]

The mode of delivery of pregnant women also influences transmission risk. Rates of vertical HIV transmission as low as 2% have been reported when the care of HIV-infected pregnant women includes both zidovudine (ZDV) and scheduled cesarean delivery (SCD).[14] Current guidelines for providing ART and SCD in the USA are shown in Box 10-1.[15] Host genetic factors are also important determinants of the susceptibility to perinatal transmission. Transmitting mothers more often carry CXCR4 tropic HIV virus than nontransmitting mothers,[16] although most transmitted virus is CCR5 tropic.[17] A genetic polymorphism in the untranslated region of the maternal stromal cell-derived factor 1 (SDF1) has been associated with an increased risk of HIV transmission.[18] Concordance between maternal and infant human leukocyte antigen (HLA) and maternal HLA homozygosity may increase the risk of mother-to-child HIV-transmission.[19] Certain maternal HLA class I alleles may increase the risk of vertical HIV transmission to the infant,[20] while some may be protective.[21]

In 1994, the Pediatric AIDS Clinical Trials Group (PACTG) 076 protocol demonstrated that a course of ZDV, when given to HIV-infected pregnant women in a regimen that included during pregnancy, peripartum, and postpartum dosing in the infant, could reduce transmission of HIV to the infant by nearly 70% in a non-breast-feeding population.[22] Based on the results of PACTG protocol 076, US Public Health Service (PHS) guidelines recommend prenatal HIV testing with consent and counseling for all

Summary of US Public Health Service Task Force Guidelines for Prevention of Mother-to-Child HIV Transmission in the United States

Maternal Antenatal Plasma HIV RNA >1000 copies/mL

- Mother: HAART* plus intrapartum ZDV[†] given via continous infusion

  Infant: ZDV for 6 weeks starting within 6 to 12 hours after delivery

- Elective cesarean delivery if plasma HIV RNA remains > 1000 copies/mL near delivery

Maternal Antenatal Plasma HIV RNA <1000 copies/mL

- Mother: HAART* plus intrapartum ZDV[†] given via continous infusion

  Infant: ZDV for 6 weeks starting within 6 to 12 hours after delivery

No ART before labor

- Mother: ZDV given via continous infusion during labor

  Infant: ZDV for 6 weeks starting within 6 to 12 hours after delivery

or

- Mother: ZDV given via continous infusion during labor, plus single dose NVP[±] at onset of labor. Consider adding 3TC[‡] during labor and maternal ZDV/3TC for 7 days postpartum to reduce development of NVP resistance.

  Infant: Single dose NVP[§], plus ZDV for 6 weeks starting within 6 to 12 hours after delivery

No ART before or during labor

- ZDV given to the infant for 6 weeks starting within 6 to 12 hours after delivery

- Some clinicians may choose to use ZDV in combination with additional antiretroviral drugs, but appropriate dosing regimens for neonates are incompletely defined

*HAART: highly active antiretroviral therapy; [†]ZDV: zidovudine; [‡]Single dose NVP (nevirapine) for mother: 200 mg given once orally at onset of labor; [‡]3TC: Lamivudine; [§]Single dose NVP for the infant: 2 mg/kg given once orally at 2 to 3 days of age if mother received intrapartum single dose NVP or given at birth if mother did not receive intrapartum single dose NVP.
See http://aidsinfo.nih.gov for updates because single dose NVP regimens have been associated with NNRTI resistance in recent studies.

pregnant women in the USA.[23] The Women and Infants Transmission Study group demonstrated a step-wise reduction in perinatal transmission rates as prevention regimens intensified from no ART (20%), to ZDV monotherapy (10%) to dual therapy (3.8%) to HAART (1.2%) in a cohort of 1542 HIV-infected women with singleton live births.[24] Use of three-drug combination HAART is the treatment standard of care recommended by PHS for HIV-infected pregnant women for both the prevention of perinatal transmission and for HIV treatment in the mother, regardless of HIV viral load or CD4+ T cell count. Recommended HAART combinations for pregnant HIV-infected women are updated and can be reviewed at PHS website.[15] In short- and long-term follow-up of large observational studies, no teratogenicity or malignancy have been reported in infants exposed to ZDV and other specific HAART.[22,25,26] Table 10-1 lists HAART medications and FDA pregnancy category and potential teratogenecity by animal studies. Perinatal exposure to HAART is associated with 20% decreases in CD8+ T cells and platelets that seem to persist for at least the first 2 years of life in uninfected, HIV-exposed infants.[27] Nucleoside reverse transcriptase inhibitors (NRTIs) have been shown to cause mitochondrial toxicity because of the affinity of these drugs for the mitochondrial gamma DNA polymerase and interference with mitochondrial replication. Clinical disorders linked to mitochondrial toxicity include cardiomyopathy, neuropathy, myopathy, hepatic steatosis, lactic acidosis, and pancreatitis. Clinically evident mitochondrial disease in children with ART exposure has only been described in Europe, with an estimated 18-month incidence of 'established' mitochondrial dysfunction of 0.26% among exposed children.[28]

Pathogenesis

HIV-1 is a lentivirus belonging to the retrovirus family. The virus contains an outer envelope and inner core proteins that surround two copies of single-stranded genomic RNA. The RNA genome encodes at least nine proteins including Gag, Pol, Env, Tat, Rev, Nef, Vif, Vpu, and Vpr of which only the former five are essential for viral replication. HIV-1 primarily infects cells that express the CD4 molecule, particularly CD4+ T lymphocytes. Other target cells include monocytes, macrophages, dendritic cells, astrocytes and microglia. The Env gene encodes a polyprotein, gp 160, which facilitates virus entry into target cells. Cleavage of gp 160 yields gp41 and gp120, a process that is essential for viral infectivity. Gp 120 is the virion surface subunit responsible for the cellular receptor (CD4) and co-receptor (CCR5 or CXCR4) binding. After virus entry, the viral RNA genome undergoes reverse transcription, and the proviral DNA then integrates into the host cell chromosome. Following translation, the viral proteins assemble at the cell membrane and the immature viral particles containing the RNA genome and viral enzymes leave the host cell. Proteolytic processing of the capsid takes place after virion budding that leads to a structural rearrangement of the virion and maturation of the viral particle (Figure 10-1).

Multiple factors acting in concert exist that contribute to severe immunodeficiency caused by HIV-1 infection. The hallmark of immunodeficiency caused by HIV-1 infection is a decrease in CD4+ T cell number and function. Recent data indicate that the depletion of CD4+ memory T cells mainly occurs in the acute phase of infection and is most profound at the gut-associated lymphoid tissue (GALT).[29] The potentially irreversible loss of immune and structural integrity at this site may permit translocation of bacteria and their products. This results in nonspecific systemic immune activation as well as lymphocyte activation-induced T lymphocyte death. Arthos and colleagues demonstrated that this assault of HIV-1 on GALT is mediated by interaction of gp 120 with the gut homing integrin $\alpha_4\beta_7$.[30] Immune activation, in concert with the host's immune response and the virulence of HIV-1 result in a set point of viremia that provides information about disease progression. HIV disease progression is faster in children compared to adults, and infants infected with HIV during the delivery manifest symptoms including developmental delay or failure to thrive within the first year of life.

HIV Infection and Allergic Diseases

Atopic diseases are frequent in HIV-infected individuals compared to the HIV-negative population. The most common atopic disease in HIV-infected patients is drug hypersensitivity which is postulated to be 100 times more common than in the general population.[31] Metabolic disturbances, polyclonal activation of B lymphocytes, dysregulation of specific immunoglobulin E (IgE) synthesis, concurrent viral or opportunistic infections, formation of toxic metabolites, increased susceptibility to oxidative stress, and genetic factors play important roles in the development of

Table 10-1 Data Relevant to the Use of Antiretroviral Agents in Pregnancy

Antiretroviral Drug	FDA Pregnancy Category[†]	Long-Term Animal Carcinogenicity Studies	Animal Teratogen Studies
Nucleoside and Nucleotide Analogue Reverse Transcriptase Inhibitors			
Zidovudine (Retrovir, AZT, ZDV)	C	Positive (rodent, noninvasive vaginal epithelial tumors)	Positive (rodent; near lethal dose)
Zalcitabine (HIVID, ddC)*	C	Positive (rodent, thymic lymphomas)	Positive (rodent; hydrocephalus at high dose)
Didanosine (Videx, ddI)	B	Negative (no tumors, lifetime rodent study)	Negative
Stavudine (Zerit, d4T)	C	Positive (mice and rats, at very high dose exposure, liver and bladder tumors)	Negative (but sternal bone calcium decreases in rodents)
Lamivudine (Epivir,3TC)	C	Negative (no tumors, lifetime rodent study)	Negative
Abacavir (Ziagen, ABC)	C	Positive (malignant and nonmalignant tumors of liver, thyroid in female rats, and preputial anc clitoral gland of mice and rats)	Positive (rodent anasarca and skeletal malformations at 1000 mg/kg (35 × human exposure) during organogenesis; not seen in rabbits)
Tenofovir DF (Viread)	B	Positive (hepatic adenomas in female mice at high doses)	Negative (osteomalacia when given to juvenile animals at high doses)
Emtricitabine (Emtriva, FTC)	B	Negative (no tumors, life time rodent study)	Negative
Non-Nucleoside Reverse Transcriptase Inhibitors			
Nevirapine (Viramune)	B	Positive (hepatocellular adenomas and carcinomas in mice and rats)	Negative
Delavirdine (Rescriptor)	C	Positive (hepatocellular adenomas and carcinoma in male and female mice but not rats, bladder tumors in male mice)	Positive (rodent; ventricular septal defect)
Efavirenz (Sustiva)	D	Positive (hepatocellular adenomas and carcinomas and pulmonary alveolar/bronchiolar adenomas in female but not male mice)	Positive (cynomologus monkey anencephaly, anophthalmia, microphthalmia)
Protease Inhibitors			
Indinavir (Crixivan)	C	Positive (thyroid adenomas in male rats at highest dose)	Negative (but extra ribs in rodents)
Ritonavir (Norvir)	B	Positive (liver adenomas and carcinomas in male mice)	Negative (but cryptorchidism in rodents)
Saquinavir (Fortovase)	B	Negative	Negative
Nelfinavir (Viracept)	B	Positive (thyroid follicular adenomas and carcinomas in rats)	Negative
Amprenavir (Agenerase)*	C	Positive (hepatocellular adenomas and carcinomas in male mice and rats)	Negative (but deficient ossification and thymic elongation in rats and rabbits)
Lopinavir/Ritonavir (Kaletra)	C	Positive (hepatocellular adenomas and carcinomas in rats and mice)	Negative (but delayed skeletal ossification and increase in skeletal variations in rats at maternally toxic doses)
Atazanavir	B	Positive (hepatocellular adenomas in female mice)	Negative
Darunavir (Prezista)	B	Not completed	Negative
Fosamprenavir (Lexiva)	C	Positive (benign and malignant liver tumors in male rodents)	Negative (deficient ossification with amprenavir but not fosamprenavir)
Tipranavir (Aptivus)	C	In progress	Negative (decreased ossification and pup weights in rats at maternally toxic doses)
Entry Inhibitors			
Enfuvirtide (Fuzeon)	B	Not done	Negative
Maraviroc (Selzentry)	B	Negative	Negative
Integrase Inhibitors			
Raltegravir (Isentress)	C	In progress	Negative (extranumerary ribs in rats at dose exposure 3-fold higher than human)

Modified from Centers for Disease Control and Prevention: Public Health Service Task Force Recommendation for Use of Antiretroviral Drugs in Pregnant Women with HIV-1 for Maternal Health and for Reducing HIV-1 Transmission in the United States, http://aidsinfo.nih.gov, July.8, 2008

*No longer available in the United States

[†]Food and Drug Administration (FDA) pregnancy categories:

A: Adequate and well-controlled studies of pregnant women fail to demonstrate a risk to the fetus during the first trimester of pregnancy (and there is no evidence of risk during later trimesters);

B: Animal reproduction studies fail to demonstrate a risk to the fetus and adequate and well-controlled studies of pregnant women have not been conducted;

C: Safety in human pregnancy has not been determined, animal studies are either positive for fetal risk or have not been conducted, and the drug should not be used unless the potential benefit outweighs the potential risk to the fetus;

D: Positive evidence of human fetal risk based on adverse reaction data from investigational or marketing experiences, but the potential benefits from the use of the drug in pregnant women may be acceptable despite its potential risks;

X: Studies in animals or reports of adverse reactions have indicated that the risk associated with the use of the drug for pregnant women clearly outweighs any possible benefit.

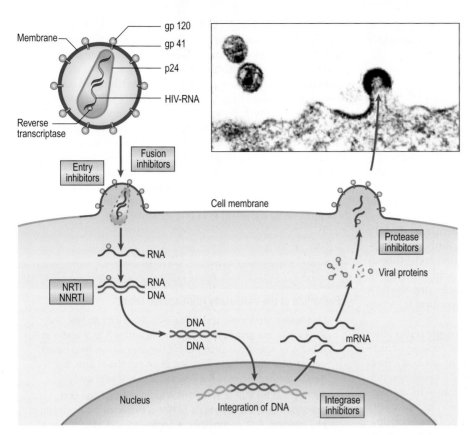

Figure 10-1 Schematic representation of human immunodeficiency virus-1 (HIV-1) life cycle and targets of currently available antiretroviral (ARV) drugs. HIV is a retrovirus that has an envelope formed of two major viral envelope proteins, gp120 and gp41, and a lipid membrane. Important core proteins are p17^{gag} matrix protein (not shown), and p24^{gag} capsid protein. Two nucleocapsid proteins, p6^{gag} and p7^{gag}, are not shown. Within the inner core are two copies of the single-stranded HIV-1 genomic viral RNA that are associated with enzymes including the reverse transcriptase, protease, and integrase enzymes. Five classes of ARV drugs are available at present. Entry and fusion inhibitors inhibit the entry of virions into the target cell. Nucleoside analogues (*NRTI*) or non-nucleoside reverse transcriptase inhibitors (*NNRTI*) blocks reverse transcription. Integrase inhibitors block integration of viral genome into DNA of the target cell. Protease inhibitors (PI) interferes with viral protein assembly and budding.

drug hypersensitivity in HIV-infected patients.[32–36] Up to 60% of HIV-infected individuals may experience hypersensitivity with trimethoprim-sulfamethoxazole (TMP-SMX) at some time during prophylaxis or treatment of *Pneumocytis jiroveci*. Antiretroviral drugs most frequently associated with hypersensivity reactions are abacavir, a nucleoside analogue; non-nucleoside reverse transcriptase inhibitors (NNRTIs); fosamprenavir, a protease inhibitor; and enfuvirtide, a fusion inhibitor.

Elevated serum IgE and increased prevalence of atopy in HIV-infected patients have been reported by several investigators. A decline in the production of interleukin (IL)-2, IL-12, and interferon gamma (IFN-γ) (type 1 cytokines) and an increase in the production of IL-4, IL-5, IL-6, and IL-10 (type 2 cytokines) by peripheral mononuclear cells of HIV-infected patients have been well documented.[37,38] Two HIV-1 proteins, gp120 and Tat, trigger the release of cytokines critical for T$_H$2 (type 2 T helper) cell polarization from immune cells containing FcεRI receptors (basophils and mast cells). This alteration in cytokine production is postulated to contribute to elevated IgE levels and increased eosinophil counts. Elevated IgE levels have also been associated with progression of HIV infection.[37] However, in a study of 122 HIV-infected children there was no correlation between serum IgE levels and the degree of immune suppression.[39]

Rhinitis and sinusitis are also common problems in HIV-infected patients. The prevalence of allergic rhinitis and sinusitis in HIV-infected individuals may be as high as 80% and 65%, respectively.[40] A correlation between immune suppression and severity of sinusitis is controversial.[40–42] Some studies report a correlation between serum IgE levels and severity of sinusitis: suggesting that sinusitis is a part of this acquired atopic state.[41]

HIV-infected patients may suffer a variety of respiratory problems including bronchitis, pneumonia, and lymphoid interstitial pneumonitis. Increased prevalence of wheezing and bronchial hyperresponsiveness to methacoline, and an elevated serum IgE

BOX 10-2 Key concepts

Differential Diagnosis

- Human immunodeficiency virus (HIV) infection should be included in the differential diagnosis of children who have recurrent infection
- Children who have undiagnosed HIV infection can present with recurrent bacterial infection
- Opportunistic infections occur at higher CD4$^+$ T cell counts for children than for adults

---

have been reported in HIV-infected men.[43] One study suggested an association between asthma and CD4$^+$ T cell count of greater than 200 cells/dL.[44] It has recently been demonstrated that incidence of asthma is greatly increased in HIV-infected children who have higher CD4$^+$ T cell percentages in the HAART era, suggesting a mechanism driven by immunoreconstitution of CD4$^+$ T cells.[45]

Differential Diagnosis

HIV infection should be in the differential diagnosis for any infant, child, or adolescent who has recurrent infections, including recurrent otitis media or bacterial pneumonia (Box 10-2). Unlike adults, recurrent bacterial infections are considered a sign of disease progression in HIV-infected children. Similar to adults, untreated HIV-infected children not uncommonly have eczematous rashes and wasting or growth failure. Therefore HIV infection should be a diagnosis considered when evaluating failure to thrive. A complete history includes discussion of maternal HIV testing during pregnancy and, for youth, obtaining drug use and sexual behavior histories. Also, opportunistic infection should trigger an evaluation for T cell immunodeficiency, including HIV infection/AIDS.

Evaluation and Management

HIV testing is recommended as part of routine care for all youths and adults aged 13 to 64 years in all clinical settings, with subsequent testing based on risks.[46] Testing for HIV infection is routinely performed in children who are older than 18 months of age and in youths using the HIV enzyme-linked immunosorbent assay (ELISA) or rapid test, which tests for the presence of specific antibody to HIV. If the HIV screening test is positive, confirmation of infection is provided most frequently by the HIV Western blot test, which also looks for specific antibody to HIV. As there is a window period between HIV infection and antibody production during which the HIV ELISA or rapid test may be negative, testing should be repeated until 6 months after the time of suspected exposure or high-risk behavior to confirm infection status.

Infants are diagnosed with HIV by using virologic tests rather than an antibody test as the test may be positive because of antibody obtained through transplacental passage of antibody from the mother (Box 10-3). The HIV DNA polymerase chain reaction (PCR) is most commonly used for diagnosis because its convenience and sensitivity in diagnosis is well known. The sensitivity and specificity of the RNA PCR test for HIV diagnosis is comparable to HIV DNA PCR testing. However, false positive results have been reported with low level HIV viral loads with HIV-1 RNA assays.[47,48] HIV cultures are more expensive and have a slower turnaround time for results, although cultures are sensitive to diagnosis when specimens are properly handled. The HIV DNA PCR was positive in 38% of 271 HIV-infected infants by age 48 hours in a meta-analysis of published data.[49] Virtually all infected infants can be definitively diagnosed by 6 months of age. Infants should be evaluated with an HIV DNA PCR within the first several days of life and at 1 to 2 and 4 to 6 months of age. Presumptive exclusion of HIV-1 infection can be based on 2 negative HIV DNA PCR tests, at 2 weeks of age and older and at 4 weeks of age and older, or 1 negative HIV DNA PCR at 8 weeks of age and older in the absence of other laboratory or clinical evidence of HIV-1 infection[49] (Box 10-3). Presumptive exclusion can be used as a means to defer prophylaxis for *Pneumocystis jiroveci* pneumonia (PJP) until HIV infection is definitively excluded. Definitive exclusion of HIV-1 infection is based on 2 negative HIV DNA PCR tests obtained at 1 month of age or older and at 4 months of age and older. Further testing at 12 to 18 months of age is required to definitively exclude HIV-1 infec-

tion by means of HIV ELISA and Western blot testing.[50] In resource-poor countries where virological tests are not available, the CD4/CD8 ratio has been shown to be an alternative method of diagnosis of HIV infection.[51]

Monitoring for disease progression and efficacy of ART is performed using CD4+ T cell count and HIV RNA PCR values; these tests are typically followed every 3 to 4 months. CD4+ T cell counts are normally 3-fold higher in infants and children than in adults and these counts decline to adult values by age 5 years.[52] Therefore CD4+ T cell counts indicating immunosuppression and risk for opportunistic infection and malignancy are higher in children than in adults and vary with age (Table 10-2).

The amount of HIV RNA in the peripheral blood is an important prognostic indicator and is a sensitive measure of treatment

---

BOX 10-3 Key concepts

Evaluation of the Perinatally HIV-Exposed Infant

- Non-breast-fed infants should be evaluated with an HIV DNA PCR within the first several days of life and at 1 to 2 and 4 to 6 months of age. If the DNA PCR is negative at two time points, one at ≥1 month of age and one at ≥4 months of age, the non-breast-fed infant is not infected with HIV perinatally.

- Prophylaxis for PJP is started at 4 to 6 weeks of age and continued until the diagnosis of HIV is excluded.* If the infant is HIV infected, PJP prophylaxis is continued until after 1 year of age at which time age-specific CD4+ T cell count or percentage thresholds are used as a guide to determine if prophylaxis should be continued or stopped with monitoring of CD4+ T cell count performed every 3 months.

- HIV antibody test followed by a confirmatory Western blot for positive screening test can be used in diagnosis of HIV infection in infants and children older than 18 months of age, after antibody that was acquired through transplacental passage from the mother has been lost.

- Infants who have been exposed to antiretroviral therapy in utero should be followed up long term.

HIV, Human immunodeficiency virus; *DNA*, deoxyribonucleic acid; *PCR*, polymerase chain reaction; *PJP*, Pneumocystis jiroveci pneumonia; *ELISA*, enzyme-linked immunosorbent assay.
*For non-breast-fed infants who have a negative virologic test at ≥14 days of age and at ≥1 month of age, HIV can be presumptively excluded forgoing the start of PJP prophylaxis. Presumptive exclusion of HIV can be done for infants with one negative virologic test at ≥2 months of age as well. HIV is definitively excluded with two negative virologic tests (at ≥1 month of age and at ≥4 months of age) or with two negative HIV antibody tests from separate specimens at ≥6 months of age.

Table 10-2 1994 Revised HIV Pediatric Classification System: Immune Categories based on Age-Specific CD4+ T Cell Count and Percentage

Immune Category	<12 Months		1–5 Years		6–12 Years	
	No./mm³	Percent	No./mm³	Percent	No./mm³	Percent
Category 1: no suppression	≥1500	(≥25)	≥1000	(≥25)	≥500	(≥25)
Category 2: moderate suppression	750–1499	(15–24)	500–999	(15–24)	200–499	(15–24)
Category 3: severe suppression	<750	(<15)	<500	(<15)	<200	(<15)

Modified from Centers for Disease Control and Prevention: MMWR 43:1–10, 1994.
HIV, Human immunodeficiency virus.

response. Viral burden is determined by quantitative HIV RNA PCR measures. HIV-infected infants typically have a rising viral load in the first several months of life that peaks in the first year and slowly declines over the next several years. The viral load peaks are typically very high; the Women and Infants Transmission study reported a mean viral load in the first year of life of 185 000 copies/mL and most infants had viral loads greater than 100 000 copies/mL.[53] Because of the effects of this high viral burden on a developing immune system, infants are usually treated aggressively with HAART in the first year of life. Adolescents are expected to behave similarly to adults following infection; that is, high viral burden is found within the first several months following infection and then, with the establishment of immune responses to HIV, viral burden declines to a lower, stable level within a year after infection. The level of the stable viral burden, or set-point, is a predictor of rapidity of disease progression.[54] The HIV Pediatric Prognostic markers Collaborative Study reported that HIV-infected children older than 2 years of age are at increased risk of disease progression or death when HIV RNA exceeded 100 000 copies (5.0 $\log_{10}$)/mL.[55] The viral set-point may be a useful value in treatment initiation decisions for older children and adolescents although newer data in adults suggest that ongoing inflammation contributes to poorer outcomes even with lower viral loads.[56,57] Figure 10-2 demonstrates factors to consider when initiating ART in children and adolescents.

Treatment

The approach to treatment of HIV infection in children differs depending upon age and mode of infection. Perinatally infected infants, children, and teens and newly HIV-infected adolescents each have unique issues to consider regarding the decision to begin ART. Perinatally infected infants should begin therapy soon after infection has been identified. This approach is taken to suppress viremia, to allow more normal maturation of immune responses, and to allow for more normal growth and development.

In adolescents, psychosocial issues must be addressed because these issues influence medication adherence. Some of these factors are family disruption resulting from loss of HIV-infected parents, and entering into adolescence with a chronic infection, one that can be transmitted to sexual partners and, for young women, to their infants; patients also may have physical stigmata, such as growth problems, which impact treatment acceptance and adherence. Clinicians should be aware of potential interactions between ART and oral contraceptives that may lower efficacy of contraception.

A total of 25 HAART medications have been approved for use in HIV-infected adults and adolescents; 17 of these have been approved for pediatric treatment and 16 are available as a pediatric formulation or capsules. These drugs include nucleoside analogue or nucleotide analogue reverse transcriptase inhibitors (NRTIs, NtRTIs), non-nucleoside reverse transcriptase inhibitors (NNRTIs), protease inhibitors (PIs), entry inhibitors (fusion inhibitors and CCR5 antagonists), and integrase inhibitors.

Combination therapy, with at least three drugs including a PI or an NNRTI plus a dual NRTI backbone, is recommended for initial treatment of HIV-infected children.

Box 10-4 shows the ART combinations that are recommended for the treatment of HIV infection in infants and children by the PHS. These medications differ somewhat from those recommended for HIV-infected adolescents and adults because of the lack of pediatric data for some medications and the formulation

- Clinical symptoms*
- Immune suppression†
  – CD4 < 25% at 1–5 years
  – CD4 < 350 cell/mm³ at ≥ 5 years
- < 12 months old††

↓ (Yes)

Initiate therapy following medication readiness preparation and patient/guardian agreement to follow treatment plan

- Asymptomatic or mild symptoms‡ and
  – CD4 ≥ 25% at 1–5 years
  – CD4 ≥ 350 cells/mm³ at ≥ 5 years and
  – HIV RNA PCR > 100 000 copies/mL

↓ (Yes)

Consider initiating therapy following medication readiness preparation and patient/guardian agreement to follow treatment plan

- Asymptomatic or mild symptoms‡ and
  – CD4 ≥ 25% at 1–5 years
  – CD4 ≥ 350 cells/mm³ at ≥ 5 years‡ and
  – HIV RNA PCR < 100 000 copies/mL

↓ (Yes)

- Consider to defer therapy§
- Follow CD4⁺ T cells counts, plasma HIV RNA level, and clinical status every 3 to 4 months and reassess need for initiation of therapy using algorithm. A repeatedly declining CD4⁺ T cell is an additional indication to initiate therapy

Figure 10-2 Algorithm for deciding when to initiate antiretroviral therapy (ART) in children and adolescents. Some experts would recommend initiating therapy in the early stages of HIV infection in most adolescents because of a theoretic advantage of reducing viral set-point, preserving immune function, and reducing the risk for viral transmission. However, the potential risks of initiating therapy in the early stages of HIV infection include indefinite need for therapy, risk for drug resistance if viral replication is not suppressed, early exposure to drugs with potential toxicities, and adverse impact on quality of life resulting from daily medication regimens. Recommendations for when to initiate therapy have been more aggressive in children than adults because of rapid HIV disease progression in children, and laboratory parameters are less predictive of risk of disease progression, particularly in young infants. *PCR*, Polymerase chain reaction;*CDC clinical category C and B (except for the following category B conditions: single episode of serious bacterial infection or lymphoid interstitial pneumonitis); †The data supporting this recommendation are stronger for those with CD4⁺ T cell percentage <20% than for those with CD4⁺ T cell percentage between 20% to 24 %. Initiation of ART is recommended for children ≥1 year with AIDS or significant symptoms (clinical category C or most clinical category B conditions) regardless of CD4⁺ T cell percentage/count or plasma HIV RNA level. Initiation of ART is also recommended for children ≥1 year who have met the age-related CD4⁺ T cell threshold for initiating treatment, regardless of symptoms or plasma HIV RNA level; ††Initiation of ART is recommended in this age group regardless of clinical status, CD4⁺ T cell percentage or viral load. It is critical that the importance of adherence to the treatment is fully discussed with the care-givers, and that potential problems are identified and resolved prior to initiation of therapy, even if this delays starting treatment; ‡CDC clinical category A or N or the following category B conditions: single episode of serious bacterial infection or lymphoid interstitial pneumonitis; ‡The data supporting this recommendation are stronger for those with CD4⁺ T cell count <200 than for those with CD⁺ T cell counts between 200 to 350 cells/mm³; §Adult HIV Guidelines suggests that the patient is at risk for disease progression. Clinical and laboratory data should be reevaluated every 3 to 4 months. However, short-term deferral of therapy may be necessary to allow for maximizing psychosocial support and medication readiness.

BOX 10-4 Therapeutic principles

Recommended Antiretroviral Regimens for Initial Therapy for Human Immunodeficiency Virus Infection in Children

Strongly Recommended

Protease inhibitor (PI)-based regimen

Two nucleoside reverse transcriptase inhibitors (NRTI) and lopinavir/ritonavir

Non-nucleoside reverse transcriptase inhibitor(NNRTI)-based regimen

Children ≥3 years old: two NRTIs and efavirenz*

Children <3 years old or who cannot swallow capsules: two NRTIs and nevirapine (NVP)*

Recommended dual NRTI combinations: abacavir (ABC) and lamivudine (3TC) or emtricitabine (FTC); dideoxyinosine (ddI) and FTC; zidovudine (ZDV) and (3TC or FTC); tenofovir and (3TC or FTC) (for Tanner stage 4 or postpubertal adolescents only)

Recommended as an Alternative

PI-based regimen

Two NRTIs and nelfinavir (children ≥2 years old)

Two NRTIs and atazanavir and low dose ritonavir (children ≥6 years old)

Two NRTIs and fosamprenavir and low dose ritonavir (children ≥6 years old)

NNRTI-based regimen

Two NRTIs and nevirapine* (children ≥3 years old)

Offered only in Special Circumstances

Two NRTIs and fosamprenavir unboosted (children ≥2 years old)

Two NRTIs and atazanavir unboosted (for treatment-naïve adolescents ≥13 years old and >39 kg)

ZDV and 3TC and ABC

From Guidelines for the Use of Antiretroviral Agents in Pediatric HIV Infection. February 23, 2009, pp. 1–139. Available at: http://aidsinfo.nih.gov. Accessed 14 Mar 2009.
*Efavirenz is currently available only in capsule form and should only be used in children ≥ 3 years old with weight ≥ 10 kg; nevirapine is preferred for children < 3 years old or who require a liquid formulation.

---

difficulties for some medications in infants and children. Efficacy of therapy is monitored by following CD4+ T cell count and viral load.

Both CD4+ T cell count and viral load are done at baseline and, after therapy is started, initial monitoring of viral load changes is usually performed at 4 weeks, although some data suggest that 1-week HIV RNA values might be predictive of long-term durability of therapy.[58] Children who start a new ART regimen or change to a new ART regimen should initially be evaluated within 2 weeks after the therapy is started to screen for side-effects and determine whether they are taking medications properly. Subsequent evaluations can be done every 3 months once adherence is established in the evidence of absence of toxicity. Children who develop ART toxicities should have appropriate laboratory tests done more frequently until the toxicities have resolved. Maximum virologic response may not occur until after 8 to 12 weeks of therapy. Virologic indications for change in therapy include less than a 1.0 $\log_{10}$ decrease from baseline after 8 to 12 weeks, HIV RNA not suppressed to <50 copies/mL after 6 months of therapy, repeated detection of HIV RNA after 12 months of therapy, and an increase in HIV RNA value after an initial response to low levels of detectable HIV RNA. Increases in HIV RNA should be confirmed by repeating the level after at least 1 week and an increase from a low level is indicated by a greater than 3-fold increase in copy number in children 2 years of age or older or a greater than 5-fold increase for children less than 2 years of age. Few data indicate that suppression to undetectable HIV RNA levels is always achievable and an immediate change in therapy may not be warranted if a 1.5 to 2.0 $\log_{10}$ decrease in baseline HIV RNA copy number is achieved, especially given the limited number of alternative regimens available for children. Substantial decline in CD4+ T cell counts indicate that a change in therapy should be considered, since CD4+ T cell count is an independent predictor of disease progression. Clinical changes such as growth failure and neurodevelopmental deterioration are also indications for a consideration of ART change.

When a change in ART is being considered, reasons for therapy failure should be assessed. The goal of therapy is to reduce plasma HIV RNA to less than 50 copies/mL to minimize the likelihood that viral resistance to ART will emerge. Measures of viral resistance while the child is still receiving the therapy, that is, before the regimen is discontinued and wild-type virus replaces resistant strains, are likely to be helpful in directing the choice of new regimens, although data are lacking in children to make recommendations regarding the use of resistance testing. The presence of resistance to a drug indicates that the drug is unlikely to suppress viremia.

Causes of drug failure include noncompliance with the regimen or subtherapeutic drug exposure; each cause should be investigated. Therapeutic drug monitoring through use of measures of plasma drug levels is increasingly becoming a routine part of care, especially when medications with drug-drug interactions caused by common elimination pathways must be used. Resistance is a serious problem given that there is cross-resistance that develops rapidly to the NNRTI medications, and resistance to one of the available PI medications may reduce sensitivity to other PIs. HIV-infected adolescents have many psychosocial barriers to antiretroviral medication adherence that must be addressed before therapy is considered or changed. Strategies should be discussed to help solve scheduling problems resulting from school, work, socializing, troubleshooting side-effects and formulation difficulties, and decreasing missed doses. The patient's transportation needs must also be met. Adolescents who are HIV infected benefit from interaction with HIV-infected peers through support groups or mentorship programs.

Adverse clinical events associated with combination ART are monitored during therapy and investigations are ongoing regarding the potential long-term effects of these therapies in children. Hyperlactatemia, possibly secondary to the mitochondrial effects of the NRTIs, discussed earlier in this chapter; hyperlipidemia, osteopenia, fat maldistribution, and hyperglycemia or diabetes mellitus, especially associated with PI use, have all been described in children on chronic ART.

The standard of care in treating HIV infection in infants, children, and adolescents includes the use of prophylaxis to prevent opportunistic infection.[59] Pneumocystis jiroveci pneumonia prophylaxis is indicated for HIV-infected or HIV-indeterminate infants aged 1 to 12 months, HIV-infected children aged 1 to 5 years with CD4+ T cell counts less than 500/mm³ or CD4+ T cell percentage less than 15%, and HIV-infected children and adolescents aged 6 years and above with CD4+ T cell percentage less than 15% (6 to 12 years old) or CD4+ T cell counts less than 200/mm³. The first choice of preventive regimens is TMP-SMX, with dapsone used as an alternative. TMP-SMX, when used daily, also protects

BOX 10-5 Key concepts

Take-Home Messages

- Human immunodeficiency virus (HIV) infection in the pediatric population occurs through perinatal infection and through new infections in adolescents resulting from sexual or intravenous drug use exposure routes.
- Testing of infants for HIV involves a direct test for virus. After 18 months of age, the screening test for HIV antibody, and Western blot can be used for diagnosis.
- Management of HIV in children and youth includes consideration of medication formulation, tolerability, and unique adherence issues.

Helpful Websites

HIV/AIDS Treatment Information Service website (http://aidsinfo.nih.gov)

Centers for Disease Control and Prevention website (http://www.cdc.org)

References

1. UNAIDS, WHO. AIDS epidemic update: December 2001. Geneva: Joint United Nations Programme on HIV/AIDS; 2001.
2. CDC. HIV/AIDS Surveillance Report 2001;13:1–41.
3. CDC. HIV/AIDS Surveillance Report, 2007. Volume 19. Atlanta: US Department of Health and Human Services, Centers for Disease Control and Prevention; 2009 (1–63). http://www.cdc.gov/hiv/topics/surveillance/resources/reports.
4. CDC. HIV prevalence estimates – United States, 2006. MMWR 2008;57(39):1073–6.
5. Mock PA, Shaffer N, Bhadrakom C, et al. Maternal viral load and timing of mother-to-child HIV transmission, Bangkok, Thailand. Bangkok Collaborative Perinatal HIV Transmission Study Group. AIDS 1999;13:407.
6. Mofenson LM. Interaction between timing of perinatal human immunodeficiency virus infection and the design of preventive and therapeutic interventions. Acta Paediatr Suppl 1997;421:1–9.
7. Rich KC, Fowler MG, Mofenson LM, et al. Maternal and infant factors predicting disease progression in human immunodeficiency virus type-1 infected infants. Women and Infant Transmission Study Group. Pediatrics 2000;105:e8.
8. Mwanyumba F, Gaillard P, Inion I, et al. Placental inflammation and perinatal transmission of HIV-1. J Acquir Immune Defic Syndr 2002;29:262–9.
9. Mandelbrot L, Le Chenadec J, Berrebi A, et al. Perinatal HIV-1 transmission: interaction between zidovudine prophylaxis and mode of delivery in the French Perinatal Cohort. JAMA 1998;280:55–60.
10. Kwiek JJ, Mwapasa V, Milner DA Jr, et al. Maternal-fetal microtransfusions and HIV-1 mother-to-child transmission in Malawi. PLoSMed 2006;3:e10.
11. WHO. HIV transmission through breastfeeding: a review of available evidence – an update from 2001 to 2007. Geneva: World Health Organization; 2007.
12. Nduati R, John G, Mbori-Ngacha D, et al. Effect of breastfeeding and formula feeding on transmission of HIV-1: a randomized clinical trial. JAMA 2000;283:1167–74.
13. Shearer WT. Breastfeeding and HIV infection. Pediatrics 2008;121:1046–7.
14. The International Perinatal HIV Group. The mode of delivery and the risk of vertical transmission of human immunodeficiency virus type 1–a meta-analysis of 15 prospective cohort studies. N Engl J Med 1999;340:977–87.
15. Perinatal HIV Guidelines Working Group. Public Health Service Task Force recommendations for use of antiretroviral drugs in pregnant HIV-infected women for maternal health and interventions to reduce perinatal HIV transmission in the United States. April 29, 2009; pp 1–90. Available at http://aidsinfo.nih.gov/ContentFiles/PerinatalGL.pdf. Accessed 15 May 2009.
16. Scarlatti G. Mother-to-child transmission of HIV-1: advances and controversies of the twentieth centuries. AIDS Reviews 2004;6:67–78.
17. Salvatori F, Scarlatti G. HIV type-1 chemokine receptor usage in mother-to-child transmission. AIDS Res Hum Retroviruses 2001;17: 925–35.
18. John GC, Rousseau C, Dong T, et al. Maternal SDF1 3'A polymorphism is associated with increased perinatal human immunodeficiency virus type 1 transmission. J Virol 2000;74:5736–9.
19. Mackelprang RD, John-Stewart G, Carrington M, et al. Maternal HLA homozygosity and mother-child HLA concordance increase the risk of vertical transmission of HIV-1. J Infect Dis 2008;197:1156–61.
20. Winchester R, Pitt J, Charurat M, et al. Mother-to-child transmission of HIV-1: strong association with certain maternal HLA-B alleles independent of viral load implicates innate immune mechanisms. J Acquir Immune Defic Syndr 2004;36:659–70.
21. Farquhar C, Rowland-Jones S, Mbori-Ngacha D, et al. Human leukocyte antigen (HLA) B*18 and protection against mother-to-child HIV type 1 transmission. AIDS Res Hum Retroviruses 2004;20:692–7.
22. Connor EM, Sperling RS, Gelber R, et al. Reduction of maternal-infant transmission of human immunodeficiency virus type 1 with zidovudine treatment. N Engl J Med 1994;331:1173.
23. CDC. US Public Health Service recommendations for human immunodeficiency virus counseling and voluntary testing for pregnant women. MMWR 1995;44:1–23.

against infection caused by *Toxoplasma gondii,* and prevention is recommended for infants, children, and adolescents who have severe immunosuppression (CD4$^+$ T cell count less than 100/mm^3; for adolescents, CD4$^+$ T cell values less than 15% for children) and positive IgG antibody to *Toxoplasma. Mycobacterium avium* complex (MAC) prophylaxis is indicated as follows: for infants less than 1 year of age, CD4$^+$ T cell count less than 750/mm^3; for children 1 to 2 years of age, CD4$^+$ T cell count less than 500/mm^3; for children 2 to 6 years of age, CD4$^+$ T cell count less than 75/mm^3; and for children at least 6 years of age and adolescents, CD4$^+$ T cell count less than 50/mm^3. Clarithromycin and azithromycin are the first-choice agents of preventive regimens for MAC and are started following documentation of a negative peripheral blood culture for mycobacterium. The tuberculin skin test (TST) is performed yearly, and antimycobacterial medication is used if the TST reaction is at least 5 mm or, in the case of contact with any case of active tuberculosis, regardless of TST result. *Varicella zoster* immune globulin should be considered for use in infants, children, or adolescents who have significant exposure to varicella or shingles with no prior history of chickenpox or shingles within 96 hours after exposure. HIV-infected children should receive routine immunizations with a few exceptions as outlined in the vaccination schedule included in the Pediatric Opportunistic Infection Guidelines.[60] All inactivated poliovirus vaccine schedules should be used for HIV-infected children and all household contacts. The measles, mumps, and rubella vaccine is not given to severely immunosuppressed (Category 3) children. Vaccination against varicella is indicated only for asymptomatic, nonimmunosuppressed children. HIV-infected children who are eligible to receive the varicella vaccine should receive two doses initially with at least a 3-month interval between doses.

Conclusions

HIV infection is a worldwide problem with tremendous impact. Although, in the USA, infection rates in the pediatric setting are markedly reduced by the use of measures to prevent perinatal transmission of HIV, young women, men, and infants continue to become infected with HIV (Box 10-5). Challenges for the future include further management difficulties caused by ART resistance that is a particular concern in the noncompliant patient; in older, treatment-experienced, perinatally infected youth; and in HIV-infected young women who are having repeated pregnancies. Newer approaches to improve compliance and prevention hold promise for the future. Practitioners impact infection risk by providing routine prevention messages to youth in their care and by promoting HIV testing in pregnant youth.

24. Cooper ER, Charurat M, Mofenson L, et al. Combination antiretroviral strategies for the treatment of pregnant HIV-1 infected women and prevention of perinatal HIV-1 transmission. J Acquir Immune Defic Syndr 2002;29:484–94.

25. Hanson IC, Antonelli TA, Sperling RS, et al. Lack of tumors in infants with perinatal HIV-1 exposure and fetal/neonatal exposure to zidovudine. J Acquir Immune Defic Syndr Hum Retrovirol 1999;20:463–7.

26. The European Collaborative Study. Exposure to antiretroviral therapy in utero or early life: the health of uninfected children born to HIV-infected women. J Acquir Immune Defic Syndr 2003;32:380–7.

27. Pacheco SE, McIntosh K, Lu M, et al. Effect of perinatal antiretroviral drug exposure on hematologic values in HIV-uninfected children: an analysis of the Women and Infants Transmission Study. J Infect Dis 2006;194:1089–97.

28. Barret B, Tardieu M, Rustin P, et al. Persistent mitochondrial dysfunction in HIV-1 exposed but uninfected infants: clinical screening in a large prospective cohort. AIDS 2003;17:1769–85.

29. Brenchley JM, Price DA, Douek DC. HIV disease: fallout from a mucosal catastrophe? Nature Immunol 2006;7:235–9.

30. Arthos J, Cicala C, Martinelli E, et al. HIV-1 envelope protein binds to and signals through integrin $\alpha 4 \beta 7$, the gut mucosal homing receptor for peripheral T cells. Nature Immunol 2008;9:301–9.

31. Carr A, Cooper DA. Adverse effects of antiretroviral therapy. Lancet 2000;356:1423–30.

32. Magnan A, Vervloet D. AIDS: a model for the sdudy of atopy? Rev Mal Respir 1995;12:177–83.

33. Davis CM, Shearer WT. Diagnosis and management of HIV drug hypersensitivity. J Allergy Clin Immunol 2008;121:826–32.

34. Phillips E, Mallal S. Drug hypersensitivity in HIV. Curr Opin Allergy Clin Immunol 2007;7:324–30.

35. Schroecksnadel K, Zangerle R, Bellmann-Weiler R, et al. Indoleamine-2,3-dioxygenase and other interferon-gamma-mediated pathways in patients with human immunodeficiency virus infection. Curr Drug Metab 2007;8:22–36.

36. Lagathu C, Eustace B, Prot M, et al. Some HIV antiretrovirals increase oxidative stress and alter chemokine, cytokine or adiponectin production in human adipocytes and macrophages. Antivir Ther 2007;12:489–500.

37. Clerici M, Fusi ML, Ruzzante S, et al. Type 1 and type 1 cytokines in HIV infection: a possible role in apoptosis and disease progression. Ann Med 1997;29:185–8.

38. Marone G, Florio G, Petraroli A, et al. Dysregulation of the IgE/FcεRI network in HIV-1 infection. J Allergy Clin Immunol 2001;107:22–30.

39. Zar HJ, Latief Z, Hughes J, et al. Serum immunoglobulin E levels in human immunodeficiency virus-infected children with pneumonia. Pediatr Allergy Immunol 2002;13:328–33.

40. Porter JP, Patel AA, Dewey CM, et al. Prevalence of sinonasal symptoms in patients with HIV infection. Am J Rhinol 1999;13:203–8.

41. Small CB, Kaufman A, Armenaka M, et al. Sinusitis and atopy in human immunodeficicnecy virus infection. J Infect Dis 1993;167:283–90.

42. Garcia-Rodriguez JF, Corominas M, Fernandez-Viladrich P, et al. Rhinosinusitis and atopy in patients infected with HIV. Laryngoscope 1999;109:939–44.

43. Poirier CD, Inhaber N, Lalonde RG, et al. Prevalence of bronchial hyperresponsiveness among HIV-infected men. Am J Respir Crit Care Med 2001;164:542–5.

44. Lin RY, Lazarus TS. Asthma and related atopic disorders in outpatients attending an urban HIV clinic. Ann Allergy Asthma Immunol 1995;74:510–5.

45. Foster SB, McIntosh K, Thompson B, et al. Increased incidence of asthma in HIV-infected children treated with highly active antiretroviral therapy in the National Institutes of Health Women and Infants Transmission Study. J Allergy Clin Immunol 2008;122:159–65.

46. CDC. Revised recommendations for HIV testing for adults, adolescents, and pregnant women in health-care settings. MMWR 2006;55:1–17.

47. Nesheim S, Palumbo P, Sullivan K, et al. Quantitative RNA testing for diagnosis of HIV-infected infants. J Acquir Immune Def Syndr 2003;32:192–5.

48. Dunn DT, Brandt CD, Kirvine A, et al. The sensitivity of HIV-1 DNA polymerase chain reaction in the neonatal period and the relative contributions of intrauterine and intrapartum transmission. AIDS 1995;9:F7–11.

49. Read JS. The Committee on Pediatric AIDS. Diagnosis of HIV-1 infection in children younger than 18 months in the United States. Pediatrics 2007;120:e1547–62.

50. CDC. Revised surveillance case definitions for HIV infection among adults, adolescents, and children aged < 18 months and for HIV infection and AIDS among children aged 18 months to < 13 years – United States, 2008. MMWR 2008;57:1–8.

51. Shearer WT, Pahwa S, Read JS, et al. CD4/CD8 T cell ratio predicts HIV infection in infants: the National Heart, Lung, and Blood Institute P2C2 Study. J Allergy Clin Immunol 2007;120:1449–56.

52. Shearer WT, Rosenblatt HM, Gelman RS, et al. Lymphocyte subsets in healthy children from birth through 18 years of age: the Pediatric AIDS Clinical Trials Group P1009 Study. J Allergy Clin Immunol 2003;112:973–80.

53. Shearer WT, Quinn TC, LaRussa P, et al. Viral load and disease progression in infants infected with human immunodeficiency virus type 1: Women and Infants Transmission Study Group. N Engl J Med 1997;336:1337.

54. Mellors JW, Kingsley LA, Rinaldo CR, et al. Quantitation of HIV-1 RNA in plasma predicts outcome after seroconversion. Ann Intern Med 1995;122:573–579.

55. HIV Paediatric Prognostic Markers Collaborative Study Group. Short-term risk of disease progression in HIV-1 infected children receiving no antiretroviral therapy or zidovudine monotherapy: a meta-analysis. Lancet 2003;362:1605–11.

56. Panel on Antiretroviral Guidelines for Adult and Adolescents. Guidelines for the use of antiretroviral agents in HIV-1-infected adults and adolescents. Department of Health and Human Services. November 3, 2008; pp 1–139. Available at http://www.aidsinfo.nih.gov/Content-Files/AdultandAdolescentGL.pdf. Accessed 27 Mar 2009.

57. Working Group on Antiretroviral Therapy and Medical Management of HIV-Infected Children. Guidelines for the use of antiretroviral agents in pediatric HIV infection. February 23, 2009; pp1–139. Available at http://aidsinfo.nih.gov/ContentFiles/PediatricGuidelines.pdf. Accessed 27 Mar 2009.

58. Polis MA, Sidorov IA, Yoder C, et al. Correlation between reduction in plasma HIV-1 RNA concentration 1 week after start of antiretroviral treatment and long-term efficacy. Lancet 2001;358:1760–1765.

59. Adult Prevention and Treatment of Opportunistic Infections Guidelines Working Group. Guidelines for prevention and treatment of opportunistic infections in HIV-infected adults and adolescents. MMWR 2009;58:1–198. Available at: http://www.cdc.gov/mmwr/preview/mmwrhtml/rr58e324a1.htm. Accessed 8 Apr 2009.

60. Working Group on Guidelines for the Prevention and Treatment of Opportunistic Infections among HIV-Exposed and HIV-Infected Children. Guidelines for prevention and treatment of opportunistic infections in HIV-exposed and HIV-infected Children (Draft). June 20, 2008; pp 1–250. Available at: http://aidsinfo.nih.gov/contentfiles/Pediatric_OI.pdf. Accessed 8 Apr 2009.

11

Complement Deficiencies

Jerry A. Winkelstein • Kathleen E. Sullivan

The complement system was first identified at the end of the 19th century as a serum activity that 'complemented' the action of antibody in the lysis of Gram-negative bacteria. During the next 100 years there was a growing appreciation that complement not only played an important role in host defense against infection but also was important in the generation of inflammation, the clearance of immune complexes and apoptotic cells, and the production of a normal humoral immune response.[1]

Deficiencies of the complement system may be genetically determined, secondary to other conditions, or the result of immaturity. In this chapter, we review deficiencies of the complement system in humans with an emphasis on pathophysiology and clinical presentation.

Pathophysiology and Clinical Expression

Patients with deficiencies of the complement system may have a variety of clinical presentations, including an increased susceptibility to infection, systemic autoimmune disorders, hemolytic uremic syndrome, and angioedema.

Pathophysiologic Basis for an Increased Susceptibility to Infection

An increased susceptibility to infection is a prominent clinical expression of most of the complement deficiency diseases.

The activation of the complement system by microorganisms results in the generation of cleavage products and macromolecular complexes that possess opsonic activity (C3b), anaphylatoxic activity (C4a, C3a, and C5a), chemotactic activity (C5a), or bactericidal/bacteriolytic activity (C5b, C6, C7, C8, and C9) (Table 11-1). All play a role in the host's defense against infection.[1,2] Experiments in complement-deficient experimental animals, whether naturally occurring or genetic 'knockouts,' have shown that the complement system plays an important role in the host's defense against a wide variety of bacteria, viruses, and fungi. Its protective effects are critical in the generation of the initial inflammatory response to infection, prevention of spread of the infection from the initial site of infection to other areas of the body, and clearance of the microorganism from the bloodstream. Furthermore, it appears to play its most important role in the early stages of infection, and the generation of opsonic activity is among its most critical functions. The opsonic function of C3b deposition on a pathogen renders the pathogen more easily phagocytosed.

The nature of the infections in complement-deficient individuals generally reflects the specific roles of the deficient component in host defense. For example, C3 is responsible for generating complement-mediated opsonic activity. Thus patients with C3 deficiency are unduly susceptible to infection from encapsulated bacteria (e.g. *Streptococcus pneumoniae, Haemophilus influenzae,* and *Streptococcus pyogenes*),[3-5] organisms for which opsonization is a critical host defense mechanism. In contrast, patients with deficiencies of C5, C6, C7, C8, or C9 possess C3 and are not susceptible to these bacteria.[3,4] They are, however, unduly susceptible to neisserial infections because the generation of bactericidal activity, mediated by C5b through C9, is critical to defense against this genus. Interestingly, although a number of Gram-negative bacteria are susceptible to the bactericidal activity of complement, the susceptibility of patients with deficiencies of C5 through C9 appears to be limited to *Neisseria* spp.[3,4] The infections seen in complement-deficient individuals can be localized (e.g. pneumonia or sinusitis), although systemic infections (e.g. bacteremia/sepsis, meningitis, or osteomyelitis) are common and often are recurrent.[3,4]

A number of studies have examined the prevalence of complement deficiencies among patients with characteristic infections. Although complement-deficient patients do not appear to be sufficiently common among patients with *single* episodes of pneumococcal, streptococcal, or *H. influenzae* sepsis and/or meningitis to justify routine screening of patients with these infections, complement deficiencies are sufficiently common among patients with systemic neisserial infections to make routine screening worthwhile.[6-8] For example, estimates of the prevalence of complement deficiencies among patients with a single episode of meningococcal sepsis have varied from 5% to 15%; the difference probably relates to differences in the populations being studied. Not unexpectedly, the prevalence is as high as 40% if the patient has had recurrent meningococcal sepsis, has an infection with an uncommon serotype, or has a positive family history of meningococcal systemic infections.[9-11]

Pathophysiologic Basis for Systemic Autoimmune Disorders

Systemic lupus erythematosus (SLE) is common in patients with deficiencies of certain specific components, namely C1, C4, C2, and C3.

A variety of pathophysiologic mechanisms exist by which complement deficiencies can lead to the development of systemic auotimmune disorders. The two most attractive relate to the role

©2010 Elsevier Ltd, Inc, BV

DOI: 10.1016/B978-1-4377-0271-2.00011-0

Table 11-1 Functions of Complement Components

Components	Functions
C4a, C2a, C3a	Anaphylatoxins, histamine release
C3b	Opsonin, costimulation of B cells
C5a	Chemotaxis
C5, C6, C7, C8, C9	Membrane attack complex, lysis

Table 11-2 Clinical Characteristics of Inherited Complement Deficiency Diseases

Component	Inheritance	Major Clinical Expression
Classical Pathway		
C1q, C1r, C1s, C4, C2	Autosomal recessive	SLE and bacterial infections with encapsulated organisms
C3	Autosomal recessive	Glomerulonephritis, severe bacterial infections
Terminal Components		
C5, C6, C7, C8, C9	Autosomal recessive	Neisseria
Regulatory Proteins		
C1 inhibitor	Autosomal dominant	Angioedema
Factor H	Variable	Infections and HUS
Factor I	Variable	Infections and HUS
MCP	Variable	Atypical HUS
Properdin	X-linked recessive	Neisseria
Factor D	Autosomal recessive	Neisseria

of the complement system in the processing and clearance of immune complexes and the processing and clearance of apoptotic cells.

The complement system participates significantly in the processing and clearance of immune complexes via a variety of mechanisms. First, immune complexes carrying C3b can be ingested by phagocytic cells. Second, the activation of C3 by immune complexes maintains them as soluble complexes.[12] Thirdly, humans possess receptors (CR1) for cleavage products of C3 on their erythrocytes, and circulating immune complexes containing C3b can reversibly bind to those receptors. As erythrocytes carrying immune complexes pass through the liver, the immune complexes are picked off the surface by Kupffer cells, ingested, and processed, thus effectively removing them from the circulation and preventing their deposition in other organs such as the kidney.[13]

The most important mechanism driving the susceptibility to systemic autoimmune disorders is the failure to clear apoptotic cells. The early components of the classical pathway, especially C1q, participate in the clearance of apoptotic cells.[14,15] As cells undergo apoptosis, intracellular constituents are reorganized and appear on the surface of the cell in blebs. Autoantigens targeted in patients with SLE, such as Sjögren's syndrome antigen A (SSA) and/or Sjögren's syndrome antigen B (SSB), are often found on the surface in these blebs, rendering a normally 'invisible' antigen 'visible.' Thus patients deficient in these components may develop SLE because they lack an important mechanism of clearance of apoptotic cells. Possibly contributing to the development of autoantibodies directed to nuclear antigens is the potential role of complement mediating B cell tolerance in the bone marrow.[16]

There are some clinical and laboratory features that are characteristic of the rheumatic diseases seen in complement-deficient individuals. For example, the SLE seen in C2-deficient patients is frequently associated with photosensitive dermatitis. It is not uncommon for C2-deficient patients to have low (or absent) titers of antibodies to antinuclear antibody (ANA) or dsDNA, whereas the prevalence of anti-Ro antibodies in C2-deficient patients with lupus is much greater than in non-C2-deficient patients with lupus.[17,18] Patients deficient in C1 or C4 usually have an early onset of clinical symptoms with prominent cutaneous manifestations.[19,20] SLE in C1 or C4 deficient individuals can be severe.

Hemolytic Uremic Syndrome (HUS)

Factor H deficiency has been found to be the underlying basis for 15–30% of patients with atypical HUS.[21] The term atypical HUS refers to the fact that there is no antecedent diarrheal illness, which is seen in most sporadic forms of HUS. The basis for the HUS in factor H deficiency is thought to be due to an inability to protect fenestrated endothelium in the glomerulus from complement-mediated damage.[22] Microtrauma arises frequently due

to the high oncotic pressure and the damaged basement membrane is able to support complement activation if not protected by factor H. Interestingly, recurrent atypical HUS has been seen in patients with antibodies to factor H, suggesting an acquired form as well. Also supporting a role for factor H in the protection of basement membranes, is the finding of a common polymorphism associated with macular degeneration.[23] The central region of the retina is gradually destroyed by a process that leaves a deposit of protein, termed drusen. These deposits contain complement components. It has been hypothesized that the abnormal factor H provides less protection to the choroidal vessels, allowing smoldering complement activation and gradual damage to the endothelium.

Inherited Complement Deficiencies

Genetically determined deficiencies have been identified for most of the individual components of complement. Most are inherited as autosomal recessive traits, although one is inherited as an X-linked recessive trait (properdin deficiency), one is inherited as an autosomal dominant trait (C1 esterase deficiency), and the defects associated with HUS have variable patterns of inheritance (Table 11-2). Except where noted, the mutations are diverse and can lead to either absent protein or dysfunctional protein.

C1q Deficiency

Molecular Biology and Pathophysiology

C1q is one of the three subcomponents of C1; the other two are C1r and C1s. C1q is composed of six identical subunits, each of which is composed of three different polypeptide chains, C1qA, C1qB, and C1qC, encoded by genes on the long arm of chromosome 1.[24] IgG or IgM, after engaging antigen and forming an immune complex, binds C1q, which then activates C1r, in turn activating C1s. Activated C1s then cleaves both C4 and C2, creating the bimolecular enzyme C4b, 2a, which activates C3 and ultimately the terminal components (C5 through C9) via the

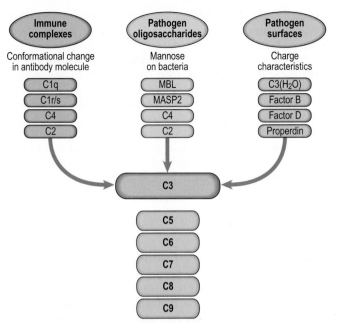

Figure 11-1 The complement cascade. The classical pathway is activated primarily by antibody while the MBL and alternative pathways are activated directly by pathogens. In each case, the activation arm leads to cleavage of C3.

classical pathway (Figure 11-1). Thus, C1q plays a critical role in activation of the classical pathway and the generation of the biologic activities of C3 and C5 through C9. In addition, recent studies have shown that C1q recognizes apoptotic cells and targets them for clearance.[14,15]

C1q-deficient individuals have markedly reduced serum total hemolytic activity and C1 functional activity. In most affected individuals, C1q protein level is also markedly reduced, but in some patients a dysfunctional immunoreactive protein is produced.[21] The disease is especially prominent in Turkey and is usually the result of a C-to-T transition in exon 2 of C1qA.[25,26]

Clinical Expression

The most prominent clinical manifestation of C1q deficiency is SLE. Although SLE is also a prominent clinical feature of patients with deficiencies of other components of the classical pathway (e.g. C1r, C1s, C4, and C2) and C3, C1q-deficient patients carry the highest risk (>90% prevalence).[3,4,27] C1q deficient patients have impaired clearance of the immune complexes and apoptotic cells. There are some differences between the SLE seen in C1q-deficient patients and that seen in complement-sufficient individuals. For example, the age of onset of the SLE tends to be earlier, usually prepubertal, and the disease tends to be more severe. In addition, although antinuclear antibodies may be present, they tend to be of low titer, and anti-double-stranded (ds) DNA antibodies are usually negative.

C1q-deficient individuals also have an increased susceptibility to encapsulated bacteria, reflecting their inability to activate the classical pathway and efficiently generate opsonically active C3b. In fact, nearly one third of C1q-deficient patients have significant bacterial infections and 10% have died of infections.[3,4,27]

C1r/C1s Deficiency

Molecular Biology and Pathophysiology

The C1 complex is composed of six C1q subunits and two subunits each of C1r and C1s. The genes for C1r and C1s are closely linked on chromosome 12 and encode highly homologous serine proteases. C1q, after it binds to an immune complex, activates C1r, which in turn activates C1s. It is C1s that cleaves C4 and C2, resulting in the assembly of the C3 cleaving enzyme C4b, 2a.

Patients with C1r deficiency have markedly reduced levels of total hemolytic complement activity and C1 functional activity. Typically, C1r levels are reduced to less than 1% of normal values, and C1s levels are between 20% and 50% of normal values.[27] Interestingly, a few patients have been described with C1s deficiency in whom C1s levels are markedly reduced. The observation that deficiency of one component leads to reduced levels of the other suggests that neither is stable in the absence of the other.

Clinical Expression

The most common clinical expression of C1r/s deficiency has been SLE.[3,4,27] Some patients have also presented with glomerulonephritis or bacterial infections.

C4 Deficiency

Molecular Biology and Pathophysiology

The fourth component of complement (C4) is encoded by two closely linked genes (C4A and C4B) located within the major histocompatibility complex (MHC) on chromosome 6. Although the protein products of the two loci share most of their structure and function, there are four amino acid differences between them that account for differences in their electrophoretic mobility, minor antigenic determinants, functional activity, and molecular weight of the alpha chain. The larger cleavage product of C4, C4b, forms part of the bimolecular enzyme C4b, 2a, which is responsible for activation of C3 and C5 through C9 via the classical pathway. It therefore plays an important role in the generation of the biologic activities of C3 and C5 through C9.

Because C4 is encoded by two distinct genes, patients with complete C4 deficiency are homozygous deficient at both loci (C4A*Q0, C4B*Q0/C4A*Q0, C4B*Q0).[19,28] In contrast to the rarity of patients with complete C4 deficiency, individuals who are heterozygous for either C4A or C4B deficiency are relatively common.[19,28] Approximately 13% to 14% of the population is heterozygous for C4A deficiency and 15% to 16% is heterozygous for C4B deficiency, with the corresponding frequencies for homozygous-deficient individuals being 1% and 3%. Individuals who have complete C4 deficiency (i.e. are homozygous deficient for both C4A and C4B) have little, if any, total hemolytic activity in their sera and markedly reduced levels of C4 protein and functional activity. As a result of the absence of C4, these individuals have a markedly decreased ability to generate serum opsonic, chemotactic, and bactericidal activities via activation of the classical pathway.[29,30]

C4A deficiency is often the result of a large gene deletion.[31] In addition, a 2-base pair (bp) insertion in exon 29 is relatively common.[32] Some instances of C4B deficiency are the result of gene deletions.[31] Finally, gene conversions can cause either C4A or C4B deficiency.[33]

Clinical Expression

Patients with complete C4 deficiency may present with SLE and/or an increased susceptibility to infection.[3,4,19] The onset of SLE is usually early in life and is characterized by prominent cutaneous features such as photosensitive skin rash, vasculitic skin ulcers, and Raynaud's phenomenon. As with other deficiencies of early components of the classical pathway, anti-DNA titers may be absent. Patients with complete C4 deficiency also have an increased susceptibility to bacterial infections; most deaths in C4-deficient patients are the result of infection.

In contrast to the rarity of complete C4 deficiency, individuals who are homozygous deficient at one but not the other locus (*C4A* or *C4B*) are relatively common in the general population.[19,28] Individuals who are homozygous deficient for C4A lack the isotype that is most efficient in interacting with proteins. The prevalence of homozygous C4A deficiency in patients with SLE is markedly elevated, approaching 10% to 15%, a frequency at least 10 times that in the population at large.[34-36] Interestingly, patients with SLE who have C4A deficiency have some clinical and laboratory features that are different from those of complement-sufficient patients with SLE. They have less neurologic and renal disease but more photosensitivity than other patients with SLE, and they have a lower prevalence of anticardiolipin, anti-Ro, anti-dsDNA, and anti-Sm antibodies.[37,38]

In contrast to individuals with homozygous C4A deficiency, homozygous C4B-deficient individuals lack the C4 isotype that interacts most efficiently with polysaccharides. There is an increased prevalence of homozygous C4B deficiency in children with bacteremia and/or bacterial meningitis.[39,40]

C2 Deficiency

Molecular Biology and Pathophysiology

The second component of complement (C2) is encoded by a gene within the MHC on chromosome 6.[1] Like C4, C2 is cleaved by C1s into two fragments, the larger of which (C2a) forms part of the C3-cleaving enzyme of the classical pathway, C4b, 2a. Thus C2, like C4, plays a critical role in generating the biologic activities of C3 and the terminal components, C5 through C9.

C2-deficient patients usually have absent total hemolytic activity and less than 1% of the normal levels of C2 protein and function.[41] Those complement-mediated serum activities that can be mediated via activation of the alternative pathway, such as serum opsonic, chemotactic, and bactericidal activities, are usually present but not generated as quickly or to the same degree as those in individuals who possess C2 and have an intact classical pathway.[42-44]

The majority of C2-deficient individuals (> 95%) have the same molecular genetic defect, a 28-bp deletion at the 3′ end of exon 6, which causes premature termination of transcription.[45,46] The deletion is associated with a conserved MHC haplotype consisting of *HLA-B18, C2*Q0, Bf*S, C4A*4, C4B*2,* and *Dr*2.*[45-47] C2 deficiency is the most common of the genetically determined complete complement deficiencies in Caucasians and the gene frequency of this deletion is between 0.05 and 0.007 in individuals of European descent, which translates into a prevalence of homozygotes of approximately 1:10 000.[47,48]

Clinical Expression

Genetically determined C2 deficiency occurs in 1 in 10 000 individuals, making it one of the most common inherited complement deficiencies.[41,48] Its clinical manifestations vary and include autoimmune disorders and an increased susceptibility to infection.[3,4,41] In addition, there are some C2-deficient individuals who are asymptomatic.

The most common clinical manifestation of C2 deficiency is lupus, most commonly either SLE or discoid lupus.[3,4,41] Patients with C2 deficiency manifest many of the typical clinical features of lupus, although photosensitive cutaneous lesions are more

common.[49,50] They also have a lower prevalence of anti-DNA antibodies than other patients with SLE, but the prevalence of anti-Ro and -La antibodies is higher.[17,18] Other autoimmune diseases have been described in C2 deficiency and have included glomerulonephritis, inflammatory bowel disease, dermatomyositis, anaphylactoid purpura, and vasculitis.

An increased susceptibility to infection is also a prominent clinical presentation of C2 deficiency.[6,7,41] The infections are usually caused by encapsulated pyogenic organisms such as *Pneumococcus, Streptococcus,* and *H. influenzae* and are bloodborne, such as in sepsis, meningitis, arthritis, and/or osteomyelitis.[3,4,51] Infection is the leading cause of death.[49,50]

C3 Deficiency

Molecular Biology and Pathophysiology

The third component of complement (C3) is encoded by a gene located on chromosome 19. Like most complement components, the majority of serum C3 is derived from hepatic synthesis, although synthesis by monocytes, fibroblasts, endothelial cells, and epithelial cells may contribute to local tissue content of C3.[52] Whether activated by the classical or alternative pathways, C3 is cleaved into two fragments of unequal sizes. The smaller, C3a, is an anaphylatoxin, whereas the larger, C3b, is an opsonin and also forms part of the classical and alternative pathway enzymes that activates C5 and the other terminal components. Thus C3 is not only critical in generating C3-mediated serum opsonizing and anaphylatoxic activities but also in generating the chemotactic and bactericidal activities of C5 through C9.

Patients with C3 deficiency usually have less than 1% of the normal level of C3 in their sera. Similarly, serum opsonic, chemotactic, and bactericidal activities are also markedly reduced.[3]

The mutations responsible for C3 deficiency in humans have been diverse.[53-55] However, there is a relatively common 800-bp deletion found among Afrikaans-speaking South Africans (gene frequency of 0.0057).[53,54]

Clinical Expression

An increased susceptibility to infection is the most prominent clinical expression of C3 deficiency.[3-5] Patients tend to present with infections in very early childhood, and recurrent infections are typical. Although the most common infections are bloodborne infections caused by pyogenic bacteria such as *Pneumococcus, H. influenzae,* and *Meningococcus,* localized infections such as pneumonia and sinusitis have also been reported.

Autoimmune diseases are also relatively common in patients with C3 deficiency.[3-5] Some patients have presented with a syndrome characterized by arthralgias and vasculitic skin rashes (similar to serum sickness), whereas others have developed a clinical picture consistent with glomerulonephritis or SLE. As with patients with deficiencies of other components of complement, they may not have the typical serologic findings of lupus.

Membranoproliferative glomerulonephritis is the most common autoimmune disease in patients with C3 deficiency.[3-5] The lesions are characterized by mesangial cell proliferation, an increase in the mesangial matrix, and electrondense deposits in both the mesangium and subendothelium of the capillary loops. Immunofluorescent studies have revealed the presence of immunoglobulins in the kidney, and circulating immune complexes may be present in the serum, suggesting that membranoproliferative glomerulonephritis in these patients is the result of immune complex deposition.

C5 Deficiency

Molecular Biology and Pathophysiology

The gene encoding the fifth component of complement (C5) is on the short arm of chromosome 9. When C5 is activated, it is cleaved into two fragments of unequal size. The smaller fragment, C5a, is a potent chemotactic fragment, and the larger, C5b, initiates assembly of the membrane attack complex, C5b through C9, and is responsible for bactericidal activity (Figure 11-1).

Affected individuals have markedly reduced levels of serum total hemolytic activity and C5. As expected, their sera are also unable to generate chemotactic or bactericidal activity.

Clinical Expression

The most common clinical expression of C5 deficiency is an increased susceptibility to systemic neisserial infections.[3,4]

C6 Deficiency

Molecular Biology and Pathophysiology

The genes for C6 and C7 are located near each other on the long arm of chromosome 5. C6 participates in the formation of the membrane attack complex and therefore plays a critical role in the generation of bactericidal activity.

The usual form of C6 deficiency is characterized by absent total serum hemolytic activity and very low levels (<1%) of serum C6. Another form of C6 deficiency, subtotal C6 deficiency (C6SD), is characterized by 1% to 2% of the normal levels of C6 and levels of total hemolytic activity that are reduced but present.[56]

The most common mutation causing C6 deficiency is a single base-pair deletion at position 879.[59,60] Interestingly, the mutations among African Americans are different from those in the African population.[57,58] C6SD is the result of a loss of the splice donor site of intron 15 and results in a truncated C6 that can support some lytic activity.[56,59]

Clinical Expression

C6 deficiency is one of the most common complement deficiencies.[3,4] Among African Americans in the USA, it is reported to be as common as 1:1600 individuals (0.062%).[58] It is thought to be uncommon among individuals of European descent. Like other terminal components, C6 deficiency is associated with systemic neisserial infections.[3,4]

C7 Deficiency

Molecular Biology and Pathophysiology

The genes for C6, C7, and C9, all members of the membrane attack complex, are clustered on the short arm of chromosome 5. C7 participates in the formation of the membrane attack complex and therefore is critical to the generation of serum bactericidal activity.

Patients who are deficient in C7 have markedly reduced serum total hemolytic activity and C7 levels. As expected, their serum bactericidal activity is similarly reduced.[60]

Clinical Expression

Like other patients with deficiencies of the terminal components (C5, C6, C7, C8, and C9), the most prominent clinical manifesta-tion of C7 deficiency is an increased susceptibility to systemic neisserial infections.[3,4] A few patients have presented with SLE, rheumatoid arthritis, pyoderma gangrenosum, and scleroderma, but it is unclear whether these are pathophysiologically related to the C7 deficiency.

C8 Deficiency

Molecular Biology and Pathophysiology

Native C8 comprises three different polypeptide chains (α, β, and γ), which are encoded by separate genes (C8A, C8B, and C8G). The genes C8A and C8B map to the short arm of chromosome 1, and the gene C8G maps to the long arm of chromosome 9. The alpha and gamma chains are covalently linked to form one chain (C8 α–γ), which is joined to the C8 β chain by noncovalent bonds. C8 is an integral part of the pore-forming membrane attack complex C5b-9 and, as such, plays a critical role in the generation of complement-mediated bactericidal activity.

There are several forms of C8 deficiency, and each is inherited as an autosomal recessive trait. In one form, patients lack the C8 β subunit, whereas in the other form the α–γ subunit is deficient.[61,62] In either form, total hemolytic activity is absent from the serum, as is functional C8 activity. However, some C8 antigen can usually be detected in C8 β deficiency because patients possess the C8 α–γ subunit. In contrast, patients with C8 α–γ deficiency usually have undetectable C8 antigen with standard immunochemical techniques. As expected, patients with either form of the deficiency have a marked reduction in serum bactericidal activity.

C8β is more common among individuals of European descent and C8 α–γ deficiency is more common among individuals of African descent. Approximately 86% of C8 β-null alleles are the result of C-to-T transition in exon 9, which results in the generation of a premature stop codon.[62–65] Only a limited number of patients with C8 α–γ deficiency have been examined, and in most instances an intronic mutation alters the splicing of exons 6 and 7 of the C8A chain and creates an insertion that generates a premature stop codon.[66]

Clinical Expression

Like deficiencies of other components of the membrane attack complex, systemic neisserial infections have been the predominant clinical presentation of C8 deficiency.[3,4]

C9 Deficiency

Molecular Biology and Pathophysiology

The gene for C9 is located on the short arm of chromosome 5, approximately 2.5 Mb from the genes for C6 and C7. The protein product has sequence homology to other members of the membrane attack complex.

Affected individuals have markedly reduced levels of both C9 antigen and functional activity. However, the hemolysis of antibody-sensitized erythrocytes can occur with the insertion of a membrane attack complex lacking C9 (i.e. C5b-8) and thus is not strictly dependent on C9. Therefore, patients with C9 deficiency have some total hemolytic activity, although it is reduced to between one third and one half of the lower limit of normal.[67–71] Similarly, their sera possess some bactericidal activity, although the rate of killing is significantly reduced.

Clinical Expression

Genetically determined C9 deficiency is uncommon among Caucasians but is relatively common among individuals of Japanese descent. A nonsense mutation in exon 4 has a gene frequency of 1 : 1000.[67,72] As with patients with deficiencies of the other components of the membrane attack complex, individuals with C9 deficiency have an increased susceptibility to systemic neisserial infections.[3,4,71]

Mannan Binding Lectin (MBL) Deficiency

Molecular Biology and Pathophysiology

MBL deficiency was initially identified in a cohort of hospitalized patients with infectious diseases. It is now known that MBL deficiency is quite common with 2–7% of people having MBL deficiency.[73] There are structural polymorphisms that destabilize the higher order complexes and several promoter mutations which compromise production.[74] The mutations/polymorphisms exist in haplotypes of varying severity.

Clinical Expression

MBL deficiency has, at most, a modest effect in isolation on infection susceptibility. In combination with other risk factors, it may contribute more substantially to infection risk. Similarly, it represents a modest risk factor or disease modifier in autoimmune diseases such as SLE or rheumatoid arthritis.[75,76]

Mannan Binding Lectin Associated Serine Protease 2 (MASP2) Deficiency

Mutations and polymorphisms in MASP2 are exceedingly common and have variable effects on function.[77] MASP2 cleaves C4 and C2 to form the same C3 convertase as the classical pathway. MASP 2 deficiency is typically associated with infection and autoimmune disease and studies suggest it is similar in effect to MBL deficiency.

C1 Esterase Inhibitor Deficiency

Molecular Biology and Pathophysiology

C1 esterase inhibitor (C1-INH) is encoded by a gene on the long arm of chromosome 11. C1-INH binds covalently to C1r and C1s, leading to dissociation of the C1 macromolecular complex and inhibition of the enzymatic actions of C1r and C1s.

Genetically determined C1 esterase inhibitor deficiency is inherited as an autosomal dominant trait. In the most common form (type I), accounting for approximately 85% of the patients, the sera of affected individuals are deficient in both C1-INH protein (5% to 30% of normal) and C1-INH function.[78-80] In the other less common form (type II), a dysfunctional protein is present in normal or elevated concentrations, but the functional activity of C1-INH is markedly reduced. The dysfunctional C1-INH molecules from different families differ not only from normal C1-INH but from each other with respect to their electrophoretic mobility, ability to bind C1s, and ability to inhibit both synthetic and natural substrates. In patients with type I C1-INH deficiency, the diagnosis can be established easily by demonstrating a decrease in serum C1-INH protein when assessed by immunochemical techniques.[81] However, in patients with type II C1-INH deficiency, the diagnosis must rest on demonstrating a

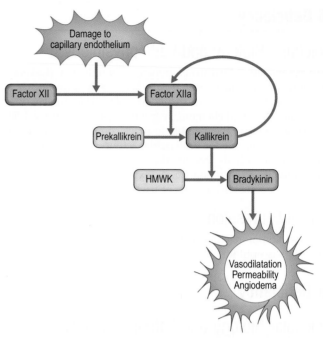

Figure 11-2 The role of C1 inhibitor in angioedema. The edema in C1 inhibitor deficiency is due primarily to activation of bradykinin. Factor XII (Hageman factor) is activated by exposure to damaged capillary vessels. Kallikrein performs two roles, it acts to cleave bradykinin from high molecular weight kininogen (HMWK), and it acts to enhance factor XIIa activation.

decrease in C1-INH functional activity. In either case, C4 levels are usually reduced below the lower limit of normal, both during and between attacks, because of the uncontrolled cleavage by C1s.[81,82]

The pathophysiologic mechanisms by which reduced C1-INH activity leads to the angioedema characteristic of the disorder are still incompletely understood. In addition to its role in inhibiting C1, C1-INH is the major inhibitor of kallikrein, and therefore diminished levels of C1-INH lead to unregulated activation of the classical pathway and kallikrein after exposure to a mild trigger (Figure 11-2).[83-85] Bradykinin and C2a appear to be the primary mediators of the angioedema.[86]

Clinical Expression

C1-INH deficiency is responsible for the clinical disorder of hereditary angioedema (HAE). The clinical symptoms of HAE are the result of submucosal or subcutaneous noninflammatory edema.[87] The three most prominent areas of involvement are the skin, upper respiratory tract, and gastrointestinal tract.[78]

Attacks involving the subcutaneous tissue may involve an extremity, the face, or genitalia. In some instances, there may be changes just preceding the edema such as subtle mottling, a transient serpiginous erythema, or frank erythema marginatum. The edema usually expands outward from a single site and may vary in size from a few centimeters to the involvement of a whole extremity. The lesions are characteristically nonpruritic. However, early in the development of the lesion, there may be a feeling of tightness in the skin because of the accumulation of subcutaneous fluid. Attacks usually progress for 1 to 2 days and resolve over an additional 2 to 3 days.

Attacks involving the upper respiratory tract represent a significant cause of morbidity, and occasionally death, in patients with HAE. In one series published in 1976, pharyngeal edema had occurred at least once in nearly two thirds of the patients.[80] The patient may initially experience a 'tightness' in the throat; swelling of the tongue, buccal mucosa, and oropharynx follows. In some instances, laryngeal edema, accompanied by hoarseness and stridor, occurs and progresses to respiratory obstruction; this is a life-threatening emergency. In fact, in that same series, tracheotomies had been performed in 1 of every 6 patients with HAE.[80]

Symptoms in the gastrointestinal tract are related to edema of the bowel wall and may include anorexia, dull aching of the abdomen, vomiting, and, in some cases, crampy abdominal pain. Abdominal symptoms are often prominent in childhood and can occur in the absence of concurrent cutaneous or pharyngeal involvement. In some instances, abdominal symptoms may be the only sypmtoms the patient has ever had, leading to difficulty in diagnosis.

Although the onset of symptoms occurs in more than half of the patients before adolescence,[80,88] in some patients their first symptoms do not occur until they are well into adult life. In just over half of the patients, no specific event can be clearly identified as initiating attacks, although anxiety or stress are frequently cited. Dental extractions and tonsillectomy can initiate edema of the upper airway, and cutaneous edema may follow trauma to an extremity. Some patients report attacks after the use of tight-fitting clothing or shoes, whereas others have related cold exposure to the onset of symptoms.

A potential source of diagnostic confusion is the association of HAE with SLE, presumably because the secondary reduction of C4 predisposes to SLE. These patients can be quite difficult to diagnose and manage.

Factor H Deficiency

Molecular Biology and Pathophysiology

The basis for the HUS in factor H deficiency is thought to be due to an inability to protect fenestrated endothelium in the glomerulus from complement-mediated damage.[22] Microtrauma arises frequently due to the high oncotic pressure and the basement membrane is able to support complement activation if not protected. Interestingly, recurrent atypical HUS has been seen in patients with antibodies to factor H suggesting an acquired form as well. This form may be slightly more amenable to therapy.

Neisserial infections are also seen in patients with factor H deficiency and the mutations in patients with HUS and neisserial infections are distinct. The infections arise due to unregulated consumption of C3.[9,23,89-91]

Clinical Expression

Factor H deficiency is responsible for 15–30% of patients with atypical HUS.[21] Both autosomal recessive and heterozygous mutations have been seen. The age of onset is quite young in most cases and the disease is recurrent.[92] Death is not uncommon although therapy with fresh frozen plasma (FFP) may be of benefit. Normal complement (C3, AH50 and factor H) levels are sometimes seen and the only way in which this disorder can be confidently identified is with direct mutation analysis.

A common tyrosine-histidine polymorphism of factor H was identified as a significant risk factor for macular degeneration in a genome-wide linkage study.[23,93] It is believed that dysfunctional factor H allows complement activation and gradual damage to the endothelium.

Factor I Deficiency

Molecular Biology and Pathophysiology

The gene for factor I is located on the long arm of chromosome 4. Factor I is a serine protease that cleaves C3b to produce iC3b, an inactive cleavage product that cannot function in the C3-cleaving enzyme of the alternative pathway.

Patients with factor I deficiency have uncontrolled activation of C3 via the alternative pathway.[94,95] There is normally a continuous low-grade generation of the alternative pathway C3-cleaving enzyme, C3b, Bb, which is inhibited by factor I. In the absence of factor I, there is no control imposed on the formation and expression of the alternative pathway C3-cleaving enzyme, and as a result, there is the continued activation and cleavage and activation of C3.[95] Patients with factor I deficiency therefore have a secondary consumption of C3 with markedly reduced levels C3 in their sera and a corresponding decrease in serum opsonic, bactericidal, and chemotactic activity.[94,95] The patients with atypical HUS have heterozygous mutations, in general, and the mutations do not localize to specific protein domain.

Clinical Expression

The most common clinical expression of factor I deficiency has been an increased susceptibility to infection.[3,4,96] Like patients with C3 deficiency, factor I deficient patients have infections caused by encapsulated pyogenic bacteria, such as *Streptococcus*, *Pneumococcus*, *Meningococcus*, and *H. influenzae*, organisms for which C3 is an important opsonic ligand. Also, like patients with C3 deficiency, some patients have had elevated levels of circulating immune complexes. In fact, there has been one report of a transient illness resembling serum sickness characterized by fever, rash, arthralgia, hematuria, and proteinuria.[97,98]

A second presentation is atypical HUS. Factor I deficiency is responsible for 5–10% of patients with atypical HUS.[21] These patients have a phenotype indistinguishable from that of patients with factor H deficiency.

Membrane Cofactor Protein (CD46) Deficiency

Deficiencies of membrane cofactor protein (MCP) are associated with atypical HUS although the presentation is usually later and milder than patients with factor H or factor I deficiencies.[92,99-101] MCP mutations account for approximately 10% of all atypical HUS. MCP is expressed on renal tissues and therefore renal transplantation can be successful. Traditional complement analyses are normal although the mechanism of disease is thought to be the same as for factor H and factor I deficiencies.

Properdin Deficiency

Molecular Biology and Pathophysiology

Properdin is the only gene of the complement system that is encoded on the X chromosome. Properdin stabilizes the alternative pathway C3 and C5 convertases by extending the half-lives of the C3 and C5 converting enzymes.

Properdin deficiency is inherited as an X-linked recessive trait. Protein may be absent or reduced in the serum depending on the specific mutation. Patients with properdin deficiency have absent function of the alternative pathway. Similarly, serum bactericidal activity for some strains of meningococci is reduced in properdin-deficient serum.

Clinical Expression

Approximately 50% of the patients described with properdin deficiency have had systemic meningococcal disease.[3,4,102] Isolated cases of SLE and discoid lupus are also seen in properdin-deficient patients.

Factor D Deficiency

Neisserial infections are seen in factor D deficiency.[3,4,103] Systemic streptococcal infections have also been seen. Other complement levels are typically normal in factor D deficiency, however, there is almost no ability to activate the alternative pathway.

Management of Genetically Determined Complement Deficiencies

Prevention of Infectious Diseases

Two strategies have been attempted to reduce susceptibility to infections and/or modify the clinical course of the infections in patients with genetically determined deficiencies of complement.

One strategy is to immunize these patients against common bacterial pathogens such as *Pneumococcus, H. influenzae,* and *Meningococcus.* Unfortunately, because the complement system participates in the generation of a normal immune response,[104,105] complement-deficient patients may not respond as well as complement-sufficient hosts.[106] Another limitation to the use of immunization in complement-deficient patients is that the vaccines may not include all of the serotypes to which complement-deficient patients are susceptible. For example, the conjugated pneumococcal conjugate vaccine is limited to seven serotypes, and the meningococcal vaccine contains only serotypes A, C, Y, and W-135. Although there are limitations, data support the use of repeated meningococcal vaccination to mitigate the risk of infection for patients with terminal complement component deficiencies.[107] It seems reasonable to consider repeated vaccination for *Pneumococcus* or *Haemophilus influenzae* for patients with defects in early complement components.

A second strategy in the prevention of infection is the use of prophylactic antibiotics. Because patients with complement deficiencies have a high risk of recurrent episodes of blood-borne infections and because immunizations may not afford them complete protection, some patients have been placed on antibiotic prophylaxis. Any recommendation for antibiotic prophylaxis must be viewed in the context of the emergence of antibiotic resistance among bacteria.

Management of Autoimmune Disorders

Regardless of the rheumatologic disorder, it is most often treated with the same immunosuppressive agents and antiinflammatory medications as one would use in a complement-sufficient patient.

Management of Angioedema

The treatment of C1-INH deficiency is different from that of other complement deficiencies in that there are specific measures available to ameliorate symptoms and to prevent recurrence. In some patients, their episodes of angioedema may be sufficiently frequent or difficult to manage to justify long-term prophylaxis. Attenuated androgens such as oxandrolone or danazol are highly effective[108,109] and act by increasing transcription of the normal allele of *C1INH*.[110] However, because of their androgenic effects, their use in children is very limited. Another class of agents historically used for long-term prophylaxis is the antifibrinolytic agents.[111,112] Tranexamic acid and aminocaproic acid act by blocking plasmin generation. Although their efficacy is less than that of attenuated androgens, the incidence of side-effects is also less than that of attenuated androgens. For this reason, these agents may be used in childhood, although they are quite difficult to obtain in the USA. The FDA recently approved the use of C1 inhibitor concentrate for use as prophylaxis.[81,113,114] Guidelines and recommendation have not yet been formulated and the twice-weekly intravenous administration and cost will be barriers for some patients.[115,116] A newer formulation available to treat acute episodes is likely to have broad acceptability. Management of angioedema also requires education of the family and cautions against estrogen-containing birth control pills, undue exposure to trauma, and use of angiotensin converting enzyme inhibitors. All of these are known to precipitate episodes.

In some instances, patients may require short-term prophylaxis for surgery or oral procedures. Attenuated androgens, fibrinolytic agents, FFP, and C1 esterase concentrate have all been used successfully for short-term prophylaxis.[81,117] Recent guidelines can be helpful.[118]

Acute attacks can be emergencies if the airway is involved. C1 esterase inhibitor concentrate is the most effective agent for the treatment of acute attacks currently licensed in the USA.[119-121] DX-88 or ecallantide, a kallikrein inhibitor, is expected to receive FDA approval in 2010 and icatibant (Firazyr or Jerini), a bradykinin B2 receptor antagonist, is also expected to receive FDA approval.[122-127] These agents, by virtue of their subcutaneous administration will be likely to find an important niche in the treatment of HAE attacks. Epinephrine, antihistamines, and corticosteroids are of no proven benefit in C1-INH deficient patients. FFP has some advocates, however, there are no clinical studies clearly demonstrating efficacy and FFP has the potential of accelerating angioedema by providing additional substrate.[128]

Management of HUS

As is done for thrombotic thrombocytopenia purpura (TTP), most patients with atypical HUS receive apheresis and FFP replacement for acute episodes.[99,129] Factor H replacement may be of benefit, and FFP may be used to replace factor H. In the case of MCP deficiency, where the affected protein is membrane-bound, it is less clear that pheresis and FFP approach would provide benefit, but it could potentially act to clear inciting agents or complement activation products. For patients with factor H or factor I deficiency and end-stage renal disease, renal transplantation is not recommended. In contrast, renal disease in MCP typically does not recur in the transplanted kidney.

Secondary Complement Deficiencies

Secondary complement deficiencies are relatively common. Any pathologic process that results in activation of the complement cascade or interferes with the synthesis of complement components can result in a secondary complement deficiency.

The Newborn

In full-term infants, the levels of most components of either the classical or alternative pathways are 50% to 80% of adult levels.[130]

However, both C8 and C9 seem to be more severely depressed, with levels in full-term newborn infants as low as 28% and 10%, respectively, of maternal levels.[131,132] The serum levels of individual components of complement in premature infants have also been studied. Significant levels of C4, C3, C7, C9, factor B, properdin, and C1 esterase inhibitor have been detected in fetal serum as early as the end of the first trimester or the beginning of the second trimester.[133] There is a general tendency for levels of these components to increase with age, and their levels in premature infants generally correlate with gestational age.[134,135]

Nephrotic Syndrome

Children with the nephrotic syndrome have an increased susceptibility to pneumococcal peritonitis and sepsis. Although they are susceptible at any point in their illness, they are at greatest risk when they have high level proteinuria. Their serum-opsonizing activity is reduced, and when factor B is added back to their sera, the defect is corrected,[136] suggesting that loss of factor B in the urine is responsible for their deficient opsonizing activity and thus may contribute to their increased susceptibility to infection.

Systemic Lupus Erythematosus

SLE is a systemic disorder in which immune complexes are generated and deposited in end organs, leading to the classical inflammatory pathologic changes in lupus. The immune complexes may activate the complement cascade, especially the classical pathway, leading to consumption of individual components such as C3 and C4. The activation and consumption of the complement system typically precedes clinical flare, and the degree of hypocomplementemia, specifically levels of C3 and C4, generally reflects the degree of clinical activity.[137-139]

Although complement activation as a result of the circulating immune complexes is particularly characteristic of lupus, it has also been described in juvenile rheumatoid arthritis, Sjögren's syndrome, a variety of vasculitides, and mixed connective tissue disease. Hypocomplementemia as a result of immune complex formation is seen less frequently in other autoimmune diseases.

Serum Sickness

Serum sickness is the consequence of immune complex formation in response to the administration of drugs (e.g. penicillin, cefaclor, and minocycline), foreign proteins (e.g. antithymocyte globulin, therapeutic monoclonal antibodies, or antivenoms), or, in some instances, infections.[140,141] Although rash, fever, and arthralgia/arthritis are the most common clinical findings, severe cases may progress to renal involvement.[142] Immune complexes are present in the circulation early in the process. Most cases have significant hypocomplementemia, and when it occurs it is characterized by low CH$_{50}$, C3, and C4 levels.[143,144]

Sepsis

Acute bacterial sepsis, specifically Gram-negative sepsis, may be associated with transient hypocomplementemia. Generally, the hypocomplementemia reflects activation of both the alternative and classical pathways and is characterized by low levels of C3 and C4, as well as total hemolytic activity (CH$_{50}$) and the generation of the cleavage products, C3a and C5a.[145-147] The hypocomplementemia is most commonly found in patients who have some degree of cardiovascular compromise and is strongly correlated with the severity of the shock and morbidity.

Cirrhosis

Patients with cirrhosis have decreased serum concentrations of C3, C4, and total hemolytic activity.[148] The presence of decreased levels of C3 and C4 correlates with the degree of liver decompensation and levels of serum proteins synthesized in the liver, such as albumin and certain coagulation factors, suggesting that decreased hepatic synthesis is the basis for the decreased levels of C4 and C3. There is a correlation between the low levels of C3 and a predisposition to spontaneous bacterial peritonitis and mortality in cirrhosis.[149,150]

Cardiopulmonary Bypass, Extracorporeal Membrane Oxygenation, and Hemodialysis

A variety of therapeutic maneuvers, such as cardiopulmonary bypass, extracorporeal membrane oxygenation, and hemodialysis, bring the patient's blood in contact with artificial surfaces or membranes. As a result, there may be activation of the complement system with concurrent decreases of individual components, such as C3, and of total hemolytic complement.[151] As a consequence of the activation of the complement system, there also is generation of biologically active cleavage products, such as C3a and C5a. A number of studies have suggested that the generation of these anaphylatoxins is responsible for the generalized inflammatory response that follows cardiopulmonary bypass (postperfusion syndrome) and hemodialysis (pulmonary neutrophil sequestration).[152]

Malnutrition

Children with malnutrition, both kwashiorkor and marasmus, have decreased levels of serum total hemolytic complement activity as well as most of the individual components of complement, such as C3 and C5.[153,154] Dietary treatment of the malnutrition results in normalization of the complement levels. The degree of the decrease in complement components, such as C3, correlates strongly with serum albumin, suggesting that the decrease is the result of poor synthetic function in the liver.

Paroxysmal Nocturnal Hemoglobinuria (PNH)

PNH is characterized by recurrent episodes of hemoglobinuria due to intravascular hemolysis and is associated with acquired somatic mutations of PIG-A or PIG-M in a clone of bone marrow progenitor cells.[155] The protein product of PIG-A is required for GPI anchored proteins and C8 binding protein, DAF and CD59 are GPI anchored proteins that protect hematopoietic cells from complement-mediated lysis.[156] The red cells are the most vulnerable because they have no ability to repair membrane damage. PNH can be associated with complement dysfunction.[157]

Laboratory Assessment of Complement

Epidemiology

Patients with recurrent sinopulmonary infections are infrequently found to have complement deficiencies. For patients with recurrent sepsis/systemic infection or sepsis on the background of autoimmune disease (or a family history of autoimmune disease), the frequency of identifying a complement defect is probably higher although there are no data to support this approach.[158] Patients with a single meningococcal infection, either meningitis or meningococcemia, probably deserve an evaluation in nonendemic areas.[8,159,160] The evaluation would include a CH50 and AH50. There is general consensus that patients with meningococcal disease with an unusual serotype, with meningococcal disease on the background of a positive family history or recurrent meningococcal disease, should have an evaluation with a CH50 and AH50. In these patient groups, the frequency of complement deficiency approaches 50%.[7,10,11,160,161] Chronic meningococcemia appears to be another condition with a high frequency of complement deficiency.[162]

Most Caucasian lupus cohorts have approximately 1–2% of patients with complement deficiency (generally C2 deficiency).[163] Given the high rate of infection, it is important to identify these patients. Patients with C1 and C4 deficiencies tend to have severe disease with early presentations and therefore testing pediatric onset severe SLE might be revealing of complement deficiencies. An additional category where a CH50 assay might be considered is in the evaluation of patients with clinical symptoms suggestive of SLE but with negative ANA and anti-dsDNA. While often thought of as important indicators of SLE, complement-deficient patients have these autoantibodies less frequently and it might support the diagnosis of SLE to know that the patient had a complement deficiency.

All patients with atypical HUS should have a complement evaluation.[99,101] A CH50, an AH50, and a C3 level should be obtained In many cases, these will be normal and mutation analysis of factor H, factor I, and MCP will most often be required. Patients with membranoproliferative glomerulonephritis type II should also be evaluated when the clinical suspicion of a complement deficiency or nephritic factor exists.

When angioedema occurs in the setting of a known allergic response, it is much less likely to be due to C1 inhibitor deficiency. Patients with recurrent angioedema in the absence of allergic reactions, patients with a family history of angioedema,

patients with angioedema preceded by a reticular rash, and patients with angioedema after trauma, should all have an evaluation. A simple but rather insensitive screen is to measure C4 levels. C4 is typically decreased at baseline but is diminished even more during an acute attack owing to consumption. A more specific strategy is to measure C1 inhibitor antigen and functional levels.

Complement Laboratory Analyses

A CH50 assay consists of adding patient serum to antibody-coated sheep red cells. Complement activation of C1 to C9 leads to lysis. A CH50 result reports out the dilution of serum capable of lysing 50% of the sheep cells. Similarly, rabbit red cells are used to measure the function of the alternative pathway. With the exception of C9 deficiency, genetic deficiencies of all the cascade components lead to a CH50 of zero or near zero. A finding of low levels of CH50 or AH50 should be repeated and appropriate handling of the serum should be ensured. Other causes of low, but not absent, CH50 results are complement consumption due to infection or autoimmune disease. Less common, but more medically important are the regulatory protein defects leading to consumption of C3 such as factor D, factor H and factor I deficiency. C9 deficiency also leads to a reduction in both the CH50 and AH50 (Figure 11-3).

Once an abnormal CH50 or AH50 has been confirmed, nephelometry is used to define the serum levels of certain components (C3 and C4 primarily) and ELISAs are available for certain other components. Individual component functional assays are not widely available but are available through reference laboratories. Once the specific diagnosis is established, the management path should be obvious.

Conclusions

Complement represents a bridge between innate and adaptive immunity. It is important for the phagocytosis of immune complexes, opsonization of bacteria, lysis of bacteria, solubilizing

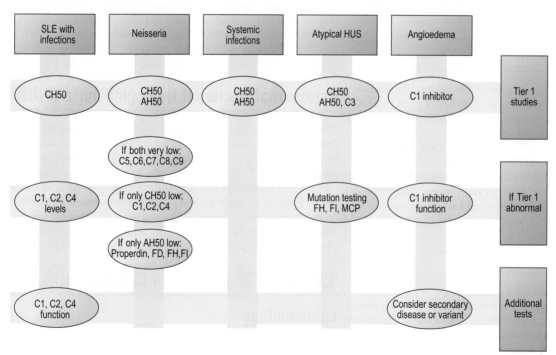

Figure 11-3 A potential algorithm for the evaluation of patients with suspected complement deficiency.

Clinical Presentation of Complement Deficiencies

- Increased susceptibility to systemic or deep bacterial infection
- Systemic lupus erythematosus
- Angioedema
- Atypical hemolytic uremic syndrome
- Specific illness depends on which complement component is involved

immune complexes, and for elimination of apoptotic cells. Complement regulatory proteins also serve to protect endothelial surfaces and hematopoietic cells. Complement deficiencies manifest themselves either as susceptibility to recurrent infections or as susceptibility to autoimmune/immune complex-mediated diseases (Box 11-1). Deficiencies of early components of the classical complement cascade (C1, C2, C4, and C3) are associated with both autoimmune/immune complex diseases and susceptibility to infections. Deficiencies of components of the alternate pathway (factor H, factor I, factor D, and properdin) and of late components of the complement system C5 to C9 are associated with susceptibility to infections, primarily to neisserial infections in the case of deficiency of C5 through C9. The diagnosis of a complement component deficiency must be entertained in all cases with recurrent severe bacterial infections, particularly in the face of elevated or upper-range levels of serum immunoglobulins and adequate antibody titers. The diagnosis of a deficiency in the early components of the classical complement cascade must be entertained in cases of SLE with a history of significant infection, and defects in regulatory proteins should be sought in cases of atypical HUS. A diagnosis of deficiency of the complement regulatory protein C1 esterase inhibitor must be considered in cases of nonpruritic angioedema in the absence of urticaria, particularly in the presence of a similar family history and in cases precipitated by trauma.

References

1. Sullivan KE, Winkelstein A, editors. Genetically determined deficiencies of complement. New York: McGraw-Hill Book; 2001.
2. Winkelstein JA. The role of complement in the host's defense against *Streptococcus pneumoniae*. Rev Infect Dis 1981;3:289–98.
3. Figueroa JE, Densen P. Infectious diseases associated with complement deficiencies. Clin Mic Rev 1991;4:359–95.
4. Ross SC, Densen P. Complement deficiency states and infection: epidemiology, pathogeneisis and consequences of neisserial and other infections in an immune deficiency. Medicine 1984;63:243–73.
5. Singer L, Colten HR, Wetsel RA. Complement C3 deficiency: human, animal, and experimental models. Pathobiology 1994;62:14–28.
6. Leggiadro RJ, Winkelstein JA. Prevalence of complement deficiencies in children with systemic meningococcal infections. Pediatr Infect Dis J 1987;6:75–9.
7. Merino J, Rodriguez-Valverde V, Lamelas JA. Prevalence of deficits of complement components in patients with recurrent meningococcal infections. J Infect Dis 1983;148:331–6.
8. Ellison RT, Kohler PH, Curd JG, et al. Prevalence of congenital and aquired complement deficiency in patients with sporadic meningococcal disease. N Engl J Med 1983;308:913–16.
9. Nielsen HE, Christensen KC, Koch C, et al. Hereditary, complete deficiency of complement factor H associated with recurrent meningococcal disease. Scand J Immunol 1989;30:711–18.
10. Nielsen HE, Koch C, Magnussesn P, et al. Complement deficiencies in selected groups of patients with meningococcal disease. Scand J Infect Dis 1989;21:389–96.
11. Fijen CA, Juijper EJ, Hannema AJ, et al. Complement deficiencies in patients over ten years old with meningococcal disease due to uncommon serogroups. Lancet 1989;ii:585–8.
12. Schifferli JA, Bartolotti SR, Peters DK. Inhibition of immune precipitation by complement. Clin Exp Immunol 1980;42:387–94.
13. Cornacoff JB, Hebert LA, Smead WL, et al. Primate erythrocyte immune complex clearing mechanism. J Clin Invest 1983;71:236–40.
14. Navratil JS, Ahearn JM. Apoptosis and autoimmunity: complement deficiency and systemic lupus erythematosus revisited. Curr Rheumatol Rep 2000;2:32–8.
15. Botto M, Dell'agnola C, Bygrave AE, et al. Homozygous C1q deficiency causes glomerulonephritis associated with multiple apoptotic bodies. Nat Genet 1998;19:56–9.
16. Shimizu I, Kawahara T, Haspot F, et al. B cell extrinsic CR1/CR2 promotes natural antibody production and tolerance induction of anti-alphaGAL-producing B-1 cells. Blood 2007;109:1773–81.
17. Meyer O, Hauptmenn G, Tappeiner G, et al. Genetic deficiency of C4, C2, or C1q and lupus syndromes. Association with anti-Ro (SS-A) antibodies. Clin Exp Immunol 1985;62:678–82.
18. Provost TT, Arnett FC, Reichlin M. Homozygous C2 deficiency, lupus erythematosus, and anti-Ro (SSA) antibodies. Arthritis Rheum 1983;26:1279–84.
19. Hauptmann G, Tappeiner G, Schifferli JA. Inherited deficiency of the fourth component of complement. Immunodeficiency Reviews 1988;1:3–22.
20. Bowness P, Davies KA, Norsworthy PJ, et al. Herditary C1q deficiency and systemic lupus erythematosus. Q J Med 1994;87:455–64.
21. Kavanagh D, Richards A, Atkinson J. Complement regulatory genes and hemolytic uremic syndromes. Annu Rev Med 2008;59:293–309.
22. Pangburn MK. Cutting edge: localization of the host recognition functions of complement factor H at the carboxyl-terminal: implications for hemolytic uremic syndrome. J Immunol 2002;169:4702–6.
23. Klein RJ, Zeiss C, Chew EY, et al. Complement factor H polymorphism in age-related macular degeneration. Science 2005;308:385–9.
24. Sellar GC, Blake DJ, Reid KBM. Characterization and organization of the genes encoding the A-, B- and C-chains of the human complement subcomponent C1q. Biochem J 1991;274:481–90.
25. Berkel AI, Birben E, Oner C, et al. Molecular, genetic and epidemiologic studies on selective complete C1q deficiency in Turkey. Immunobiology 2000;201:347–55.
26. Petry F, Berkel AI, Loos M. Repeated identification of a nonsense mutation in the C1qA-gene of deficient patients in south-east Europe. Mol Immunol 1996;33(Suppl. 1):9.
27. Loos M, Colomb M. C1, the first component of complement: structure-function-relationship of C1q and collectins (MBP, SP-A, SP-D, conglutinin), C1-esterases (C1r and C1s), and C1-inhibitor in health and disease. Behring Inst Mitt 1993;1–5.
28. Truedsson L, Awdeh Z, Yunis EJ, et al. Quantitative variation of C4 variant proteins associated with many MHC haplotypes. Immunogen 1989;30:414–21.
29. Mascart-Lemone F, Hauptmann G, Goetz J, et al. Genetic deficiency of C4 presenting with recurrent infections and a SLE-like disease. Genetic and immunologic studies. Am J Med 1983;75:295–304.
30. Clark RA, Klebanoff SJ. Role of the classical and alternative complement pathways in chemotaxis and opsonization: studies of human serum deficient in C4. J Immunol 1978;120:1102–8.
31. Kemp ME, Atkinson JP, Skanes VM, et al. Deletion of C4 genes in patients with systemic lupus erythematosus. Arthritis Rheum 1987;30:1015–22.
32. Barba G, Rittner C, Schneider PM. Genetic basis of human complement C4A deficiency. J Clin Invest 1993;91:1681–6.
33. Braun L, Schneider PM, Carroll MC, et al. Null alleles of human complement C4. Evidence for psuedogenes at the C4A locus and gene conversion at the C4B locus. J Exp Med 1990;171:129–40.
34. Howard PF, Hochberg MC, Bias WB, et al. Relationship between C4 Null Genes, HLA-D Region Antigens, and Genetic Susceptibility to Systemic Lupus Erythematosus in Caucasian and Black Americans. Am J Med 1986;81:187–93.
35. Fiedler AHL, Walport MJ, Batchelor JR, et al. Family study of the major histocompatibility complex in patients with systemic lupus erythematosus: importance of null alleles of C4A and C4B in determining disease susceptibility. Brit Med J 1983;286:425–8.
36. Christiansen FT, Dawkins RL, Uko G, et al. Complement allotyping in SLE: association with C4A null. Aust NZ J Med 1983;13:483–8.
37. Welch TR, Brickman C, Bishof N, et al. The phenotype of SLE associated with complete deficiency of complement isotype C4A. J Clin Immunol 1998;18:48–51.
38. Petri M, Watson R, Winkelstein JA, et al. Clinical expression of systemic lupus erythematosus in patients with C4A deficiency. Medicine 1993;72:236–44.
39. Biskof NA, Welch TR, Beischel LS. C4B deficiency: a risk factor for bacteremia with encapsulated organisms. J Infect Dis 1990;162:248–54.
40. Rowe PC, McLean RH, Wood RA, et al. Association of C4B deficiency with bacterial meningitis. J Infect Dis 1989;160:448–51.
41. Ruddy S. Component deficiencies: the second component. Prog All 1986;39:250–60.

42. Repine JE, Clawson CC, Friend PS. Influence of a deficiency of the second component of complement on the bactericidal activity of neutrophils in vitro. J Clin Invest 1977;59:802–9.

43. Giebink GS, Verhoef J, Peterson PK, et al. Opsonic requirements for phagocytosis of *Streptococcus pneumoniae* types VI, XVIII, XXIII, and XXV. Infect Immun 1977;18:291–7.

44. Friend P, Repine JE, Clawson CC, et al. Deficiency of the second component of complement (C2) with chronic vasculitis. Ann Intern Med 1975;83:813–16.

45. Johnson CA, Densen P, Wetsel RA, et al. Molecular heterogeneity of C2 deficiency. N Engl J Med 1992;326:871–4.

46. Sullivan KE, Petri MA, Schmeckpeper BJ, et al. Prevalence of a mutation causing C2 deficiency in systemic lupus erythematosus. J Rheumatol 1994;21:1128–33.

47. Truedsson L, Alper CA, Awdeh ZL, et al. Characterization of type I complement C2 deficiency MHC haplotypes. J Immunol 1993;151:5856–63.

48. Sullivan KE, Petri MA, Schmeckpeper BJ, et al. The prevalence of a mutation which causes C2 deficiency in SLE. J Rheumatol 1994;21:1128–33.

49. Jonsson G, Sjoholm AG, Truedsson L, et al. Rheumatological manifestations, organ damage and autoimmunity in hereditary C2 deficiency. Rheumatology (Oxford) 2007;46:1133–9.

50. Jonsson G, Truedsson L, Sturfelt G, et al. Hereditary C2 deficiency in Sweden: frequent occurrence of invasive infection, atherosclerosis, and rheumatic disease. Medicine (Baltimore) 2005;84:23–34.

51. Fasano MB, Densen P, McLean RH, et al. Prevalence of homozygous C4B deficiency in patients with deficiencies of terminal complement components and meningococcemia. J Infect Dis 1990;162:1220–1.

52. Colten HR, Rosen FS. Complement deficiencies. Ann Rev Immunol 1992;10:809–34.

53. Botto M, Fong KY, So AK, et al. Homozygous hereditary C3 deficiency due to a partial gene deletion. Proc Natl Acad Sci U S A 1992;89:4957–61.

54. Botto M, Fong KY, So AK, et al. Molecular basis of hereditary C3 deficiency. J Clin Invest 1990;86:1158–63.

55. Singer L, Whitehead WT, Akama H, et al. Inherited human complement C3 deficiency: an amino acid substitution in the beta-chain (ASP549 to ASN) impairs C3 secretion. J Biol Chem 1994;269:28494–9.

56. Wurzner R, Hobart MJ, Fernie BA, et al. Molecular basis of subtotal complement C6 deficiency. J Clin Invest 1995;95:1877–83.

57. Hobart MJ, Fernie BA, Fijen KA, et al. The molecular basis of C6 deficiency in the western Cape, South Africa. Hum Genet 1998;103:506–12.

58. Zhu Z, Atkinson TP, Hovanky KT, et al. High prevalence of complement component C6 deficiency among African-Americans in the south-eastern USA. Clin Exp Immunol 2000;119:305–10.

59. Orren A, O'Hara AM, Morgan BP, et al. An abnormal but functionally active complement component C9 protein found in an Irish family with subtotal C9 deficiency. Immunology 2003;108:384–90.

60. Rameix-Welti MA, Regnier CH, Bienaime F, et al. Hereditary complement C7 deficiency in nine families: subtotal C7 deficiency revisited. Eur J Immunol 2007;37:1377–85.

61. Tedesco F, Roncelli L, Petersen BH, et al. Two distinct abnormalities in patients with C8 alpha-gamma deficiency. Low level of C8 beta chain and presence of dysfunctional C8 alpha-gamma subunit. J Clin Invest 1990;86:884–8.

62. Kojima T, Horiuchi T, Nishizaka H, et al. Genetic basis of human complement C8 alpha-gamma deficiency. J Immunol 1998;161:3762–6.

63. Kotnik V, Luznik-Bufon T, Schneider PM, et al. Molecular, genetic, and functional analysis of homozygous C8 b-chain deficiency in two siblings. Immunopharmacology 1997;38:215–21.

64. Saucedo L, Ackerman L, Platonov AE, et al. Delineation of additional genetic bases for C8b deficiency. J Immunol 1995;155:5022–8.

65. Kaufmann T, Hansch G, Rittner C, et al. Genetic basis of human complement C8 beta deficiency complement component C4 deficiencies and gene alterations in patients with systemic lupus erythematosus. J Immunol 1993;150:4943–7.

66. Densen P, Ackerman L, Saucedo L, et al. The genetic basis of C8a-g deficiency. Mol Immunol 1996;33(Suppl. 1):68.

67. Kira R, Ihara K, Takada H, et al. Nonsense mutation in exon 4 of human complement C9 gene is the major cause of Japanese complement C9 deficiency. Hum Genet 1998;102:605–10.

68. Kira R, Ihara K, Watanabe K, et al. Molecular epidemiology of C9 deficiency heterozygotes with an Arg95Stop mutation of the C9 gene in Japan. J Hum Genet 1999;44:109–111.

69. Witzel-Schlomp K, Hobart MJ, Fernie BA, et al. Heterogeneity in the genetic basis of human complement C9 deficiency. Immunogen 1998;48:144–7.

70. Inai S, Kitamura H, Hiramatsu S, et al. Deficiency of the ninth component of complement in man. J Clin Lab Immunol 1979;2:85–90.

71. Lint TF, Zeitz HJ, Gewurz H. Inherited deficiency of the ninth component of complement in man. J Immunol 1980;125:2252–8.

72. Horiuchi T, Nishizaka H, Kojima T, et al. A non-sense mutation at Arg95 is predominant in complement 9 deficiency in Japanese. J Immunol 1998;160:1509–13.

73. Thiel S, Frederiksen PD, Jensenius JC. Clinical manifestations of mannan-binding lectin deficiency. Mol Immunol 2006;43:86–96.

74. Garred P, Larsen F, Seyfarth J, et al. Mannose-binding lectin and its genetic variants. Genes Immun 2006;7:85–94.

75. Garred P, Voss A, Madsen HO, et al. Association of mannose-binding lectin gene variation with disease severity and infections in a population-based cohort of systemic lupus erythematosus patients. Genes Immun 2001;2:442–50.

76. Graudal N. The natural history and prognosis of rheumatoid arthritis: association of radiographic outcome with process variables, joint motion and immune proteins. Scand J Rheumatol 2004;(Suppl.):1–38.

77. Thiel S, Kolev M, Degn S, et al. Polymorphisms in mannan-binding lectin (MBL)-associated serine protease 2 affect stability, binding to MBL, and enzymatic activity. J Immunol 2009;182:2939–47.

78. Cicardi M, Bergamaschini L, Cugno M, et al. Pathogenetic and clinical aspects of C1 inhibitor deficiency. Immunobiology 1998;199:366–76.

79. Donaldson VH, Rosen FS, Bing DH. Kinin generation in hereditary angioneurotic edema (H.A.N.E.) plasma. Adv Exp Med Biol 1983;156:183–91.

80. Frank MM, Gelfand JA, Atkinson JP. Hereditary angioedema: the clinical syndrome and its management. Ann Intern Med 1976;84:580–91.

81. Cugno M, Zanichelli A, Foieni F, et al. C1-inhibitor deficiency and angioedema: molecular mechanisms and clinical progress. Trends Mol Med 2009;15:69–78.

82. Cugno M, Zanichelli A, Bellatorre AG, et al. Plasma biomarkers of acute attacks in patients with angioedema due to C1-inhibitor deficiency. Allergy 2009;64:254–7.

83. Schapira M, Silver LD, Scott CF, et al. Prekallikrein activation and high-molecular-weight kininogen consumption in hereditary angioedema. N Engl J Med 1983;308:1050–3.

84. Curd JG, Progais LJ Jr, Cochrane CG. Detection of active kallikrein in induced blister fluids of hereditary angioedema patients. J Exp Med 1980;152:742–8.

85. Klemperer MR, Donaldson VH, Rosen FS. Effect of C1 esterase on vascular permeability in man: studies on normal and complement deficient individuals and in patients with hereditary angioneurotic edema. J Clin Invest 1968;47:604–10.

86. Cugno M, Nussberger J, Cicardi M, et al. Bradykinin and the pathophysiology of angioedema. Int Immunopharmacol 2003;3:311–17.

87. Sheffer AL, Craig JM, Willms-Kretschmer K, et al. Histopathological and ultrastructural observations on tissues from patients with hereditary angioneurotic edema. J Allergy 1971;47:292–7.

88. Cicardi M, Zingale L, Zanichelli A, et al. C1 inhibitor: molecular and clinical aspects. Springer Semin Immunopathol 2005;27:286–98.

89. Sanchez-Corral P, Perez-Caballero D, Huarte O, et al. Structural and functional characterization of factor H mutations associated with atypical hemolytic uremic syndrome. Am J Hum Genet 2002;71:1285–95.

90. Amar L, Lidove O, Kahn JE, et al. Hereditary angio-oedema: effective treatment with the progestogen-only pill in a young woman. Br J Dermatol 2004;151:713–14.

91. Reis ES, Falcao DA, Isaac L. Clinical aspects and molecular basis of primary deficiencies of complement component C3 and its regulatory proteins factor I and factor H. Scand J Immunol 2006;63:155–68.

92. Caprioli J, Peng L, Remuzzi G. The hemolytic uremic syndromes. Curr Opin Crit Care 2005;11:487–92.

93. Haines JL, Hauser MA, Schmidt S, et al. Complement factor H variant increases the risk of age-related macular degeneration. Science 2005;308:419–21.

94. Vyse TJ, Spath PJ, Davies KA, et al. Hereditary complement factor I deficiency. Q J Med 1994;87:385–401.

95. Abramson N, Alper CA, Lachmann PJ, et al. Deficiency of C3 inactivator in man. J Immunol 1971;107:19–25.

96. Vyse TJ, Morley BJ, Bartok I, et al. The molecular basis of hereditary complement factor I deficiency. J Clin Invest 1996;97:925–33.

97. Genel F, Sjoholm AG, Skattum L, et al. Complement factor I deficiency associated with recurrent infections, vasculitis and immune complex glomerulonephritis. Scand J Infect Dis 2005;37:615–18.

98. Solal-Celigny P, Laviolette M, Hebert J, et al. C3b inactivator deficiency with immune complex manifestations. Clin Exp Immunol 1982;47:197–205.

99. Caprioli J, Noris M, Brioschi S, et al. Genetics of HUS: the impact of MCP, CFH, and IF mutations on clinical presentation, response to treatment, and outcome. Blood 2006;108:1267–79.

100. Richards A, Kemp EJ, Liszewski MK, et al. Mutations in human complement regulator, membrane cofactor protein (CD46), predispose to development of familial hemolytic uremic syndrome. Proc Natl Acad Sci U S A 2003;100:12966–71.

101. Zimmerhackl LB, Besbas N, Jungraithmayr T, et al. Epidemiology, clinical presentation, and pathophysiology of atypical and recurrent hemolytic uremic syndrome. Semin Thromb Hemost 2006;32:113–20.

102. Fijen CA, van den Bogaard R, Schipper M, et al. Properdin deficiency: molecular basis and disease association. Mol Immunol 1999;36:863–7.

103. Kluin-Nelemans H, van Velzen-Blad H, van Helden HPT, et al. Functional deficiency of complement factor D in a monozygous twin. Clin Exp Immunol 1984;58:724–30.

104. Carroll MC. The complement system in regulation of adaptive immunity. Nat Immunol 2004;5:981–6.

105. Carroll MC, Fischer MB. Complement and the immune response. Curr Opin Immunol 1997;9:64–9.

106. Biselli R, Casapollo I, D'Amelio R, et al. Antibody response to meningococcal polysaccharides A and C in patients with complement defects. Scand J Immunol 1993;37:644–50.

107. Platonov AE, Beloborodov VB, Pavlova LI, et al. Vaccination of patients deficient in a late complement component with tetravalent meningococcal capsular polysaccharide vaccine. Clin Exp Immunol 1995;100:32–9.

108. Church JA. Oxandrolone treatment of childhood hereditary angioedema. Ann Allergy Asthma Immunol 2004;92:377–8.

109. Gelfand JA, Sherins RJ, Alling DW, et al. Treatment of hereditary angioedema with danazol: reversal of clinical and biochemical abnormalities. N Engl J Med 1976;295:1444–50.

110. Agostoni A, Cicardi M, Cugno M, et al. Clinical problems in the C1-inhibitor deficient patient. Behring Inst Mitt 1993;93:306–12.

111. Sheffer AL, Austen KF, Rosen FS. Tranexamic acid therapy in hereditary angioneurotic edema. N Engl J Med 1972;287:452–9.

112. Frank MM, Sergent JS, Kane MA, et al. Epsilon aminocaproic acid therapy of hereditary angioneurotic edema. A double-blind study. N Engl J Med 1972;286:808–12.

113. Waytes AT, Rosen FS, Frank MM. Treatment of hereditary angioedema with vapor-heated C1 inhibitor concentrate. N Engl J Med 1996;334:1630–4.

114. Levi M, Choi G, Picavet C, et al. Self-administration of C1-inhibitor concentrate in patients with hereditary or acquired angioedema caused by C1-inhibitor deficiency. J Allergy Clin Immunol 2006;117:904–8.

115. Bowen T, Cicardi M, Bork K, et al. Hereditary angiodema: a current state-of-the-art review, VII: Canadian Hungarian 2007 international consensus algorithm for the diagnosis, therapy, and management of hereditary angioedema. Ann Allergy Asthma Immunol 2008;100:S30–40.

116. Bowen T, Cicardi M, Farkas H, et al. Canadian 2003 International consensus algorithm for the diagnosis, therapy, and management of hereditary angioedema. J Allergy Clin Immunol 2004;114:629–37.

117. Cicardi M, Zingale LC. The deficiency of C1 inhibitor and its treatment. Immunobiology 2007;212:325–31.

118. Szema AM, Paz G, Merriam L, et al. Modern preoperative and intraoperative management of hereditary angioedema. Allergy Asthma Proc 2009.

119. Zuraw BL. Diagnosis and management of hereditary angioedema: an American approach. Transfus Apher Sci 2003;29:239–45.

120. Bork K, Barnstedt SE. Treatment of 193 episodes of laryngeal edema with C1 inhibitor concentrate in patients with hereditary angioedema. Arch Intern Med 2001;161:714–18.

121. Bork K, Siedlecki K, Bosch S, et al. Asphyxiation by laryngeal edema in patients with hereditary angioedema. Mayo Clin Proc 2000;75:349–54.

122. Reshef A, Leibovich I, Goren A. Hereditary angioedema: new hopes for an orphan disease. Isr Med Assoc J 2008;10:850–5.

123. Cruden NL, Newby DE. Therapeutic potential of icatibant (HOE-140, JE-049). Expert Opin Pharmacother 2008;9:2383–90.

124. Frank MM. Hereditary angiodema: a current state-of-the-art review, VI: novel therapies for hereditary angioedema. Ann Allergy Asthma Immunol 2008;100:S23–9.

125. Bernstein JA. Hereditary angioedema: a current state-of-the-art review, VIII: current status of emerging therapies. Ann Allergy Asthma Immunol 2008;100:S41–6.

126. Epstein TG, Bernstein JA. Current and emerging management options for hereditary angioedema in the US. Drugs 2008;68:2561–73.

127. Lehmann A. Ecallantide (DX-88), a plasma kallikrein inhibitor for the treatment of hereditary angioedema and the prevention of blood loss in on-pump cardiothoracic surgery. Expert Opin Biol Ther 2008;8:1187–99.

128. Prematta M, Gibbs JG, Pratt EL, et al. Fresh frozen plasma for the treatment of hereditary angioedema. Ann Allergy Asthma Immunol 2007;98:383–8.

129. Goodship TH. Factor H genotype-phenotype correlations: lessons from aHUS, MPGN II, and AMD. Kidney Int 2006;70:12–13.

130. Johnston RB Jr, Altenburger KM, Atkinson AW Jr, et al. Complement in the newborn infant. Pediatrics 1979;64:781–6.

131. Adinolfi M, Beck SE. Human complement C7 and C9 in fetal and newborn sera. Arch Dis Child 1975;50:562–4.

132. Ballow M, Fang F, Good RA, et al. Developmental aspects of complement components in the newborn. The presence of complement components and C3 proactivator (properdin factor B) in human colostrum. Clin Exp Immunol 1974;18:257–66.

133. Gitlin D, Biasucci A. Development of gamma G, gamma A, gamma M, beta IC-beta IA, C 1 esterase inhibitor, ceruloplasmin, transferrin, hemopexin, haptoglobin, fibrinogen, plasminogen, alpha 1-antitrypsin, orosomucoid, beta-lipoprotein, alpha 2-macroglobulin, and prealbumin in the human conceptus. J Clin Invest 1969;48:1433–46.

134. Sawyer MK, Forman ML, Kuplic LS, et al. Developmental aspects of the human complement system. Biol Neonate 1971;19:148–62.

135. Fireman P, Zuchowski DA, Taylor PM. Development of human complement system. J Immunol 1969;103:25–31.

136. McLean RH, Forsgren A, Bjorksten B, et al. Decreased serum factor B concentration associated with decreased opsonization of Escherichia coli in the idiopathic nephrotic syndrome. Pediatr Res 1977;11:910–16.

137. Swaak AJG, Aarden LA, Statious van Eps LW, et al. Anti-dsDNA and complement profiles as prognostic guides in systemic lupus erythematosus. Arthritis Rheum 1979;22:226–35.

138. Lloyd W, Schur PH. Immune complexes, complement, and anti-DNA in exacerbations of systemic lupus erythematosus (SLE). Medicine 1981;60:208–17.

139. Buyon JP, Tamerius J, Belmont HM, et al. Assessment of disease activity and impending flare in patients with systemic lupus erythematosus: comparison of the use of complement split products and conventional measurements of complement. Arthritis Rheum 1992;35:1028–36.

140. Parshuram CS, Phillips RJ. Retrospective review of antibiotic-associated serum sickness in children presenting to a paediatric emergency department. Med J Aust 1998;169:116.

141. Heckbert SR, Stryker WS, Coltin KL, et al. Serum sickness in children after antibiotic exposure: estimates of occurrence and morbidity in a health maintenance organization population. Am J Epidemiol 1990;132:336–42.

142. Border WA, Noble NA. From serum sickness to cytokines: advances in understanding the molecular pathogenesis of kidney disease. Lab Invest 1993;68:125–8.

143. Bielory L, Gascon P, Lawley TJ, et al. Human serum sickness: a prospective analysis of 35 patients treated with equine anti-thymocyte globulin for bone marrow failure. Medicine (Baltimore) 1988;67:40–57.

144. Bielory L, Gascon P, Lawley TJ, et al. Serum sickness and haematopoietic recovery with antithymocyte globulin in bone marrow failure patients. Br J Haematol 1986;63:729–36.

145. Sprung CL, Schultz DR, Marcial E, et al. Complement activation in septic shock patients. Crit Care Med 1986;14:525–8.

146. Fust G, Petras G, Ujhelvi E. Activation of the complement system during infections due to gram-negative bacteria. Clin Immunol Immunopathol 1976;5:293–302.

147. Fearon DT, Ruddy S, Schur PH, et al. Activation of the properdin pathway of complement in patients with gram-negative bacteremia. N Engl J Med 1975;292:937–40.

148. Ellison RT 3rd, Horsburgh CR Jr, Curd J. Complement levels in patients with hepatic dysfunction. Dig Dis Sci 1990;35:231–5.

149. Homann C, Varming K, Hogasen K, et al. Acquired C3 deficiency in patients with alcoholic cirrhosis predisposes to infection and increased mortality. Gut 1997;40:544–9.

150. Andreu M, Sola R, Sitges-Serra A, et al. Risk factors for spontaneous bacterial peritonitis in cirrhotic patients with ascites. Gastroenterology 1993;104:1133–8.

151. Jacob HS. Complement-induced vascular leukostasis: its role in tissue injury. Arch Pathol Lab Med 1980;104:617–20.

152. Amadori A, Candi P, Sasdelli M, et al. Hemodialysis leukopenia and complement function with different dialyzers. Kidney Int 1983;24:775–81.

153. Sakamoto M, Fujisawa Y, Nishioka K. Physiologic role of the complement system in host defense, disease, and malnutrition. Nutrition 1998;14:391–8.

154. Mishra OP, Agrawal S, Usha, et al. Levels of immunoglobulins and complement C3 in protein-energy malnutrition. J Trop Pediatr 1999;45:179–81.

155. Shichishima T, Noji H. Heterogeneity in the molecular pathogenesis of paroxysmal nocturnal hemoglobinuria (PNH) syndromes and expansion mechanism of a PNH clone. Int J Hematol 2006;84:97–103.

156. Shichishima T. Glycosylphosphatidylinositol (GPI)-anchored membrane proteins in clinical pathophysiology of paroxysmal nocturnal hemoglobinuria (PNH). Fukushima J Med Sci 1995;41:1–13.

157. Villaescusa R, Santos MN, Garcia Y, et al. Circulating immune complexes in paroxysmal nocturnal hemoglobinuria. Acta Haematol 1982;68:136–41.

158. Ekdahl K, Truedsson L, Sjoholm AG, et al. Complement analysis in adult patients with a history of bacteremic pneumococcal infections or recurrent pneumonia. Scand J Infect Dis 1995;27:111–17.

159. Ernst T, Spath PJ, Aebi C, et al. Screening for complement deficiency in bacterial meningitis. Acta Paediatrica 1997;86:1009–10.

160. Fijen CA, Kuijper EJ, te Bulte MT, et al. Assessment of complement deficiency in patients with meningococcal disease in The Netherlands. Clin Infect Dis 1999;28:98–105.

161. Cremer R, Wahn V. Deficiency of late complement components in patients with severe and recurrent meningococcal infections. Eur J Pediatr 1996;155:723–4.

162. Nielsen HE, Koch C, Mansa B, et al. Complement and immunoglobulin studies in 15 cases of chronic meningococcemia: properdin deficiency and hypoimmunoglobulinemia. Scand J Infect Dis 1990;22:31–6.

163. Collins TC, Winkelstein JA, Sullivan KE. Regulation of early complement components C3 and C4 in the synovium. Clin Diagn Lab Immunol 1996;3:5–9.

12

White Blood Cell Defects

Sergio D. Rosenzweig • Steven M. Holland

White blood cells (WBCs) can be easily classified into lymphoid (T, B, NK and NKT) and myeloid (neutrophils, eosinophils, basophils, and monocytes/macrophages) by virtue of their lineage-restricted progenitor's origin. This chapter focuses especially on neutrophils and monocytes and the disorders that arise from their quantitative or functional defects.

Mature neutrophils develop in the bone marrow from a myeloid stem cell over about 14 days, during which time proliferation, differentiation, and maturation take place. Mature neutrophils, with their load of primary, secondary, and tertiary granules, are released into the bloodstream where they stay 6 to 10 hours before exiting by diapedesis. In the tissues they may work in ways that are primarily phagocytic, bactericidal, fungicidal, or in the removal of damaged tissue. Neutrophil disorders can be divided into quantitative disorders, marked typically by neutropenias, and functional disorders, marked by failures in specific metabolic or interactive pathways. Quantitative disorders include neutrophilia (>7000 neutrophils per microliter in adult patients), and neutropenia (mild: <1500 neutrophils per microliter, moderate: 1500 to 1000 neutrophils per microliter, severe: <500 neutrophils per microliter). With very few exceptions (e.g. chronic idiopathic neutrophilia, leukocyte adhesion deficiencies, myeloproliferative diseases) neutrophilia is dependent on causes extrinsic to the neutrophils (e.g. acute or chronic infection, steroids, epinephrine). On the other hand, the causes of neutropenia are multiple and can be intrinsic or extrinsic to neutrophils or their progenitors (Box 12-1). Neutropenia usually falls into categories of decreased production or increased destruction, or a combination of these two. Qualitative myeloid disorders include defects in motility (adhesion, chemotaxis), defects in phagocytosis, defects of granule synthesis and release, and defects in killing (see Box 12-1).

A neutrophil disorder should be suspected in patients with recurrent, severe, bacterial or fungal infections, especially those caused by unusual organisms (e.g. *Chromobacterium violaceum*) or in uncommon locations (e.g. liver abscess; Table 12-1). Viral and parasitic infections are not apparently increased in these patients, and should direct attention elsewhere. Initial laboratory evaluation should take into account the clinical presentation to direct where the defect is likely to be. Some assays, such as repeated WBC counts with differentials or microscopic evaluation of neutrophils, are relatively simple and can readily exclude neutropenia or some granule defects. Flow cytometry requires a careful consideration of which markers to examine. Functional assays, such as oxidative burst testing, phagocytosis, or chemotaxis are the most challenging because so few laboratories do them routinely (Table 12-2). We will consider some of the clinical, diagnos-

tic, and management aspects of a few of the best characterized myeloid disorders.

Severe Congenital Neutropenia

Severe congenital neutropenia (SCN) comprises a heterogeneous group of disorders with variable inheritance patterns that share the common characteristics of bone marrow granulocytic maturation arrest at the promyelocyte or myelocyte stage, severe chronic neutropenia (fewer than 200 neutrophils per microliter), and increased susceptibility to acute myeloid leukemia.

The clinical manifestations of SCN appear promptly after birth: 50% of affected infants are symptomatic before the first month of life, and 90% within the first 6 months; omphalitis, upper and lower respiratory tract infections, and skin and liver abscesses are common. Subcutaneous recombinant granulocyte-colony stimulating factor (G-CSF; 5 µg/kg/day) has dramatically changed the prognosis of these patients.[1] Since the advent of recombinant G-CSF, reductions in the number of infections and hospitalization days, and an increase in life expectancy have been described.[1]

In 1956 Kostmann described a Swedish kindred with severe congenital neutropenia inherited in an autosomal recessive pattern.[2] More than half a century elapsed before its genetic cause was found. Using linkage analysis and a candidate gene sequencing approach, Klein and colleagues identified homozygous mutations in the antiapoptotic molecule HAX1 in patients with autosomal recessive SCN, which was confirmed to be the cause in the original Kostmann pedigree, as well.[3] HAX1 is critical for maintaining the inner mitochondrial membrane potential and protects myeloid cells from apoptosis, as well as signal transduction and cytoskeletal control. Some patients with HAX1 deficiency also suffer from mild to severe cognitive problems ranging to epilepsy. Two isoforms of HAX1 have been identified: those carrying mutations affecting exclusively isoform A present with SCN, while those carrying mutations affecting both isoforms display SCN plus neurological symptoms.[4]

Among patients with SCN, single allele mutations in the G-CSF receptor (GCSFR, 1p35-p34.3), have been described associated with the development of acute myeloid leukemia.[5] However, not all patients with SCN syndrome show mutations in the G-CSF receptor, suggesting that these mutations are epiphenomena that occur in the setting of severe congenital neutropenia but do not cause it.[6] Autosomal recessive mutations in the glucose-6-phosphatase catalytic subunit 3 (G6PC3) also cause congenital neutropenia along with cardiac and urogenital malformations.[7]

©2010 Elsevier Ltd, Inc, BV

DOI: 10.1016/B978-1-4377-0271-2.00012-2

BOX 12-1

Neutrophil Disorders: Causes

Neutrophilia

Usually dependent on causes *extrinsic* to the neutrophils (e.g. acute or chronic infection)

Neutropenia

Caused by defects *intrinsic* to the neutrophils or their progenitors (severe congenital neutropenia, cyclic neutropenia, neutropenia associated to other well-defined syndromes [e.g. Schwachman syndrome, Fanconi's syndrome, dyskeratosis congenita, Chédiak-Higashi syndrome, reticular dysgenesis, WHIM syndrome])

Caused by defects *extrinsic* to the neutrophil or their progenitors (infections, drugs, immune mediated, metabolic diseases, nutritional deficiencies, bone marrow infiltration)

Motility Disorders

Adhesion: Leukocyte adhesion deficiency 1, 2, or 3.

Chemotaxis: Leukocyte adhesion deficiency 1, 2, or rac2; localized juvenile periodontitis, neutrophil β-actin deficiency, secondary to extensive burns, secondary to alcohol consumption

Phagocytosis Disorders

Leukocyte adhesion deficiency 1 (complement-mediated only); secondary to antibody deficiencies; complement deficiencies; mannose binding protein deficiency

Disorders of Granule Formation and Content

Chédiak-Higashi syndrome; specific granule deficiency

Microbicidal Disorders

Chronic granulomatous disease; myeloperoxidase deficiency; glucose-6-phosphate dehydrogenase deficiency, glutathione pathway deficiencies

Horwitz and colleagues[8] and Dale and colleagues[9] found that 22 out of 25 patients with dominant or spontaneous SCN had heterozygous mutations in the gene encoding neutrophil elastase (ELA2, 19p13.3). Interestingly, mutations in this same gene are also responsible for cyclic neutropenia. The mutations in ELA2 that cause cyclic neutropenia tend to be clustered around the catalytically active site of ELA2, whereas the mutations that are associated with SCN are located in a different part of the gene that winds up on a different side of the three-dimensional structure of the protein. The mechanism by which ELA2 mutations lead to SCN is thought to be due to the 'unfolded protein response', an apoptotic signal delivered to the cell when a specific protein is folded incorrectly. ELA2 mutations are responsible for more than 50% of SCN cases in Caucasian patients.[10]

Devriendt and colleagues[11] described a family with an X-linked form of severe congenital neutropenia (XLN) caused by mutations in the Wiskott-Aldrich syndrome protein (WASP). In contrast to the WASP mutations that produce classical Wiskott-Aldrich syndrome or X-linked thrombocytopenia, most of which are caused by mutations resulting in reduced WASP transcription or translation, the mutation causing XLN (L270P) disrupts a WASP autoinhibitory domain, thereby creating a constitutively active mutant protein.

Two families with heterozygous mutations in GFI1 and congenital neutropenia and monocytosis have been described.[12] GFI1 mutations act in a dominant-negative way and cause dysregulation of several target genes such as C/EBP epsilon, ELA2, and the monocytopoietic cytokine CSF1.

Reticular dysgenesis is an autosomal recessive form of severe combined immunodeficiency in which early myeloid arrest, neutropenia, lymphopenia, and sensorineural loss occur. Mutations in adenylate kinase 2 (AK2), localized in the mitochondrial intermembrane space (similar to HAX1), cause reticular dysgenesis.[13,14] AK2 may be important in mitochondrial energy metabolism and control of apoptosis. Importantly, the neutropenia in reticular dysgenesis is not responsive to G-CSF. Hematopoietic stem cell transplantation is the only successful therapeutic option for these patients.

Table 12-1 Infections and WBC Defects: Features Highly Suspicious of Phagocyte Disorders. (A) Severe Infections, (B) Recurrent Infections, (C) Infections Due to Specific Microorganisms, (D) Unusually Located Infections

(A) Severe Infections		(B) Recurrent Infections		(C) Specific Infections		(D) Unusually Located Infections	
Type of Infection	Diagnosis to Consider	Site of Infection	Diagnosis to Consider	Microorganism	Diagnosis to Consider	Site of Infection	Diagnosis to Consider
Cellulitis	Neutropenia, LAD CGD, HIES	Cutaneous	Neutropenia, CGD, LAD, HIES	S. epidermidis	Neutropenia, LAD	Umbilical cord	LAD
Colitis	Neutropenia, CGD	Gums	LAD, neutrophil motility disorders	S. marscecens, C. violaceum, Nocardia, B. cepacia	CGD	Liver abscess	CGD
Osteomyelitis	CGD, MSMD pathway defects	Upper and lower respiratory tract	Neutropenia, HIES, functional neutrophil disorders	Aspergillus	Neutropenia, CGD, HIE	Gums	LAD, neutrophil motility disorders
		GI tract	CGD, MSMD pathway defects (salmonella)	Nontuberculous mycobacteria, BCG	MSMD pathway defects, SCID, CGD		
		Lymph nodes	CGD, MSMD pathway defects (mycobacteria)	Candida	Neutropenia, CGD, MPO		
		Osteomyelitis	CGD, MSMD				

Table 12-2 Laboratory Evaluation of Patient with Suspected Neutrophil Disorder*

Test	If Normal, It Excludes ...
WBC count and differential (repeated)	All forms of neutropenia
Neutrophil morphologic evaluation	Specific granule deficiency; Chédiak-Higashi syndrome
Flow cytometry	
CD18	LAD 1 (complete)
CD15s (sialyl Lewis^x)	LAD 2
Dihydrorhodamine (DHR) oxidation	CGD (severe G6PD deficiencies and glutathione pathway deficiencies have abnormal DHR oxidation as well)
STAT-1 phosphorylation	IFNGR1, IFNGR2 deficiency
STAT-4 phosphorylation	IL-12Rβ1 and Tyk2 deficiency
Bone marrow aspirate	
Neutrophil maturation	Severe congenital neutropenia; cyclic neutropenia
Neutrophil retention	WHIM syndrome
Nitroblue tetrazolium reduction	CGD (severe G6PD deficiencies and glutathione pathway deficiencies have abnormal NBT reduction as well)

*Patients should be evaluated considering their familial history, physical examination, and associated co-morbid factors.

Cyclic Neutropenia/Cyclic Hematopoiesis

Cyclic neutropenia/Cyclic hematopoiesis is typically inherited as an autosomal dominant trait and characterized by regular cyclic fluctuations in all hematopoietic lineages. However, clinical manifestations are almost exclusively associated with variations in neutrophils. Neutrophil counts cycle on an average of every 21 days (range 14 to 36 days), including periods of severe neutropenia (< 200/μL) that last from 3 to 10 days.[15,16] Different single-base heterozygous substitutions in ELA2 (neutrophil elastase 2, 19p13.3) have been identified in all pedigrees analyzed.[9,10] Most patients have clinical manifestations of neutropenia in early childhood. Oral ulcerations, gingivitis, lymphadenopathy, pharyngitis/tonsillitis, and skin lesions are the most frequently reported findings. Early loss of permanent teeth as a consequence of chronic gingivitis and periapical abscesses is common.[17] Bone marrow aspirates obtained during periods of neutropenia show maturation arrest at the myelocyte stage, or, less frequently, bone marrow hypoplasia.[18]

Granulocyte-colony stimulating factor (G-CSF) dramatically improves peripheral neutrophil counts and decreases morbidity in cyclic neutropenia patients. Interestingly, infections and hospitalizations appear to naturally lessen with age.[17]

Myelokathexis/Warts, Hypogammaglobulinemia, Infections, and Myelokathexis Syndrome

Myelokathexis (from the Greek, meaning 'retained in the bone marrow') is a congenital disorder associated with severe chronic neutropenia. Unlike other forms of congenital neutropenia, bone marrow aspirates from myelokathexis patients show myeloid hypercellularity with increased numbers of granulocytes at all stages of differentiation. A significant number of patients with myelokathexis also have warts, hypogammaglobulinemia, and infections, with different degrees of severity. The acronym WHIM (warts, hypogammaglobulinemia, infections and myelokathexis) tries to capture the clinical hallmarks of this syndrome. Most WHIM patients have single heterozygous C-terminus deletion mutations of the intracellular carboxy terminus of the chemokine receptor CXCR4.[19] These mutations lead to enhanced responses to CXCL12, its cognate ligand, which is expressed on bone marrow stromal cells. Enhanced activity of CXCR4 delays release of mature neutrophils from bone marrow, resulting in peripheral neutropenia and apoptosis of the mature neutrophils retained in the marrow.[20,21] Recurrent sinopulmonary infections are frequent. During episodes of infection neutrophil counts are typically increased compared to baseline levels. Steroids, subcutaneous epinephrine, intravenous endotoxin, as well as G-CSF and GM-CSF, have all been shown to mobilize mature neutrophils from the bone marrow. Sustained therapy with G-CSF or GM-CSF increases the number of neutrophils in the peripheral blood and decreases the number of infections. The presence of warts and hypogammaglobulinemia, although not severe, indicate a broader immunologic defect including T and the B cells.[22]

Immune-Mediated Neutropenias

Alloimmune Neonatal Neutropenia

Alloimmune neonatal neutropenia (ANN) is a form of immune-mediated neutropenia produced by the transplacental transfer of maternal antibodies against NA1 and NA2, two isotypes of the immunoglobulin receptor FcγRIIIb, causing immune destruction of neonatal neutrophils.[23-27] This problem typically arises in otherwise normal children of apparently normal healthy mothers. Several of the healthy mothers did not express FcγRIIIb on their own neutrophils, leading to the elaboration of antibodies against FcγRIIIb expressed on fetal neutrophils. These complement activating antineutrophil antibodies can be detected in 1 in 500 live births, making the potential incidence of ANN high. This disease should be considered in the evaluation of all infants with neutropenia, with or without infection. Antibody-coated neutrophils in ANN are phagocytosed in the reticuloendothelial system and removed from the circulation, leaving the neonate neutropenic and prone to infections. Omphalitis, cellulitis, and pneumonia may be the presenting infections within the first 2 weeks of life. The diagnosis can be made by detection of neutrophil specific alloantibodies in maternal serum. Parenteral antibiotics (even in the absence of other signs of sepsis) and G-CSF, should be included in the initial management of ANN. As expected, ANN tends to spontaneously improve with the waning of maternal antibody levels, but this process may take months.[27]

Primary and Secondary Autoimmune Neutropenia

Autoimmune neutropenia (AIN) is a rare disorder, caused by peripheral destruction of neutrophils and/or their precursors by autoantibodies present in patient serum or mediated by large granular lymphocytes (CD3$^+$/CD8$^+$/CD57$^+$ T cells) in the bone marrow. Autoimmune neutropenia can be either primary or secondary. When the neutropenia is an isolated clinical entity it is primary AIN, and when associated with another disease, it is secondary AIN.

Primary Autoimmune Neutropenia

Primary AIN is the most common cause of chronic neutropenia (absolute neutrophil count <1500/µL lasting at least 6 months) in infancy and childhood. There is a slight female predominance and it has been reported in about 1:100000 live births, ten times more frequent than severe congenital neutropenia. Antibodies directed against different neutrophil antigens can be detected in almost all patients. Approximately one third of these autoantibodies are anti-NA1 and NA2, two of the glycosylated isoforms of FcγRIIIb (the same targets recognized in ANN). Almost 85% of these antibodies are IgG. Other antigens toward which autoantibodies can be found are CD11b/CD18 (Mac-1); CD32 (FcγRII); and CD35 (C3b complement receptor). The average age at diagnosis for primary AIN is 8 months. The majority of patients present with either skin or upper respiratory tract infections. Infrequently, some patients may suffer from severe infections such as pneumonia, meningitis, or sepsis. The diagnosis may be incidental, as patients may remain asymptomatic despite low neutrophil counts. Monocytosis is also frequent. Neutrophil counts are usually below 1500/µL, with the majority of patients having >500 neutrophils/µL at the time of diagnosis. The neutrophil count may transiently increase 2-fold to 3-fold during severe infections and return to neutropenic levels following resolution. Bone marrow findings may be normal or hypercellular. The cause of this disease remains unknown. Detection of granulocyte-specific antibodies is key to the diagnosis of primary AIN and may require repeated testing.[28]

The prognosis of primary AIN is very good because it is usually a self-limited disease. The neutropenia remits spontaneously within 7 to 24 months in 95% of patients, preceded by the disappearance of autoantibodies from the circulation. Symptomatic treatment with antibiotics for infections is usually sufficient. Treatment for severe infections or in the setting of emergency surgery often now includes G-CSF.[28]

Secondary Autoimmune Neutropenia (Secondary AIN)

Secondary AIN can be seen at any age but is more common in adults and has a more variable clinical course. Various systemic and autoimmune diseases such as systemic lupus erythematosus, Hodgkin's disease, large granular lymphocyte proliferation or leukemia, Epstein-Barr virus infection, cytomegalovirus infection, HIV infection, and Parvovirus B19 infection have been associated with secondary AIN.[28] These patients are predisposed to the development of other autoimmune problems as well. Antineutrophil antibodies typically have pan-FcγRIII specificity, rather than specificity to the FcγRIII subunits, making the resulting neutropenia more severe. Anti-CD18/11b antibodies have been detected in a subset of patients. Secondary AIN responds best to therapy directed at the underlying cause.[28]

Defects of Granule Formation and Content

Chédiak-Higashi Syndrome

Chédiak-Higashi syndrome (CHS) is a rare and life-threatening autosomal recessive disease, clinically characterized by oculocu-

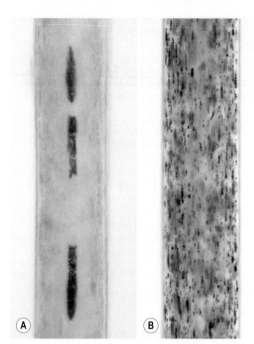

Figure 12-1 Pigment distribution in hair. Normal hair **(A)** shows opacity typically located in the cortex of the hair shaft. In Chédiak-Higashi syndrome **(B)** small aggregates of clumped melanin are haphazardly distributed all along the hair shaft. (20 × magnification).

taneous albinism, frequent pyogenic infections, neurologic abnormalities, and a relatively late-onset lymphoma-like 'accelerated phase'. The disease is caused by mutations in the lysosomal trafficking regulator gene, LYST or CHS1 (1q42.1-q42.2).[29,30] Affected patients show hypopigmentation of the skin, iris, and hair because of giant and aberrant melanosomes (macromelanosomes). Hair color is light brown to blonde, with a characteristic metallic silver-gray sheen. Under light-microscopy, CHS hair shafts shows pathognomonic small aggregates of clumped pigment (Figure 12-1).[31-33]

Giant azurophil granules formed from the fusion of multiple primary granules are seen in neutrophils, eosinophils, and basophils. In fact, enlarged cytoplasmic granules are found in all granule-containing cells. Neutropenia is also frequently seen. Neurologic involvement of the peripheral and central nervous systems is common. Progressive neuropathy of the legs, cranial nerve palsies, seizures, mental retardation, and autonomic dysfunction are reported.

The accelerated phase, one of the main causes of death in CHS, is clinically indistinguishable from other hemophagocytic syndromes, with fever, hepatosplenomegaly, lymphadenopathy, cytopenias, hypertriglyceridemia, hypofibrinogenemia, hemophagocytosis, and tissue lymphohistiocytic infiltration. Etoposide (VP16), steroids, and intrathecal methotrexate (when the CNS is involved) have been effective treatments. However, without successful bone marrow transplantation, the accelerated phase usually recurs.

Neutrophil-Specific Granule Deficiency

Neutrophil-specific granule deficiency is a rare, heterogeneous, autosomal recessive disease characterized by the profound reduction or absence of neutrophil-specific granules and their contents.[34] In several cases a homozygous, recessive, mutation was found in C/EBP ε (14q11.2).[35] However, other cases do not have mutations in C/EBP ε, suggesting genetic heterogeneity.

C/EBP ε is a member of the CCAAT/enhancer binding proteins, transcription factors that play critical roles in myelopoiesis and cellular differentiation.[36]

In neutrophil-specific granule deficiency: there is a paucity of neutrophil-specific granules, neutrophils with bilobed nuclei predominate (pseudo-Pelger-Huët anomaly), eosinophils may not be detected in peripheral smears, and there is increased susceptibility to pyogenic infections of the skin, ears, lungs, and lymph nodes. Neutrophils have very low specific granule contents (e.g. lactoferrin) and low to absent defensins, a primary granule product. Hemostasis abnormalities, caused by reduced levels of platelet-associated high molecular-weight von Willebrand factor and platelet fibrinogen and fibronectin, have been reported.[37]

Aggressive diagnosis of infection, prolonged and intensive therapy, and early use of surgical excision and debridement are necessary. Unrelated bone marrow transplantation corrected neutrophil-specific granule deficiency (C/EBP ε mutation negative) in a 13-month-old patient with intractable diarrhea and severe infections.[38]

Defects of Oxidative Metabolism

Chronic Granulomatous Disease

Chronic granulomatous disease (CGD) predisposes to recurrent life-threatening infections caused by catalase-positive bacteria and fungi, and exuberant granuloma formation due to defects in the NADPH oxidase.[39] Before assembly the NADPH oxidase exists as a heterodimeric membrane-bound complex embedded in the walls of secondary granules, and four distinct cytosolic proteins. The structural components are referred to as *phox* proteins (*ph*agocyte *ox*idase). The secondary granule membrane complex is cytochrome b_{558}, composed of a 91-kd glycosylated β chain (gp91^{phox}) and a 22-kd nonglycosylated α chain (p22^{phox}), which binds heme and flavin. The cytosol contains the structural components p47^{phox}, p67^{phox}, and the regulatory components p40^{phox} and rac. On cellular activation the cytosolic components p47^{phox} and p67^{phox} are phosphorylated and bind tightly together. In association with p40^{phox} and rac, these proteins combine with the cytochrome complex (gp91^{phox} and p22^{phox}) to form the intact NADPH oxidase. An electron is taken from NADPH and donated to molecular oxygen, leading to the formation of superoxide. In the presence of superoxide dismutase, this is converted to hydrogen peroxide, which, in the presence of myeloperoxidase and chlorine, is converted to bleach. Until recently, the metabolites of superoxide themselves were thought to be the critical mediators of bacterial killing. However, it is now believed that phagocyte production of reactive oxygen species is most critical for microbial killing through the activation of certain primary granule proteins inside the phagosome.[40] This new paradigm for NADPH oxidase-mediated microbial killing suggests that the reactive oxidants are most critical as intracellular signaling molecules, leading to activation of other pathways, rather than exerting a microbicidal effect per se.

Mutations in five genes of the NADPH oxidase have been found to cause CGD. Mutations in the X-linked gp91^{phox} account for about two thirds of cases; the remainder are autosomal recessive; there are no autosomal dominant cases of CGD.[39] A single case of p40^{phox} deficiency has recently been identified.[41] The frequency of CGD in the USA is higher than 1 : 200 000. Clinically, CGD is quite variable but the majority of patients are diagnosed as toddlers and young children.[42] Infections and granulomatous lesions are the usual first manifestations. The lung, skin, lymph

Table 12-3 Prevalence of Infection by Site in 368 Patients with Chronic Granulomatous Disease*

Type of Infection (Most Frequent Microorganisms Isolated)	Total (N = 368) No. (%)
Pneumonia (*Aspergillus* spp; *Staphylococcus* spp; *Burkholderia* cepacia; *Nocardia* spp; *Mycobacteria* spp)	290 (79%)
Abscess (*Staphylococcus* spp; *Serratia* spp; *Aspergillus* spp)	250 (68%)
Suppurative adenitis (*Staphylococcus* spp; *Serratia* spp; *Candida* spp)	194 (53%)
Osteomyelitis (*Serratia* spp; *Aspergillus* spp; *Paecilomyces* spp; *Staphylococcus* spp)	90 (25%)
Bacteremia/fungemia (*Salmonella* spp; *Burkholderia cepacia*; *Candida* spp; *Staphylococcus* spp; *Pseudomonas* spp)	65 (18%)
Cellulitis (*Chromobacterium violaceum* and *Serratia marsescens* were identified in one case each)	18 (5%)
Meningitis (*Candida* spp was identified in three cases)	15 (4%)
Other†	112 (30%)

Modified from Winkelstein JA, Marino MC, Johnston RB Jr, et al. Medicine (Baltimore) 2000;79:155–169.
*These data include patients on variable prophylactic regimens, if any, and are meant to portray the natural history of disease over the last 20 years.
†Includes impetigo, sinusitis, otitis media, septic arthritis, urinary tract infection/pyelonephritis, gingivitis/periodontitis, chorioretinitis, gastroenteritis, paronychia, conjunctivitis, hepatitis, epididymitis, empyema, epiglottitis, cardiac empyema, mastoiditis, and suppurative phlebitis.

nodes, and liver are the most frequent sites of infection (Table 12-3). The overwhelming majority of infections in CGD in North America are caused by only five organisms: *S. aureus*, *Burkholderia cepacia*, *Serratia marcescens*, *Nocardia*, and *Aspergillus*.[53] Trimethoprim/sulfamethoxazole prophylaxis has reduced the frequency of bacterial infections in general and staphylococcal infections in particular. On prophylaxis, staphylococcal infections are essentially confined to the liver and cervical lymph nodes.[42] Staphylococcal liver abscesses encountered in CGD are dense, caseous, and difficult to drain, requiring surgery in almost all cases.[43]

The gastrointestinal (GI) (Figure 12-2A) and genitourinary tracts (GU) (Figure 12-2B), are frequently affected by inflammatory and granulomatous manifestations in CGD patients. The retinas and lungs also develop inflammatory lesions in CGD. Gastrointestinal inflammatory manifestations occur in up to 43% of X-linked and 11% of autosomal recessive cases.[44] Abdominal pain is the most common gastrointestinal symptom; diarrhea, nausea and vomiting, also occur. Colonic granulomatous lesions mimic Crohn's-like inflammatory bowel disease (IBD), but oral ulcers, esophagitis, gastric outlet obstruction, villous atrophy, intestinal strictures, fistulae and perirectal abscesses occur. The extraintestinal manifestations of Crohn's (pyoderma, arthritis) are typically absent. Most CGD-associated IBD manifestations are responsive to steroids. Prednisone (1 mg/kg/day for several weeks followed by progressive tapering) usually resolves the symptoms. Unfortunately, relapses occur in nearly 70% of patients.[44] Low-dose maintenance prednisone may control symptoms without an apparent increase in serious infections. Sulfasalazine, mesalazine, 6-mercaptopurine, azathioprine, and cyclosporine are effective second-line treatment options.

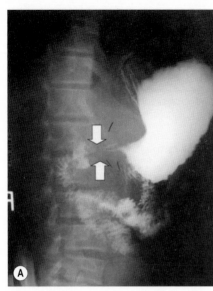 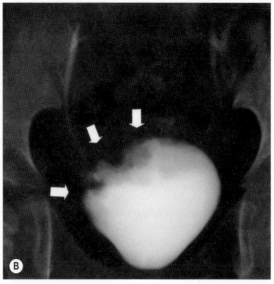

Figure 12-2 Gastrointestinal and genitourinary obstructive lesions in chronic granulomatous disease. **(A)** High-grade obstruction of the gastric outlet in a 17-year-old boy with gp91^{phox} deficient CGD *(arrows)*. He had early satiety, weight loss, and intermittent vomiting for several weeks. He improved rapidly on steroid therapy. **(B)** Extensive bladder granuloma formation in the superior aspect of the bladder in a 3-year-old boy with gp91^{phox} deficient CGD *(arrows)*. Note the mildly dilated ureter on the obstructed side. This child presented with dysuria and right hydronephrosis that responded promptly to steroids.

Anecdotal reports of the use of TNFα blocking antibodies in severe cases of IBD in CGD patients have been associated with symptom control but also severe infections with typical CGD pathogens. Therefore, intensified prophylaxis and vigilance for intercurrent infections are needed in the setting of these potent immunosuppressives. Other anecdotal case reports suggest that CGD-associated colitis may respond to G-CSF and GM-CSF, respectively.

GU strictures and granulomas occur in up to 18% of CGD patients, mostly limited to cytochrome b558-mutated patients.[45] Steroid therapy similar to that used for GI manifestations usually controls these complications.[46,47]

Inflammatory retinal involvement is found in up to 24% of X-linked CGD cases with well-circumscribed asymptomatic 'punched out' retinal scars localized along the retinal vessels and associated with pigment clumping. Interestingly, these same lesions were also detected in three X-linked CGD female carriers. These lesions are typically nonprogressive, asymptomatic and need no specific treatment. However, two CGD patients needed enucleation for painful retinal detachments.[48,49]

Autoimmune disorders are more common in CGD than in the general population. Discoid and systemic lupus erythematosus occur in CGD and in X-linked CGD female carriers. Idiopathic thrombocytopenic purpura and juvenile rheumatoid arthritis are also more frequent in CGD than in the general population.[42,50,51]

The X-linked carriers of gp91^{phox} have one population of phagocytes that produces superoxide and one that does not, giving carriers a characteristic mosaic pattern on oxidative testing. Infections are not usually seen in these female carriers unless the normal neutrophils are below 10%, in which case these carriers are at risk for CGD type infections.[42,52]

The diagnosis of CGD is usually made by direct measurement of superoxide production, ferricytochrome c reduction, chemiluminescence, nitroblue tetrazolium (NBT) reduction, or dihydrorhodamine oxidation (DHR). Currently, we prefer the latter assay because of its relative ease of use, its ability to distinguish X-linked from autosomal patterns of CGD on flow cytometry, and its sensitivity to even very low numbers of functional neutrophils.[53,54] Of note, several other conditions, such as glucose-6-phosphate dehydrogenase deficiency, myeloperoxidase

deficiency, and synovitis, acne, pustulosis, hyperostosis and osteitis (SAPHO) can also affect the respiratory burst.[55,56]

Male sex, earlier age at presentation, and increased severity of disease suggest X-linked disease, but the precise gene defect should be determined in all cases for genetic counseling and prognosis. Autosomal recessive forms of CGD (mostly p47^{phox} deficient) have a significantly better prognosis than X-linked disease.[42]

Prophylactic trimethoprim/sulfamethoxazole (5 mg/kg/day based on trimethoprim) reduces the frequency of major infections from about once every year to once every 3.5 years.[57] It reduces staphylococcal and skin infections without increasing the frequency of serious fungal infections in CGD.[57] Itraconazole prophylaxis prevented fungal infection in CGD (100 mg daily for patients <13 years or <50 kg; 200 mg daily for those ≥13 years or ≥50 kg).[58] IFN-γ also reduces the number and severity of infections in CGD by 70% compared to placebo, regardless of the inheritance pattern of CGD, sex, or use of prophylactic antibiotics.[59] Interestingly, no significant difference could be detected in terms of in vitro superoxide generation, bactericidal activity, or cytochrome b levels.[59] Systemic IFN-γ also augmented neutrophil activity against *Aspergillus conidia* in vitro. Therefore, our current recommendation is to use prophylaxis with trimethoprim/sulfamethoxazole, itraconazole, and interferon gamma (50 µg/m²) in CGD. Because the differential diagnosis for a given process in these patients includes bacteria, fungi, and granulomatous processes, a microbiologic diagnosis is critical. Leukocyte transfusions are often used for severe infections, but their efficacy is anecdotal.

Winkelstein and colleagues reported American mortality from the 1970s through 1990s for the X-linked form of the disease was around 5% per year and 2% per year for the autosomal recessive varieties.[42] The European experience cumulated from 1954 to 2003 found that autosomal recessive CGD patients had an average life expectancy of 50 years, while X-linked cases had an average life expectancy of close to 38 years.[60] Mortality in CGD correlates with noncirrhotic portal hypertension and progressive damage of the hepatic microvasculature. Local or systemic infections, in addition to drug-induced liver injury may be underlying conditions. A history of liver abscess, alkaline phosphatase elevations, and platelet count decrease over time were individually associated with mortality in CGD patients.[61]

Successful hematopoietic stem cell transplantation (HSCT) provides a cure for CGD. Seger and colleagues reported on 27 mostly pediatric European CGD patients transplanted with unmodified marrow grafts from human leukocyte antigen (HLA)-identical siblings (25/27) or unrelated (2/27) donors. Absence of preexisting overt infection was the single best prognostic factor for HSCT.[62] Since as few as 5–10% of normal cells are sufficient to prevent and control infections as shown in Lyonized females, stable mixed hematopoietic chimerism is sufficient to prevent infection, but most centers now perform HSCT in CGD patients after somewhat myeloablative conditioning regimens.

CGD is a group of single gene defects that almost exclusively affect the hematopoietic system. Vectors providing normal phox genes can reconstitute NADPH oxidase activity in deficient cells, establishing the proof-of-principle for gene therapy in CGD. Two adults with X-linked CGD were successfully treated with retrovirus-based gene therapy performed on autologous hematopoietic stem cells after nonmyeloablative ablative bone marrow conditioning. Clinical response was observed after transplantation, but one of the patients died 27 months after the procedure due to infection. The long-term risks and effectiveness of gene therapy remain to be determined.[63,64]

Myeloperoxidase Deficiency

Myeloperoxidase (MPO) deficiency is an autosomal recessive disease with variable expressivity. It is also the most common primary phagocyte disorder: 1/4000 individuals have complete MPO deficiency, and 1/2000 have a partial defect.[65] Myeloperoxidase (17q23) is synthesized in neutrophils and monocytes, packaged in the azurophilic granules, and released either into the phagosome or the extracellular space where it catalyzes the conversion of H_2O_2 to hypohalous acid (in neutrophils the halide is Cl^- and the acid is bleach). Of the MPO-deficient patients who have had clinical findings, infections caused by different *Candida* strains were the most common: mucocutaneous, meningeal, and bone infections, as well as sepsis, have been described.[66–69] Diabetes mellitus appears to be a critical cofactor for *Candida* species infections in the context of MPO deficiency. Definitive diagnosis is established by neutrophil/monocyte peroxidase histochemical staining or specific protein detection. There is no specific treatment for MPO deficiency; diabetes should be sought and controlled, and infections should be treated.

Leukocyte Adhesion Deficiencies

Leukocyte movement from the bloodstream toward inflamed sites is crucial in fighting infections. Adhesion to the endothelium, other leukocytes, and bacteria is critical for leukocytes to travel, communicate, inflame, and fight. The integrin and selectin adhesion molecules mediate these processes.

Leukocyte Adhesion Deficiency, Type 1 (LAD1)

LAD1 is an autosomal recessive disorder produced by mutations in the common β2 chain (CD18) of the β2 integrin family (ITGB2, 21q22.3; Table 12-4).[70] Each of the β2 integrins is a heterodimer composed of an α chain (CD11a, CD11b, or CD11c), noncovalently linked to the common β2 subunit (CD18). The α-β heterodimers of the β2 integrin family include CD11a/CD18 (lymphocyte-function-associated antigen-1, LFA-1), CD11b/CD18 (macrophage antigen-1, Mac-1 or complement receptor-3, CR3), and CD11c/CD18 (p150,95 or complement receptor-4, CR4). CD18 is required for normal expression of the α-β heterodimers. Therefore mutations resulting in failure to produce a functional β2 subunit lead to either very low or no expression of CD11a, CD11b, and/or CD11c, causing LAD1.[70]

The severe phenotype of LAD1 is caused by less than 1% of normal expression of CD18 on neutrophils whereas the moderate phenotype shows from 1% to 30% of normal expression.[71] However, patients with normal β2 integrin expression but without functional activity were described. Therefore expression of CD18 alone is not sufficient to exclude the diagnosis of LAD1: functional assays must be performed if the clinical suspicion is high.[72,73]

Patients with the severe phenotype of LAD1 characteristically have delayed umbilical stump separation and omphalitis, persistent leukocytosis (>15000/μL) even in the absence of obvious active infection, and severe, destructive gingivitis and periodontitis with associated loss of dentition and alveolar bone. Recurrent infections of the skin, upper and lower airways, bowel, and perirectal area, are common and usually caused by *S. aureus* or Gram-negative bacilli, but not by fungi. Infections tend to be

Table 12-4 Leukocyte Adhesion Deficiency Syndromes

Leukocyte Adhesion Deficiency (LAD)	Type 1 (LAD1)	Type 2 (LAD2 or CDG-IIc)	Type 3 (LAD3)	E-Selectin Deficiency	Rac2 Deficiency
OMIM*	116920	266265	612840	131210	602049
Inheritance pattern	Autosomal recessive	Autosomal recessive	Autosomal recessive	Unknown	Autosomal dominant
Affected protein(s)	Integrin β2 common chain (CD18)	Fucosylated proteins (e.g., sialyl-Lewisˣ, CD15s)	Kindlin 3	Endothelial E-selectin expression	Rac2
Neutrophil function affected	Chemotaxis, tight adherence	Rolling, tethering	Chemotaxis, adhesion, superoxide production	Rolling, tethering	Chemotaxis, superoxide production
Delayed umbilical cord separation	Yes (severe phenotype only)	Yes	Yes	Yes	Yes
Leukocytosis/ neutrophilia	Yes	Yes	Yes	No (mild neutropenia)	Yes

*OMIM, Online Mendelian Inheritance in Man

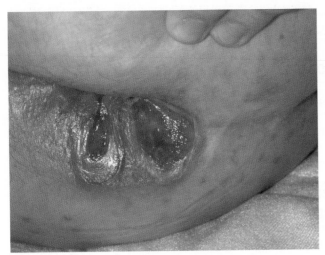

Figure 12-3 Ulcerative perirectal lesion in an 18-year-old boy with LAD1. No pus was seen and there was poor inflammation in the surrounding tissues.

necrotizing and may progress to ulceration (Figure 12-3). Typically, no pus is seen in these lesions and there is almost complete absence of neutrophil invasion on histopathology. Aggressive medical management with antibiotics, neutrophil transfusions, and prompt surgery, when indicated, are required. Impaired healing of infectious, traumatic, or surgical wounds is also characteristic of LAD1 patients. Scars tend to acquire a dystrophic 'cigarette-paper' appearance. Patients with the moderate phenotype tend to be diagnosed later in life, have normal umbilical separation, have fewer life-threatening infections, and live longer. However, leukocytosis, periodontal disease, and delayed wound healing are still common.[71]

Flow cytometry of LAD1 blood samples shows reduction (moderate phenotype) or near absence (severe phenotype) of CD18 and its associated molecules CD11a, CD11b and CD11c on neutrophils and other leukocytes. LAD1 patients show diminished neutrophil migration and in vitro.[71] Adherence of affected granulocytes to glass, plastic, nylon, wool, and to other LAD neutrophils is greatly reduced and does not improve after stimulation. Complement-mediated phagocytosis is severely impaired because of the absence of the complement receptor CD18/CD11b (CR3/Mac-1).

Somatic reversion of the mutation has been reported in LAD1 involving cytotoxic T lymphocytes.[74] However, bone marrow transplantation is the only definitive treatment.[75] Laboratory and animal gene-therapy studies in LAD1 are provocative.[76]

Leukocyte Adhesion Deficiency, Type 2 (LAD2) or Congenital Disorder of Glycosylation Type IIc (CDG-IIc)

LAD2, or CDG-IIc, is a very rare autosomal recessive inherited disease in which fucose metabolism is primarily affected because of mutations in the GDP-fucose transporter gene, FUCT1, located at 11p11-q11[77,78] (see Table 12-4). Lack of the GDP-fucose transporter leads to a lack of expression of sialyl-Lewis[x] and other fucosylated proteins, impairing leukocyte rolling adhesion as well as other pathways. The clinical phenotype is characterized by infections of the skin, lung, and gums; leukocytosis; and poor pus formation, as well as mental retardation, short stature, distinctive facies, and the Bombay (hh) blood phenotype. The frequency and severity of infections tend to decline with time.[79]

Fucose supplementation has had variable results in LAD2 patients.[80,81]

Leukocyte Adhesion Deficiency, Type 3 (LAD3)

LAD3 deficiency (previously known as LAD1 variant) resembles LAD1 on the one hand, but is associated with a syndrome like Glanzmann's thrombasthenia (a β3 integrin-related bleeding disorder) on the other. LAD3 is due to mutations in *KINDLIN3*, a molecule responsible for β1, β2 and β3 integrin activation in leukocytes and platelets.[82,83]

Rac2 Deficency

Ambruso and colleagues[84] and Williams and colleagues[85] reported a male patient with an autosomal dominant mutation in the Rho GTPase RAC2 gene (RAC2, 22q12.13-q13.2; see Table 12-4). This molecule, comprising more than 96% of Rac in neutrophils, is a member of the Rho family of GTPases and is critical to the regulation of the actin cytoskeleton and superoxide production. The patient had delayed umbilical cord separation, perirectal abscesses, failure to heal surgical wounds, and absent pus in infected areas despite neutrophilia. Chemotaxis and superoxide production were impaired. In addition, the patient's neutrophils showed defective azurophilic granule release and impaired phagocytosis. Four months after a matched related bone marrow transplantation, the patient was thriving, showing 100% donor cells in his bone marrow, and normalized superoxide production.

Mendelian Susceptibility to Mycobacterial Diseases (MSMD): Interferon-γ/IL-12/IL-23 Pathway Deficiencies (Interferon-γ Receptor 1 Deficiency, Interferon-γ Receptor 2 Deficiency, IL-12 Receptor β1 Deficiency, IL-12 p40 Deficiency, STAT1 Deficiency, NEMO Deficiency)

The mononuclear phagocyte is crucial for protection against intracellular infections and for antigen presentation. It is also necessary for lymphocyte stimulation, lymphocyte proliferation, cytokine production, and response. Mycobacteria infect macrophages leading to the production of interleukin 12 p70, a heterodimer of IL-12 p40 and IL-12 p35 and IL-23, a heterodimer of IL-12p40 and p19. IL-12 and IL-23 stimulate T cells and NK cells through their receptors to phosphorylate STAT4 and produce IFN-γ. IFN-γ acts through its heterodimeric receptor to phosphorylate STAT1 and turn on interferon responsive genes. (Figure 12-4). NFkB essential modulator (NEMO) hypomorphic mutations are also associated with MSMD in hemizygous males. Affected males may have a complex phenotype including hypohydrotic ectodermal dysplasia, immune deficiency, and more rarely, lymphedema and osteopetrosis. Almost 40% of males with hypomorphic mutations in NEMO develop mycobacterial infections, mostly with environmental organisms.[86] In heterozygous females, NEMO mutations are associated with *incontinentia pigmenti*.[87]

Patients with defects in IFNGR1 (6q23-q24), INFGR2 (21q22.1-q22.2), IL-12 receptor β1 (19p13.1), IL-12 p40 (5q31.1-33.1), and STAT1 (2q32.2-q32.3) have been identified through their suscep-

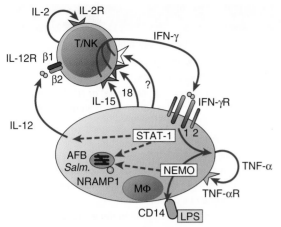

Figure 12-4 Schematic representation of the interferon-γ/interleukin-12 pathway. Ingested pathogens such as acid-fast bacilli (*AFB*) or salmonella (salm.) stimulate interleukin-12 (*IL-12*) production by macrophages (*MΦ*). Acting through its cognate IL-12 receptor, composed of the IL-12 receptor β1 chain (IL-12Rβ1) and the IL-12 receptor β2 chain (IL12Rβ2), IL-12 stimulates T and NK cells to produce interferon-γ (*IFN-γ*) and interleukin-2 (*IL-2*). Homodimeric IFN-γ binds to the interferon γ receptor complex (*IFN-γR*). Interferon γ receptor 1 (*IFN-γR1*) is the binding chain whereas interferon γ receptor 2 (*IFN-γR2*) is necessary to transmit the signal intracellularly through the signal transduction and activator of transcription 1 (*STAT1*). The mechanisms by which IFN-γ stimulates intracellular microorganism killing are not fully understood, but are likely to be numerous (e.g. upregulation of MHC expression and IL-12 production, enhancing of antigen processing and reactive oxygen species production, reducing the phagosomal pH). IFN-γ also stimulates tumor necrosis factor-α (*TNF-α*) production. TNF-α, acting through the TNF-α receptor (*TNF-αR*), also shows effects against intracellular infections. Patients with mutations in the NF-κB essential modulator (*NEMO*), a protein critical in the TNF-α signaling pathway, have enhanced susceptibility to mycobacterial disease as well as other infections. IL-12 is not the only cytokine that stimulates IFN-γ production: interleukin-15 (*IL-15*), interleukin-18 (*IL-18*), and probably other factors have the same effect. Lipopolysaccharide (*LPS*) stimulation through the CD14/Toll-like receptor 2 (TLR2) complex can also stimulate IL-12 production.

tibility to mycobacteria as well as to *Salmonella* infections.[88,89] Although these patients have a common infection susceptibility, there are phenotypic distinctions for the different genotypes.

Patients with autosomal recessive mutations leading to abolition of IFNGR1, IFNGR2 or STAT1 expression or function have the most severe phenotypes. They present early in life, especially if they receive BCG vaccination. In contrast, patients with an autosomal dominant mutation in IFNGR1 as a result of a recurrent 4 base deletion (named 818del4), have a truncation of the molecule that preserves the ligand-binding aspects but removes its recycling domain.[90] The incapable mutant IFNGR1 product remains stuck on the cell surface, where it binds IFN-γ but also interferes with the normal function of the wild type allele. Therefore, this is a dominant negative mutant. These patients usually present before the age of 7 years with pulmonary nontuberculous mycobacterial infection but then may go on to develop recurrent multifocal nontuberculous osteomyelitis. Patients with IL-12p40, IL-12 receptor β1, and dominant STAT1 mutations usually have a phenotype not as severe as complete IFNGR1, IFNGR2 or STAT1 deficiency. For IL-12 receptor β1 deficiency, the infection risk for nontuberculous mycobacteria is high in childhood but wanes after age 12.[91]

Defects in this pathway can be detected in several ways. Flow cytometry is very efficient for IFNGR1 defects, as this protein is expressed on all nucleated cells all the time, to varying extents. In the case of the autosomal dominant form of IFNGR1 deficiency, the protein is overabundant on the cell surface and therefore very easy to detect.[92] In contrast, detection of IFNGR2 and

Table 12-5 Clinical Characteristics of Hyper IgE Syndrome with STAT3 Mutations

Clinical Findings in HIES	
Eczema	100%
Peak IgE > 2000 IU/mL	97%
Eosinophilia	93%
Recurrent pneumonias	87%
Characteristic face	83%
Mucocutaneous candidiasis	83%
Pneumatoceles	77%
Retarined primary teeth	72%
Pathologic fractures	71%
Focal brain hyperintensities	70%
Scoliosis (>16 years, >10°)	63%

IL-12Rβ1 require cell culture and proliferation. Detection of intracellular phosphorylated STAT1 after IFNγ stimulation, or phosphorylated STAT4 after IL-12 stimulation, are indirect means of demonstrating functional integrity of the interferon gamma and IL-12 receptors, respectively.[92,93] Direct detection of IL-12p40 or IL-12 p70 can be used for the diagnosis of patients who are deficient in IL-12 p40. Defects in STAT1 require research techniques.

Treatment of infections in these patients poses special problems. For the patients with complete IFNGR defects IFN-γ is of no help in the clearance of mycobacterial disease. However, in patients with autosomal dominant IFNGR1 deficiency, IL-12 defects, or IL-12R defects, IFN-γ is effective. Bone marrow transplantation for IFNGR defects has been disappointing overall, for reasons that are still unclear. Long-term prophylaxis against environmental mycobacterial infections with a macrolide such as azithromycin or clarithromycin seems advisable.

Hyper-IgE Syndrome (HIES; Job's Syndrome)

The hyper-IgE syndrome (HIES or Job's) is characterized by elevated serum immunoglobulin E (IgE), eczema, recurrent skin and lung infections, and somatic features including characteristic facies, scoliosis, and fractures[94] (Table 12-5). Job's syndrome is a multisystem disease caused by STAT3 mutations.[95,96] All human mutations found thus far have been heterozygous missense or in-frame deletion mutations predominantly in the SH2 domain (mediating protein–protein interactions) and the DNA-binding domains (mediating the interaction of protein with DNA). These protein positive mutants allow the production of full-length mutant STAT3 protein, which exerts dominant negative effects.

A newborn rash is usually the first manifestation of Job's syndrome. About one fifth have the rash at birth, and one quarter develop it in the first week of life. Although mucocutaneous candidiasis is common, typically as oral thrush, vaginal candidiasis, or onychomycosis, systemic *Candida* infections are very rare.[94] Cutaneous 'cold' abscesses are common and due to *Staphylococcus aureus* infections. Antistaphylococcal antibiotics or topical antiseptics, such as bleach, are effective.

Recurrent pneumonias caused by *S. aureus, Streptococcus pneumoniae,* and *Haemophilus influenzae* typically start in childhood, with fewer symptoms than would be expected in a immune competent person. Pneumatoceles and bronchiectasis form during the healing process and usually persist once the infection has cleared. These anatomic abnormalities predispose the patient to Gram-negative bacterial infection (typically *Pseudomonas*) and fungal infections (typically *Aspergillus* or *Scedosporium* species). The decision to resect the large pneumatoceles that sometimes form following pneumonia is complex. These large cysts may become secondarily infected and be a source of infection, bleeding, and possibly death. On the other hand, thoracic surgery can be complicated by poor expansion of the remaining lung, often resulting in thoracoplasty. Antimicrobial prophylaxis to prevent *S. aureus* skin and lung infection (e.g., trimethoprim/sulfamethoxazole) may be broadened if Gram-negative lung infections occur. Antifungal prophylaxis to prevent pulmonary aspergillosis remains attractive but unproven, but it is highly effective in treating and preventing mucocutaneous candidiasis.

Scoliosis, osteopenia, minimal trauma fractures, hyperextensibility, degenerative joint disease, craniosynostosis and Chiari 1 malformations also occur fairly frequently; craniosynostosis and Chiari 1 seldom need surgical correction.[97] The general mechanism underlying bone abnormalities is unknown, and the role of bisphosphonates in treating the osteoporosis and minimal trauma fractures in HIES is undefined.

Starting in childhood and adolescence, most Job's or HIES patients develop characteristic facial features including facial asymmetry, broad nose, and deep-set eyes with a prominent forehead. Most patients retain some, if not all, of their primary teeth past the age of normal primary dental exfoliation; at times, layers of both primary and secondary teeth coexist.[94,97] Vascular abnormalities are common in Job's or HIES, including: coronary artery aneurysms,[98] dilatations and tortuosities; carotid artery berry aneurysms; and early onset MRI T2-weighted hyperintensities (unidentified bright objects or UBOs).[99]

As reported in other primary immunodeficiency diseases affecting lymphocytes, both Hodgkin and non-Hodgkin lymphomas are significantly increased in Job's syndrome.[100]

An autosomal recessive IgE elevation syndrome has also been described which has predominant clinical manifestations of severe eczema and recurrent skin and lung infections, as well as cutaneous viral infections (molluscum contagiosum, herpes simplex, and varicella zoster viruses).[101] Severe eczematoid rashes start early in life, although not necessarily in the newborn period. Unlike Job's syndrome, pneumonias due to *S aureus, H influenzae, Proteus mirabilis, Pseudomonas aeruginosa,* and *Cryptococcus* typically heal without pneumatocele formation. Neurologic manifestations range from facial paralysis to hemiplegia and are more prevalent than in STAT3 deficiency.[101] This distinct entity, previously referred to as autosomal recessive HIES, is now known to be due to recessive mutations in dedicator of cytokinesis 8 (DOCK8).[102,103] DOCK8 deficiency lacks the connective tissue, skeletal, tooth exfoliation, fracture, and characteristic facial features of Job's syndrome.

Another autosomal recessive syndrome with IgE elevation and infection susceptibility is due to Tyk2 deficiency, in which a man had BCG and herpes and molluscum susceptibility due to the loss of Tyk2.[104]

Mucocutaneous Candidiasis

Genetic conditions predisposing to predominantly mucocutaneous candidiasis have been identified. Mutations in dectin-1, the

cell surface receptor for beta-D-glucan, a fungal cell wall component, have been associated with severe vulvovaginal, oral, and nail infections.[105] An apparently more serious form of severe candidiasis is due to mutations in CARD9, one of the downstream signal transducers for dectin-1, which also transduces signal for some Toll-like receptors.[106]

Conclusions

Various defects of phagocytes have been painstakingly elucidated over the last several decades. Despite the fact that profound neutropenia predisposes patients to essentially all members of the bacterial and fungal kingdoms, metabolic defects in neutrophils and monocytes have relatively narrow spectra of infection. Some of these disorders have almost pathognomonic infection profiles (e.g. CGD, IFN-γ/IL-12 pathway defects). We have now put genetic faces to some of the names of these puzzling diseases. The simple recognition of genes and pathways should not be confused with careful and complete understanding of mechanism. The latter, despite all the complex diagrams, remains elusive (Boxes 12-2 and 12-3). Although we have been very successful at identifying rare and flagrant defects affecting white cells that lead to severe infections, the more subtle defects that cause recurrent staphylococcal infections, common causes of mucocutaneous candidiasis, and hydradenitis, to name only a few of the vexing problems that frequently confront the clinical immunologist, remain to be determined. Careful study of the known pathways, assiduous following of the ramifications of those pathways to the points where they merge with new pathways, and conscientious characterization of clinical phenotypes will lead to the discovery of these remaining immune defects. In the process we will gain new insights into exactly how we remain

- In general, attenuated or inactivated viral vaccines are not contraindicated in individuals with primary phagocyte disorders, as antiviral cell-mediated immunity is intact.

- BCG vaccination should be avoided in individuals with CGD or MSMD pathway defects, as well as in their newborn close relatives, until the defect is ruled out.

- Mulching and gardening should be avoided by individuals with increased susceptibility to aspergillus infections, such as patients with CGD, HIES, or neutropenia.

- Patients with white blood cell defects often fail to mount a normal inflammatory response, so clinicians and parents must keep a high index of suspicion for asymptomatic or hyposymptomatic infection.

- Standard recommendations for duration of therapy of infections are based on assumptions in normal specimens. In the patient with a white cell defect, the host contribution to resolution of infection may be relatively small, leading to a need for longer or more intensive antibiotic or antifungal therapy.

- When infections are necrotizing or poorly responsive to antibiotic therapy, surgery may be needed, even in situations in which it would not be needed in unaffected individuals (e.g. liver abscesses and lymphadenitis in CGD almost always need operative removal).

- Obtain experienced expert advice whenever possible.

so remarkably healthy in the face of so many daily microbial challenges.

References

1. Dale DC, Cottle TE, Fier CJ, et al. Severe chronic neutropenia: treatment and follow-up of patients in the Severe Chronic Neutropenia International Registry. Am J Hematol 2003;72:82–93.

2. Kostmann R. Infantile genetic agranulocytosis. Acta Paediatr Scand [suppl] 1956;45:1–178.

3. Klein C, Grudzien M, Appaswamy G, et al. HAX1 deficiency causes autosomal recessive severe congenital neutropenia (Kostmann disease). Nat Genet 2007;39:86–92.

4. Germeshausen M, Grudzien M, Zeidler C, et al. Novel HAX1 mutations in patients with severe congenital neutropenia reveal isoform-dependent genotype-phenotype associations. Blood 2008;111:4954–7.

5. Dong F, Brynes R, Tidow N, et al. Mutations in the gene for the granulocyte colony-stimulating-factor receptor in patients with acute myeloid leukemia preceded by severe congenital neutropenia. N Engl J Med 1995;333:487–93.

6. Germeshausen M, Skokowa J, Ballmaier M, et al. G-CSF receptor mutations in patients with congenital neutropenia. Curr Opin Hematol 2008;15:332–7.

7. Boztug K, Appaswamy G, Ashikov A, et al. A syndrome with congenital neutropenia and mutations in G6PC3. N Engl J Med 2009;360:32–43.

8. Horwitz M, Benson KF, Person RE, et al. Mutations in ELA2, encoding neutrophil elastase, define a 21-day biological clock in cyclic haematopoiesis. Nat Genet 1999;23:433–6.

9. Dale DC, Person RE, Bolyard AA, et al. Mutations in the gene encoding neutrophils elastase in congenital and cyclic neutropenia. Blood 2000;96:2317–22.

10. Horwitz MS, Duan Z, Korkmaz B, et al. Neutrophil elastase in cyclic and severe congenital neutropenia. Blood 2007;109:1817–24.

11. Devriendt K, Kim AS, Mathijs G, et al. Constitutively activating mutation in WASP causes X-linked severe congenital neutropenia. Nat Genet 2001;27:313–7.

12. Person RE, Li FQ, Duan Z, et al. Mutations in proto-oncogene GFI1 cause human neutropenia and target ELA2. Nat Genet 2003;34:308–12.

13. Pannicke U, Honig M, Hess I, et al. Reticular dysgenesis (aleukocytosis) is caused by mutations in the gene encoding mitochondrial adenylate kinase 2. Nat Genet 2009;41:101–5.

14. Lagresle-Peyrou C, Six EM, Picard C, et al. Human adenylate kinase 2 deficiency causes a profound hematopoietic defect associated with sensorineural deafness. Nat Genet 2009;41:106–11.

15. Wright DG, Dale DC, Fauci AS, et al. Human cyclic neutropenia: clinical review and long-term follow-up of patients. Medicine (Baltimore) 1981;60:1–13.

16. Dale DC, Hammond WP. Cyclic neutropenia: a clinical review. Blood Rev 1988;2:178–85.

17. Palmer SE, Stephens K, Dale DC. Genetics, phenotype, and natural history of autosomal dominant cyclic hematopoiesis. Am J Med Genet 1996;66:413–22.

18. Souid AK. Congenital cyclic neutropenia. Clin Pediatr (Phila) 1995;34:151–5.

19. Hernandez PA, Gorlin RJ, Lukens JN, et al. Mutations in the chemokine receptor gene CXCR4 are associated with WHIM syndrome, a combined immunodeficiency disease. Nat Genet 2003;34:70–4.

20. Balabanian K, Lagane B, Pablos JL, et al. WHIM syndromes with different genetic anomalies are accounted for by impaired CXCR4 desensitization to CXCL12. Blood 2005;105:2449–57.

21. Balabanian K, Levoye A, Klemm L, et al. Leukocyte analysis from WHIM syndrome patients reveals a pivotal role for GRK3 in CXCR4 signaling. J Clin Invest 2008;118:1074–84.

22. Gulino AV, Moratto D, Sozzani S, et al. Altered leukocyte response to CXCL12 in patients with warts hypogammaglobulinemia, infections, myelokathexis (WHIM) syndrome. Blood 2004;104:444–52.

23. Dale DC. Immune and idiopathic neutropenia. Curr Opin Hematol 1998;5:33–6.

24. Huizinga TW, Kuijpers RW, Kleijer M, et al. Maternal genomic neutrophil FcRIII deficiency leading to neonatal isoimmune neutropenia. Blood 1990;76:1927–32.

25. Stroncek DF, Skubitz KM, Plachta LB, et al. Alloimmune neonatal neutropenia due to an antibody to the neutrophil Fc-gamma receptor III with maternal deficiency of CD16 antigen. Blood 1991;77:1572–80.

26. Fromont P, Bettaieb A, Skouri H, et al. Frequency of the polymorphonuclear Fc-gamma receptor III deficiency in the French population and its involvement in the development of neonatal alloimmune neutropenia. Blood 1992;79:2131–4.

27. Maheshwari A, Christensen RD, Calhoun DA. Immune-mediated neutropenia in the neonate. Acta Paediatr Suppl 2002;91:98–1.

28. Akhtari M, Curtis B, Waller EK. Autoimmune neutropenia in adults. Autoimmun Rev 2009;9:62–6.

29. Barbosa MD, Nguyen QA, Tchernev VT, et al. Identification of the homologous beige and Chediak-Higashi syndrome genes. Nature 1996;382:262–5.

30. Nagle DL, Karim MA, Woolf EA, et al. Identification and mutation analysis of the complete gene for Chediak-Higashi syndrome. Nat Genet 1996;14:307–11.

31. Introne W, Boissy RE, Gahl WA. Clinical, molecular, and cell biological aspects of Chediak-Higashi syndrome. Mol Genet Metab 1999;68:283–303.

32. Huizing M, Helip-Wooley A, Westbroek W, et al. Disorders of lysosome-related organelle biogenesis: clinical and molecular genetics. Annu Rev Genomics Hum Genet 2008;9:359–86.

33. Blume RS, Wolff SM. The Chédiak-Higashi syndrome: studies in four patients and a review of the literature. Medicine (Baltimore) 1972;51:247.

34. Gallin JI, Fletcher MP, Seligmann BE, et al. Human neutrophil-specific granule deficiency: a model to assess the role of the neutrophil-specific granules in the evolution of the inflammatory response. Blood 1982;59:1317–29.

35. Lekstrom-Himes JA, Dorman SE, Kopar P, et al. Neutrophil-specific granule deficiency results from a novel mutation with loss of function of the transcription factor CCAAT/enhancer binding protein epsilon. J Exp Med 1999;189:1847–52.

36. Lekstrom-Himes J, Xanthopoulos KG. Biological role of the CCAAT/enhancer-binding protein family of transcription factors. J Biol Chem 1998;273:28545–8.

37. Gombart AF, Koeffler HP. Neutrophil specific granule deficiency and mutations in the gene encoding transcription factor C/EBP(epsilon). Curr Opin Hematol 2002;9:36–4.

38. Wynn RF, Sood M, Theilgaard-Monch K, et al. Intractable diarrhoea of infancy caused by neutrophil specific granule deficiency and cured by stem cell transplantation. Gut 2006;55:292–6.

39. Segal BH, Leto TL, Gallin JI, et al. Genetic, biochemical, and clinical features of chronic granulomatous disease. Medicine (Baltimore) 2000;79:170–200.

40. Reeves EP, Lu H, Jacobs HL, et al. Killing activity of neutrophils is mediated through activation of proteases by K^+ flux. Nature 2002;416:291–7.

41. Matute J, Arias A, Wright N, et al. A new genetic subgroup of chronic granulomatous disease with autosomal recessive mutations in p40 phox and selective defects in neutrophil NADPH oxidase activity. Blood 2009;114:3309–15.

42. Winkelstein JA, Marino MC, Johnston RB Jr, et al. Chronic granulomatous disease: report on a national registry of 368 patients. Medicine (Baltimore) 2000;79:155–69.

43. Lublin M, Bartlett DL, Danforth DN, et al. Hepatic abscess in patients with chronic granulomatous disease. Ann Surg 2002;235:383–91.

44. Marciano BE, Rosenzweig SD, Kleiner DE, et al. Gastrointestinal involvement in chronic granulomatous disease. Pediatrics 2004;114:462–8.

45. Walther MM, Malech HL, Berman A, et al. The urologic manifestations of chronic granulomatous disease. J Urol 1992;147:1314–8.

46. Chin TW, Stiehm ER, Faloon J, et al. Corticosteroids in treatment of obstructive lesions of chronic granulomatous disease. J Pediatr 1987;111:349–52.

47. Quie PG, Belani KK. Corticosteroids for chronic granulomatous disease. J Pediatr 1987;111:393–4.

48. Goldblatt D, Butcher J, Thrasher AJ, et al. Chorioretinal lesions in patients and carriers of chronic granulomatous disease. J Pediatr 1999;134:780–3.

49. Kim SJ, Kim JG, Yu YS. Chorioretinal lesions in patients with chronic granulomatous disease. Retina 2003;23:360–5.

50. Manzi S, Urbach AH, McCune AB, et al. Systemic lupus erythematosus in a boy with chronic granulomatous disease: case report and review of the literature. Arthritis Rheum 1991;34:101–5.

51. Cale CM, Morton L, Goldblatt D. Cutaneous and other lupus-like symptoms in carriers of X-linked chronic granulomatous disease: incidence and autoimmune serology. Clin Exp Immunol 2007;148:79–84.

52. Anderson-Cohen M, Holland SM, Kuhns DB, et al. Severe phenotype of chronic granulomatous disease presenting in a female with a de novo mutation in gp91-phox and a non familial, extremely skewed X chromosome inactivation. Clin Immunol 2003;109:308–17.

53. Vowells SJ, Sekhsaria S, Malech HL, et al. Flow cytometric analysis of the granulocyte respiratory burst: a comparison study of fluorescent probes. J Immunol Methods 1995;178:89–97.

54. Vowells SJ, Fleisher TA, Sekhsaria S, et al. Genotype-dependent variability in flow cytometric evaluation of reduced nicotinamide adenine dinucleotide phosphate oxidase function in patients with chronic granulomatous disease. J Pediatr 1996;128:104–7.

55. Mauch L, Lun A, O'Gorman MR, et al. Chronic granulomatous disease (CGD) and complete myeloperoxidase deficiency both yield strongly reduced dihydrorhodamine 123 test signals but can be easily discerned in routine testing for CGD. Clin Chem 2007;53:890–6.

56. Ferguson PJ, Lokuta MA, El-Shanti HI, et al. Neutrophil dysfunction in a family with a SAPHO syndrome-like phenotype. Arthritis Rheum 2008;58(10):3264–9.

57. Margolis DM, Melnick DA, Alling DW, et al. Trimethoprim-sulfamethoxazole prophylaxis in the management of chronic granulomatous disease. J Infect Dis 1990;162:723–6.

58. Gallin JI, Alling DW, Malech HL, et al. Itraconazole to prevent fungal infections in chronic granulomatous disease. N Engl J Med 2003;348(24):2416–22.

59. International Chronic Granulomatous Disease Cooperative Study Group: A controlled trial of interferon gamma to prevent infection in chronic granulomatous disease. N Engl J Med 1991;324:509–16.

60. van den Berg JM, van Koppen E, Ahlin A, et al. Chronic granulomatous disease: the European experience. PLoS One 2009;4:e5234.

61. Feld JJ, Hussain N, Wright EC, et al. Hepatic involvement and portal hypertension predict mortality in chronic granulomatous disease. Gastroenterology 2008;134:1917–26.

62. Seger RA, Gungor T, Belohradsky BH, et al. Treatment of chronic granulomatous disease with myeloablative conditioning and an unmodified hemopoietic allograft: a survey of the European experience, 1985–2000. Blood 2002;100:4344–50.

63. Ott MG, Schmidt M, Schwarzwaelder K, et al. Correction of X-linked chronic granulomatous disease by gene therapy, augmented by insertional activation of MDS1-EVI1, PRDM16 or SETBP1. Nat Med 2006;12:401–9.

64. Ott MG, Seger R, Stein S, et al. Advances in the treatment of chronic granulomatous disease by gene therapy. Curr Gene Ther 2007;7:155–61.

65. Nauseef WM. Myeloperoxidase deficiency. Hematol Oncol Clin North Am 1988;2:135.

66. Okuda T, Yasuoka T, Oka N. Myeloperoxidase deficiency as a predisposing factor for deep mucocutaneous candidiasis: a case report. J Oral Maxillofac Surg 1991;49:183–6.

67. Ludviksson BR, Thorarensen O, Gudnason T, et al. Candida albicans meningitis in a child with myeloperoxidase deficiency. Pediatr Infect Dis J 1993;12:162–4.

68. Nguyen C, Katner HP. Myeloperoxidase deficiency manifesting as pustular candidal dermatitis. Clin Infect Dis 1997;24:258–60.

69. Chiang AK, Chan GC, Ma SK, et al. Disseminated fungal infection associated with myeloperoxidase deficiency in a premature neonate. Pediatr Infect Dis J 2000;19:1027–9.

70. Notarangelo LD, Badolato R. Leukocyte trafficking in primary immunodeficiencies. J Leukoc Biol 2009;85:335–43.

71. Anderson DC, Schmalsteig FC, Finegold MJ, et al. The severe and moderate phenotypes of heritable Mac-1, LFA-1 deficiency: their quantitative definition and relation to leukocyte dysfunction and clinical features. J Infect Dis 1985;152:668–89.

72. Kuijpers TW, van Lier RAW, Hamann D, et al. Leukocyte adhesion deficiency type 1 (LAD/1)/variant. J Clin Invest 1997;100:1725–33.

73. Hogg N, Stewart MP, Scarth SL, et al. A novel leukocyte adhesion deficiency caused by expressed but nonfunctional beta2 integrins Mac-1 and LFA-1. J Clin Invest 1999;103:97–106.

74. Uzel G, Tng E, Rosenzweig SD, et al. Reversion mutations in patients with leukocyte adhesion deficiency type-1 (LAD-1). Blood 2008;111(1):209–18.

75. Thomas C, Le Deist F, Cavazzana-Calvo M, et al. Results of allogeneic bone marrow transplantation in patients with leukocyte adhesion deficiency. Blood 1995;86:1629–35.

76. Bauer TR Jr, Gu YC, Creevy KE, et al. Leukocyte adhesion deficiency in children and Irish setter dogs. Pediatr Res 2004;55:363–7.

77. Lübke T, Marquardt T, Etzioni A, et al. Complementation cloning identifies CDG-IIc, a new type of congenital disorders of glycosylation, as a GDP-glucose transporter deficiency. Nat Genet 2001;28:73–6.

78. Lühn K, Wild MK, Eckhardt M, et al. The gene defective in leukocyte adhesion deficiency II encodes a putative GDP-fucose transporter. Nat Genet 2001;28:69–72.

79. Etzioni A, Gershoni-Baruch R, Pollack S, et al. Leukocyte adhesion deficiency type II: long-term follow-up. J Allergy Clin Immunol 1998;102:323–4.

80. Marquardt T, Luhn K, Srikrishna G, et al. Correction of leukocyte adhesion deficiency type II with oral glucose. Blood 1999;94:3976–85.

81. Etzioni A, Tonetti M. Glucose supplementation in leukocyte adhesion deficiency type II (letter). Blood 2000;95:3641–2.

82. Mory A, Feigelson SW, Yarali N, et al. Kindlin-3: a new gene involved in the pathogenesis of LAD-III. Blood 2008;112:2591.

83. Kuijpers TW, van de Vijver E, Weterman MA, et al. LAD-1/variant syndrome is caused by mutations in FERMT3. Blood 2009;113:4740–6.

84. Ambruso DR, Knall C, Abell AN, et al. Human neutrophil immunodeficiency syndrome is associated with an inhibitory Rac2 mutation. Proc Natl Acad Sci U S A 2000;97:4654–9.

85. Williams DA, Tao W, Yang F, et al. Dominant negative mutation of the hematopoietic-specific Rho GTPase, Rac2, is associated with a human phagocyte immunodeficiency. Blood 2000;96:1646–54.

86. Hanson EP, Monaco-Shawver L, Solt LA, et al. Hypomorphic nuclear factor-kappaB essential modulator mutation database and reconstitution system identifies phenotypic and immunologic diversity. J Allergy Clin Immunol 2008;122:1169–77.e16.

87. Smahi A, Courtois G, Vabres P, et al. Genomic rearrangement in NEMO impairs NF-kappaB activation and is a cause of incontinentia pigmenti. The International Incontinentia Pigmenti (IP) Consortium. Nature 2000;405:466–72.

88. Haverkamp MH, van Dissel JT, Holland SM. Human host genetic factors in nontuberculous mycobacterial infection: lessons from single gene disorders affecting innate and adaptive immunity and lessons from molecular defects in interferon-gamma-dependent signaling. Microbes Infect 2006;8(4):1157–66.

89. Al-Muhsen S, Casanova JL. The genetic heterogeneity of mendelian susceptibility to mycobacterial diseases. J Allergy Clin Immunol 2008;122(6):1043–51.

90. Jouanguy E, Lamhamedi-Cherradi S, Lammas D, et al. A human IFNGR1 small deletion hotspot associated with dominant susceptibility to mycobacterial infection. Nat Genet 1999;21:370–8.

91. Fieschi C, Dupuis S, Catherinot E, et al. Low penetrance, broad resistance, and favorable outcome of interleukin 12 receptor beta1 deficiency: medical and immunological implications. J Exp Med 2003;197:527–35.

92. Fleisher AT, Dorman SE, Anderson JA, et al. Detection of intracellular phosphorylated STAT-1 by flow cytometry. Clin Immunol 1999;90:425–30.

93. Uzel G, Frucht DM, Fleisher A, et al. Detection of intracellular phosphorylated STAT-4 by flow cytometry. Clin Immunol 2001;100:270–6.

94. Grimbacher B, Holland SM, Gallin JI, et al. Hyper-IgE syndrome with recurrent infections: an autosomal dominant multisystem disorder. N Engl J Med 1999;340:692–702.

95. Minegishi Y, Saito M, Tsuchiya S, et al. Dominant negative mutations in the DNA-binding domain of STAT3 cause hyper-IgE syndrome. Nature 2007;448:1058–62.

96. Holland SM, DeLeo FR, Elloumi HZ, et al. STAT3 mutations in the hyper-IgE syndrome. N Engl J Med 2007;18:1608–19.

97. Freeman AF, Holland SM. The hyper-IgE syndromes. Immunol Allergy Clin N Am 2008;28:277–91.

98. Ling JC, Freeman AF, Gharib AM, et al. Coronary artery aneurysms in patients with hyper IgE recurrent infection syndrome. Clin Immunol 2007;122:255–8.

99. Freeman AF, Collura-Burke CJ, Patronas NJ, et al. Brain abnormalities in patients with hyperimmunoglobulin E syndrome. Pediatrics 2007;119: e1121–e1125.

100. Leonard GD, Posadas E, Herrmann PC, et al. Non-Hodgkin's lymphoma in Job's syndrome: a case report and review of the literature. Leuk Lymphoma 2004;45:2521–5.

101. Renner ED, Puck JM, Holland SM, et al. Autosomal recessive hyper-immunoglobulin E syndrome: a distinct disease entity. J Pediatr 2004;144:93–9.

102. Zhang Q, Davis JC, Lamborn IT, et al. Combined immunodeficiency associated with DOCK8 mutations. N Engl J Med 2009;361.

103. Engelhardt KR, McGhee S, Winkler S, et al. Large deletions and point mutations involving the dedicator of cytokinesis 8 (DOCK8) in the autosomal-recessive form of hyper-IgE syndrome. J Allergy Clin Immunol 2009;124:1289–302.

104. Minegishi Y, Saito M, Morio T, et al. Human tyrosine kinase 2 deficiency reveals its requisite roles in multiple cytokine signals involved in innate and acquired immunity. Immunity 2006;25(5): 745–55.

105. Ferwerda B, Ferwerda G, Plantinga TS, et al. Human dectin-1 deficiency and mucocutaneous fungal infections. N Engl J Med 2009;361: 1760–7.

106. Glocker EO, Hennigs A, Nabavi M, et al. A homozygous CARD9 mutation in a family with susceptibility to fungal infections. N Engl J Med 2009;361:1727–35.

CHAPTER 12

White Blood Cell Defects

13

Rheumatic Diseases of Childhood: Therapeutic Principles

J. Roger Hollister

The rheumatic diseases of childhood encompass a wide spectrum of symptomatology. As a group, these illnesses are considered to be autoimmune disorders, implying that pathogenesis involves the host's immune system producing inflammation in the affected organs. Important disease differentials include those caused by a specific agent (e.g. septic arthritis, Lyme disease), malignancy (e.g. solid tumors or hematologic neoplasia), and allergic disorders (e.g. chronic sinusitis, chronic urticaria, or serum sickness). Box 13-1 lists the disease differential. Figure 13-1 is an algorithm for an approach to the evaluation of musculoskeletal pain in childhood.

Juvenile Idiopathic Arthritis

Juvenile idiopathic arthritis (JIA) is the most common rheumatic disease of childhood.[1] It affects approximately one in a thousand children under the age of 16 years. There is a three to one female predominance except for the systemic-onset type, which is more gender neutral. The cause of JIA remains unknown. The most promising research suggests a multigene predisposition in combination with an unknown environmental agent. Diet, trauma, person-to-person transmission, and geographic locale have been eliminated as potential causes. The pathogenesis involves chronic inflammation of synovial tissue with infiltration of neutrophils and activated macrophages and lymphocytes. Many cytokines are locally active, and tumor necrosis factor (TNF) may play a central regulatory role.[2,3] There are three disease-onset patterns that have been recognized, and the natural history and complications are sufficiently unique to each type to merit the distinction.

Diagnosis

Oligoarticular JIA is the most common type. There are two peaks of onset: one between the ages of 1 and 5 years and the other between 12 and 16 years. Most patients present with a gradual onset of pain and swelling in one to four joints. The pattern is frequently asymmetric. The knee is most commonly affected, followed by the ankle, wrist, and elbow. The role of trauma as the triggering event for the chronic inflammatory process is difficult to analyze because children frequently experience mild extremity trauma as a result of their normal daily activities. Although there may be a history of such minor trauma, joint swelling lasting more than 24 hours is distinctly unusual from orthopedic causes. Similarly, internal mechanical derangements such as torn menisci are very uncommon in childhood.

The pain may range from being quite severe to extremely mild, where only the joint swelling is manifest. Morning stiffness or gelling during the day is very characteristic and suggests an inflammatory cause to the joint swelling. It is important to obtain a history with regard to limping or failure to use an upper extremity in judging the severity of joint pain, particularly in individuals whose joint swelling may not be apparent.

It is unusual for JIA to begin in a single hip, and such onset requires a wider differential diagnosis, particularly of orthopedic conditions within the hip. With onset below the age of 3 years, particularly with involvement of a single knee, there is the possibility of leg-length discrepancy over time and significant muscle atrophy.[4] There is evidence that a local steroid injection may prevent these sequelae.[5]

The oligoarticular pattern of JIA onset defines a type of arthritis that is uniquely at risk for chronic, asymptomatic anterior uveitis. This may occur in up to 30% of such children if they are antinuclear antibody (ANA) positive. Detection of the uveitis is not possible with a routine ophthalmoscope, and therefore these children need to be in a screening program with an ophthalmologist for slit-lamp evaluation of the earliest signs of inflammation. Early detection of the uveitis is important in preventing sequelae, which may lead to decreased visual acuity or even blindness.[6]

Oligoarticular presentation in males over the age of 10 years, particularly with lower-extremity involvement, suggests the possibility of a spondyloarthropathy (see the section 'Spondyloarthropathies').

Polyarticular Juvenile Idiopathic Arthritis

Polyarticular JIA affects many joints, large and small, and frequently manifests a symmetric pattern. This type of JIA most resembles adult rheumatoid arthritis in its clinical presentation. It is important to obtain both a history and physical evidence of joint swelling in defining these individuals because there are other causes of only arthralgias (see Figure 13-1). It is this group of patients who may manifest rheumatoid nodules over areas of dermal trauma such as the elbows or feet. Systemic features are more common in this group of patients and include afternoon fatigue and anemia.

A subgroup of polyarticular JIA patients has positive tests for rheumatoid factor, most often in the older-age onset children. In long-term follow-up studies, the presence of rheumatoid factors

©2010 Elsevier Ltd, Inc, BV
DOI: 10.1016/B978-1-4377-0271-2.00013-4

BOX 13-1

Differential Diagnosis of Musculoskeletal Pain

I. Autoimmune diseases
   A. Arthritides
      Juvenile idiopathic arthritis
      Spondyloarthropathies
      Reactive, acute rheumatic fever
         Postdysentery
         Transient synovitis
   B. Collagen vascular disorders
      Systemic lupus erythematosus
      Juvenile dermatomyositis
      Vasculitis: Henoch-Schönlein purpura, polyarteritis nodosa, Kawasaki disease, Wegener's granulomatosis

II. Infections
   A. Bacterial septic arthritis
   B. Lyme disease
   C. Viral: Parvo B19

III. Malignancy
   A. Solid tumors
   B. Leukemia
   C. Neuroblastoma

IV. Orthopedic
   A. Trauma
   B. Aseptic necrosis (Legg-Calvé-Perthes disease)
   C. Slipped capital femoral epiphysis
   D. Stress fracture
   E. Spondylolysis and spondylolisthesis
   F. Osteochondroses (Osgood-Schlatter disease, Sever's disease)

V. Pain syndromes
   A. Growing pains
   B. Fibromyalgia
   C. Overuse syndrome
   D. Hypermobility syndrome
   E. Complex regional pain syndrome

---

in serum connotes more aggressive disease with a greater possibility of joint damage and disability.[1] Antibodies to cyclic citrullinated peptide (CCP) are new antibodies identified in children with polyarticular JIA which are also associated with long-term joint damage.[7] Therefore, seropositive children with polyarticular JIA should be treated early with second-level antiinflammatory or immunosuppressive medications.

The third type of JIA, *systemic-onset JIA* (called *Still's disease* in Europe), is the least common form. It presents to the physician as a fever of unknown origin (FUO). The fevers are prolonged, lasting from weeks to months. They are high-grade fevers reaching 104° to 105° F on a daily basis, often at the same time each day.[8] They have a quotidian or double quotidian pattern with normal or subnormal temperature levels in between. Sustained fevers throughout a 24-hour period are not characteristic. Patients may experience chills and toxicity with the fevers, which improve during afebrile intervals. Appetite is frequently decreased, and weight loss may occur.

A diagnostic rash occurs in 90% of patients with systemic-onset JIA[9] (Figure 13-2). The rash consists of an evanescent 3- to 5-mm erythematous macular or barely papular lesion occurring most commonly on the trunk and proximal extremities; however, the rash can involve the face and hands and feet as well. A rash located in a single area for more than 24 hours is incompatible with the diagnosis. The rash may be asymptomatic or occasionally pruritic and is frequently found during fever elevations. The rash may demonstrate the Koebner phenomenon of rash induction with dermal trauma. In patients with a diagnostic rash, extensive evaluation for other causes of an FUO may not be necessary.

Less specific symptoms or findings include lymphadenopathy, hepatosplenomegaly, or serositis. Joint symptoms may be lacking in the first several weeks of the FUO in these patients. Arthralgia may be more prominent than arthritis.

Laboratory assessment of systemic-onset JIA shows striking evidence of inflammation. The white blood cell count is frequently elevated in the 20 000 to 30 000 range with a left shift. Sedimentation rate is always elevated, usually between 60 to 80 mm/hr. A normal sedimentation rate excludes the diagnosis of systemic-onset JIA. Anemia may be significant, with hemoglobin as low as 7 g/dL but rarely lower. Platelet counts should be normal and are frequently significantly elevated. Thrombocytopenia is a worrisome finding and suggests an alternative diagnosis such as malignancy, lupus, or macrophage activation syndrome.

Laboratory Assessment

The laboratory assessment of JIA should include a complete blood cell count (CBC), sedimentation rate, ANA, rheumatoid factor, and anti-CCP antibodies (the last two tests in older-age children with polyarticular presentation); the results may be nondiagnostic. Oligoarticular JIA with a single involved joint may demonstrate a normal sedimentation rate, which does not mitigate against the diagnosis in a patient who, by history and physical examination, demonstrates chronic synovitis. A positive ANA in a patient with oligoarticular disease increases the risk of uveitis from 10% to 30%. All ANA-positive oligoarticular patients need 3-month ophthalmologic screening, whereas ANA-negative patients can be screened every 6 months. The duration of the ophthalmologic screening should be for 4 years after the onset of the arthritis regardless of whether the joint disease enters remission. Systemic-onset JIA patients never have a positive ANA or rheumatoid factor. In older-age onset males with lower-extremity presentation, a human leukocyte antigen (HLA)-B27 test may be positive in support of the diagnosis of a spondyloarthopathy.

X-rays of involved joints show little more than soft tissue swelling. Bone scans in perplexing patients usually show tracer uptake on both sides of the joint, which is consistent with arthritis and not indicative of osteomyelitis. Magnetic resonance imaging (MRI) scans are rarely indicated but, when performed, show increased joint fluid with evidence of synovial inflammation.

Differential Diagnosis

Pain in a single extremity requires that infection and malignancy be excluded. With either of these conditions, the pain is usually progressive and severe. If a joint is not swollen, osteomyelitis, bone tumor, or hematologic malignancy are possible. An X-ray and blood count with sedimentation rate can help to distinguish these entities. In questionable cases, an MRI can help

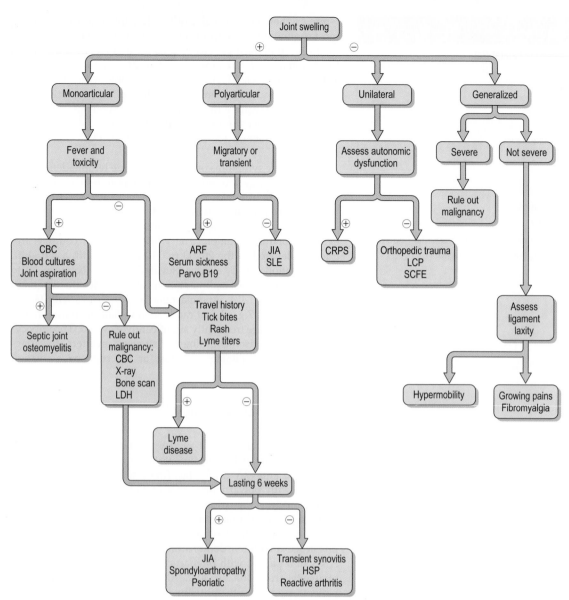

Figure 13-1 Algorithm for evaluation of musculoskeletal pain in childhood. *CBC*, complete blood cell count; *ARF*, acute rheumatic fever; *JIA*, juvenile idiopathic arthritis, *SLE*, systemic lupus erythematosus; *CRPS*, complex regional pain syndrome. *LCP*, Legg-Calvé-Perthes disease; *SCFE*, slipped capital femoral epiphysis; *LDH*, lactic dehydrogenase; *HSP*, Henoch-Schönlein purpura.

differentiate osteomyelitis, and serum lactate dehydrogenase (LDH) can discriminate conditions with rapid cell turnover such as malignancy.[10]

If a joint is acutely swollen with progressive pain, fever, toxicity, and erythema over the joint, septic arthritis must be excluded by aspiration of the joint (see Figure 13-1). A septic hip will not, however, demonstrate joint swelling, but patients are usually systemically ill, the pain is rapidly progressive, and the white blood count and sedimentation rate are markedly elevated. *Staphylococcus* accounts for the vast majority of septic joints, and in acute situations, treatment with the appropriate antibiotic is reasonable until the results of the cultures are known. With monoarticular involvement of the lower extremity and a preceding history of viral infection and only moderate pain, a reactive arthritis or transient synovitis may be the most likely explanation; blood work and sedimentation rates will be normal.

With polyarticular joint complaints and swelling, the differential diagnosis includes rheumatic fever, systemic lupus erythematosus (SLE), disseminated gonococcal infection, and in the

adolescent population Parvo B19 viral arthritis. The arthritis of rheumatic fever is frequently migratory and quite painful. Evidence of rheumatic carditis should be carefully sought with auscultation for a regurgitant heart murmur. Markedly elevated sedimentation rates are the hallmark of rheumatic fever and poststreptococcal arthritis. Evidence of recent streptococcal infection with antibody titers is essential to the diagnosis. The polyarthralgia and polyarthritis of SLE is usually accompanied by other evidence of multi-organ involvement with that disease. Disseminated gonococcal infection with polyarthralgia and eventual monoarthritis is usually accompanied by embolic skin lesions, onset during menstruation, and a history of recent unprotected sex. Parvovirus B19 polyarthritis may be distinguished by exposure to children with fifth disease, skin rash, and low-grade fever.

Lyme arthritis resembles oligoarticular JIA; however, it occurs as discrete, recurrent episodes of arthritis lasting 2 to 6 weeks.[11] It appears primarily in five states, all of which are endemic for Lyme disease. A negative test for antibodies to *Borrelia burgdorferi* excludes this diagnosis.

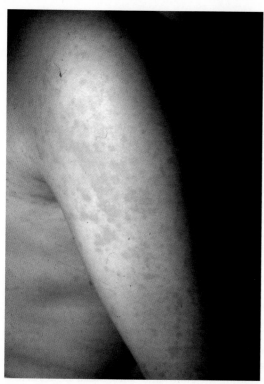
Figure 13-2 Skin eruption in systemic juvenile idiopathic arthritis.

Juvenile Idiopathic Arthritis

Antiinflammatory Medications

Nonsteroidal antiinflammatory drugs

COX2 inhibitor

Steroids

Analgesics

Rehabilitation Techniques

Physical therapy

Occupational therapy

Psychologic support

Exercise

Advanced Therapies

Immunosuppressants

Biologic agents

Treatment

The treatment principles for JIA are shown in Box 13-2. The treatment of JIA begins with nonsteroidal antiinflammatory drugs (NSAIDs). For younger children who require liquid medications, naprosyn (7.5 mg/kg twice daily) or ibuprofen (10 mg/kg two or three times daily) and meloxicam (0.125 mg/kg) are available. For older children, naprosyn 250 to 375 mg twice daily, diclofenac 50 to 75 mg twice daily, tolmetin (30 mg/kg/day) or meloxicam 15 mg once a day should provide symptomatic relief. The COX2 inhibitor, celecoxib, 6 mg/kg twice a day has been approved for children over the age of 2 years. Celecoxib produces less gastric irritation, and it does not affect platelet function. Temporary symptomatic relief using steroids such as prednisone 5 mg daily

or twice daily should be done in consultation with a pediatric rheumatologist.

Second-line therapy of JIA begins with methotrexate in a low dose, administered on a weekly basis. Newer agents, including TNF inhibitors (etanercept and infliximab), are available for patients in whom methotrexate therapy fails.[12] The newest biologic agents approved for the treatment of JIA are adalimumab[13] and abatacept.[14] Anakinra is an IL1 receptor antagonist which is uniquely effective in systemic-onset JIA.

Prognosis

Overall, the prognosis for patients with JIA is markedly better than it was in the late 1990s. Treatment with second-line agents has reduced disability and the need for total joint replacement; 80% to 90% of children should have a favorable course and be able to maintain a largely normal lifestyle. Less favorable prognosis is associated with systemic-onset JIA that becomes chronic arthritis, chronic uveitis, and rheumatoid factor-positive polyarticular JIA.[1]

Spondyloarthropathies

Diagnosis

The spondyloarthropathies are a group of inflammatory disorders in childhood, which at disease onset and over the course of time are distinguishable from the more common JIA.[15] Several characteristics of these patients set them apart and, with proper classification, should suggest somewhat different treatments and follow-up protocols. As a group, these patients have an older age of onset (usually over the age of 9 years), males are much more affected than females, and pauciarticular lower-extremity synovitis is most typical. The history frequently reveals evidence of enthesitis (inflammation at the insertion of tendons and ligaments on bone), most often at the heel or at the knee over the tibial tuberosity; enthesitis is very uncommon in children with JIA. Furthermore, the history frequently reveals other members of the family in preceding generations with ankylosing spondylitis, psoriasis, inflammatory bowel disease, or Reiter's disease. These individuals, in particular those with a strong family history, may be HLA-B27 positive. Axial involvement (sacroiliitis or lumbosacral pain) may not be present at disease onset but may evolve over time, which allows better classification of these individuals.

Extraarticular manifestations include acute iritis (a hot, red, photophobic process markedly different from the silent, chronic uveitis seen in JIA patients). Psoriatic skin lesions, symptoms of inflammatory bowel disease, or the quite rare triad of Reiter's syndrome (conjunctivitis, urethritis, and arthritis) may be found.

As with other inflammatory arthritic conditions, the history may indicate morning stiffness and fatigue, which may be helpful in distinguishing these entities from the osteochondroses (Osgood-Schlatter disease or Sever's disease).

Laboratory Assessment

Laboratory assessment may reveal an elevated sedimentation rate or C-reactive protein (CRP) indicative of inflammation as the source of the patient's symptoms as opposed to trauma or overuse. ANA is rarely positive and rheumatoid factors are absent. Positive tests for HLA-B27 provide supportive information but are not diagnostic.[16] The test is positive in approximately 80% to 90% of patients as opposed to 6% to 8% in the general Caucasian population. Therefore, a negative HLA-B27 does not exclude the diagnosis if the clinical symptomatology is characteristic.

Radiologic techniques are not especially useful early in the disease course. Routine X-rays may show swelling of peripheral joints. MRI, which is expensive, may show the same inflammatory process at the enthesis or tendon sheath, which is evident on physical examination.

Differential diagnosis includes patients with oligoarticular JIA, overuse syndromes such as plantar fasciitis, and the osteochondroses.

Pathology

Pathologic specimens from affected areas reveal chronic inflammation indistinguishable from JIA. The pathogenesis of these diseases in patients who are HLA-B27 positive may relate to specific environmental triggers (see a fuller discussion in Chapter 14).

Treatment

Patients identified as having a spondyloarthopathy do not need to undergo long-term screening slit-lamp examinations as JIA patients would need to do because their eye symptoms are dramatic and lead to early referral to an ophthalmologist.

In patients with axial involvement of the lumbosacral spine or sacroiliac joints, physical therapy to maintain good posture is very important. Should a child's illness evolve into typical ankylosing spondylitis, fusion of axial joints is possible, and physical therapy should ensure that this is done in the most functional position possible. Orthotics may be of some benefit in managing the enthesitis in the foot.

Although no control trials in children have been conducted, naproxen 20 mg/kg/day), tolmetin (20 to 30 mg/kg/day), and indomethacin (2 to 4 mg/kg/day) are more effective than other nonsteroidal agents. Refractory cases may benefit from treatment with sulfasalazine.[17] Response to methotrexate is less impressive than it is in JIA patients. Treatment with the new anti-TNF agents appears effective in adult series and may well be applied to children with these disorders.

Systemic Lupus Erythematosus

SLE is the prototypic autoimmune disease with the most diverse clinical presentation resulting from multiorgan disease.[18] Disease pathogenesis is related to the deposition in tissue of soluble immune complexes. The spectrum of manifestations is not caused by tissue-specific autoantibodies but rather by immune complex deposition with subsequent inflammatory events with neutrophils, lymphocytes, complement activation, and cytokine production. Initiation and perpetuation of the disease may be caused by autoreactive T lymphocytes that have escaped clonal deletion and poorly regulated B lymphocytes producing autoantibodies. Integral to the activation of these T and B cells may be a defect in apoptosis and handling of self antigens in these patients.[19]

SLE is not a common disease. Various estimates from several different series have concluded that the annual incidence is approximately 0.36 cases per 100 000 children under the age of 16 years; SLE under the age of 6 years is rare. The female-to-male ratio is approximately 8:1, depending on the series. SLE appears to be both more common and more severe in the African-American and Hispanic populations.

Diagnosis

The diagnosis of SLE has benefited from criteria developed and validated by the American College of Rheumatology and these are listed in Box 13.3. If 4 of the 11 criteria are fulfilled in an individual patient, there is a 90% probability that SLE is the correct diagnosis.

Musculoskeletal symptoms of joint pain and swelling are the most common organ system manifestations of SLE. They are present at onset or during disease evolution in more than 90% of patients.[20] If patients present with only constitutional symptoms such as fatigue, malaise, subjective weakness, or a weight loss, one should not seriously consider SLE or an ANA unless arthritic symptoms are part of the history. The pain of the arthritis, although it is a 'nonerosive' process, may be more striking than the degree of swelling in the individual joints found on physical examination.

Rashes in SLE may take many forms (Figure 13-3). Vasculitic rashes appear as 3- to 4-mm erythematous, non-blanching macular, or macular/papular, which may be seen on many parts of the body, including the palms and soles. Malar rashes across the cheeks and over the bridge of the nose, which gave the disease its name because it was felt to resemble the mask or bite of the wolf, are present in fewer than 50% of SLE patients. Besides erythema in that distribution, there should be evidence of scaling and follicular plugging. Photosensitive rashes may be seen in other parts of the body besides the malar distribution, where ultraviolet light exposure occurs. However, true photosensitivity occurs in only 30% of SLE patients. These individuals must protect the skin from ultraviolet exposure, as a flare of the skin

---

BOX 13-3

American College of Rheumatology 1997 Criteria for Systemic Lupus Erythematosus

Malar (butterfly) rash

Discoid–lupus rash

Photosensitivity

Oral or nasal mucocutaneous ulceration

Nonerosive arthritis

Nephritis

    Proteinuria 0.5 g/day

    Cellular casts

Encephalopathy

    Seizures

    Psychosis

Pleuritis or pericarditis

Cytopenias

Positive immunoserology

    Antibodies to dsDNA

    Antibodies to Smith nuclear antigen

    Positive tests for antiphospholipid antibodies (lupus anticoagulant or anticardiolipin antibodies)

Positive antinuclear antibody

From Hochberg MC. Arthritis Rheum 1997;40:1725.

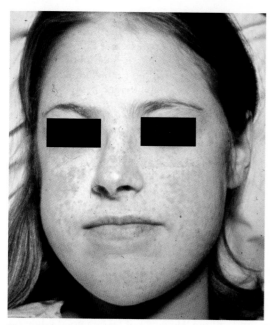

Figure 13-3 Rash in systemic lupus erythematosus.

disease may lead to a generalized autoimmune activation of the symptoms in many other organs. Urticaria as a skin manifestation is very uncommon in SLE. Evidence of other organ involvement should be sought in urticarial patients before ordering an ANA because there is a considerable false-positive ANA rate in chronic urticaria patients.

Chest pain may suggest lung or heart involvement in SLE. Pleuritis is the most common lung manifestation in SLE. Pleuritic chest pain and shortness of breath are the usual symptoms. Physical examination may reveal diminished breath sounds indicating a pleural effusion, which can be documented by a chest X-ray. Pulmonary hemorrhage, a rare but potentially lethal manifestation of SLE, should be suspected in patients with cough, hypoxia, and rapid fall in hemoglobin. Hemoptysis may not be present. Costochondritis may mimic pleuritic chest pain, but on physical examination there are discrete tender areas at the costochondral junctions along the sternum.

Pericarditis is the most common cardiac manifestation of SLE. The chest pain is usually precordial and it is worse in the recumbent position. A chest X-ray will show cardiomegaly, and an echocardiogram can ascertain that this is caused by pericardial fluid as opposed to cardiac dilation. Electrocardiogram changes are a less sensitive way of detecting pericarditis. Liebman-Sachs endocarditis is an unusual finding in the pediatric population; when it occurs, it most often involves the mitral value with a new onset of a systolic regurgitant heart murmur.

Gastrointestinal involvement in SLE is uncommon; however, acute pancreatitis with severe left upper quadrant pain penetrating to the back can be an emergent situation. Liver involvement may produce mild elevation of hepatocellular enzymes but rarely causes symptoms.

Lupus nephritis produces no symptoms at disease onset. Microscopic hematuria, proteinuria, and cellular casts are indications of lupus nephritis. Hypertension, which requires treatment, is a frequent concomitant of lupus nephritis, especially when steroid therapy is initiated. In the past, lupus nephritis was a major cause of death, and in the modern era it is still capable of producing end-stage renal disease. Therefore aggressive therapy is indicated, although patients rarely experience symptoms directly attributable to the nephritis.

Anemia and thrombocytopenia reflect other aspects of this autoimmune diathesis. Autoimmune Coombs' positive hemolytic anemia is less common than an inflammatory anemia of chronic disease with decreased red cell production. Teenagers with the new onset of idiopathic thrombocytopenic purpura should be screened for wider evidence of an autoimmune process.

Neuropsychologic involvement in SLE patients is rare as a presenting symptom, with the exception of chorea. Seizures, stroke, and peripheral neuropathies are manifestations that are easy to discern. The more difficult issues arise with psychologic symptoms such as affective disorders, organic brain syndromes, and psychosis. Radiologic imaging is most helpful in patients with focal neurologic findings, but when the manifestations are primarily psychologic, computed tomography (CT) scans and MRIs are frequently normal.[21] Headaches are common in lupus patients and frequently have the characteristics of a vascular headache, but their occurrence does not necessarily parallel other manifestations of the disease and may exist when the rest of the patient's lupus is in excellent control.

Constitutional symptoms, which are not specific for lupus but nonetheless trouble the patient, include fever, weight loss, and fatigue. The organic fatigue of SLE tends to occur in the afternoon and evening, and it interferes with activities that patients enjoy doing. The fatigue may also be the last symptom to improve once therapy has been initiated.

Laboratory Assessment

A CBC will frequently show an anemia, leukopenia, or thrombocytopenia. Anemia is Coombs' positive in 15% of patients but it is often indicative of the anemia of chronic disease. The leukopenia most often shows a relative lymphopenia. Thrombocytopenia may manifest large platelets, suggesting autoimmune destruction.

The sedimentation rate is elevated in 90% of patients with SLE.[20] Although it is not specific, this test is very useful in discerning patients with inflammatory causes for their symptomatology. In many settings it may be worthwhile to measure the sedimentation rate before an ANA is ordered.

Because the ANA test is positive in more than 95% of SLE patients, a negative ANA effectively excludes the diagnosis of SLE. In SLE the titer of ANA is usually high (>1:160). The fluorescent pattern reported on the ANA is not very helpful.

False-positive ANAs are seen more in the pediatric population. These are usually of low titer (<1:320). In patients in whom the sedimentation rate is normal and the ANA is of low titer, further laboratory assessment is frequently not necessary. The reasons for the false-positive ANA incidence in pediatric patients may relate to frequent viral or streptococcal infections. Repetition of low titer positive ANAs is not recommended because they are likely to remain positive.

In patients in whom there is a high titer-positive ANA, an ANA profile provides increased disease specificity if it is positive. Table 13.1 lists the elements of the ANA profile and their disease associations. Only 60% of patients fulfilling the diagnostic criteria for SLE will have elements positive on the ANA profile. Anti-DNA antibodies reflect disease activity; the other antibodies do not.

With successful treatment of SLE, the anti-DNA antibody levels should fall. Recrudescence of disease may be heralded by increases in anti-DNA levels.

In patients with lupus nephritis, the routine urinalysis is the most sensitive indicator of both disease activity and response to

Table 13-1 Antinuclear Antibody Profile

Test	Disease Association
Anti-DNA	Systemic lupus erythematosus (SLE) with nephritis
Anti-SM (Smith)	SLE
Anti-SSA/anti SSB	SLE with photosensitivity Sjögren's syndrome Neonatal SLE
Antiribonuclear protein	SLE and mixed connective tissue disease
Anticentromere or anti-SCL70	Scleroderma

therapy. Hematuria is usually microscopic. Cellular casts are helpful but depend on the freshness of the specimen. Proteinuria can be quantitated and followed with a spot, protein-to-creatinine ratio. Values less than 0.2 are normal, and values greater than 2.0 are indicative of nephrotic levels of proteinuria. Timed collections of urine to quantitate proteinuria are both tedious and frequently inaccurate. Similarly, serum creatinine levels provide accurate information; however, the glomerular filtration rate must be below 50% of normal before seeing an elevation in the serum creatinine. In questionable cases, timed creatinine clearances can provide additional information.

The serum C3 level is useful both for SLE diagnosis and monitoring disease activity.[22] Total hemolytic complement values correlate well in lupus patients with the C3 and are technically more difficult. However, in patients in whom a complement deficiency leading to SLE is a strong consideration, a single CH50 value can be obtained, and if the result is zero, individual complement factor levels can be measured to ascertain the complement deficiency. Measurements of complement split products (C3a, C5a, and others) have not been proven to improve the laboratory reflection of disease activity more than the C3 level itself. As with anti-DNA antibodies, C3 values that are low in untreated disease, indicating complement consumption, will improve with therapy and disease control. C3 levels that fall during therapy may herald a disease flare. However, some patients maintain low C3 levels, and therapy should be adjusted to the degree of patient symptomatology. C4 levels are not useful in the diagnosis or management of SLE. The frequency of various C4 null genes in the population is sufficiently frequent that this will result in persistently low C4 levels regardless of therapy and disease control.

In patients with SLE, measurements of antiphospholipid antibodies are important because these antibodies contribute to an increased risk of venous and arterial thromboses.[23] Anticardiolipin antibodies detect one type of prothrombotic antibody. The presence of a lupus anticoagulant (a different epitope) is most often detected with a prolonged partial tissue prothrombin time, which does not correct when mixed with fresh plasma. A Russell viper venom time should also be measured as a sensitive indicator of a lupus anticoagulant. Patients who have antiphospholipid antibodies should be treated with one baby aspirin per day (see 'Treatment' section). Unfortunately, these antibodies are relatively steroid resistant and are likely to exist for long periods of time regardless of disease therapy.

Treatment

Successful management of SLE begins with education of the patients and their families. SLE is a complicated disease, and it is to be anticipated that it will take two or three education sessions for them to feel comfortable with the information. It is important that all those involved realize that SLE is a lifelong condition. They also need to know that the possibility of a drug-free remission occurs in only a small percentage of patients; the remainder can be expected to do well but remain on medication. At disease onset, fatigue and decreased endurance occur in the majority of patients, and they should modify their schedules to include adequate amounts of rest. There is no proof that any specific diet is beneficial to the disease. Patients treated with steroids should take a diet adequate in calcium (1500 mg/day), and the diet should be a no-salt-added diet to reduce the cosmetic puffiness associated with salt and water retention.

In mild SLE nonsteroidal medications can provide significant benefit to the musculoskeletal symptomatology. In the absence of renal disease, most nonsteroidal medications are safe.

Antimalarial therapy has been a cornerstone for the management of certain aspects of SLE. These medications exert a significant antiinflammatory effect. Hydroxychloroquine is used in a dose of 5 to 7 mg/kg/day, with a maximum of 400 mg once a day, and has been shown to be beneficial for the skin disease, joint symptoms, and fatigue. However, it takes a good while for the benefits to be realized by the patient, so a trial of 8 to 12 weeks should be envisioned. The side-effects include occasional nausea, rare skin pigment change, and the possibility of a retinopathy for which ophthalmologic supervision is necessary at 12-month intervals.

Steroid therapy is the cornerstone of acute management of SLE with major organ involvement or cytopenias. High-dose steroid therapy is necessary at disease onset at a dose of 2 mg/kg/day divided into doses every 12 hours. For seriously ill children, more rapid control of symptoms can be achieved with intravenous Solu-Medrol (30 mg/kg with a maximum dose of 1000 mg) given once a day for 3 days followed on the fourth day with prednisone at 2 mg/kg/day. The long-term goal in steroid therapy for the management of SLE is to reduce the dose to a nontoxic level.

With control of symptomatology and laboratory improvement (i.e. normal erythrocyte sedimentation rate, improved C3 levels, and clearing of urinary sediment), the dose of prednisone is reduced and condensed to a single daily dose. The legion of steroid side-effects (see Chapter 41) mandates a dose reduction to the lowest level that will keep the patient well. In children, there are unique steroid side-effects seen with very low levels of daily prednisone administration. Growth suppression and osteoporosis can occur with doses in the 3- to 5-mg range if taken on a daily basis. However, up to 15 mg of prednisone can be taken every other day without these side-effects occurring,[24] so the goal of therapy is to get to every-other-day management.

Anticoagulation therapy is necessary in patients who have antiphospholipid antibodies (anticardiolipin antibodies or a lupus anticoagulant). In patients who have not had a thrombotic event, treatment with one baby aspirin per day is indicated. If a thrombotic event has occurred, anticoagulation over several years is necessary with warfarin or subcutaneous heparin. With warfarin, an international normalized ratio should be maintained between 2 and 3.

In patients who fail to achieve the goal of every-other-day steroid management, addition of immunosuppressant medications is necessary. Azathioprine is most often the initial immunosuppressant at a dose of 2 to 3 mg/kg/day. Side-effects include bone marrow suppression, opportunistic infections, nausea, and liver function abnormalities. Mycophenolate mofetil is a newer immunosuppressive agent that inhibits the enzyme inosine monophosphate dehydrogenase, leading to a reduced synthesis of guanosine nucleosides. The dose is 15 to 50 mg/kg/day divided twice daily with a maximum of 1 to 1.5 g twice a day. Side-effects include bone marrow suppression, opportunistic infections, and diarrhea. Methotrexate administered once a week may be beneficial for the arthritic manifestations of SLE; however, it is not an effective agent to treat major organ involvement such as kidney disease. Patients who fail management with azathioprine or mycophenolate mofetil are candidates for treatment with cyclophosphamide with a monthly intravenous pulse protocol or daily basis. Consultation with a pediatric rheumatologist is indicated should that be the case.

Many biologic agents are currently under study to modify aspects of the immune response in patients with SLE; unfortunately, animal studies with anti-TNF medications, which have proven to be so successful in managing JIA, have suggested disease worsening with these agents in SLE patients. Rituximab has shown promise but more studies are necessary.[25] Also new combinations of existing medications appear to be achieving remissions in patients.[26]

Prognosis

The disease course with SLE is waxing and waning. The first year after diagnosis may be the most difficult because new organ system involvement is frequently seen. By the end of the second year, most patients will have set their individual disease manifestations and organ system involvement. For instance, new onset of renal disease or central nervous system disease is unusual if not seen in the first 2 years. In most patients, disease control can be achieved over the first year with lowering medications to nontoxic levels.

The prognosis for survival with SLE has improved markedly since the 1980s.[27] Most series have shown a 10-year survival of 85% to 90%. Over this same interval, the causes of death in SLE patients have changed. Although end-stage renal disease was previously the major cause of death, with modern management including dialysis and kidney transplant, renal deaths are now rare, and serious systemic infections now count for most of the mortality in lupus. These infections are caused by both the underlying disease and its immune disregulation and the effects of steroidal and immunosuppressive medications that are necessary for disease control. Immunization against pneumococcus and meningococcus is indicated in all patients. Pneumocystis prophylaxis should be used in patients on high-dose steroid and immunosuppressant therapy.

There is the second increase in mortality caused by accelerated arteriosclerosis in patients who have survived the acute autoimmune phase of the disease.[27]

Kawasaki Disease

Kawasaki disease (formerly known as *mucocutaneous lymph node syndrome*) is an acute, dramatic type of vasculitis seen primarily in young children.[28] Although uncommon, it is the second most common form of vasculitis after Henoch-Schonlein purpura (HSP). The cause of the vasculitis is unknown, and morbidity and mortality were significant prior to treatment with intravenous immunoglobulin (IVIG). The disease description was published first in Japan in 1967 where the disease remains more common, but it is seen worldwide. It is most common in children less than 2 years of age, and the majority of cases occur in children less than 5 years of age. Many series suggest it is somewhat more common in males. In the USA it is estimated to have an annual incidence of 5.95 per 100 000 children in the Chicago area under the age of 5 years; familial occurrence is unusual, and concordance in twins is low.

Criteria	Characteristics
Fever	>39° C for >5 days
Conjunctivitis	Bilateral, nonsuppurative
Lymphadenopathy	Cervical, > 1.5 cm nonpurulent
Rash	Polymorphous
Changes in lips or oral mucosa	Red, cracked lips; 'strawberry' tongue, erythematous oropharynx
Changes in extremities	Erythema and edema of palms and soles, desquamation of fingertips

Table 13-2 Kawasaki Disease Criteria*

From Centers for Disease Control: MMWR 1985;34:33.
*Diagnosis requires five of six criteria or four criteria plus coronary aneurysm on echocardiography.

Diagnosis

The criteria for the diagnosis have been created and validated and are summarized in Table 13.2. Three phases of the disease have been identified; in the acute febrile phase the children become abruptly ill with high-grade fever (>39° C) and an unusual degree of irritability. Over the next 3 or 4 days (but in no particular order) other manifestations develop, including red eyes, red and cracked lips, swollen lymph nodes, a pleomorphic rash, and redness and edema of the hands and feet. In the subacute phase, defined as the interval of 3 to 4 weeks (if untreated) when the fever resolves, peeling of the digits and perineum occurs and arthritis may be seen in some children, but most importantly this is the period that coronary artery aneurysms are most frequently found on echocardiography. Finally, in the convalescent phase the acute-phase reactants in the laboratory have normalized, and the children are basically asymptomatic.

Clinical characteristics of the illness at presentation may appear unique and classic; however, atypical cases are frequently seen. The fever is high grade and unresponsive to antibiotics. The conjunctivitis appears as nonpurulent erythema. Uveitis may be found on slit-lamp examination, contributing further to the diagnosis. The oral manifestations include red and cracked lips, mucosal erythema, and, frequently, a 'strawberry tongue'. Lymphadenopathy, although sometimes dramatic, in other cases is not greatly different from that in other viral causes of fever. The rash is erythematous, occurring primarily on the trunk and the perineum and progressing to the extremities. The rash is never vesicular or crusting. Changes in the extremities are primarily manifested by edema of the hands and feet, often with erythema of the palms and soles. A tachycardia out of proportion to the fever or degree of anemia should raise concern about myocarditis in the acute phase of the illness.

Other manifestations seen in some patients include sterile pyuria, aseptic meningitis, and hydrops of the gallbladder.

Laboratory Assessment

Laboratory assessment shows evidence of significant inflammation in the first few days of the disease. The white blood count is frequently elevated and shifted to the left, often with toxic granulations; there may be a mild anemia. The platelet count is often elevated, but in atypical cases the evolution to a characteristic thrombocytosis with platelet counts greater than 700 000 may be delayed into the second or third week of the illness. Sedimentation rates and CRP values are elevated. The initial evaluation should also include an electrocardiogram and echocardiography. Coronary artery dilatations but not true aneurysms are found early on.

In the differential diagnosis of Kawasaki disease, scarlet fever mimics the disease most closely but the rash has a dry 'sandpaper' texture, throat cultures are positive for *Streptococcus*, and elevated antistreptolysin O titers are found. Adenoviral infection may also mimic Kawasaki disease. In doubtful cases, the response to IVIG and the evolution of symptoms over time may allow a more accurate diagnosis. Among other collagen vascular diseases, systemic-onset JIA also presents with dramatic fevers, but the rash is totally different. Infantile polyarteritis nodosa may present many of the same features and in autopsy series shares the same pathology as that found in Kawasaki disease.

Pathology

The pathology of Kawasaki disease is characterized by a narcotizing vasculitis of medium-sized arteries, with the coronary arteries being most often involved. In subacute and convalescent stages, aneurysms may develop as the inflammation diminishes. These aneurysms may regress over time, but they may also be the sites of future thrombosis causing myocardial ischemia.

The cause of Kawasaki disease is unknown.[29] Although seasonality and clustering of new cases are observed, no person-to-person spread has been found. Many features of Kawasaki disease are seen in patients with toxic shock syndrome caused by *Streptococcus* or *Staphylococcus*, but proof of this mechanism has been difficult to reproduce. A recent multicenter study of Kawasaki patients found bacterial isolates of streptococci and staphylococci that produced certain exotoxins capable of producing a 'superantigen' response in these children.[30] Genetic predisposition is inconclusive across various ethnic populations. Although IgA may be found in affected vessels, the responsible antigen has not been identified.

Treatment

The introduction of IVIG as a treatment for Kawasaki disease has dramatically changed the natural history and outcome of this condition. Patient response is often dramatic with: defervescence of fever; reduction in irritability; and diminishment of rash, edema, and lymphadenopathy. The dose of IVIG is 2 g/kg administered over 10 to 12 hours.[31] With a conclusively favorable response, the patient can be discharged. If symptoms recur, a second dose of IVIG at 2 g/kg may produce a permanent cessation of acute symptoms. With the occasional failure of IVIG, treatment with steroids (2 mg/kg/day or pulse intravenous Solu-Medrol 30 mg/kg)[32,33] will frequently control the inflammation. The newest treatment to be used in refractory cases is infliximab, 5–10 mg/kg.[34]

In the acute inflammatory phase, salicylates (100 mg/kg/day in divided doses) are used for their antiinflammatory and anticoagulant effects. With the resolution of fever, the dose is changed to 5 mg/kg/day as an anticoagulant measure.

Follow-up echocardiography is a mandatory part of the treatment sequence. If no aneurysms are detected during this subacute phase, the prognosis should be very good and the salicylates can be discontinued. In patients with persistent aneurysm, long-term anticoagulation to prevent thrombosis is indicated.

Prognosis

Overall, the prognosis today for Kawasaki disease is largely favorable; however, there are patients in whom late morbidity and mortality are found because of progressive coronary artery disease.[35]

Juvenile Dermatomyositis

Juvenile dermatomyositis (JDMS) is a unique autoimmune disease in childhood. It is characterized by a pathognomonic rash and proximal muscle weakness.[36] The disease has a remarkably stable incidence worldwide at approximately 0.4 case per 100 000 children under the age of 16 years; girls are more often affected than boys. The rash frequently begins before the symptoms of muscle weakness. JDMS is considered a separate type of inflammatory myopathy based on the original classification by Bohan and Peters in the early 1970s. It is distinguished from adult dermatomyositis by the absence of associated malignancy, a unique vascular pathology, and a tendency to run a self-limited course.

Diagnosis

The muscle disease presents most often as the subacute onset of proximal muscle weakness. The hips are more affected than the shoulders, with symptoms of difficulty with stairs, getting out of a chair, and other lower-extremity functions. Shoulder girdle manifestations may include difficulty doing the hair or reaching for items over the head. Untreated, the weakness may progress to difficulty in getting off the floor, lifting the head off the bed, and inability to perform a sit-up. The weakness is usually out of proportion to degree of soreness or tenderness in the affected muscles. The distal muscles of the hands and feet are spared until very late in the course of the disease. In severely involved patients, there may be a history of difficulty swallowing or dysphonia (a new nasal quality to the voice). On physical examination, patients demonstrate weakness of the proximal muscles including the neck flexors, shoulder girdle, abdominal muscles, and hip muscles. In younger children, evidence of this may be gained by asking them to lift their heads off the examination table, perform a sit-up, and rise from the floor from a supine position. In this latter example, evidence of the Gower maneuver may be obtained as children appear to 'climb up their legs' while using shoulder girdle musculature to substitute for weakness in the hip girdle. Deep tendon reflexes and other aspects of the neurologic examination should be normal.

In most patients the pathognomonic rash has a unique distribution on the body not seen with any other rash of childhood (Figure 13-4). The most commonly affected areas are the extensor surfaces of the knuckles, elbows, and knees. The rash begins initially as an erythematous, scaling eruption that may form papules known as *Gottron's papules*. The cheeks may also develop the rash, with a malar distribution similar to lupus; the upper chest may develop a rash in a 'shawl' distribution; and lastly, the

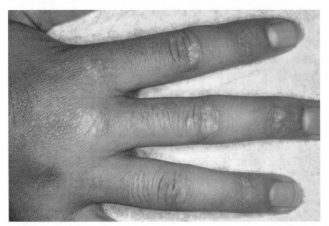

Figure 13-4 Rash in juvenile dermatomyositis.

upper eyelids may manifest a rash that produces a faint purple discoloration referred to as *heliotrope*, so named for the purple flower. The rash may be photosensitive. Although the rash is necessary for diagnosis, its extent and severity may not parallel the course of the muscle weakness.

Other symptoms may include fever, weight loss, fatigue, and abdominal pain. If the abdominal pain is severe and cramping, vasculitis of the gastrointestinal tract may be present, which can be dangerous because it includes a risk of perforation.

The cause of JDMS is unknown. Familial cases are rare, but some studies have indicated a genetic predisposition to the disease with an increase carriage of HLA-B8 and DQA 1*0501.[37-39]

The diagnosis is established with five elements: proximal muscle weakness, characteristic rash, elevated muscle enzymes, myopathic electromyelogram, and occasionally a muscle biopsy. Most authorities would omit the latter two criteria if the other elements were met. Laboratory tests may include evidence of acute inflammation with an elevated sedimentation rate, anemia, and elevated acute-phase reactants. However, evidence of muscle injury with elevated muscle enzymes in the serum is the most useful test. In addition, these enzymes can be used to follow the response to treatment. At onset, a full panel of muscle enzymes, including LDH, SGOT, SGPT, CPK, and aldolase, should be obtained. The last test has been most sensitive and useful. Aldolase values may be the last to normalize with treatment, indicating full disease control. The ANA may be positive but is nonspecific. Antimyositis-specific antibodies have not been useful in JDMS.

Differential Diagnosis

The differential diagnosis includes other rheumatic diseases such as SLE and mixed corrective tissue disease. Viral myositis demonstrates more muscle pain than does JDMS, although muscle enzymes may be very high in the acute phase. The calf musculature is always involved in viral myositis. Neuropathic causes such as weakness are important to rule out. In conditions such as Guillain-Barré syndrome, distal muscle weakness is found. In difficult cases, an electromyelogram is helpful in distinguishing a myopathy from a neuropathy.

MRI of the involved musculature has provided new and useful information, although it should be reserved for selected cases. In JDMS, abnormalities are demonstrated in a patchy distribution characteristic of the disease. If a muscle biopsy is necessary,

involved areas can be selected (with MRI) and the chance of the sampling error giving a normal biopsy result can thereby be reduced. In addition, late in the course of JDMS when muscle enzymes may no longer reflect disease activity, an abnormal MRI indicates continuing disease activity.

Pathology

The pathology of the rash shows epidermal atrophy, hydropic degeneration of basal cells, and moderate dermal infiltrate with vascular dilation; immunofluorescence is negative. The muscle pathology shows evidence of vascular inflammation in the muscle with muscle fiber degeneration, necrosis, and regeneration. Perifascicular atrophy in the muscles is believed to be highly characteristic of JDMS even in the absence of inflammation in the particular biopsy sample.

The autoimmune pathogenesis of JDMS appears to involve both humoral and cell-mediated immunity. Although antibodies to muscle are not demonstrated in JDMS, the vasculature of the involved muscle demonstrates immunoglobulin and complement deposits. Cellular immune mechanisms have been suggested from studies showing that lymphocytes with JDMS are stimulated to blast formation on exposure to muscle antigens in vitro. Similarly, studies have indicated that patients' lymphocytes are capable of destroying cultured fetal muscle cells in vitro.

The cause of this autoimmune attack on skin and muscles is unknown. Because some series have shown seasonality at onset and there are viral models of myositis in experimental animals, there continues to be interest in trying to identify a viral cause of JDMS. However, a recent study examining muscle biopsy specimens with active disease prior to treatment was unsuccessful in identifying a viral cause.[40] This study used polymerase chain reaction technology with primers to more than 20 viruses and controls, which demonstrated that two or three DNA copies could be detected. Importantly, cancers that had been identified in adults with dermatomyositis have not been found in children with JDMS.

The disease course in JDMS may be quite heterogeneous.[36] Three distinct patterns have been identified. The first is monocyclic, in which the patient has the illness for approximately 2 years, requiring treatment during that interval, but thereafter has a return to normal health. In the polycyclic pattern there can be periods of disease activity that alternate with remission and the patient can be taken off all medications; remissions may be as long as 5 years in duration. The third course is described as chronic, where patients require therapy past the 2-year point. These patients may be detected at disease onset by capillary, nail-fold microscopy showing capillary dropout, dilatation, tortuosity, and telangiectasia.

Calcinosis is a postinflammatory sequela, which may be limited to one or two deposits in some patients or extensive debilitating deposits in rare cases. No effective preventive treatments have been developed. Surgical removal should be used only when the calcium deposits produce functional difficulties.

Although no control studies have been performed, the usual standard of therapy is with high-dose steroids. In severely weak patients, treatment may be initiated with pulse Solu-Medrol intravenously in a dose of 30 mg/kg/day for 3 days. Muscle enzyme levels should begin to fall with that therapy, and then prednisone (2 mg/kg/day in split dose) is given by mouth until disease control is achieved. Many authors have attributed treatment failures to underdosing with steroids or premature withdrawal of medication. Disease control is reflected in normalization of muscle enzymes and return of strength. With normalization of the muscle enzymes, a steroid taper is initiated with laboratory monitoring so that reductions in steroid dose cannot lead to return of disease activity. Elevations of muscle enzymes during steroid therapy may herald disease recurrence before a patient becomes clinically ill. In uncomplicated patients, alternate-day dosing of prednisone should be possible within 3 to 4 months. The dose of alternate-day steroids should be decreased to 10 mg every other day, which is essentially a nontoxic dose. Cushingoid side-effects will regress, and linear growth will resume. This dose of steroid should be continued for 2 years. Calcium supplementation should be administered during steroid therapy, as steroid-induced osteoporosis is compounded by reduced physical activity.

Physical therapy modalities are employed to reverse contractures should they occur. Resistive exercises may be prescribed in children over the age of 8 years to aid in muscle strength recovery. Plaquenil and sunscreens may be used for treatment of the rash.

Immunosuppressant therapy may be necessary in patients who are not improving on prednisone or those in whom the steroid burden is too great. Again, control studies are lacking for this rare disease, but the current standard of care is to use steroid-sparing agents beginning with methotrexate at a dose of 1 mg/kg (maximum dose 50 mg) administered subcutaneously once a week.[41] Cyclosporin A has provided additional benefit in patients who achieve inadequate disease control with steroids and methotrexate.[42]

IVIG has been reported to be beneficial in a series of patients with resistant skin disease.[43] This adjunctive therapy may be used early in the treatment of the disease, when immunosuppressive medication is begun.

Treatment with new biologic agents in refractory cases has included rituximab[44] and infliximab.[45]

Wegener's Granulomatosis

Wegener's granulomatosis is a rare form of vasculitis that is lethal if untreated; it frequently presents with chronic upper respiratory symptoms suggestive of more benign entities.[46] Wegener's granulomatosis as a distinct disease entity was first recognized in the German literature in the 1930s as a triad of upper and lower respiratory disease and glomerulonephritis.

The granulomatous inflammation affects medium-sized vessels. Left untreated, the disease may have a 90% mortality 5 years after disease onset; 3% of patients with Wegener's granulomatosis have disease onset at less than 20 years. The disease prevalence may approximate 0.1 per 100 000 individuals under the age of 16 years. The cause of Wegener's granulomatosis is unknown, but research continues to focus on the role of infection, given the unusual distribution of the vasculitic inflammation.

Upper respiratory involvement is characterized by inflammation of the nasal mucosa, sinuses, and middle ear. Sinusitis or otitis media unresponsive to aggressive antibiotic or surgical management should raise a suspicion of Wegener's granulomatosis, especially if there are constitutional symptoms such as fever and weight loss.

Lower respiratory symptoms include cough, dyspnea, hemoptysis, and stridor. Wegener's granulomatosis should be suspected in patients presenting with pulmonary hemorrhage characterized by hypoxia, pulmonary infiltrates, and rapid development of anemia. The stridor is caused by tracheal involvement with granulomas.

The renal disease of Wegener's granulomatosis is that of a glomerulonephritis with proteinuria, hematuria, and cast formation. Azotemia at disease diagnosis is an ominous sign because the glomerulonephritis is a necrotizing process with early, irreversible crescent formation, whereas other aspects of Wegener's granulomatosis may be fully reversible with treatment. The crescentic glomerulonephritis may be stabilized but not fully reversed.

Less common manifestations of Wegener's granulomatosis are purpuric skin lesions resembling those of HSP, arthralgias, and arthritis. Fever, weight loss, and fatigue, which are nonspecific symptoms, should nonetheless alert the physician that a more benign diagnosis may need further investigation.

Central nervous system lesions and involvement of the eye are late manifestations of disease activity.

Diagnosis

The differential diagnosis of Wegener's granulomatosis includes chronic, allergic upper respiratory disease. Patients presenting with pulmonary hemorrhage may have SLE, idiopathic pulmonary hemosiderosis, Goodpasture's syndrome, or Churg-Strauss syndrome, but the latter two entities are extremely rare in childhood. Lower-extremity purpura may be seen in HSP and SLE.

X-rays of the sinuses show chronic mucosal thickening. Chest X-ray demonstrates scattered pulmonary infiltrates that may be transient or segmental, suggestive of pulmonary hemorrhage. CT scans of the lungs frequently demonstrate the nodular inflammatory process indicative of Wegener's granulomatosis.

Laboratory Assessment

Initial laboratory tests are indicative of systemic inflammation. Anemia, leukocytosis, and thrombocytosis are nonspecific indicators of inflammation. Similarly, an elevated sedimentation rate and CRP are usually found. An elevated level of carbon monoxide diffusion in the lung is suggestive of pulmonary hemorrhage. The urinalysis demonstrates hematuria, proteinuria, and casts.

The development of the antineutrophilic cytoplasmic antibody (ANCA) test has provided greater than 90% sensitivity and greater than 90% specificity for Wegener's granulomatosis.[47] The usual antibody detected is the c-ANCA, which can be further elucidated by enzyme-linked immunosorbent assay (ELISA) techniques for antibody to the cytoplasmic PR3 antigen.[48] A p-ANCA antibody may occasionally be found but is also seen in patients with polyarteritis nodosum, crescentic glomerulonephritis, and inflammatory bowel disease. This antibody can be confirmed by an ELISA technique with myeloperoxidase as antigen. In patients with refractory otitis media, sinusitis, or lower-extremity purpura, a negative ANCA serves to eliminate the diagnosis of this very serious disease.

Pathology

Pathologic specimens demonstrate a granulomatous vasculitis of vessel walls or the interstitium with collections of macrophages, neutrophils, and giant cells; however, obtaining diagnostic tissue is frequently difficult. Sinus tissue biopsies may only show chronic inflammation without the diagnostic findings. Similar sampling problems are found with transbronchial lung biopsies or needle kidney biopsies. The ANCA test has supplanted the necessity for aggressively pursuing pathologic tissue. The pathogenesis of Wegener's granulomatosis is incompletely understood. There is evidence to suggest that an ANCA antibody is capable of enhancing neutrophilic release of tissue-damaging enzymes.[47]

Treatment

Unless Wegener's granulomatosis is limited to the upper respiratory tract, treatment should be aggressive. High-dose steroid therapy (1 to 2 mg/kg/day) in a split dose or with initial pulse Solu-Medrol (30 mg/kg/day) in severely ill patients produces the most rapid improvement in symptoms. However, cyclophosphamide (2 mg/kg/day) should be started immediately because there is some lag time in its effect on the disease, and treatment with steroids alone has no effect on disease mortality.[37] The potential for sterility caused by cyclophosphamide, which must be given for 1 to 2 years, may be ameliorated by using testosterone in males and Lupron in females. Methotrexate may be considered in limited disease and as maintenance therapy in patients who have achieved excellent disease control with cyclophosphamide. However, relapses of patients on methotrexate are not uncommon and may lead to reinstitution of cyclophosphamide therapy.

Rituximab is showing early promise in the treatment of Wegener's.[49]

Prognosis

Wegener's granulomatosis is highly lethal if untreated. Drug-free remissions are rare, but with modern therapy many patients are able to lead a normal life. In children the incidence of subglottic stenosis is five times more common than in adults.[46] Chronic inflammation of the nasal mucosa may lead to cartilage collapse in the nose and a 'saddle' deformity. The renal lesion of Wegener's granulomatosis is the most difficult to reverse, but patients can be maintained for many years with only mild renal insufficiency; some patients, however, may progress to end-stage renal disease.

Henoch-Schönlein Purpurea

HSP is the most common form of leukocytoclastic vasculitis in children.[50] It is uniquely mediated by IgA immune complex deposition. The annual incidence is 13.5 per 100 000 children under the age of 16 years. Boys are more commonly affected than girls (1.5:1). It is more common in winter and often is preceded by a viral upper respiratory infection. Beta-hemolytic streptococcal bacteria may be important in recurrent HSP but not in population-based studies.[51]

Diagnosis

The clinical manifestations include lower extremity purpura, arthralgia, arthritis, abdominal pain, and hematuria, which may be grossly apparent.

The skin lesions begin as macular, papular, or urticarial lesions but progress to a nonblanching purpura. The majority of lesions are on the lower extremities and buttocks, although they may be scattered elsewhere. Arthralgias and arthritis are most commonly in the lower extremities and are often associated with edema of the hands and feet; in young children the edema may involve the scalp, scrotum, and the back.

Gastrointestinal involvement is suggested by abdominal pain that becomes colicky or cramping. Submucosal vasculitis and hemorrhage produce hematest-positive stools. Vasculitic involvement of the intestine may lead to intussusception (4.5% in some series) or, more rarely, to intestinal perforation.

Renal involvement is usually silent with microscopic hematuria and proteinuria; occasionally gross hematuria may be found. A nephritic presentation with hypertension and azotemia increases the risk of a persistent IgA nephropathy.

Laboratory Assessment

There is no diagnostic test for HSP. A CBC should not show thrombocytopenia, which would indicate other important disease entities. The sedimentation rate is usually normal or only slightly elevated. Sedimentation rates greater than 40 mm/hr may suggest other disease entities, such as SLE or Wegener's granulomatosis, and appropriate tests for these entities should be ordered. The serum IgA level is elevated in 50% of patients during the acute phase. In doubtful cases or cases with prolonged disease activity (seen particularly in the adolescent population), a skin biopsy of a fresh lesion will demonstrate diagnostic IgA deposits.[52]

Prognosis

In the majority of young children the disease runs a self-limited course, lasting 2 to 4 weeks with full recovery. Older children (above 10 years) may have a more protracted course, but their outcome remains nonetheless good. Recurrences are not uncommon (15% to 40% in some series). They are most common within the first 2 years following the initial episode.

Treatment

In the majority of patients, the treatment is supportive. Non-steroidal antiinflammatory agents can be helpful for the arthritic manifestations. Steroids are indicated (1 to 2 mg/kg/day in split dose) in patients who present with cramping abdominal pain in order to prevent the complications of intussusception or perforation.[50] Steroid therapy may be required for 2 to 3 weeks with a tapering schedule, depending on the recurrence of abdominal pain as the steroids are tapered. Treatment with steroids does not prevent the development of kidney disease in HSP patients.[53] The treatment for a nephritic renal presentation remains controversial, although most authors use steroids and a combination of immunosuppressant agents. The proteinuria of persistent IgA nephropathy in HSP patients may also improve when treatment with angiotensin-converting enzyme inhibitors is instituted.

The vast majority of children make a full recovery from HSP. Long-term morbidity is caused by IgA nephropathy with progression to end-stage renal disease. Patients with a nephritic or nephrotic presentation should be referred to a renal specialist.

Conclusions

The panoply of illnesses included in the rheumatic diseases of childhood accounts for a major segment of chronic disease. Although proximate causes for these diseases are not known,

> **BOX 13-4 Key concepts**
>
> **Diagnosis of Rheumatic Diseases of Childhood**
>
> - The diagnosis of the rheumatic diseases of childhood is based on history and physical examination.
> - Laboratory tests add supportive information but seldom produce diagnoses not indicated by the history and physical examination.
> - Most autoimmune diseases demonstrate evidence of inflammation in laboratory tests, which guides the clinician away from trauma, allergy, or emotions as possible causes.

increasing evidence indicates that genetic predisposition together with environmental influences will explain disease expression. Treatment advances since the 1990s have improved the outcome for the majority of patients Box 13-4.

References

1. Ravelli A, Martini A. Juvenile idiopathic arthritis. Lancet 2007;369:767–78.
2. Jarvis JN. Pathogenesis and mechanisms of inflammation in the childhood rheumatic diseases. Curr Opin Rheumatol 1998;10:459–67.
3. Glass DN, Giannini EH. JRA as a complex genetic trait. Arthritis Rheum 1999;42:2261–8.
4. Vostrejs M, Hollister JR. Muscle atrophy and leg length discrepancies in pauciarticular juvenile rheumatoid arthritis. Am J Dis Child 1988;142:343–5.
5. Sherry DD, Stein LD, Reed AM, et al. Prevention of leg length discrepancy in young children with pauciarticular juvenile rheumatoid arthritis by treatment with intraarticular steroids. Arthritis Rheum 1999;42:2330–4.
6. Chylack Jr TL. The ocular manifestations of juvenile rheumatoid arthritis. Arthritis Rheum 1977;20:217–23.
7. Ferucci ED, Majka DS, Parrish LA, et al. Antibodies against cyclic citrullinated peptide are associated with HLA-DR4 in simplex and multiplex polyarticular-onset juvenile rheumatoid arthritis. Arthritis Rheum 2005;52:239–46.
8. McMinn FJ, Bywaters EGL. Differences between the fever of Still's disease and that of rheumatic fever. Ann Rheum Dis 1959;18:293.
9. Isdale IC, Bywaters EGL. The rash of rheumatoid arthritis and Still's disease. Q J Med 1956;5:377–9.
10. Wallendahl M, Stork L, Hollister JR. The discriminating value of serum LDH values in children with malignancy presenting as joint pain. Arch Pediatr Adolesc Med 1996;150:70–3.
11. Szer IS, Taylor E, Steere AC. The long-term course of Lyme arthritis in children. N Engl J Med 1991;325:159–63.
12. Lovell DJ, Giannini EH, Reiff A, et al. Efficacy and safety of etanercept (tumor necrosis factor receptor p75 Fc fusion protein; Enbrel) in children with polyarticular-course juvenile rheumatoid arthritis. N Engl J Med 2000;342:1703–10.
13. Lovell DJ, Ruperto N, Goodman S, et al. Adalimumab with or without methotrexate in juvenile rheumatoid arthritis. New Eng. J Med 2008;359:810–20.
14. Ruperto N, Lovell DJ, Quartier P, et al. Abatacept in children with juvenile idiopathic arthritis: a randomized double blind, placebo controlled withdrawl trial. Lancet 2008;372:383–91.
15. Cabral DA, Malleson PN, Petty RE. Spondyloarthropathies of childhood. Pediatr Clin North Am 1995;42:1051–70.
16. Cassidy JT, Petty RS. Juvenile ankylosing spondylitis. In: Cassidy JT, Petty RE, Laxer RM, Lindsley CB, editors. Textbook of pediatric rheumatology, 5th edition. Philadelphia, PA: Elsevier Saunders; 2005.
17. Dougados M, Boumier P, Amor B. Sulphasalazine in ankylosing spondylitis: a double blind control study in 60 patients. Br Med J 1986;293:911–4.
18. Gottlieb, BS, Ilowite NT. Systemic lupus erythematosus in children and adolescents. Pediatr Rev 2006;37:323–9.
19. D'Cruz DP, Khamashta MA, Hughes GRV. Systemic lupus erythematosus. Lancet 2007;369:587–96.
20. Iqbal S, Sher MR, Good RA, et al. Diversity in presenting manifestations of systemic lupus erythematosus in children. J Pediatr 1999;135:500–5.
21. West SG. Lupus and the central nervous system. Curr Opin Rheumatol 1996;8:408–14.
22. Singsen BH, Berstein BH, King KK, et al. Systemic lupus erythematosus in childhood: correlation between change in disease activity and serum complement levels. J Pediatr 1976;89:358–64.
23. Petri M. Pathogenesis and treatment of the antiphospholipid syndrome. Med Clin North Am 1997;81:151–77.
24. Auerbach HS, Williams M, Kirkpatrick JA, et al. Alternate-day prednisone reduces morbidity and improves pulmonary function in cystic fibrosis. Lancet 1985;2:686–8.
25. Garcia-Carrasco M, Jimenez-Hernandez M, Escarcega RO, et al. Use of rituximab in patients with systemic lupus erythematosus: an update. Autoimmun Rev 2009;8:343–8.
26. Bao H, Liu Z, Xie H, et al. Successful treatment of Class V and IV lupus nephritis with multitarget therapy. J Am Soc Nephrol 2008;19:2001–10.
27. Ippolito A, Petrie M. An update on mortality in systemic lupus erythematosus. Clin Exp Rheumatol 2008;26(Suppl. 51):S72–9.
28. Burns JC. Kawasaki disease. Adv Pediatr 2001;48:157–77.
29. Yeung R. Pathogenesis and treatment of Kawasaki's disease. Cur. Opin. In Rheumatology 2005;17:617–23.
30. Leung DYM, Meissner H, Shulman ST, et al. Prevalence of superantigen-secreting bacteria in patients with Kawasaki disease. J Pediatr 2002;140:742–6.
31. Newburger JW, Takahashi MT, Beiser AS, et al. A single intravenous infusion of gamma globulin as compared with four infusions in the treatment of acute Kawasaki syndrome. N Engl J Med 1991;324:1633–9.
32. Wright DA, Newburger JW, Baker A, et al. Treatment of immune globulin-resistant Kawasaki disease with pulsed doses of corticosteroids. J Pediatr 1996;128:146–9.
33. Dale RC, Saleem MA, Daw S, et al. Treatment of severe complicated Kawasaki disease with oral prednisolone and aspirin. J Pediatr 2000;137:723–6.
34. Burns JC, Mason WH, Hauger SB, et al. Infliximab treatment of refractory Kawasaki syndrome. J Pediatr 2005;146:662–7.
35. Fulton DR, Newburger JW. Long-term cardiac sequelae of Kawasaki disease. Curr Rheum Reports 2000;2:324–9.
36. Feldman BM, Rider LG, Reed AM, et al. Juvenile dermatomyositis and other idiopathic inflammatory myopathies. Lancet 2008;371:2201–12.
37. Reed AM, Pachman LM, Hayford J, et al. Immunogenetic studies in families of children with juvenile dermatomyositis. J Rheumatol 1998;25:1000–2.
38. Pachman LM, Fedezyna TO, Lechman TS, et al. Juvenile dermatomyositis: the association of the TNF alpha-308A allele and disease chronicity. Curr Rheumatol Reports 2001;3:379–86.
39. Tezak Z, Hoffman EP, Lutz JL, et al. Gene expression profiling in DQA1*0501 + children with untreated dermatomyositis: a novel model of pathogenesis. J Immunol 2002;168:4154–63.
40. Pachman LM, Litt DL, Rowley AH, et al. Lack of detection of enteroviral or bacterial DNA in magnetic resonance imaging-directed muscle biopsies from twenty children with active untreated juvenile dermatomyositis. Arthritis Rheum 1995;38:1513–8.
41. Miller LC, Sisson BA, Tucker LB, et al. Methotrexate treatment of recalcitrant childhood dermatomyositis. Arthritis Rheum 1992;35:1143–9.
42. Reiff A, Rawlings DJ, Shaham B, et al. Preliminary evidence for cyclosporin A as an alternative treatment of recalcitrant juvenile rheumatoid arthritis and juvenile dermatomyositis. J Rheumatol 1997;24:2436–43.
43. Al-Mayouf SM, Laxer RM, Schneider R, et al. Intravenous immunoglobulin therapy for juvenile dermatomyositis. J Rheumatol 2000;27:2498–503.
44. Cooper MA, Willingham DL, Brown DE, et al. Rituximab for the treatment of juvenile dermatomyositis: a report of four pediatric patients. Arthritis Rheum 2007;55:3107–11.
45. Riley P, McCann LJ, Maillard SM, et al. Effectiveness of infliximab in the treatment of refractory juvenile dermatomyositis with calcinosis. Rheumatology 2008;47:877–80.
46. Rottem M, Fauci AS, Hallahan CW, et al. Wegener granulomatosis in children and adolescents: clinical presentation and outcome. J Pediatr 1993;122:27–31.
47. Duna GF, Galperin C, Hoffman GS. Wegener's granulomatosis. Rheum Dis Clin North Am 1995;21:949–86.
48. Jenne DE, Tschopp J. Wegener's autoantigen decoded. Nature 1990;346(6284):520.

49. Aouba A, Pagnoux C, Bienvenu B, et al. Analysis of Wegener's granulomatosis responses to rituximab: current evidence and therapeutic prospects. Clin Rev Allerg Immunol 2008;34:65–73.

50. Tizard EJ, Hamilton-Ayres MJJ. Henoch-Schlonlein purpura. Arch Dis Child Educ Pract Ed 2008;93:1–8.

51. Nielsen HE. Epidemiology of Schonlein-Henoch purpura. Acta Paediatr Scand 1988;77:125–31.

52. Faille-Kuyber EH, Kater L, Kooiker CJ, et al. IgA-deposits in cutaneous blood-vessel walls and mesangium in Henoch-Schonlein syndrome. Lancet 1973;1:892–3.

53. Chartapisak W, Opastiraku S, Willis NS, et al. Prevention and treatment of renal disease in Henoch-Schonlein purpura: a systematic review. Arch Dis Child 2009;94:132–7.

CHAPTER 14

Autoimmune Diseases

Erin Janssen • Andrew Shulman • Robert P. Sundel

The immune system's defenses against the outside world are predicated upon the ability to discriminate self from nonself. In practice, however, distinguishing exogenous pathogens and environmental exposures from chemically and structurally similar bodily constituents is an extraordinarily complex and exacting task. When the process fails, autoreactive lymphocytes, autoantibodies, and/or dysregulated inflammation in the absence of infection or other external factors are the result; autoimmunity is the consequence. The process, termed 'horror autotoxicus' by Ehrlich more than 100 years ago, affects approximately 5% of the Western population, making it a significant public health concern.[1] Nonetheless, given the challenge of 'self'-'nonself' discrimination, it is remarkable that pathologic self-directed responses do not occur more commonly. This is scant comfort for the more than 50 000 000 Americans with autoimmune diseases, in whom a breakdown in tolerance leads to some of the most vexing and complex conditions that physicians can face.

An understanding of autoimmune disease requires characterization of several factors, ranging from self-tolerance, the mechanism that prevents damaging self-directed immunity, to environmental and infectious triggers that can subvert normal homeostasis. In this chapter, we will attempt to use current understanding of how tolerance is maintained and details of how it fails to understand the initiation and progression of auto-immunity. We will also review current approaches to treating autoimmune diseases, as well as novel targets that may one day expand the options.

Immune Recognition and Maintenance of Self-Tolerance

Multicelled organisms use a two-tiered defense in their battle against foreign invaders. The first layer provides an immediate nonspecific inflammatory response that limits the extent of infection at the site of exposure. The second level is a delayed but long-lived adaptive response that is able to identify and target repeated or persistent infection.[2]

Receptors capable of sensing the presence of pathogen-derived molecules are the first requirement for protection from infection. Innate immune receptors are highly conserved across species and represent an evolutionarily ancient strategy for pathogen defense. They bind to structural and chemical motifs shared by pathogens and absent from the host, known as pathogen-associated molecular patterns (PAMPs). PAMPs are ligands for innate immune receptors and include lipids, peptidolgycans, nucleic acids, enzymes, and structural proteins common to bacteria, parasites, and viruses. Innate immune receptors are present at the cell-surface, on the membranes of lysosomes containing endocytosed extracellular contents, and in the cytoplasm of diverse cell types including macrophages, dendritic cells, epithelial cells, and lymphocytes. Stimulation of innate receptors leads to activation of inflammatory pathways and elaboration of cytokines, chemokines, vasoactive amines, and eicosanoids. These, in turn, recruit effector cells for the neutralization of infections, and facilitate antigen presentation and priming of the adaptive immune response. Complex controls limit the degree to which this response is perpetuated. These may be subverted when innate immune receptors are triggered through a non-pathogen response, as in autoinflammatory syndromes, or when an inflammatory response is not extinguished normally.

Dysregulated Innate Immunity and the Autoinflammatory Syndromes

Inflammatory pathways are capable of sensing tissue stress or cellular malfunction through endogenous signals unrelated to infection, such as protein release from necrotic cells or decreased secretory protein quality in the endoplasmic reticulum. The response of resident tissue macrophages to these signals results in an intermediate inflammatory state, which has evolved to maintain tissue homeostasis under conditions of stress. Pathological consequences of this 'para-inflammatory' state have been hypothesized to play a central role in chronic inflammation associated not only with autoimmune disease, but also with common acquired conditions such as Type 2 diabetes mellitus (DM) and cardiovascular disease.[2]

The autoinflammatory syndromes (previously known as periodic fever syndromes) are examples of diseases resulting from dysregulated inflammation (Table 14-1). These syndromes are rare inherited diseases characterized by episodic inflammation in the absence of infection, autoantibody production, or autoreactive lymphocytes. Familial Mediterranean fever (FMF) is the prototypic autoinflammatory disorder. It is characterized by recurrent fever episodes associated with polyserositis, erysipeloid erythema, monoarthritis, and splenomegaly.[3] Systemic amyloidosis due to the accumulation of a misfolded acute phase reactant, serum amyloid A, is a life-threatening complication of FMF and other periodic fever syndromes.

Human genetic and biochemical investigations have identified mutations within the 'inflammasome' as the cause of autoinflammatory disorders. The inflammasome protein complex

©2010 Elsevier Ltd, Inc, BV
DOI: 10.1016/B978-1-4377-0271-2.00014-6

Table 14-1 Features of Periodic Fever Syndromes

Features	FMF	HIDS	Autosomal dominant periodic fever syndrome	PFAPA
Inheritance	AR	AR	AD	Not familial
Locus	MEFV	MEVK	TNFRSF1A	Unknown
Age of onset	90% by age 20 years	96% by age 10 years	Usually childhood	Usually < 5 years
Lymphadenopathy	Uncommon	Very common	Common	Common
Abdominal involvement	Common; constipation more frequent	Common with vomiting and diarrhea	Common with either diarrhea or constipation	Uncommon
Pleural involvement	Common	Very rare	Common	Very rare
Rash	Erysipeloid erythema, usually below knee	Erythematous macules and papules common	Tender erythematous patches common	Rare
Arthritis	Common, usually monoarticular	Usually symmetric oligoarthritis	True arthritis rare, oligoarthralgia common	Not characteristic
Conjunctivitis	Uncommon	Uncommon	Frequent with unilateral periorbital edema	Uncommon
Amyloidosis	Common	Not associated	Very rare	Not associated
Treatment	Colchicine to prevent attacks and amyloidosis	None	High-dose steroids	Single dose of steroid; cimetidine; tonsillectomy

FMF, familial Mediterranean fever; *HIDS*, hyperimmuneglobulin-D syndrome; *PFAPA*, periodic fever, aphthous stomatitis, pharyngitis and adenitis syndrome.

controls IL-1β processing and secretion through activation of the upstream protease caspase-1.[4] Mutations in the *MEFV* gene encoding pyrin, a novel death-domain fold-containing protein, cause FMF.[5,6] Polymorphisms or mutations of the related nucleotide-binding oligomerization domain (NOD)-containing protein, NOD2 (CARD15), confer an increased risk for the development of Crohn's disease. NOD2 mutations have also been identified in Blau syndrome, an inherited disorder of multiorgan granulomatous inflammation.[5]

Three autosomal dominant and clinically heterogeneous autoinflammatory syndromes, Muckle-Wells syndrome (MWS), familial cold autoinflammatory syndrome (FCAS), and neonatal-onset multisystem inflammatory disease (NOMID), are due to mutations in another gene of the inflammasome, the gene encoding cryopyrin (also known as NALP3 [NACHT-, leucine-rich-repeat, and pyrin-domain-containing protein]).[6–8] In addition to fever episodes of short duration (24–48 hours), FCAS is characterized by a cold-induced urticarial rash. MWS can be distinguished from other periodic fever syndromes by the occurrence of sensorineural hearing loss. NOMID is a disorder of nearly continuous systemic inflammation that presents in infancy with urticarial rash, chronic aseptic meningitis, arthropathy, and sensorineural hearing loss.

Cryopyrin/NALP3 serves as a cytoplasmic receptor for multiple chemical irritants including uric acid crystals, silica, and alum in addition to being a key regulator of the inflammasome. Thus, autonomous activation leads to the autoinflammatory conditions MWS, FCAS, and NOMID, while exogenous activation of IL-1-mediated inflammation through NALP3 appears to play a central role in the pathogenesis of gout, silicosis, and the inflammatory activity of adjuvants.[9,10] As understanding of autoinflammatory syndromes increases, so too does the list of conditions potentially related to abnormalities of the inflammasome. For example, gene expression analysis suggests that the IL-1 pathway also may be dysregulated in systemic-onset juvenile idiopathic arthritis, a form of childhood arthritis characterized by fever, rash, and systemic inflammation. This, in turn, has had signifi-

cant therapeutic implications, providing support for the clinical use of the IL-1 receptor antagonist, anakinra, in both juvenile idiopathic arthritis (JIA) and gout.[11] The possibility that other common diseases involving pathogenic inflammation, from coronary artery disease and malaria to Alzheimer's disease, may benefit from inflammatory cytokine inhibition, is an area of active investigation.

Innate immune receptors for nucleic acids allow for cytoplasmic recognition of viral genomic intermediates and the activation of a protective type I interferon response. Transfection of double-stranded DNA (dsDNA) in macrophages is sufficient to activate an interferon response. This suggests that DNA translocation out of the nucleus in damaged or apoptotic cells, or endogenous dsDNA produced from genomic retrotransposon elements, has the potential to act as an autoinflammatory trigger.[12,13] The interferon-inducible HIN200 protein family member AIM2 has recently been found to be a cellular dsDNA receptor that activates the IL-1 inflammasome. Intriguingly, AIM2 maps to a known systemic lupus erythematosus (SLE) susceptibility locus, suggesting that increased AIM2 activity in lupus-predisposed individuals may lead to an exaggerated inflammatory and type I interferon response to cytoplasmic dsDNA.[14,15] Providing further evidence of the importance of cytoplasmic nucleic acid surveillance in the pathogenesis of autoimmunity is the recent finding that a 3′ to 5′ repair exonuclease (Trex1) which metabolizes single-stranded DNA and inhibits nucleic acid-mediated inflammation is mutated in familial chilblain lupus and Aicardi-Goutieres syndrome, an infantile disease of severe encephalitis with elevated cerebrospinal fluid interferon levels.[12]

Adaptive Immunity

Adaptive immunity is the second, lymphocyte-mediated arm of the immune response characterized by a specific and long-lasting reaction to infection. It also has the capacity to recognize a vast array of antigens, even many that have not yet been encountered.

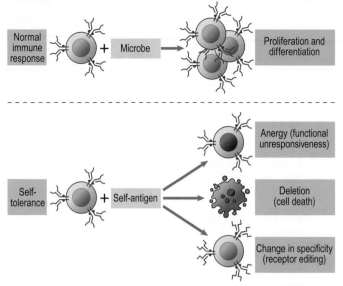

Figure 14-1 Self-tolerance. Fates of lymphocytes after encounter with antigens. In a normal immune response, microbes stimulate the proliferation and differentiation of antigen-specific lymphocytes. (Microbial antigens are typically recognized by lymphocytes in the presence of costimulators and innate immune responses, which are not shown.) Self-antigens may induce functional unresponsiveness or death of antigen-specific lymphocytes or a change in the specificity of the receptors, making these cells incapable of responding to the antigen (self-tolerance). Some antigens elicit no response (ignorance), but the lymphocytes are able to respond to subsequent antigen challenge (not shown). This illustration depicts B lymphocytes; the same general principles apply to T lymphocytes. Redrawn from Abbas AK, Lichtman AH, and Shiv P. Cellular and Molecular Immunology, 6th edition, Saunders, Philadelphia, PA, 2007.

The molecules responsible for this diverse repertoire are the T cell receptors (TCRs) and B cell receptors (BCRs). The capacity for broad antigen recognition results from V(D)J recombination of gene segments, as well as random nucleotide additions and mutations that introduce even more variability. Overall, an estimated 10^9 to 10^{11} antigenic determinants may be recognized as a result of antigen receptor reassortment.[16] During this random rearrangement, receptors that bind self-antigens are generated at a high frequency – up to 20–50% of the total number of receptors.[17-19] *Tolerance* is the term used for the process that eliminates or suppresses such potentially autoreactive cells. When tolerance breaks down, whether in the central lymphoid organs or in the periphery, autoimmunity results (Figure 14-1).

T Cell Tolerance

T cells orchestrate adaptive immunity against infectious agents with protein determinants recognized by specific T cell receptors. These receptors trigger direct effector and cytotoxic responses, refine antibody production though B cell costimulation, and promote cytokine and chemokine signaling to the innate immune system. Central tolerance mechanisms mediated in the thymus govern the development of T cells expressing specific TCRs. Peripheral tolerance mechanisms inhibit potential autoimmune effects of self-reactive T cells that have escaped the thymus (Figure 14-2).

Central T Cell Tolerance

Immature T lymphocytes migrate from the bone marrow to the thymus, where they undergo further maturation. In the thymus, the T cell repertoire is shaped through a process often termed 'T cell education'. This education involves exposure to a wide array of antigens. T cells with very low affinity for self major histocom-

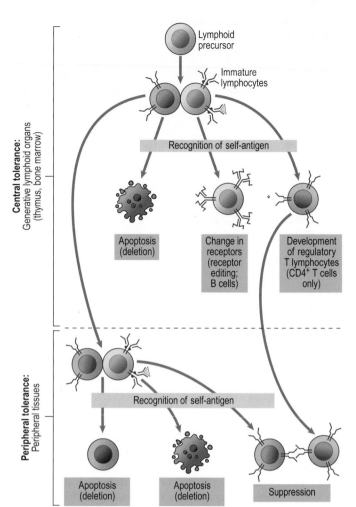

Figure 14-2 Central and peripheral tolerance to self-antigens. Immature lymphocytes specific for self-antigens may encounter these antigens in the generative lymphoid organs and are deleted, change their specificity (B cells only), or (in the case of CD4+ T cells) develop into regulatory lymphocytes (central tolerance). Some self-reactive lymphocytes may mature and enter peripheral tissues and may be inactivated or deleted by encounter with self-antigens in these tissues, or are suppressed by the regulatory T cells (peripheral tolerance). (Note that T cells recognize antigens presented by antigen-presenting cells, which are not shown.) Redrawn from Abbas AK, Lichtman AH, and Shiv P. Cellular and Molecular Immunology, 6th edition, Saunders, Philadelphia, PA, 2007.

patibility complex (MHC) molecules and self-peptides do not receive survival signals; they die from 'neglect'. Positive selection occurs for cells that have an intermediate affinity for self-peptide-MHC complexes. Finally, those cells with high affinity for self-peptide MHC complexes undergo negative selection and receive signals to undergo apoptosis.

A breakdown in self-peptide expression leads to impaired negative selection and autoimmunity. This is seen in autoimmune polyendocrinopathy-candidiasis-ectodermal dystrophy (APECED), a condition marked by a failure of central T cell tolerance.[20] T cells in the thymic medulla are vulnerable to negative selection.[21] Medullary thymic epithelial cells (mTECs) express a wide array of ubiquitous and tissue specific antigens in addition to MHC class II molecules. Through positional cloning, mutations in the *AIRE* gene were found to be responsible for the development of APECED.[22,23] AIRE is expressed in mTECs, and mTECs deficient in AIRE have reduced expression of tissue specific antigens[20,24,25] AIRE-deficient mice develop autoimmunity with autoantibodies targeting multiple organs by 6 months of life.[24,26] Typical features of patients with APECED are an aberrant immune response to *Candida* and high titer autoantibodies that primarily target endocrine organs.[27]

mTECs are also implicated in the genesis of myasthenia gravis. Patients with myasthenia gravis have easy muscle fatigability and ptosis, as well as antibodies directed against the acetylcholine receptor (AchR). Differences in promoter sequences alter the amount of AchR subunits expressed by mTECs.[28] This altered expression is likely to lead to abnormal peptide presentation and central tolerance induction. In patients with thymomas, dysplastic mTECs also contribute to disrupted selective processes and T cell priming in the thymus.

Peripheral T Cell Tolerance

The importance of preventing autoimmunity is demonstrated by the redundant mechanisms available for thwarting its development. Thus, several processes hamper potentially autoreactive T cells that escape thymic deletion from initiating an autoimmune sequence.

1. *Ignorance.* Potentially autoreactive T cells may remain ignorant of their antigens due to protein expression levels below the threshold for detection.

2. *Anergy.* The requirement for a second, costimulatory signal for T cell activation is a critical factor in integrating information regarding the inflammatory context with the encounter of an antigenic peptide. In addition to the primary signal mediated by the interaction of the TCR expressed on an autoreactive T cell with a self-peptide loaded on the MHC class II molecule of an antigen-presenting cell (APC), interactions between costimulatory ligands and receptors are required for effective TCR signaling and T cell activation. Autoreactive T cells that encounter an antigenic peptide in the absence of costimulation fail to produce IL-2, which in turn is essential for driving T cell proliferation through positive autocrine and paracrine feedback loops. These potentially self-reactive T cells are termed 'anergic' and encounter self-antigens without triggering autoimmunity. Recent work suggests that AIRE is central to this process as well: secondary lymphoid organs that express self-antigens contain AIRE-expressing cells that make stable antigen specific interactions with autoreactive T cells and induce peripheral tolerance.[29] This highlights the effect on T cell tolerance of regulated expression of key self-antigens in peripheral cells. Importantly, an inflammatory trigger, such as an intercurrent viral infection, may lead to activation of dendritic cells and other professional APCs. The result could be the generation of a costimulatory environment in which previously anergic autoreactive T cells become activated.

3. *Deletion.* Engagement of T cell surface receptors that induce apoptotic pathways can lead to the deletion of autoreactive T cells via programmed cell death. The interaction of Fas (CD95) on T cells with Fas-ligand (Fas-L) on adjacent cells triggers T cell apoptosis. Genetic lesions in Fas or Fas-L result in the autoimmune lymphoproliferative syndrome (ALPS). ALPS is characterized by lymphadenopathy, splenomegaly, hypergammaglobulinemia, and cell- and antibody-mediated autoimmunity directed against multiple organs including the GI tract and hematopoietic lineages.[30] A dramatic increase in the number of TCRαβ positive, CD4/8 double negative naïve thymocytes is a hallmark of this disorder. Family members of ALPS patients can have Fas or Fas-L mutations in the absence of clinical lymphoproliferative disease, demonstrating the importance of both Fas-Fas-L signaling and modifier genes or environmental factors in the generation of pathogenic autoreactive T cells.[31]

   Mutations in other apoptotic signal transducers are also associated with the ALPS phenotype. ALPS type II is due to dysfunction of the caspase-10 gene, an initiator of apoptosis.[32,33] Another patient with features of ALPS (ALPS IV) was found to have a heterozygous mutation in the N-RAS gene which led to increased activation of N-RAS and the downstream mitogen-activated protein (MAP) kinase pathway.[34] This pathway is important in down-regulating BIM (BCL-2-interacing mediator of cell death) protein expression and subsequent mitochondrial apoptosis. More recently, compound heterozygotes for the Fas and caspase-10 mutations have been identified with ALPS.[35]

4. *Regulation.* It has been known for more than 3 decades that thymic manipulation or sublethal radiation can cause a break of tolerance and autoimmune disease in normal animals. These results suggested the existence of a thymus-derived subset of T cells capable of suppressing the activation of autoreactive T cells. Multiple lines of evidence have substantiated this previously controversial hypothesis and identified regulatory T cells (Tregs) as key mediators of peripheral tolerance.[36] 'Natural' regulatory T cells are produced in the thymus and can be identified by expression of CD4 and CD25, the IL-2 receptor α chain. Transfer of T cells depleted with anti-CD25 antibodies into athymic mice results in systemic autoimmunity, indicating that the small population of peripheral regulatory T cells is important in suppressing T cell autoreactivity. Foxp3 (forkhead box P3), a member of the forkhead/winged-helix family of transcription factors, was identified as the master regulator of Treg development. The essential role of Tregs in the maintenance of self-tolerance was confirmed by the discovery that the human disease IPEX (Immune dysregulation, Polyendocrinopathy, Enteropathy, X-linked syndrome) is due to mutations in *FOXP3*.[37]

   T cells with higher affinity for MHC-self-peptide complexes appear to be preferentially recruited to the Treg lineage. Tregs may in part exert their suppressive activity by out-competing autoreactive T cells for interactions with APCs expressing self-antigens. Other proposed mechanisms for Treg-mediated suppression include inhibition of self-antigen presentation by reducing APC expression of costimulatory proteins, secretion of inhibitory cytokines, and direct killing of effector T cells with granzyme and perforin.

   IL-2, TGF-β, and retinoic acid can induce the expression of Foxp3 and its downstream target genes, converting naïve T cells to an induced Treg (iTreg) phenotype. These cells may function in down-regulating the T cell-mediated response during resolution of infections, a function necessary for homeostatic control and blocking of collateral immunopathology. The presence of autoreactive T cells with specificity for disease-associated self-antigens in the peripheral blood of healthy individuals depleted of Tregs suggests that Treg dysfunction may occur in particular autoimmune diseases.[37] For example, the centrality of T cells recognizing glutamic acid decarboxylase suggests a possible role for Tregs in the pathogenesis of Type I DM.

T Cell Mediation of Inflammation

Naïve CD4[+] T cells differentiate into effector subsets characterized by the secretion of certain cytokines. T helper type 2 (T$_H$2) cells produce IL-4, IL-5, and IL-13; they are responsible for many allergic phenomena. T$_H$1 cells produce interferon-γ and are essential for the clearance of intracellular pathogens. T$_H$1 cells have been implicated in autoimmune conditions, though in certain animal models autoimmunity develops despite deficient production of T$_H$1 cells or type 1 cytokines.[31,38]

Under certain conditions, CD4[+] naïve cells can also develop into IL-17 producers (T$_H$17 cells).[39] TGF-β and IL-6 together inhibit Foxp3 expression leading to T_H17 generation. Expression of the transcription factor, RORγt, is also important for T_H17 differentiation.[40] T_H17 cells regulate tissue inflammation through IL-17-induced expression of other proinflammatory cytokines, chemokines, and matrix metalloproteases. IL-17 is also an important factor for neutrophil maturation and chemotaxis, and thus tissue infiltration and destruction.[41]

IL-17 and, by extension, T_H17 cells, have been implicated in various autoimmune conditions. High levels of IL-17 have been found in the sera and tissues of patients with conditions such as rheumatoid arthritis (RA),[42] multiple sclerosis,[43] SLE,[44] and inflammatory bowel disease.[45] In certain murine models, IL-17 deficiency can protect from induced autoimmunity.[46]

B Cell Tolerance

For B cells, development and central tolerance occur in the bone marrow. More than half of all BCRs on immature B cells are autoreactive.[18] If an immature B cell expresses a self-reactive BCR on its surface, strong intracellular signals lead to deletion. Intermediate signals cause receptor internalization and a block in the maturation process. Lymph node homing receptors are also not expressed, stranding the B cell in the bone marrow.[47] The recombination activating gene (RAG) proteins are re-expressed, and a replacement BCR light chain can be rearranged through receptor editing.[48] Autoreactive B cells may also become anergic and enter a state of antigen insensitivity.

There is no known mechanism in the bone marrow for expression of tissue-specific antigens, and a large proportion of B cells leave the bone marrow with self-directed specificities. These cells are regulated in the periphery through various signaling pathways. There is an ill-defined second checkpoint in the periphery that functions to remove autoreactive B cells. In addition, interactions with Tregs dampen the effects of autoreactive B cells.

Naïve B cells activated by antigen through T cell dependent mechanisms journey to germinal centers. There they undergo somatic hypermutation, where random nucleotide substitutions are introduced at the BCR locus. While self-reactivity can be reversed through somatic hypermutation, it can also be gained. Selective mechanisms in the germinal center also operate to suppress most autoreactive cells.[49]

B cell checkpoints may be circumvented in autoimmune conditions. Once activated, rogue autoreactive B cells foster autoimmunity in several ways. These B cells not only produce pathogenic antibodies, but they also secrete inflammatory cytokines and act as antigen-presenting cells for self-peptide specific T cells. Both SLE and RA are characterized by high-affinity IgG autoantibodies. Early B cell checkpoint defenses are thwarted in both conditions.[50,51] In SLE patients, early germinal center checkpoints are also subverted.[52]

Disease Modifiers

Genetic Disease Modifiers

While much can be learned from monogenic disorders, most autoimmune conditions are polygenic; genome-wide association studies have elucidated dozens of loci that confer susceptibility to a wide variety of autoimmune conditions. The most commonly cited modifier genes encode MHC molecules in the human leukocytes antigen (HLA) super-locus. Variable patterns of gene expression in the HLA complex have been identified in conditions such as psoriasis, SLE, and RA. Expression profiles also have been applied to subclassifying patients within disease conditions, providing insight into disease pathogenesis.[53]

The contribution of MHC genes to autoimmune disease is perhaps best illustrated in ankylosing spondylitis (AS). AS is a chronic, inflammatory arthritis primarily affecting the spine and sacroiliac joints. More than 4 decades ago, AS was noted to run in families, leading to the identification of the HLA-B27 allele as a susceptibility factor for AS. More than 90% of Caucasians with AS carry the HLA-B27 allele.[54] More recently, two additional non-MHC loci were identified in AS association studies. One is the locus for the receptor of IL-23, a cytokine that amplifies the T_H17 inflammatory responses. Another marker was found in the ARTS1 loci.[55] ARTS1 is a transmembrane aminopeptidase that functions in trimming peptides for MHC class I loading. ARTS1 may amplify HLA-B27 susceptibility due to an interaction of its trimmed peptides with HLA-B27 molecules.

Genes that encode costimulatory molecules also are frequently cited as modifiers of autoimmune diseases. There are a wide variety of costimulatory molecules. Some impart positive signals while others dampen activation. For example, signaling through cytotoxic T lymphocyte antigen 4 (CTLA-4) imparts a negative costimulatory signal. Vulnerability to autoimmune conditions, such as Graves' disease, autoimmune hypothyroidism, and Type 1 diabetes mellitus, has been mapped to a noncoding region of the CTLA-4 gene.[56] Mutations in this region may lead to decreased expression of CTLA-4 and abnormal regulation of T cells.[57] Subtle variations in costimulatory molecules can enhance autoimmunity or, conversely, protect from it. Ultimately, modifier gene data may be used to predict disease occurrence, determine prognosis, and also individualize treatment plans.

Environmental Factors

Complex modifier genes only partially explain the genesis of autoimmunity. Twin studies report a concordance rate between 24–50% for a variety of autoimmune conditions.[58] This discrepancy and the delayed onset of most autoimmune diseases suggest that additional factors are also at play. Determinants as varied as psychosocial stressors, smoking, exogenous hormone exposures, medications, and infections have been invoked to explain nongenetic differences in the incidence of autoimmunity.

Hormonal Factors

There is a skewing of the sex ratio in many autoimmune diseases. Overall, women are at a 2.7 times greater risk for acquiring an autoimmune condition.[1] The bias towards women is particularly striking in SLE. Explanations for this distribution include both sex-linked genes and hormonal factors.

B cells express estrogen receptors. In murine models, estrogen administration leads to an increase in serum B cell activating factor (BAFF). Estrogen also binds receptors on B cells, causing up-regulation of the antiapoptotic factor Bcl-2 and downstream BCR signaling components. Engagement of this estrogen-dependent pathway can lead to rescue of high affinity anti-DNA B cells from negative selection. Meanwhile, prolactin has a role in the activation of autoreactive B cells. Peripheral blood mononuclear cells (PBMCs) from SLE patients produce more prolactin than healthy controls. In addition, secretion of autoantibodies including anti-dsDNA is augmented by the incubation of prolactin with PBMCs from SLE patients.[59] These effects may partially explain the increased incidence of B cell dependent autoimmune conditions in women.

Stress, both physical and psychological, has been recognized as a risk factor for autoimmunity. The human stress response involves activation of the hypothalamic-pituitary-adrenal axis.

There is release of neurotransmitters and hormones, as well as activation of immune system components. Prolonged stress may activate inflammatory pathways without subsequent down-modulation of these responses. Glucocorticoids are decreased in many chronic diseases, which may partially explain their usefulness in the treatment of autoimmune conditions. In a study of patients with RA, a good response to anti-TNF therapy was associated with increased endogenous cortisol levels. Conversely, poor responders continued to have reduced serum cortisol.[60]

Vitamin D is another immunomodulatory hormone. Low vitamin D levels have been associated with an increased incidence of autoimmune disease.[61,62] Vitamin D can skew CD4+ T cell towards T_H2 and Treg differentiation.[63,64] Vitamin D also inhibits autoantibody production and secretion by B cells. Incubation of PBMCs from SLE patients with vitamin D resulted in decreased proliferation of B cells and diminished production of antibodies against dsDNA.[65]

Epigenetic and Epitope Modifications

Gene expression can be significantly altered via methylation, best studied in patients with SLE. Cells from patients with SLE and RA have reduced methylation compared with aged matched controls.[64,65] This may cause over-expression of certain genes as well as unmasking of latent viral genomes. Drugs may trigger autoimmunity through methylation changes as well. Hydralazine and procainamide are among the drugs most strongly implicated in the onset of drug-induced lupus. Both induce hypomethylation of T cell DNA. Hydralazine exerts its effect through inhibition of the extracellular-signal-regulated kinases (ERK) signaling pathways, thereby blocking up-regulation of methytransferases in activated T cells. Procainamide acts more directly as a competitive inhibitor of DNA methyltransferase.[66]

Alteration of self-epitopes is another mechanism for drug-induced autoimmunity. In certain cases of drug-induced autoimmune hemolytic anemia, the drug binds intrinsic red cell proteins. These complexes are recognized by the immune system as foreign antigens, triggering an immune response. Two medications associated with such haptenization, α-methyldopa and penicillin, were at one time associated with more than 10% of all cases of autoimmune hemolytic anemia.[67]

Infectious Triggers

Infectious agents have been long implicated in the triggering of autoimmunity and disease flares. This may occur in a variety of ways, including molecular mimicry, in which microorganisms and host antigens share expression of common epitopes. One specific BCR or TCR can recognize both host and foreign proteins, leading to both protective immunity and damaging autoimmunity. One example of molecular mimicry is Guillian-Barré syndrome (GBS), in which patients have weakness, abnormal reflexes, and sensory disturbances due to deposition of antibodies and complement along peripheral nerve axons. In GBS, there is cross-reactivity between antigens of *Campylobacter jejuni* and components of peripheral nerves. However, since only about 0.1% of the population infected with *C. jejuni* develops GBS, susceptibility factors such as impaired peripheral tolerance also play a major role.[68]

Other infectious agents also have been implicated in the induction of autoimmunity through molecular mimicry. The hepatitis B and coxsackie B4 viruses have been incriminated in the development of multiple sclerosis.[69] Group A streptococcal infections and rheumatic fever is another well known association. Recently, patients afflicted with pauci-immune necrotizing glomerulo-

phritis were shown to have autoantibodies directed against the lysosomal protein LAMP-2 which cross-react with epitopes from bacterial adhesion proteins.[70]

Other mechanisms by which infections may induce autoimmunity involve polyclonal activation of lymphocytes, whereby microbial components act as adjuvants to enhance immune responses. Alternatively, expression of potent costimulatory molecules also may be induced by these infectious agents, the so-called 'bystander effect'.[69] For example, mixed cryoglobulinemia is a systemic vasculitis mediated by immune complex deposition, often in the setting of infection with the hepatitis C virus (HCV). In this case, HCV chronically stimulates antibody-secreting B cell clones, leading to lymphocyte activation.[71]

Therapeutic Strategies

Inadequate understanding of fundamental disease mechanisms has limited treatment options for autoimmune diseases. Since the initial use of corticosteroids almost 60 years ago, clinicians could offer little more than global nonspecific immunosuppresion plus supportive care to mitigate end-organ damage from ongoing tissue destruction (e.g. insulin therapy for Type 1 DM). Fortunately, advances in molecular immunology have coincided with theoretical and practical demonstration of the utility of early, aggressive treatment of inflammatory disorders.[72] The potential to reverse or control autoimmunity before maturation and progression of the immune response has offered new approaches for reducing long-term disability and total exposure to immunosuppressive therapy.[73,74] Current practice has evolved to stress utilization of aggressive immunomodulatory therapy as soon as possible after diagnosis. Prominent treatments for autoimmune disease are reviewed in Table 14-2.

Systemic Immunosuppression

The mainstay of treatments for systemic autoimmune diseases remains immunosuppressive medications. These ameliorate the clinical and serologic effects of disease activity by targeting the effectors of the immune response. Adverse effects of immunosuppression result from interfering with protective immunity as well as pathologic autoimmunity. These include the ongoing risk of infection and the cumulative potential for increased malignancy due to diminished immune surveillance.

Corticosteroids, perhaps the least discriminating tool in the armamentarium, are used in doses ranging from daily low-dose oral regimens to 'pulsed' high-dose intravenous therapy.[75] Traditional disease-modifying antirheumatic drugs (DMARDs) such as methotrexate, leflunomide, hydroxychloroquine, and sulfasalazine are mildly immunosuppressive, and as such, cause minimally increased risks of infection. Their benefits are likely to be mediated through antiinflammatory and immunomodulatory effects rather than through immunosuppression per se.[76] More potent immunosuppressive agents such as azathioprine, cyclosporine A, mycophenolate mofetil, and cyclophosphamide are often necessary for treating more severe conditions, such as vasculitis and SLE.

Plasmapheresis is an important treatment utilized to remove pathogenic antibodies from the circulation. It is employed when urgent measures are needed to stabilize a patient before longer-term interventions take effect, for example cases of acute hemorrhage from the pulmonary-renal syndromes, Wegener's granulomatosis, and Goodpasture's syndrome.[77] Intravenous immunoglobulin (IVIG) has immunomodulatory properties

Table 14-2 Common Current Therapeutic Options for Treating Autoimmune Disease

	Mechanism of Action	Diseases Treated	Dosage	Principal Toxicities	Monitoring and Precautions
Disease-Modifying Antirheumatic Drugs					
Methotrexate	Blocks folate metabolism and purine synthesis Increases adenosine levels (antiinflammatory mediator)	Arthritis (rheumatoid, psoriatic) Ankylosing spondylitis	10 mg/m^2 qwk PO/SQ/IV, escalate as tolerated	Hepatitis, nausea, oral ulcers, bone marrow suppression, pneumonitis (rare in children)	LFTs q4–8 wks, periodic CBCs; folate can limit gastrointestinal and hematologic toxicity
Hydroxychloroquine	? Blocks lysosomal acidification and antigen processing. Regulation of autophagy	SLE	≤7.0 mg/kg/d PO, maximum 400 mg/d, divided qd to bid	Retinopathy, nausea, rash, agranulocytosis	Ophthalmologic evaluation q6mos, CBCs, LFTs q3–6 mos
Sulfasalazine	? Increases adenosine levels	Psoriatic arthritis Reactive arthritis Inflammatory bowel disease	Goal: 40–70 mg/kg/d PO divided bid/tid, maximum 3 g, start slowly	Rash, nausea, leukopenia, hepatitis, headache, photosensitivity, Stevens-Johnson syndrome	CBCs + LFTs qmo × 3–4 mos then periodically
Leflunomide	Blocks pyrimidine synthesis	Rheumatoid arthritis	Adult: 10–20 mg/d	Diarrhea, hepatitis, bone marrow suppression, alopecia/rash	LFTs qmo until stable, then q4–8 wks
Biologic Response Modifiers					
TNF-α inhibitors (etanercept, infliximab, adalimumab, certolizumab)	Blocks TNF-α	Arthritis (rheumatoid, psoriatic), ankylosing spondylitis, inflammatory bowel disease	Variable dosing regimens	Injection site reactions if given SC, infections, cytopenias, increased risk of cancers	Screening PPD before starting, monitor CBCs. May use with low-dose methotrexate to inhibit development of antibodies against drug
Abatacept	Modulates costimulatory signaling	Arthritis (rheumatoid and juvenile idiopathic)	10 mg/kg IV Q2 weeks × 2 weeks then Q4 weeks	Increased risk of infections	CBC
Anakinra	IL-1 receptor antagonist, blocks IL-1 action	Systemic onset arthritis and some autoinflammatory conditions	1–2 mg/kg daily SC injections up to a maximum of 100 mg daily	Painful local injection reactions, increased risk of infection	
Rituximab	B cell depletion	Autoimmune cytopenias, SLE	375 mg/m^2 per dose	Infusion reactions, hypogammaglobulinemia, increased risk of infection	Monitor immunoglobulin levels and for B cell recovery
Immunosuppressive Agents					
Azathioprine	Active metabolite 6-MP, blocks purine synthesis	Rheumatoid arthritis SLE Dermatomyositis	1–3+ mg/kg/d PO	Bone marrow suppression, infection (especially zoster), nausea, hepatitis, rash	CBC, LFTs
Cyclosporine A	Blocks synthesis of IL-2 and other cytokines by inhibiting calcineurin	Arthritis (rheumatoid, psoriatic) Macrophage activation syndrome	5–10 mg/kg/d divided bid	Hypertension, nephrotoxicity, hyperlipidemia, diabetes, tremor, seizures, gingival hyperplasia, hirsutism, skin cancer, lymphoma	Blood pressure, UA, CBC, BUN/Cr, glucose, LFTs, K, Mg q2 wks × 3 mos then q2–3 mos; multiple drug interactions
Mycophenolate mofetil	Blocks purine synthesis	SLE	600 mg/m^2/dose bid, maximum 1 g bid	Bone marrow suppression, infections, nausea, diarrhea	CBC
Cyclophosphamide	Alkylate DNA, leading to strand breakage	Lupus nephritis Systemic vasculitis (e.g. Wegener's granulomatosis) Goodpasture's syndrome	Monthly IV: 500–1000 mg/m^2, maximum 1.2 g (with concurrent mesna) PO: 50–100 mg/m^2/d	Bone marrow suppression, nausea, alopecia, bladder toxicity, infertility, cardiotoxicity	Whole blood cell count; periodic UA, BUN/Cr; long-term monitoring for leukemia and bladder cancer; PCP prophylaxis if on steroids

LFTs, Liver function tests; *CBCs,* complete blood counts; *SLE,* systemic lupus erythematosus; *TNF,* tumor necrosis factor; *UA,* urinalysis; *BUN/Cr,* blood urea nitrogen/creatinine; *K,* serum potassium; *Mg,* serum magnesium; *PCP, Pneumocystis carinii* pneumonia.

without the risks of immunosuppression, useful in the treatment of conditions such as dermatomyositis. IVIG is superior to any other therapy in arresting acute inflammation and preventing target-organ damage in cases of Kawasaki disease, an inflammatory vasculitis of childhood.[78] There is not yet a convincing explanation for this unique situation.

Targeted Molecular Therapies

During the past decade, a new generation of drugs targeting cytokines and lymphocyte receptors has dramatically altered the therapeutic landscape of rheumatology. These so-called 'biologic response modifiers' (BRMs) are recombinant monoclonal antibodies and receptor antagonists that inhibit specific targets following parenteral administration. Anti-TNFα therapies were the first of these 'biologic' therapies, and they have become routine options for treating a variety of autoimmune diseases including RA, JIA, inflammatory bowel disease, and psoriasis. Interestingly, these drugs were first used for treating patients with sepsis, in whom levels of TNF are massively elevated. The medications were not beneficial, however, and they subsequently found their niche in the treatment of RA and other inflammatory disorders as a result of basic investigations revealing a central role for TNF in the activation of macrophages, endothelial cells, and synoviocytes.[79,80] Today, anti-TNF biologics are often used in combination with methotrexate. Although they share the potential toxicities of all immunosuppressive medications, the precise targeting afforded by inhibition of TNF affords these medications a high degree of safety and efficacy during extended use in pediatric patients.[81]

Another target for inhibiting self-directed immunity is costimulatory interactions between T cells and APCs. CTLA-4 is a T cell surface protein that binds to CD80 and CD86 on activated APCs and modulates costimulatory activation signaling mediated by CD28.[82] Abatacept (Orencia) is a fusion protein of the extracellular domain of human CTLA-4 with a fragment of the Fc portion of human IgG1. This approach has the theoretical advantage of targeting only activated cells, and in fact, abatacept appears to increase risk of infections less than TNF inhibitors. Abatacept is currently approved for use in the treatment of RA and JIA that is refractory to anti-TNF therapy.[83,84]

B cell depletion using monoclonal antibodies directed against B cell surface markers is a relatively specific means of targeting a central mediator of the immune response. Rituximab (Rituxan) is a chimeric monoclonal antibody generated against the B cell protein CD20. A single dose rapidly reduces numbers of mature B cells in the peripheral circulation to unmeasureable levels. Rituximab was originally approved for the use of B cell non-Hodgkin lymphoma in 1997. Since that time, it has been evaluated in a variety of rheumatologic diseases associated with B cell dysregulation and autoantibody production. Thus far, rituximab has been shown to be effective in the treatment of autoimmune cytopenias in pediatric lupus patients without exposing them to significant risk of infection.[85] Further, because B cells are also important for antigen presentation, rituximab is effective in a variety of inflammatory disorders thought to be driven by cellular immunity, including RA and multiple sclerosis.

Just as unexpected benefits of medications like rituximab are revealing new aspects of autoimmune pathogenesis, biologic response modifiers occasionally demonstrate unexpected toxicity as well. Thus, the potential for activation of costimulatory molecules on platelets was only recognized when SLE patients treated with an anti-CD40 ligand (CD154) monoclonal antibody unexpectedly developed severe thromboembolic complica-

tions.[86] Similarly, a trial of an anti-CD28 monoclonal antibody had to be halted when patients developed circulatory collapse from cytokine storm.[87] These experiences underline the importance of introducing new biologic agents in the context of well-controlled clinical trials, not ad hoc individual experiments.

Novel Therapeutic Targets

Novel targeted therapies for autoimmune disease will continue to exploit cytokines and lymphocyte cell surface molecules involved in mediating inflammation and lymphocyte activation. Not only monoclonal antibodies, but small molecule inhibitors and interfering RNA are being investigated. IL-6 is a potent inflammatory cytokine that is inhibited by tocilizumab (Actemra), a humanized monoclonal antibody directed against the IL-6 receptor. It has shown greater efficacy than methotrexate as monotherapy in RA and has been approved for this indication in Europe.[88] Additional cytokine targets currently in preclinical investigation include IL-17 and IL-23, cytokines implicated in the action of T_H17 cells. Drugs targeting B cell activation molecules such as BAFF and APRIL (a proliferation-inducing ligand) are also under investigation.[89]

Proteosome inhibition and pharmacologic regulation of autophagy, a cellular recycling pathway in which intracellular contents are sequestered within double-lipid membrane-enclosed autophagosomes and delivered to lysosomes for degradation, represent additional autoimmune disease targets of interest. Plasma cells rely on high rates of protein synthesis for immunoglobulin secretion. Multiple myeloma cells have been shown to be susceptible to inhibition of the proteosome, a molecular machine involved in protein degradation. Bortezomib, a drug approved for the treatment of multiple myeloma, depletes short and long-lived plasma cells by activation of the terminal unfolded protein response, leading to reduced autoantibody production. It can protect lupus-prone mouse strains from the development of nephritis.[90] Hydroxychloroquine, a drug used to treat malaria for more than half a century, also blocks acidification of phagolysosomes. It is known to prolong remissions in SLE, and may exert beneficial effects in other autoimmune disease by modulating autophagy-mediated antigen presentation and innate immune receptor activation.[91] Future work may lead to therapies that capitalize on immune cell requirements for cellular recycling and unfolded protein response pathways in order to inhibit autoreactive responses without causing significant immunosuppresion.

Small molecule protein kinase inhibitors developed for the treatment of malignancies may have utility in autoimmune diseases. For example, patients with systemic sclerosis (SSc) demonstrate increased activity of the PDGFR (platelet-derived growth factor receptor), possibly due to stimulatory autoantibodies.[92] Studies have focused attention on imatinib (Gleevec), a drug that inhibits multiple tyrosine kinases including PGDFR, as a possible therapy for SSc. This kinase inhibitor has already revolutionized the treatment of chronic myelogenous leukemia and gastrointestinal stromal tumors.

When all else fails, patients with severe immune dysregulation and autoimmune disease may be treated by 'resetting' of the immune system in an attempt to restore normal tolerance. Treatment of severe autoimmunity with stem cell transplantation remains experimental, largely because of the significant morbidity and mortality that still accompany this approach. Nonetheless, this approach has been used in uncontrolled systemic JRA, SSc, and SLE, among other conditions. For example, a recent report documented sustained clinical remission in seven patients with severe refractory SLE treated with immunoablation and autologous hematopoietic stem cell transplantation. Further, after transplantation the patients demonstrated evidence of normalization of naïve lymphocyte populations and generation of thymic-derived regulatory T cells.[93] Safer methods for reconstituting the bone marrow compartment, such as autologous stem cell reconstitution protocols, could provide a therapeutic alternative for the most difficult to treat patients.

Conclusions

All autoimmune diseases, despite their diversity and tissue heterogeneity, can be traced to a breakdown in self-tolerance or dysregulation of innate immunity. As in other acquired diseases, autoimmunity results from a complex interplay of genetic predisposition, environmental influences, and ill-defined stochastic effects. Although targeted therapies have already revolutionized the care of patients with autoimmune disease, immunosuppressive treatment remains a necessary evil. With a more nuanced understanding of the mechanisms regulating self-tolerance and innate immunity, improved therapies are on the horizon. Formerly fatal diseases may soon be successfully managed, and chronic conditions that currently require life-long therapy may be susceptible to cures.

Acknowledgment

This work was supported by the Samara Jan Turkel Center for Pediatric Autoimmune Disease.

References

1. Jacobson DL, et al. Epidemiology and estimated population burden of selected autoimmune diseases in the United States. Clin Immunol Immunopathol 1997;84:223–43.
2. Medzhitov R. Origin and physiological roles of inflammation. Nature 2008;454:428–35.
3. Stojanov S, Kastner DL. Familial autoinflammatory diseases: genetics, pathogenesis and treatment. Curr Opin Rheumatol 2005;17:586–99.
4. Franchi L, et al. The inflammasome: a caspase-1-activation platform that regulates immune responses and disease pathogenesis. Nat Immunol 2009;10:241–7.
5. Miceli-Richard C, et al. CARD15 mutations in Blau syndrome. Nat Genet 2001;29:19–20.
6. Aksentijevich I, et al. De novo CIAS1 mutations, cytokine activation, and evidence for genetic heterogeneity in patients with neonatal-onset multisystem inflammatory disease (NOMID): a new member of the expanding family of pyrin-associated autoinflammatory diseases. Arthritis Rheum 2002;46:3340–8.
7. Feldmann J, et al. Chronic infantile neurological cutaneous and articular syndrome is caused by mutations in CIAS1, a gene highly expressed in polymorphonuclear cells and chondrocytes. Am J Hum Genet 2002;71:198–203.
8. Hoffman HM, et al. Mutation of a new gene encoding a putative pyrin-like protein causes familial cold autoinflammatory syndrome and Muckle-Wells syndrome. Nat Genet 2001;29:301–5.
9. Dostert C, et al. Innate immune activation through Nalp3 inflammasome sensing of asbestos and silica. Science 2008;320:674–7.
10. Marrack P, McKee AS, Munks MW. Towards an understanding of the adjuvant action of aluminium. Nat Rev Immunol 2009;9:287–93.
11. Pascual V, et al. Role of interleukin-1 (IL-1) in the pathogenesis of systemic onset juvenile idiopathic arthritis and clinical response to IL-1 blockade. J Exp Med 2005;201:1479–86.
12. Stetson DB, et al. Trex1 prevents cell-intrinsic initiation of autoimmunity. Cell 2008;134:587–98.
13. Stetson DB, Medzhitov R. Recognition of cytosolic DNA activates an IRF3-dependent innate immune response. Immunity 2006;24:93–103.
14. Burckstummer T, et al. An orthogonal proteomic-genomic screen identifies AIM2 as a cytoplasmic DNA sensor for the inflammasome. Nat Immunol 2009;10:266–72.
15. Roberts TL, et al. HIN-200 proteins regulate caspase activation in response to foreign cytoplasmic DNA. Science 2009;323:1057–60.
16. Delves PJ, Roitt IM. The immune system. First of two parts. N Engl J Med 2000;343:37–49.
17. Zerrahn J, Held W, Raulet DH. The MHC reactivity of the T cell repertoire prior to positive and negative selection. Cell 1997;88:627–36.
18. Wardemann H, et al. Predominant autoantibody production by early human B cell precursors. Science 2003;301:1374–7.
19. Laufer TM, et al. Unopposed positive selection and autoreactivity in mice expressing class II MHC only on thymic cortex. Nature 1996;383:81–5.
20. Liston A, et al. Aire regulates negative selection of organ-specific T cells. Nat Immunol 2003;4:350–4.
21. Kishimoto H, Sprent J. Negative selection in the thymus includes semimature T cells. J Exp Med 1997;185:263–71.
22. Nagamine K, et al. Positional cloning of the APECED gene. Nat Genet 1997;17:393–8.
23. Finnish-German APECED Consortium. An autoimmune disease. APECED, caused by mutations in a novel gene featuring two PHD-type zinc-finger domains. Nat Genet 1997;17:399–403.
24. Anderson MS, et al. Projection of an immunological self shadow within the thymus by the aire protein. Science 2002;298:1395–401.
25. Anderson MS, et al. The cellular mechanism of Aire control of T cell tolerance. Immunity 2005;23:227–39.
26. Ramsey C, et al. Aire deficient mice develop multiple features of APECED phenotype and show altered immune response. Hum Mol Genet 2002;11:397–409.
27. Ahonen P, et al. Clinical variation of autoimmune polyendocrinopathy-candidiasis-ectodermal dystrophy (APECED) in a series of 68 patients. N Engl J Med 1990;322:1829–36.
28. Kyewski B, Taubert R. How promiscuity promotes tolerance: the case of myasthenia gravis. Ann N Y Acad Sci 2008;1132:157–62.
29. Gardner JM, et al. Deletional tolerance mediated by extrathymic Aire-expressing cells. Science 2008;321:843–7.
30. Fleisher TA. The autoimmune lymphoproliferative syndrome: an experiment of nature involving lymphocyte apoptosis. Immunol Res 2008;40:87–92.
31. Jones LS, et al. IFN-gamma-deficient mice develop experimental autoimmune uveitis in the context of a deviant effector response. J Immunol 1997;158:5997–6005.
32. Kischkel FC, et al. Death receptor recruitment of endogenous caspase-10 and apoptosis initiation in the absence of caspase-8. J Biol Chem 2001;276:46639–46.
33. Wang J, et al. Inherited human Caspase 10 mutations underlie defective lymphocyte and dendritic cell apoptosis in autoimmune lymphoproliferative syndrome type II. Cell 1999;98:47–58.
34. Oliveira JB, et al. NRAS mutation causes a human autoimmune lymphoproliferative syndrome. Proc Natl Acad Sci U S A 2007;104:8953–8.
35. Cerutti E, et al. Co-inherited mutations of Fas and caspase-10 in development of the autoimmune lymphoproliferative syndrome. BMC Immunol 2007;8:28.
36. Sakaguchi S, et al. Regulatory T cells and immune tolerance. Cell 2008;133:775–87.
37. Danke NA, et al. Autoreactive T cells in healthy individuals. J Immunol 2004;172:5967–72.
38. Ferber IA, et al. Mice with a disrupted IFN-gamma gene are susceptible to the induction of experimental autoimmune encephalomyelitis (EAE). J Immunol 1996;156:5–7.
39. Park H, et al. A distinct lineage of CD4 T cells regulates tissue inflammation by producing interleukin 17. Nat Immunol 2005;6:1133–41.
40. Yang XO, et al. T helper 17 lineage differentiation is programmed by orphan nuclear receptors ROR alpha and ROR gamma. Immunity 2008;28:29–39.
41. Kolls JK, Linden A. Interleukin-17 family members and inflammation. Immunity 2004;21:467–76.
42. Chabaud M, et al. Contribution of interleukin 17 to synovium matrix destruction in rheumatoid arthritis. Cytokine 2000;12:1092–9.
43. Matusevicius D, et al. Interleukin-17 mRNA expression in blood and CSF mononuclear cells is augmented in multiple sclerosis. Mult Scler 1999;5:101–4.
44. Wong CK, et al. Elevation of proinflammatory cytokine (IL-18, IL-17, IL-12) and Th2 cytokine (IL-4) concentrations in patients with systemic lupus erythematosus. Lupus 2000;9:589–93.
45. Fujino S, et al. Increased expression of interleukin 17 in inflammatory bowel disease. Gut 2003;52:65–70.
46. Bettelli E, et al. Loss of T-bet, but not STAT1, prevents the development of experimental autoimmune encephalomyelitis. J Exp Med 2004;200:79–87.
47. Hartley SB, et al. Elimination of self-reactive B lymphocytes proceeds in two stages: arrested development and cell death. Cell 1993;72:325–35.
48. Goodnow CC, et al. Cellular and genetic mechanisms of self tolerance and autoimmunity. Nature 2005;435:590–7.
49. Tiller T, et al. Autoreactivity in human IgG+ memory B cells. Immunity 2007;26:205–13.
50. Yurasov S, et al. Defective B cell tolerance checkpoints in systemic lupus erythematosus. J Exp Med 2005;201:703–11.

51. Samuels J, et al. Impaired early B cell tolerance in patients with rheumatoid arthritis. J Exp Med 2005;201:1659–67.

52. Cappione A 3rd, et al. Germinal center exclusion of autoreactive B cells is defective in human systemic lupus erythematosus. J Clin Invest 2005;115:3205–16.

53. Shiina T, et al. The HLA genomic loci map: expression, interaction, diversity and disease. J Hum Genet 2009;54:15–39.

54. Brown MA, Breakthroughs in genetic studies of ankylosing spondylitis. Rheumatology (Oxford) 2008;47:132–7.

55. Burton PR, et al. Association scan of 14,500 nonsynonymous SNPs in four diseases identifies autoimmunity variants. Nat Genet 2007;39:1329–37.

56. Ueda H, et al. Association of the T cell regulatory gene CTLA4 with susceptibility to autoimmune disease. Nature 2003;423:506–11.

57. Yamada A, Salama AD, Sayegh MH. The role of novel T cell costimulatory pathways in autoimmunity and transplantation. J Am Soc Nephrol 2002;13:559–75.

58. Dooley MA, Hogan SL. Environmental epidemiology and risk factors for autoimmune disease. Curr Opin Rheumatol 2003;15:99–103.

59. Cohen-Solal JF, et al. Hormonal regulation of B cell function and systemic lupus erythematosus. Lupus 2008;17:528–32.

60. Straub RH, et al. Increased cortisol relative to adrenocorticotropic hormone predicts improvement during anti-tumor necrosis factor therapy in rheumatoid arthritis. Arthritis Rheum 2008;58:976–84.

61. Cantorna MT, Mahon BD. Mounting evidence for vitamin D as an environmental factor affecting autoimmune disease prevalence. Exp Biol Med (Maywood) 2004;229:1136–42.

62. Munger KL, et al. Vitamin D intake and incidence of multiple sclerosis. Neurology 2004;62:60–5.

63. Boonstra A, et al. 1alpha,25-Dihydroxyvitamin d3 has a direct effect on naive CD4(+) T cells to enhance the development of Th2 cells. J Immunol 2001;167:4974–80.

64. Mahon BD, et al. The targets of vitamin D depend on the differentiation and activation status of CD4 positive T cells. J Cell Biochem 2003;89:922–32.

65. Linker-Israeli M, et al. Vitamin D(3) and its synthetic analogs inhibit the spontaneous in vitro immunoglobulin production by SLE-derived PBMC. Clin Immunol 2001;99:82–93.

66. Richardson B, DNA methylation and autoimmune disease. Clin Immunol 2003;109:72–9.

67. Gehrs BC, Friedberg RC. Autoimmune hemolytic anemia. Am J Hematol 2002;69:258–71.

68. Ang CW, Jacobs BC, Laman JD. The Guillain-Barre syndrome: a true case of molecular mimicry. Trends Immunol 2004;25:61–6.

69. Bach JF, Infections and autoimmune diseases. J Autoimmun 2005; 25(Suppl):74–80.

70. Kain R, et al. Molecular mimicry in pauci-immune focal necrotizing glomerulonephritis. Nat Med 2008;14:1088–96.

71. De Vita S, Quartuccio L, Fabris M. Hepatitis C virus infection, mixed cryoglobulinemia and BLyS upregulation: targeting the infectious trigger, the autoimmune response, or both? Autoimmun Rev 2008;8: 95–9.

72. Rantalaiho V, et al. The good initial response to therapy with a combination of traditional disease-modifying antirheumatic drugs is sustained over time: the eleven-year results of the Finnish rheumatoid arthritis combination therapy trial. Arthritis Rheum 2009;60:1222–31.

73. Albers HM, et al. Time to treatment as an important factor for the response to methotrexate in juvenile idiopathic arthritis. Arthritis Rheum 2009;61:46–51.

74. Fisler RE, et al. Aggressive management of juvenile dermatomyositis results in improved outcome and decreased incidence of calcinosis. J Am Acad Dermatol 2002;47:505–11.

75. Parker BJ, Bruce IN. High dose methylprednisolone therapy for the treatment of severe systemic lupus erythematosus. Lupus 2007;16: 387–93.

76. Cespedes-Cruz A, et al. Methotrexate improves the health-related quality of life of children with juvenile idiopathic arthritis. Ann Rheum Dis 2008;67:309–14.

77. Sugimoto T, et al. Pulmonary-renal syndrome, diffuse pulmonary hemorrhage and glomerulonephritis, associated with Wegener's granulomatosis effectively treated with early plasma exchange therapy. Intern Med 2007;46:49–53.

78. Newburger JW, et al. Diagnosis, treatment, and long-term management of Kawasaki disease: a statement for health professionals from the Committee on Rheumatic Fever, Endocarditis and Kawasaki Disease, Council on Cardiovascular Disease in the Young, American Heart Association. Circulation 2004;110:2747–71.

79. Choy EH, Panayi GS. Cytokine pathways and joint inflammation in rheumatoid arthritis. N Engl J Med 2001;344:907–16.

80. O'Shea JJ, Ma A, Lipsky P. Cytokines and autoimmunity. Nat Rev Immunol 2002;2:37–45.

81. Lovell DJ, et al. Safety and efficacy of up to eight years of continuous etanercept therapy in patients with juvenile rheumatoid arthritis. Arthritis Rheum 2008;58:1496–504.

82. Bayry J, Autoimmunity: CTLA-4: a key protein in autoimmunity. Nat Rev Rheumatol 2009;5:244–5.

83. Lovell DJ, et al. Adalimumab with or without methotrexate in juvenile rheumatoid arthritis. N Engl J Med 2008;359:810–20.

84. Ruperto N, et al. Abatacept in children with juvenile idiopathic arthritis: a randomised, double-blind, placebo-controlled withdrawal trial. Lancet 2008;372:383–91.

85. Kumar S, et al. B cell depletion for autoimmune thrombocytopenia and autoimmune hemolytic anemia in pediatric systemic lupus erythematosus. Pediatrics 2009;123:e159–63.

86. Kawai T, et al. Thromboembolic complications after treatment with monoclonal antibody against CD40 ligand. Nat Med 2000;6:114.

87. Suntharalingam G, et al. Cytokine storm in a phase 1 trial of the anti-CD28 monoclonal antibody TGN1412. N Engl J Med 2006;355: 1018–28.

88. Jones G, et al. Comparison of tocilizumab monotherapy versus methotrexate monotherapy in patients with moderate to severe rheumatoid arthritis: the AMBITION study. Ann Rheum Dis 2009;Mar 17 (Epub ahead of print).

89. Waldburger JM, Firestein GS. Garden of therapeutic delights: new targets in rheumatic diseases. Arthritis Res Ther 2009;11:206.

90. Neubert K, et al. The proteasome inhibitor bortezomib depletes plasma cells and protects mice with lupus-like disease from nephritis. Nat Med 2008;14:748–55.

91. Rubinsztein DC, et al. Potential therapeutic applications of autophagy. Nat Rev Drug Discov 2007;6:304–12.

92. Baroni SS, et al. Stimulatory autoantibodies to the PDGF receptor in systemic sclerosis. N Engl J Med 2006;354:2667–76.

93. Alexander T, et al. Depletion of autoreactive immunologic memory followed by autologous hematopoietic stem cell transplantation in patients with refractory SLE induces long-term remission through de novo generation of a juvenile and tolerant immune system. Blood 2009;113: 214–23.

15

Congenital Immune Dysregulation Disorders

Thomas A. Fleisher • Joao Bosco Oliveira • Troy R. Torgerson

Down-regulation of the immune response has become a subject of increased focus as immunologists look for regulatory mechanisms that may play a role in the prevention of chronic inflammatory disorders. This emerging area of investigation complements extensive work done to characterize the differentiation and activation of immune cells. Primary lymphoid immune deficiency diseases have provided critical insights into these processes including an improved understanding of lymphocyte development, antigen recognition, and cell activation. In a similar fashion, recently described prototypic human disorders that affect various immunoregulatory pathways have provided important insights into mechanisms required for tolerance and the control of immune responses. In this chapter we will discuss congenital disorders that impact central deletion of autoreactive T cells in the thymus as well as those that impact other mechanisms involved in the maintenance of tolerance in the periphery. In all of these disorders the clinical phenotype includes autoimmunity together with other manifestations.

Autoimmune Polyendocrinopathy, Candidiasis, Ectodermal Dystrophy (APECED)

APECED (OMIM #240300) is the prototypic disorder of defective central immune tolerance. It is an autosomal recessive disorder characterized by systemic autoimmunity that primarily affects endocrine organs, particularly the parathyroid and adrenal glands.[1,2] Hypoparathyroidism, adrenal insufficiency, and chronic mucocutaneous candidiasis typically characterize the syndrome but patients may also have type 1 diabetes, gonadal failure, pernicious anemia (secondary to atrophy of gastric parietal cells), autoimmune hepatitis, and cutaneous manifestations.[1,2]

Genetics and Immunopathogenesis

APECED is caused by mutations in the gene encoding the autoimmune regulator (AIRE), a transcription factor that plays a role in ectopic expression of tissue-specific antigens on medullary thymic epithelial cells (mTECs). In mice, AIRE-mediated self-antigen expression in the thymus has been shown to play a significant role in negative selection of autoreactive T cell clones thus preventing their escape into the periphery where they may cause autoimmunity.[3,4] The mechanism by which AIRE causes expression of tissue-specific gene products is unknown but recent evidence suggests that it may do so by regulating large-scale access to chromatin.

Since naturally arising T regulatory (T_{REG}) cells are also thymically derived, it has been hypothesized that AIRE may also play a role in generation of T_{REG} cells. Recent investigations, using a transgenic mouse model with a monospecific T cell receptor, suggest that the autoimmunity seen in $Aire^{-/-}$ mice results from a combination of defective negative selection of autoreactive effector T cells and defective generation of antigen-specific T_{REG} cells.[5]

The role of AIRE in generation and function of T_{REG} cells has also been investigated in humans. Two studies have evaluated patients with APECED by flow cytometry and quantitative real-time PCR for the presence of T_{REG} cells expressing the forkhead DNA-binding protein, FOXP3, in the peripheral blood. In each study, patients were found to have a decreased percentage of $CD4^+CD25^{high}$ T cells. In addition, $CD4^+CD25^{high}$ T cells from patients expressed less FOXP3 than similar cells from normal controls.[6,7] Coincident with the decreased FOXP3 expression in the $CD4^+CD25^{high}$ cells, isolated T_{REG} cells from APECED patients had a decreased ability to suppress proliferation of effector T cells in response to anti-CD3 or mitogen in vitro.[6] These data suggest that AIRE plays a significant role in the generation of functional T_{REG} cells in humans.

Diagnosis and Treatment (Box 15-1)

APECED is typically suspected in patients who have two of the three basic symptoms: hypoparathyroidism (usually manifested by hypocalcemia), adrenal insufficiency, and mucocutaneous candidiasis. Suspicion is raised further by the presence of other autoimmune manifestations including diabetes, gonadal insufficiency, hepatitis, pernicious anemia, etc. A definitive diagnosis can be made by sequencing the AIRE gene.

Despite the impressive autoimmune phenotype, most of the therapy for APECED has focused on symptomatic treatment, including calcium supplementation, steroid replacement, and the management of diabetes and other endocrinopathies. Particularly problematic is the mucocutaneous candidiasis which may be related to autoantibodies to IL-17 and causes significant morbidity and increases the risk of oral malignancies.[8] In many patients, the candidal species develop reduced sensitivity to azole antifungals over time, making long-term management very challenging.[9]

Immunosuppressants are not routinely used in APECED unless patients develop autoimmune hepatitis or renal disease, in which case, azathioprine and cyclosporine A have shown benefit.[2] Recent studies in $Aire^{-/-}$ mice have demonstrated a sig-

©2010 Elsevier Ltd, Inc, BV
DOI: 10.1016/B978-1-4377-0271-2.00015-8

BOX 15-1 Key concepts
Autoimmune Polyendocrinopathy, Candidiasis, Ectodermal Dystrophy (APECED)
Typical clinical triad:
• Hypoparathyroidism
• Adrenal insufficiency
• Chronic mucocutaneous candidiasis

BOX 15-2 Key concepts
Immunodysregulation, Polyendocrynopathy, Enteropathy, X-Linked Syndrome (IPEX)
Characteristic clinical findings:
• Very early onset, typically first year of life
• Watery diarrhea
• Type 1 diabetes
• Dermatitis

nificant role for B cells and autoantibodies in the pathogenesis of disease, suggesting a potential role for B cell depletion therapy in this disorder.[10] Bone marrow transplantation generally has not been considered for APECED, even in severe cases.

Immune Dysregulation, Polyendocrinopathy, Enteropathy, X-linked (IPEX)

IPEX syndrome (OMIM #304930) is the prototypic disease resulting from a loss of peripheral immune tolerance. The basic clinical triad of IPEX includes autoimmune enteropathy, early onset endocrinopathy, and dermatitis.[11-13] The enteropathy typically presents very early in life as watery diarrhea, frequently resulting in malnutrition and failure to thrive. Type 1 diabetes is the most common endocrinopathy but clinical and/or laboratory evidence of thyroiditis is common as well. Eczema is the most common dermatitis in IPEX but erythroderma, psoriasiform dermatitis, and pemphigoid nodularis have also been observed.[14-16]

In addition to the 'IPEX-triad', most patients with IPEX also have other associated autoimmune disorders including autoimmune hemolytic anemia, thrombocytopenia, neutropenia, nephropathy, or hepatic disease (Torgerson & Ochs, unpublished data). These conditions contribute substantially to the morbidity of patients with IPEX and increase the risk of death from disease. Patients with the classical form of the disease typically die secondary to malnutrition, electrolyte imbalances, or infection before the age of 2 years, if not treated with aggressive immunosuppression.[16]

Genetics and Immunopathogenesis

IPEX is caused by mutations in FOXP3, a 431 amino acid protein expressed by CD4+CD25high regulatory T cells.[17-19] Recent studies have demonstrated that FOXP3 is required for T_{REG} cells to develop suppressor function.[20,21] This has been demonstrated in two separate knock-in mouse models in which CD4+ T cells destined to become T_{REGS} were unable to express functional FOXP3 but rather expressed green fluorescent protein. Despite this, the cells still acquired the expected cell surface phenotype of a T_{REG} (CD25high CTLA-4high GITRhigh) but had no suppressive function. Instead, they developed a gene expression profile suggestive of an effector/cytotoxic T cell and the animals developed evidence of systemic autoimmunity similar to $Foxp3^{-/-}$ mice.[21]

Under quiescent conditions, FOXP3 expression is restricted primarily to T_{REG} cells, however, recent data has demonstrated that FOXP3 can be inducibly expressed in a large percentage of activated human T cells.[22-25] Originally shown to be a transcriptional repressor acting on key cytokine genes,[26-28] recent genome-wide screening approaches suggest that it functions more commonly as a transcriptional enhancer.[29,30] A great deal of work remains to identify the key FOXP3-regulated gene (or genes) that that confers suppressor function on T cells.

Most pathologic mutations in FOXP3 cluster in three important functional domains of the protein: the C-terminal forkhead DNA-binding domain, the leucine zipper and the N-terminal repression domain.[31] Recent studies suggest that FOXP3 physically and functionally interacts with other transcription factors including NFAT, NF-κB, AML-1/RUNX1, and the retinoic acid receptor-related orphan receptors RORα and RORγt to modulate gene transcription at key cytokine promoters.[27,28,32-35]

Diagnosis and Treatment (Box 15-2)

IPEX is generally suspected in any patient who demonstrates at least two of the three basic clinical features of IPEX including enteropathy, endocrinopathy (Type 1 diabetes or thyroiditis), and dermatitis. Flow cytometry using intracellular staining for the FOXP3 protein in order to identify FOXP3+ T_{REG} cells is a valuable tool to rapidly screen for the absence of T_{REG}. In our hands, approximately 5–7% of the CD4+ T cell population is positive for FOXP3 expression in controls and a marked decrease suggests a diagnosis of IPEX which can be confirmed by sequencing the FOXP3 gene (Figure 15-1). Currently, the gold standard for diagnosis is identification of a mutation in FOXP3; however, in the cohort of patients that we have evaluated, mutations are identified in only 25–30% of those in whom there is a clinical suspicion of disease (Torgerson, unpublished data).

From a clinical laboratory standpoint, the most consistent abnormality among patients with IPEX is markedly elevated immunoglobulinum E (IgE) which is present in the majority of cases. IgA is also modestly elevated in more than 50% of patients (Torgerson & Ochs, unpublished data). There are no consistent abnormalities in absolute lymphocyte numbers, including CD4+, CD8+, CD19+, or CD16/56+ cells. T cells usually respond normally to proliferative stimuli with either mitogens or antigen.

Adoptive transfer studies in mice have demonstrated that the CD4+ T cells from an affected $Foxp3^{-/-}$ male are capable of recapitulating the entire disease phenotype in a lymphopenic recipient.[36] Treatment of IPEX has therefore focused primarily on suppression of unregulated, auto-aggressive T cells using cyclosporine, tacrolimus (FK506), or sirolimus (rapamycin).[12,13,37,38] These are often combined with steroids and/or other immunomodulatory agents, including methotrexate or azathioprine in an effort to control symptoms.[38,39] In cases where there is evidence for pathogenic autoantibodies, rituximab (anti-CD20) has proven effective.[15] These therapies are often effective initially and there is one report of a patient with IPEX being maintained for a prolonged period with aggressive immunosuppression; however, most patients ultimately fail therapy.[40] Currently, bone marrow transplantation holds the only hope for a long-term cure.[41-43] Both complete and reduced intensity conditioning protocols have been reported as successful although reduced intensity regimens seem to be associated with better survival.[42,43] In many of the cases transplanted thus far, patients are successfully

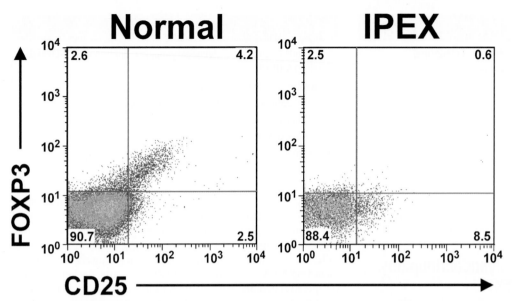

Figure 15-1 Absence of FOXP3 + regulatory T cells in IPEX. Peripheral blood mononuclear cells (PBMCs) from a normal individual and a patient with IPEX were fixed, permeabilized, and stained for the presence of CD4, CD25, and FOXP3. After gating on the CD4+ T cell population, two-dimensional analysis demonstrates the absence of CD25+ *FOXP3*+ regulatory T cells in the PBMCs of a patient with IPEX syndrome due to a mutation in the polyadenylation site of the *FOXP3* gene.

engrafted and have resolution of all IPEX symptoms except for the diabetes. Rapid diagnosis and transplantation early in the course of disease, before the pancreatic islets are destroyed, should therefore be the goal in order to avoid the long-term sequellae of diabetes in these patients.

Defects in IL-2 Signaling

Since the realization that mice lacking CD25 (the α-chain of the IL-2 receptor) have a phenotype similar to *Foxp3*[-/-] mice, there has been a suspicion that defects that blunt IL-2 signaling in T cells might lead to an IPEX-like presentation in humans.

CD25 Deficiency

Two unrelated patients with CD25 deficiency (OMIM #606367) have now been described in the literature. Similar to the clinical manifestations of IPEX, both patients developed severe, chronic diarrhea and villous atrophy in infancy (one at 6 weeks and the other at 8 months of age).[44,45] One also developed early onset insulin-dependent diabetes and later developed eczema.[44] Subsequently, both patients developed autoantibodies, hepatosplenomegaly, lymphadenopathy, and lymphocytic infiltrates in various organs (gut, liver, etc.) indicative of ongoing immune dysregulation.[44–46] Unlike patients with *FOXP3* mutations, serum IgE levels were only mildly elevated in one patient and normal in the other.[44,45]

In addition to autoimmune features, both CD25-deficient patients had infectious complications suggestive of a more extensive defect in cellular immunity. Most prominent in both patients was early onset, recurrent CMV pneumonitis, although persistent thrush, candidal esophagitis, chronic gastroenteritis, and EBV infection were also seen.[44,45] One patient even failed to reject an allogeneic skin graft.[47]

Genetics and Immunopathogenesis

In each case, inheritance was found to be autosomal recessive leading to a complete lack of CD25 protein expression on acti-

vated T cells. One patient, the product of consanguinuous parents, was homozygous for a four base pair deletion in the coding region of *CD25* that causes a frameshift and early termination codon within the CD25 protein.[45,47] The other patient had compound heterozygous mutations in the *CD25* gene that led to a frameshift on one allele and a premature stop codon on the other.[44]

Recent studies in *Cd25*[-/-] mice have demonstrated that T$_{REG}$ cell development is normal in the thymus and these cells have normal suppressive function in vitro. There is, however, a defect in the survival, maintenance, and competitive fitness of mature T$_{REG}$ cells, which appears to underlie the immune dysregulation observed[48,49] (Figure 15-2). Future efforts to assess T$_{REG}$ cells in CD25-deficient patients will hopefully help to determine whether a similar mechanism is at play in humans.

Diagnosis and Treatment

As noted above, CD25 deficiency has been inherited in an autosomal recessive manner in both of the described cases. Both patients also lacked CD25 expression on T cells suggesting that flow cytometry is an effective screening tool to identify CD25-deficient patients. Sequencing of the *CD25* gene is, however, recommended to confirm the diagnosis.

Because of the 'SCID-like' features of this syndrome, one patient underwent a successful bone marrow transplant from a matched sibling donor and has done well.[46,47] It is possible, however, that patients may respond to IL-2 therapy since the T cell proliferative defect was overcome in one patient by ex vivo treatment with high dose IL-2 or IL-15. Exogenous IL-2 may provide enough stimulation through the remaining 'intermediate-affinity' IL-2 receptor beta and gamma chains to allow T$_{REG}$ cells to survive and control autoreactive effector T cells.

STAT5b Deficiency

Deficiency of STAT5b (OMIM #245590) causes a rare autosomal recessive disorder reported in only a handful of patients.[50–52] Since STAT5b mediates signaling from various growth factors, the most recognizable clinical features of the syndrome are

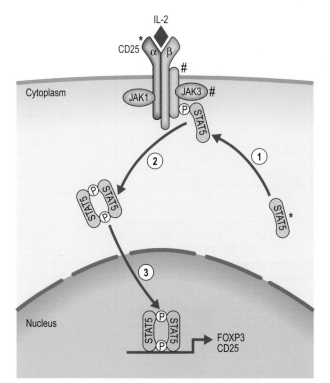

Figure 15-2 The role of CD25 and STAT5b in the IL-2 signaling pathway. The illustration demonstrates the relative positions of CD25 and STAT5 (marked by *) in the IL-2 signaling pathway. Binding of IL-2 to the IL-2 receptor (made up of an alpha chain [CD25], a beta chain and a gamma chain [γc]) causes cross-phosphorylation of receptor chains on tyrosine by receptor-associated JAK1 and JAK3 kinases. Unphosphorylated STAT5 binds to phosphotyrosine residues on the activated receptor using its SH2 domain (1). STAT5 is then phosphorylated on tyrosine by the JAK kinases and released from the receptor where it dimerizes through binding of the SH2 domain on one subunit to the phosphotyrosine residue on the adjacent subunit and vice versa (2). Dimerized STAT5 accumulates in the nucleus where it directly binds to specific sites in the *FOXP3* and *CD25* promoters causing sustained expression of these two proteins in regulatory T cells (3). In contrast to deficiency in CD25 and STAT5b which causes an IPEX-like phenotype, mutations in the IL2 receptor gamma chain or in JAK3 (both marked with #) cause a phenotype of severe combined immunodeficiency (SCID).

dwarfism, a prominent forehead, saddle nose, and a high-pitched voice. STAT5b is also the primary transcription factor that mediates IL-2 stimulated gene transcription in T cells (Figure 15-2). Consequently, most patients also have a marked immunodeficiency, with recurrent varicella virus, herpes virus, and *Pneumocystis jiroveci* infections.[51,52]

In addition to frank immunodeficiency, most patients who lack functional STAT5b also have symptoms suggestive of immune dysregulation including chronic, early onset diarrhea, eczema and lymphocytic interstitial pneumonitis.[50-52] Murine models have demonstrated that Stat5b is a critical transducer of IL-2-mediated signals required to sustain FOXP3 expression and to maintain T_{REG} cells.[53,54] Mice lacking Stat5b have a significant reduction in the number of FOXP3+ T_{REG} cells in thymus and spleen and as a consequence, develop splenomegaly and have a marked increase of activated T cells in the periphery.[54,55]

Like other members of the Signal Transducer and Activator of Transcription (STAT) protein family, STAT5b is present as a monomer in the cytoplasm of quiescent cells. It is recruited to IL-2 receptors following activation where it is phosphorylated by receptor-associated tyrosine kinases (Figure 15-2). The phosphorylated STAT5b subunits dimerize through their SH2 domains, translocate to the nucleus, and bind DNA to regulate gene transcription.[56]

Genetics and Immunopathogenesis

To evaluate the effect of STAT5b deficiency on T_{REG} cells in humans, two patients have been studied; one, with a homozygous missense mutation (A630P) in the SH2 domain of *STAT5b* and the second, with a homozygous nonsense mutation (R152X). Both resulted in markedly reduced or absent STAT5b protein expression.[51,57] In both cases, the patients had significantly fewer CD4+CD25high cells than normal individuals and these cells expressed much less FOXP3 than normal CD4+CD25high T_{REG} cells and had no in vitro suppressive activity.[51,57] Decreased CD25 expression (≈20% of normal) on the patient's T cells in response to activation was shown to be a direct consequence of STAT5b deficiency and is thought to synergize with the underlying STAT5b mutation to effectively abrogate IL-2 signals required for the maintenance of FOXP3 expression and T_{REG} function. Interestingly, signaling pathways required for IL-2 induced expression of other effector molecules such as perforin, remained intact in STAT5b-deficient T cells.[57]

Diagnosis and Treatment

Diagnosis of STAT5b deficiency is suspected in patients with the overt physical features of dwarfism combined with evidence of a significant immunodeficiency. Patients typically have normal serum growth hormone levels but very low insulin-like growth factor-1 (IGF-1) levels.[51,52] Immunologically, patients generally have low γδ T cell and NK cell numbers and modest T cell lymphopenia with a normal CD4/CD8 ratio.[51,57] Sequencing of the *STAT5b* gene can be done to confirm the diagnosis.

Treatment of patients with STAT5b deficiency is generally focused on symptomatic therapy and prophylaxis against infections. We are unaware of any patients with STAT5b deficiency who have undergone bone marrow transplantation although it would be predicted that this would correct the significant immunodeficiency and immune dysregulation typically associated with this disorder.

Autoimmune Lymphoproliferative Syndrome

In 1967, Canale and Smith described a group of patients who presented in early childhood with generalized lymphadenopathy and hepatosplenomegaly associated with autoimmune anemia, thrombocytopenia and increased gammaglobulins.[58] In 1992, Sneller and colleagues reported two patients with similar features and noted that there was a marked increase in circulating α/β-TCR+CD3+ T cells that did not express either CD4 or CD8.[59] These T cells are referred to as α/β–double-negative T (DNT) cells and constitute less than 1% of peripheral blood lymphocytes in normal adults (Figure 15-3). The presence of autoimmunity, lymphadenopathy, and expansion of α/β-DNT cells in these patients led Sneller and colleagues to suggest that this could represent the human equivalent to the *lpr* and *gld* murine models of autoimmunity.

Following the discovery that mutations in the genes encoding FAS and FAS ligand caused disease in these murine models, two studies identified heterozygous *Fas* (TNFRSF6) mutations in many patients diagnosed with ALPS.[60,61] Since 1995, an increasing number of patients with mutations in *FAS* have been identified worldwide, including some patients originally described by Canale and Smith.[62] In addition, a substantial number of patients with typical features of ALPS have been found without mutations in *FAS*. Investigation of the genes encoding FASL and intracellular proteins involved in the apoptotic pathway identified patients with mutations in the FASL (TNFSF6), caspase 10

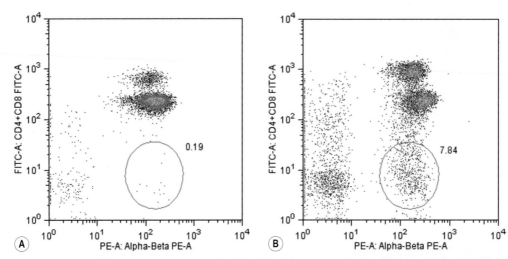

Figure 15-3 Double negative T cells in ALPS. Flow cytometric evaluation of peripheral blood from a control patient **(A)** and an ALPS patient **(B)** demonstrating the increase of mature lymphocytes expressing the T cell receptor αβ (X axis), that lack CD4 and CD8 co-receptor expression (Y axis) in ALPS.

(*CASP10*) and caspase 8 (*CASP8*) genes.[63–65] Recently, a somatic mutation in the gene encoding NRAS has been found in a patient with ALPS who also demonstrated defective intrinsic, mitochondria-mediated lymphocyte apoptosis.[66] However, there remain patients with an ALPS phenotype who have none of the known genetic defects.

The typical clinical course in ALPS (OMIM #601859) begins within the first 5 years of life with nonmalignant peripheral lymphadenopathy.[67,68] This is often associated with splenomegaly and hypersplenism that may necessitate splenectomy (Figure 15-4). Hepatomegaly is also quite common. Clinically apparent autoimmunity is seen in about 50% of the patients, most commonly presenting as autoimmune hemolytic anemia either alone or in concert with idiopathic thrombocytopenic purpura (ITP). Typically, the direct Coombs' test is positive and thrombocytopenia can be significant with platelet counts below 20000/mm³. Some ALPS patients may also develop neutropenia that can be immunologically mediated or secondary to hyperesplenism. Dermatologic findings are seen in ALPS, with urticarial rashes being the most common. Although less common, other autoimmune disorders may be present in ALPS including glomerulonephritis, polyneuropathy, autoimmune hepatitis and Guillain-Barré syndrome. Perhaps the most life-threatening manifestation of ALPS is the dramatically increased incidence of lymphoma in individuals with *FAS* mutations, with an increased relative risk of 51 for Hodgkin disease and 14 for non-Hodgkin lymphoma[69] (Box 15-3).

The laboratory findings in ALPS are summarized in Box 15-4. Immunophenotyping usually reveals peripheral lymphocytosis with expansion of α/β-DNT cells. Other frequent abnormalities include an expansion of HLA-DR⁺ T cells, a decrease in the CD3⁺CD25⁺ T cells, and very low numbers of circulating CD20⁺CD27⁺ (memory) B cells.[70] A polyclonal increase in serum immunoglobulins is seen in virtually all patients. Autoantibodies directed to platelets and neutrophils, as well as antiphospholipid antibodies, are present in 70–80% of the patients, but bear no relationship to the clinical manifestations of thrombocytopenia or neutropenia.[71] Interestingly, serum Vitamin B12 levels are elevated in most ALPS patients, for unknown reasons.[68] There also are markedly elevated serum levels of IL-10 in ALPS patients; this appears to be at least in part a product of the DNT cells and the circulating monocytes.[72,73] Histologically, the enlarged lymph nodes in ALPS show follicular hyperplasia and marked paracortical expansion, with immunoblasts and plasma cells. In addition, the paracortical areas demonstrate large numbers of infiltrating α/β-DNT cells.[74]

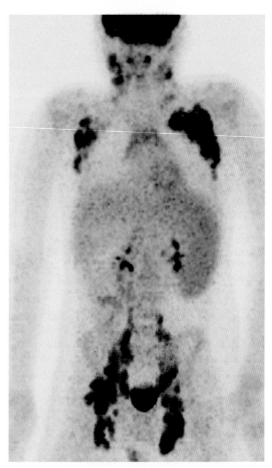

Figure 15-4 Lymphoid accumulation in ALPS. Positron emission tomography demonstrating increasing fluorodeoxyglucose uptake on cervical, axillary and inguinal lymph nodes as well as an enlarged spleen in ALPS.

BOX 15-3 Key concepts

Autoimmune Lymphoproliferative Syndrome (ALPS): Differential Diagnosis

- Lymphoid malignancy
- Chronic viral infection
- Primary autoimmune hemolytic anemia
- Primary idiopathic thrombocytopenic purpura

BOX 15-4

Laboratory Findings in Autoimmune Lymphoproliferative Syndrome

Immunologic

Lymphocytes

   Increase: α/β-double-negative T cells, CD8 T cells, B cells

   Decrease: CD4/CD25 T cells, CD27+ B cells

Immunoglobulins: increased IgG, IgA, and IgE

Cytokines: increased levels of serum IL-10

Autoantibodies: directed at blood cells and platelets

Hematologic

Lymphocytosis

Anemia

Thrombocytopenia

Neutropenia

Eosinophilia

Chemistry

Increased vitamin B_{12} level

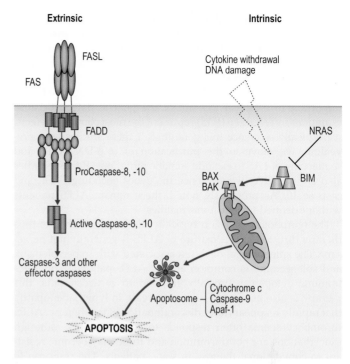

Figure 15-5 Lymphocyte apoptosis pathways. Lymphocytes have two main pathways of apoptosis, regulated either by surface receptors of the TNF superfamily (extrinsic pathway) or proteins of the BCL-2 family (intrinsic pathway). The majority of ALPS patients have a defect in the extrinsic pathway involving FAS but some ALPS patients also have been reported with a defect in the intrinsic pathway.

Genetic and Immunopathogenesis

The majority (≈65%) of ALPS patients have germline heterozygous mutations in *FAS*.[75] A review of the clinical and genetic information in ALPS pedigrees revealed that the site of the *FAS* mutation has a direct impact on the development of disease manifestation.[76] Specifically, mutations in the intracellular domain of *FAS* are correlated with higher penetrance and more severe clinical manifestations, as compared to extracellular mutations.[77]

Recently, somatic mutations in *FAS*, affecting primarily DNT cells with variable presence in other leukocyte subtypes have been described in a group of six patients with sporadic ALPS.[78] Evaluation of the NIH cohort revealed 11 additional cases (Rao K & Dowdell K, personal communication), making somatic *FAS* mutations the second most common genetic cause of ALPS. A minority of ALPS patients, however, do not have mutations affecting *FAS*. Evaluation of the gene encoding FASL established that two patients with typical findings of ALPS have a heterozygous defect affecting *FASL*.[65,79] In addition, two patients with normal *FAS* and *FASL* have been demonstrated to have a defect in caspase 10, an intracellular protease downstream of FAS in the apoptotic pathway (Figure 15-5).[64] Recent work from our group has also identified a somatic mutation in the *NRAS* gene that can cause the clinical and laboratory findings of ALPS, associated with defective lymphocyte apoptosis.[66] These findings form the basis of the current classification scheme for ALPS:

- ALPS type Ia: germline mutation in the gene encoding FAS (*TNFRSF6*)
- ALPS type Im (mosaic): somatic mutation in the gene encoding FAS
- ALPS type Ib: mutation in the gene encoding FASL (*TNFSF6*)
- ALPS type II: mutation in the gene encoding caspase 10 (*CASP10*)
- ALPS type III: no known mutation
- ALPS type IV: mutation in the gene encoding NRAS (*NRAS*)

Diagnosis and Treatment

The constellation of clinical and laboratory findings in ALPS patients is rather unique. However, the initial presentation of

BOX 15-5 Key concepts

Diagnostic Criteria for Autoimmune Lymphoproliferative Syndrome (ALPS)

Required

- Nonmalignant chronic lymphadenopathy (>6 months)
- Increased percentage (>1% of lymphocytes) and/or numbers (>17 cells/uL) of alpha-beta T cell receptor double negative T cells
- Defective in vitro anti-FAS or cytokine withdrawal-induced lymphocyte apoptosis or mutation on *FAS*, *FASL*, *CASP10*, *CASP8* or *NRAS*

Supportive

- Coombs positive hemolytic anemia or immune thrombocytopenia or autoimmune leucopenia
- Compatible family history

lymphadenopathy often raises the issue of malignancy which generally requires a biopsy to differentiate between these two diagnoses. The initial findings can also be suggestive of a chronic viral infection such as Epstein-Barr virus, although there are no serologic studies or in situ hybridization data to support this. The autoimmunity seen in ALPS patients is most commonly directed against red blood cells and platelets. The laboratory findings associated with the autoimmunity do not distinguish patients with ALPS from those who do not have this disorder in that there is a broad range of autoantibody specificities observed (Box 15-5).

The diagnostic triad for ALPS is nonmalignant lympho-accumulation, defective in vitro FAS-mediated lymphocyte apoptosis, and increased levels of α/β-DNT cells. Clearly, after a history and physical examination, flow cytometric evaluation of peripheral blood lymphocytes is necessary to evaluate increased levels of α/β-DNT cells (Box 15-4). The assessment of FAS-mediated lymphocyte apoptosis must be performed to establish this diagnosis. Once ALPS has been diagnosed, it is important to establish the site of the genetic defect. Because mutations in *TNFRSF6* (*FAS*) represent the most common defects, we typically sequence this gene first. If these studies are unrevealing, we move to the purification of α/β-DNT cells and sequencing of *FAS* to exclude somatic mutations. If these studies also are negative, we sequence the genes encoding FASL and caspase 10. As previously noted, there remain ALPS patients without defined genetic abnormalities.

The lymphoid expansion typically diminishes with age; thus therapy directed at this feature of ALPS is generally not necessary. The splenomegaly is often associated with hypersplenism, and splenectomy is common among ALPS patients. The autoimmune cytopenias typically respond to corticosteroids; this therapy is also associated with a decrease in lymphadenopathy that rapidly reappears after discontinuation of the therapy. ALPS thrombocytopenia often responds to corticosteroids, although exacerbations are not uncommon and these may become resistant to conventional therapy in some patients. The response to intravenous immunoglobulin therapy is less satisfactory than in childhood ITP cases. Preliminary data suggest that mycophenolate mofetil may be useful in the treatment of ALPS patients with ITP who are unresponsive to standard therapy.[80] Fansidar (sulfadoxine-pyrimethamine) was suggested to improve autoimmune cytopenias and diminish lymphadenopathy in certain ALPS patients, but this was not confirmed in additional studies employing pirimethamine alone.[81-83] Importantly, the increased risk for the development of lymphoma appears to be life-long and careful vigilance is required to monitor for this complication in all family members known to have *FAS* mutations.

Conclusions

In recent years, identification of the gene defects in a handful of clinical syndromes with congenital systemic autoimmunity has led to the definition of a new class of primary immunodeficiency disorders in which the defect involves specific features of the regulatory compartment of the immune system. Lessons learned from these disorders have clarified aspects of thymic selection, T_{REG} function and FAS-mediated apoptosis. There are a number of unresolved issues that include defining other contributing genetic and/or environmental factors and clarifying the basis for the specific patterns of autoimmunity seen in these disorders. In addition, defining the molecular basis that contributes to other findings in these various disorders will further our understanding of the immune system. Certainly, studying these experiments of nature will continue to be a fertile field of investigation over the coming years as we strive to uncover the basic mechanisms of immune tolerance.

References

1. Halonen M, Eskelin P, Myhre AG, et al. AIRE mutations and human leukocyte antigen genotypes as determinants of the autoimmune polyendocrinopathy-candidiasis-ectodermal dystrophy phenotype. J Clin Endocrinol Metab 2002;87:2568–74.
2. Perheentupa J. Autoimmune polyendocrinopathy-candidiasis-ectodermal dystrophy. J Clin Endocrinol Metab 2006;91:2843–50.
3. Liston A, Lesage S, Wilson J, et al. Aire regulates negative selection of organ-specific T cells. Nat Immunol 2003;4:350–4.
4. Anderson MS, Venanzi ES, Klein L, et al. Projection of an immunological self shadow within the thymus by the aire protein. Science 2002;298:1395–401.
5. Aschenbrenner K, D'Cruz LM, Vollmann EH, et al. Selection of Foxp3(+) regulatory T cells specific for self antigen expressed and presented by Aire(+) medullary thymic epithelial cells. Nat Immunol 2007;8:351–8.
6. Kekalainen E, Tuovinen H, Joensuu J, et al. A defect of regulatory T cells in patients with autoimmune polyendocrinopathy-candidiasis-ectodermal dystrophy. J Immunol 2007;178:1208–15.
7. Ryan KR, Lawson CA, Lorenzi AR, et al. CD4+CD25+ T-regulatory cells are decreased in patients with autoimmune polyendocrinopathy candidiasis ectodermal dystrophy. J Allergy Clin Immunol 2005;116:1158–9.
8. Puel A, Doffinger R, Natividad A, et al. Autobodies against IL-17A, IL-17F and IL-22 in patients with chronic mucocutaneous candidiasis and polyendocrinopathy syndrome type 1. J Exp Med 2010;207:291–7.
9. Rautemaa R, Richardson M, Pfaller M, et al. Reduction of fluconazole susceptibility of Candida albicans in APECED patients due to long-term use of ketoconazole and miconazole. Scand J Infect Dis 2008;40:904–7.
10. Gavanescu I, Benoist C, Mathis D. B cells are required for Aire-deficient mice to develop multi-organ autoinflammation: a therapeutic approach for APECED patients. Proc Natl Acad Sci U S A 2008;105:13009–14.
11. Powell BR, Buist NR, Stenzel P. An X-linked syndrome of diarrhea, polyendocrinopathy, and fatal infection in infancy. J Pediatr 1982;100:731–7.
12. Levy-Lahad E, Wildin RS. Neonatal diabetes mellitus, enteropathy, thrombocytopenia, and endocrinopathy: further evidence for an X-linked lethal syndrome. J Pediatr 2001;138:577–80.
13. Wildin RS, Smyk-Pearson S, Filipovich AH. Clinical and molecular features of the immunodysregulation, polyendocrinopathy, enteropathy, X linked (IPEX) syndrome. J Med Genet 2002;39:537–45.
14. Nieves DS, Phipps RP, Pollock SJ, et al. Dermatologic and immunologic findings in the immune dysregulation, polyendocrinopathy, enteropathy, X-linked syndrome. Arch Dermatol 2004;140:466–72.
15. McGinness JL, Bivens MM, Greer KE, et al. Immune dysregulation, polyendocrinopathy, enteropathy, X-linked syndrome (IPEX) associated with pemphigoid nodularis: a case report and review of the literature. J Am Acad Dermatol 2006;55:143–8.
16. Torgerson TR, Ochs HD. Immune dysregulation, polyendocrinopathy, enteropathy, X-linked: forkhead box protein 3 mutations and lack of regulatory T cells. J Allergy Clin Immunol 2007;120:744–50; quiz 751–742.
17. Chatila TA, Blaeser F, Ho N, et al. JM2, encoding a fork head-related protein, is mutated in X-linked autoimmunity-allergic disregulation syndrome. J Clin Invest 2000;106:R75–81.
18. Bennett CL, Christie J, Ramsdell F, et al. The immune dysregulation, polyendocrinopathy, enteropathy, X-linked syndrome (IPEX) is caused by mutations of FOXP3. Nat Genet 2001;27:20–1.
19. Wildin RS, Ramsdell F, Peake J, et al. X-linked neonatal diabetes mellitus, enteropathy and endocrinopathy syndrome is the human equivalent of mouse scurfy. Nat Genet 2001;27:18–20.
20. Gavin MA, Rasmussen JP, Fontenot JD, et al. Foxp3-dependent programme of regulatory T cell differentiation. Nature 2007;445:771–5.
21. Lin W, Haribhai D, Relland LM, et al. Regulatory T cell development in the absence of functional Foxp3. Nat Immunol 2007;8:359–68.
22. Gavin MA, Torgerson TR, Houston E, et al. Single-cell analysis of normal and FOXP3-mutant human T cells: FOXP3 expression without regulatory T cell development. Proc Natl Acad Sci U S A 2006;103:6659–64.
23. Allan SE, Crome SQ, Crellin NK, et al. Activation-induced FOXP3 in human T effector cells does not suppress proliferation or cytokine production. Int Immunol 2007.
24. Pillai V, Ortega SB, Wang CK, et al. Transient regulatory T cells: a state attained by all activated human T cells. Clin Immunol 2007;123:18–29.
25. Wang J, Ioan-Facsinay A, van der Voort EI, et al. Transient expression of FOXP3 in human activated nonregulatory CD4+ T cells. Eur J Immunol 2007;37:129–38.
26. Schubert LA, Jeffery E, Zhang Y, et al. Scurfin (FOXP3) acts as a repressor of transcription and regulates T cell activation. J Biol Chem 2001;276:37672–9.
27. Bettelli E, Dastrange M, Oukka M. Foxp3 interacts with nuclear factor of activated T cells and NF-kappa B to repress cytokine gene expression and effector functions of T helper cells. Proc Natl Acad Sci U S A 2005;102:5138–43.

28. Wu Y, Borde M, Heissmeyer V, et al. FOXP3 controls regulatory T cell function through cooperation with NFAT. Cell 2006;126: 375–87.

29. Zheng Y, Josefowicz SZ, Kas A, et al. Genome-wide analysis of Foxp3 target genes in developing and mature regulatory T cells. Nature 2007;445:936–40.

30. Marson A, Kretschmer K, Frampton GM, et al. Foxp3 occupancy and regulation of key target genes during T cell stimulation. Nature 2007;445:931–5.

31. Lopes JE, Torgerson TR, Schubert LA, et al. Analysis of FOXP3 reveals multiple domains required for its function as a transcriptional repressor. J Immunol 2006;177:3133–42.

32. Ichiyama K, Yoshida H, Wakabayashi Y, et al. Foxp3 inhibits RORgammat-mediated IL-17A mRNA transcription through direct interaction with RORgammat. J Biol Chem 2008;283:17003–8.

33. Zhou L, Lopes JE, Chong MM, et al. TGF-beta-induced Foxp3 inhibits T(H)17 cell differentiation by antagonizing RORgammat function. Nature 2008;453:236–40.

34. Ono M, Yaguchi H, Ohkura N, et al. Foxp3 controls regulatory T cell function by interacting with AML1/Runx1. Nature 2007.

35. Du J, Huang C, Zhou B, et al. Isoform-specific inhibition of ROR alpha-mediated transcriptional activation by human FOXP3. J Immunol 2008;180:4785–92.

36. Blair PJ, Bultman SJ, Haas JC, et al. CD4+CD8- T cells are the effector cells in disease pathogenesis in the scurfy (sf) mouse. J Immunol 1994;153:3764–74.

37. Ferguson PJ, Blanton SH, Saulsbury FT, et al. Manifestations and linkage analysis in X-linked autoimmunity-immunodeficiency syndrome. Am J Med Genet 2000;90:390–7.

38. Bindl L, Torgerson T, Perroni L, et al. Successful use of the new immune-suppressor sirolimus in IPEX (immune dysregulation, polyendocrinopathy, enteropathy, X-linked syndrome). J Pediatr 2005;147: 256–9.

39. Kobayashi I, Nakanishi M, Okano M, et al. Combination therapy with tacrolimus and betamethasone for a patient with X-linked auto-immune enteropathy. Eur J Pediatr 1995;154:594–5.

40. Taddio A, Faleschini E, Valencic E, et al. Medium-term survival without haematopoietic stem cell transplantation in a case of IPEX: insights into nutritional and immunosuppressive therapy. Eur J Pediatr 2007;166: 1195–7.

41. Mazzolari E, Forino C, Fontana M, et al. A new case of IPEX receiving bone marrow transplantation. Bone Marrow Transplant 2005;35: 1033–4.

42. Lucas KG, Ungar D, Comito M, et al. Submyeloablative cord blood transplantation corrects clinical defects seen in IPEX syndrome. Bone Marrow Transplant 2007;39:55–6.

43. Rao A, Kamani N, Filipovich A, et al. Successful bone marrow transplantation for IPEX syndrome after reduced-intensity conditioning. Blood 2007;109:383–5.

44. Caudy AA, Reddy ST, Chatila T, et al. CD25 deficiency causes an immune dysregulation, polyendocrinopathy, enteropathy, X-linked-like syndrome, and defective IL-10 expression from CD4 lymphocytes. J Allergy Clin Immunol 2007;119:482–7.

45. Sharfe N, Dadi HK, Shahar M, et al. Human immune disorder arising from mutation of the alpha chain of the interleukin-2 receptor. Proc Natl Acad Sci U S A 1997;94:3168–71.

46. Aoki CA, Roifman CM, Lian ZX, et al. IL-2 receptor alpha deficiency and features of primary biliary cirrhosis. J Autoimmun 2006;27: 50–3.

47. Roifman CM. Human IL-2 receptor alpha chain deficiency. Pediatr Res 2000;48:6–11.

48. D'Cruz LM, Klein L. Development and function of agonist-induced CD25+Foxp3+ regulatory T cells in the absence of interleukin 2 signaling. Nat Immunol 2005;6:1152–9.

49. Fontenot JD, Rasmussen JP, Gavin MA, et al. A function for interleukin 2 in Foxp3-expressing regulatory T cells. Nat Immunol 2005;6: 1142–51.

50. Hwa V, Little B, Adiyaman P, et al. Severe growth hormone insensitivity resulting from total absence of signal transducer and activator of transcription 5b. J Clin Endocrinol Metab 2005;90:4260–6.

51. Bernasconi A, Marino R, Ribas A, et al. Characterization of immunodeficiency in a patient with growth hormone insensitivity secondary to a novel STAT5b gene mutation. Pediatrics 2006;118: e1584–92.

52. Kofoed EM, Hwa V, Little B, et al. Growth hormone insensitivity associated with a STAT5b mutation. N Engl J Med 2003;349:1139–47.

53. Yao Z, Kanno Y, Kerenyi M, et al. Nonredundant roles for Stat5a/b in directly regulating Foxp3. Blood 2007;109:4368–75.

54. Burchill MA, Goetz CA, Prlic M, et al. Distinct effects of STAT5 activation on CD4+ and CD8+ T cell homeostasis: development of CD4+CD25+ regulatory T cells versus CD8+ memory T cells. J Immunol 2003;171: 5853–64.

55. Antov A, Yang L, Vig M, et al. Essential role for STAT5 signaling in CD25+CD4+ regulatory T cell homeostasis and the maintenance of self-tolerance. J Immunol 2003;171:3435–41.

56. Kim HP, Imbert J, Leonard WJ. Both integrated and differential regulation of components of the IL-2/IL-2 receptor system. Cytokine Growth Factor Rev 2006;17:349–66.

57. Cohen AC, Nadeau KC, Tu W, et al. Cutting edge: decreased accumulation and regulatory function of CD4+ CD25(high) T cells in human STAT5b deficiency. J Immunol 2006;177:2770–4.

58. Canale VC, Smith CH. Chronic lymphadenopathy simulating malignant lymphoma. J Pediatr 1967;70:891–9.

59. Sneller MC, Straus SE, Jaffe ES, et al. A novel lymphoproliferative/autoimmune syndrome resembling murine lpr/gld disease. J Clin Invest 1992;90:334–41.

60. Fisher GH, Rosenberg FJ, Straus SE, et al. Dominant interfering Fas gene mutations impair apoptosis in a human autoimmune lymphoproliferative syndrome. Cell 1995;81:935–46.

61. Rieux-Laucat F, Le Deist F, Hivroz C, et al. Mutations in Fas associated with human lymphoproliferative syndrome and autoimmunity. Science 1995;268:1347–9.

62. Drappa J, Vaishnaw AK, Sullivan KE, et al. Fas gene mutations in the Canale-Smith syndrome, an inherited lymphoproliferative disorder associated with autoimmunity. N Engl J Med 1996;335: 1643–9.

63. Chun HJ, Zheng L, Ahmad M, et al. Pleiotropic defects in lymphocyte activation caused by caspase-8 mutations lead to human immunodeficiency. Nature 2002;419:395–9.

64. Wang J, Zheng L, Lobito A, et al. Inherited human Caspase 10 mutations underlie defective lymphocyte and dendritic cell apoptosis in autoimmune lymphoproliferative syndrome type II. Cell 1999;98: 47–58.

65. Bi LL, Pan G, Atkinson TP, et al. Dominant inhibition of Fas ligand-mediated apoptosis due to a heterozygous mutation associated with autoimmune lymphoproliferative syndrome (ALPS) Type Ib. BMC Med Genet 2007;8:41.

66. Oliveira JB, Bidere N, Niemela JE, et al. NRAS mutation causes a human autoimmune lymphoproliferative syndrome. Proc Natl Acad Sci U S A 2007;104:8953–8.

67. Bleesing JJ, Straus SE, Fleisher TA. Autoimmune lymphoproliferative syndrome: a human disorder of abnormal lymphocyte survival. Pediatr Clin North Am 2000;47:1291–310.

68. Fleisher TA, Oliveira JB. Autoimmune lymphoproliferative syndrome. Isr Med Assoc J 2005;7:758–61.

69. Straus SE, Jaffe ES, Puck JM, et al. The development of lymphomas in families with autoimmune lymphoproliferative syndrome with germline Fas mutations and defective lymphocyte apoptosis. Blood 2001;98: 194–200.

70. Bleesing JJ, Brown MR, Straus SE, et al. Immunophenotypic profiles in families with autoimmune lymphoproliferative syndrome. Blood 2001;98:2466–73.

71. Kwon SW, Procter J, Dale JK, et al. Neutrophil and platelet antibodies in autoimmune lymphoproliferative syndrome. Vox Sang 2003;85: 307–12.

72. Lopatin U, Yao X, Williams RK, et al. Increases in circulating and lymphoid tissue interleukin-10 in autoimmune lymphoproliferative syndrome are associated with disease expression. Blood 2001;97: 3161–70.

73. Magerus-Chatinet A, Stolzenberg MC, Loffredo MS, et al. FAS-L, IL-10, and double-negative CD4- CD8- TCR alpha/beta+ T cells are reliable markers of autoimmune lymphoproliferative syndrome (ALPS) associated with FAS loss of function. Blood 2009;113:3027–30.

74. Lim MS, Straus SE, Dale JK, et al. Pathological findings in human autoimmune lymphoproliferative syndrome. Am J Pathol 1998;153: 1541–50.

75. Su HC, Lenardo MJ. Genetic defects of apoptosis and primary immunodeficiency. Immunol Allergy Clin North Am 2008;28: 329–51, ix.

76. Jackson CE, Fischer RE, Hsu AP, et al. Autoimmune lymphoproliferative syndrome with defective Fas: genotype influences penetrance. Am J Hum Genet 1999;64:1002–14.

77. Patey-Mariaud de Serre N, Canioni D, Ganousse S, et al. Digestive histopathological presentation of IPEX syndrome. Mod Pathol 2009;22: 95–102.

78. Holzelova E, Vonarbourg C, Stolzenberg MC, et al. Autoimmune lymphoproliferative syndrome with somatic Fas mutations. N Engl J Med 2004;351:1409–18.

79. Del-Rey M, Ruiz-Contreras J, Bosque A, et al. A homozygous Fas ligand gene mutation in a patient causes a new type of autoimmune lymphoproliferative syndrome. Blood 2006;108:1306–12.

80. Rao VK, Dugan F, Dale JK, et al. Use of mycophenolate mofetil for chronic, refractory immune cytopenias in children with autoimmune lymphoproliferative syndrome. Br J Haematol 2005;129:534–8.

81. van der Werff Ten Bosch J, Schotte P, Ferster A, et al. Reversion of autoimmune lymphoproliferative syndrome with an antimalarial drug: preliminary results of a clinical cohort study and molecular observations. Br J Haematol 2002;117:176–88.

82. van der Werff ten Bosch JE, Demanet C, Balduck N, et al. The use of the anti-malaria drug Fansidar (pyrimethamine and sulphadoxine) in the treatment of a patient with autoimmune lymphoproliferative syndrome and Fas deficiency. Br J Haematol 1998;102:578–81.

83. Rao VK, Dowdell KC, Dale JK, et al. Pyrimethamine treatment does not ameliorate lymphoproliferation or autoimmune disease in MRL/lpr-/- mice or in patients with autoimmune lymphoproliferative syndrome. Am J Hematol 2007;82:1049–55.

16

Epstein-Barr Virus Infections

James F. Jones

All viral illnesses are identified by the combination of their clinical components and specific laboratory parameters. The clinical components are dictated by the characteristics of the infectious agent, its predilection for binding to certain cell types, its mode of replication, and the types of host responses that are genetically controlled by the host. The laboratory parameters detect representations of the host response, isolate the infective agent, or identify its presence by protein or nucleic acid identification. Epstein-Barr virus (EBV) infections, in particular, must be understood by pediatricians and allergist-immunologists because of the cellular targets of the virus and the orchestrated immune responses required to control the infection. One of the three primary targets for infection is the B lymphocyte. Other primary targets are epithelial cells in a variety of anatomic sites. A recent study suggests that B lymphocytes are actually required in order for a person to become infected.[1] The previous hypothesis supported initial infection of oropharyngeal epithelial cells followed by spread to B cells with establishment of latent infection in both cell types. This study could not identify the virus in oropharyngeal cells obtained from patients who totally lack B cells (Bruton thymidine kinase deficiency). T lymphocytes are also a target, but little is known about either the process of such infections or the clinical consequences, except for the development of T cell lymphomas.[2]

The immunologic response is required to control active replication (production of new virions) and to control reactivation of an active infection once the typical herpesvirus latent state is achieved.[3] The immune response must also be tempered because the proliferation of noninfected lymphoid cells that accompanies the infection needs to be controlled. The immune response is then required to control infection of one or more of its constituent members and at the same time to prevent exaggerated host responses that could cause injury.[4,5]

As discussed further, the clinical expression of EBV infections is extraordinarily variable.[6,7] This variability is dictated by genetically controlled host responses that induce the clinical illness. It is also dependent on the presence or absence of appropriate 'restraint' of the active response. Although multiple attempts have been made, no specific relationships between various viral genome structures and differing clinical states have been identified.

Antibodies to the virus are present in populations throughout the world. In the not too distant past it was found that a majority of younger children in developed countries are specific antibody negative.[8] One can hypothesize that with the advent of a higher percentage of children below school age receiving care during the day outside of the home, exposure to the virus occurs at a younger age. Unfortunately, this question has not been formally addressed. It should be clear, however, that infectious mononucleosis (IM) is not the only clinical entity of importance in childhood and adolescence. Diagnosis requires recognition of symptoms, signs, and laboratory findings that constitute the spectrum of EBV infections, not just the IM syndrome. The nonspecific heterophile test should not be the procedure relied upon to diagnose all infections with this virus as it has been in the past.[9]

Epidemiology/Etiology

Epidemiology

The prevalence of EBV antibodies (demonstrating exposure to the virus with replication as evidence of infection) in children and adolescents does not correspond to the prevalence of EBV-associated illness. The incidence of IM as reported in 1972 in adolescents and young adults was 45 cases/100 000/year.[10] As recently as in the early 1980s the majority of children in the USA and other western countries remained free of specific anti-EBV antibodies until adolescence.[8] At that time, if a child developed classic IM, a syndrome consisting of pharyngitis and cervical lymphadenopathy, hepatosplenomegaly, an increased lymphocyte count with a high percentage of atypical lymphoid cells, a positive heterophile test, and generalized malaise, there was an 85% chance that the infection was caused by EBV. This illness presentation was assumed to be the first exposure to the virus as acquired in adolescence. The determinants of the expression of EBV infection as IM in adolescents are unclear. It may be that there are indeed factors relating to adolescence per se that influence the presentation of classic IM. For example, familial factors may be as important in expression of illness as is the age of onset. Typically, in a family of five susceptible persons, if one individual develops IM, only one of the remaining four susceptible persons will also demonstrate illness after the exposure. If the family member first presenting with IM is a child, however, the development of IM in other family members occurs at a higher rate.[11]

The prevalence of specific antibodies in young children throughout the world varies with socioeconomic status more than it does with identifiable illnesses. In countries, cities, and rural living sites that lack modern hygienic conditions, most children are seropositive for EBV by the age of 2 years; no clinical illness is common among these children. In the USA, children with illnesses such as nonspecific upper respiratory

DOI: 10.1016/B978-1-4377-0271-2.00016-X

tract infections, pharyngitis, isolated hepatosplenomegaly, cough, vomiting, and diarrhea were found to have antibody patterns consistent with primary disease in a prospective study of acute hospitalizations.[12] A different approach was taken by Roberts and colleagues[13] who examined hospital records of children with EBV infections to determine the range of clinical illnesses. These researchers found that 16 of 41 patients ranging from 4 weeks to 13 years of age had 'serious' problems, including pneumonia, chronic active hepatitis, gastrointestinal hemorrhage, prolonged intermittent fever, failure to thrive, and bone marrow failure; the remainder had typical IM. Clinical illnesses consistent with IM in younger children (under 15 years) vary in symptom patterns from those in adolescents according to Rehse and Helwig.[14] The younger children were more likely to display exudative pharyngitis, exanthems, and hepatosplenomegaly than were the adolescents, but the remaining syndromic components were similar.

It is interesting to note that virtually no new population-based epidemiologic studies have been published in the last 15 years. One recent study of 66 infants from China, beginning at birth with samples every 4 months until 2 years of age, found that all children were positive at birth, but 8 of them remained seropositive at 8 months of age.[15] However, 60% were positive by the end of the study. One factor influencing this observation is that EBV infections are not reportable diseases. Secondly, it is generally assumed that IM is the 'only' infection with this virus and that it is a self-limited process with minor consequences. Unfortunately, the latter issue has not been formally studied. A third known factor that may influence epidemiologic studies is the fact that 90% of adults over 30 years of age are EBV seropositive, but only one third of them have had an illness identified as being caused by an EBV infection.

IM, however, is not the only illness associated with infection.[6,16] The initial illness may obviously be totally asymptomatic or it may include the following organ systems: central and peripheral nervous systems, hematologic system, eyes, skin, cardiovascular system, respiratory tract, gastrointestinal tract (including oral cavity and salivary glands), genitourinary tract, and breast tissue.[17] Severe infections that may be short-lived if responsive to treatment or prolonged if unresponsive to treatment or left untreated have also been described.[18] Box 16-1 lists some of the established clinical consequences associated with EBV infection.

Another category of EBV-associated diseases that deserves particular emphasis is cancer. Tumors that carry the virus include Burkitt's lymphoma (cell lines from this tumor were found to have the virus by electron microscopy); nasopharyngeal carcinoma; Hodgkin's and non-Hodgkin's lymphomas of B cell origin; NK and T cell lymphomas; leiomyomas in a variety of anatomic sites; and primarily B cell tumors that occur in patients with posttransplantation lymphoproliferative disorder (PTLD), human immunodeficiency virus (HIV), and other types of immunosuppression.[19] The most recent entry into the EBV-associated cancer arena is breast cancer, in which tumor cells were found by several independent investigators to contain the viral genome.[20]

More recently, old questions regarding a potential role for EBV in triggering autoimmune diseases have resurfaced; one such illness is systemic lupus erythematosus.[21]

Etiology

The reader is referred to a recent virology text for a detailed description of the virus and its replication.[22] For this discussion,

---

BOX 16-1

Clinical Illnesses Caused by Epstein-Barr Virus Infection

Nervous System

Meningitis

Encephalitis

Acute hemoplagia

Cerebellar ataxia

Alice-in-Wonderland syndrome

Psychoses

Guillain-Barré syndrome

Acute transverse myelitis

Sleep disorders

Peripheral neuropathies

Pulmonary System

Lymphoid interstitial pneumonia

Pulmonary lymphomatoid granulomatosis

Pneumonia

Follicular bronchitis-bronchiolitis

Hematologic System

Anemia

Thrombocytopenia

Neutropenia

Aplastic anemia

Leukopenia

Hemophagocytic syndrome

Skin

Chronic urticaria

Ampicillin-associated exanthem

Gianotti-Crosti syndrome

Gastrointestinal System

Hepatitis

Vanishing bile duct syndrome

Congenital Infection

Immunologic System

X-linked lymphoproliferative syndrome (sphingolipid activator protein deficiency)

Acquired hypogammaglobulinemia

Oral Cavity

Hairy leukoplakia

Parotiditis

Opthalmologic System

Uveitis

Conjunctival lymphoid infiltrates

Genitourinary System

Vaginal ulcers

Penile ulcers

Interstitial nephritis

---

it is important to review a few facts. The virus is a double-stranded DNA member of the herpesvirus family (herpesvirus 4). In its infectious and new virion production state the structure of the virion is linear. New virion production is associated with expression of a variety of replicative and structural proteins. Once infected, certain B cells somehow become the reservoir of the virus in its latent state (approximately 1 in 10^6 infected cells). These cells carry the viral DNA in closed, circular extrachromosomal episomes that replicate only with cell division and express a small number of latent proteins. The virus has been completely sequenced and contains approximately 100 open reading frames, but all the potential proteins have not been identified. Infection begins with binding of the virus to the CR2 or C3d complement receptors.

The production of symptoms in healthy persons requires levels of assumed normal immune function, as seen in Table 16-1.[23-25] A study by Svedmyr and colleagues[26] attempting to evaluate the early immunologic events in IM in teenagers observed that symptoms coincided with the immune response. Perhaps surprisingly, there appeared to be little, if any, host response during the 4- to 6-week incubation period. Two general types of responses are required for control of the primary infection: cellular responses directed against the infected cells and humoral responses directed against free virions. These responses vary with active replication (new virion production) and the latent stage. The majority of the information describing these processes has thus far been generated from in vitro studies.[27]

Although antibody responses are the primary method of identifying infection, it is important to note that those antibodies are not functional in resolution of the illness; they are simply markers of the response, albeit important ones. The antibody responses identified in clinical laboratories identify responses to the viral capsid antigen (VCA), early antigen(s) (EA[s]), and the Epstein-Barr nuclear antigen (EBNA). Using assay systems that include the 'gold standard' immunofluorescent antibody (IFA) technique or an enzyme-based recognition technique, IgM, IgA, and IgG isotype antibodies to the various proteins or protein complexes can be detected.[28] Antibodies that detect membrane antigen (gp 350/220) are associated with virus neutralization, but measurement of these antibodies is not standard clinical practice.

Cell-mediated responses include natural killer activity, lymphokine-activated cell cytotoxicity, and specific EBV protein-directed T cell cytotoxicity, appearing in that order as detected in vitro.[29] The last process is determined by the genetic makeup of the host.[30] Specific T cell receptor sequences (Vβ) bind to specific viral peptides expressed on the infected cells during both latent replication and new virion replication. One study suggests that IM is associated with selective Vβ utilization.[31]

The consequences of this recognition process then lead to a litany of inflammatory events producing the illness and controlling the infection.[25] Through Class I human leukocyte antigen (HLA) restriction, certain individuals have selective patterns of viral peptide recognition that are in part associated with the two different stages of viral replication. Early evaluations of these processes concentrated on the genetics of T cell responses to proteins expressed during latent infection.[4] Similar work identified an important role for restrictions in recognition of proteins expressed in new virion replication.

Possible Role of Allergy in EBV Infections

Assignment of IM to an allergic origin was suggested in the 1940s by Randolph and Hettig[32] before EBV was identified as the causative agent of the classic syndrome in adults. The clinical symptoms allowing this assignation were fatigue, swollen lymph nodes, and a history of allergy.

Preliminary observations comparing the history of the presence or the absence of clinical IM in EBV-seropositive subjects with or without immunoglobulin (IgE) allergy demonstrated a history of IM in 77% of patients with allergy, but only in 25% of those without allergy (Jones J, unpublished observations). Because the frequency of allergy in the general population is approximately 30%, it may be that the presence of allergy may then predispose the patient to the expression of the EBV IM that occurred in one third of individuals found to be seropositive.

Several studies from Sweden have shown that both children and adults with allergies have higher anti-VCA antibody titers than nonallergic individuals.[33,34] A general elevation in serum immunoglobulin levels is typically seen in acute IM as part of the proliferation, stimulation, and increased stimulation

Table 16-1 Signs and Symptoms of EBV Infection and Possible Mechanisms

Signs/Symptoms	Possible Mechanisms

Nonspecific symptoms
  Malaise
  Headache
  Anorexia
  Myalgia
  Chills
  Arthralgia
  Nausea
	Mediators of inflammation: IFN-α, IL-1, TNF-α, and others

Lymphadenopathy	IFN-α, proliferation of infected and noninfected lymphoid cells
Fever	IL-1, TNF-α
Pharyngitis	Direct infection of epithelial cells; mediators of inflammation: bradykinin; immune-cell injury of infected cells
Splenomegaly	Cellular proliferation in response to mediators; infected lymphoid cells
Palatal exanthem	Lymphoid follicle infection; mediators of inflammation
Jaundice	Unknown
Rash	Unknown
Encephalitis/meningitis (other neurologic problems)	Mediators of inflammation; infiltrating lymphocytes
Pneumonia	Infected lymphoid cells
Hematologic	IFN-α; direct infection; viral transformation of B cells
Cardiac	Unknown; possibly IFN
Pancreas	Unknown
Vestibular, other otologic problems	Unknown
Ocular (including palpebral edema)	Unknown
Hairy leukoplakia	Direct infection of epithelial cells in immunocompromised patients
Tumors	Possible EBV-genome induced alteration of cell growth

From Jones J, Katz B. Epstein-Barr virus infections in normal and immunosuppressed patients. In: Glaser R, Jones J, eds. Herpesvirus infection. Philadelphia, WB Saunders; 1994
EBV, Epstein-Barr virus; IFN, interferon; TNF, tumor necrosis factor; IL, interleukin.

of B cells, but IgE levels are particularly increased to high levels.[35] The increased production of IgE appears to be due to dysregulation rather than altered numbers of IgE-producing cells in the allergic subjects.[36] In addition, although less frequent than IgM- and IgG-bearing B cells, IgE-expressing B cell clones can be established by infection with EBV.[37] Regardless of the surface isotype, some of these clones actually produce antibodies, including autoantibodies with specificity for endogenous hormones, particularly antithyroid antibodies.[38]

An ongoing issue is whether EBV infection protects a child from developing overt allergy or predisposes the individual to these conditions. Studies support each outcome.[39-41] Nilsson and colleagues have recently shown that, in 2-year-old children, an inverse realtionship exists between EBV seropositivity and IgE sensitization, but there were no relationships between INF-γ, IL-4, Il-10, and Il-12 expressing cell numbers.[42] The same group also found that, in the same children, EBV serpositivity was associated with reduced moncyte-induced NK cell INF-γ production along with a decreased proportion of INF-γ + NK cells and cognate intracellular INF-γ levels.[43] In both studies, cytomegalovirus (CMV) seropositivity enhanced the findings.

The mechanisms by which presumed benefit of EBV infection inhibits IgE sensitization are unclear, but ongoing studies regarding the role(s) of T regulatory cells in allergy may offer some insight.

Three additional rare clinical observations regarding EBV and 'allergy' are worth mentioning. The first is hypersensitivity to mosquito bites. This illness is most common in Asia and Mexico. This syndrome consists of intense local skin reactions and high fever, lymphadenopathy, and hepatosplenomegaly. The skin responses are not IgE-mediated allergy as first thought. The skin lesions represent NK cell infiltration with cells containing EBV, with some being malignant. It is thought that CD4 cells recognize mosquito antigens and cause triggering of NK migration and proliferation that in turn contribute to EBV proliferation and oncogene expression.[44]

The second condition is indirectly linked to the immunology of allergy by having elevated, rather than diminished levels of IFN-γ. The condition is hemophagocytic lymphohistiocytosis (HLH), where T cells are the primary site of infection with the virus. HLH is characterized by hemophagocytosis and results in fever, splenomegaly, cytopenia, hypertriglyceridemia or hypofirinogenemia.[45,46] The third condition is the drug-induced hypersensitivity syndrome that occurs following 3 to 6 weeks of expossure to drugs such as anticonvulsants, allopurinol, and sulfasalazine. It usually is accompanied by eosinophilia, high fever, erythema, facial swelling, lymphadenopathy, and a follicular maculopapular eruption. Along with the eosinophilia, atypical lymphocytes and abnormal liver function tests are typical.[47]

Differential Diagnosis

Although classic IM is frequently caused by EBV, similar conditions are perhaps too often incorrectly labeled EBV mononucleosis even though they are not causally related to an EBV infection. Typical examples include (1) patients with malaise with or without fever, a sore throat, and mildly enlarged cervical lymph nodes but no hematologic changes or hepatosplenomegaly and with a positive heterophile spot test; (2) patients with malaise and a positive spot test; and (3) patients with a compatible clinical illness whose spot tests are negative but whose specific antibody patterns are simply those of past infection and are interpreted by the performing laboratory or treating physician as being consistent with active infection. The use of tables that

outline antibody patterns and are reported along with numerical values by the performing laboratory may lead to faulty interpretations of disease activity. These tables were originally described on the basis of IFA results and formulated based on long-term (at least 10-year) studies. Similar studies using the more sensitive but less quantitative enzyme-associated tests have been published. For example, anti-EA antibodies may persist in healthy patients and therefore do not always indicate an active or convalescent infection; thus some reevaluation of the usefulness of such tables is appropriate.

Since all systemic infections share the same basic symptoms, the differential diagnosis of EBV infections must start with a blank slate. Some infections are more likely than others to be considered 'mono-like illnesses' and therefore can be mistaken for an EBV infection. These include cytomegalovirus, HHV-6/7, adenovirus, and HIV infections. All these infections share infection of cells associated with the immune system. An additional virus yielding overlapping symptoms is parvovirus B19. All these agents are capable of establishing prolonged or latent infections and, except for HIV, are all DNA viruses. A parasite, *Toxoplasmosis gondii*, also produces an infection with similar clinical components plus a positive heterophile test.[48] In each of these instances the proper diagnosis is achieved by virtue of specific laboratory testing. An EBV infection may be considered by the presence of problems that are common to clinical presentations that are not typically considered in the IM category; for example, a patient with chronic urticaria unresponsive to standard therapy with antithyroid antibodies[49] was subsequently found to have an active EBV infection. Another example is that of chronic thrombocytopenia and/or chronic neutropenia, each of which and their consequences may be the only heralds of an EBV infection. As mentioned in the introduction, the heterophile antibody test in one form or another, particularly those used in small laboratories, is often positive in clinical situations that are caused by EBV infections. Other infectious agents that may trigger the production of this antibody are malaria, rubella, and, not unusually, *T. gondii*. Heterophile antibodies that can be absorbed with sera from different species are also present in serum sickness.[9]

The question of complications of IM needs to be discussed. If one considers IM as the disease caused by EBV, conditions that are not always present in IM have been considered to be 'complications'; such conditions could include hepatitis or meningitis.[50] But in the broader universe of EBV diseases, both these conditions can be direct components of the infection. On the other hand, a relatively common feature is neutropenia. A true complication would then be a bacterial infection, such as subcutaneous abscesses that would only occur in the presence of neutropenia. Peritonsillar abscesses and subcapsular splenic hematomas are considerations for other true complications, as is enlargement of the oral lymphoid mass, which creates airway obstruction and requires intervention.

Evaluation and Management

Diagnosis of any EBV infection in 2010 starts with a high level of suspicion for this agent as the cause of a very wide spectrum of clinical problems. Any patient even suspected of any of the clinical entities listed in Box 16-1 should be assumed to have an EBV infection unless there is a clear alternative explanation. The importance of identification of EBV-related diseases is not merely academic and there are several methods of approaching treatment of these problems. The first laboratory test is determination of the presence or absence of specific EBV antibodies. Depending on the results of such tests and the clinical status of

Table 16-2 Diagnostic Levels of Anti-EBV Antibody Titers (Immunofluorescent Titers)

	Stage of Infection			
	Active Primary	**Reactivated**	**Severe**	**Past**
Anti-VCA				
IgM	1:10–1:40	Negative	Negative	Negative
IgG	1:20–1:5120	1:80–1:5120	≥1:10000	1:80–1:5120
Anti-EA	1:20–1:320*	1:20–1:320	>1:640	1:20–1:320
Anti-EBNA	Negative†	<1:40	<1:40	≥1:40
Heterophile Ab	Positive‡	N/A	N/A	Negative

EBV, Epstein-Barr virus; *VCA*, viral capsid antigen; *EA*, early antigen; *EBNA*, Epstein-Barr nuclear antigen; *N/A*, not applicable.
*May be only positive titer very early in infection.
†May remain positive for 12 months with resolution of illness and positive anti-EBNA.
‡85% positive in classic infectious mononucleosis; magnitude of response is not meaningful.

the patient, testing for viral DNA or expressed RNA may be recommended.

The antibody pattern seen in acute primary infections as determined by both IFA and enzyme tests is positive IgM and IgG anti-VCA and positive anti-EA but negative anti-EBNA. The latter is thought only to appear once the active infection is under control and the virus has assumed its latent state, during which EBNA proteins are being produced. The magnitude of the response is not as important as the pattern, except when anti-VCA and anti-EA titers are more than 1:10000 and 1:640, respectively, and anti-EBNA titers are 1:40 or lower. Comparable quantitative statements cannot be made about levels generated by the family of enzyme-linked assays.

How the host first 'sees' EBNA proteins, however, remains unclear and there are variations on the antibody pattern when patients are first evaluated. Very early in the infection one may observe only anti-EA antibodies. The EA proteins are seen during the early stages of productive replication and may generate specific responses before the production of structural proteins identified by the anti-VCA antibodies. Perhaps the most useful finding to suggest an active infection, either a primary or reactivated state, is the absence of anti-EBNA.[6] Table 16-2 addresses the pattern and magnitude of antibody responses that are typically seen at various stages of clinical EBV infections and is based on IFA titers because there are no experimentally determined observations using the enzyme-linked systems.

The exception to reliance on antibodies for identification of EBV infection per se is a severe infection in infants. As with other infectious illnesses, overwhelming infections in these children may not be associated with specific antibody production. This situation is one indication for the use of nucleic acid or a viral protein presence in tissues, peripheral blood cells, or fluids such as serum, plasma, ascites, and effusions or transudates from a variety of sources.[51,52]

The presence of viral DNA in any of these specimens confirms an EBV infection, but does its presence support a cause-and-effect relationship for the clinical situation under evaluation? This question must be asked because of the presumed permanence of the latent state in B cells. It is possible that the viral genome as identified by the presence of DNA in lymph node cells is simply such a finding. If viral DNA, however, is found free in serum or plasma in an ill patient who has not mounted an anti-EBNA response, the likelihood of an ongoing active infection is very high Box 16-2). In the normal course of a primary EBV infection typified by IM, free viral DNA is usually not found in serum

---

BOX 16-2 Key concepts

Evaluation and Management

- Consider Epstein-Barr virus (EBV) in patients with clinical features seen in spectrum of EBV-associated diseases.
- Specific EBV antibody testing is second step.
- Absence of anti–Epstein-Barr nuclear antigen antibodies supports an active infection, particularly accompanied by IgM antiviral capsid antigen and antiearly antigen antibodies.
- Viral DNA, RNA, and proteins in tissue support an EBV infection.
- Quantitative and semiquantitative assays assist in determination of reactivated infection in immunosuppressed patients.

---

or plasma after 2 weeks of illness.[53] The same can be said for the presence of viral DNA in tumor cells that have undergone genomic rearrangements.

Several methodologic issues need to be addressed at this time. If sufficient viral DNA can be found in tissue or saliva by Southern blotting, it suggests a high copy number and not simply the presence of virus at the lower limits of detection. But which components of the viral genome might be optimum targets for such an assay? There are a number of inherent repeat areas of the viral genome that have served as natural amplification factors. For instance, the BAM H1 W restriction fragment sequence may be repeated more than 10 times in a specific virus isolate but only a few times in others. Use of this fragment in identifying new EBV disease associations has been recorded.[2] This fragment was also useful when applied to in situ hybridization techniques in the same report.

More recently, gene amplification techniques, such as polymerase chain reaction (PCR), have assumed prominence in identification of viral nucleic acids. The sensitivity of these procedures makes them naturally useful as diagnostic tools. The use of quantitative testing approaches some of the questions raised by the query of whether one is simply identifying latent infections. This issue has been particularly important in evaluation of PTLD states.[54] The sensitivity of PCR allows use of virtually any portion of the viral genome as long as the genomic sequence is known to be consistently present in all isolates.[55]

The application of PCR for identification of messenger RNA (RT-PCR) as representative of viral genes undergoing active replication was an important advance.[45] In latent infections two small RNAs known as EBERs are abundantly expressed (over 10^5 copies), making such infections an excellent target for this technique and for in situ hybridization studies. The use of EBERs is ideal for the detection of latent infection; however, they are not present in situations where the tissue in question hosts an active infection associated with new virion production, such as hairy leukoplakia, or in T cell lymphomas where there might be incomplete replication but no detectable establishment of a latent infection.[56]

The use of identification of viral proteins in cells or tissues also commonly depends on the presence of latent stage proteins such as latent membrane protein (LMP). This protein is not expressed in cells in which the virus is actively replicating. Again, reliance on detection of this protein or other latent state proteins as the only approach or in conjunction with EBER identification may prevent detection of the virus and lead to faulty conclusions that may prevent therapeutic intervention.

Choice of the technique used for identification of the virus will be guided by the reason or reasons for needing to know of its presence. For instance, the number of copies of latent transcripts in lymphoid cells in patients with PTLD may be of prognostic value and indicators for therapy[54] (see Box 16-2).

Treatment

Treatment (Box 16-3) is based on the clinical circumstance and varies, whether the virus is actively producing new virions or is in the latent state, but cell proliferation is out of control. Treatment of IM is usually supportive and requires adequate rest, fluids, and the avoidance of contact sports if hepatosplenomegaly is significant. A circumstance that arbitrarily requires intervention is classic IM in a high school or college student at the time of final examinations where school absence would be costly. Oral steroid therapy has been described as helpful with lessening symptoms without adverse effect on the duration of the infection or inhibition of antibody production.[57] The use of intravenous and/or oral antiviral therapy with viral thymidine kinase inhibitors, such as acyclovir, in acute IM demonstrated a mild shortening of the acute illness and fever with no adverse effects.[58,59] The results, however, did not generate overwhelming enthusiasm for routine therapy with this group of compounds. Although there have been no formal studies, clinical experience with individuals in this age group who have prolonged (arbitrarily defined as >2 weeks) active disease with systemic complaints accompanied by pharyngitis preventing normal fluid intake, persistently elevated liver function test values, absence of anti-EBNA antibodies, and presence of viral DNA in serum or plasma by semiquantitative PCR, demonstrated marked improvement over a few days with a combination of oral corticosteroids and oral acyclovir or related compounds (Jones, unpublished observations).

BOX 16-3 Key concepts

Treatment

- Infectious mononucleosis: supportive; corticosteroids for airway obstruction (possibly combined with antiviral drugs)
- Severe infections: corticosteroids (or cyclosporin A), antiviral drugs, intravenous immunoglobulin, cytotoxic T cells
- Posttransplantation lymphoproliferative disorder: initial decrease in immunosuppression; same as for severe infections; antimetabolites
- Prevention: future immunizations

In the case of severe disease, defined by multisystem involvement, IgG anti-VCA antibody titers greater than 1:10000, anti-EA titers greater than 1:640, and anti-EBNA titers ranging from 0 to less than 1:40, intravenous immunoglobulin (IVIG) has been given to provide neutralizing and antibody dependent cell cytotoxicity (ADCC) antibodies along with corticosteroids and antiviral drugs (J. Jones, unpublished observations). No trials of this combination have been performed because these patients are infrequently seen, but the responses have been dramatic when accompanied by standard or heroic supportive care. Monitoring of serum and plasma-free viral DNA and changes in the abnormal antibody titers along with clinical responses are required; however, one should not consider this approach without the nucleic acid data.

The standard initial therapy for PTLD is to decrease the amount of immunosuppressive therapy. This approach is usually effective when the proliferative response is polyclonal in nature or the copy number of latent viral genomes in the proliferating cells is not considered to be dangerously elevated. If the proliferating cell population is oligoclonal, more vigorous intervention is required and may include alteration of the type of immunosuppressive therapy and addition of antiviral agents. The presence of monoclonal cells indicates tumor development and requires cytotoxic therapy. A detailed discussion of the pathophysiology and treatment of PTLD is provided by Davis.[60]

Two relatively recent approaches to the more serious PTLD state include the use of cloned T cells derived in vitro and directed against patient B cell lines[61] and treatment with the monoclonal anti-CD20 antibody rituximab.[62] These clones may be derived from the patient or matched or even unmatched donors. The goal of therapy is cytotoxic T cell control of the proliferating B cells. This mode of therapy has recently been applied to patients with chronic active infections determined by persistent viral DNA in serum or plasma and abnormal antibody responses.[63]

Since rutixamab was used successfully for treatment of many types of lymphoma expressing CD20,[64] it was successfully used to lower high copy numbers of EBV as measured by real-time PCR in proliferating B cells, but not necessarily EBV-containing tumor cells.[65] Rutixamab was then given with conditioning regimens prior to stem cell transplants (SCT) with the aim of preventing PTLD.[66] Even though EBV containing cell proliferation was altered, functional B cell engraftment was markedly delayed requiring replacement IVIG administration for several years.[67] Obviously, pre-SCT treatment requires further analysis based on the status of the primary tumor and EBV-associated proliferation and the delay in replacement of B cells.

A most intriguing concept of therapy reported by Slobod and colleagues[68] is based upon laboratory observations made by Chodosh and colleagues.[69] These researchers found that maintenance of the latent state in EBV-transformed cell lines could be inhibited in vitro in the presence of hydroxyurea. This chemical (drug) prevents the formation of new deoxynucleotides, among other actions. The chemical process by which linear EBV genomes become closed circles is not entirely clear, but based on this work, the production of new deoxynucleotides is required. Two AIDS patients had central nervous system B cell lymphomas known to carry the EBV genome in the latent state. The patients were treated with low-dose hydroxyurea and had marked clinical response, including shrinkage of the tumor mass. Perhaps this mode of therapy needs further evaluation because the persistence of the virus in its latent state is a major source of morbidity in EBV infections.

Treatment of EBV-associated malignancies in general and other syndromes associated with abnormal proliferative responses (i.e. HLH) is beyond the scope of this discussion. Suffice it to say, however, that early recognition of these conditions is imperative if therapy is to be successful.

The best therapy in infectious disease practice is prevention. EBV immunization has been proposed for several years. Possible candidate vaccines include structural protein preparations and DNA vaccines. Because viral vaccines that undergo replication induce long-lasting immunity, development of an EBV vaccine that would undergo active partial replication but not establish latency would be worthy of consideration (see Box 16-3).

Conclusions

According to most practitioners, IM remains the primary illness associated with EBV infection; one of the aims of this chapter is to dispel this belief. The spectrum of illness is broad and it is deep in terms of potential disease severity. EBV infections in general cannot be reliably diagnosed by depending on the use of the heterophile antibody test in any of its forms. The only time that it is associated with EBV infection is in classic IM, and in that instance the syndrome per se with the typical white blood cell (WBC) changes and increases in liver enzymes negates a need for the test. If heterophile antibodies are present, they are simply present; if they are not present, they are simply not present. There is no such thing as a false-positive or false-negative heterophile test, at least in terms of EBV infections. Specific antibody testing is the starting point for establishing an infection with this virus. Improvements are required in recommendations regarding interpretation of serologic test results. When in doubt about antibody test values in a patient, requesting that the tests be performed by the IFA method is often beneficial.

Another aim is to broaden the reader's understanding of diagnosis and treatment. EBV infections do not have to be considered 'just a virus infection that will go away with time.' In most cases, this statement is true but in situations in which resolution of the active process does not occur within the expected 1 to 2 weeks, steps can be taken to determine if therapy is required. The rite of passage through childhood no longer requires suffering through an EBV infection.

References

1. Faulkner G, Burrows S, Khanna R, et al. X-linked agammaglobulinemia patients are not infected with Epstein-Barr virus: implications for the biology of the virus. J Virol 1999;73:1555–64.
2. Jones J, Shurin S, Abramowsky C, et al. T cell lymphomas containing Epstein-Barr viral DNA in patients with chronic Epstein-Barr virus infections. N Engl J Med 1988;318:733–41.
3. Rickinson A, Moss D. Human cytotoxic T lymphocyte responses to Epstein-Barr virus infection. Ann Rev Immunol 1997;15:405–31.
4. Khanna R, Burrows SR, Moss DJ. Immune regulation in Epstein-Barr virus-associated diseases. Microbiol Rev 1995;59:387–405.
5. Cohen J. The biology of Epstein-Barr virus: lessons learned from the virus and the host. Curr Opin Immunol 1999;11:365–70.
6. Okano M. Epstein-Barr virus infection and its role in the expanding spectrum of human diseases. Acta Paediatr 1998;87:11–8.
7. Schuster V, Kreth H. Epstein-Barr virus infection and associated diseases in children. Eur J Pediatr 1992;1:718–25.
8. Henle W, Henle G. Epidemiologic aspects of Epstein-Barr virus (EBV)-associated diseases. Ann N Y Acad Sci 1980;80:326–31.
9. Sumaya C, Ench Y. Epstein-Barr virus infectious mononucleosis in children: II. Heterophil antibody and viral-specific responses. Pediatrics 1985;75:1011–9.
10. Heath CJ, Brodsky A, Potodsky A. Infectious mononucleosis in a general population. Am J Epidemiol 1972;95:46.
11. Sumaya C, Ench Y. Epstein-Barr virus infections in families: the role of children with infectious mononucleosis. J Infect Dis 1986;154:842–50.
12. Fleisher G, Henle W. Primary Epstein-Barr virus infection in American infants. J Infect Dis 1979;139:553–8.
13. Roberts W, Wotherspoon R, Herrod HG. Morbidity of Epstein-Barr virus infection in children. In: Ablashi DV, Levine PH, Pagano JS, editors. Epstein-Barr virus and human disease. Clifton, NJ: Humana Press; 1987.
14. Rehse C, Helwig H. Das krankheitsbild der infektiosen mononucleose imkindesalter. Monatsschr Kinderheilkd 1985;133:806–10.
15. Chan K, Tam S, Peiris JS, et al. Epstein-Barr virus (EBV) infection in infancy. J Clin Virol 2001;21:57–62.
16. Kawa K. Epstein-Barr virus-associated diseases in humans. Int J Hematol 2000;71:108–17.
17. Jones J, Katz B. Epstein-Barr virus infections in normal and immunosuppressed patients. In: Glaser R, editor. Herpesvirus infection. Philadelphia: WB Saunders; 1994.
18. Kimura H, Hoshino Y, Kanegane H, et al. Clinical and virologic characteristics of chronic active Epstein-Barr virus infection. Blood 2001;98:280–6.
19. Pagano J. Epstein-Barr virus: the first human tumor virus and its role in cancer. Proc Assoc Am Physicians 1999;111:573–80.
20. Bonnet M, Guinebretiere J, Kremmer E, et al. Detection of Epstein-Barr virus in invasive breast cancers. J Natl Cancer Inst 1999;91:1376–81.
21. James J, Kaufman K, Farris A, et al. An increased prevalence of Epstein-Barr virus infection in young patients suggests a possible etiology for systemic lupus erythematosus. J Clin Invest 1997;100:3019–26.
22. Ascherio A, Munch M. Epstein-Barr virus and multiple sclerosis. Epidemiology 2000;11:220–4.
23. Wright-Browne V, Schnee A, Jenkins M, et al. Serum cytokine levels in infectious mononucleosis at diagnosis and convalescence. Leuk Lymphoma 1998;30:583–9.
24. Crawford DH. Biology and disease associations of Epstein-Barr virus. Philos Trans R Soc Lond B Biol Sci 2001;356:461–73.
25. Andersson J. Clinical and immunological considerations in Epstein-Barr virus-associated diseases. Scand Univ Press 1996;100:S72–82.
26. Svedmyr E, Ermberg O, Seeley K. Virologic, immunologic, and clinical observations on a patient during the incubation, acute and convalescent phases of infectious mononucleosis. Clin Immunol Immunopathol 1984;30:437–50.
27. Apolloni A, Moss D, Stumm R, et al. Sequence variation of cytotoxic T cell epitopes in different isolates of Epstein-Barr virus. Eur J Immunol 1992;22:183–9.
28. Linde A. Diagnosis of Epstein-Barr virus-related diseases. Scand J Infect Dis 1996;100:S83–88.
29. Konttinen Y, Bluestein H, Zvaifler N. Regulation of the growth of Epstein-Barr virus-infected B cells: temporal profile of the in vitro development of three distinct cytotoxic cells. Cell Immunol 1986;103:84–95.
30. Rickinson A, Wallace L, Epstein M. HLA-restricted T cell recognition of Epstein-Barr virus-infected B cells. Nature 1980;283:865–7.
31. Steven NM, Annels NE, Kumar A, et al. Immediate early and early lytic cycle proteins are frequent targets of the Epstein-Barr virus-induced cytotoxic T cell response. J Exp Med 1997;185:1605–17.
32. Randolph TG, Hettig RA. The coincidence of allergic disease, unexplained fatigue, and lymphadenopathy: possible diagnostic confusion with infectious mononucleosis. Am J Med Sci 1945;306:14.
33. Rystedt I, Strannegard I, Strannegard O. Increased serum levels of antibodies to Epstein-Barr virus in adults with history of atopic dermatitis. Int Arch Allergy Immunol 1984;75:179–83.
34. Strannegard I, Strannegard O. Epstein-Barr virus antibodies in children with atopic disease. Int Arch Allergy Immunol 1981;64:314–9.
35. Bahna S, Heiner D, Horwitz C. Sequential changes of the five immunoglobulin classes and other responses in infectious mononucleosis. Int Arch Allergy Immunol 1984;74:1–8.
36. Martinez-Maza O, Guilbert B, David B, et al. The Epstein-Barr virus-induced production of IgE by human B cells. Clin Immunol Immunopathol 1986;39:405–13.
37. Thyphronitis G, Max E, Finkelman FD. Generation and cloning of stable human IgE-secreting cells that have rearranged the C epsilon gene. J Immunol 1991;146:1496–502.
38. Robinson J, Stevens K. Production of autoantibodies to cellular antigens by human B cells transformed by Epstein-Barr virus. Clin Immunol Immunopathol 1984;33:339–50.
39. Okudaira H, Mori A. Concepts of the pathogenesis of allergic disease: possible roles of Epstein-Barr virus infection and interleukin-2 production. Int Arch Allergy Immunol 1999;120:177–84.
40. Sidorchuk A, Wickman M, Pershagen G, et al. Cytomegalovirus infection and development of allergic diseases in early childhood: Interaction withEBV infection. J Allergy Clin Immunol 2004;114:1434–40.
41. Nilsson C, Linde A, Montgomery SM, et al. Does EBV infection protect against IgE sensitization? J Allergy Clin Immunol 2005;116:438–44.
42. Nilsson C, Sigfrinius A-KL, Montgomery SM, et al. Epstein-Barr virus and cytomegalovirus are differentially associated with numbers of cytokine-producing cells and early atopy. Clin Exp Allergy 2009;39: 509–17.

43. Saghafian-Hedengren S, Sundstrom Y, Sohlberg E, et al. Herpesvirus seropositivity in childhood associates with decreased monocyte-induced NK cell IFN-γproduction. J Immunol 2009;182:2511–7.

44. Asada H. Hypersensitivity to mosquito bites: a unique pathogenic mechanism linking Epstein-Barr virus infection, allergy, and oncogenesis. J Dermatol Sci 2007;45:153–60.

45. Mischler M, Fleming GM, Shanley TP, et al. Epstein-Barr virus-induced hemophagocytic lymphohistiocytosis and X-linked lymphoproliferative disease: a mimicker of sepsis in the pediatric intensive care unit. Pediatrics 2007;119:e1212–8.

46. Janka GE. Hemophagocytic syndromes. Blood Reviews 2007;21: 245–53.

47. Seishima M, Yamanaka S, Fujisawa T, et al. Reactivation of human Herpesvirus (HHV) family members other than HHV-6 in drug-induced hypersensitivity syndrome. Br J Dermatol 2006;155:344–9.

48. Sayre M, Jehle D. Elevated toxoplasma IgG antibody in patients tested for infectious mononucleosis in an urban emergency department. Ann Emerg Med 1988;84:383–6.

49. Dreyfus D, Schocket A, Milgrom H. Steroid-resistant chronic urticaria associated with anti-thyroid microsomal antibodies in a nine-year-old boy. J Pediatr 1996;128:576–8.

50. Alpert G, Fleisher G. Complications of infection with Epstein-Barr virus during childhood: a study of children admitted to the hospital. Pediatr Infect Dis 1984;3:304–6.

51. Ambinder RF, Mann RB. Detection and characterization of Epstein-Barr virus in clinical specimens. Am J Pathol 1994;145:239–52.

52. Fan H, Gullery M. Epstein-Barr viral load measurement as a marker of EBV-related disease. Molec Diag 2001;6:279–89.

53. Yamamoto M, Kimura H, Hironaka T, et al. Detection and quantification of virus DNA in plasma of patients with Epstein-Barr virus-associated diseases. J Clin Microbiol 1995;33:1765–8.

54. Rowe D, Qu L, Reyes J, et al. Use of quantitative competitive PCR to measure Epstein-Barr virus genome load in the peripheral blood of pediatric transplant patients with lymphoproliferative disorders. J Clin Microbiol 1997;35:1612–5.

55. Gulley M. Molecular diagnosis of Epstein-Barr virus-related diseases. J Molec Diag 2001;3:1–10.

56. Raab-Traub N, Webster-Cyriaque J. Epstein-Barr virus infection and expression in oral lesions. Oral Dis 1997;3:S164–70.

57. Brandfonbrener A, Epstein A, Wu S. Corticosteroid therapy in Epstein-Barr virus infection: effect on lymphocyte class, subset, and response to early antigen. Arch Intern Med 1986;146:337–9.

58. Andersson J, Britton S, Ernberg I, et al. Effect of acyclovir on infectious mononucleosis: a double-blind, placebo-controlled study. J Infect Dis 1986;153:283–90.

59. Yao Q, Ogan P, Rowe M, et al. The Epstein-Barr virus: host balance in acute infectious mononucleosis patients receiving acyclovir anti-viral therapy. Int J Can 1989;43:61–6.

60. Davis C. The antiviral prophylaxis of post-transplant lymphoproliferative disorder. Springer Semin Immunopathol 1998;20:437–53.

61. Liu Z, Savoldo B, Huls H, et al. Epstein-Barr virus (EBV)-specific cytotoxic T lymphocytes for the prevention and treatment of EBV-associated post-transplant lymphomas. Recent Results Cancer Res 2002;159:123–33.

62. Savoldo B, Huls M, Liu Z, et al. Autologous Epstein-Barr virus (EBV)-specific cytotoxic T cells for the treatment of persistent active EBV infection. Blood 2002;100:4059–66.

63. Savoldo B, Huls M, Liu Z, et al. Autologous Epstein-Barr virus (EBV)-specific cytotoxic T cell therapy treatment of persistent active EBV infection. Blood 2002;100:4059–66.

64. Coiffier B. Rituximab therapy in malignant lymphoma. Oncogene 2007;26:3603–13.

65. Yang J, Tao Q, Flinn IW, et al. Characterization of Epstein-Barr virus-infected B cells in patients with posttransplantation lymphoproliferative disease: disappearance after rituximab therapy does not predict clinical response. Blood 2000;96:4055–63.

66. Comoli P, Basso S, Zecca M, et al. Pre-emptive therapy of EBV-related lymphoproliferative disease after pediatric haploidentical stem cell transplantation. Am J Transplant 2007;7:1648–55.

67. Hicks LK, Woods A, Buckstein R, et al. Rituximab purging and maintenance combined with auto-SCT: long-term molecular remissions and prolonged hypogammaglobulinemia in relapsed follicular lymphoma. Bone Marrow Transplant 2009;43:701–8.

68. Slobod K, Taylor G, Sandlund J, et al. Epstein-Barr virus-targeted therapy for AIDS-related primary lymphoma of the central nervous system. Lancet 2000;356:1493–4.

69. Chodosh J, Holder VP, Gan Y, et al. Eradication of latent Epstein-Barr virus by hydroxyurea alters the growth-transformed cell phenotype. J Infect Dis 1998;177:1194–201.

Intravenous Immune Serum Globulin (IVIG) Therapy in Patients with Antibody Immune Deficiency

Mark Ballow • Heather K. Lehman

Introduction

At the beginning of World War II, Cohn and colleagues from Harvard University developed an ethanol fractionation method to separate plasma proteins into stable fractions.[1] Fraction II was an antibody rich fraction that could be administered in small amounts intramuscularly and had a protective effect against measles and Hepatitis A. In 1952, Bruton described the first case of agammaglobulinemia, and showed that replacement with Cohn's fraction II immunoglobulin was effective in the treatment of these patients[2] However, the replacement could be done only intramuscularly; administration intravascularly caused serious side-effects. In the early 1960s the Swiss Red Cross Laboratories developed methods to adapt the Cohn fraction II immunoglobulin for intravenous use. In 1981 the first commercial intravenous immunoglobulin became available in the USA.

Immunoglobulin Replacement Therapy in Primary Immunodeficiency

The goal of immunoglobulin replacement therapy in patients with primary immunodeficiency is to provide adequate antibodies to prevent infections and long-term complications, especially pulmonary disease. Any patient with recurrent infections and profound hypogammaglobulinemia and/or defective antibody production may be a candidate for intravenous immune serum globulin (IVIG).[3] It is very important to evaluate the ability of the patient to produce specific antibodies to polysaccharide or protein antigens. Immunoglobulin replacement therapy should be considered only in patients with deficiencies in antibody formation, but not necessarily in patients with low levels of immunoglobulin or in IgG subclasses. The FDA approved uses for IVIG as replacement or adjunct therapy in patients with immune deficiency, recurrent infections, or autoimmune and inflammatory disorders is shown in Box 17-1.

Preparation of Intravenous Immunoglobulin

Most of the IVIG preparations are derived from plasma by Cohn's ethanol fractionation method or its Cohn-Oncley modification.[4] This fractionation process obtains four fractions. Fraction II is the immunoglobulin-rich fraction containing 95 to 99% IgG.

There are small varying amounts of IgM, IgA, and other proteins.[5] Cohn fraction II can only be given intramuscularly. The side-effects of Cohn fraction II when given intravenously is thought to result from aggregation of the IgG molecules and its anticomplementary activity, which can produce a severe, anaphylactoid reaction. A number of approaches have been used to further purify the IgG fraction including capyralate precipitation, octanoic acid precipitation, anion chromatography, or polyethylene glycol (Table 17-1). Other additions, such as an amino acid, stabilize the IgG molecules from reaggregation making it suitable for intravenous use. Almost all products available today in the USA are liquids, either 5 or 10%. One liquid 16% product is only suitable for the subcutaneous route (Table 17-1). Incubation at low pH or treatment with solvent and detergent, pasteurization, depth filtration and nanofiltration are important steps for viral removal and inactivation.

IVIG is made from pooled plasma from at least 10 000 donors, but each pool by FDA guidelines may contain up to 60 000 donors, and contains a broad spectrum of antibodies with biological activities especially for infectious pathogens. It contains at least 90% intact monomeric IgG with a normal ratio of subclasses, and is free of aggregates. The biologic activity of the IgG is maintained especially for Fc-mediated function; and it contains no infectious agents or other potentially harmful contaminants. Although there is no standardization for the titer of antibodies against common organisms such as *Streptococcus pneumoniae* and *Haemophilus influenzae*, each lot must contain adequate levels of antibody to certain microbial agents, e.g. measles. These IVIG products may vary slightly from manufacturer to manufacturer and from lot to lot but they are generally comparable.[6] Some products containing very low amounts of IgA may be beneficial in some immune deficiency patients with immunoglobulin E (IgE) antibodies to IgA to minimize the risk of possible anaphylactic reactions[7] (Box 17-2). All current preparations are essentially equivalent, and are selected on the basis of tolerability, cost, or availability. The characteristics of IVIG preparations available in the United States are shown in Table 17-1.

The half-life of antibodies varies. It depends on the isotype and the subclass of the antibody. Total IgG has a half-life of approximately 17 to 30 days.[8,9] However, the half-life of IgG3 is much shorter (7.5 to 9 days)[9,10] compared to IgG1 and IgG2 which have a half-life of approximately 27 to 30 days. Generally, it should take about 3 months after beginning monthly IVIG infusions or a dosage change to reach equilibration (steady state)[5] Infusing increased amounts of IVIG results in a more rapid

DOI: 10.1016/B978-1-4377-0271-2.00017-1

FDA-approved Uses of Intravenous Immunoglobulin (IVIG) Therapy in Patients with Immunodeficiency Disorders, Infection, and Inflammatory Processes

Primary immunodeficiency disease or primary antibody immunodeficiency

Idiopathic thrombocytopenic purpura (ITP)

Kawasaki disease

B cell chronic lymphocytic leukemia (CLL) with reduced IgG and recurrent bacterial infections

Bone marrow transplantation to decrease the risk of infection, interstitial pneumonia, and acute GVHD

Pediatric HIV-1 infection to decrease the frequency and severity of bacterial infections

Chronic inflammatory demyelinating polyneuropathy (CIDP)

catabolic rate since the catabolism of IgG is concentration dependent.[10] This process is mediated by the Fc receptors on phagocytic cells.[11]

Dosage

The recommended dose for IVIG as replacement therapy is generally 400–600 mg/kg/month given every 3 to 4 weeks in patients with primary immune deficiency. A higher dose of immunoglobulin can lead to higher peak and trough levels of serum IgG.[12] On average, peak serum IgG levels increase approximately 250 mg/dL,[12] and trough levels increase 100 mg/dL[13] for each 100 mg/kg of IVIG infused. Several trials had been conducted to compare the efficacy of immunoglobulin given intramuscularly vs intravenously, and low dose (less than 200 mg/kg) vs high dose (usually more than 250 mg/kg). In 1987, Bernatowska and colleagues[14] compared 150 mg/kg with 500 mg/kg, and showed that the higher dose decreased the days of fever, and days on antibiotics, and improved pulmonary function. The benefits of the higher dose of IVIG were more significant in children who had severe clinical symptoms. In a randomized cross-over study, Roifman and colleagues[15] administered either 200 mg/kg or 600 mg/kg of IVIG to 12 patients with antibody deficiency and chronic lung disease. Pulmonary function improved on the higher doses of IVIG therapy.[15] In 1992, Liese and colleagues[16] reported that 29 patients with X-linked agammaglobulinemia who received immunoglobulin replacement therapy between 1965 and 1990 showed a significant decrease in the incidence of pneumonias and the number of hospitalized days in patients receiving 350–600 mg/kg/IVIG every 3 weeks compared with patients receiving less than 200 mg/kg/IVIG every 3 weeks or 100 mg/kg of IM gamma globulin every 3 weeks. The improvements were more evident when the high dose IVIG was initiated before the age of 5 years. Eijkhout and colleagues[17] studied the effects of two different doses of IVIG on the incidence of recurrent infections in patients with primary immune deficiency in a randomized, double-blinded, multi-center cross-over study. Standard doses of IVIG included 300 mg/kg every 4 weeks for adults, and 400 mg/kg every 4 weeks for children. The administration of high IVIG doses (600 mg/kg for adults, and 800 mg/kg for children) significantly reduced the number (3.5 vs 2.5 per patient) and duration (median, 33 days vs 21 days) of infections. Trough levels also increased during high-dose therapy. Importantly, the incidence and type of side-effects did not differ between the standard and high-dose therapies.

In 1999, Kainulainen and colleagues[18] published data on 22 patients with primary hypogammaglobulinemia and pulmonary abnormalities who were treated with IVIG. Despite adequate trough serum IgG levels (>500 mg/dL), silent and asymptomatic pulmonary changes occurred. Quartier and associates[19] performed a retrospective study of the clinical features and outcomes of 31 patients with X-linked agammaglobulinemia (XLA) receiving replacement IVIG therapy between 1982 and 1997. IVIG was given at doses of >250 mg/kg every 3 weeks with a mean serum trough level between 500 and 1140 mg/dL (median – 700 mg/dL). The incidence of bacterial infections requiring hospitalizations fell from 0.4 to 0.06 per patient per year. However, enteroviral meningoencephalitis still developed in 3 patients. Of 23 patients evaluated by pulmonary function tests and chest CT, 3 had obstructive disease, 6 had bronchiectasis and 20 had chronic sinusitis. The authors concluded that although early treatment with IVIG and achieving a trough serum IgG level of >500 mg/dL was effective in preventing severe acute bacterial infections; these levels may not prevent pulmonary disease and sinusitis. The authors suggested that more intensive therapy to maintain a higher serum IgG level, e.g. >800 mg/dL, may improve pulmonary outcome in patients with XLA. In a more recent retrospective study of patients with common variable immunodeficiency, Busse and colleagues[20] reported that treatment with IVIG significantly decreased the incidence of pneumonia from 84% to 22%. Pulmonary abnormalities are the most important factors associated with morbidity and mortality in patients with primary immunodeficiencies. All newly diagnosed patients placed on IVIG replacement therapy should have pulmonary function testing and high-resolution chest computed tomography (CT) as baseline, and periodically thereafter. Chest CT may show evidence of lung damage even without clinical evidence of lung infection. The number of infections, days missed from school or work, and hospitalized days may not be sufficient indicators of adequate treatment. Improvement or maintenance of pulmonary function is an important measure of the success of therapy.

Administration

In patients with primary immune deficiency the replacement dose of IVIG is generally 400–600 mg/kg. The dose, manufacturer, and lot number should be recorded for each infusion in order to perform look-back procedures for adverse events or other consequences. It is crucial to record all side-effects that occur during the infusion. It is also recommended to monitor liver and renal function tests periodically, approximately every 6 months. Antigen detection for hepatitis B and polymerase chain reaction (PCR) for hepatitis C should be performed, if clinically indicated. There are several routes of administration of immunoglobulin.

Intravenous Administration

The recommended rates of IVIG infusion were determined in early studies using reduced and alkylated IgG. Such preparations led to rate-related side-effects in more than 50% of patients. Newer preparations are more tolerable but manufacturers still recommend starting rates of 0.8 mg/kg/min up to rates of 8 mg/kg/min. With some preparations much higher rates (12–14 mg/kg/min)[22,23] can be tolerated in selected patients who have had no adverse reactions with conventional rates.[21] The FDA recommends that for patients at risk of renal failure, e.g. pre-existing renal insufficiency, diabetes, age greater than 65 years, volume

Table 17-1 Commercial Intravenous Immunoglobulin Preparations

Brand (Manufacturer)	Manufacturing Process	pH	Additives	Parenteral Form and Final Concentrations	IgA Content µg/mL	Antiviral Steps
Gammagard S/D (Baxter Healthcare Corp)	Cohn-Oncley cold ethanol fractionation, followed by ultrafiltration and ion exchange chromatography; solvent detergent treated	6.4–7.2	5% solution: 0.3% albumin, 2.25% glycine, 2% glucose	Lyophilized powder 5%, or 10%	<2.2 (5% solution)	Solvent/detergent
Gammagard Liquid 10% (Baxter Healthcare Corp)	Cohn-Oncley cold ethanol fractionation and ion exchange chromatography followed by ultrafiltration; solvent detergent treated, nanofiltration, low pH incubation	4.6–5.1	10% solution, no sugars – stabilized with glycine	Liquid 10%	37	Solvent/detergent, low pH, nanofiltration
Flebogamma NF 5% (Instituto Grifols, Spain)	Cohn-Oncley cold ethanol fractionation and ion exchange chromatography followed by PEG precipitation, heat pasteurization	5–6	5% solution, 2 µg/mL albumin, 5% D-sorbitol	5% liquid	13	Heat pasteurization, PEG precipitation, nanofiltration
Carimune NF (CLS Behring, LLC)	Kistler-Nitschmann, pH 4.0 plus pepsin, nanofiltration	6.4–6.8	5% sucrose (3% solution)	Lyophilized powder – reconstitute to 3, 6, 9 or 12%	720 (6% solution)	pH 4.0/pepsin, nanofiltration
Gamunex (Talecris Biotherapeutics)	Cohn-Oncley cold ethanol fractionation, caprylate chromatography purified, low pH incubation	4.0–4.5	10% solution no sugar, stabilized with glycine	10% liquid	46	Caprylate treatment, low pH incubation, depth filtration
Octagam 5% (Octapharma Pharmazeutika)	Cohn-Oncley cold ethanol fractionation, and ion exchange chromatography followed by ultrafiltration, solvent/detergent treated	5.1–6.0	5% solution, maltose 100 mg/mL	5% liquid	≤200	Solvent/detergent, pH 4
Privigen 10% (CLS Behring, LLC)	Cold ethanol fractionation, octanoic acid precipitation, anion exchange chromatography	4.8	No sugars, stabilized with L-proline	Liquid 10%	8.6	Low pH incubation, depth filtration, nanofiltration
Vivaglobin (CLS Behring, LLC)	Cold ethanol fractionation, pasteurization	6.4–7.2	No sugar, stabilized with glycine	16% liquid for subcutaneous administration only	≤1700	Ethanol, low pH, pasteurization

Source: manufacturers' package inserts and product publications.

BOX 17-2 Key concepts

Intravenous Immune Serum Globulin (IVIG)

- Cold ethanol fractionation (Cohn fraction II)
- >95% IgG; >90% monomeric IgG
- Traces of other immunoglobulins, e.g. IgA and IgM, and serum proteins
- Addition of an amino acid to stabilize IgG from aggregation
- Intact Fc receptor biological function
  - opsonization and phagocytosis
  - complement activation
- Normal half life for serum IgG
- Normal proportion of IgG subclasses
- Broad spectrum of antibodies to bacterial and viral agents

---

during the initial treatment is much higher. It is generally associated with the presence of infections and formation of immune complexes. In patients with active infection, the dose should be halved, i.e. 200–300 mg/kg, and the dose repeated 2 weeks later to achieve a full dose. Thereafter, adverse reactions are uncommon unless patients have active infection.

To minimize cost and inconvenience, self-administration and home treatment have been studied and used successfully.[24,25] For home therapy, patients need to be selected carefully. Patients must have several uneventful treatments in the hospital and be trained under close supervision to assure correct techniques, and be able to recognize and treat side-effects. Infusions should be done only in the presence of a responsible adult who is knowledgeable and ready to respond to an adverse event. Patients receiving home treatment should be seen regularly to monitor clinical status, liver function, renal function, and trough serum IgG levels.[26] A better choice for those patients who want to self-infuse is the subcutaneous (SC) route of administration.

Subcutaneous Immunoglobulin (SCIg) Administration

Berger and colleagues[27] were the first to describe the use of the subcutaneous route for immunoglobulin replacement therapy in

depletion, sepsis, paraproteinemia, and use of nephrotoxic drugs, or patients at risk of thromboembolic complications, should be gradually increased to a more conservative 3–4 mg/kg/min.

The initial treatment should be administered in the hospital or a blood product infusion center under the close supervision of experienced personnel. The risk of developing adverse reactions

1980. It was reported as safe, well tolerated, and effective in achieving adequate serum IgG levels. Although subcutaneous administration was used successfully,[28] it was not very popular because it was time consuming due to the slow rate of infusion (1–2 mL/hr). SCIg infusions (100 mg/kg) reach a steady state after 6 months if given weekly, or in a week if patients are first loaded with IVIG or given daily SC infusions for 5 days, and thereafter weekly.[29] Before infusion, the line needs to be checked to ensure that there is no blood return. Infusions need to be given weekly between 2 to 6 sites. Infusion sites are usually on the abdominal wall and thigh. The rate of infusion on the pump is set initially at 10 mL/hr and may be increased 1 mL/hr every month up to 15–20 mL/hr, if no adverse reactions occur. A general guideline is 0.1 to 0.25 mL/kg/site/hr.[30] In the USA a 16% immunoglobulin product for intravenous use is available although any 10% liquid IVIG product can also be used by the subcutaneous route. Local tissue reactions include swelling, soreness, redness, induration, local heat, itching, and bruising, and are often transient. The severity and frequency of these local reactions decrease as the patient continues SCIg. In general, the SCIg route has been remarkably free from severe systemic reactions. Higher and more stable trough levels have been seen with the subcutaneous administration of immunoglobulin, alleviating the fatigue and general constitutional symptoms patients have on IVIG towards the end of their 3–4 weeks dosing interval. The FDA has recommended a dosage adjustment of a 37% increase when transitioning patients from IV to SCIg, although the dosing recommendation by the European regulatory agency is a 1:1 equivalence. Rates of infection in patients with primary immune deficiency have shown similar efficacy between IVIG and SCIg.[31,32] Before home treatment, patients need to be instructed on the correct technique under close supervision, and the recognition of possible side-effects. SCIg infusion is safer, less expensive, better tolerated and preferred by some patients. It should be considered as an alternative in selected patients, especially those with frequent adverse reactions by the intravenous route.

Adverse Effects of IVIG Associated with Administration

Rate-related Adverse Reactions

Most adverse reactions of IVIG are related to the administration of IVIG and are rate related. Common adverse events include tachycardia, chest tightness, back pain, arthralgia, myalgia, hypertension or hypotension, headache, pruritus, rash or low-grade fever (Box 17-3). More serious reactions included dyspnea, nausea, vomiting, circulatory collapse and loss of consciousness. Patients with more profound immunodeficiency or patients with active infections have more severe reactions. The reactions are related to the anticomplementary activity of IgG aggregates in the IVIG.[33] In addition, the formation of oligomeric or polymeric IgG complexes can interact with Fc receptors and trigger the release of inflammatory mediators.[34] These adverse reactions occurred less frequency (10–15%), and with less severity in the more recent preparations of IVIG. These reactions most commonly occur in newly diagnosed patients with hypogammaglobulinemia and in those patients who have chronic underlying infections, such as sinusitis and bronchitis. One possible etiology is the binding of the infused antibodies to pathogen component antigens of the underlying chronic infection or inflammatory process. In a large prospective study of 459 antibody-deficient patients by Brennan and colleages[35] of 13 508 infusions, the reaction rate was only 0.8%. There were no severe reactions; 0.1%

were moderate and 0.6% were mild. There was a greater number of adverse events in those patients receiving home infusion. However, the highest rate was in those patients who had active infection, e.g. 5.1%.

Fatigue, myalgia and headache may be delayed and may last several hours after the infusion. Slowing the infusion rate or discontinuing therapy until symptoms subside may diminish the reaction. Pretreatment with a nonsteroidal antiinflammatory agent, e.g. ibuprofen (10 mg/kg/dose), acetaminophen (15 mg/kg/dose), diphenhydramine (1 mg/kg/dose) and/or hydrocortisone (6 mg/kg/dose, maximum 100 mg)[13,33,36] 1 hour before the infusion may prevent the adverse reactions. If the patient continues to have moderate to severe adverse effects from IGIV, physicians should consider changing the route of administration to subcutaneous.

BOX 17-3

Adverse Effects of IVIG Administration

Common

Chills

Headache

Backache

Myalgia

Malaise, fatigue

Fever

Pruritis

Rash, flushing

Nausea, vomiting

Tingling

Hypo- or hypertension

Fluid overload

Uncommon (Multiple Reports)

Chest pain or tightness

Dyspnea

Severe headaches

Aseptic meningitis

Renal failure

Rare (Isolated Reports)

Anaphylaxis

Arthritis

Thrombosis/cerebral infarction

Myocardial infarction

Acute encephalopathy

Cardiac rhythm abnormalities

Coagulopathy

Hemolysis – alloantibodies to blood type A/B

Neutropenia

Alopecia

Uveitis

Noninfectious hepatitis

Hypothermia

Lymphocytic pleural effusion

Potential (No Reports)

New variant Creutzfeldt-Jakob (prion) disease

HIV infections

Parvovirus B19

Aseptic meningitis can occur with large doses, rapid infusions, and in the treatment of patients with autoimmune or inflammatory diseases.[37-40] Interestingly, this adverse reaction rarely occurs in immunodeficient subjects.[36] Symptoms, including headache, stiff neck, and photophobia, usually develop within 24 hours after completion of the infusion and may last 3 to 5 days. Spinal fluid pleocytosis occurs in most patients.[37,38,40] Long-term complications are minimal.[40] The etiology of aseptic meningitis is unclear but migraine has been reported as a risk factor and may be associated with recurrence despite the use of different IVIG preparations and slower rates of infusion.[37]

Renal Adverse Reactions

Acute renal failure is a rare but significant complication of IVIG treatment. Histopathologic findings of acute tubular necrosis, vacuolar degeneration and osmotic nephrosis, are suggestive of osmotic injury to the proximal renal tubules. Fifity five percent of the cases were patients treated for idiopathic thrombocytopenic purpura, and less than 5% involved patients with primary immunodeficiency.[41] This complication may relate to the higher doses of IVIG used in ITP. The majority of the cases were treated successfully with conservative treatment, but deaths were reported in 17 patients who had serious underlying conditions. Preliminary reports suggest that IVIG products using sucrose as a stabilizer may have a greater risk for this renal complication. As stated above, the infusion rate for sucrose-containing IVIG should not exceed 3 mg/kg/min. Risk factors for this adverse reaction include preexisting renal insufficiency, diabetes mellitus, dehydration, age greater than 65 years, sepsis, paraproteinemia and concomitant use of nephrotoxic agents. For patients at increased risk, monitoring blood urea nitrogen and creatinine before starting the treatment, and periodically thereafter, are necessary. If renal function deteriorates, the product should be changed to a nonsucrose containing IVIG. Eventually nonsucrose containing IVIG products will be commercially available.

Thromboembolic Events

This adverse effect is likely to be due to increased serum viscosity in patients receiving large doses of IGIV for autoimmune diseases. Patients with elevated serum viscosity, e.g. cryoglobulinemia, hypergammaglobulinemia, and hypercholesterolemia are at risk of developing a critical increase in serum viscosity with IGIV, especially high doses that predispose them to thromboembolic events. These changes can result in myocardial infarction, stroke, or pulmonary embolism. Besides cerebral infarction, reversible posterior leukoencephalopathy syndrome has also been seen in several patients receiving high-dose IGIV.[42]

Anaphylactic Reactions

IgE antibodies to IgA have been reported to cause severe transfusion reactions in IgA-deficient patients.[7,43] Symptoms were typical of an IgE-mediated anaphylactic reaction. The severity ranges from mild reactions to death. The serum levels of IgE antibody against IgA were found to correlate with anaphylaxis.[7] However, several patients with antibodies against IgA did not have anaphylactic reactions when treated with IVIG preparations containing very low concentrations of contaminating IgA (Table 17-1).[7,44] Thus, if replacement of immunoglobulin is needed in these patients, IVIG products containing minimal amounts of IgA should be used. Other patients may have more of a serum sickness-like reaction from IgG antibodies to IgA. However, this is uncommon with estimates of 1.3 reactions in 10⁶ infusions.[45]

Infectious Complications

Hepatitis C infection in patients receiving IVIG products was initially reported in experimental lots in Europe and the USA. Hepatitis C infection occurred in clusters associated with contaminated lots[46-48] and specific manufacturing procedures. The clinical course of HCV infection in patients with immune deficiency is not well defined. Routine screening of plasma donors for hepatitis C RNA by RT-PCR and the addition of a viral inactivation process in the final manufacturing step, e.g. treatment with solvent/detergent and/or pasteurization, has drastically reduced the risk of transmission of hepatitis C and other viruses.

In addition to these approaches in donor and plasma screening and testing, there have been new innovative steps incorporated during the manufacturing process that include viral inactivation and vial removal stages. Some of the more common processes include solvent-detergent treatment of the final IGIV product to destroy potential lipid-envelope viruses, incubation at low pH, pasteurization, caprylate treatment, and viral removal steps with depth filtration and nanofiltration. In aggregate, all these steps lead to a potential removal of 10–20 (depending on the virus) log 10 reduction values.[49,50] Thus, today's IGIV products are considered safe from a number of potential viral pathogens that were of concern in the early and mid 1990s. However, one potential pathogen that is still of potential concern is prions, which can cause transmissible spongiform encephalopathies, a fatal degenerative disease of the brain.[51] Although there are many regulations that prevent the transmission of the sporadic type of Creutzfeldt-Jakob Disease (CJD), there have been concerns about new-variant CJD (vCJD), which is an emerging pathogen in the UK and some parts of Europe.[52,53] To address this potential risk, the FDA has imposed very strict guidelines for blood donation of any individual spending time or traveling in England and Europe. IGIV manufacturers have recognized vCJD as a potential problem and have initiated testing steps, and IGIV purification and treatment steps, e.g. nanofiltration to address this issue, although not presently required by the FDA.[54]

Other Adverse Reactions

There are other more uncommon or rare complications of IVIG treatment (Box 17-3). Since IVIG preparations are prepared from large numbers of donors, antibodies against A/B blood-group antigens are present. Nonagglutinating antibodies in the IVIG may cause hemolytic reactions, especially if large amounts are infused.[55] Patients receiving large doses of IVIG may also develop fluid overload or hyperviscosity that can compromise cardiac function.

IVIG as an Immune Modulating Agent in Patients with Autoimmune or Inflammatory Disorders

Since the first report by Imbach and colleagues[56] on the use of intravenous immune globulin (IVIG) in childhood idiopathic thrombocytopenia purpura (ITP), IVIG has been used for the treatment of a variety of inflammatory and autoimmune disorders (Box 17-4). A number of mechanisms have been postulated for the immunomodulatory effects of IVIG (Box 17-5).[57] Platelet counts rise rapidly in children with ITP following the administration of IVIG 1–2 g/kg.[58] The mechanisms for platelet destruction is from FcγR-mediated phagocytic clearance of autoantibody-opsonized platelets in the spleen and liver.[59] Fehr and colleagues[60] and Bussel[61] suggested that the rapid responses following IVIG treatment in ITP were caused by a blockade of

IVIG in the Treatment of Patients with Autoimmune and Inflammatory Diseases

Proven Benefit

Idiopathic thrombocytopenia purpura*

Kawasaki disease*

Chronic inflammatory demyelinating polyradiculoneuropathy*

Graves ophthalmopathy

Guillain-Barré syndrome

Multifocal motor neuropathy

Probable Benefit

Dermatomyositis/polymyositis

Autoimmune uveitis

Lambert-Eaton myesthenic syndrome

Myesthenia gravis

Stiff-man syndrome

Toxic epidermal necrolysis/Stevens-Johnson syndrome

Might Provide Benefit

Multiple sclerosis

Rheumatoid arthritis

Autoimmune diabetes mellitus

Posttransfusion purpura

Autoimmune neutropenia

Autoimmune hemolytic anemia

Autoimmune hemophilia

Systemic lupus erythematosus

Fetomaternal alloimmune thrombocytopenia

Neonatal isoimmune hemolytic jaundice

ANCA-positive vasculitis

High-dose steroid-dependent asthma

Chronic urticaria

Autoimmune blistering skin diseases

Autoimmune liver disease

Intractable childhood epilepsy

Rasmussen syndrome

Pediatric autoimmune neuropsychiatric disorders associated with streptococcal infections

Cerebral infarcts in antiphospholipid antibody syndrome

Unlikely Benefit

Inclusion body myositis

Antiphospholipid antibody syndrome in pregnancy

Amyotrophic lateral sclerosis

POEMS syndrome

Adrenoleukodystrophy

Chronic fatigue syndrome

Atopic dermatitis

Non-steroid-dependent asthma

Autism

*FDA-approved indication

Adapted from Orange, JS et al. J Allergy Clin Immunol 2006; 117:S525–553.

Antiinflammatory Mechanisms Intravenous Immunoglobulin Action

1. Neutralization of autoantibodies by antiidiotypic antibodies in intravenous immunoglobulin

2. Enhancement of autoantibody clearance through FcRn blockade

3. Inhibition of complement uptake on target tissues and attenuation of complement-mediated tissue damage

4. Fc receptor blockade of the reticuloendothelial system

5. Inhibition of Fas-mediated cell death by Fas-blocking antibodies in the IVIG

6. Modulation of dendritic cell maturation and function

7. Modulation of macrophage activation and B cell activity through upregulation of the inhibitory FcγRIIB receptor

8. Neutralization of proinflammatory cytokines by anticytokine antibodies (IL-1, TNF-α, IFN-α, IFN-γ, IL-6)

9. Neutralization of staphylococcal and streptococcal exotoxins

10. Interaction of sialylated IgG with DC-SIGN, leading to inhibition of effector cell function

the reticuloendothelial system (RES). Clarkson and colleagues[62] demonstrated a marked increase in platelet count in patients with ITP using a monoclonal antibody directed against the low-affinity FcγRIIIA receptor found on neutrophils, NK cells and macrophages, suggesting that this effect might be related to the specific blockade of Fc fragment binding on macrophages in the spleen and in other parts of the RES system. Debre and colleagues[63] reported that children with acute ITP treated with intravenous Fcγ fragments from a preparation of IVIG showed a rapid increase in platelet counts. These studies strengthen the hypothesis that Fcγ receptor blockade is an important mechanism of action of IVIG in ITP, although other immune regulatory mechanisms are present.

As in childhood ITP, Kawasaki disease (KD) is an FDA approved therapeutic indication for IVIG administration.[64] KD is an acute multisystem disease of unknown etiology that primarily affects young children. Although the acute illness is generally self-limited, coronary artery abnormalities related to inflammation and immune activation of small and medium sized blood vessels develop in up to 25% of untreated patients. Geographical clustering, epidemics and even pandemics in Japan, and seasonal variations, e.g. late winter and spring, suggest an infectious etiology. The observation that children less than 6 months or more than 8 years of age are rarely affected suggests that the lack of a protective antibody against the putative KD agent may be an important risk factor for development of the disease. Leung and colleagues[65,66] have proposed that enterotoxin producing *Staphylococcus* and *Streptococcus* acting as superantigens may be responsible for the inflammatory and immunologic changes seen in patients with KD. IVIG contains high titers of antibodies that inhibit T cell activation by staphylococcal and streptococcal superantigens.[67] IVIG suppresses the immune activation associated with KD[68,69] and more importantly, prevents the development of coronary artery aneurysms.[65,70] Some patients require re-treatment[71] and this suggests that IVIG contains variable antitoxin titers.[72]

Other potential mechanisms of IVIG in KD include immunomodulation of cytokine effects, and inhibition of vascular endothelial cell activation. It has been demonstrated that IVIG inhibits the production of IL-1, TNF-α, TNF-β and IFN-γ by peripheral blood mononuclear cells stimulated with bacterial superantigens or lipopolysaccharide, while increasing production of IL-1 receptor antagonist (IL-1ra), an antiinflammatory cytokine that counteracts the effects of IL-1.[73] Furthermore, Xu and colleagues,[74] using human umbilical vein endothelial cells, demonstrated that IVIG inhibits endothelial cell proliferation, and down-regulates the mRNA expression of adhesion molecules (ICAM-1, VCAM-1), chemokines (MCP-1), growth factors (M-CSF and GM-CSF), and proinflammatory cytokines (TNF-α, IL-1α, IL-6). Thus, IVIG may exert its antiinflammatory effects in KD by interrupting or modifying a number of different steps in the inflammatory cascade, from the inhibition of effector cell function to reduction in cytokine-induced endothelial cell activation.

Another proposed antiinflammatory mechanism of IVIG is that it may increase the clearance of pathogenic autoantibodies by competing with the autoantibody for the neonatal Fc receptor (FcRn).[11] FcRn protects IgG from degradation, and is critical for its long half-life in the serum.[75] In mouse models of bullous pemphigoid and arthritis, IVIG treatment results in a reduction in pathogenic antibodies to levels beneath the disease-causing threshold, and this effect is attenuated in FcRn-deficient mice.[76,77] Hansen and Balthasar[78] reported that high dose IVIG in a rat model of immune thrombocytopenia enhanced the clearance of antiplatelet antibodies by the saturation of the FcRn receptor for IgG.

IVIG binds to activated C3b and C4b and prevents the tissue deposition of these activated complement proteins.[79] Several diseases and animal models have been reported in which inhibition of complement has been suggested as the mechanism of IVIG's antiinflammatory activity. Frank and his coworkers,[79] using an animal model of Forssman shock, demonstrated that high-dose IVIG prevented the death of guinea pigs. The inflammatory process in this guinea pig model is mediated by complement uptake and activation on endothelial cells that results in tissue damage. These investigators postulated that very high levels of serum IgG from IVIG therapy prevent active C3 and C4 fragments from binding to target cells, resulting in the modulation of acute complement-dependent tissue injury. Basta and colleagues[80] showed that IVIG not only inhibited the uptake of C3 fragments onto antibody-sensitized cells, but also C4, an early complement component.

Dermatomyositis (DM) is an autoimmune disease characterized by the subacute onset of muscle weakness, affecting predominantly the proximal muscle groups, is often accompanied or preceded by a characteristic skin rash, and is associated with circulating autoantibodies to endothelial cells and histidyl-tRNA synthetase (Jo-1).[81,82] A humoral immune process directed against the intramuscular capillaries characterizes the immunopathogenesis of DM. This process leads to a complement-mediated endomysial microangiopathy with deposition of the membrane attack complex (MAC) consisting of activated complement components C5b-9 on the intramuscular capillaries.[82] The endomysial capillary damage as a result of MAC deposition leads to microinfarcts within the muscle fascicles, muscle ischemia, inflammation, and eventually perifascicular atrophy.[83] The expression of ICAM-1 is increased on the endomysial blood vessels and muscle cells, which further facilitates the infiltration of inflammatory cells, mainly CD4+ T cells and some B cells.[83,84] The efficacy of IVIG treatment in adult DM has been demonstrated in a double-blinded, placebo-controlled study by Dalakas and colleagues.[82,85] Smaller, uncontrolled studies and case reports suggest that IVIG may also be efficacious in juvenile DM.[86,87] Muscle biopsies of patients improving after IVIG showed the disappearance of MAC deposits from the endomysial capillaries as well as decreased ICAM-1 expression in muscle tissues.[82,88]

The pathophysiology of a number of autoimmune diseases may be related to perturbations of the idiotype network.[89] Several groups have postulated that IVIG contains antiidiotypic antibodies that down-regulate the immune response.[90,91] A number of diseases may serve as models for this mechanism of IVIG, including patients with circulating autoantibody inhibitors to Factor VIII coagulant activity, systemic lupus erythematosus, and antineutrophil cytoplasmic antibodies (ANCA)-associated vasculitis. The presence of antiidiotypic antibodies in IVIG was first suggested by the response to IVIG therapy in a patient with hemophilia and inhibitory autoantibodies to Factor VIII.[92] The treatment with high-dose IVIG in two patients with high-titer autoantibodies to Factor VIII resulted in rapid and prolonged suppression of this inhibitory autoantibody.[93] Sultan and co-workers[92] showed that IVIG can also reduce Factor VIII inhibitor activity in vitro, and that this immunomodulatory effect resided within the F(ab')$_2$ fragment. Dietrich and Kazatchkine[91] prepared F(ab')$_2$ fragments from commercial IVIG preparations that could neutralize or bind to known autoantibodies, such as anti-Factor VIII, antithyroglobulin, anti-DNA, antiintrinsic factor, and ANCA. IVIG has also been shown to contain antibodies with idiotypic specificities that can bind and neutralize potentially pathogenic autoantibodies such as antibodies to GM1 ganglioside (anti-GM1) in patients with Guillain-Barré syndrome (GBS) and chronic inflammatory demyelinating polyradiculoneuropathy (CIDP), and antiacetylcholine receptor (AChR) antibodies in myasthenia gravis (MG).[94–97] Malik and coworkers[98] showed that antiidiotypic antibodies in the IVIG directed against idiotopes located on the anti-GM$_1$ immunoglobulin molecule blocked the binding of the anti-GM$_1$ antibodies to their target antigen, suggesting that an idiotype/antiidiotype interaction is a possible mechanism by which IVIG modifies the immune-mediated disease process and contributes to remyelination in patients with GBS and CIDP. Support for a similar mechanism in MG comes from the fact that IgG or F(ab')$_2$ fragments in the IVIG preparations are capable of binding to AChR antibodies in vitro.[99] Vassilev and colleagues[100] showed that normal human IVIG could suppress experimental MG in severe combined immunodeficiency disease (SCID) mice. Further studies are necessary to determine the significance of these antiidiotypic antibodies in IVIG as immune modulators in the pathogenesis of these autoimmune neurological diseases. Most experimental systems have shown that the active component of IVIG lies within the Fc fragments rather than the F(ab)$_2$ component, implicating Fc receptor effects rather than neutralization mechanisms.

While IVIG has been shown to have suppressive effects on effector T cells,[101,102] IVIG has been shown to expand and enhance the function of Fox p 3+ regulatory T cells (Tregs). In a mouse model of multiple sclerosis, the protective effect of IVIG was lost in mice that were depleted of Tregs.[103] In patients with Kawasaki disease and Guillain-Barré syndrome, clinical improvement with IVIG therapy correlated with increased Treg number and function.[104] De Groot and colleagues[105] proposed that IVIG has a positive effect on Tregs because of the presence of T cell epitopes in the Fc fragment which, when presented by antigen-presenting cells, specifically activate CD4+ CD25+ Fox p 3+ Tregs, and that this expansion of Tregs mediates the immunomodulatory effects of IVIG.

In ITP patients treated with IVIG, several studies have shown a decrease in antiplatelet antibody production.[61,106] Changes in the immunoregulatory function of T and B cells have been proposed as a mechanism for this decrease in antiplatelet antibodies following IVIG therapy. IVIG may have other immune modulating effects in addition to blockade of the Fcγ receptor. Studies have shown that the addition of IVIG in vitro suppresses lymphocyte proliferative responses to a variety of T cell mitogens.[107,108] This suppressive activity was dependent on the Fc portion of IVIG in that the F(ab')$_2$ fragments had no effect. Other studies have suggested that the target cell for inhibition of antibody production was the B lymphocyte rather than the T cell,[109,110] and that IVIG inhibits B cell proliferation in vitro.[111] In severe oral steroid-dependent asthmatic children treated with high dose IVIG, Mazer and colleagues[112] demonstrated a decrease in total serum IgE and allergen specific IgE antibodies. Sigman and colleagues[113] showed that IVIG in vitro could modulate IgE production. High concentrations of IVIG, in a dose-dependent manner, inhibited IgE production in anti-CD40/IL-4 stimulated B cells. This effect was not due to a blocking antibody in the IVIG, but impairment of IgE synthesis. The inhibitory effect on IgE production was associated with a decrease in Cε mRNA transcripts.

Bayry and colleagues demonstrated that IVIG can inhibit dendritic cell (DC) maturation and the ability of DCs to stimulate T cells.[114] This effect may have significance in the immune-modulating effects of IVIG in some diseases. Siragam and colleagues described a murine model of immune thrombocytopenic purpura (ITP) in which the therapeutic effect of IVIG could be replicated by adoptive transfer of IVIG-treated DCs.[115] It has recently been proposed that the effects of IVIG on DC function may be due to enhanced antibody-dependent cell-mediated cytotoxicity of mature DCs by NK cells.[116]

Macrophages, B cells and a subpopulation of T cells express a low-affinity inhibitory Fcγ receptor (FcγRIIB).[117,118] This receptor provides an inhibitory signal to cells through a pathway mediated by an immunoregulatory tyrosine-based inhibition motif, e.g. ITIM. Similar inhibitory Fcγ receptors are present on basophils and mast cells. Samuelsson and colleagues[119] investigated a murine model of immune thrombocytopenia. They found that the protective effects of IVIG required the inhibitory Fcγ receptor, e.g. Fcγ RIIB, since either disruption of the receptor or blocking with a monoclonal antibody reversed the therapeutic effects. In addition, IVIG therapy results in the up-regulation of the inhibitory FcγRIIB on effector macrophages.[119,120] This immune-modulatory action of IVIG may work in concert with the antiidiotypic antibodies in IVIG discussed above by coligation of the B cell receptor by a Fcγ RIIB antiidiotypic antibody. The observations on the effects of IVIG in patients with steroid-dependent asthma[112,121] may be related to similar Fcγ RIIB regulatory receptors on basophils and mast cells.

Another mechanism of action of IVIG related to specific antibodies in the IVIG is its effects on apoptosis. Viard et al. and colleagues[122] reported that IVIG could inhibit the apoptotic process, e.g. program cell death in patients with toxic epidermal necrolysis (TEN or Lyell's syndrome), a severe drug-induced bullous skin reaction. In in vitro studies IVIG was demonstrated to protect the keratinocytes from apoptosis by blocking the effects of FasL on the Fas receptor. These investigators also determined that the depletion of anti-Fas antibodies from the IVIG abrogated the ability of IVIG to inhibit FasL-mediated apoptosis. In an open, uncontrolled trial of IVIG (0.2–0.75 g/kg/day for 4 consecutive days) in 10 patients with TEN, skin progression was halted within 1–2 days that was followed by rapid skin healing and a favorable outcome. This immune modulating effect of IVIG in patients with TEN represents another unique mechanism by which IVIG can modify the disease process, and may prove to be useful in other Fas-mediated inflammatory or autoimmune diseases.

IVIG therapy has been tried in many different inflammatory diseases (Box 17-4) and this list is continuing to expand.[123] One disease in which the role of IVIG is just beginning to be investigated is the acute vaso-occlusive crisis of sickle cell disease (SCD). In SCD, abnormal sickle red blood cells (RBCs) have an increased propensity to adhere to each other and to vascular endothelial cells, resulting in vascular occlusion. Sickled RBCs have also been shown to adhere to other blood cells, including leukocytes. Chang and colleagues[124] investigated the effect of IVIG on a mouse model of sickle cell acute vaso-occlusive crisis, in which the adhesion of sickle RBCs to leukocytes is known to cause the vaso-occlusive pathology. In this model, high-dose IVIG given after the onset of a crisis resulted in improved blood flow and prolonged survival. The investigators demonstrated that the mechanism of IVIG in this model was a rapid reduction in neutrophil adhesion to vascular endothelium and decreased interaction between RBCs and leukocytes. Clinical trials are now being conducted to determine if IVIG offers therapeutic benefit in sickle cell patients during acute vaso-occlusive crises.

Recent studies by Keneko and colleagues[120] showed that that a component moiety of the IVIG molecule responsible for its antiinflammatory activity is the part of the IgG molecule that contains a sialylation site on the glycan linked to asparagine at position 297 on the Fc fragment (only 1–2% of the total IgG in IVIG). Desialylation of the sialic acid residues with neuraminidase was demonstrated to blunt the protective effect of an IVIG preparation in a mouse model of rheumatoid arthritis. In the same K/BxN arthritis model, sialic acid-enriched fractions of IVIG with the 2,6-sialylated linkage at Asn297 on the Fc portion showed a 10-fold increase in protection against immune-mediated arthritis. Anthony and colleagues[125,126] have demonstrated that greatly reduced doses of a recombinant, sialylated Fc fragment can completely recapitulate the antiinflammatory effects of IVIG in this same mouse model. These investigators have shown that the action of sialylated Fc in the rheumatoid arthritis mouse model is mediated through the interaction of sialylated Fc with the SIGN-R1 receptor on macrophages.[125] The authors propose that the interaction between sialylated Fc and SIGN-R1 produces an antiinflammatory state that results in an up-regulation of inhibitory FcγRIIB receptors on effector cells, making these cells more resistant to triggering by immune complexes. They suggest that DC-SIGN, the human homologue of SIGN-R1, may have a comparable role in the antiinflammatory effects of IgG Fcs. These new findings may explain many of the observed effects of IVIG, and have the potential to tie together several of the proposed antiinflammatory actions into a more cohesive model for the mechanism of IVIG activity in many autoimmune diseases.[127]

Conclusions

Immunoglobulin replacement is the mainstay of treatment for patients with primary humoral immune deficiency. The goal of the treatment is to provide a broad spectrum of antibodies to prevent infections and chronic long-term complications. The usual dose is 400–600 mg/kg/mo but this may vary individually and actually may require higher doses during active infection. A serum trough level above 500 mg/dL has been shown to be effective in the prevention of infections. However, recent studies have suggested that even higher doses and achieving trough levels of IgG >700 mg/dL may be desirable. Recently, SCIg has gained acceptance as an alternative route for the administration of replacement therapy in patients with immune deficiency. Generally, IVIG replacement therapy is considered safe in the majority of patients. Side-effects are usually mild and treatable by premedication. Improvements in good manufacturing practices, closer screening of plasma donors, testing of the source plasma with sensitive nucleic acid assays, e.g. PCR, and additional viral

BOX 17-6 Therapeutic principles

Principles of IVIG Treatment

Patients with Primary Immune Deficiency

Initial dosage: 300–400 mg/kg every 4 weeks for replacement therapy

– maintain a serum trough level of >500 mg/dL

– some patients may benefit from trough levels of 700–900 mg/dL

– may adjust the dose and/or dosing interval depending on clinical response

– record manufacturer, lot number and dose with each infusion

Equilibration takes several months even when dosage changes made

– check trough levels if patient continues to have infections or prior to dose change

– increase dose to 400–600 mg/kg to obtain clinical improvement

For patients with adverse effects or poor venous access, the subcutaneous route may be a better option

Monitor:

– liver and renal function tests every 6 months

– nucleotide testing for viral pathogens, e.g. hepatitis C when indicated

– pulmonary function testing; high resolution chest tomography

Patients with Autoimmune Disorders

Dosage: 1–2 g/kg over 1–2 days or 400 mg/kg × 4–5 days

Monitor very carefully during infusion for side-effects

Caution in patients at risk for adverse reactions, e.g. Over 65 years, underlying renal or cardiovascular disease, hyper-coagulation state, diabetes, volume depletion, paraproteinemia

Do not use hyperosmolar IVIG preparations, or preparations containing sucrose

---

inactivation steps has made IVIG a better and safer plasma-derived product. The majority of the utilization of IVIG therapy is in patients with autoimmune disorders. The use of IVIG in these patient groups has not only led to a new treatment modality but has enhanced our understanding of the disease pathogenesis and the mechanisms by which IVIG may modulate the immune and inflammatory processes (Box 17-6).

References

1. Cohn EJ, Luetscher Jr JA, Oncley JL, et al. Preparation and properties of serum and plasma proteins. III. Size and charge of proteins separating upon equilibration across membranes with ethanol-water mixtures of controlled pH, ionic strength and temperature. J Am Chem Soc 1940;62:3396–400.

2. Bruton OC. Agammaglobulinemia. Pediatrics 1952;9:722–8.

3. Ballow M. Primary immunodeficiency disorders: antibody deficiency. J Allergy Clin Immunol 2002;109:581–91.

4. Cohn EJ. The history of plasma fractionation. In: Andrus EC, Bronk DW, Carden Jr GA, Keefer CS, Lockwood JS, Wall JT, et al. editors. Advances in military medicine. Volume 1. Boston: Little, Brown; 1948. p. 364–443.

5. Eibl MM, Wedgwood RJ. Intravenous immunoglobulin: a review. Immunodef Rev 1989;1(suppl):1–42.

6. Mikolajcyk M, Concepcion N, Wang T, et al. Characterization of antibodies to capsular polysaccharide antigens of Hemophilus influenza Type b and Streptococcus pneumoniae in human immune globulin intravenous preparations. Clin Diagn Lab Immunol 2004;11:1158–64.

7. Burks A, Sampson H, Buckley R. Anaphylactic reactions after gamma-globulin administration in patients with hypogammaglobulinemia. Detection of IgE antibodies to IgA. N Engl J Med 1986;314:560.

8. Fischer SH, Ochs HD, Wedgwood RJ, et al. Survival of antigen-specific antibody following administration of intravenous immunoglobulin in patients with primary immunodeficiency diseases. Monogr Allergy 1988;23:225–35.

9. Mankarious S, Lee M, Fischer S, et al. The half-lives of IgG subclasses and specific antibodies in patients with primary immunodeficiency who are receiving intravenously administered immunoglobulin. J Lab Clin Med 1988;112:634–40.

10. Waldmann TA, Strober W. Metabolism of immunoglobulins. Prog Allergy 1969;13:1–110.

11. Yu Z, Lennon VA. Mechanism of intravenous immune globulin therapy in antibody-mediated autoimmune diseases. N Engl J Med 1999;340(3):227–8.

12. Ochs HD, Fischer SH, Wedgewood RJ, et al. Comparison of high-dose and low-dose intravenous immunoglobulin therapy in patients with primary immunodeficiency diseases. Am J Med 1984;76:78–82.

13. Stiehm ER. Immunodeficiency disorders general conditions. In: Stiehm ER, editor. Immunologic disorders in infants and children. 4th Ed. Philadelphia: Saunders; 1996. p. 201–52.

14. Bernatowska E, Madalinski K, Janowicz W, et al. Results of a prospective controlled two-dose crossover study with intravenous immunoglobulin and comparison (retrospective) with plasma treatment. Clin Immunol Immunopathol 1987;43:153–62.

15. Roifman CM, Schaffer FM, Wachsmuth SE, et al. Reversal of chronic polymyositis following intravenous immune serum globuin therapy. JAMA 1987;258:513–5.

16. Liese JG, Wintergerst U, Tympner KD, et al. High- vs low-dose immunoglobulin therapy in the long-term treatment of x-linked agammaglobulinemia. AJDC 1992;146:335–9.

17. Eijkhout HW, van der Meer JWM, Kallenberg CGM, et al. The effect of two different dosages of intravenous immunoglobulin on the incidence of recurrent infections in patients with primary hypogammaglobulinemia: a randomized, double-blind, multicenter crossover trial. Ann Int Med 2001;135:165–74.

18. Kainulainen L, Varpula M, Liippo K, et al. Pulmonary abnormalities in patients with primary hypogammaglobulinemia. J Allergy Clin Immunol 1999;104:1031–6.

19. Quartier P, Debre M, DeBlie J, et al. Early and prolonged intravenous immunoglobulin replacement therapy in childhood agammaglobulinemia: a retrospective survey of 31 patients. J Pediatrics 1999;134:589–96.

20. Busse PJ, Razvi S, Cunningham-Rundles C. Efficacy of intravenous immunoglobulin in the prevention of pneumonia in patients with common variable immunodeficiency. J Allergy Clin Immunol 2002;109:1001–4.

21. Schiff RI. Individualizing the dose of intravenous immune serum globulin for therapy of patients with primary humoral immunodeficiency. Vox Sanguinis 1985;49(Suppl 1):15–24.

22. Gelfand EW, Hanna K. Safety and tolerability of increased rate of infusion of intravenous immunoglobulin G, 10% in antibody-deficient patients. J Clin Immunol 2006;26:284–90.

23. Church J, Nelson R, Wasserman R, et al. Safety and tolerability of a new intravenous immunoglobuiln product (Privigen™) adminsitered at high infusion rates. J Allergy Clin Immunol 2008;121:S165.

24. Kobayashi RH, Kobayashi AD, Lee N, et al. Home self-administration of intravenous immunoglobulin therapy in children. Pediatrics 1990;85:705–9.

25. Daly PB, Evans JH, Kobayashi RH, et al. Home-based immunoglobulin infusion therapy: quality of life and patient health perceptions. Ann Allergy 1991;67:504–410.

26. Schiff R. Transmission of viral infections through intravenous immune globulin. N Engl J Med 1994;331:1649–50.

27. Berger M, Cupps TR, Fauci AS. Immunoglobulin replacement therapy by slow subcutaneous infusion. Ann Intern Med 1980;93:55–66.

28. Roord JJ, van der Meer JW, Kuis W, et al. Home treatment in patients with antibody deficiency by slow subcutaneous infusion of gamma-globulin. Lancet 1982;1:689–90.

29. Waniewski J, Gardulf A, Hammarstrom L. Bioavailability of gamma-globulin after subcutaneous infusions in patients with common variable immunodeficiency. J Clin Immunol 1994;14:90–7.

30. Radinsky S, Bonagura V. Subcutaneous immunoglobulin infusion as an alternative to intravenous immunoglobulin. J Allergy Clin Immunol 2003;112:630–3.

31. Chapel HM, Spickett GP, Ericson D, et al. The comparison of the efficacy and safety of intravenous versus subcutaneous immunoglobulin replacement therapy. J Clin Immunol 2000;20(2):94–100.

32. Ochs HD, Gupta S, Kiessling P, et al. Safety and efficacy of self-administered subcutaneous immunoglobulin in patients with primary immunodeficiency diseases. J Clin Immunol 2006;26:265–73.

33. Lederman H, Roifman T, Lavi S, et al. Corticosteroids for prevention of adverse reactions to intravenous immune serum globulin infusions in hypogammaglobulinemic patients. Am J Med 1986;81:443–6.

34. Camussi G, Aglietta M, Coda R, et al. Release of platelet activating factor (PAF) and histamine. II. The cellular origin of human PAF monocytes, polymorphonuclear neutrophils and basophils. Immunology 1981;42: 191–9.

35. Brennan VM, Salome-Bentley NJ, Chapel HM. Prospective audit of adverse reactions occurring in 459 primary antibody-deficient patients receiving intravenous immunoglobulin. Clin Exp Immunol 2003;133: 247–51.

36. Roberton DM, Hosking CS. Use of methylprednisolone as prophylaxis for immediate adverse infusion reactions in hypogammaglobulinaemic patients receiving intravenous immunoglobulin: a controlled trial. Aust Paediatr J 1988;24:174–7.

37. Sekul EA, Cupler EJ, Dalakas MC. Aseptic meningitis associated with high-dose intravenous immunoglobulin therapy: frequency and risk factors. Ann Intern Med 1994;121:259–62.

38. Scribner CL, Kapit RM, Phillips ET, et al. Aseptic meningitis and intravenous immunoglobulin therapy. Ann Intern Med 1994;121:305–6.

39. Kato E, Shindo S, Eto Y, et al. Administration of immune globulin associated with aseptic meningitis. JAMA 1988;259:3269–71.

40. Brannagan TH, Nagle KJ, Lange DJ, et al. Complications of intravenous immune globulin treatment in neurologic disease. Neurology 1996;47: 674–7.

41. Centers for Disease Control and Prevention. Renal insufficiency and failure associated with immune globulin intravenous therapy – United States, 1986–1998. MMWR Morb Mortal Wkly Rep 1999;48:518–21.

42. Ziegner U, Kobayashi R, Cunningham-Rundles C, et al. Progressive neurodegeneration in patients with primary immunodeficiency disease on IVIG treatment. Clin Immunol 2002;102:19–24.

43. Cunningham-Rundles C. Intravenous immune serum globulin in immunodeficiency. Vox Sanguinis 1985;49 (Suppl 1):8–14.

44. Apfelzweig R, Piszkiewicz D, Hooper JS. Immunoglobulin A concentrations in commercial immune globulins. J Clin Immunol 1987;7:46–50.

45. de Albuquerque Campos R, Sato MN, da Silva Duarte AJ. IgG Anti-IgA subclasses in common variable immunodeficiency and association with severe adverse reactions to intravenous immunoglobulin therapy. J Clin Immunol 2000;20:77–82.

46. Bjoro K, Froland SS, Yun Z, et al. Hepatitis C infection in patients with primary hypogammaglobulinemia after treatment with contaminated immune globulin. N Engl J Med 1994;331:1607–11.

47. Yap PL, McOmish F, Webster ADB, et al. Hepatitis C virus transmission by intravenous immunoglobulin. Journal of Hepatology 1994;21: 455–60.

48. Bresee JS, Mast Ee, Coleman PJ, et al. Hepatitis C virus infection associated with administration of intravenous immune globulin. JAMA 1996;276:1563–7.

49. Ballow M. Intravenous immunoglobulins: clinical experience and viral safety. J Am Pharm Assoc 2002;42:449–59.

50. Ballow M. Safety of IGIV therapy and infusion-related adverse events. Immunologic Research 2007;38:122–32.

51. Johnson RT, Gibbs Jr CJ. Creutzfeldt-Jakob disease and related transmissible spongiform encephalopathies. N Engl J Med 1998;339:1994–2004.

52. Brown P. Can Creutzfeldt-Jakob disease be transmitted by transfusion? Curr Opin Hematol 1995;2:472–7.

53. Wroe SJ, Pal S, Siddique D, et al. Clinical presentation and pre-mortem diagnosis of variant Creutzfeldt-Jakob disease associated with blood transfusion. Lancet 2006;368:2061–7.

54. Trejo SR, Hotta JA, Lebing W, et al. Evaluation of virus and prion reduction in a new intravenous immunoglobulin manufacturing process. Vox Sanguinis 2003;84:176–87.

55. Robertson VM, Dickson LG, Romond EH, et al. Positive antiglobulin tests due to intravenous immunoglobulin in patients who received bone marrow transplant. Transfusion 1987;27:28–31.

56. Imbach P, Barandun S, d'Apuzzo V, et al. High dose intravenous gammaglobulin for idiopathic thrombocytopenic purpura in childhood. Lancet 1981;1:1228–132.

57. Ballow M. Mechanisms of action of intravenous immune serum globulin in autoimmune and inflammatory diseases. J Allergy Clin Immunol 1997;100:151–7.

58. Blanchette VS, Luke B, Andrew M, et al. A prospective, randomized trial of high-dose intravenous immune globulin G therapy, oral prednisone therapy, and no therapy in childhood acute immune thrombocytopenic purpura. J Pediatr 1993;123:989–95.

59. Clynes R, Ravetch JV. Cytotoxic antibodies trigger inflammation through Fc receptors. Immunity 1995;3:21.

60. Fehr J, Hofmann V, Kappeler U. Transient reversal of thrombocytopenia in idiopathic thrombocytopenic purpura by high-dose intravenous gammaglobulin. N Engl J Med 1982;306:1254–8.

61. Bussel J. Modulation of Fc receptor clearance and antiplatelet antibodies as a consequence of intravenous immune globulin infusion in patient with immune thrombocytopenic purpura. J Allergy Clin Immunol 1989;84:566–78.

62. Clarkson SB, Bussel JB, Kimberly RP, et al. Treatment of refractory immune thrombocytopenic purpura with an anti-Fcg receptor antibody. N Engl J Med 1986;314:1236–9.

63. Debre M, Bonnet MC, Fridman WH, et al. Infusion of Fc gamma fragments for treatment of children with acute immune thrombocytopenic purpura. Lancet 1993;342:945–9.

64. Newburger JW, Takahashi M, Burns JC, et al. The treatment of Kawasaki syndrome with intravenous gamma globulin. N Engl J Med 1986;315: 341–7.

65. Leung DY. Kawasaki syndrome: immunomodulatory benefit and potential toxin neutralization by intravenous immune globulin. Clin Exp Immunol 1996;104(Suppl 1):49–54.

66. Leung DY, Schlievert PM, Meissner HC. The immunopathogenesis and management of Kawasaki syndrome. Arthritis Rheum 1998;41: 1538–47.

67. Takei S, Arora YK, Walker SM. Intravenous immunoglobulin contains specific antibodies inhibitory to activation of T cells by staphylococcal toxin superantigens. J Clin Invest 1993;91:602–7.

68. Leung DY, Burns JC, Newburger JW, et al. Reversal of immunoregulatory abnormalities in Kawasaki syndrome by intravenous gammaglobulin. J Clin Invest 1987;79:468–72.

69. Leung DYM, Cotran RS, Kurt-Jones EZ, et al. Endothelial cell activation and increased interleukin 1 secretion in the pathogenesis of acute Kawasaki disease. Lancet 1989;2:1298–302.

70. Newburger JW, Takahashi M, Beiser AS, et al. A single intravenous infusion of gamma globulin as compared with four infusions in the treatment of acute Kawasaki syndrome. N Engl J Med 1991;324:1633–9.

71. Burns JC, Capparelli EV, Brown JA, et al. Intravenous gamma-globulin treatment and retreatment in Kawasaki disease. US/Canadian Kawasaki Syndrome Study Group. Pediatr Infect Dis J 1998;17:1144–8.

72. Norrby-Teglund A, Basma H, Andersson J, et al. Varying titers of neutralizing antibodies to streptococcal superantigens in different preparations of normal polyspecific immunoglobulin G: implications for therapeutic efficacy. Clin Infect Dis 1998;26(3):631–8.

73. Gupta M, Noel GJ, Schaefer M, et al. Cytokine modulation with immune g-globulin in peripheral blood of normal children and its implications in Kawasaki disease treatment. J Clin Immunol 2001;21:193–9.

74. Xu C, Poirier B, Van Huyen JPD, et al. Modulation of endothelial cell function by normal polyspecific human intravenous immunoglobulins. Am J Pathol 1998;153:1257–66.

75. Junghans RP, Anderson CL. The protection receptor for IgG catabolism is the β2–microglobulin-containing neonatal intestinal transport receptor. Proc Natl Acad Sci U S A 1996;93:5512–6.

76. Akilesh S, Petkova S, Sproule TJ, et al. The MHC class I-like Fc receptor promotes humorally mediated autoimmune disease. J Clin Invest 2004;113:1328–33.

77. Li N, Zhao M, Hilario-Vargas J, et al. Complete FcRn dependence for intravenous Ig therapy in autoimmune skin blistering diseases. J Clin Invest 2005;115:3440–50.

78. Hansen RJ, Balthasar JP. Effects of intravenous immunoglobulin on platelet count and antiplatelet antibody disposition in a rat model of immune thrombycytopenia. Blood 2002;100:2087–93.

79. Basta M, Kirshbom P, Frank MM, et al. Mechanism of therapeutic effect of high-dose intravenous immunoglobulin: attenuation of acute, complement-dependent immune damage in a guinea pig model. J Clin Invest 1989;84:1974–81.

80. Basta M, Fries LF, Frank MM. High doses of intravenous Ig inhibit in vitro uptake of C4 fragments onto sensitized erythrocytes. Blood 1991;77:376–80.

81. Dalakas MC. Polymyositis, dermatomyositis, and inclusion-body myositis. New Eng J Med 1991;325:1487–98.

82. Dalakas MC, Illa I, Dambrosia JM, et al. A controlled trial of high-dose intravenous immunoglobulin infusions as treatment for dermatomyositis. N Engl J Med 1993;329:1993–2000.

83. Dalakas MC. Clinical relevance of IVIg in the modulation of the complement-mediated tissue damage: implications in dermatomyositis, Guillain Barre syndrome and myasthenia gravis. In: Kazatchkine M MA, editor. Intravenous immunoglobulin research and therapy. London: Parthenon Publishing; 1996, p. 89–93.

84. Soueidan SA, Dalakas MC. Treatment of autoimmune neuromuscular diseases with high-dose intravenous immune globulin. Pediatr Res 1993;33(Suppl):S95–100.

85. Dalakas MC. Controlled studies with high-dose intravenous immunoglobulin in the treatment of dermatomyositis, inclusion body myositis, and polymyositis. Neurology 1998;51(Suppl 5):S37–45.

86. Lang BA, Laxer RM, Murphy G, et al. Treatment of dermatomyositis with intravenous gammaglobulin. Am J Med 1991;91:169–72.

87. Sansome A, Dubowitz V. Intravenous immunoglobulin in juvenile dermatomyositis: four year review of nine cases. Arch Dis Child 1995;72:25–8.

88. Basta M, Dalakas MC. High-dose intravenous immunoglobulin exerts its beneficial effect in patients with dermatomyositis by blocking endomysial deposition of actiated complement fragments. J Clin Invest 1994;94:1729–35.

89. Shoenfeld Y. Idiotypic induction of autoimmunity: a new aspect of the idiotypic network. FASEB J 1994;8:1296–301.

90. Rossi F, Kazatchkine MD. Antiidiotypes against autoantibodies in pooled normal human polyspecific IgG. J Immunol 1989;143:4104–9.

91. Dietrich G, Kazatchkine MD. Normal immunoglobulin G (IgG) for therapeutic use (intravenous Ig) contain antiidiotypic specificities against an immunodominant, disease-associated, cross-reactive idiotype of human anti-thyroglobulin autoantibodies. J Clin Invest 1990;85:620.

92. Sultan Y, Rossi F, Kazatchkine MD. Recovery from anti-VIIIc (antihemophilic factor) autoimmune disease is dependent on generation of anti-idiotypes against anti VIIIc autoantibodies. Proc Natl Acad Sci U S A 1987;84:828–31.

93. Sultan Y, Kazatchkine MD, Maisonneuve P, et al. Anti-idiotypic suppression of autoantibodies to factor VIII (antihaemophilic factor) by high-dose intravenous gammaglobulin. Lancet 1984;2:765–8.

94. Dalakas MC. Mechanism of action of intravenous immunoglobulin and therapeutic considerations in the treatment of autoimmune neurologic diseases. Neurology 1998;51(6 Suppl 5):S2–8.

95. Van Der Meché FGA. The Guillain-Barré syndrome: pathogenesis and treatment. Rev Neurol (Paris) 1996;152:355–8.

96. van der Meché FGA, Visser LH, Jacobs BC, et al. Guillain-Barré Syndrome: multifactorial mechanisms versus defined subgroups. J Infect Dis 1997;176(Suppl 2):S99–S102.

97. Yuki N, Miyagi F. Possible mechanism of intravenous immunoglobulin treatment on anti-GM1 antibody-mediated neuropathies. J Neurol Sci 1996;139:160–2.

98. Malik U, Oleksowicz L, Latov N, et al. Intravenous g-globulin inhibits binding of anti-GM1 to its target antigen. Ann Neurol 1996;39:136–9.

99. Liblau R, Gajdos PH, Bustarret A, et al. Intravenous g-globulin in myasthenia gravis: interaction with anti-acetylcholine receptor autoantibodies. J Clin Immunol 1991;11:128–31.

100. Vassilev T, Yamamoto M, Aissaoui A, et al. Normal human immunoglobulin suppresses experimental myasthenia gravis in SCID mice. Eur J Immunol 1999;29:2436–42.

101. Amran D, Renz H, Lack G, et al. Suppression of cytokine-dependent human T cell proliferation by intravenous immunoglobulin. Clin Immunol Immunopathol 1994;73:180–6.

102. Aukrust P, Muller F, Nordoy I, et al. Modulation of lymphocyte and monocyte activity after intravenous immunoglobulin administration in vivo. Clin Exp Immunol 1997;107:50–6.

103. Ephrem A, Chamat S, Miquel C, et al. Expansion of CD4+CD25+ regulatory T cells by intravenous immunoglobulin: a critical factor in controlling experimental autoimmune encephalomyelitis. Blood 2008;111:715–22.

104. Furuno K, Yuge T, Kusuhara K, et al. CD25+CD4+ regulatory T cells in patients with Kawasaki disease. J Pediatrics 2004;145:385–90.

105. De Groot AS, Moise L, McMurry JA, et al. Activation of natural regulatory T cells by IgG Fc-derived peptide 'Tregitopes'. Blood 2008;112(8):3303–11.

106. Bussel J, Pahwa S, Porges A. Changes in the vitro antibody synthesis in ITP treated with intravenous gamma globulin are closely linked to long-term outcome. J Clin Immunol 1986;6:50–6.

107. Antel J, Medof M, Oger J, et al. Generation of suppressor cells by aggregated human globulin. Clin Exp Immunol 1981;43:351–6.

108. Hashimoto F, Sakiyama Y, Matsumoto S. The suppressive effect of gamma globulin preparations on in vitro pokeweed mitogen-induced immunoglobulin production. Clin Exp Immunol 1986;65:409.

109. Kondo N, Ozawa T, Mushiake K, et al. Suppression of immunoglobulin production of lymphocytes by intravenous immunoglobulin. J Clinical Immunol 1991;11(3):152–8.

110. Stohl W. Cellular mechanisms in the in vitro inhibition of pokeweed mitogen induced B cell differentiation by immunoglobulin for intravenous use. J Immunol 1986;136:1407–13.

111. de Grandmont M, Racine C, Roy A, et al. Intravenous immunoglobulins induce the in vitro differentiation of human B lymphocytes and the secretion of IgG. Blood 2003;101:3065–71.

112. Mazer BD, Gelfand EW. An open-label study of high-dose intravenous immunoglobulin in severe childhood asthma. J Allergy Clin Immunol 1991;87:976–83.

113. Sigman K, Ghibu F, Sommerville W, et al. Intravenous immunoglobulin inhibits IgE production in human B lymphocytes. J Allergy Clin Immunol 1998;102:421–7.

114. Bayry J, Lacroix-Desmazes S, Carbonneil C, et al. Inhibition of maturation and function of dendritic cells by intravenous immunoglobulin. Blood 2003;101:758–65.

115. Siragam V, Crow AR, Brinc D, et al. Intravenous immunoglobulin ameliorates ITP via activating Fc gamma receptors on dendritic cells. Nat Med 2006;12:688–92.

116. Tha-In T, Metselaar HJ, Tilanus HW, et al. Intravenous immunoglobulins suppress T cell priming by modulating the bidirectional interaction between dendritic cells and natural killer cells. Blood 2007;110(9):3253–62.

117. Daeron M. Fc receptor biology. Annu Rev Immunol 1997;15:203–34.

118. Kimberly RP, Salmon JE, Edberg JC. Receptors for immunoglobulin G. Arthritis Rheum 1995;38:306–14.

119. Samuelsson A, Towers TL, Ravetch JV. Antiinflammatory activity of IVIG mediated through the inhibitory Fc receptor. Science 2001;291:484–6.

120. Kaneko Y, Nimmerjahn F, Madaio MP, et al. Pathology and protection in nephrotoxic nephritis is determined by selective engagement of specific Fc receptors. J Exp Med 2006;203:789–97.

121. Salmun LM, Barlan I, Wolf HM, et al. Effects of intravenous immunoglobulin on steroid consumption in patients with severe asthma: a double-blind, placebo-controlled, randomized trial. J Allergy Clin Immunol 1999;103:810–5.

122. Viard I, Wehrli P, Bullanim R, et al. Inhibition of toxic epidermal necrolysis by blockade of CD95 with human intravenous immunoglobulin. Science 1998;282:490–3.

123. Orange JS, Hossny M, Weiler CR, et al. Use of intravenous immunoglobulin in human disease: a review of evidence by members of the Primary Immunodeficiency Committee of the American Academy of Allergy, Asthma and Immunology. J Allergy Clin Immunol 2006;117:S525–53.

124. Chang J, Shi PA, Chiang EY, et al. Intravenous immunoglobulins reverse acute vaso-occlusive crises in sickle cell mice through rapid inhibition of neutrophil adhesion. Blood 2008;111(2):915–23.

125. Anthony RM, Nimmerjahn F, Ashline DJ, et al. Recapitulation of IVIG Antiinflammatory activity with a recombinant IgG Fc. Science 2008;18:373–6.

126. Anthony RM, Wermeling F, Karlsson MC, et al. Identification of a receptor required for the antiinflammatory activity of IVIG. Proc Natl Acad Sci U S A 2009;10:19571–8.

127. Kaveri SV, Lacroix-Desmazes S, Bayry J. The antiinflammatory IgG. N Engl J Med 2008;359(3):307–9.

Intravenous Immune Serum Globulin Therapy

18

Bone Marrow Transplantation

Luigi D. Notarangelo • Evelina Mazzolari

Attempts to employ marrow for therapeutic purposes began in 1939.[1] In 1959, the first cases of autologous marrow transplantation in patients with metastatic malignancy whose marrow was collected and frozen at the time of remission were reported: after intensive radiation-chemotherapy, the marrow was thawed and infused intravenously, and one of the patients treated by this approach achieved long-term survival.[2] But it was only in 1968, after almost 30 years of scientific endeavors, that allogeneic marrow transplantation from a sibling donor was successfully used to restore immune function in infants with immune deficiency.[3-5] Knowledge of the human leukocyte antigen (HLA) system and appreciation of the inability of immunodeficient hosts to reject the graft were essential to realize this pioneering experience.

Until 1980, hematopoietic cell transplantation (HCT) in children was restricted to use of HLA-identical related donors (usually siblings). In fact unfractionated HCT from an HLA-mismatched related donor (such as a haploidentical parent) was inevitably followed by reaction of the donor T lymphocytes against the recipient (graft-versus-host disease, GvHD), with fatal outcome. In the late 1970s, studies in animal models showed that mature T lymphocytes depletion (TCD) from HLA nonidentical donor marrow restored lymphohematopoietic function upon injection into lethally irradiated recipients, without causing fatal GvHD reaction.[6,7] Because only about 20% of the patients had a matched related donor (MRD), this important achievement opened the way to the use of haploidentical parents as donors. However, despite significant improvement in methods to prevent both GvHD and graft failure, the results with mismatched-related donor (MMRD)-HCT remain inferior to those obtained with MRD. This reflects a slower kinetics of immune reconstitution following TCD haploidentical HCT, leading to an increased susceptibility to infections. In addition, MMRD-HCT is also associated with a higher rate of graft failure and recurrence of malignancies.

In an attempt to overcome these problems, alternative sources of hematopoietic stem cells (HSCs) have been explored. In the 1970s, the first experiences documenting the use of bone marrow transplant from a volunteer matched unrelated donors (URDs) to cure pediatric diseases were reported.[8-10] Later on, a patient with Fanconi's anemia was successfully transplanted by means of HLA-identical umbilical cord blood (UCB), opening the way for unrelated donors UCB-HCT.[11] Availability of high resolution HLA-typing and establishment of cooperating unrelated donor registries around the globe have led to a progressive increase in the use of HCT from alternative donors.

More recently, the demonstration that hematopoietic progenitor cells can be collected from peripheral blood, after in vivo mobilization upon administration of growth factors, has allowed the diffusion of peripheral blood HCT.[12,13]

So far, several thousands of children have been cured by HCT. At the same time, a better understanding of the molecular bases of inherited disorders on the one hand, and of the basic mechanisms of immune recognition and cell differentiation on the other hand, have expanded clinical indications to HCT and permitted earlier intervention. Finally, gene transfer into hematopoietic progenitor cells has been explored and is becoming a promising therapeutic option for inherited disorders.[14,15] In this chapter, we will review the fundamentals of HCT in childhood (Box 18-1).

Immunological Issues Related to Allogeneic HCT

Histocompatability

The HLA major histocompatibility complex plays a critical role in determining the reactivity of donor-recipient cells. In particular, donor-recipient HLA differences may cause host-versus-graft (HvG) reaction (leading to graft rejection), GvHD, and graft-versus-leukemia (GvL) (Box 18-2). Therefore, analysis of HLA alleles in the recipient and in the prospective donor is of great importance in selecting optimal donors for allogeneic HCT.[16,17] It is widely accepted that the most important HLA loci influencing outcome of HCT are HLA class I A, B and C loci, and class II DRB1 locus.[18,19] In addition, differences between minor histocompatibility antigens can also influence donor-recipient compatibility, but for practical reasons these differences are not considered in the selection of potential donors.

HLA class I (HLA-A, B, C) and class II (HLA-DR, DQ, DP) antigens can be serologically defined on peripheral blood mononuclear cells. Low resolution DNA typing provides the same level of HLA characterization as serologic typing. High-resolution molecular techniques have made it possible to better define the extremely polymorphic nature of HLA molecules, and to optimize strategies for the identification of optimal unrelated donors for HCT. At present, more than 11 million HLA-typed volunteer donors have been registered in an international database of volunteer bone marrow donors, and more than 300 000 UCB units have been typed and made available for transplantation purposes.

©2010 Elsevier Ltd, Inc, BV
DOI: 10.1016/B978-1-4377-0271-2.00018-3

BOX 18-1 Key concepts and steps in HCT

HCT Corrects Congenital or Acquired Defects in Blood Cell Production/Function and Restores Hematopoiesis after High-Dose Chemo-Radiotherapy for Malignancy

- The identification of allele-matched donors is the primary goal of histocompatibility testing for patients referred for allogeneic hematopoietic cell transplantation (HCT). A related matched sibling donor can be identified for about 20% of the patients. An unrelated donor can be identified for more than 80% of Caucasian recipient patients. For patients who lack an HLA-matched related or unrelated donor, there is a progressive improvement of outcome following partially mismatched, T cell-depleted HCT.

- In general, the infusion of hematopoietic stem cells is preceded by intensive immune suppressive and/or cytotoxic therapy (conditioning regimen), aimed at eliminating malignant cells (in the case of malignancy) and host immune cells that mediate immunologic recipient reaction. Recently, reduced intensity conditioning (RIC) regimens have been developed, that may allow successful engraftment with less toxicity.

- Hematopoietic stem cells can be obtained from different sources (bone marrow, peripheral blood, umbilical cord blood). The stem cells can be transplanted the same day they are collected, or can be cryopreserved for future use. The collected hematopoietic cells are given to the recipient as a blood transfusion; minimal (plasma volume reduction, RBCs depletion) or extensive (T cell depletion, purging) manipulation of the stem cells sample may be required.

- Obtaining durable engraftment (chimerism) of donor cells, that may provide long-term immune reconstitution and hematopoiesis, is the ultimate goal of allogeneic HCT. With the use of genetic markers, the presence and distribution of engrafted donor-derived cells can be traced throughout the entire life of the recipient from the time of post-transplant hematological reconstitution. Full or mixed chimerism is possible.

- GvHD and infections remain the major determinants of morbidity and mortality post-HCT.

- Life-long surveillance of engraftment and of clinical complications is necessary.

BOX 18-2

Immunological Aspects of HCT

Understanding of the Immunology of Hematopoietic Cell Transplantation has Provided the Basis for the Ongoing Development of Clinical Applicability of HCT

- HCT differs from solid organ transplantation, where the graft contains only limited numbers of cells with immunologic function, and life-long administration of immunosuppressive drugs is typically required to prevent graft rejection by the host's immune system. In contrast, the preparative regimen administered before HCT eliminates most recipient immune cells, and a new immune system is generated by the donor graft. If immunologic tolerance is achieved, immunosuppressive drugs can be discontinued 3 to 6 months post HCT.

- The HLA system plays a central role in determining donor/recipient cell reactivity. The identification of methods that allow definition of HLA genes at the allele level has enhanced our ability in typing HLA and identifying optimal donors. This has also largely facilitated the development of HCT from unrelated bone marrow donors and with the use of umbilical cord blood.

- Graft rejection may manifest early or late after allogeneic HCT, and is characterized by a lack of donor cells, associated with the presence of recipient T cells. Use of genetic markers facilitates detection of graft rejection. Risk factors for graft rejection include genetic donor-recipient HLA disparity and transfusion-induced sensitization.

- Acute GvHD is a distinctive syndrome of dermatitis, hepatitis and enteritis developing within 100 days after allogeneic HCT. Donor T lymphocytes recognize disparate HLA antigens expressed by recipient cells, and cause significant tissue infiltration and damage. Chronic GvHD is a disorder of immune regulation. It shares many biological similarities with various autoimmune disease, has highly variable clinical manifestations, and develops beyond 100 days after HCT. The past 4 decades have witnessed considerable progress in the understanding and control of GvHD.

- The persistence of donor cell engraftment in the absence of GvHD, together with recovery of host immune defenses, indicate that immunologic tolerance has been achieved between the donor and recipient. This may occur regardless of full or mixed chimerism. Immune tolerance is essential to permit long-term persistence of donor-derived cells.

Engraftment and Induction of Tolerance

Durable engraftment of donor cells is essential to achieve successful HCT. The term 'chimerism' describes the presence of engrafted donor cells in the recipient of the HCT, and can be traced by using of genetic markers. Full chimerism is achieved when all hematopoietic cells are derived from the allogeneic donor; mixed chimerism represents the situation when both donor- and recipient-derived hematopoietic cells are detected. Even in the case of mixed hematopoietic chimerism, donor and host HSCs continuously give rise to both host-derived and donor-derived antigen presenting cells (APCs), which home to the thymus and, through the process of negative selection, mediate deletion of auto- and allo-reactive T cell clones. Immune tolerance is essential to permit long-term persistence of donor-derived cells.[20,21] Critical factors to induce permanent immune tolerance and persistent chimerism include: (a) donor-recipient matching at the most important HLA loci (A, B, C, DRB1); (b) infusion of adequate doses of stem cells; (c) strategies to avoid graft rejection, by overcoming host immunity. Myeloablative and immunosuppressive drugs are typically used to achieve this goal. Nonetheless, graft failure, graft rejection and GvHD remain major barriers to successful HCT.

Acute Graft Versus Host Disease

Acute GvHD (aGvHD) can be considered an amplified, undesirable inflammatory reaction that follows an encounter between donor lymphocytes and host antigens. Three sequential steps have been recognized in the pathophysiology of aGvHD.[22] In the *first phase*, the myeloablative chemo- and/or radiotherapy (conditioning regimen) used to facilitate engraftment leads to damage of host tissues, release of inflammatory cytokines (IL-1, IL-6, TNF-α) and activation of antigen-presenting cells (APCs). In the *second phase*, both donor and recipient APCs present alloantigens to the donor T cells, triggering their activation and differentiation into effector cells. Th1 cells secreting IL-2, IL-12 and interferon

Table 18-1 Strategies Aimed at Prevention and Treatment of aGvHD

Phase of aGvHD	Pathophysiology Mechanisms	Preventive and/or Therapeutic Approaches
I	Conditioning regimen-related tissue damage	Reduced-intensity conditioning (RIC)[112] Administration of growth factors (e.g. KGF)[113]
II	APC-mediated antigen presentation and activation of Th1 effector cells	Ex-vivo T cell depletion Selective in vivo depletion of activated T lymphocytes Inhibition of lymphocyte activation (calcineurin inhibitors, mycophenolate mofetil, rapamycin) Inhibition of DCs function[114] In vivo administration of alemtuzumab (anti-CD52 mAb) to deplete T, B, NK cells, monocytes and DCs[115] In vivo administration of ATG Transfusion of marrow mesenchymal stem cells
III	T cell-mediated cytotoxicity and tissue damage	Glucocorticoids Photopheresis Use of mAbs to target T cells and inflammatory cytokines

APC: antigen-presenting cells; *KGF*: keratinocyte growth factor; *mAb*: monoclonal antibody; *DC*: dendritic cells; *ATG*: antithymocyte globulin.

γ (INFγ) appear, and potentiate the inflammatory response.[23] In this activation phase, minor HLA antigens play a central role, particularly in the setting of matched sibling transplants. In the *third phase*, activated donor T cells mediate citotoxicity against target host cells through Fas-Fas ligand interactions, perforin-granzyme B. Production of inflammatory cytokines such as IL-1, TNF-α and mediators such as nitric oxide contribute to tissue damage. A variety of preventive strategies have been envisaged to counteract the molecular mechanisms involved in the three phases of aGvHD (Table 18-1).

Although aGvHD is typically seen in recipient of allogeneic HCT, it can also be observed following autologous stem cell transplantation. In this case, dysregulation of the central and peripheral mechanisms that control tolerance play a key role.

Despite prophylaxis, 30% to 50% of patients who receive HCT from MRD, and 50% to 80% of recipients of URD-HCT may develop aGvHD. Donor-recipient HLA disparity remains the greatest predictor of aGvHD in pediatric HCT, but additional risk factors include: older donor age, sex mismatch (female donor into a male recipient) and an underlying malignant disease.

Typically, the clinical presentation of aGVHD occurs before day 100 after HCT but may also occur later (Figure 18-1). It is characterized by appearance of an erythematous maculopapular rash, vomiting and/or diarrhea, and hepatitis with elevation of bilirubin and/or liver enzymes. Grading of the severity has been defined (Table 18-2),[24] to subdivide patients into categories at different risk for complications and mortality.[25] Skin, liver or gut biopsies may be required to confirm the diagnosis of aGvHD.

Treatment of aGvHD is largely based on the use of steroids (Table 18-1). Photopheresis has been used to treat steroid-resistant disease. Monoclonal antibodies (mAb) targeted to T lymphocytes and to cytokines have also been used, although with limited results. More recently, bone marrow-derived mesenchymal stem cells (MSCs) have been explored to prevent and treat aGvHD.[26] MSCs display immunosuppressive effects on T, B lymphocytes, dendritic cells (DCs) and NK cells.[27] Moreover, MSCs inhibit alloantigen-induced DC differentiation and APC maturation, and favor the differentiation of CD4+ CD25+ regulatory T cells.

GvHD remains the major cause of mortality and morbidity after pediatric HCT, even if it is less common in children than in adults. Although few outcome studies have been performed in children, response to primary therapy represents the most

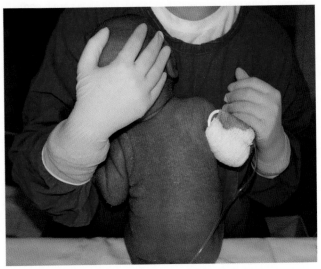

Figure 18-1 Generalized erythroderma and desquamation consistent with acute graft-versus-host disease (aGvHD) in a 5-month-old boy after HCT from an HLA-phenotypically identical parent.

important predictor. Patients with a complete response to therapy have about a 50% 5-year survival rate, as opposed to about 30% 5-year survival in patients with no or incomplete response.[28]

Chronic Graft Versus Host Disease

Chronic graft versus host disease (cGvHD) is a disorder of immune regulation, and is characterized by a variety of clinical manifestations that reflect the multiple underlying pathophysiology mechanisms.[29] The disease is initiated by donor T cells that recognize recipient alloantigens. Thymic damage, with deletion of marrow-derived dendritic cells and medullary epithelial cells caused by acute GvHD and/or a conditioning regimen, results in impaired negative selection of nascent T cells. Furthermore, several lines of evidence indicate that B cells also play a role in the pathogenesis of cGvHD. In particular, clinical improvement after administration of anti-CD20 mAb, altered Toll-like receptor 9 (TLR9) responses in circulating B cells, and high serum levels

Table 18-2 Extent of Organ Involvement in Acute GvHD

Stage	Skin	Liver (bilirubin)	Gut (stool output per day)
0	No GvHD rash	<2 mg/dL	<500 mL/day or persistent nausea (child: <10 mL/kg/day)
1	Maculopapular rash <25% BSA	2–3 mg/dL	500–999 mL/day (child: 10–19.9 mL/kg/day) or persistent nausea, vomiting or anorexia, with a positive upper GI biopsy
2	Maculopapular rash 25–50% BSA	3.1–6 mg/dL	1000–1500 mL/day (child: 20–30 mL/kg/day)
3	Maculopapular rash 50–100% BSA	6.1–15 mg/dL	Adult >1500 mL/day (child: >30 mL/kg/day)
4	Generalized erythroderma plus bullae formation and desquamation	>15 mg/dL	Severe abdominal pain with or without ileus formation and desquamation
Grade			
I	Stages 1–2	None	None
II	Stages 1–3	Stage 1	Stage 1
III	Stages 2–3	Stages 2–3	Stages 2–3
IV	Stages 1–4	Stages 2–4	Stages 2–4

BSA: body surface area; *GI*: gastrointestinal; *GvHD*: graft-versus-host disease.

of B cell activating factor (BAFF) which promotes the survival and differentiation of activated B cells, have been described in patients with cGvHD. Conflicting results have been reported with respect to the role of regulatory T cells in preventing the development of cGVHD.

Chronic GvHD occurs generally between 3 and 24 months after allogeneic HCT and has an incidence of 25% in pediatric patients. Risk factors for cGvHD in children include: recipient age greater than 15 years, donor age greater than 5 years, female donor into male recipient, conditioning with total body irradiation (TBI), underlying malignant disease, and previous grade II–IV aGvHD.[30] Use of alternative sources of stem cells has also been correlated with an increased incidence of GvHD.

The clinical manifestations of cGvHD resemble a systemic autoimmune disease, and include lichenoid and sclerodermatous skin lesions, malar rash, sicca syndrome, arthritis and fasciitis, obliterative bronchiolitis, weight loss, lower gastrointestinal tract disease, and bile duct degeneration with cholestasis. While thrombocytopenia is the most common hematological manifestation, any kind of cytopenia can occur and eosinophilia is often seen in children.

Recommendations have begun to standardize the diagnosis and clinical assessment of the disease.[31] These criteria have emphasized the importance of qualitative differences, as opposed to time of onset after HCT, in making the distinction between acute and chronic GvHD. More recently, studies have tried to develop a prognostic grading scale, showing that thrombocytopenia, extensive skin involvement, low Karnofsky performance status, and gastrointestinal involvement, clearly decrease survival.

At present, single-agent prednisone or calcineurin inhibitors remain the mainstay of treatment, although other agents such as mycophenolate mofetil, thalidomide, pentostatin, hydroxychloroquine and photopheresis have also been employed. A better understanding of the pathophysiological mechanisms of cGvHD might help improve treatment. Use of specific monoclonal antibodies, tyrosine kinase inhibitors, and adoptive transfer of regulatory T cells have been proposed.

Increased susceptibility to infections, caused both by cGvHD itself and by immunosuppressive treatment, requires life-long prophylaxis against encapsulated organisms, *Pneumocystis jiroveci*, and fungal infections. Immunoglobulin replacement therapy is often necessary.

Graft Versus Leukemia

The immune-mediated destruction of recipient leukemic blasts by donor lymphocytes is known as graft-versus-leukemia (GvL) effect. Both T cells and NK cells are involved. The influence of donor T lymphocytes is supported by the strong correlation between the development of GvHD and in particular cGvHD and lower relapse rate of leukemia, and by the higher relapse rate associated with T cell depleted graft.[32] Post-HCT donor lymphocyte infusion (DLI) is used as immunotherapy to improve antileukemia activity.[33,34]

A role for NK in GvL was suggested by studies in mismatched transplants.[35] A donor vs recipient NK-cell alloreactivity is elicited by the allelic difference of MHC molecules that NK cells can discriminate via killer immunoglobulin-like receptors (KIR). This NK cell-mediated alloreactivity can control the relapse of acute myeloid leukemia without causing GvHD. KIR genotyping assures that a 'perfect mismatch' is found in the case of a noncompatible transplant.

Graft Failure

Graft failure after HCT may be manifested as either lack of initial engraftment if severe granulocytopenia persists for 21 days after transplantation (primary graft failure) or the development of pancytopenia and marrow aplasia after initial engraftment (late graft failure). Chimerism analysis is necessary to formally document the absence of donor cells. Functional studies indicate alloimmune-mediated rejection as the predominant mechanism for graft failure. Residual host T lymphocytes may mediate cytotoxicity against donor alloantigens. Furthermore, allospecific antibodies may favor antibody-dependent cell-mediated cytotoxicity against donor cells.[36,37] NK cells might also be involved.

Risk factors for graft failure include donor-recipient genetic disparity at HLA loci and previous sensitization to alloantigens. The latter is more common in patients who have received multiple blood transfusions because of acquired or congenital marrow aplasia or hemoglobinopathies. The risk for graft failure is also related to the underlying diagnosis and is lower in patients with congenital immunodeficiency. In other diseases, incorporation of immunosuppressive drugs in the conditioning regimen reduces the risk of graft failure.

After graft failure, recovery of autologous myeloid cells can occur, especially if the patient is treated with granulocyte colony-stimulating factor (G-CSF). If there is no recovery of myeloid function despite treatment with G-CSF, a second transplant may become necessary.

Sources and Manipulation of Hematopoietic Stem Cells

Bone Marrow

The objective of allogeneic HCT is to replace defective, absent or malignant cells of the recipient with normal donor hematopoietic stem cells.

Pioneering studies in the 1960s showed that the bone marrow contains stem cells capable of self-renewal and full differentiation to blood cell lineages.[38,39] These cells were then identified as CD34+ Thy-1+ Lin−[44], and were shown to provide long-term reconstitution of all myeloid and lymphoid lineages after transplantation.[40,41]

The bone marrow is generally harvested through the posterior iliac crests under regional or general anesthesia. Needles are inserted 50 to 100 times on each side (but usually with only two sky entry points) to aspirate the cells required (Figure 18-2). Successful engraftment requires 2 to 3×10^8 nucleated marrow cells/kg of the recipient's weight (or a minimal dose of 1×10^8 cells/kg in autologous grafts), containing 1 to 5×10^6 CD34+ cells/kg. Typically, the volume of bone marrow collected corresponds to 10–20 mL/kg of donor's body weight.

In the case of allogeneic transplant, the collected marrow is given to the recipient as a blood transfusion the same day of the collection. If necessary, red blood cell depletion and/or volume reduction can be applied.

Importantly, in the case of HLA-mismatched HCT, ex vivo mature T cell depletion (TCD) from the graft is required to avoid the high risk of GvHD. It has been demonstrated that when the number of HLA-mismatched T cells infused with the graft is below 2×10^4 cells/kg, the risk of GvHD is virtually eliminated, even in the absence of pharmacological immunosuppression.[42-45] Methods to achieve robust TCD by negative selection include E-rosetting with soybean lectin agglutination, and use of mAb that are targeted to T cell surface antigens.[46-49] The development of anti-CD34 antibody-coated columns to select hematopoietic progenitors has provided an alternative to TCD.[50,51] Since 1999, the automated Clinimacs device (Myltenyi Biotech, Bergisch Gladbach, Germany) has ensured a median of 4.5 log T cell depletion and 3.2 log B cell depletion, which also helps prevent EBV-related lymphoproliferative disorders in recipients of an extensively T cell depleted HCT. Although TCD is effective in reducing the risk of aGvHD, additional concerns related to TCD are represented by graft failure, increased risk of relapse of leukemia, and delayed immune reconstitution, leading to higher risk of opportunistic infections. Furthermore, positive selection and in vitro expansion of bone marrow CD4+ CD25+ regulatory T cells, appear to reduce the risk of GvHD without affecting the GvL effect and the ability of antigen-specific T cells to fight against viral infections.[52,53] In addition, DLI is also used with the purpose of providing additional donor T cells in TCD transplants as adoptive immunotherapy against tumor or infections.[33,34]

In the case of an autologous transplant for malignancies, the bone marrow is harvested and cryopreserved when the patient is in complete remission, and autologous HSCs are then reinfused as a rescue treatment after administration of high-dose radio- or chemotherapy, in order to achieve hematological reconstitution. Polymerase chain reaction (PCR) with oligonucleotide primers to detect tumor-specific genes or transcripts may be used to detect low numbers of contaminating tumor cells in the bone marrow. Immunologic purging (using mAbs to target tumor cells) and pharmacologic purging (with use of drugs at appropriate concentrations to kill tumor cells without significant HSC toxicity) can be used to deplete the marrow of cancer cells. Even better results can be obtained with a combination of positive selection of CD34+ cells and tumor cell purging by negative selection. However, purging has a different impact on outcome of autologous HCT, depending on the underlying malignant disorder. A long-term follow-up analysis in patients with stage IV neuroblastoma showed significantly better 5-year event-free survival (EFS) and overall survival (OS) for myeloablative therapy with purged autologous HCT.[54] In vivo purging with tumor-specific mAbs, and infusion of tumor antigen-loaded DCs as therapeutic vaccines represent new areas of investigation.[55,56]

Peripheral Blood

Peripheral blood can also be a source of HSC.[57] However, under normal conditions the number of circulating peripheral blood stem cells (PBSCs) is inadequate to achieve robust engraftment. In vivo administration of recombinant G-CSF for 5 days to donors results in mobilization of bone marrow HSCs into the periphery. Furthermore, chemotherapy-induced mobilization (usually with cyclophosphamide) is used to collect autologous PBSCs in patients with malignancies. PBSCs are concentrated by leukapheresis. Enumeration of peripheral CD34+ cells (>10–20 cells/μL) is used to define optimal time to initiate collection of PBSCs.[58] In allogeneic peripheral blood stem cell transplantation (PBSCT), 5×10^6 CD34+/kg of recipient's body weight need to be

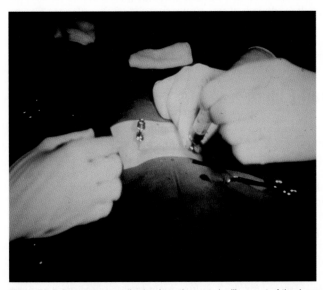

Figure 18-2 Bone marrow collection from the posterior iliac crest of the donor under general anesthesia. The iliac crest is entered through a skin puncture and marrow is aspirated through large needles into plastic heparinized syringes.

collected to achieve robust engraftment. In autologous PBSCT, the minimal acceptable dose is 1 to 2×10^6/kg. While collection of PBSC has become the standard procedure for autologous HCT in children,[59] its use in allogeneic HCT from child donors is controversial. In particular, the need to place pheresis catheters, to use G-CSF to mobilize HSCs, to prime the apheresis machine with red cells for smaller children, and the risk of symptomatic hypocalcemia limit its use.[60]

To avoid GvHD in the setting of allogeneic HCT, PBSCs can be processed ex vivo and depleted of contaminating mature T cells by TCD[61-63] or by CD34$^+$/CD133$^+$ cells positive selection.[64,65] Positive selection of CD34$^+$ cells and tumor-specific mAbs can also be used to purge tumors cells from PBSC, provided that the tumor does not express the CD34 antigen.[66,67]

Umbilical Cord Blood

Umbilical cord blood (UCB) was demonstrated to contain HSC with the ability to result in sustained engraftment, despite relatively small numbers.[68] Thus, UCB is now established as a viable alternative source to bone marrow, particularly in pediatric recipients, and in some settings, even as a preferable source.

UCB is harvested immediately following a healthy infant's birth, by collecting the infant's blood that remains in the cord and placenta after the cord is clamped. After collection, UCB is cryopreserved without any manipulation until infusion.

Successful clinical outcome after UCB-HCT correlates with the number of nucleated cells/kg of the recipient, with a recommended cell dose $\geq 3.7 \times 10^7$ nucleated cells/kg (or $>2 \times 10^5$ CD34$^+$/kg).[69-71] In large size recipients, this UCB cell dose could be a limiting factor. New approaches, such as ex vivo expansion of UCB stem cells and pooling of two UCB units, have been employed to overcome this limitation.[72,73]

Clinical Indications for HCT According to the Donor

HCT is the treatment of choice for children with congenital or acquired defects in blood cell production, severe congenital immune deficiencies and certain malignancies (Box 18-3). As improvements in supportive therapy have become available, survival and long-term outcome after HCT for these disorders have also improved. In addition, advances in the characterization of the molecular and cellular bases of these disorders, and gene transfer technologies have expanded the spectrum of diseases that can be treated by transplantation of unmodified or gene-corrected HSCs.

HCT from an HLA-Identical Matched Related Donor (MRD)

Allogeneic HCT from an HLA-identical sibling is the optimal treatment for several hematologic disorders. The best results, with low transplant-related mortality, are achieved in congenital or acquired nonmalignant disorders.

Primary Immunodeficiencies

Primary immunodeficiencies and severe combined immunodeficiency (SCID), in particular, are ideal candidates for HCT. In fact, these disorders are characterized by a strong selective differentiative and/or proliferative advantage of donor-derived cells within the cell lineage(s) that is (are) missing in the affected patient. Accordingly, full donor chimerism is often not strictly required to achieve correction of the disease. Furthermore, graft

---

BOX 18-3

Indications for Allogenic Hematopoietic Transplant for Pediatric Diseases

Nonmalignant

Severe acquired aplastic anemia
Inherited bone marrow failure syndrome
  Fanconi anemia
  Shwachmann-Diamond syndrome
  Dyskeratosis congenita
  Amegakaryocitic thrombocytopenia
  Diamond-Blackfan anemia
Hemoglobinopathies (thalassemia, sickle cell disease)
Primary immunodeficiency diseases
  Combined immunodeficiencies
  Wiskott-Aldrich syndrome
  CD40 ligand and CD40 deficiency
  Phagocytic cell disorders (CGD,LAD, SCN)[b]
  Hemophagocytic lymphohistiocytosis and cytotoxicity defects
  Immune dysregulation disorders
Autoimmune disorders unresponsive to treatments
Metabolic diseases
  Infantile malignant osteopetrosis
  Types of mucopolysaccharidoses
  Types of lisosomal/peroxisomal disorders

Malignant

Acute lymphoblastic leukemia
  First complete remission for very high risk relapse[a]
  Second or later complete remission
Acute myeloid leukemia
Philadelphia chromosome-positive chronic myeloid leukemia
Myelodysplastic syndromes
Non-Hodgkin's and Hodgkin's lymphoma
Selected solid tumors
  Stage IV neuroblastoma
  Renal cell carcinoma
  Very high-risk Ewing sarcoma

[a] First complete remission for very high-risk relapse: translocation t(9;22) or t(4;11); non responder after 1 week of steroid therapy and T immunophenotype or >100000 cells/μL; high level of minimal residual disease
[b] Chronic granulomatous disease, leukocyte adhesion deficiency, severe congenital neutropenia

failure is very uncommon in this setting. Overall survival is reported >80% after MRD-HCT for immunodeficiencies, and is even >90% in the case of SCID.

Bone Marrow Failure Syndromes

Bone marrow failure (BMF) syndromes are treated with MRD-HCT when cytopenia is significant (ANC: <500/µL; platelet count: <20,000/µL; reticulocyte count: <200/µL, and anemia with hypoplasic bone marrow, i.e. with total bone marrow cellularity <25%). A low number (<20) of previous blood transfusions and younger age (<10 years) at transplantation are positive prognostic factors.[74] Careful clinical and laboratory examination, including appropriate genetic testing, must be performed in order to prevent the selection of a sibling donor who is also affected.

The best results are reported in Fanconi Anemia (FA).[75] Initially, unusually severe tissue damage and GvHD were observed using classical myeloablative conditioning in FA patients, because of the underlying chromosomal instability. The development of reduced intensity conditioning (RIC) regimens, such as those based on low-dose cyclophoshamide (one-tenth the standard dose) and limited field irradiation (TAI 400 to 500 cGy) with or without antithymocyte globulin (ATG) has permitted the achievement of a 10-year actuarial survival of 89%, with aGvHD occurring in 23%, and cGVHD in 12% of the cases, respectively.[76] More recently, radiation has been eliminated from preparative regimens because of the high risk for cancer in these DNA damage-sensitive patients. In particular, fludarabine-based preparative regimens have been employed, with good engraftment and without significant toxicity or GvHD.[77] However, RIC typically results in mixed chimerism. In theory, the presence of residual autologous hematopoietic cells might result in development of late malignancies. Long-term follow-up studies after HCT for FA are therefore needed. Furthermore, genotype-phenotype correlation studies may be important to indicate which patients are more likely to benefit from HCT.

The indications for HCT in other BMF syndromes remain less well defined, because of the rarity of diseases. The decision as to whether or not to perform HCT should be individualized for each child. In dyskeratosis congenita (DC), the chromosomal instability predisposing to toxicity and cancer, and the underlying tendency to develop restrictive pulmonary disease, require an approach similar to that used for FA. However, the results are less encouraging and longer follow-up studies are needed to establish the consequence of RIC on late cardiac, hepatic and pulmonary complications that have been observed in these patients.[78] In Shwachman-Diamond syndrome (SDS), only 20% of the patients develop aplastic anemia, myelodysplasia or cytogenetic abnormalities (eventually leading to acute leukemia) and hence require HCT. Survival using a fully myeloablative preparative regimens is 60%.[79] Improved outcome has been recently demonstrated with RIC.[80] In Diamond-Blackfan anemia, steroid-resistant and transfusion-dependent patients may be considered for HCT. A 5-year survival rate of 72.7% is reported after a conventional preparative regimen.[81] As the risk of malignancy is lower in comparison to other hereditary BMF syndromes, but greater than in the general population, a fludarabine-based RIC preparative regimen should be considered. Although few examples are reported in the literature,[82] HCT represents the treatment of choice in amegakaryocytic thrombocytopenia, because of the very poor prognosis of the disease. Transplantation should be performed early to avoid allosensitization related to use of platelet transfusions and to prevent the development of marrow aplasia.

HCT is the treatment of choice for patients with acquired aplastic anemia with an available MRD. The survival rate in children is excellent (85%) and is even higher in some series in which a preparative regimen based on cyclophosphamide and ATG was used.[83] Younger age, a low number of previous transfusions and high stem cell dose have a positive impact on outcome, reducing the rate of rejection and graft failure. The use of cyclosporine prophylaxis and short-term methotrexate has resulted in a 94% overall survival rate, showing that adequate control of GvHD is also essential for a successful outcome.[84]

Thalassemia

Thalassemia is very common in some areas of the world (the Mediterranean region and South Asia). Although conservative treatment has dramatically improved both the survival and the quality of life of patients, changing an early fatal disease into a chronic disorder, HCT remains the only curative treatment available. Thus, patients with an HLA-identical donor should be offered HCT, also in the light of recent advances in transplantation. In children, older age at HCT, state of iron overload and concomitant viral hepatitis represent risk factors for transplant-related mortality. Currently, three classes of risk have been identified which include the presence of hepatomegaly, hepatic fibrosis on liver biopsy and inadequate chelation therapy. Using a conventional myeloablative regimen with busulfan and cyclophosphamide, the disease-free survival probability is of 87%, 85% and 82% in patients classed as 1, 2 and 3, respectively.[85] The cumulative incidence of aGvHD in patients treated with cyclosporine and methotrexate was 17% and the incidence of cGvHD was 27%.[86] Mixed chimerism is not uncommon. Although some of these patients may develop late graft failure, most remain stable with mixed chimerism that is sufficient to allow transfusion independence.[87] Because mixed chimerism may allow for disease correction, RIC regimens have been advocated in thalassemia. Gene therapy may represent a solid perspective in the future.

Autoimmune Diseases

Certain autoimmune diseases of childhood (e.g. juvenile idiopatic arthritis, systemic lupus erythematosus, Crohn's disease, and juvenile dermatomyositis) that are unresponsive to treatment, or have an unacceptable drug-related toxicity, can be considered for MRD-HCT.[88] In this case, the objective is to induce a donor/recipient mixed chimerism that reduces the genetic susceptibility to autoimmunity and elicits a 'graft versus autoimmunity' at the same time, without causing GvHD. However, allogeneic HCT for autoimmune diseases remains an experimental procedure. In contrast, a larger number of patients have been treated with autologous HCT, with the goal of eliminating immune cells that are responsible for autoimmune reactions, while building on the patient's stem cells ability to regenerate a naïve immune system tolerogenic to self-antigens.

Metabolic Diseases

Metabolic diseases are often characterized by multi-organ enzyme deficiency associated with storage disease. In selected cases, HCT from an HLA-identical sibling may support production of the defective enzyme by donor-derived cells of the monocyte/macrophage lineage, including tissue-restricted specialized cells, such as glial cells in the central nervous system.[89,90] While early HCT has been advocated to prevent or slow progression of signs of the disease, the potential benefits of HCT for metabolic storage diseases are still controversial.

Infantile malignant osteopetrosis (IMO) includes a variety of genetic disorders with impaired osteoclast development and/or function. Recent advances in genotype-phenotype correlation in IMO have permitted identification of which forms are more likely to benefit from HCT, and which ones, on the other hand, are characterized by disease progression (especially of neurological symptoms) even if stable donor stem cell engraftment is achieved. For the former group of patients, HCT from MRD results in a 5-year EFS of 73%, using standard conditioning regimens.[91] However, growth retardation and vision impairment and preexisting neurological problems may not be improved by HCT. Therefore, early diagnosis and intervention are important to minimize the risk of these complications.

Malignancies

Allogeneic HCT in patients with malignancies can restore hematopoiesis after high-dose myeloablative therapy and may provide potent anticancer adoptive immunotherapy. For patients with acute lymphoblastic leukemia (ALL) at very high risk of relapse, HCT is indicated in the first complete remission (CR1); in the remaining cases, HCT should be considered in second complete remission (Box 18-3). The long-term survival for patients transplanted in CR1 or CR2 is 60–70% and 50%, respectively. Patients transplanted after the second remission have both high transplant-related morbidity/mortality and high relapse rates. The use of total body irradiation (TBI) during the preparative regimen offers an advantage in terms of longer EFS compared to conditioning with busulfan and cyclophosphamide. Consistent with a therapeutic role for GvL activity, intensive GvHD immunosuppression has been shown to influence the risk of relapse.[92] For patients with acute myeloid leukemia (AML), HCT from an HLA-identical donor is considered as the mainstay of treatment during the first complete remission (CR1) for children with intermediate or high-risk cytogenetics or who have achieved CR1 after the second course of induction therapy.[93,94] Disease-free survival is 60–70% using preparative regimens containing total body irradiation or chemotherapy. For the remaining patients with AML, HCT provides a disease-free survival of 45% when performed in CR2. Allogeneic HCT is also considered the only curative approach for children with Philadelphia-positive chronic myeloid leukemia. Outcome is related to the phase of the disease, recipient age and time interval between diagnosis and HCT; disease free-survival is 45–80%. The development of imatinib and other tyrosine kinase inhibitors that permit long-term cytogenetic responses could modify indications to transplant. In juvenile myelomonocytic leukemia, characterized in 75% of cases by genetic mutations of the Ras pathway signaling, HCT is the only intervention that can control the disease long term. An EFS of 55% has been reported using preparative regimens with busulfan, cyclophosphamide and melphalan.[95] Myelodysplastic syndromes are clonal disorders characterized by ineffective hematopoiesis and a propensity to transform into AML. Allogeneic HLA-identical HCT is the only curative therapy, and for patients with monosomy 7 or with complex somatic karyotypic clonal aberrancies, it should be performed early in the course of the disease. EFS is 78% using busulfan-based conditioning regimens.[95]

HCT from Unrelated Donors

For many patients who lack an MRD, transplantation from URD has become an option. Bone Marrow Donors Worldwide (BMDW) is the international organization that collects the HLA phenotype of prospective volunteer bone marrow donors and cord blood units, and is responsible for the coordination of their distribution worldwide.

At present, 3 to 5 months represents the median time required to identify a suitable bone marrow URD. The likelihood of finding such a donor depends, especially, on the ethnic group of the patient: for Caucasians, the probability of finding at least one potential HLA-A, HLA-B, and HLA-DR matched URD is more than 85%; whereas it is 60% and 10% for African-Americans and for other ethnic groups poorly represented in the BMDW registry, respectively. For all donors, serological typing of HLA class I loci is available, and for almost one-third of these donors there is information on DRB1 typing. Search criteria are often based only on the HLA A-B-C and DR loci, the role played by other class II loci (DQB1 and DPB1) remaining controversial. Matching by high-resolution HLA typing for both HLA class I and II loci has reduced the risk of post-transplant immune complications such as graft rejection and GvHD. When a fully-matched URD is identified, results of HCT may be expected to compare well with those of HCT from an HLA-identical sibling.[96] In contrast, multiple disparities at major HLA loci are associated with a higher risk of GvHD and transplantation-related mortality, and therefore with reduced survival. Single disparities at the HLA loci B and C appear to be better tolerated than mismatches at the loci A and DRB1. To decrease the risk of aGvHD, ex vivo T cell depletion has been attempted, however, the outcome was similar to the outcome observed with unmanipulated graft with pharmacological GvHD prophylaxis. Other variables may also affect the outcome of HCT from URD. In particular, transfusion of a larger number of stem cells correlates with a better outcome, whereas use of peripheral blood instead of bone marrow as the source of stem cells may result in increased risk of cGvHD. Related to the increased risk of GvHD, a higher risk of late infections has been observed in recipients of URD-HCT, even if the advent of prophylactic and preemptive therapy has reduced mortality associated with this complication.

Because of the time required to identify optimal URD and to harvest stem cells, alternative sources of stem cells should be considered in patients who need HCT urgently, because of complications or disease progression.

The demonstration of efficacy of UCB as a source of stem cells for HLA-identical sibling transplantation has provided the clinical basis for starting large programs of collection, characterization, cryopreservation and storage of UCB units, and this has allowed the performance of more than 3000 UCB-HCTs worldwide. The search is based on low-resolution typing for HLA-A, HLA-B and allele typing for DRB1. Relative to other sources of stem cells, UCB has revealed certain advantages. As compared to availability of URD (which requires 3 to 5 months on average), UCB can be obtained in less than 1 month. Furthermore, UCB-HCT is associated with a reduced risk of transmitting viral infection, particularly cytomegalovirus (CMV). In addition, most of the T lymphocytes in cord blood have a naïve phenotype and display a lower alloreactive potential. Accordingly, mismatches of up two HLA antigens may be accepted for UCB-HCT, because of a lower risk of developing GvHD than following URD-HCT.[97] Despite the decreased incidence of GvHD, the GvL effect is maintained and the risk of leukemia recurrence is not increased.

On the other hand, compared with children transplanted from matched, unrelated bone marrow donors, recipients of UCB-HCT have a reduced probability of sustained donor engraftment and show a slower hematopoietic recovery. Finally, the slow kinetics of neutrophil recovery and the lack of antigen memory T cells contained in the UCB unit, may expose recipients of UCB-HCT to an increased risk of infection in the early post-transplant period. Overall, similar results have been obtained using 1- or 2-HLA antigens-mismatched UCB-HCT vs HLA matched bone marrow HCT.[98] UCB-HCT has been proposed as the optimal source of stem cells for transplantation in children with acute leukemia who lack an MRD.[99]

Preliminary studies show efficacy of UCB-HCT also in certain nonmalignant disease, such as thalassemia and certain immuno-deficiencies. However, further studies are required to address the efficacy of UCB-HCT in diseases associated with a higher risk of graft failure, such as aplastic anemia, or for which good results have been reported with marrow URD-HCT.

HCT from Haploidentical Related Donors

Haploidentical parents represent a readily available source of stem cells for children who require HCT. In this allogeneic mis-matched setting, donor and recipient HLA disparity increases the risk of developing GvHD and graft failure. T cell depletion techniques have been developed to overcome these risks.[46-51] At present, the risk of aGvHD and cGvHD after haploidentical HCT ranges between 0–24% and between 0–19%, respectively, and is therefore comparable with that observed after URD-HCT. To overcome the risk of graft failure, whenever an increasing signal of autologous cells is observed in patients who have attained mixed chimerism, low-dose DLI[33,34] infusions or cessation of immunosuppression are recommended. The possible role of co-transplanting mesenchymal stem cells (MSCs) to prevent graft failure is also being explored.[100]

Importantly, in patients given a TCD-HCT (such as those who receive transplantation from a haploidentical parent), a delayed immune reconstitution is observed that increases the risk of life-threatening infections of viral or fungal origins. The initial popu-lation of donor-derived lymphocytes seen as early as 14 days post transplant is comprised mainly of NK cells, while CD3$^+$ T lymphocytes (most of which initially have a CD8$^+$ phenotype) appear 120–180 days after TCD-HCT and normal in vitro lym-phocyte proliferative responses to mitogens are detected, on average, 7 to 8 months after HCT.[101,102] Thus, to protect the recipi-ent in the early post-transplant period, screening for viral detec-tion, preemptive antiviral therapy and adoptive immunotherapy with donor T cells specific against CMV, adenovirus, EBV or Aspergillus, has been successfully employed.[103,104] Interestingly, a lesser number of infectious deaths are reported in children, prob-ably reflecting a thymic function not as impaired as in the older patients. In the long term, the immune recovery of children given a haploidentical HCT with myeloablative conditioning, does not differ from that of patients given a graft from other alternative donors. T cell depleted haploidentical HCT without any condi-tioning regimen has been used in patients with SCID, because of their predicted intrinsic inability to reject the graft. However, in this case, engraftment of donor-derived cells is often restricted to T lymphocytes, and many patients fail to achieve functional B cell reconstitution, and hence require life-long administration of immunoglobulins.

Overall, 3-year survival after haploidentical HCT for diseases other than SCID ranges from 18 to 48% in various series.[105,106] In patients with malignancies, relapse remains the major cause of death, and a better disease-free survival is observed in patients who receive a mega dose of CD34$^+$ cells[107,108] and who are transplanted in centers that have specific experience with this type of HCT. Ongoing studies are aimed at addressing the potential benefits of post-transplant immunotherapy, such as the infusion of donor-derived effector cells (alloreactive NK cells or T cells) with antileukemic potential.[33-58] Moreover, possible graft-versus-tumor effects after haploidentical HCT are being currently evaluated in children with relapsed solid tumor.[109]

Time Course of Infections and Hematological Recovery

Infections continue to be the major cause of failure following HCT. The post-transplant period can be divided into three phases that correlate with the initial ablation (pre-engraftment period) and the recovery of hematopoietic and immunological function (early and late post-engraftment periods) (Figure 18-3).[110] During the pre-engraftment period (0 to 30 days) the predominant risk factors for infection are represented by profound neutropenia and damage to mucosal surfaces that result from the preparatory regimen. The type of transplant affects the length of this period: unrelated bone marrow and UCB transplants typically have delayed engraftment, whereas PBSC transplants provide more rapid engraftment. In addition, nonmyeloablative conditioning regimens may avoid severe neutropenia and significant toxicity. Infectious complications that occur early after HCT are predomi-nantly of bacterial origin, and are most often due to Gram-positive organisms and enteric species. Fungal infections (Candida, Aspergillus) also typically occur during the pre-engraft-ment period of neutropenia, whereas viral infections other than herpes simplex (HSV) and human herpes virus (HHV)-6 are uncommon. Advances in supportive care (central venous line, HEPA air filtration, laminar air flow rooms) (Figure 18-4), along with reinforced hygiene (hand washing) and low microbial diet have been crucial to reduce the risk of early infections. Further-more, antifungal prophylaxis (fluconazole, voriconazole) and acyclovir for preventing HSV reactivation are now universal practice to control infections, while an antibiotic prophylaxis regimen has not been shown to alter survival. More recently, better techniques of early fungal detection (Aspergillus galacto-mannan or Candida DNA) have also contributed to improved survival. The risk of severe bacterial and fungal infections becomes significantly lower when hematologic reconstituion (defined as the first three consecutive days that absolute neu-trophil count exceeds 500/μL) is achieved.

In the early post-engraftment period (30–100 days), life-threat-ening infections with opportunistic viral, fungal and protozoal pathogens predominate, reflecting abnormalities of donor T and B lymphocyte number and/or function. NK cells (CD56$^+$, CD16$^+$) are the first lymphoid cells that appear post transplant. A normal number of NK cells is reached within the first 2 months post-HCT, with very little difference among different types of trans-plant. NK cells offer the first line of defense against viral infection.

In contrast, several months are usually required to attain T cell reconstitution. The only exception is represented by SCID patients who receive unconditioned and unmanipulated MRD-HCT; in these subjects, donor-derived mature T cells contained in the graft expand after infusion. In all other cases, a prolonged and profound CD4$^+$ lymphopenia (especially following TCD-HCT), a predominance of T cells expressing a memory/activated phenotype (CD45R0), limited T cell receptor diversity and low numbers of TRECs (T cell receptor excision circles) characterize the early post-engraftment period.[111] Transplantation at a young age, a higher dose of total nucleated cells/kg, and transplant from HLA-matched sibling or UCB, are associated with faster T cell recovery. In the early post-transplant period, most patients remain with significant defects of humoral immunity and require immunoglobulin supplementation.

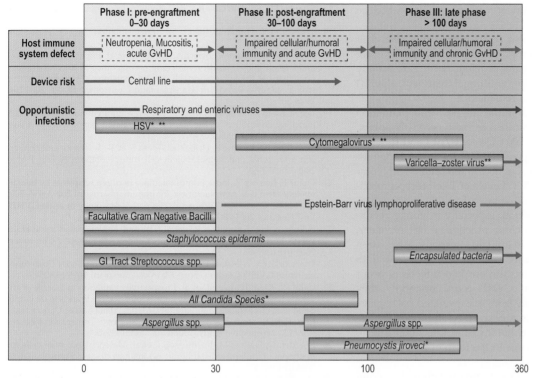

	Phase I: pre-engraftment 0–30 days	Phase II: post-engraftment 30–100 days	Phase III: late phase > 100 days
Host immune system defect	Neutropenia, Mucositis, acute GvHD	Impaired cellular/humoral immunity and acute GvHD	Impaired cellular/humoral immunity and chronic GvHD
Device risk	Central line →		
Opportunistic infections	Respiratory and enteric viruses →		

HSV* **

Cytomegalovirus* **

Varicella–zoster virus** →

Epstein-Barr virus lymphoproliferative disease

Facultative Gram Negative Bacilli

Staphylococcus epidermis

GI Tract Streptococcus spp.

Encapsulated bacteria →

*All Candida Species**

Aspergillus spp.

Aspergillus spp.

*Pneumocystis jiroveci**

0   30   100   360

* Without standard prophylaxis   ** Primarily among persons who are seropositive before transplant

High incidence (>10%)   → Low incidence (<10%)   → Episodic and endemic   → Continuous risk

Figure 18-3 The three phases of opportunistic infection after hematopoietic cell transplantation. (Adapted from Shah AJ, Kapoor N, Crooks GM, et al. Biol Blood Marrow Transplant 2007;13:584–593.)

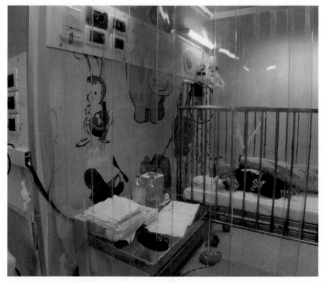

Figure 18-4 Laminar air flow room for isolation of allogeneic HCT recipients with primary immunodeficiency.

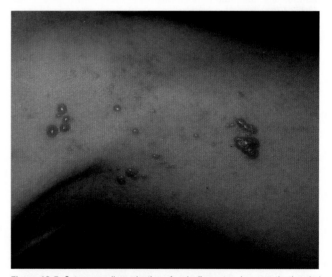

Figure 18-5 Cutaneous dissemination of varicella zoster virus reactivation during the late period after hematopoietic cell transplantation.

Infection due to CMV is common in this phase, and although it does not inevitably lead to clinical symptoms, disease occurs in 5% of recipients of allogeneic grafts. The risk of CMV infection and reactivation is increased in patients with aGvHD. Current strategies to prevent CMV disease are based on preemptive use of ganciclovir or foscarnet when CMV antigenemia or viremia are detected. Adenovirus is another important viral pathogen (with 20% infection rate in pediatric recipients of HCT). Risk factors for adenoviral infection include T cell depleted HCT,

alemtuzumab as part of the conditioning regimen, GvHD and severe lymphopenia (<100/μL). Promising results have been reported with cidofovir. Epstein-Barr virus (EBV) viremia can be detected in >60% of allogeneic HCT recipients. The most significant risk factors are unrelated donor graft, selective T cell-depletion sparing B lymphocytes, use of ATG and treatment for aGvHD. EBV-related post-transplant lymphoproliferative disease (LPD) occurs in <2% of allogeneic transplants: treatment with rituximab and/or infusion of EBV-specific cytotoxic lymphocytes have significantly reduced the severity of this complication. Preemptive treatment with rituximab, based on viral load can also be effective.

P. jiroveci pneumonia may also occur during this period, if patients are not maintained on appropriate prophylaxis. Invasive aspergillosis remains a significant problem, with case-fatality rates of 80–90% despite aggressive antifungal treatment; aGvHD and use of steroids are the main risk factors.

Serious infections are unusual in the late post-transplantation period (>100 days). In fact, regardless of the type of transplant, an increase in T cell number (>200 CD4$^+$ cells/μL) and function (proliferative response to mitogens >80% of the lower range for normals) are achieved at a median of 5 to 6 months, with complete recovery at 1 year post HCT. Levels of T cell receptor excision circles (TRECs), a marker of de novo T cell generation, also rapidly increase during this period, especially in young recipients, demonstrating effective thymic function. B cell recovery, with ability to mount protective antibody responses, has been demonstrated by 6 months after transplant. Consistent with these kinetics of immune reconstitution, late infections occur predominantly in patients with cGvHD. More commonly, they are of bacterial origin (especially from encapsulated pathogens) and involve skin and the respiratory tract. As immunosuppression is increased, invasive and noninvasive infections due to *Aspergillus* or varicella-zoster virus in the form of herpes zoster, can also occur (Figure 18-5).

The initiation of routine childhood immunizations is recommended when immunological recovery is documented.

References

1. Osgood EE, Riddle MC, Mathews TJ. Aplastic anaemia treated with daily transfusions and intravenous marrow. Ann Intern Med 1939;13:357–67.

2. Haurani FI. Thirty-one-year survival following chemotherapy and autologous bone marrow in malignant lymphoma. Am J Hematol 1997;55:35–8.

3. Bach FH, Albertini RJ, Joo P, et al. Bone marrow transplantation in a patient with the Wiskott-Aldrich syndrome. Lancet 1968;2:1364–6.

4. Gatti RA, Meuwissen HJ, Allen HD, et al. Immunological reconstitution of sex-linked lymphopenic immunological deficiency. Lancet 1968;2:1366–9.

5. Bortin MM, Bach FH, van Bekkum DW, et al. Twenty-fifth anniversary of the first successful allogeneic bone marrow transplants. Bone Marrow Transplant 1994;14:211–2.

6. Muller-Ruchholtz W, Wottge HU, Muller-Hermelink HK. Bone marrow transplantation in rats across strong histocompatibility barriers by selective elimination of lymphoid cells in donor marrow. Transplant Proc 1976;8:537–41.

7. Reisner Y, Itzicovitch L, Meshorer A, et al. Hematopoietic stem cell transplantation using mouse bone marrow and spleen cells fractionated by lectins. Proc Natl Acad Sci USA 1978;75:2933–6.

8. Speck B, Zwan FE, Rood JJV, et al. Allogeneic bone marrow transplantation in a patient with aplastic anemia using a phenotypically HLA-identical unrelated donor. Transplantation 1973;16:24–8.

9. Horowitz SD, Bach FH, Groshong T, et al. Treatment of severe combined immunodeficiency with bone marrow from an unrelated, mixed leucocyte culture non reactive-donor. Lancet 1975;2:432–3.

10. Foroozonfar N. Bone marrow transplant from un unrelated donor for chronic granulomatous disease. Lancet 1977;1:210–3.

11. Gluckman E, Broxmeyer HA, Auerbach AD, et al. Hematopoietic reconstitution in a patient with Fanconi's anemia by means of umbilical-cord blood from an HLA-identical sibling. N Engl J Med 1989;321:1174–8.

12. Reifers J, Bernard P, David B, et al. Successful autologous transplantation with peripheral blood haemopoietic cells in a patient with acute leukaemia. Exp Hematol 1986;14:312–5.

13. Besinger WI, Weaver CH, Appelbaum FR, et al. Transplantation of allogeneic peripheral blood stem cells mobilized by recombinant human granulocyte colony-stimulating factor. Blood 1995;85:1655–8.

14. Kohn DB, Candotti F. Gene therapy fulfilling its promise. N Engl J Med 2009;360(5):518–21.

15. Aiuti A, Cattaneo F, Galimberti S, et al. Gene therapy for immunodeficiency due to adenosine deaminase deficiency. N Engl J Med 2009;360(5):447–58.

16. Thomas ED, Storb R, Clift RA, et al. Bone-marrow transplantation. N Eng J Med 1975;292:895–902.

17. Terasaki PI. Humoral theory of transplantation. Am J Transplant 2003;3:665–73.

18. Flomenberg N, Baxter-Lowe LA, Confer D, et al. Impact of HLA class I and class II high-resolution matching on outcomes of unrelated donor bone marrow transplantation. HLA-C mismatching is associated with a strong adverse effect on transplantation outcome. Blood 2004:104:1923–30.

19. Lee SJ, Klein J, Haagenson M, et al. High resolution donor-recipient HLA matching contributes to the success of unrelated donor marrow transplantation. Blood 2007:110:4576–83.

20. Scandling JD, Busque S, Dejbakhsh-Jones S, et al. Tolerance and chimerism after renal and hematopoietic-cell transplantation. N Eng J Med 2008;358:353–61.

21. Ophir E, Reisner Y. Induction of tolerance in organ recipients by hematopoietic stem cell transplantation. Int Immunopharmacol 2009;9:694–700.

22. Ferrara JL, Cooke KR, Teshima T. The pathophysiology of acute GVHD. Int J Hematol 2003;78:181–7.

23. Nikolic B, Lee S, Bronson RT, et al. Th1 and Th2 mediated acute graft-versus-host disease, each with distinct end-organ targets. J Clin Invest 2000;105:1289–98.

24. Przepiorka D, Wiesdorf D, Martin P, et al. 1994 Consensus Conference on Acute GVHD Grading. Bone Marrow Transplant 1995;15:825–8.

25. Cahn JY, Klein JP, Lee SJ, et al. Prospective evaluation of 2 acute graft-versus-host (GVHD) grading system: a joint Societe Francaise de Greffe de Moelle et Therapie Cellulaire (SFGM-TC), Dana Farber Cancer Institute (DFCI), and International Bone Marrow Transplant Registry (IBMTR) prospective study. Blood 2005;106:1495–500.

26. Ringden O, Uzunel M, Rasmusson I, et al. Mesenchymal stem cells for treatment of therapy-resistant graft-versus-host disease. Transplantation 2006;81:1390–7.

27. Uccelli A, Pistoia V, Moretta L. Mesenchymal stem cells: a new strategy for immunosuppression? Trends Immunol 2007;28:219–26.

28. Weisdorf D, Haake R, Blazar B, et al. Treatment of moderate/severe acute graft-versus-host disease after allogeneic bone marrow transplantation: an analysis of clinical risk features and outcome. Blood 1990;75:1024–30.

29. Martin PJ. Biology of chronic graft-versus-host disease: implications for a future therapeutic approach. Keio J Med 2008;57:177–83.

30. Zecca M, Prete A, Rondelli R, et al. Chronic graft-versus-host disease in children: incidence, risk factors, and impact on outcome. Blood 2002;100:1192–200.

31. Filipovich AH, Wiesdorf D, Pavletic S, et al. National Institutes of Health Consensus Development Project on Criteria for Clinical Trials in Chronic Graft-Versus-Host disease: I. Diagnosis and staging working group report. Biol Blood Marrow Transplant 2005;11:945–56.

32. Horowitz MM, Gale RP, Sondel PM, et al. Graft-versus-leukemia reactions after bone marrow transplantation. Blood 1990;75:555–62.

33. Kolb HJ, Schattenberg A, Goldman JM, et al. Graft-versus-leukemia effect of donor lymphocyte transfusions in marrow grafted patients. Blood 1995;86:2041–50.

34. Collins RH, Goldstein S, Giralt S, et al. Donor leukocyte infusions in acute lymphocytic leukemia. Bone Marrow Transplant 2000;26:511–16.

35. Ruggeri L, Capanni M, Casucci M, et al. Role of natural killer cell alloreactivity in HLA-mismatched hematopoietic stem cell transplantation. Blood 1999;94:333–39.

36. Kernan NA, Folmberg N, Dupont B, et al. Graft rejection in recipient of T depleted HLA-nonidentical marrow transplants for leukemia: identification of host-derived antidonor allocytotoxic T lymphocytes. Transplantation 1987;43:842–7.

37. Barge AJ, Johnson G, Witherspoon R, et al. Antibody-mediated marrow failure after allogeneic bone marrow transplantation. Blood 1989;74:1477–80.

38. Becker A, McCulloch E, Till J. Cytological demonstration of the clonal nature of spleen colonies derived from transplanted mouse marrow cells. Nature 1963;197:452–4.

39. Wu A, Till J, Siminovitch L, et al. Cytological evidence for a relationship between normal hematopoietic colony-forming cells and cells of the lymphoid system. J Exp Med 1963;127:455–64.

40. Baum CM, Weissman IL, Tsukamoto AS, et al. Isolation of a candidate human hematopoietic stem-cell population. Proc Natl Acad Sci U S A 1992;89:2804–8.

41. DiGiusto D, Chen S, Combs J, et al. Human fetal bone marrow early progenitors for T, B, and myeloid cells are found exclusively in the population expressing high level of CD34. Blood 1994;84:421–32.

42. Muller S, Schulz A, Reiss U, et al. Definition of a critical T cell threshold for prevention of GvHD after HLA non-identical PBPC transplantation in children. Bone Marrow Transplant 1999;24:575–81.

43. Alyea EP, Weller E, Fisher DC, et al. Comparable outcome with T cell depleted unrelated donor versus related donor allogeneic bone marrow transplant. Biol Blood Marrow Transplant 2002;8:601–7.

44. Aversa F, Tabilio A, Velardi A, et al. Treatment of high-risk acute leukemia with T cell-depleted stem cells from related donors with one fully mismatched HLA haplotype. N Engl J Med 1998;339:1186–93.

45. Antoine C, Muller S, Cant A, et al. Long-term survival and transplantation of haemopoietic stem cells for immunodeficiencies: report of the European experience 1968–1999. Lancet 2003; 361:553–60.

46. Reisner Y, Kapoor N, Kirkpatrick D, et al. Transplantation for severe combined immunodeficiency with HLA-A, B, D, DR incompatible parental marrow cells fractionated by soybean agglutinin and sheep red blood cells. Blood 1983;61:341–8.

47. Waldmann H, Polliak A, Hale G, et al. Elimination of graft-versus-host disease by in-vitro depletion of alloreactive lymphocytes with a monoclonal rat anti-human lymphocyte antibody (CAMPATH-1). Lancet 1984;2:483–6.

48. O'Reilly RJ. Immunologic aspects of hematopoietic stem-cell transplantation. Cytotherapy 2002;4:431–2.

49. Collins NH, Fernandez JM. T cell depletion and manipulation in allogeneic hematopoietic cell transplantation. Immunomethods 1994;5:189–96.

50. Tabilio A, Falzetti F, Zei T, et al. Graft engineering for allogeneic haploidentical stem cell transplantation. Blood Cells Mol Dis 2004;33:274–80.

51. Aversa F, Martelli MF. Transplantation of haploidentically mismatched stem cells for the treatment of malignant diseases. Springer Semin Immunophatol 2004;26:155–68.

52. Blazar BR, Taylor PA. Regulatory T cells. Biol Blood Marrow Transplant 2005;11:46–49.

53. Peggs KS, Mackinnon S. Augmentation of virus-specific immunity after hematopoietic stem cell transplantation by adoptive T cell therapy. Hum Immunol 2004;65:550–7.

54. Matthay KK, Reynolds CP, Seeger RC, et al. Long term results for children with high-risk neuroblastoma treated on a randomized trial of myeloablative therapy followed by 13-cis-retinoic acid: a Children's Oncology Group Study. Journal of Clin Oncol 2009;27:1007–13.

55. Fujii S, Fujimoto K, Shimizu K, et al. Presentation of tumor antigens by phagocytic dentritic cell clusters generated from human CD34+ hematopoietic progenitor cells: induction of autologous cytotoxic T lymphocytes against leukemic cells in acute myelogenous leukemia patients. Cancer Res 1999;59:2150–8.

56. Gilboa E. DC-based cancer vaccines. J Clin Invest 2007;117:1195–203.

57. Kessinger A, Armitage JO, Landmark JD, et al. Reconstitution of human hematopoietic function with autologous cryopreserved circulating stem cells. Exp Hematol 1986;14:192–96.

58. Yu J, Leisenring W, Bensinger WI, et al. The predictive value of white cell or CD34+ cell count in the peripheral blood for timing apheresis and maximizing yield. Transfusion 1999;39:442–50.

59. Grupp SA, Stern JW, Bunin N, et al. Rapid-sequence tandem transplant for children with high-risk neuroblastoma. Med Oncol 2000;35:696–700.

60. Pulsipher MA, Nagler A, Iannone R, et al. Ethical and safety considerations regarding risks for normal pediatric bone marrow donors: the use of G-CSF prior to stem cell harvest. Pediatric Blood Cancer 2006;46:422–33.

61. Aversa F, Terenzi A, Felicini R, et al. Mismatched T cell-depleted hematopoietic stem cell transplantation for children with high-risk acute leukemia. Bone Marrow Transplant 1998;22(Suppl 5):S29–32.

62. Bader P, Soerensen J, Koehl U, et al. Excellent engraftment and rapid immune recovery in haplo-identical stem cell transplantation using CD3/CD19 depleted peripheral stem cell grafts after reduced intensity conditioning. Bone Marrow Transplant 2007;39:S11.

63. Chen X, Hale GA, Barfield R, et al. Rapid immune reconstitution after a reduced-intensity conditioning regimen and a CD3-depleted haploidentical stem cell graft for paediatric refractory haematological malignancies. Br J Haematol 2006;135:524–32.

64. Lang P, Bader P, Schumm M, et al. Transplantation of a combination of CD133+ and CD34+ selected progenitor cells from alternative donors. Br J Haematol 2004;124:72–9.

65. Marks DI, Khattry N, Cummins M, et al. Haploidentical stem cell transplantation for children with acute leukaemia. Br J Haematol 2006;134:196–201.

66. Donovan J, Temel J, Zuckerman A, et al. CD34 selection as a stem cell purging strategy for neuroblastoma: pre-clinical and clinical studies. Med Ped Oncol 2000;35:677–82.

67. Reynolds CP, Seeger RC, Vo DD, et al. Model system for removing neuroblastoma cells from bone marrow using monoclonal antibodies and magnetic immunobeads. Cancer Res 1986;5:5882–6.

68. Broxmeyer HE, Srour EF, Hangoc G, et al. High-efficiency recovery of functional hematopoietic progenitor and stem cells from human cord blood cryopreserved for 15 years. Proc Natl Acad SCI USA 2003;100:645–50.

69. Rubinstein P, Carrier C, Scaradavou A, et al. Outcomes among 562 recipients of placental-blood transplants from unrelated donors. N Engl J Med 1998;339:1565–77.

70. Wagner JE, Barker JN, DeFor TE, et al.Transplantation of unrelated donor umbilical cord blood in 102 patients with malignant and nonmalignant diseases: influence of CD34 cell dose and HLA disparity on treatment-related mortality and survival. Blood 2002;100:1611–8.

71. Gluckman E, Rocha V, Arcese W, et al. Factors associated with outcomes of unrelated cord blood transplant: guidelines for donor choice. Exp Hematol 2004;32:397–407.

72. Shpall EJ, Quinone R, Giller R, et al. Transplantation of ex vivo expanded cord blood. Biol Blood Marrow Transplant 2002;8:368–376.

73. Barker JN, Weisdorf DJ, DeFor TE, et al. Transplantation of 2 partially HLA-matched umbilical cord blood units to enhance engraftment in adults with hematologic malignancy. Blood 2005;105:1343–7.

74. Meyers KC, Davies SM. Hematopoietic stem cell transplantation for bone marrow failure syndrome. Biol Blood Marrow Transplant 2009;15:279–92.

75. Dalle JH. HSCT for Fanconi anemia in children: factors that influence early and late results. Bone Marrow Transplant 2008;42:51–3.

76. Farzin A, Davies SM, Smith FO, et al. Matched sibling donor haemotopoietic stem cell transplantation in Fanconi anaemia: an update of the Cincinnati Children's experience. Br J Haematol 2007;136:633–40.

77. Tan PL, Wagner JE, Auerbach AD, et al. Successful engraftment without radiation after fludarabine-based regimen in Fanconi anemia patients undergoing genotypically identical donor hematopoietic cell transplantation. Pediatr Blood Cancer 2006;46:630–6.

78. De la Fuente J, Dokal I. Dyskeratosis congenita: advances in the understanding of the telomerase defect and the role of stem cell transplantation. Pediatr Transplant 2007;11:584–94.

79. Cesaro S, Onero R, Messina C, et al. Haematopoietic stem cell transplantation for Shwachman-Diamond disease: a study from the European Group for Blood and Marrow Transplantation. Br J Haematol 2005;131:231–6.

80. Bhatla D, Davies SM, Shenoy S, et al. Reduced intensity conditioning is effective and safe for transplantation of patients with Shwachman-Diamond syndrome. Bone Marrow Transplant 2008;42(3):159–65.

81. Lipton JM, Atsidaftos E, Zyskind I, et al. Improving clinical care and elucidating the pathophhysiology of Diamond-Blackfan anemia: an update from the Diamond-Blackfan Anemia Registry. Pediatr Blood Cancer 2006;46:558–64.

82. Lackner A, Basu O, Biering ML, et al. Haematopoietic stem cell transplantation for amegakaryocyte thrombocytopenia. Br J Haematol 2000;109:773–5.

83. Locasciulli A. Oneto R, Bacigalupo A, et al. Outcome of patients with acquired aplastic anemia given first line bone marrow transplantation or immunosuppressive treatment in the last decade: a report from the European Group for Blood and Marrow Transplantation. Haematologica 2007;92:11–8.

84. Locatelli F, Bruno B, Zecca M, et al. Cyclosporine A and short-term methotrexate versus cyclosporin A as graft-versus-host disease prophylaxis in patients with severe aplastic anemia given allogeneic bone marrow transplantation from an HLA-identical sibling: results of a GITMO/EBMT randomized trial. Blood 2000;96:1690–7.

85. Gaziev J, Sodani P, Lucarelli G. Hematopoietic stem cell transplantation in thalassemia. Bone Marrow Transplant 2008;42(Suppl 1):S41.

86. Graziev D, Polchi P, Galimberti M, et al. Graft- versus- host disease after bone marrow transplantation for thalassemia: an analysis of incidence and risk factor. Transplantation 1997;63:854–60.

87. Lisini D, Zecca M, Giorgiani G, et al. Donor/recipient mixed chimerism does not predict graft failure in children with β-thalassemia given an allogeneic cord blood transplant from an HLA-identical sibling. Haematologica 2008;93:1780–4.

88. Daikeler T, Hugle T, Farget D, et al. Allogeneic hematopoietic SCT for patients with autoimmune diseases. Bone Marrow Transplant 2009;44:27–33.

89. Peter C, Steward C. Hematopoietic cell transplantation for inherited metabolic diseases: an overview of outcome and practice guidelines. Bone Marrow Transplant 2003;31:229–39.

90. Lange MC, Teive HG, Troiano AR, et al. Bone marrow transplantation in patients with storage diseases. Arq Neuropsiquiatr 2006;64:1–4.

91. Driessen GJA, Gerritsen EJA, Fischer A, et al. Long-term outcome of haematopoietic stem cell transplantation in autosomal recessive osteopetrosis: an EBMT report. Bone Marrow Transplant 2003;32:657–63.

92. Locatelli F, Zecca M, Rondelli R, et al. Graft versus host disease prophylaxis with low-dose cyclosporine-A reduces the risk of relapse in children with acute leukemia given an HLA-identical sibling bone marrow transplantation: results of a randomized trial. Blood 2000;95:1572–9.

93. Morra E, Barosi G, Bosi A, et al. Clinical management of primary non acute promyelocytic leukemia acute myeloid leukemia: practice guidelines by the Italian Society of Hematology, the Italian Society of Experimental Hematology and the Italian Group for Bone Marrow Transplantation. Haematologica 2008;94:102–12.

94. Shenoy S, Smith FO. Hematopoietic stem cell transplantation for childhood malignancies of myeloid origin. Bone Marrow Transplant 2008;41: 141–8.

95. Nyemeyer CM, Kratz CP. Paediatric myelodysplastic syndrome and juvenile myelomonocytic leukemia: molecular classification and treatment options. Br J Haematol 2008;140:610–24.

96. Saarinen-Pihkaka UM, Gustafsson G, Ringden O, et al. No disadvantages in outcome of using matched unrelated donors as compared with matched sibling donors for bone marrow transplantation in children with acute lymphoblastic leukemia in second remission. J Clin Oncol 2001;19:3406–14.

97. Gluckman E, Rocha V, Arcese W, et al. Factors associated with outcomes of unrelated cord blood transplant: guidelines for donor choice. Exp Hematol 2004;32:397–407.

98. Hwang WY, Samuel M, tan D, et al. A meta-analysis of unrelated donor umbilical cord blood transplantation versus unrelated donor bone marrow transplantation in adult and pediatric patients. Biol Blood Marrow Transplant 2007;13:444–53.

99. Gluckman E, Rocha V, EBMT Paediatric, Acute Leukemia Working Parties and Eurocord. Indications and results of cord blood transplant in children with leukemia. Bone Marrow Transplant 2008;41(S2): S80–2.

100. Ball LM, Bernardo ME, Roelofs H, et al. Cotransplantation of ex vivo expanded mesenchymal stem cells accelerates lymphocyte recovery and may reduce the risk of graft failure in haploidentical hemopoietic stemcell transplantation. Blood 2007;110:2764–7.

101. Eyrich M, Lang P, Lal S, et al. A prospective analysis of the pattern of immune reconstitution in a pediatric cohort following transplantation of positively selected human leucocyte antigen-disparate haematopoietic stem cells from parental donors. Br J Haematol 2001;114: 422–32.

102. Ball LM, Lankester AC, Bredius RG, et al. Graft dysfunction and delayed immune reconstitution following haploidentical peripheral blood hematopoietic stem cell transplantation. Bone Marrow Transplant 2005; 35(Suppl1):S35–8.

103. Perruccio K, Tosti A, Burchielli E, et al. Transferring functional immune responses to pathogens after haploidentical hematopoietic transplantation. Blood 2005;106:4397–406.

104. Comoli P, Basso S, Zecca M, et al. Preemptive treatment of EBV-related post-transplant lymphoproliferative disorders after pediatric haploidentical stem cell transplantation. Am J Transplant 2007;7: 1648–55.

105. Lang P, Greil J, Bader P, et al. Long-term outcome after haploidentical stem cell transplantation in children. Blood Cells Mol Dis 2004;33: 281–7.

106. Marks DI, Khattry N, Cummins M, et al. Haploidentical stem cell transplantation for children with acute leukemia. Br J Haematol 2006;134: 196–201.

107. Reisner Y, Martelli MF. Tolerance induction by 'megadose' transplants of CD34+ stem cells: a new option for leukemia patients without an HLA-matched donor. Curr Opin Immunol 2000;12:536–41.

108. Lang P, Handgretinger R. Haploidentical SCT in children: an update and future perspective. Bone Marrow Transplant 2008;425:54–9.

109. Lang P, Pfeiffer M, Muller I, et al. Haploidentical stem cell transplantation in patients with pediatric solid tumors: preliminary results of a pilot study and analysis of graft versus tumor effects. Klin Padiatr 2006;218: 321–6.

110. Center for International Blood and Marrow Transplant Research (CIBMTR), National Marrow Donor Program (NMDP), European Blood and Marrow Transplant Group (EBMT), et al. Guidelines for preventing infectious complications among hematopoietic cell transplant recipients: a global perspective. Bone Marrow Transplant 2009;44: 453–8.

111. Inoue H, Yasuda Y, Hattori K, et al. The kinetics of immune reconstitution after cord blood transplantation and selected CD34+ stem cell transplantation in children: comparison with bone marrow transplantation. Int J Hematol 2003;77:399–407.

112. Jacobsohn DA, Duerst R, Tse W, et al. Reduced intensity haemopoietic stem-cell transplantation for treatment of non-malignant diseases in children. Lancet 2004;364:156–62.

113. Spielberg R, Stiff P, Bensinger W, et al. Palifermin for oral mucositis after intensive therapy for hematologic cancers. N Engl J Med 2004;351: 2590–8.

114. Shlomchik WD, Couzens MS, Tang CB, et al. Prevention of graft versus host disease by inactivation of host-antigen-presenting cells. Science 1999;285:412–5.

115. Shah AJ, Kapoor N, Crooks GM, et al. The effects of Campath 1H upon graft-versus-host disease, infection, relapse, and immune reconstitution in recipients of pediatric unrelated transplants. Biol Blood Marrow Transplant 2007;13:584–93.

Gene Therapy and Allergy

Catherine M. Bollard • Conrad Russell Y. Cruz • Malcolm K. Brenner

Introduction

When investigators first considered using gene therapy to treat human disease, it was assumed that monogenic disorders would be the target, with the intent of restoring a functional gene to a defective cell. Moreover, because of the unknown risks of this novel therapeutic approach, these disorders had to be both immediately life-threatening and lacking in safe, effective alternative treatments. The allergic disorders do not meet these guidelines. While a strong genetic component is doubtless present, allergic diseases are a complex, heterogeneous group of maladies with an equally complex and heterogeneous polygenic basis. And while allergic responses certainly may be fatal, the great majority of patients live with, rather than die from, their condition, and it has been difficult to identify subgroups who might justifiably be exposed to the unknown risks of gene therapy. Gradually, however, these requirements have become less rigid. First of all, it has become appreciated that gene therapy may be of considerable value even for the treatment of complex genetic disorders. Cancer, for example, is a complex (albeit acquired) genetic disorder and yet represents by far the commonest clinical setting for trials of gene transfer, and although there have been well-publicized severe adverse events attributed to the administration of viral vectors, the safety profile overall has been excellent: many thousands of other patients have received treatment with gene transfer vectors or gene modified cells, apparently without associated severe toxicity or mortality.

For the above reasons, serious consideration of gene therapy approaches to the treatment of allergic disorders is now justified. Since this proposed application represents an embryonic usage for a field that is itself in a highly rudimentary stage of development, the major purpose of this chapter is to explain the principles of gene therapy, and to illustrate what it can and cannot do. We will show how it may be possible to use gene transfer, either directly as therapy for allergic disorders, or as a tool to validate target molecules and pathways whose function may later be modified by more conventional therapeutics. The examples and suggestions we make will, where possible, be backed by published experimental data. But since this chapter is intended to be provocative and not just didactic, we have not entirely omitted unsupported speculation!

Vectors

A prerequisite for any gene therapy approach is the ability to transduce the desired target cell. Several viral and nonviral gene transfer systems have entered, or are about to enter, clinical practice, and they are summarized in Table 19-1 and discussed in more detail below and elsewhere in the literature.[1–5] Each of these systems has its advantages and disadvantages, but for the moment none possess the generally desirable characteristics of wide biodistribution, high transduction efficiency, specific cell targeting, and high levels of gene expression. For many gene therapy approaches, including those intended to modulate the immune response to allergens, it would also be useful to control the transgene product. Several different regulatory systems have been described and tested successfully in animal models,[6,7] and a phase I clinical trial of a radiation-inducible gene in an adenovirus vector has been well tolerated in patients with treatment-refractory solid tumors.[8]

Because no available vector systems yet come close to meeting the requirements for a truly effective agent, the choice has to be based on the 'least bad' or best available alternative for the specific application proposed. Hence, no vector system can be considered universal. Since cells of the immune response play a major role in pathology in allergic disorders these need to be effective targets for gene modification. Each of the vector systems described below should thus be considered in the context of their effects on these cells.

Viral Vectors

Murine Retroviral Based

Retroviruses, most of them based on the Moloney murine leukemia virus (MoMuLV), are vectors that are capable of integrating in host cell DNA. The ability to guarantee the expression of the transgene in every daughter cell has led to their extensive use in clinical settings where the target cell undergoes extensive division. These clinical applications have included gene marking studies and the correction of severe combined immune deficiency syndromes.[9–12] Along with adenoviral vectors, retroviral vectors account for a majority of all gene therapy clinical trials to date.[13] MoMuLV are single-stranded, enveloped RNA viruses that are transcribed by reverse transcriptase into double-stranded DNA. In a clinical vector, the packaging signal and long terminal repeats (LTRs) of the wild-type virus are retained, while its structural and replicative genes (gag, pol and env) are replaced by one or more genes of interest, driven either by the retroviral promoter in the 5′ LTR, or by an internal promoter. The retroviral constructs are made in cell lines that express the missing retrovirus genes in trans, and thus reproduce and package a replication-incompetent vector. After production of viral

Table 19-1 Key Concepts Advantages and Disadvantages of Vector Systems

Vector	Advantages	Disadvantages	Current Clinical Applications
Murine retrovirus	Stable integration into dividing cells Minimal immunogenicity Stable packaging system	Low titer Only integrates in dividing cells Limited insert size Risk of silencing Risk of insertional mutagenesis	Marker studies Gene therapy approaches using hematopoietic stem cells or T cells (e.g. to treat immunodeficiency syndromes and malignancies) Transduction of tumor cell lines
Lentivirus	Integrates into dividing cells Expressed in nondividing cells Larger insert size than murine retroviruses	No stable packaging system Complex safety issues	No approved trials as yet
Self inactivating (SIN-Lenti) and replication incompetent	Incapable of replications post transfection Increased safety Stable packaging system	?safety concerns remain	Gene therapy approaches using hematopoietic stem cells T cells (e.g. to treat aquired and congenital immunodeficiency syndromes and inherited metabolic disorders)
Adenovirus	Infects wide range cell types Infects nondividing cells High titers High level of expression Accepts 12–15kb DNA inserts	Highly immunogenic Non-integrating	Direct in vivo applications Transduction of tumor cells Transduction of antigen-presenting cells for in vitro and in vivo use
Adeno-associated virus (AAV)	Integrates into dividing cells Infects wide range cell types	No stable packaging cell line Very limited insert size	Gene therapy approaches targeting muscle, liver, eye, and brain
Herpesvirus	High titers Transduces some target cells at high efficiency Accepts large DNA inserts	No packaging cell lines Non-integrating May be cytotoxic to target cell	Transduction of tumor cells Neurologic disorders
Liposomes and other physical methods using plasmid DNA (e.g. sleeping beauty)	Easy to prepare in quantity Virtually unlimited size Limited immunogenicity	Inefficient entry into target cell Variable integration	Transduction of tumor cells Gene therapy approaches for vascular diseases Gene modification of T cell for cancer

particles and infection of target cells, the vector is uncoated in the cytosol and the RNA is transcribed via reverse transcriptase into DNA, which integrates into the host genome (Figure 19-1). The host range of MoMuLV viruses is determined by the gp70 envelope protein, which interacts with the target cells' receptors.[14] The envelope also affects the sensitivity of the vector to primate complement, and hence determines the feasibility of using the virus for in vivo as well as ex vivo transduction of target cells. It is possible to modify the target cell range and to increase the physical stability and complement resistance of MoMuLV particles simply by growing the vector in packaging cell lines that supply a different envelope in trans. For example, retroviruses with the Gibbon Ape Leukemia Virus (GALV) envelope more efficiently transduce T lymphocytes compared with the same retrovirus expressing an amphotropic envelope,[15] and viruses with the feline leukemia virus envelope may have an enhanced capacity to transduce human hematopoietic stem cells.[16]

Merely modifying the viral envelope cannot, however, overcome one of the main limitations of Moloney-based vectors: the inability to transduce nondividing cells. The unstable pre-integration complex of the virus cannot penetrate the small nuclear membrane pores present in resting cells.[17] This requirement for cell division has been a major limitation when human hematopoietic stem cells are the targets, because so few of these cells are in cycle at any one time. Efforts to increase the cycling fraction with growth factors may lead to differentiation and loss of stem cell activity.[18] Combining MoMuLV with improved cytokine cocktails (e.g. adding Flt 3 ligand, IL-3 and stem cell factor [SCF]) and bringing the vector and target cell into close apposition through physical entrapment (e.g. with fibronectin) have produced more satisfactory levels of transduction of human stem cells[19] but may have increased concerns regarding safety as discussed below.[20]

Lentiviral Vectors

The inability of murine retroviruses to transduce resting, non-dividing cells refocused attention onto human and feline lentiviral vectors.[1,21] Lentiviral vectors readily transduce hematopoietic progenitor cells[22] primarily because they form a more stable pre-integration complex than MoMuLV. As such, they are able to infect quiescent subsets of primitive hemopoietic stem cells, such as the CD34$^+$ CD38$^-$ or the CD38$^-$ lineage negative population, where they persist and integrate once these cells enter cycle.[23] The well-characterized human lentivirus, HIV, can also efficiently infect terminally differentiated cells such as neurons[24] where high levels of gene expression have been reported.

Although lentiviral vectors have clear advantages over murine retroviruses, several technical and safety problems complicate their entry into general clinical usage. At the technical level, the toxicity of some HIV proteins has made generation of stable packaging cells difficult.[1] In terms of safety, there is justifiable public health concern that HIV-derived vector systems will recombine in vivo to form mutant infectious HIV particles, for example by recombination with lentiviral sequences embedded in the human genome. Efforts to address the latter have resulted in the development of third and fourth generation self-inactivating lentiviral (SIN-L) vectors, where the parental HIV-1 enhancer and promoter sequences from the lentivirus 3'LTR have been

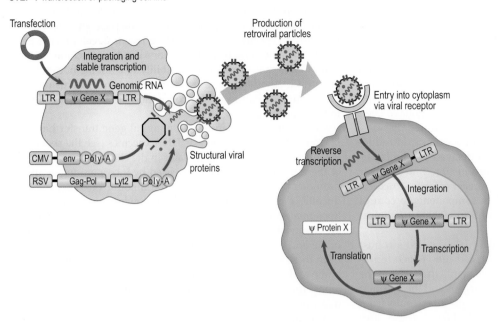

Figure 19-1 Production of an infectious retroviral particle and transduction of a target cell.

deleted.[25] When the SIN vector infects its target cells, it is incapable of transcribing vector-length RNA, reducing the likelihood of recombination to generate replication-competent retroviruses. Accumulating evidence from preclinical studies suggest that SIN vectors will have a good safety profile[5] and initial reports from the first clinical trial using lentiviral vectors are encouraging. Patients who were enrolled in the study using lentivirus-transduced T cells for the treatment of HIV infection had sustained gene transfer, improved immune function (in four of five), and no evidence of insertional mutagenesis.[26] To date, there are 21 clinical trials using lentiviral vectors, which is still only a small fraction (1.4%) of the total.[13]

Adenoviral Vectors

Adenoviral vectors infect a wide range of cell types within and outside the immune system. Unlike retroviruses, these vectors are nonintegrating and express their genes in nondividing cells. The vectors can be used to transduce cells ex vivo but are also stable in vivo and so can be used to infect cells in situ. Adenoviruses are a suitable delivery system for gene therapy approaches for allergic disorders, if the strategy chosen requires high level but short-term transgene expression by the target cell, and if an immune response directed against the adenovector or its infected target cell is unlikely to be problematic.

First generation adenoviral vectors are El (early protein) and/or E3 deletion mutants and are therefore replication incompetent. These viruses have been used for transfer of immunostimulatory genes into cancer cells to enhance the immune response, for transfer of pro-drug metabolizing enzymes in an effort to sensitize normal and/or malignant cells to killing, and in gene correction studies, for example in cystic fibrosis and hemophilia.[27,28] Subsequent vector 'generations' involved the deletion of additional genes (E4 and E2 for the second generation, and eventually of all viral genes to form helper dependent or 'gutless' adenoviral vectors, with supposedly reduced immunogenicity and increased transgenic cargo capacity).[29]

Adenoviral vectors have many limitations. Because they are nonintegrating, the gene products are expressed from episomal DNA, and are lost after cell division; indeed they can be inactivated even in nondividing cells.[30] Adenoviral vectors are therefore unsuited to long-term expression in a rapidly turning-over cell population. The vectors themselves also induce an acute inflammatory response, with release of cytokines including tumor necrosis factor-alpha (TNFα), and interleukins (IL) such as IL-6 and IL-8. Indeed, the acute phase response to injected adenoviral vectors has been fatal in humans.[31] Subsequent to this acute phase response, adenoviral vectors induce antibodies that can neutralize subsequent adenoviral vectors administered to the patient, and T cell responses directed to adenoviral and transgenic proteins. Since wild-type infections with adenovirus are widespread in the general population, these immune reactions are probable, even if not always predictable.[32] Unfortunately, cell-mediated immunity may recognize and eliminate cells expressing low levels of adenoviral proteins directly derived from the infecting vector, so that even vectors that translate little or no viral proteins from their endogenous structural genes may still provoke an immune response against the cells they enter.

In an effort to reduce the immunogenicity of adenoviral vectors, still further, a helper-dependent vector system has been developed in which one virus (helper) contains all viral replication genes and the other contains only the therapeutic gene sequence, the viral inverted terminal repeats (ITRs) and the packaging recognition signal.[33] In principle, only the therapeutic virus is packaged, although a small number of helper particles do in fact contaminate the final product. The process is currently labor intensive and difficult to scale-up and there is a continued problem with contaminating helper virus, although the amounts have now been reduced to less than 0.1%.[34] Nevertheless, these helper-dependent vectors may be less likely to trigger a cellular response against the transduced target cell, allowing for more persistent transgene expression.

Adeno-Associated Viral Vectors

Adeno-associated viruses (AAVs) are integrating parvoviruses that normally depend on a helper virus (adeno or herpes virus) for productive infection.[35] They can, however, exist as a latent provirus in the absence of the helper virus. Vectors based on AAV have been developed as gene transfer vehicles able to transduce a wide variety of cells including nondividing cells.[36] The target cell range depends on the AAV subtype,[37,38] but none are associated with any known disease, and the AAV vector genome lacks viral coding sequences. Hence, the vector itself has not been associated with toxicity. Nonetheless, neutralizing antibodies are produced in vivo so that repeat administration of AAV may require the use of a different serotype. AAV vectors have been used in various animal models of genetic and acquired diseases. Despite the advantages of low toxicity and persistence, introduction of these viruses into the clinic was delayed by the labor-intensive nature of large-scale vector production, and by their limited transgene capacity, precluding transfer of large structural genes, or of incorporation of regulatory components to control transgene expression. Nonetheless, as of Spring 2009, 67 clinical trials are in progress.[13]

Results from some early AAV clinical trials showed a robust T cell-mediated response against transduced cells which terminated gene expression. This outcome was unanticipated from the animal data. The use of alternative target organs and the addition of immunosuppression has produced more positive results from two clinical trials, renewing optimism in this class of vectors after disappointments associated with the unexpected immunogenicity in patients treated for hemophilia B.[39] Leber's congenital amaurosis is an inherited form of retinal degeneration causing progressive visual loss. Patients injected in their retinas with an AAV vector carrying the RPE65 gene had objective and subjective improvements in their visual function. Because the eye can be an immunologically 'privileged' site, a damaging immune response was not observed.[40,41] In a second study in patients with Parkinson's disease, AAV expressing glutamic acid decarboxylase, which increases the concentration of the inhibitory neurotransmitter gamma-amino butyric acid (GABA), was injected into the subthalamic region of one cerebral hemisphere, with the contralateral side serving as a control. Subjective improvements in symptoms were associated with objective improvements in thalamic metabolism, measured by positron emission tomography.[42]

Herpes Viruses

Herpes viruses have been proposed as high-efficiency vectors for many cell types. Although they usually do not integrate in the host cell, they have the potential to persist after primary infection in a latent state.[43] Deletion of the five immediate early (IE) genes allows herpes simplex virus (HSV) vectors to be grown in high titers in complementing cell lines without the production of replication competent virus.[44] In fact, up to half of the HSV genes are nonessential for virus replication in culture and can be removed. This allows insertion of a large payload, which may be multiple structural genes or structural and regulatory elements in combination.[45] The large insert size allowed by HSV may be of particular advantage in allergic disorders, in which a multiplicity of immunomodulatory genes may need to be expressed simultaneously.

HSV vectors have now been used in numerous animal models including those in which peripheral[46] or central nervous system disorders are targeted,[47] and in cancer as well.[48,49] Clinical experience with these vectors is beginning to accrue, and it is likely that they will have wider application in human disease over the next few years.

Nonviral Vectors

Because of the complexities associated with the manufacture of viral vectors and concerns over their immunogenicity and toxicity, increasing attention has been paid to nonviral vector systems. Until recently these systems were profoundly limited for clinical applications because of their extreme inefficiency and lack of targeting to specific cell types. More recent developments have begun to show how these limitations can be overcome. Of particular interest is our increasing ability to combine nonviral and physical methods of gene transfer, for example, by using plasmids coupled with local electroporation of target tissues in situ to favor gene uptake.

Most clinical experience with nonviral gene transfer has used plasmids injected primarily as DNA vaccines (see the section on 'Producing a Soluble Protein' later in the chapter). The efficiency of these plasmids has been increased by incorporating synthetic promoters, which may enhance the amount of transgene produced.[50] Plasmids are also given following incorporation into liposomal complexes.[51,52] Cationic liposome/DNA complexes, are the most widely used of these; they fuse with the cell membrane and enter the endosomal uptake pathway. DNA released from these endosomes may then pass through the nuclear membrane and be expressed. Liposomal delivery of plasmid DNA is more efficient than direct injection, and since liposomes are relatively nontoxic, they can be given repeatedly. Although levels of gene expression comparable to viral vectors have been obtained in some cellular targets, the DNA transferred by liposomes does not integrate into the genome. Moreover, the ability to target these vectors is still relatively limited despite the incorporation of a variety of ligands into the liposome-DNA complex.[52]

Plasmids may also be successfully coupled with other physical methods of gene transfer. For example, successful gene transfer in vivo has been reported with use of a bioballistic ('gene gun') technique in which DNA coated onto colloidal gold particles is driven at high velocity by gas pressure into the cell.[53] Alternatively, increased cellular uptake of plasmid may be obtained locally by application of an electrical charge (electroporation)[52,54] that induces reversible holes in the cell membrane. Laser light and ultrasonic transducers (optoporation and sonoporation, respectively) may have identical effects. Electroporation techniques have been successfully used to transfer the cytotoxic drug bleomycin into human tumors in situ, and the first clinical protocols using this approach for plasmid gene transfer are now under consideration by regulatory bodies.

A nonviral strategy, termed 'transkaryotic implantation' was recently employed in a clinical trial for the treatment of patients with severe hemophilia A. Somatic cells are isolated from a patient, transfected with a therapeutic gene using physical means, and then a rare transduced clone is isolated, expanded ex vivo and reimplanted in vivo. An early study of this approach has shown some promise, but it remains cumbersome.[55]

Nonviral gene delivery would be more attractive if the transgene were able to integrate with higher efficiency in the host cell genome. Transposon technology,[56] in which these mobile genetic elements are used to integrate transgenes into host cell genomes, may afford such an opportunity. If a plasmid encoding a therapeutic gene (Factor IX, for example) and portions of a transposon, is co-injected with a second plasmid encoding an enzyme that activates those transposon elements, there is chromosomal integration and transposition that leads to long-term expression (>5 months) of factor IX at levels therapeutic for a mouse model of hemophilia B. Both the Sleeping Beauty and, more recently, the piggyBac transposon systems are being explored for human gene therapy studies, since each may have a lower frequency of integration proximate to functional genes and their control sequences than do conventional retroviruses.[57] It is not yet clear whether the use of transposons will safely improve the duration of plasmid-dependent gene expression in gene-modified human cells.[58]

In summary, advances in the technology of the components of nonviral vector systems will likely lead to a progressive increase in their effectiveness and a corresponding increase in their usage in human gene therapy studies.

Vector Safety Concerns

Adverse publicity has sensitized investigators and public alike to the potential dangers of gene transfer vectors. Every new therapeutic agent must, of course, be carefully monitored for adverse effects, and gene transfer vectors are no different. Beyond these general concerns, however, there are more specific issues that must be considered.

Insertional mutagenesis is a potential consequence of any integration event, regardless of the vector used.[59] Investigators from European severe combined X-linked immunedeficiency studies, in which the deficient cytokine common gamma chain was transferred into CD34[+] selected stem cells by a Moloney-based vector, recently reported the development of T cell leukemia in 5[20,60] of 17 patients who were successfully cured of their primary immune disorder.[61] Four of these cases resulted from insertions near the LMO2 proto-oncogene,[20,60] while the fifth resulted from insertions near the BMI1 proto-oncogene. Of these patients, four achieved remissions after treatment with chemotherapy.[20,60]

A clinical trial reported the successful cure of X-linked chronic granulomatous disease (CGD) in two patients who received autologous CD34[+] cells transduced with a gammaretroviral vector expressing gp91[phox] (the defective gene causing the lack of superoxide production in CGD). Cells from the patients were observed to produce therapeutic levels of superoxide, and the gene-corrected cells contributed to the eradication of preexisting bacterial and fungal infections. However, clones containing insertions in MDS1-EVI1, PRDM16, and SETBP1 were noted to emerge[62] and these genes are associated with the development of myelodysplasia and leukemia.[62]

It is unclear whether the risks of tumorigenesis due to insertional mutagenesis are influenced by the transgene carried by the retroviral vector. While it can be argued that the IL2RG transgene in the SCID-X1 trials conferred a survival advantage to transduced cells (an advantage that is lacking in cells from CGD patients when they express transgenic gp91[phox]),[63] a recent study argues that the γ-C gene is not oncogenic, and that an underlying predisposition in severe combined immunodeficiency (SCID) patients may interact with insertional mutagenesis leading to the development of cancer.[64] This seems an unlikely generalization, however, as correction of adenosine deaminase (ADA)-deficient SCID patients by gene transfer has not been associated with any malignant manifestations.[65]

These outcomes emphasize that, as with any medical therapy, the risk:benefit ratio of the disease and its treatment must be carefully considered. It is noteworthy, however, that even for patients with X-linked SCID, gene therapy still has a considerably superior safety and efficacy outcome than the alternative of stem cell transplantation from an HLA (the name for the human major histocompatability complex, the 'human leukocyte antigen') mismatched donor. Although well over a thousand other individuals have received cells modified by retroviral vectors, no further cases of leukemia or myelodysplasia have been noted. Nonetheless, all recipients of retroviral vectors or of cells modified by these vectors require 15-year follow-up, including genetic analysis of any tumors that may appear.

Although nonintegrating vectors should not cause significant genotoxicity, many are highly immunogenic, a characteristic that may be particularly unwelcome in the allergic host. Immunity to adenoviral vectors is perhaps the best studied, and

illustrates the complex innate and adaptive immune host defense mechanisms that viral vectors may trigger. Inflammatory and adaptive humoral immune responses are generated against the vector proteins themselves, while T cell responses appear against the low levels of adenoviral proteins expressed, even when cells are transduced by defective viruses.[66] The death of a teenager injected with an adenoviral vector encoding ornithine transcarbomylase transgene was almost certainly attributable to the systemic inflammatory response and disseminated intravascular coagulation due to his innate immune response to viral proteins.[67] That such reactions are idiosyncratic does not minimize their importance, and this outcome still serves as an important guideline for the maximum doses of vectors that it will be safe to give.[32]

It is unlikely that it will ever be possible to safely ablate the multiplicity of immune defenses that we have developed against viruses and viral vectors. The ultimate need will be to develop synthetic vectors that combine the efficiency and targeting ability of viruses with the more benign physical characteristics of current plasmids.

Principles and Mechanisms of Disease – The Effector Cells and Effector Molecules of the Immune System and Their Roles in Allergy

To devise successful gene therapy interventions for allergic responses, we require an understanding of the cellular and molecular mechanisms involved in generating and regulating these phenomena. A detailed description of all that is known about this subject is beyond the scope of this chapter. However, a basic overview of the effector cells and molecules of the immune system is provided in Figure 19.2 and in the section that follows, which are offered only as a basis for explaining how components of the allergic response could in principle become targets for genetic manipulation.

Inflammation in Allergy

The effector phase of the allergic response is composed of several events: mucus production by surface epithelial cells, increased adhesion receptor expression by endothelial cells that facilitates leukocyte adhesion and subsequent extravasation, smooth muscle cell contraction, eosinophilia, secretion of active proteases and vasodilators following mast cell degranulation, and inflammatory cell recruitment.[68] These events, in turn, are mediated by a complex interplay of immune cells and their cytokines, any of which can, in principle, be modulated by genetic manipulation, for sustained benefit.

Cells Involved in the Allergic Response

B lymphocytes and IgE

A subset of B cells release immunoglobulin E (IgE), and elevated amounts of this immunoglobulin class are often present in the serum of patients with allergic disease. The Fc region of the IgE molecule binds at its C-3 domain with receptors such as CD23 and with the high affinity receptor FcεRI (present on tissue mast cells, basophils, B cells and other antigen-presenting cells [APCs] including dendritic cells). When the host is exposed to the specific antigen, cross-linking of cell bound IgE occurs and produces mast cell degranulation and release of inflammatory mediators such as histamine, prostaglandin D2, thromboxane A2, the

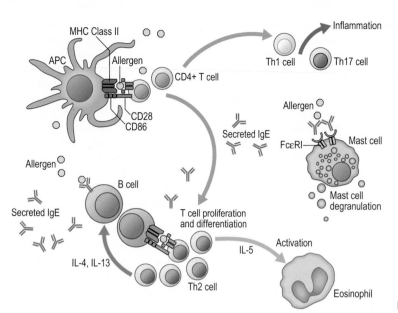

Figure 19-2 The effector response in allergy.

leutkotrienes C4 and B4 and Th2 cytokines. The biological effects of these mast cell mediators and cytokines result in the clinical allergic response.

Interleukin-4 (IL-4), produced by Th2 cells (see below 'T Cells and the T Helper Response') is one important cytokine that favors IgE synthesis from B cells,[69] but interleukin-13 (IL-13) release plays an additional role.[70] Engagement of the C40 antigen on B cells by T cells or APC expressing the CD40 ligand (CD154) also promotes IgE class switching.[71]

T cells and the T helper (Th) Response

Naïve CD4 T cells can differentiate into at least five functional classes – Th0, Th1, Th2, Th17, and Tregs – depending on the signals they acquired from the APC and the existing cytokine environment. *Th0 cells* secrete interleukin 4 (IL-4), IL-13 and gamma interferon (IFNγ), *Th1 cells* favor induction of cytotoxic/ antiviral effector cells and produce cytokines such as IL-12 and IFNγ, which tend to antagonize the allergic response. *Th2 cells* favor induction of an inflammatory and antibody response, producing cytokines such as IL-4, IL-5, IL-6, IL-10, IL-13 and granulocyte macrophage colony stimulating factor. By promoting B cell synthesis of IgE, Th2, cells can effectively arm basophils, mast cells and eosinophils, which are also capable of releasing Th2-like proinflammatory cytokines in response to antigen. *Th17 cells* have been implicated in the induction of proinflammatory microenvironments in tissues. They secrete IL-17, IL-17F, IL-6, TNFα, and IL-22 on activation, which promote granulopoiesis and maintain active homeostasis of neutrophils. Neutrophil inflammation has been shown to associate with severe asthma,[72] and sputum IL-17 mRNA positively correlates with airway neutrophilia, which in turn negatively correlates with the degree of bronchial reactivity.[73] *Regulatory T cells* (Tregs) are important components of antigen-specific immune tolerance, and will be discussed in greater detail in the section on immune tolerance below.

Antigen-Presenting Cells

For an antigen to stimulate a T cell response, it requires presentation by antigen-presenting cells (APC) such as dendritic cells (DCs). APC take up antigen, process it to peptides and present it in association with class I and class II molecules of the major histocompatibility complex (MHC). If these cells encounter T lymphocytes expressing an appropriate, specific CD3 receptor for the MHC-peptide complex they are presenting, CD80 and CD86 surface molecules on the APC engage the CD28 molecule on T cells and provide signals crucial for T cell survival and cytokine secretion.[74] The T cell's interaction with peptide and APC helps determine whether a CD8 (recognizes antigen and class I MHC molecules) or a CD4 (recognizes antigen and class II MHC molecules) response is generated, and whether a CD4 response is predominantly Th0, Th1, Th2, Th17 or T regulatory (Treg). The population of T cells recruited, in turn, modifies the immunoglobulin (Ig) class of the antibody response made by antigen-specific B cells, and the class of Ig determines which downstream effector mechanisms are recruited. For example, activation of Th2 cells favors recruitment of IgE-producing B cells, with subsequent arming of basophils and mast cells for an acute hypersensitivity response.[75,76]

Inducing Tolerance in the Effector Cells of the Allergic Response

While antigen-specific tolerance had predominantly been considered to be a passive process involving inactivation or death of clones of antigen-specific cells following exposure to the specific antigen, it is now widely accepted that active peripheral mechanisms underlie tolerance to self-antigens, and that these comprise a fundamental property of the immune system (Figure 19-3). As a consequence, gene transfer may also be capable of favorably modulating the complex processes involved in producing tolerance to an antigen that had previously induced a potent allergic response.

Immature or developing lymphocytes are more susceptible to tolerance induction than mature, competent cells. During their development, all lymphocytes go through a stage in which self-antigen recognition leads to their death or inactivation and failure of this mechanism may lead to autoimmune disease. Elimination takes place in the generative lymphoid organs and is known as central tolerance. Of greater relevance to control of the allergic response, is the phenomenon of peripheral tolerance, which affects mature lymphocytes. Such tolerance may be due to passive unresponsiveness, or anergy, but it is now increasingly accepted that it may also be a more active process, in which antigen-specific regulatory T cells produce inhibitory signals that

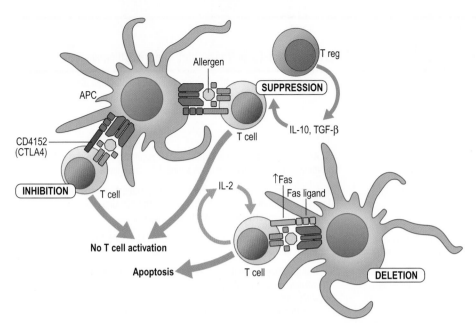

Figure 19-3 Mechanisms of peripheral tolerance induction.

down-regulate the activity of antigen-specific T helper cells that would otherwise induce an inflammatory or cytotoxic T cell response.

Anergy can be induced if the APCs presenting the antigen lack, or have had blocked, one or more of the critical costimulatory molecules involved during antigen-activation of T cells. Lacking appropriate costimulation, T cells are rendered incapable of responding to the antigen, even if the antigen is later presented by competent APCs. Peripheral tolerance may also be induced by activation-induced cell death, in which repeated stimulation of T lymphocytes by antigens induces IL-2 release and up-regulates Fas ligand, increasing the sensitivity of the T cells to Fas-mediated apoptosis, although the physiological importance of 'clonal exhaustion' is unclear.

Tregs also help regulate peripheral tolerance by actively suppressing other effector cells including Th1, Th2 and Th17 CD4+ T cells. Tregs also suppress IgE production by B cells and favor instead the production of IgG4 antibodies. They inhibit effector T cell migration to the tissues by interacting with blood vessel endothelial cells, suppress inflammatory dendritic cells and induce tolerogenic IL-10 producing DCs. Finally, they inhibit other effector cells within the allergic inflammatory cascade, including mast cells, basophils and eosinophils by both direct and indirect mechanisms.[77]

What Can Gene Therapy Do for the Allergic Patient?

Based on the cellular and molecular mechanisms underlying the immune response outlined above, it is possible to define several types of gene transfer intervention that could modify the nature of the allergic response. These are summarized in Table 19-2, and examples are illustrated below.

1. Correcting a Genetic Defect to Restore Cellular Function

A strong genetic component involved in allergic disorders has been observed in the clinic, but it was only recently that several genes playing a role in the susceptibility of individuals to developing these diseases have been identified.[78] Genes that direct CD4 T cell differentiation have been associated with asthma and asthma-like diseases.[78]

Unfortunately, we do not yet have a hierarchy of potency that can tell us which of these genes has the greatest effect, or how they are influenced by environmental triggers.[79] Although it is therefore premature to suggest specific gene modification or replacement targets for the treatment of allergic diseases, immune deficiency disorders provide an excellent model of the way gene replacement therapies might work, and also illustrate very clearly the limitations of the approach. Since the principles learned from these immunodeficiency studies will doubtless ultimately apply to gene correction efforts for allergic disorders, we will briefly describe the outcomes in one such trial.

Severe combined immunodeficiency diseases (SCID) due to common γ-chain deficiency or to adenosine deaminase (ADA) deficiency were amongst the first disorders treated by gene therapy. They were chosen not just because they were life-threatening diseases in which the relevant genes were well characterized, but also because studies of carriers showed that even a low level of correction could be beneficial, and/or that gene-corrected cells had a proliferative and survival advantage over the uncorrected population. (See 'Vector Safety Concerns' earlier in the chapter.)

ADA deficiency is a fatal immunodeficiency disorder resulting from abnormalities in purine metabolism. Autologous CD34+ bone marrow cells infected with a retrovirus encoding the ADA gene were infused in 10 patients, all of whom remained alive after a median follow-up of 4 years. Eight of these patients no longer require ADA enzyme-replacement therapy, and their blood cells have been demonstrated to express ADA with no signs of abnormal purine degradation.[65] No abnormal proliferative events have been observed in any hemopoietic lineage.

2. Changing the Effector Function of the Cell

One of the best examples of this approach in allergy is the modification of antigen-presenting cells so that they induce a tolerizing rather than an activating immune response. In the treatment of allergic disorders, one can envision modifying the effector

Table 19-2 Key Concepts What Gene Therapy Can Do

What Gene Therapy Can Do	General Examples	Examples for Gene Therapy of Allergic Disease
Restore cell function/correcting cell deficits	Transduction of target cells with deficient gene as in SCID common γchain deficiency → hematopoietic stem cells (HSCs) transduced with γc-retroviral vector	No example yet in view of the polygenic nature of the allergic diseases
Change the function of the cell	Indirect modification of DC/APC – resulting in immune-inhibition	CTLA4 gene transfer expands CD4+CD25+ regulatory T cells and induces production of the inhibitory indoleamine 2,3-dioxygenase in murine models
Produce a protein	Transduction of protein gene into target cells	Adenoviral transfer of allergen gene to sensitize subjects → state of tolerance Mucosal transfer of IL-12 and IFNγ to reduce Th2 cytokine expression Transfer of glucocorticoid receptor to epithelial cells
Produce an altered protein	Transduction of a mutant protein into cells to modify function of target cells	Administration of mutated versions of allergens to induce anergy in T cells specific for native allergen
Remove a protein	Administration of ribozymes, intracellular antibodies (intrabodies), antisense oligonucleotides, or siRNA	The use of ribozymes and antisense oligonucleotides targeting transcripts of cytokines mediating allergic response Intrakines that down-regulate chemokine receptors on T cells and reduce their ability to migrate in response to inflammatory signals
Provide insights into cell biology	Gene modification and/or marking of cells critical in cellular pathways to track function	Potentially could simulate activation or blockade of specific molecular pathways in specific cell types as a means to analyze components of the allergic response

function of CD4 T cells (allowing them to differentiate along the Treg pathway) or antigen-presenting cells (from stimulatory to tolerogenic DCs).

The exact mechanisms of Treg cell generation in vivo are still unknown. However, in theory, it would be feasible to adoptively transfer ex vivo generated T cells that have been cultured in the presence of transforming growth factor beta (TGFβ) to allow differentiation along the Treg pathway,[80] or Treg expanded from peripheral blood by culture in low dose IL-2.[81]

It may not be necessary to modify a DC directly, since T lymphocytes can also deliver negative regulatory signals to antigen-presenting cells, for example through the CTLA4 ligand. CTLA4 prevents the proinflammatory response of antigen-presenting cells by competing with stimulatory signals from CD28. Forced expression of this ligand in a proportion of T cells can mediate profound, generalized immune-inhibition[82] and this ability to antagonize positive costimulatory signals, could be used to inhibit allergen-specific responses.[83] This approach illustrates one of the important principles of gene transfer into immune system cells: modification of the behavior of even a small percentage of cells of a single subpopulation may influence not just the behavior of the modified cell, but the entire immune system, and produce distant actions on unmodified and apparently unrelated components.

Direct genetic modification of cellular behavior is also feasible. Transfer of the glucocorticoid receptor to epithelial cells is one such possibility. NFκB is a transcription factor, which is constitutively present within the cytoplasm bound to IκB molecules, which retain NFκB in an inactive state. Proinflammatory stimuli induce phosphorylation of the IκB molecules, leading to their degradation and transfer of NFκB to the nucleus where it is activated, and induces transcription of components that induce synthesis of the cytokine cascade. When corticosteroids bind their cytoplasmic receptor, the complex inhibits NFκB release. In vitro overexpression of the glucocorticoid receptor on the epithelial cell line A549, leads to repression of transcription factor-mediated cytokine gene transcription, an effect that might be of value in treatment of resistant asthma.[84] This type of approach would be likely to require a high proportion of cells to be gene

corrected in situ if there was to be any clinical benefit. It is not yet clear how this could be accomplished with our current vector systems.

3. Producing a Soluble Protein with Immunomodulating Activity

DNA plasmid-mediated gene transfer may be used to vaccinate patients with allergen genes, in a modified form of specific immunotherapy (SIT).[85,86] Conventional SIT using gradually increasing doses of standardized allergen extracts has been effective for many antigens, but is sometimes a high risk approach where potent allergens (e.g. latex) are used.[87] In addition, SIT requires inconveniently frequent injections over a prolonged period of time. In animal models, DNA vaccination appears to offer an alternative. Allergen encoding vectors consisting either of naked plasmid DNA or of recombinant mycoplasma[88–91] have been successfully used for the prophylaxis of atopic responses, reducing IgE titers, and shifting the immune response from Th2 to Th1. These actions lead to a decrease in airway hyper-responsiveness and anaphylactic hypersensitivity. Because this approach is less effective at modifying a pre-existing IgE response, efforts were made to boost its potency by substituting an adenoviral vector as the gene delivery system. For example, adenoviral vectors expressing the β-galactosidase enzyme can be given to mice intraperitoneally and the animals subsequently inoculated with β-galactosidase itself, using a route and schedule that normally induces a high level of IgE Ab and anaphylaxis. In the Ad β-gal mice, the development of specific IgE antibodies is blocked and the immune response shifted from a Th2 to a Th1 phenotype. Although it is unknown whether or not this approach would be significantly more effective at modulating a pre-existing IgE response than a simple plasmid, the approach is being investigated using several different allergenic protein genes.[92] Even if this immunization method can be effectively implemented for pre-existing immune responses, the approach has the fundamental limitation that it can only be effective when a small number of well-defined protein antigens are the cause of the allergic response. This criterion is met by some, but by no means all, of the atopy inducing allergens.

Plasmids have also been explored for use in food allergies, where SIT is considered to be excessively risky.[93] In the AKR/J mouse the main peanut allergen is Arah2. Anaphylaxis can be induced by combined oral and intraperitoneal sensitization with peanut extracts, followed by intraperitoneal challenge with recombinant Arah2. Chitosan, a natural polysaccharide found in crustacean shells, is nontoxic and biodegradable. It can be complexed with plasmid DNA to form stable nanoparticles that can be endocytosed by gastrointestinal epithelial cells. If an Arah2 plasmid is complexed with chitosan and fed to the AKR/J mice, there is an increase in serum IgG2a titers and a decrease in IgE titers compared to control mice. When the mice are sensitized and challenged there is substantial blunting of response in the plasmid/chitosan group versus the controls.[94] Further investigations and modifications of the latter strategy (the administration of chitosan and IFN-γ-DNA nanoparticles to OVA-sensitized mice) demonstrate that it can effectively reduce established allergen-induced airway inflammation and hyperresponsiveness.[95]

Distinct from the vaccination approach, transgenic production of soluble proteins may also be used to modify patterns of cytokine expression, in an effort to favor a less inflammatory immune response. This can be achieved either by increasing expression of the cytokines themselves or by changing expression of their receptors (see also 'Changing the Effector Function of the Cell' above). For example, in a mouse model of asthma, mucosal transfer of IL-12 and IFN-γ genes significantly reduced Th2 cytokine expression and bronchial hyperresponsiveness.[96,97]

Finally, it has been shown that a lactose-intolerant rat can be rendered lactose tolerant following oral administration of an adeno-associated viral vector encoding the beta-galactosidase (β-gal) transgene, which is expressed in both gut epithelial and lamina propria cells.[98] One highly speculative possibility, therefore, is that it might be possible to use gene transfer of an appropriate metabolizing enzyme so that potential allergens are simply destroyed before they have a chance to induce an immune response.

4. Express a Novel Engineered Protein

Until now we have focused on transfer of 'naturally occurring' genes, but of course it is also possible to transfer genes that have been bioengineered to have specific properties lacking in their natural counterparts. The availability of such genes affords a number of therapeutic opportunities. For example, the balance between a desirable and undesirable immune response in an allergic patient is determined in part by the pattern of cytokines produced. In the illustrations in section three above, we briefly outlined how transgenic cytokines or cytokine receptors could be used to alter the prevailing balance. A related alternative is to render cells more or less sensitive to a given cytokine by introducing genes for mutant receptors which have higher or lower affinity than the native receptor and which, ideally, have a dominant phenotype. As yet, there are no examples where this application has been used in allergy, but there are several cancer applications that are conceptually relevant. When patients with relapsed Epstein Barr virus (EBV) positive Hodgkin disease are treated with EBV-specific cytotoxic T lymphocytes (CTL), the activity of these cells is diminished by the high level of TGFβ the Hodgkin tumor cells produce.[99] To overcome this problem, CTL can first be transduced with a retrovirus vector expressing a mutant dominant-negative TGFβ type II receptor (DNR) which blocks TGFβ signal transduction and renders the CTL resistant

to the anticytolytic and antiproliferative effects of TGFβ.[100] If related effects were obtained following transduction of T cells from atopic patients with mutant IL-4 or IL-10 receptors, the prediction would be that generation of a Th2 response would now be less favored.

A novel engineered protein could also serve as a vaccine comprising the amino acid sequences of known allergens while restricting their epitope specificity to those recognized by T cells – effectively avoiding an IgE response. Such an approach using a recombinant protein (made of three different bee venom allergens modified to elicit T and not B cell responses) has been shown to prevent the secretion of IgE antibodies in chimeric protein-vaccinated mice after administration of a protein challenge. This chimeric protein also demonstrated reduced allergenicity in a skin-prick test when given to patients with bee venom allergy,[101] indicating clear potential for clinical application.

5. Removing a Function

While gene transfer can add or modify a pre-existing function in the immune system, it can also be used to remove an activity. One example given in section four above is the transfer of mutant cytokine receptors that are dominant negative inhibitors of the response. Much broader classes of 'function-removing agents' exist, of which the best studied are ribozymes, intrabodies, intrakines, and RNAi oligonucleotides.

Ribozymes are a unique class of RNA molecules that can catalytically cleave specific target mRNA leading to its degradation.[102] Intrabodies are single chain antibodies with Golgi retention signals incorporated into their sequence that can trap intracellular proteins before they reach their place of intracellular activity or are secreted by the cell.[103] Intrakines are chemokine fragments, again with Golgi retention signals, that trap cellular chemokine receptors before they appear on the cell surface. Antisense oligonucleotides hybridize with target mRNAs which mark them for destruction by activated RNAse H.[104] RNA interference (RNAi) is mediated by the action of small interfering RNAs (siRNAs) which are supplied by exogenously administered oligonucleotides, expressed by viral vectors or plasmids, or generated by the Dicer enzyme from long double-stranded RNA. siRNA is incorporated into a complex called RISC, which targets and binds mRNAs specific to the siRNA. These mRNAs are 'marked' for destruction, effectively ceasing its translation of proteins.[104]

These 'loss of function' molecules could therefore be used to prevent or treat allergic disorders. Ribozymes could destroy the transcripts for cytokines or cytokine receptors, and intrabodies could trap the equivalent proteins. Expression of intrakine genes would down-regulate chemokine receptors on T cells and reduce their ability to migrate in response to inflammatory or atopy-inducing signals. Unfortunately, however, the in vivo instability and limited biodistribution of all these molecules has largely precluded clinical development, and it is likely that additional technological advances will be necessary before this conceptual approach can be exploited.

6. Providing Insights into Cell Biology and Target Validation for Small Molecules

Gene transfer ultimately may have much to offer the treatment of the allergic disorders, but it is probable that for the next several years, its most important role will be to help us identify the

What Gene Therapy Cannot Do

- Produce a functional change in every cell
- Correct a deficit in every cell
- Produce tightly regulated transgenes
- Produce very high levels of products

cellular and molecular mechanisms underlying the allergic response and to help us to validate particular molecular targets for other therapeutic interventions. The ability to simulate activation or blockade of specific molecular pathways in specific cell types represents a powerful tool for analyzing the constituents of the allergic response, and over the next decade we can expect our knowledge of the molecular and cellular basis of allergic diseases to improve. We can also anticipate an improvement in the technology for efficiently transferring genes in a targeted, safe, and controlled manner. As our knowledge and our practical capabilities both increase, we can expect to see gene transfer making a significant contribution to the alleviation and cure of allergic diseases.

Conclusions

It is too early to assign a role for gene therapy in the treatment of allergic diseases, and we have outlined instead, the potential strengths and current weaknesses of this technology (Table 19-2 and Box 19-1). We have offered potential examples of how gene transfer can be applied to the allergic disorders. Our prediction is that the transfer of antiinflammatory/immunomodulatory genes will provide a convenient way of controlling the allergic response, while exploitation of effective oral gene therapy, in combination with the mucosal route of antigen presentation, will be valuable for induction of antigenic tolerance. But although a dismayingly large gap remains between the theory and potential application of gene therapy to allergic disorders and the clinical reality, our improved understanding of the molecular basis of the allergic response and its regulation, coupled to improvements in vector production and cell culture technology, should allow at least some of the promise to be fulfilled.

References

1. Buchschacher GL Jr, Wong-Staal F. Development of lentiviral vectors for gene therapy for human diseases. Blood 2000;95:2499–504.
2. High KA. Gene therapy: a 2001 perspective. Haemophilia 2001;7 (Suppl 1):23–7.
3. Hitt MM, Graham FL. Adenovirus vectors for human gene therapy. Adv Virus Res 2000;55:479–505.
4. Kay MA, Glorioso JC, Naldini L. Viral vectors for gene therapy: the art of turning infectious agents into vehicles of therapeutics. Nat Med 2001;7:33–40.
5. Xu K, Ma H, McCown TJ, et al. Generation of a stable cell line producing high-titer self-inactivating lentiviral vectors. Mol Ther 2001;3: 97–104.
6. Rossi FM, Blau HM. Recent advances in inducible gene expression systems. Curr Opin Biotechnol 1998;9:451–6.
7. Wang Y, O'Malley BWJ, Tsai SY, et al. A regulatory system for use in gene transfer. Proc Natl Acad Aci USA 1994;91:8180–4.
8. Senzer N, Mani S, Rosemurgy A, et al. TNFerade biologic, an adenovector with a radiation-inducible promoter, carrying the human tumor necrosis factor alpha gene: a phase I study in patients with solid tumors. J Clin Oncol 2004;22:592–601.
9. Hacein-Bey-Abina S, Le Deist F, Carlier F, et al. Sustained correction of X-linked severe combined immunodeficiency by ex vivo gene therapy. N Engl J Med 2002;346:1185–93.
10. Brenner MK. Gene marking. Gene Ther 1996;3:278–9.
11. Bollard CM, Heslop HE, Brenner MK. Gene-marking studies of hematopoietic cells. Int J Hematol 2001;73:14–22.
12. Wivel NA, Wilson JM. Methods of gene delivery. Hematol Oncol Clin North Am 1998;12:483–501.
13. Journal of Gene Medicine. Gene therapy clinical trials worldwide. 2009.
14. Miller AD. Cell-surface receptors for retroviruses and implications for gene transfer. Proc Natl Acad Sci USA 1996;93:11407–13.
15. Lam JS, Reeves ME, Cowherd R, et al. Improved gene transfer into human lymphocytes using retroviruses with the gibbon ape leukemia virus envelope. Hum Gene Ther 1996;7:1415–22.
16. Kelly PF, Vandergriff J, Nathwani A, et al. Highly efficient gene transfer into cord blood nonobese diabetic/severe combined immunodeficiency repopulating cells by oncoretroviral vector particles pseudotyped with the feline endogenous retrovirus (RD114) envelope protein. Blood 2000;96:1206–14.
17. Miller DG, Adam MA, Miller AD. Gene transfer by retrovirus vectors occurs only in cells that are actively replicating at the time of infection [published erratum appears in Mol Cell Biol 1992 Jan;12:433]. Mol Cell Biol 1990;10:4239–42.
18. Tisdale JF, Hanazono Y, Sellers SE, et al. Ex vivo expansion of genetically marked rhesus peripheral blood progenitor cells results in diminished long-term repopulating ability. Blood 1998;92:1131–41.
19. Pollok KE, Hanenberg H, Noblitt TW, et al. High-efficiency gene transfer into normal and adenosine deaminase-deficient T lymphocytes is mediated by transduction on recombinant fibronectin fragments. J Virol 1998;72:4882–92.
20. Hacein-Bey-Abina S, Garrigue A, Wang GP, et al. Insertional oncogenesis in 4 patients after retrovirus-mediated gene therapy of SCID-X1. J Clin Invest 2008;118:3132–42.
21. Amado RG, Chen IS. Lentiviral vectors: the promise of gene therapy within reach? Science 1999;285:674–6.
22. Sutton RE, Wu HT, Rigg R, et al. Human immunodeficiency virus type 1 vectors efficiently transduce human hematopoietic stem cells. J Virol 1998;72:5781–8.
23. Case SS, Price MA, Jordan CT, et al. Stable transduction of quiescent CD34(+)CD38(–) human hematopoietic cells by HIV-1-based lentiviral vectors. Proc Natl Acad Sci USA 1999;96:2988–93.
24. Naldini L, Blomer U, Gallay P, et al. In vivo gene delivery and stable transduction of nondividing cells by a lentiviral vector. Science 1996;272:263–7.
25. Yu SF, Von Ruden T, Kantoff PW, et al. Self-inactivating retroviral vectors designed for transfer of whole genes into mammalian cells. Proc Natl Acad Sci USA 1986;83:3194–8.
26. Levine BL, Humeau LM, Boyer J, et al. Gene transfer in humans using a conditionally replicating lentiviral vector. Proc Natl Acad Sci USA 2006;103:17372–7.
27. Alton E, Kitson C. Gene therapy for cystic fibrosis. 1. Expert Opin Investig Drugs 2000;9:1523–35.
28. Balague C, Zhou J, Dai Y, et al. Sustained high-level expression of full-length human factor VIII and restoration of clotting activity in hemophilic mice using a minimal adenovirus vector. Blood 2000;95: 820–8.
29. Gardlik R, Palffy R, Hodosy J, et al. Vectors and delivery systems in gene therapy. Med Sci Monit 2005;11:RA110–21.
30. Michou AI, Santoro L, Christ M, et al. Adenovirus-mediated gene transfer: influence of transgene, mouse strain and type of immune response on persistence of transgene expression. Gene Ther 1997;4:473–82.
31. Ferber D. Gene therapy: safer and virus-free? Science 2001;294: 1638–42.
32. Thomas CE, Ehrhardt A, Kay MA. Progress and problems with the use of viral vectors for gene therapy. Nat Rev Genet 2003;4:346–58.
33. Morsy MA, Caskey CT. Expanded-capacity adenoviral vectors: the helper-dependent vectors. Mol Med Today 1999;5:18–24.
34. Morral N, O'Neal W, Rice K, et al. Administration of helper-dependent adenoviral vectors and sequential delivery of different vector serotype for long-term liver-directed gene transfer in baboons. Proc Natl Acad Aci USA 1999;96:12816–21.
35. Inoue N, Russell DW. Packaging cells based on inducible gene amplification for the production of adeno-associated virus vectors. J Virol 1998;72:7024–31.
36. Miao CH, Nakai H, Thompson AR, et al. Nonrandom transduction of recombinant adeno-associated virus vectors in mouse hepatocytes in vivo: cell cycling does not influence hepatocyte transduction. J Virol 2000;74:3793–803.
37. Buning H, Perabo L, Coutelle O, et al. Recent developments in adeno-associated virus vector technology. J Gene Med 2008;10:717–73.
38. Rabinowitz JE, Samulski RJ. Building a better vector: the manipulation of AAV virions. Virology 2000;278:301–8.
39. Manno CS, Pierce GF, Arruda VR, et al. Successful transduction of liver in hemophilia by AAV-Factor IX and limitations imposed by the host immune response. Nat Med 2006;12:342–7.

40. Maguire AM, Simonelli F, Pierce EA, et al. Safety and efficacy of gene transfer for Leber's congenital amaurosis. N Engl J Med 2008;358: 2240–8.

41. Bainbridge JW, Smith AJ, Barker SS, et al. Effect of gene therapy on visual function in Leber's congenital amaurosis. N Engl J Med 2008;358: 2231–9.

42. Feigin A, Kaplitt MG, Tang C, et al. Modulation of metabolic brain networks after subthalamic gene therapy for Parkinson's disease. Proc Natl Acad Sci USA 2007;104:19559–64.

43. Wolfe D, Goins WF, Kaplan TJ, et al. Herpesvirus-mediated systemic delivery of nerve growth factor. Mol Ther 2001;3:61–9.

44. Samaniego LA, Neiderhiser L, DeLuca NA. Persistence and expression of the herpes simplex virus genome in the absence of immediate-early proteins. J Virol 1998;72:3307–20.

45. Krisky DM, Marconi PC, Oligino TJ, et al. Development of herpes simplex virus replication-defective multigene vectors for combination gene therapy applications. Gene Ther 1998;5:1517–30.

46. Chancellor MB, Yoshimura N, Pruchnic R, et al. Gene therapy strategies for urological dysfunction. Trends Mol Med 2001;7:301–6.

47. Martino G, Poliani PL, Marconi PC, et al. Cytokine gene therapy of autoimmune demyelination revisited using herpes simplex virus type-1-derived vectors. Gene Ther 2000;7:1087–93.

48. Burton EA, Glorioso JC. Multi-modal combination gene therapy for malignant glioma using replication-defective HSV vectors. Drug Discov Today 2001;6:347–56.

49. Dilloo D, Rill D, Entwistle C, et al. A novel herpes vector for the high efficiency transduction of normal and malignant human hemopoietic cells. Blood 1997;89:119–27.

50. Li X, Eastman EM, Schwartz RJ, et al. Synthetic muscle promoters: activities exceeding naturally occurring regulatory sequences. Nat Biotechnol 1999;17:241–5.

51. Nabel GJ, Nabel EG, Yang ZY, et al. Direct gene transfer with DNA-liposome complexes in melanoma: expression, biologic activity, and lack of toxicity in humans. Proc Natl Acad Sci USA 1993;90(23):11307–11.

52. Templeton NS, Lasic DD. New directions in liposome gene delivery. Mol Biotechnol 1999;11:175–80.

53. Seemann S, Hauff P, Schultze-Mosgau M, et al. Pharmaceutical evaluation of gas-filled microparticles as gene delivery system. Pharm Res 2002;19:250–7.

54. Seemann S, Hauff P, Schultze-Mosgau M, et al. Pharmaceutical evaluation of gas-filled microparticles as gene delivery system. Pharm Res 2002;19:250–7.

55. Roth DA, Tawa NE Jr, O'Brien JM, et al. Nonviral transfer of the gene encoding coagulation factor VIII in patients with severe hemophilia A. N Engl J Med 2001;344:1735–42.

56. Yant SR, Meuse L, Chiu W, et al. Somatic integration and long-term transgene expression in normal and haemophilic mice using a DNA transposon system. Nat Genet 2000;25:35–41.

57. Liu H, Visner GA. Applications of Sleeping Beauty transposons for non-viral gene therapy. IUBMB Life 2007;59:374–9.

58. Glover DJ, Lipps HJ, Jans DA. Towards safe, non-viral therapeutic gene expression in humans. Nat Rev Genet 2005;6:299–310.

59. Donahue RE, Kessler SW, Bodine D, et al. Helper virus induced T cell lymphoma in nonhuman primates after retroviral mediated gene transfer. J Exp Med 1992;176:1125–35.

60. Howe SJ, Mansour MR, Schwarzwaelder K, et al. Insertional mutagenesis combined with acquired somatic mutations causes leukemogenesis following gene therapy of SCID-X1 patients. J Clin Invest 2008;118(9): 3143–50.

61. Fischer A, Cavazzana-Calvo M. Gene therapy of inherited diseases. Lancet 2008;371:2044–7.

62. Ott MG, Schmidt M, Schwarzwaelder K, et al. Correction of X-linked chronic granulomatous disease by gene therapy, augmented by insertional activation of MDS1-EVI1, PRDM16 or SETBP1. Nat Med 2006;12:401–9.

63. Dave UP, Jenkins NA, Copeland NG. Gene therapy insertional mutagenesis insights. Science 2004;303:333.

64. Scobie L, Hector RD, Grant L, et al. A novel model of SCID-X1 reconstitution reveals predisposition to retrovirus-induced lymphoma but no evidence of gammaC gene oncogenicity. Mol Ther 2009;17:1031–8.

65. Aiuti A, Cattaneo F, Galimberti S, et al. Gene therapy for immunodeficiency due to adenosine deaminase deficiency. N Engl J Med 2009;360: 447–58.

66. Brenner M. Gene transfer by adenovectors. Blood 1999;94:3965–7.

67. Raper SE, Chirmule N, Lee FS, et al. Fatal systemic inflammatory response syndrome in a ornithine transcarbamylase deficient patient following adenoviral gene transfer. Mol Genet Metab 2003;80:148–58.

68. Holgate ST, Polosa R. Treatment strategies for allergy and asthma. Nat Rev Immunol 2008;8:218–30.

69. Coffman RL, Carty J. A T cell activity that enhances polyclonal IgE production and its inhibition by interferon-gamma. J Immunol 1986; 136:949–54.

70. Minty A, Chalon P, Derocq JM, et al. Interleukin-13 is a new human lymphokine regulating inflammatory and immune responses. Nature 1993;362:248–50.

71. Kawabe T, Naka T, Yoshida K, et al. The immune responses in CD40-deficient mice: impaired immunoglobulin class switching and germinal center formation. Immunity 1994;1:167–78.

72. Wenzel SE, Schwartz LB, Langmack EL, et al. Evidence that severe asthma can be divided pathologically into two inflammatory subtypes with distinct physiologic and clinical characteristics. Am J Respir Crit Care Med 1999;160:1001–8.

73. Sun YC, Zhou QT, Yao WZ. Sputum interleukin-17 is increased and associated with airway neutrophilia in patients with severe asthma. Chin Med J (Engl) 2005;118:953–6.

74. Schwartz RH. Costimulation of T lymphocytes: the role of CD28, CTLA-4, and B7/BB1 in Interleukin-2 production and immunotherapy. Cell 1992;71:1065–8.

75. Keane-Myers AM, Gause WC, Finkelman FD, et al. Development of murine allergic asthma is dependent upon B7-2 costimulation. J Immunol 1998;160:1036–43.

76. Kuchroo VK, Das MP, Brown JA, et al. B7-1 and B7-2 costimulatory molecules activate differentially the Th1/Th2 developmental pathways: application to autoimmune disease therapy. Cell 1995;80:707–18.

77. Akdis CA, Akdis M. Mechanisms and treatment of allergic disease in the big picture of regulatory T cells. J Allergy Clin Immunol 2009;123: 735–46.

78. Vercelli D. Discovering susceptibility genes for asthma and allergy. Nat Rev Immunol 2008;8:169–82.

79. Isidoro-Garcia M, vila-Gonzalez I, Pascual de PM, et al. Interactions between genes and the environment: epigenetics in allergy. Allergol Immunopathol (Madr) 2007;35:254–8.

80. Eghtesad S, Morel PA, Clemens PR. The companions: regulatory T cells and gene therapy. Immunol 2009;127:1–7.

81. Godfrey WR, Ge YG, Spoden DJ, et al. In vitro-expanded human CD4(+) CD25(+) T-regulatory cells can markedly inhibit allogeneic dendritic cell-stimulated MLR cultures. Blood 2004;104:453–61.

82. Li W, Li B, Fan W, et al. CTLA4Ig gene transfer alleviates abortion in mice by expanding CD4(+)CD25(+) regulatory T cells and inducing indoleamine 2,3-dioxygenase. J Reprod Immunol 2009;80:1–11.

83. Wan H, Zhou M, Xu Q, et al. The role of CTLA4-Ig in a mouse model against allergic asthma. Chin Med J (Engl) 2003;116:462–4.

84. Mathieu M, Gougat C, Jaffuel D, et al. The glucocorticoid receptor gene as a candidate for gene therapy in asthma. Gene Ther 1999;6: 245–52.

85. Durham SR, Walker SM, Varga EM, et al. Long-term clinical efficacy of grass-pollen immunotherapy. N Engl J Med 1999;341:468–75.

86. Bousquet J, Michel FB. Specific immunotherapy in asthma. Allergy Proc 1994;15:329–33.

87. Leynadier F, Herman D, Vervloet D, et al. Specific immunotherapy with a standardized latex extract versus placebo in allergic healthcare workers. J Allergy Clin Immunol 2000;106:585–90.

88. Janssen R, Kruisselbrink A, Hoogteijling L, et al. Analysis of recombinant mycobacteria as T helper type 1 vaccines in an allergy challenge model. Immunol 2001;102:441–9.

89. Raz E, Tighe H, Sato Y, et al. Preferential induction of a Th1 immune response and inhibition of specific IgE antibody formation by plasmid DNA immunization. Proc Natl Acad Sci USA 1996;93:5141–5.

90. Hsu CH, Chua KY, Tao MH, et al. Immunoprophylaxis of allergen-induced immunoglobulin E synthesis and airway hyperresponsiveness in vivo by genetic immunization. Nat Med 1996;2:540–4.

91. Horner AA, Nguyen MD, Ronaghy A, et al. DNA-based vaccination reduces the risk of lethal anaphylactic hypersensitivity in mice. J Allergy Clin Immunol 2000;106:349–56.

92. Sudowe S, Montermann E, Steitz J, et al. Efficacy of recombinant adenovirus as vector for allergen gene therapy in a mouse model of type I allergy. Gene Ther 2002;9:147–56.

93. Moffatt MF, Cookson WO. Gene therapy for peanut allergy. Nat Med 1999;5:380–1.

94. Roy K, Mao HQ, Huang SK, et al. Oral gene delivery with chitosan–DNA nanoparticles generates immunologic protection in a murine model of peanut allergy. Nat Med 1999;5:387–391.

95. Kumar M, Kong X, Behera AK, et al. Chitosan IFN-gamma-pDNA Nanoparticle (CIN) Therapy for allergic asthma. Genet Vaccines Ther 2003;1:3.

96. Hogan SP, Foster PS, Tan X, et al. Mucosal IL-12 gene delivery inhibits allergic airways disease and restores local antiviral immunity. Eur J Immunol 1998;28:413–23.

97. Dow SW, Schwarze J, Heath TD, et al. Systemic and local interferon gamma gene delivery to the lungs for treatment of allergen-induced airway hyperresponsiveness in mice. Hum. Gene Ther 1999;10: 1905–14.

98. During MJ, Xu R, Young D, et al. Peroral gene therapy of lactose intolerance using an adeno-associated virus vector. Nat Med 1998;4:1131–5.

99. Poppema S, Potters M, Visser L, et al. Immune escape mechanisms in Hodgkin's disease. Ann Oncol 1998;9(Suppl 5):S21–4.

100. Bollard CM, Rossig C, Calonge MJ, et al. Adapting a transforming growth factor beta-related tumor protection strategy to enhance antitumor immunity. Blood 2002;99:3179–87.

101. Sudowe S, Ludwig-Portugall I, Montermann E, et al. Prophylactic and therapeutic intervention in IgE responses by biolistic DNA vaccination primarily targeting dendritic cells. J Allergy Clin Immunol 2006;117: 196–203.

102. Lewin AS, Hauswirth WW. Ribozyme gene therapy: applications for molecular medicine. Trends Mol Med 2001;7:221–8.

103. Marasco WA, Dana JS. Antibodies for targeted gene therapy: extracellular gene targeting and intracellular expression. Adv Drug Deliv Rev 1998;31:153–70.

104. Popescu FD. Antisense- and RNA interference-based therapeutic strategies in allergy. J Cell Mol Med 2005;9:840–53.

Hematopoietic Stem Cell Transplantation and Gene Therapy for Primary Immune Deficiency Diseases

Alan K. Ikeda • Donald B. Kohn

Primary Immune Deficiencies and Hematopoietic Stem Cell Transplantation

The primary immune deficiencies (PIDs) result from mutations of genes involved in the production, function, or survival of leukocytes. Therefore, PIDs can be treated by performing hematopoietic stem cell transplantations (HSCTs) that provide these patients with a new source of genetically normal leukocytes. The first successful clinical allogeneic bone marrow transplant (BMT) was performed in 1968 for a patient with severe combined immune deficiency (SCID), resulting in sustained reconstitution of immunity lasting for a decade.[1] Since that time, allogeneic HSCT has become the standard of care for patients with SCID, and is often used for patients with other severe, life-threatening forms of PID, including Wiskott-Aldrich syndrome (WAS), X-linked hyper-IgM (CD154 or gp39 deficiency), leukocyte adhesion deficiency (LAD), X-linked lymphoproliferative syndrome (XLP), chronic granulomatous disease (CGD), hemophagocytic lymphohistiocytosis (HLH), and immune dysregulation, polyendocrinopathy, enteropathy, X-linked syndrome (IPEX). Patients with less severe PID, especially those primarily affecting antibody production that can be replaced with intravenous gammaglobulin administration, generally are not treated with HSCT.

The major barriers to allogeneic HSCT are immunologic. In solid organ transplantation, a recipient's T cells can reject the organ donor's cells. Graft rejection is less of a problem in severely immune deficient recipients, such as patients with SCID who lack T, B and NK cell function. In some of the PIDs that retain partial function of the immune system, a significant risk for graft rejection remains. In most cases, transplant recipients need partial or essentially complete ablation of their endogenous immune and hematopoietic systems to achieve enduring engraftment of donor HSCs.

The flip-side of graft rejection, which is mostly limited to HSCT and only rarely encountered in solid organ transplant, is graft versus host disease (GvHD) where the T cells from the donor that are given with the allogeneic bone marrow can, in effect, reject the recipient's cells. GvHD can be severe, chronic and even fatal, with these complications increasing in frequency and severity with increasing degree of mismatch between the donor and the recipient. Efforts to prevent or suppress GvHD, by administration of immune suppressive medications or by depleting the donor's mature T lymphocytes from the graft, often result in prolonged immune deficiency, which poses high risks for

opportunistic infections, especially beyond the infant period when patients may bear latent herpesviruses (e.g. cytomegalovirus [CMV], human herpes virus [HHV]-6).

Severe Combined Immune Deficiency (SCID)

Severe combined immune deficiency (SCID) is the most severe of the PIDs, with inherited absence of T and B cell function (and variable NK activity). In the absence of medical intervention, infants with SCID suffer a high rate of early mortality from infections. SCID is a clinical phenotype which may result from defects in any one of more than 12 genes (Box 20-1), including the receptors or downstream-signaling molecules for lymphoid cytokines (the common cytokine receptor γ chain {γc} in the X-linked form [XSCID], Jak3 kinase, IL-7 receptor chain α, Zap70 kinase, CD45, CD3δ, CD3ε), the genes involved in the DNA recombinatorial events leading to generation of diverse immunoglobulin and T cell receptors (Rag-1/2, Artemis, DNA PKcs), and enzymes of purine metabolism (adenosine deaminase [ADA] and purine nucleoside phosphorylase [PNP]). The clinical research associated with the treatment of human SCID has produced many of the major advances in the field of HSCT[1-6] (Box 20-2).

Allogeneic BMT can be curative for SCID when bone marrow from a human leucocyte antigen (HLA)-matched sibling donor (MSD) is used, with most centers reporting greater than 90% long-term survival. PID patients who receive an allogeneic HSC transplant from an HLA-MSD in general, achieve high rates of immune reconstitution and good quality of life. For patients with SCID, HLA-MSD marrow can be infused without 'conditioning' with chemotherapy or total body irradiation and will appropriately restore T cell function in most patients. Most other PIDs require full or partial marrow 'conditioning' for proper engraftment of donor cells without rejection.

Methods to deplete T lymphocytes from bone marrow in order to limit GvHD risks were developed in the mid-1970s. T cell depletion allowed the use of marrow from donors other than fully matched siblings (Box 20-3). Using approaches to deplete T cells, marrow from parental donors, who are only matched by one HLA haplotype and therefore mismatched for a full HLA haplotype, have been frequently used for SCID patients lacking an HLA-matched donor. Without T cell depletion, severe GvHD would be likely, from the high frequency of T cells from the parent that would react against the HLA proteins inherited from the other parent. Using T cell-depleted haploidentical transplants,

thereof, of pretransplant conditioning with chemotherapy or other immune suppressive medications to facilitate long-term engraftment of donor HSCs. In the absence of conclusive data from randomized clinical trials, there are strong advocates of either of these approaches. Rebecca Buckley and colleagues at Duke University have performed haploidentical transplants for SCID patients for more than 3 decades, giving T cell depleted bone marrow from a parent without any conditioning therapy or immune suppressive medicines to prevent graft versus host disease.[8] They have reported 78% survival in 77 SCID patients treated by this technique, with most having clinically protective T cell reconstitution. Needless to say, none of these patients experienced any of the complications associated with chemotherapy. However, more than half of them have had inadequate B cell reconstitution and were reported to still require regular administration with intravenous gammaglobulin, possibly indicating a failure to engraft sufficient numbers of HSCs in the absence of marrow conditioning. Some of these patients have had successful T cell immune reconstitution lasting decades, although it will take longer observation to assess the longevity of T cell function.

Use of cytoreductive conditioning prior to HSCT for SCID typically leads to donor cell chimerism in all lineages, indicating replacement of the endogenous HSCs with those of the donor. This full donor engraftment may lead to more sustained production of new T cells and may lead to increased numbers and activity of B and NK cells. However, the acute and long-term toxicities of the chemoablative regimens may lead to increased toxicity and mortality in the initial period, especially in patients with preexisting infections, and may cause long-term growth, endocrinological and neurocognitive abnormalities.[9,10]

Historically, less has been done using matched unrelated donor marrow (MUD) or cord blood for transplantation of SCID patients who do not have an HLA-MSD. As the National Marrow Donor Program has developed an increasingly large database of potential MUD donors of marrow and cord blood, the availability of this treatment option has grown for patients with PID. HSC transplantation using MUD or cord blood carries increased risks for GvHD, compared to the use of marrow from an MSD. The frequency of severe GvHD in MUD marrow and cord blood HSC transplantation is in the range of 25–50% and 20–40%, respectively. In addition, HSC transplantation with cord blood has a risk for nonengraftment between 10–20%. These increased complication risks are likely to be due to more mismatches for non-HLA (minor) antigens. Generally, full cytoablation and GvHD prophylaxis (i.e. posttransplant immune suppression) are needed to prevent graft rejection or GvHD. Recent advances in HLA typing methods that utilize precise determination of the HLA genotypes, rather than the earlier less discriminative determination of serological phenotype, improves the quality of matching and the resultant outcomes and may benefit patients with PID.[11]

One large series compared the outcomes of BMT for SCID who received haploidentical or MUD donors.[12] This was a retrospective analysis of 94 patients with SCID receiving BMT between 1990–2004 at the Hospital for Sick Children in Toronto, Ontario, and the Department of Pediatrics at the University of Brescia, Italy (Table 20-1). Survival was significantly higher in recipients of MUD marrow (80.5%) than haploidentical transplants (52.5%), although a high percentage of the MUD recipients developed GvHD. At present, in the absence of a clear-cut optimal approach, the experience of individual centers with a specific approach is likely the most important factor in determining outcome. An effort in the USA to formally combine data from major transplant centers may provide additional guidance.[13]

50–80% of SCID patients have realized long-term survival.[7,8] While this transplant option has been invaluable for the successfully treated patients, nevertheless, haploidentical donor transplants have relatively poorer outcomes compared to MSD transplants. For example, in a comprehensive review on the outcome of HSCT for PIDs in Europe that analyzed 475 SCID patients, 3-year survival with sustained engraftment was significantly better after HLA-identical than after mismatched transplantation (77% vs 54%; p = 0.002).[7] The lower success rate with haploidentical transplants may reflect the morbidity and mortality associated with: (1) the increased risks of graft rejection and/or GvHD, (2) the T cell depletion that is utilized to prevent GVHD which slows immune reconstitution and prolongs the period of increased susceptibility to infections, and (3) the adverse effects that are secondary to the use of chemotherapy to make space and eliminate residual immunity.

One of the ongoing controversies about the optimal approach to haploidentical HSCT for SCID concerns the necessity, or lack

Table 20-1 Comparison of Outcomes by Donor Sources Used in HSCT for SCID

Donor Source	Matched Sibling (n = 13)	Haploidentical (n = 40)	Matched Unrelated (n = 41)
Survival	12/13 (92.3%)	21/40 (52.5%)	33/41 (80.5%)
Engraftment	13/13 (100%)	28/40 (70%)	38/41 (92.7%)
aGVHD	4/13 (30.7%)	18/40 (45%)	30/41 (73.1%)

Grunebaum E, Mazzolari E, Porta F, et al. JAMA 2006;295:508.

Wiskott-Aldrich Syndrome

Wiskott-Aldrich syndrome (WAS) is an X-linked immune deficiency characterized by the triad of recurrent infections, thrombocytopenia, and eczema. The gene that encodes for the WAS protein is located on Xp11.22-23. WAS protein is an integral part of actin polymerization. As a result, defects in the protein result in problems with cellular signaling and the cytoskeleton. Mortality is a consequence of increased risk of severe infections, autoimmune disorders, malignancies, and hemorrhage. Bach and colleagues performed the first sibling HSCT for WAS.[14] MSD HSCT provides the best outcome for WAS patients and is established as the standard of care when available. WAS patients treated with HSCT (n = 170) between the years 1980–1996 were evaluated by the CIBMTR.[15] MSD (n = 55), other related donor (n = 48), and unrelated donor (n = 67) HSCT resulted in an overall 5-year probability of survival of 70%. It is difficult to know if this exceeds the natural history with conservative medical care. As a whole, donor sources had an obvious effect on 5-year survival, which were HLA-MSDs 87% (74–93%), other related donors (mostly haploidentical) 52% (37–65%), and unrelated donors 71% (58–80%). The patients who were less than 5 years old and received an HLA-MUD HSCT had survival rates similar to those who received an HLA-MSD HSCT. The European experience has also shown a significant difference in outcome based on the donor source. The 7-year event-free survival rates after HSCT for WAS were: HLA-MSD 88%, other related donor 55% (p = 0.003), and HLA-MUD 71% (p = 0.03). A post-HSCT complication, relatively unique to WAS, is post-HSCT autoimmune disease, not attributed to GvHD. The frequency of this was as high as 28% in the MUD group and 26% in the other related group, but just 11% in the HLA-MSD group. 71% of the patients who had mixed chimerism of donor engraftment and retained some of their endogenous hematopoietic systems exhibited autoimmunity, while those who achieved full donor chimerism had significantly less at 8% (p = 0.001).[7] Overall, HLA-MSD HSCT in patients who are less than 5 years of age and achieve full donor chimerism have the best outcome, but if an MSD is unavailable, a matched unrelated donor HSCT is a viable option.

Chronic Granulomatous Disease

Chronic granulomatous disease (CGD) is a genetic syndrome that may be inherited in an autosomal recessive or X-linked pattern and subsequently leads to an error in one of the four protein subunits responsible for mounting an antimicrobial oxidative burst. Due to dysfunctional NADPH oxidase in phagocytes, patients with CGD are susceptible to severe infections, especially *Staph. aureus* and *Aspergillus*. T cell and B cell functions are intact. Although these patients are classified under one syndrome, the natural course is quite heterogeneous. It is estimated that the median lifespan is 20 to 25 years and the mortality rate is 2–5% per year.[16]

Since many CGD patients live into their adulthood, in contrast to the near certain early mortality of SCID, they often choose against the risks and complications that are associated with a myeloablative HSCT. One study evaluated 27 (25 pediatric) CGD patients who received an HLA-MSD HSCT. 23/27 patients were conditioned using a myeloablative busulfan-based regimen. Overall survival was 85% and 22/23 were cured of CGD. There was survival in all 18 of the patients who received an HLA-MSD HSCT while they were free of infection. Those patients who engrafted did not show any evidence of ongoing infections nor the inflammatory lesions that were present prior to HSCT.[17,18] A group in the UK has shown that umbilical cord transplant can be curative for patients with CGD.[19] However, nonengraftment rates with cord blood have historically been greater in comparison to peripheral blood and bone marrow transplants. Two patients have been successfully transplanted with a second cord transplant after failed engraftment of the first.[20]

As previously mentioned, the toxicities of myeloablative HSCT may outweigh the risks of a disease that allows many patients to live into their adulthood. Theoretically, reduced intensity conditioning decreases the toxicity associated with the conditioning regimen and T cell depletion decreases the risks for GvHD. Horwitz and colleagues performed HLA-MSD peripheral blood stem cell transplants (PBSCT) for 5 adults and 5 children with CGD. The infused product was T cell depleted (> 5.0×10^6 CD34+ cells/kg with 1.0×10^5 CD3+ T cells/kg) and the conditioning regimen was a nonmyeloablative (mainly immune suppressive) regimen that consisted of Cytoxan 120 mg/kg, fludarabine 125 mg/m^2, and ATG 160 mg/kg. If donor T cells were less than 60% of the total circulating CD3+ T cells after transplant, then donor lymphocyte infusions (DLI) were administered every 30 days and decreased to every 90 days after the cessation of cyclosporine to attempt to sustain donor engraftment. At a median of 17 months (8 to 26), 8 of 10 patients showed at least 33% donor chimerism with 6 having full donor chimerism. Two patients did not engraft and died. One patient with mixed chimerism died secondarily to complications of a second HSCT 1 year after the first transplant. While 3 of the 4 adult patients who engrafted exhibited grade II–IV acute GvHD, none of the pediatric patients had any significant GvHD. For the 7 surviving patients, preexisting granulomatous lesions resolved.[21] These outcomes are not markedly better than those with fully ablative HSCT.

Hemophagocytic Lymphohistiocytosis

Hemophagocytic lymphohistiocytosis (HLH) is a rare disorder that is characterized by highly activated macrophages and lymphocytes. Primary or familial HLH is an autosomal recessive disease, while secondary HLH is an acquired form that is usually associated with a viral illness. While initially considered to be a malignant disorder of histiocytes, more recent understanding of HLH classifies it as a PID, with defects in T cell effector function, such as perforin, leading to a failure to control activated macrophages. The diagnosis of HLH can be made on the presence of hemophagocytosis and 5 of 8 of the following: fever, splenomegaly, bicytopenia, hypertriglyceridemia, hypofibrinogenemia, low/absent NK-cell-activity, hyperferritinemia, and high-soluble interleukin-2-receptor levels. If there is a strong family history or molecular diagnosis, then fulfillment of the criteria is not necessary. The first curative HSCT for HLH was performed in 1986.[22] Currently, standard treatment according to the HLH-2004 protocol developed by the Histiocyte Society is induction immunochemotherapy with etoposide, dexamethasone, and cyclosporine A, followed by HSCT for the familial type. HSCT is reserved for persistent or relapsed disease in the acquired form of the disease. An earlier clinical trial, HLH-94, showed that the outcomes with MUD HSCT were equivalent to those with HLA-MSD HSCT (67 vs 68%). Patients who received transplants from related donors (usually haploidentical) had a survival rate of 43%.[23,24]

Other Primary Immune Deficiencies Amenable to Hematopoietic Stem Cell Transplantation

HSCTs have been done for many of the other severe PIDs, including X-linked hyper IgM, XLP, IPEX, etc. with similar findings of immune restoration, but risks from conditioning and GvHD. Less severe PIDs, such as X-linked agammaglobulinemia, common variable immune deficiency, selective antibody defects, etc. have not been routinely subjected to HSCT, since the risks of HSCT may exceed those of the underlying disorders. When HSCT advances to a state where the associated risks are further reduced (e.g. more selective immune modulation or effective gene therapy), these conditions may also be benefited.

Gene Therapy Using HSCs

Gene Therapy for ADA Deficient SCID

Gene therapy was conceived as an alternative to allogeneic HSCT in which a patient's own HSCs would have a normal copy of the disease-related gene inserted into their HSCs (Figure 20-1). Autologous gene therapy should avoid the immunological complications of allogeneic HSCT (graft rejection and GvHD), but could yield the same clinical benefits. Although initial plans for gene therapy considered the hemoglobin disorders as first candidates, it was soon recognized that the gene transfer efficiency to hematopoietic stem cells was likely to be too low to improve those diseases. Based on the known therapeutic effects from nonmyeloablated MSD transplants for SCID with only low engraftment of donor HSCs, it was postulated that in SCID there would be selective lymphoid expansion from a small number of gene-corrected HSCs that could amplify the effects of low efficiency gene transfer (Figure 20-2).

ADA-deficiency was the first etiological form of human SCID for which the responsible genetic lesion was identified.[25] The normal human ADA cDNA was cloned in the 1980s, enabling the development of retroviral vectors to transfer it into cells. Six clinical trials of gene therapy for ADA-deficient SCID were performed in the 1990s.[5,6,26–30] All of these studies used retroviral vectors to transfer a normal ADA cDNA, targeting either mature T lymphocytes that developed after PEG-ADA therapy, or CD34+

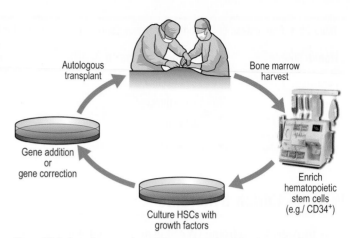

Figure 20-1 Gene therapy using autologous hematopoietic stem cells. Bone marrow is harvested from the PID patient. In the laboratory, the HSCs are enriched by immune-affinity with a monoclonal antibody to the CD34 antigen. The CD34 enriched cells are cultured with hematopoietic growth factors to activate the cells and then gene addition or gene correction is performed. The HSCs are then transplanted by intravenous infusion back into the patient.

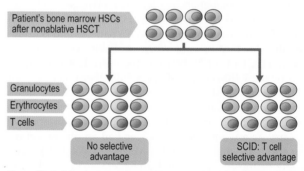

Figure 20-2 Selective expansion of T lymphocytes after HSCT for SCID. Patients undergoing HSCT with nonmyeloablative conditioning may have only a small percentage of donor or gene-corrected HSCs in their marrow (top). In the absence of a selective advantage for the growth of any specific lineage, low levels of all blood cell types will be seen (lower left). In SCID, the selective advantage for T lymphocyte proliferation in the lymphopenic hosts will lead to their expansion and the repopulation of the lymphoid system (lower right). The cells with purple nuclei represent recipient cells, while cells with red nuclei are genetically modified.

HSCs from autologous bone marrow or umbilical cord blood. The methods that were used to culture the T cells or CD34+ cells for gene transfer are now recognized to have been suboptimal. In addition, all subjects remained on PEG-ADA, which is now known to blunt the selective advantage of corrected T cells. Furthermore, cytoreductive conditioning was not used to 'make space' in the recipient marrow. While pretransplant conditioning was expected to increase engraftment of gene corrected HSCs, the risks associated with chemotherapy for an experimental therapy of unproven benefit were considered unacceptable for these initial studies. While there were no serious adverse events from the gene transfer in any of the subjects, there were also no significant clinical benefits. In recipients of gene–modified mature T cells, these cells have been shown to persist in circulation for more than a decade.[31] But, the diversity of the immune repertoire of these cells was uncertain and the patients remained on PEG-ADA enzyme replacement. In the recipients of gene-modified HSCs, only low levels of gene transfer and engraftment of HSCs were observed. Overall, the survival and immune function in these subjects was comparable to patients receiving only PEG-ADA therapy.

During the 1990s, incremental progress was made with the methods for gene transfer to HSCs, including the development

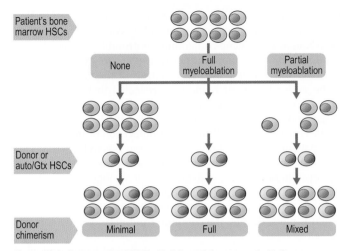

Figure 20-3 Outcome after HSCT with full, partial or no myeloablative conditioning. If HSCs are transplanted from an allogeneic donor or as gene-corrected autologous cells with no pretransplant conditioning, only minimal chimerism of donor cells will occur (lower left). If full myeloablation is given, essentially complete donor cell chimerism will be achieved (lower middle). If partial myeloablation is administered, as has been done in some gene therapy clinical trials, mixed chimerism will be achieved with a significant fraction of donor or gene-corrected cells engrafted (lower right).

of better vectors made to higher titers, the identification of hematopoietic growth factors better able to induce cycling of pluripotent HSCs (e.g. *ckit* ligand, flt-3 ligand), and optimization of in vitro culture conditions using recombinant fibronectin and serum-free medium.[32,33,34] These approaches led to increased levels of stable gene transfer to HSCs in large animal transplant models (e.g. 1–10%), indicating that they achieved greater gene transfer to HSCs which retained their ability to engraft in vivo.[35,36] Additionally, the use of reduced intensity conditioning prior to allogeneic HSCT was shown to allow a moderate degree of engraftment of donor cells, with significantly reduced acute toxicity.[37,38] Such nonmyeloablative conditioning was postulated to be beneficial in the autologous gene therapy setting (Figure 20-3). Based on these advances, second-generation clinical trials of gene therapy for SCID were begun in the late 1990s.

The investigators at the San Raffaele Telethon Institute for Gene Therapy in Milan, Italy made a major advance in the field with their clinical trial of gene therapy for ADA-deficient SCID.[39] Initial results were reported in 2002 on two ADA-SCID infants treated using retroviral-mediated ADA gene transfer to bone marrow CD34[+] cells.[30,40] Two important variables were changed, compared to prior trials. First, the patients were given nonmyeloablative conditioning, using a moderate dosage of busulfan (4 mg/kg) to eliminate some of the endogenous HSCs prior to infusion of the gene-corrected bone marrow cells. Secondly, the patients were *not* given PEG-ADA enzyme replacement therapy, which was expected to allow the maximum selective advantage of gene-corrected T cells to manifest. Indeed, over the first 6 to 9 months, their immune function was largely restored, with the development of antigen-specific T cell responses and antibody production. Measurements of gene-marking showed that 75–100% of T, B, and NK cells contained the transferred gene, consistent with the strong purported selective advantage for ADA expressing lymphocytes. At the same time, 1–10% of myeloid cells contained the gene, which was a level significantly higher than that seen in prior studies in which cytoreductive chemotherapy was not given. Further results of this approach have now been reported from Milan, with 8 of 10 subjects realizing excellent and sustained immune reconstitution.[30,40,41] Similar studies in London, England and in the USA at Children's Hospital Los

Angeles and the National Human Genome Research Institute, NIH have led to similar clinically beneficial results.[28,29,42,43] Thus, for ADA-deficient SCID patients lacking an HLA-MSD, gene therapy has become a proven therapeutic modality.

Gene Therapy for XSCID

One of the next PIDs approached by gene therapy was the X-linked form (XSCID), caused by deficiencies of the common cytokine receptor γ chain (γc). Investigators at the Hopital Necker-Enfants Malades in Paris, France instituted a clinical trial of retroviral-mediated transfer of a normal human γc cDNA into CD34[+] cells from bone marrow of infants with XSCID.[44] In this trial, the transduced CD34[+] cells were re-infused without prior cytoreduction, counting on the very potent selective survival advantage of the γc-corrected lymphoid cells to repopulate the immune system from a low level of gene-modified HSCs. No adverse events were noted in the initial years in 9 treated subjects. The γc gene was present and expressed in T, NK and B cells. Over the initial 2 to 5 months, 9 of 10 infants developed normal numbers of T and NK cells, with good immune function. While B cell numbers remain low, protective levels of antibodies were produced and most subjects were removed from routine gammaglobulin treatment. The subjects were in good health over the first 1 to 2 years, without opportunistic infections and were growing and developing without protective isolation. Four XSCID infants were treated in a similar clinical trial by investigators at the Institute of Child Health, University College London, London, England with similar good outcome.[45]

However, 5 subjects from these two trials subsequently developed a leukemia-like complication, with escalating white blood cell counts, 2.5 to 5 years after the gene therapy procedures. Four of these subjects have been successfully treated for the lymphoproliferative syndrome and have retained the benefits of the gene therapy on immune reconstitution, but 1 died as a result of this complication. Investigations have implicated the process of insertional oncogenesis, in which the retroviral vector integrates semirandomly into different chromosomal sites in each transduced cell; integrants adjacent to cellular genes that mediate proliferation or survival may be inappropriately activated by transcriptional elements of the vector, such as the potent enhancers present in the long terminal repeats (LTRs). In fact, in 4 of the 5 patients with this complication, the leukemia cells had at least one copy of the vector integrated on chr11p13, near the first of the LMO-2 gene.[46,47] LMO-2 encodes a protein involved in stem cell growth which is normally not expressed in mature T cells. LMO2 is a known proto-oncogene that is inappropriately activated in some spontaneous cases of T cell leukemia, through activating translocations. LMO2 is likely to be expressed in the targeted CD34[+] HSCs and would thus be susceptible to nearby vector insertions, as the Moloney leukemia virus (MLV)-based vectors have been shown to integrate preferentially into the 5′ end of genes that are actively expressed in target cells.[48]

It remains uncertain why the complication of insertional oncogenes with lymphoproliferation was seen in 25% of the XSCID subjects, but in none of the more than 20 subjects with ADA-deficient SCID. Various hypotheses suggest that the marrow of XSCID subjects has an expanded target cell pool of lymphoid progenitors that would support the proliferative effects of LMO2 transactivation, or that the severely lymphopenic environment in XSCID patients supports a highly robust lymphoid expansion which is conducive to transformation, or that the constitutive expression of the γc gene per se may play a role. In fact, it has subsequently been appreciated that transactivation of adjacent

Hematopoietic Stem Cell Transplantation and Gene Therapy

cellular proto-oncogenes may occur even without the development of overt lymphoproliferation; vector integrants near the evi-1 gene have been found to be present at a disproportionately high frequency and transactivation of evi-1 may provide a selective survival or expansion advantage to cells, allowing them to predominate in the HSC that reconstitute hematopoiesis after gene transfer/transplantation.

Faced with these mixed results with life-savings immune reconstitution in the majority of XSCID subjects using gene therapy, but a severe treatment-related complication in a significant fraction of these, the relative risks and benefits need to be compared to the current therapeutic alternative for these subjects, allogeneic HSCT from a haploidentical or MUD donor. The outcomes for SCID patients with allogeneic donors other than HLA-matched siblings have led to survival rates of 50–80% with restored T cell immunity, as discussed previously. But, more than half of these patients may fail to produce protective antibodies, and there are risks of GvHD and post-transplant Epstein-Barr virus (EBV)-driven lymphoproliferative disease (LPD). Gene therapy for XSCID using retroviral vectors led to immune restoration in 95% (19/20) of patients, but with a 25% incidence of LPD. The way forward for gene therapy for XSCID will involve the evaluation of new vectors that have been shown by in vitro and murine transplant studies to have significantly lowered risks for causing insertional oncogenesis.[49-51] Ideally, these improved vectors will lead to similar levels of immune reconstitution, with minimal or absent occurrences of insertional oncogenesis.

Notably, this same approach for gene therapy has been applied in two studies to older subjects, most of whom had undergone unsuccessful HSCT from haploidentical donors. These adolescent subjects showed minimal responses to the gene therapy, suggesting that their older age was associated with inadequate thymic function to support de novo lymphopoiesis; it is uncertain if the prior transplants were associated with GvHD, which is known to impair thymic function.[52,53]

Gene Therapy for CGD

The other major PID that has been approached in several gene therapy clinical trials is chronic granulomatous disease (CGD). The cDNA for the oxidases responsible for the X-linked form (gp91phox), and most common autosomal forms (p47 phox, p67 phox, or p22 phox) were cloned and placed into retroviral vectors. Preclinical studies using patient-derived cells and murine gene knock-out models provided evidence that gene transfer could restore the defective oxidase function in myeloid cells, although the absolute amounts of the oxidase proteins produced were often less than fully normal.[54,55] Initial trials used MLV-based retroviral vectors, targeted G-CSF mobilized CD34+ PBSC and did not administer cytoreductive chemotherapy. Neutrophils were produced in vivo in multiple subjects that had their functional activity restored, based upon sensitive flow cytometric assays, but these were present at very low frequencies and only transiently.[56]

A later study performed at the German Cancer Research Center added the use of cytoreductive conditioning with 8 mg/kg of busulfan (approximately 2 × higher than the dose used in the ADA-deficient SCID studies) and used a retroviral vector derived from the murine spleen focus forming virus (SFFV) which has LTRs that are highly potent in myeloid progenitor cells expressing the normal human gp91phox.[57] Two young men in their 20s with X-CGD and life-long histories of chronic infections, poorly responsive to intensive medical therapy, were treated. They had clinically beneficial responses to the treatment with resolution of the long-standing infections. The production of gene-corrected, oxidase(+) neutrophils was readily detected; the frequencies of gene-containing neutrophils increased from 20% in the first few months after transplant to levels exceeding 60% over the next few months. Analysis of the insertional sites of the vector into their blood cells revealed that up to 80% of the cells had vector integrated near one of three genes (common integration sites). These genes (MDS1-EVI1, PRDM16 and SETBP1) have been implicated in proliferation of myeloid cells. Both patients developed monosomy 7 and myelodysplasia. This polyclonal myeloid expansion progressed in both patients to a myeloproliferative state, with emergence of monosomy 7. One of these patients died as a result of gastrointestinal (GI) infection, at a time when there was loss of expression of oxidase activity in neutrophils, despite the continued presence of gene-containing cells.

The highly dichotomous outcome of clinical benefit followed by severe adverse event in these CGD patients is highly reminiscent of the XSCID studies. For CGD, the use of a vector with a potent myeloid-type LTR promoter led to myeloproliferation, while there was lymphoproliferation in the XSCID studies where the MLV LTR is more active in lymphoid cells. It is known from research on wild-type retroviruses that the virus's LTRs may play a major role in defining the disease tropism.[58] Retroviral vectors used to drive high-level expression of a transgene in a specific lineage may predispose that lineage to insertional oncogenic effects. The unexpected complications that occurred in these patients treated for PID led to major increases in the understanding of these risks, their underlying mechanisms, and potential ways to overcome them. Some of these improved approaches will be discussed below.

Other PIDs that are under extensive study and have entered, or will enter, gene therapy clinical trials, include Wiskott-Aldrich syndrome, leukocyte adhesion deficiency, and hereditary lymphocytic histiocytosis. Other diseases that involve cytokine and signaling pathway components, such as the Jak3 kinase and Zap70 kinase deficient forms of SCID, CD40 ligand deficiency (X-linked hyper-IgM syndrome), IPEX, IL-7 receptor, and X-linked agammaglobulinemia will require new approaches to gene therapy to achieve more sophisticated control of the expression of the responsible gene than occurs using constitutive promoters, such as viral LTRs.

New Approaches to Gene Therapy using HSCs

Gene therapy for PIDs has progressed from an essentially ineffective state a decade ago to the present status, when clear-cut efficacy can be achieved for several disorders, albeit with a risk for significant degree of side-effects. Further advances will be based upon new insights into HSC biology and new methods for gene transfer. New understandings may eventually support efforts for ex vivo expansion of HSCs, which would allow the selective use of HSCs with favorable vector integration sites. Elements such as the HoxB4 homeodomain protein, and the β-catenin and Notch ligand pathways may be capable of driving proliferation of HSCs, without causing irreversible differentiation and loss of stem cell function.

New major alternatives to the murine γ-retroviral vectors are vectors derived from lentiviruses or Foamy viruses.[59-61] These latter types of retroviruses are of primate origin (HIV-1 lentiviruses from humans and the Simian Foamy virus from nonhuman primates) and are more efficient for transferring genes into human cells, and can do so needing less activation of the

HSCs. These vectors can be made lacking the strong LTR enhancers that are problematic in the γ-retroviral vectors, using the promoters from cellular genes that have weaker transactivation activity. Another important tactic being explored is the addition to vectors of 'insulator' sequences, which are DNA sequences that act as boundaries to prevent transcriptional cross-talk between adjacent genes in the chromosomes.[62] Lentiviral vectors have entered clinical trials for T cells and CD34+ HSCs and are likely to be applied to several PIDs in the near future.[63,64] A study in a canine model of leukocyte adhesion deficiency showed excellent clinical response using a Foamy viral vector to transfer the relevant CD18 cDNA.[65]

Gene Correction

All of the gene therapy efforts discussed so far have involved the use of methods for *adding* a new copy of a gene to cells. A promising new approach to gene therapy under investigation seeks to *correct* the disease-causing mutation in a patient's own gene, rather than adding a new copy of the relevant gene. Effective gene correction may have key advantages over gene addition. The corrected therapeutic gene would be in its normal location in the chromosomes and so should be expressed in the normal developmental and quantitative pattern. Gene correction should avoid the problems from gene addition due to random insertion throughout the genome, resulting in activation of nearby genes.

Cells have multiple ways to repair damage to their chromosomal DNA, including homologous recombination (HR) that can lead to the genetic information on one strand being copied into a homologous, but nonidentical sequence. Flooding cells with high concentrations of nucleic acids complementary to an endogenous gene sequence can cause the HR pathways to introduce corrective sequences into a cellular gene, for example to correct the single base pair change in the human β-globin gene responsible for sickle cell disease.[66] However, efforts to direct gene repair by HR were limited by very low efficiency. More recently, the efficiency of HR has been markedly improved by the use of transiently-expressed endonucleases targeted to introduce double-stranded DNA breaks near the intended site of HR. For example, so-called 'zinc-finger endonucleases' (ZFNs) can be designed to have DNA recognition domains that bind to unique sites in the genome and introduce a double-stranded break to induce HR, guided by a 'donor' oligonucleotide.[67,68] ZFNs targeting the CCR5 HIV-1 co-receptor are moving toward a clinical trial for AIDS and may be developed to achieve correction of the genes involved in PIDs. It will need to be determined whether the efficacy and safety of gene correction provides a better therapeutic window than gene addition methods.

A futuristic approach to gene therapy for these disorders may make use of the ability to 're-program' somatic cells to a pluripotent state (Figure 20-4). These induced pluripotent stem cells (iPS) could be produced from patient cells that are efficiently gene corrected in vitro. Then, the iPS could be directed to differentiate to HSCs for transplantation. This process has been demonstrated in a murine model of sickle cell disease, although several key steps have not been advanced to sufficient efficacy for human cells.[69]

Conclusions

Although advances in supportive therapy and enzyme therapy have made improvements in the treatment of primary immune

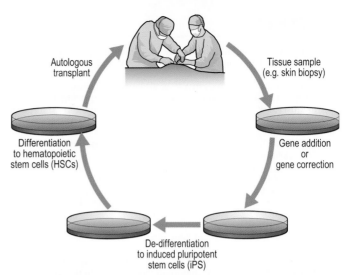

Figure 20-4 Gene therapy using autologous HSCs made from induced pluripotent stem cells. Somatic cells from a PID patient, such as skin fibroblasts or keratinocytes, can be obtained from a skin biopsy. These cells can be cultured and genetically corrected by gene addition or gene correction methods. The cells can then be de-differentiated to produce induced pluripotent stem cells (*iPS*). The iPS can then be directed to differentiate to hematopoietic stem cells that can then be used to transplant the PID patient. The gene correction of the cultured somatic cells can be analyzed and selected for clones with complete appropriate gene correction and safe gene integration sites for use in the production of HSCs.

deficiencies, they are not curative for these life-threatening illnesses. The cost of these treatments can provide a financial burden for many families and become insurmountable over time. HSCT and gene therapy provide the only curative options at this time. Matched sibling donor hematopoietic stem cell transplantation remains the gold standard of treatment for many of these patients, but further data and experience have shown that closely matched unrelated bone marrow, peripheral blood stem cell and umbilical cord blood transplantation have satisfactory results in these disorders. Hematopoietic stem cell transplantation carries its own morbidities, some of which are fatal, including GvHD, infections, toxicity associated with chemotherapy, and nonengraftment. Gene therapy utilizes autologous cells, so there is no risk for GvHD nor graft rejection and immune suppressive therapies are not needed. In addition, gene therapy may be successful and potentially have less toxicity due to the use of pretransplant conditioning regimens that are less than fully myeloablative and therefore less toxic. However, unexpected genotoxicity has occurred in some patients with the retroviral vectors used in previous trials.

The research in gene therapy has reached the clinical setting. Retroviral-mediated gene transfer to HSCs has restored immunity in patients with ADA(-) SCID, XSCID, and CGD. There was a setback in the progress of gene therapy when 5 of 20 XSCID patients treated with gene therapy developed T-lymphoproliferative disease as a late complication from insertional oncogenesis. However, there have since been no further reports of similar events. Improvements in gene transfer to HSCs are under development that should increase clinical efficacy and decrease the risks. Lentiviral or Foamy viral vectors are being studied and have the potential to be superior for gene transfer to HSCs, compared to the γ-retroviral vectors used to date. There are ongoing and upcoming trials for several PIDs as well as β-thalassemia, sickle cell disease, metachromatic leukodystrophy, X-linked adrenoleukodystrophy, and mucopolysaccharidosis type I. Furthermore, direct gene correction may offer advantages over gene addition, if sufficient efficiency can be achieved.

References

1. Gatti RA, Meuweisen HJ, Allen HD, et al. Immunological reconstitution of sex-linked lymphopenic immunological deficiency. Lancet 1968;2: 1366–9.

2. Dupont B, Andersen V, Ernst P, et al. Immunologic reconstitution in severe combined immunodeficiency with HL-A-incompatible bone marrow graft: donor selection by mixed lymphocyte culture. Transplant Proc 1973;5:905–8.

3. Park BY, Biggar WD, Good RA. Transplantation of incompatible bone marrow in infants with severe combined immunodeficiency disease. Birth Defects Orig Artic Ser 1975;11:380–4.

4. The ADA human gene therapy clinical protocol. Hum Gene Ther 1990;1:327–62.

5. Blaese RM, Culver KW, Miller AD, et al. T lymphocyte-directed gene therapy for ADA- SCID: initial trial results after 4 years. Science 1995;270:475–80.

6. Bordignon C, Notarangelo LD, Nobili N, et al. Gene therapy in peripheral blood lymphocytes and bone marrow for ADA- immunodeficient patients. Science 1995;270:470–5.

7. Antoine C, Muller S, Cant A, et al. European Group for Blood and Marrow Transplantation; European Society for Immunodeficiency. Long-term survival and transplantation of haemopoietic stem cells for immunodeficiencies: report of the European experience 1968–99. Lancet 2003;361:553–60.

8. Buckley RH, Schiff SE, Schiff RI, et al. Hematopoietic stem-cell transplantation for the treatment of severe combined immunodeficiency. N Engl J Med 1999;340:508–16.

9. Titman P, Pink E, Skucek E, et al. Cognitive and behavioral abnormalities in children after hematopoietic stem cell transplantation for severe congenital immunodeficiencies. Blood 2008;112:3907–13.

10. Ozsahin H, Cavazzana-Calvo M, Notarangelo LD, et al. Long-term outcome following hematopoietic stem-cell transplantation in Wiskott-Aldrich syndrome: collaborative study of the European Society for Immunodeficiencies and European Group for Blood and Marrow Transplantation. Blood 2008;111:439–45. Epub 2007 Sep 27.

11. Flomenberg N, Baxter-Lowe LA, Confer D, et al. Impact of HLA class I and class II high-resolution matching on outcomes of unrelated donor bone marrow transplantation: HLA-C mismatching is associated with a strong adverse effect on transplantation outcome. Blood 2004;104: 1923–30.

12. Grunebaum E, Mazzolari E, Porta F, et al. Bone marrow transplantation for severe combined immune deficiency. JAMA 2006;295:508–18.

13. Griffith LM, Cowan MJ, Kohn DB, et al. Allogeneic hematopoietic cell transplantation for primary immune deficiency diseases: current status and critical needs. J Allergy Clin Immunol 2008;122:1087–96.

14. Bach FH, Anderson JL, Albertini RJ, et al. Bone Marrow transplantation in a patient with the Wiskott-Aldrich syndrome. Lancet 1968;292: 1364–6.

15. Filipovich AH, Stone JV, Tomany SC, et al. Impact of donor type on outcome of bone marrow transplantation for Wiskott-Aldrich syndrome. Blood 2001;97:1598–603.

16. Winkelstein JA, Marino MC, Johnston RB, et al. Chronic granulomatous disease: report on a national registry of 368 patients. Medicine 2000;79:155–69.

17. Horwitz ME, Barrett AJ, Brown MR, et al. Treatment of Chronic Granulomatous Disease with Nonmyeloablative Conditioning and a T cell–Depleted Hematopoietic Allograft. New Engl J Med 2001;344: 881–8.

18. Seger RA, Gungor T, Belohradsky BH, et al. Treatment of chronic granulomatous disease with myeloablative conditioning and an unmodified hemopoietic allograft: a survey of the European experience, 1985–2000. Blood 2002;100:4344–50.

19. Bhattacharya A, Slatter M, Curtis A, et al. Successful umbilical cord blood stem cell transplantation for chronic granulomatous disease. Bone Marrow Transplantation 2003;31:403–5.

20. Parikh SH, Szabolcs P, Prasad VK, et al. Correction of chronic granulomatous disease after second unrelated-donor umbilical cord blood transplantation. Pediatr Blood Cancer 2007;49:982–1046.

21. Horwitz ME, Barrett AJ, Brown MR, et al. Treatment of chronic granulomatous disease with nonmyeloablative conditioning and a T cell-depleted hematopoietic allograft. N Engl J Med 2001;344:881–8.

22. Fischer A, Cerf-Bensussan N, Blanche S, et al. Allogeneic bone marrow transplantation for erythrophagocytic lymphohistiocytosis. J Pediatr 1986;108:267–70.

23. Henter JI, Samuelsson-Horne A, Arico M, et al. Treatment of hemophagocytic lymphohistiocytosis with HLH-94 immunochemotherapy and bone marrow transplantation. Blood 2002;100:2367–73.

24. Henter JI, Horne A, Arico M, et al. HLH-2004: diagnostic and therapeutic guidelines for hemophagocytic lymphohistiocytosis. Pediatr Blood Cancer 2007;48:124–31.

25. Giblett ER, Anderson JE, Cohen F, et al. Adenosine deaminase deficiency in two patients with severely impaired cellular immunity. Lancet 1972:1067–9.

26. Onodera M, Ariga T, Kawamura N, et al. Successful peripheral T lymphocyte-directed gene transfer for a patient with severe combined immune deficiency caused by adenosine deaminase deficiency. Blood 1998;91:30–6.

27. Hoogerbrugge PM, van Beusechem VW, Fischer A, et al. Bone marrow gene transfer in three patients with adenosine deaminase deficiency. Gene Ther 1996;3:179–83.

28. Kohn DB, Hershfield MS, Carbonaro D, et al. T lymphocytes with a normal ADA gene accumulate after transplantation of transduced autologous umbilical cord blood CD34+ cells in ADA-deficient SCID neonates. Nat Med 1998;4:775–80.

29. Kohn DB, Weinberg KI, Nolta JA, et al. Engraftment of gene-modified umbilical cord blood cells in neonates with adenosine deaminase deficiency. Nat Med 1995;1:1017–23.

30. Aiuti A, Vai S, Mortellaro A, et al. Immune reconstitution in ADA-SCID after PBL gene therapy and discontinuation of enzyme replacement. Nat Med 2002;8:423–5.

31. Muul LM, Tuschong LM, Soenen SL, et al. Persistence and expression of the adenosine deaminase gene for 12 years and immune reaction to gene transfer components: long-term results of the first clinical gene therapy trial. Blood 2003;101:2563–9.

32. Miller AD, Garcia JV, von Suhr N, et al. Construction and properties of retrovirus packaging cells based on gibbon ape leukemia virus. J Virol 1991;65:2220–4.

33. Moritz T, Patel VP, Williams DA. Bone marrow extracellular matrix molecules improve gene transfer into human hematopoietic cells via retroviral vectors. J Clin Invest 1994;93:1451–7.

34. Dao MA, Shah AJ, Crooks GM, et al. Engraftment and retroviral marking of CD34+ and CD34+CD38- human hematopoietic progenitors assessed in immune-deficient mice. Blood 1998;91:1243–55.

35. Kiem HP, McSweeney PA, Bruno B, et al. Improved gene transfer into canine hematopoietic repopulating cells using CD34-enriched marrow cells in combination with a gibbon ape leukemia virus-pseudotype retroviral vector. Gene Ther 1999;6:966–72.

36. Wu T, Kim HJ, Sellers SE, et al. Prolonged high-level detection of retrovirally marked hematopoietic cells in nonhuman primates after transduction of CD34+ progenitors using clinically feasible methods. Mol Ther 2000;1:285–93.

37. McSweeney PA, Storb R. Mixed chimerism: preclinical studies and clinical applications. Biol Blood Marrow Transplant 1999;5: 192–203.

38. Carella AM, Champlin R, Slavin S, et al. Mini-allografts: ongoing trials in humans. Bone Marrow Transplant 2000;25:345–50.

39. Laboratory of Hematology, Istituto Scientifico H.S. Raffaele, Milano, Italy. Hum Gene Ther 1990;1:327–62.

40. Aiuti A, Slavin S, Aker M, et al. Correction of ADA-SCID by stem cell gene therapy combined with nonmyeloablative conditioning. Science 2002;296:2410–3.

41. Aiuti A, Cattaneo F, Galimberti S, et al. Long-term safety and efficacy of gene therapy for adenosine deaminase (ADA)-deficient severe combined immunodeficiency. New Engl J Med 2009;360:447–58.

42. Gaspar HB, Bjorkegren E, Parsley K, et al. Successful reconstitution of immunity in ADA-SCID by stem cell gene therapy following cessation of PEG-ADA and use of mild preconditioning. Mol Ther 2006;14: 505–13.

43. Sokolic R, Podsakoff G, Muul L, et al. Myelosuppression and withdrawal of PEG-ADA lead to superior results after gene therapy for adenosine deaminase deficiency (ADA-SCID). Mol Ther 2008;16:S111. (Abstract).

44. Cavazzana-Calvo M, Hacein-Bey-Abina S, Fischer A. Gene therapy of X-linked severe combined immunodeficiency. Curr Opin Allergy Clin Immunol 2002;2:507–9.

45. Gaspar HB, Parsley KL, Howe S, et al. Gene therapy of X-linked severe combined immunodeficiency by use of a pseudotyped gammaretroviral vector. Lancet 2004;364:2181–7.

46. Hacein-Bey-Abina S, von Kalle C, Schmidt M, et al. A serious adverse event after successful gene therapy for X-linked severe combined immunodeficiency. N Engl J Med 2003;348:255–6.

47. Hacein-Bey-Abina S, von Kalle C, Schmidt M, et al. LMO2-associated clonal T cell proliferations in two patients after gene therapy for SCID-X1. Science 2003;302:415–9.

48. Howe SJ, Mansour MR, Schwarzwaelder K, et al. Insertional mutagenesis combined with acquired somatic mutations causes leukemogenesis following gene therapy of SCID-X1 patients. J Clin Invest 2008;118: 3143–50.

49. Dave UP, Jenkins NA, Copeland NG. Gene therapy insertional mutagenesis insights. Science 2004;303:333.

50. Bonini C, Grez M, Traversari C, et al. Safety of retroviral gene marking with a truncated NGF receptor. Nat Med 2003;9:367–9.

51. Rivella S, Lisowski L, Sadelain M. Globin gene transfer: a paradigm for transgene regulation and vector safety. Gene Ther Reg 2003;2: 149–75.

52. Thrasher AJ, Hacein-Bey-Abina S, Gaspar HB, et al. Failure of SCID-X1 gene therapy in older patients. Blood 2005;105:4255–7.

53. Chinen J, Davis J, De Ravin SS, et al. Gene therapy improves immune function in preadolescents with X-linked severe combined immunodeficiency. Blood 2007;110:67–73.

54. Dinauer MC, Li LL, Bjorgvinsdottir H, et al. Long-term correction of phagocyte NADPH oxidase activity by retroviral-mediated gene transfer in murine X-linked chronic granulomatous disease. Blood 1999;94: 914–22.

55. Mardiney M 3rd, Jackson SH, Spratt SK, et al. Enhanced host defense after gene transfer in the murine p47phox-deficient model of chronic granulomatous disease. Blood 1997;89:2268–75.

56. Malech HL, Maples PB, Whiting-Theobald N, et al. Prolonged production of NADPH oxidase-corrected granulocytes after gene therapy of chronic granulomatous disease. Proc Natl Acad Sci USA 1997;94: 12133–8.

57. Ott MG, Schmidt M, Schwarzwaelder K, et al. Correction of X-linked chronic granulomatous disease by gene therapy, augmented by insertional activation of MDS1-EVI1, PRDM16 or SETBP1. Nat Med 2006;12:401–9.

58. Celander D, Haseltine WA. Tissue-specific transcription preference as a determinant of cell tropism and leukaemogenic potential of murine retroviruses. Nature 1984;312:159–62.

59. Naldini L, Blomer U, Gallay P, et al. In vivo gene delivery and stable transduction of nondividing cells by a lentiviral vector. Science 1996; 272:263–7.

60. Naldini L. Lentiviruses as gene transfer agents for delivery to non-dividing cells. Curr Opin Biotechnol 1998;9:457–63.

61. Hirata RK, Miller AD, Andrews RG, et al. Transduction of hematopoietic cells by foamy virus vectors. Blood 1996;88:3654–61.

62. Ramezani A, Hawley TS, Hawley RG. Combinatorial incorporation of enhancer-blocking components of the chicken beta-globin 5′HS4 and human T cell receptor alpha/delta BEAD-1 insulators in self-inactivating retroviral vectors reduces their genotoxic potential. Stem Cells 2008;26:3257–66.

63. Levine BL, Humeau LM, Boyer J, et al. Gene transfer in humans using a conditionally replicating lentiviral vector. Proc Natl Acad Sci U S A 2006;103:17372–7.

64. Cartier N. Gene therapy strategies for X-linked adrenoleukodystrophy. Curr Opin Mol Ther 2001;3:357–61.

65. Bauer TR Jr, Allen JM, Hai M, et al. Successful treatment of canine leukocyte adhesion deficiency by foamy virus vectors. Nat Med 2008;14:93–7.

66. Goncz KK, Prokopishyn NL, Abdolmohammadi A, et al. Small fragment homologous replacement-mediated modification of genomic beta-globin sequences in human hematopoietic stem/progenitor cells. Oligonucleotides 2006;16:213–24.

67. Urnov FD, Miller JC, Lee YL, et al. Highly efficient endogenous human gene correction using designed zinc-finger nucleases. Nature 2005;435:646–51.

68. Lombardo A, Genovese P, Beausejour CM, et al. Gene editing in human stem cells using zinc finger nucleases and integrase-defective lentiviral vector delivery. Nat Biotechnol 2007;25:1298–306.

69. Hanna J, Wernig M, Markoulaki S, et al. Treatment of sickle cell anemia mouse model with iPS cells generated from autologous skin. Science 2007;318:1920–3.

CHAPTER 21

Autoinflammatory Disorders

Fatma Dedeoglu • Susan Kim

One of the hallmarks of the new millennium has been the discovery of the 'familial Mediterranean fever' gene, which triggered the exponential discovery of other genes, and more importantly, new inflammatory pathways. These have shed light on our understanding of inflammation and led to more effective treatment in many patients with 'periodic fever' syndromes. This area of medicine is one of the best examples of bench-to-bedside innovation and translational research.

Formerly poorly understood periodic fever syndromes are now grouped under the term 'autoinflammatory disorders', adapted in the last decade to reflect the improved understanding of these conditions, which present with heightened inflammatory responses.[1] While periodicity and fever are the cardinal features of many of these conditions, some may have a more chronic and/or afebrile course. The inflammatory response is typically localized to serosa, joints and skin. Unlike autoimmune conditions, autoantibodies or antigen specific T cells are lacking, and monocytes and neutrophils are the major effector cells rather than lymphocytes. These syndromes are now considered inborn errors of innate immunity.[2]

Most of the known mutations found involve proteins that modulate inflammation and apoptosis. The majority of these mutations are monogenic, such as familial Mediterranean fever (FMF), TNF receptor-associated periodic fever syndrome (TRAPS), familial cold autoinflammatory syndrome (FCAS) and hyper IgD syndrome (HIDS). Other conditions share features and inflammatory pathways with monogenic diseases, but appear to be polygenic, acquired and multifactorial, such as systemic onset juvenile idiopathic arthritis (SOJIA), Crohn's Disease and gout. There are other conditions that are phenotypically similar to autoinflammatory syndromes, such as periodic fevers, apthous stomatitis, pharyngitis and adenitis (PFAPA), without known mutations, that remain under investigation. A genotyping database, called Infevers (http://fmf.igh.cnrs.fr/infevers) was established in 2002 and more than 540 sequence variants of these monogenic diseases have been registered at present.[3]

This chapter gives an overview of autoinflammatory disorders with a focus on the monogenic types.

Common Features

The majority of autoinflammatory disorders present with recurrent episodes of inflammatory states, generally with fever and elevated inflammatory markers (CRP, ESR, SAA: Table 21-1 summarizes the typical features of these disorders). Patients are usually asymptomatic between the attacks, though in the severe forms, longer duration of symptoms may occur without complete resolution[4,5] Patients usually experience similar symptoms with each attack. Variability of features is seen within each syndrome, between different patients, and even within affected members of the same family. There may be a prodromal period with nonspecific features, such as fatigue and headaches.

When a patient presents with recurrent fevers, the differential remains broad: from infectious to rheumatologic to oncologic/lymphoproliferative causes, as well as immunodeficiencies. The longer the duration of these typical recurrent episodes, the greater the likelihood of an autoinflammatory disorder. Since the penetrance of the mutations is not 100%, and de novo mutations may occur, a negative family history does not exclude a particular diagnosis.

After careful history, physical examination and exclusion of other etiologies, when autoinflammatory disorders are considered, genetic testing may be helpful in confirming the diagnosis. However, it should be noted that depending on the syndrome, up to 60% of patients may have negative genetic testing, despite clinical features consistent with a particular syndrome.[5] This suggests the presence of yet unknown genetic defects in the same inflammatory pathways causing a similar phenotype.

In recent years, based on the inheritance pattern, age of onset, duration, frequency and associated features of the attacks and ethnicity, *decision-making trees* have been proposed in evaluation of patients with periodic inflammatory episodes. With this approach, diagnostic possibilities may be narrowed down to two or three syndromes. In these situations, further genetic testing usually has a low yield.[6,7] These algorithms are more applicable in areas of higher prevalence, and genetic testing might be considered more liberally outside these regions.

The fundamental problem in autoinflammatory disorders appears to be an exaggerated inflammatory response, due to increased sensitivity to a normal or insignificant stimuli or due to the inability of the immune system to dampen normal responses in an efficient and timely manner. Most of the mutated proteins in these disorders are members of the death-domain fold (DDF) family, which are involved in apoptosis, NF-κB activation and proinflammatory cytokine production. Despite significant progress, the exact roles of these proteins and the effects of the mutations are not well understood: there have been conflicting results of studies that may be related to differences in experimental models. It is also possible that these proteins assume different roles under different situations.[2,8]

©2010 Elsevier Ltd, Inc, BV
DOI: 10.1016/B978-1-4377-0271-2.00021-3

Table 21-1 Typical Features in Autoinflammatory Disorders

	Blau Syndrome	FCAS	MWS	NOMID	PAPA	TRAPS	FMF	HIDS	Majeed Syndrome	PFAPA
Typical age	<5 years	<1 year	Variable, usually <20 years	<1 year	<16 years	<20 years	<20 years	<1 year	<2 years	Preschool age
Fever duration	Continuous	1–2 days	1–3 days	Continuous	3–7 days	7 + days	1–3 days	3–7 days	3–4 days	3–5 days
Frequency	Continuous	Based on cold exposure	1 month to continuous	Continuous	1–2 months	Variable	Variable	1–2 months	1–2 months	1 month
Ethnic/cultural/regional predilection	None	Western European	Western European	Western European	None	Western European	Middle Eastern, Armenian, Turkish, Arab, Jewish	Western European	Arab	None
Common clinical findings	Granulomatous uveitis, arthritis, lymphadenopathy	Conjunctivitis, headache, arthralgia, myalgia, nausea	Conjunctivitis, uveitis, headache, deafness, arthralgia/arthritis, myalgia	Papilledema, uveitis, optic disc edema/vision loss, headache, aseptic meningitis, deafness, frontal bossing, epiphyseal overgrowth, mental retardation	Arthralgia, destructive arthritis	Periorbital edema, conjunctivitis, arthralgia, migratory myalgia, serositis, abdominal pain	Serositis (peritonitis, pleuritis), monoarthritis, oligoarthritis, arthralgia	Lymph node enlargment, abdominal pain, vomiting, diarrhea, oral sores, arthralgia, splenomegaly, headache	Deforming arthritis, growth retardation, osteomyelitis, hepatosplenomegaly	Stomatitis, pharyngitis, cervical lymph node enlargement, fatigue, headache
Skin manifestations	Maculopapular nodular rash	Urticarial rash	Urticarial rash	Urticarial rash	Pyoderma gangrenosum, cystic acne	Migratory erythematous rash	Erysipeloid erythema	Maculopapular, nodular rash	Sweet syndrome, pustulosis	Rare
Amyloidosis		Rare	30%	Rare		25%	Up to 75% (before colchicine)	Rare		
Inheritance	AD and de novo NOD2/CARD15 encoding NOD2	AD CIAS1/NLRP3, encoding cryopyrin	AD CIAS1/NLRP3, encoding cryopyrin	AD and de novo CIAS1/NLRP3, encoding cryopyrin	AD PSTPIP1	AD TNFSF1A-encoding p55 TNF receptor	AR MEFV, encoding pyrin	AR MVK, encoding mevalonate kinase	AR	Unknown
Treatment	Steroids, anti-TNF therapy	Anti-IL-1 therapy	Anti-IL-1 therapy	Anti-IL-1 therapy	Steroids and possibly anti-TNF therapy, anti-IL-1 therapy	Steroids and possibly anti-TNF therapy, anti-IL-1 therapy	Colchicine daily and possibly anti IL-1 therapy	Steroids and possibly anti-TNF therapy, anti-IL-1 therapy, statins	Steroids, NSAIDs and possibly anti-TNF, anti IL-1 therapy	Tonsillectomy, steroids, cimetidine

FCAS: familial cold autoinflammatory syndrome; *MWS:* Muckle Wells syndrome; *TRAPS:* TNF receptor-associated periodic fever syndrome; *FMF:* familial Mediterranean fever; *HIDS:* hyper IgD syndrome

Familial Mediterranean Fever (FMF)

Familial Mediterranean fever (FMF) was the first described periodic fever syndrome and is the most common. In1908, Janeway and Rosenthal described a Jewish girl with recurrent fevers and abdominal pain, and it was described as a separate entity in 1945 by Siegal.[9,10]

The majority of the patients' ancestry is from the Mediterranean basin, particularly in the Middle East (Turks, Arabs, Jews, Armenians) with a prevalence of 1:250–1:1000. Recently, it has been reported throughout the world, and is likely to be related to worldwide migration.[11] With the help of haplotype analysis, the initial spread of FMF can be traced back to Mesopotamia 2500 years ago. It is an autosomal recessive condition with a carrier frequency as high as 1 in 3–5 in the Middle East, suggesting a survival advantage against possible infectious agents via an enhanced innate immune response. Carriers of the FMF gene have a heightened inflammatory response supporting this hypothesis.[12] After mapping the FMF susceptibility locus to chromosome 16p in 1992,[13] the mutated gene, named MEFV (MEditerranean FeVer) was discovered by two independent groups, using positional cloning in 1997.[14,15] The deduced protein was named *pyrin* (from the Greek for 'fever') by one group and *Marenostrin* (from the Latin 'Mare Nostrum' for 'our sea') by the other. Pyrin is 781aa long, and is primarily expressed in the cytoplasm of neutrophils but is also found in eosinophils, monocytes, dendritic cells and fibroblasts. Via its N-terminal death domain (pyrin domain-PYD), pyrin interacts with the pyrin domain of ASC, an adaptor protein, to assemble and activate inflammatory complexes, known as inflammasomes. These proteins have been found to play a role in controlling IL-1β production by regulating caspase-1.[8] It has also been shown that pyrin interacts with caspase-1 directly via its C-terminal, B30.2 domain, modulating IL-1β activation[16] Despite extensive research in this field, the exact physiologic role and underlying mechanisms of mutated pyrin are not well understood. There are studies supporting both proinflammatory and antiinflammatory effects of pyrin, via either inhibition or induction of apoptosis, as well as activation or inhibition of NF-κB.[17]

The majority of MEFV mutations are on the last exon (exon 10, B30.2 domain). Mutations in position 694 usually cause a more severe phenotype, especially M694V, suggesting an important role for methionine at this position in the function of pyrin. Low penetrance mutations such as E148Q, are also described. Allele frequency of E148Q is 10–20% in Asians and 1–2% in Caucasians.[18,19]

FMF episodes may be triggered by physical or emotional stress, menstruation and diet. Major features are fever and serositis, mostly peritonitis (95%), recurrent attacks of which may cause adhesions. Pleuritis, which is usually unilateral, is seen in about 40% patients, while pericarditis is rare in FMF. Orchitis occurs in about 5% and is more common in children. Arthritis/arthralgia affects primarily the lower extremities and is transient, resolving without any sequelae, though some patients may develop chronic destructive arthritis. The erysipelas-like rash, commonly seen around the ankles, is a relatively unique feature of FMF and occurs in about 20–30% of the patients. Rarely, prolonged, severe muscle pain affecting lower extremities and abdominal muscles, known as protracted febrile myalgia, may occur, and is responsive to steroid therapy. Occasionally, there is an accompanying vasculitic rash.[20,21] Laboratory investigation reveals leukocytosis and elevated inflammatory markers. Peritoneal fluid analysis is positive for neutrophil predominance and low levels of C5a inhibitor.[22]

Diagnosis is still primarily clinical, since about 25% of the patients have a negative genetic analysis for MEFV mutation. Furthermore, a significant number of patients with homozygosity never develop clinical features, while about 30–40% of the patients with FMF are heterozygotes. Clinical criteria have been proposed by Livneh in 1997 for diagnosis, which are very specific and sensitive in areas of high prevalence, but may have a lower specificity in areas where it is not as prevalent. Certain vasculitides such as Henoch- Schonlein purpura (HSP) and polyarteritis nodosa (PAN) are shown to have increased frequency in FMF patients.[20]

Colchicine is the mainstay of the treatment of FMF, which eliminates or substantially decreases the symptoms in about 95% of the patients. More importantly, regular use of colchicine prevents the development of amyloidosis, the major contributor to morbidity and mortality in patients.[19] The favorable results of colchicine in FMF were reported simultaneously by Dr Goldfinger in the USA and by Dr Ozkan in Turkey in 1972.[23] Before the use of colchicine, up to 75% of patients would develop amyloidosis after the age of 40 years. Risk factors for amyloidosis include M694V mutation, male gender, SAA α/α genotype and family history of amyloidosis.[21] In addition, environmental factors also play a crucial role in the development of amyloidosis.

To date, the mechanism of action of colchicine in FMF is not well understood. Colchicine accumulates primarily in neutrophils and is postulated to affect neutrophil adhesion and mobility by binding to the cytoskeleton of the cells.[21,23] It is generally well tolerated with minimal side-effects, diarrhea being the most common (10–20%) though acute toxicity from an overdose can be very serious. Studies have suggested that it is safe to use during pregnancy and lactation and does not cause infertility. Colchicine has no effect in the treatment of an acute attack. It is a preventative medication, therefore intermittent use or increasing the dose during attacks has no role in management of FMF. True colchicine resistance is rare (< 5%), therefore in nonresponsive patients, an alternative diagnosis or compliance should be considered. In truly colchicine-resistant patients, newer biologics such as anti-IL-1 receptor antagonist (anakinra) and etanercept have been shown to be beneficial. Infliximab has shown mixed results.

TNF Receptor-Associated Periodic Fever Syndrome (TRAPS)

TNF receptor-associated periodic fever syndrome (TRAPS), an autosomal dominant autoinflammatory disorder, was formerly known as 'Hibernian fever'. It was first described in Ireland in 1982[24] and is most common in Irish and Scottish populations but has recently been reported from all around the world.

Fevers in TRAPS generally last longer compared to other forms of periodic fever syndromes, ranging from one week to several weeks. Attacks occur with irregular intervals from once to twice a year to 6 to 7 times a year. In a subset of patients, the symptoms are present continuously.[25] Median age of onset is about 3 years (ranging from 1 to 53 years). Common features of TRAPS include: severe abdominal pain (92%) due to serositis with risk of adhesion formation, painful centrifugally migrating myalgia (due to monocytic fasciitis) sometimes with an overlying erythematous rash, ocular inflammation with conjunctivitis, uveitis, unilateral periorbital edema and arthralgia (less commonly arthritis) primarily affecting large joints. Less common findings include chest pain due to pleuritis and scrotal swelling from the inflammation of tunuca vaginalis testis. Similar to other autoinflammatory disorders, elevated inflammatory markers are found. In addition, some patients have low soluble TNF receptor levels between episodes.[5] The risk of development of amyloidosis is 10–25%, especially in patients with mutations involving cysteine substitutions, which have a higher penetrance.[4,25]

The association of this syndrome to mutations in the TNFRSF1A gene on chromosome 12p13 was discovered in 1999.[1] This gene encodes the TNF receptor type 1 (also known as p55TNFR), which is a member of the TNF receptor superfamily. It is a transmembrane protein with an intracellular death domain and four extracellular cysteine-rich domains.

Binding of TNF-α to the receptor initiates the intracellular activation cascade through the DD, leading to the activation of both NF-κB and apoptosis pathways. Once activated, TNFR1 is shed from the cell surface and becomes soluble, and binds to circulating TNF-α. This binding competitively prevents the binding of TNF-α to cell bound receptor, leading to a decrease in the inflammatory response.

The decreased shedding of the mutated TNFR1 was found in the initial TRAPS patients studied, and was implicated as the underlying mechanism of the prolonged inflammatory response. However, later work has shown that this is not the case for a significant group of the patients. Other research has shown non-ligand binding activation of the intracellular events via misfolded intracellular TNFR1 protein which triggers the unfolded protein response causing cytokine activation such as IL-1β. Aggregates of TNFR1 have been found in the cytoplasm and in the endoplasmic reticulum, supporting these hypotheses. This may be why some patients with TRAPS respond to anti-IL-1 treatment.[2] To date, more than 50 mutations have been described. Among these mutations R92Q (in Caucasians) and P46L (in African-Americans) have been found in chromosomes of 1–2.5% of the general population. These mutations may have reduced penetrance leading to atypical presentations of TRAPS[8]

Steroids have been the mainstay of therapy. Unfortunately, prolonged use is usually necessary, leading to significant side-effects. After the discovery of the gene, etanercept has been administered to patients with TRAPS. Etanercept is a dimeric fusion protein consisting of the p75 portion of TNFR linked to Fc portion of IgG1. It is beneficial in some but not all patients in decreasing the severity of the attacks. Another anti-TNF-α agent, infliximab, a chimeric IgG1 monoclonal antibody to TNF-α, has not been shown to be beneficial in TRAPS. Furthermore, it has induced exacerbations in some patients. Recently, it has been reported that some of the etanercept nonresponders respond to the IL-1 receptor antagonist, anakinra.[5]

Hyper IgD Syndrome (HIDS)

The first description of HIDS was in 1984 in 6 Dutch patients.[26] Its onset is often in infancy (90%) and is characterized by fevers recurring every 4–8 weeks, accompanied by painful cervical lymphadenopathy (90%), abdominal pain and vomiting (70%), often maculopapular, occasionally urticarial, purpuric and E. nodosum type skin rash (60%), arthralgia/myalgia (80%), apthous and/or genital ulcers (50%), and hepatosplenomegaly (30%). Chills and sweating are also common. Arthritis affecting large joints and pleuritis are less common.[27] Immunizations usually trigger attacks. HIDS features resemble that of PFAPA, which is also discussed later in this chapter.

It was unexpected when the gene affecting HIDS was found to encode mevalonate kinase, an enzyme in the cholesterol biosynthesis pathway,[28,29] already known to be implicated in mevalonic aciduria (MA), which is a metabolic disorder that presents in infancy with devastating neurologic abnormalities (mental retar-dation, cerebellar ataxia, cataracts, hypotonia, dysmorphic features) and eventually leads to early death, but also carries many of the features of HIDS.

How abnormal functioning of an enzyme in the cholesterol biosynthesis pathway caused heightened inflammatory response was initially unknown. This led to new areas of research, ultimately showing a connection with IL-1β pathway, similar to many of the periodic fever syndromes.[30] It appears that HIDS and MA are a phenotypic continuum of mevalonate kinase deficiency, from mild to severe disease[31]

The most common mutation in HIDS is at position V377I, a founder effect from a common ancestor. Urine mevalonic acid level increases during the episodes in HIDS, while it is persistently high in MA. 1–10% of enzyme activity is found in HIDS but < 1% in MA. The mutated enzyme activity decreases even further with fevers. With reduced enzyme activity, mevalonic acid accumulates and there is a decrease in the end products of the pathway, which are important in isoprenylation of proteins, hence increasing their ability to be membrane bound. It has been shown that the shortage of some of these end products, especially geranlygeranylated proteins, are involved in increased IL-1β production. Despite the nomenclature, not every patient with HIDS has elevated IgD levels, especially children, putting the role of elevated IgD in HIDS under further questioning.[27] Elevated IgD levels are not unique to this syndrome: it has been described in infections, such as tuberculosis and other inflammatory conditions, including other periodic fever syndromes. Polyclonal IgA elevation may also be seen in HIDS.

Effective treatment for HIDS is not available. Steroids, etanercept and colchicine, are only beneficial in small group of patients. Lately anakinra has shown some promise. Simvastatin, an HMG-CoA reductase inhibitor, may help in some patients with HIDS but it may exacerbate the condition in some patients with MA. There are also anecdotal reports of benefit from leukotriene inhibitor, montelukast.

Cryopyrin-Associated Periodic Syndromes (CAPS)

Cryopyrin-associated periodic syndromes (CAPS) include a spectrum of conditions that share a similar genotype with mutations in the gene encoding for cryopyrin (also known as: NLRP3, NALP3 or PYPAF1). Cryopyrin belongs to the NLR (nucleotide-binding domain and leucine rich repeat) protein family[32] and is found primarily in activated T cells, monocytes, neutrophils, and chondrocytes. These conditions are autosomal dominant, but de novo mutations may occur, and over 80 mutations have been described to date. Due to the association with cold exposure and development of fever, the protein was named as 'cryopryin' and familial cold-induced urticaria was named as familial cold autoinflammatory syndrome.

From most to least in severity of the CAPS are: neonatal onset multisystem inflammatory disease (NOMID), Muckle Wells syndrome (MWS) and FCAS. Though these have 'classic' presentations, as detailed further below, CAPS represent a spectrum of pathology, and there may be a clinical overlap among these conditions.

The first CAPS to be described was FCAS, as early as 1940.[33] Twenty three of 47 family members were affected and developed fever, urticaria, pain and arthritis after exposure to the cold. Muckle Wells syndrome was first described in 1962 with a triad of urticaria, deafness and amyloidosis in nine members of a family over five generations[34] Neonatal onset multisystem inflammatory disease (NOMID), was probably first reported in the literature in 1975:[35] two siblings, born to nonconsanguineous parents, were described as having a Still's disease-like rash, deforming arthopathy, mental retardation and uveitis.

These conditions were originally considered to be separate disease entities, based on their phenotypic differences, but clinical similarities led to the discovery that the underlying mutations were homologous. The mutations for CAPS, were first reported in 1996[36] and later confirmed in 2000 and 2001.[37]

Cryopyrin contains three domains: an N-terminal pyrin domain (PYD), a nucleotide-binding oligomerization domain (NOD or NLRP3) and a leucine-rich repeat (LRR) region. Cryopyrin functions as an intracellular pattern recognition receptor and recognizes pathogen-associated molecular patterns and danger-associated molecular patterns (PAMPS and DAMPS) via LRR. Cryopyrin is integral in the activation of the cryopyrin inflammasome: cryopyrin interacts with ASC (apoptosis-associated speck-like protein) and CARDINAL to form the activated complex with two procaspase molecules, generating active caspase-1, leading to IL-1β and IL-18 activation. The mechanism that leads to inflammation with CIAS1 mutation is not entirely understood, but studies suggest that it is a *gain-of-function mutation*, likely to be via the loss of the autoinhibition or regulatory step associated with initial NOD/NLRP3/NALP3 activation. These mutations, found on chromosome 1q, appear to lead to increased caspase-1 activation, and thus increased IL-1β secretion.

All three phenotypes of CAPS, are associated with urticaria-like skin rash that is characterized by interstitial and perivascular infiltrates of primarily neutrophils.[38]

FCAS patients typically present at less than 6 months of age. Symptoms usually occur several hours following exposure to generalized cold. The urticarial rash is the most common feature, which can be associated with swelling. The majority of patients will have arthralgia and myalgia, fever, conjunctivitis, fatigue, headache, and nausea. The duration of these attacks is typically 24 hours or less.

MWS patients typically present during adolescence with attacks that last 24 to 48 hours at irregular intervals, every few weeks. Patients have fevers and rash during typical attacks, with associated arthralgia and myalgia. Progressive sensorineural hearing loss commonly occurs in about 75% of patients and about a third of patients may develop secondary amyloidosis with nephropathy.

NOMID, also known as chronic infantile neurologic cutaneous and articular syndrome (CINCA), typically presents at less than 6 months of age and also is usually associated with significant neurologic symptoms, including: chronic meningitis, increased intracranial pressure with associated developmental delay, seizures, blindness, sensorineural hearing loss, daily fevers, and significant morbidity. These patients also have major bony abnormalities, with dysmorphic features, including: frontal bossing, erosive arthritis with severe arthropathy and joint deformity. Without treatment, patients suffer significant morbidity, and early mortality before adulthood in 20% of affected individuals.

The development of therapies for CAPS[39] is an excellent example of bench-to-bedside innovation that have greatly improved the morbidity of patients with CAPS. Steroids and NSAIDs generally do not adequately treat these conditions though steroids may have some limited benefit. IL-1 Trap, or rilonacept, a fully human dimeric fusion protein administered via weekly injection, binds soluble IL-1 and prevents its interaction with cell surface receptors[40] It was approved by the FDA in 2008 for CAPS under orphan drug status. Another option is interleukin-1 receptor antagonist, known as anakinra, administered as a daily injection which competitively inhibits the binding of IL-1α and IL-1β to the IL-1 receptor. It is approved in moderate to severe rheumatoid arthritis (RA), and is efficacious in patients with CAPS.[39] A fully human anti IL-1β monoclonal antibody with no cross reactivity to other members of the IL-1 family, known as canakinumab, is administered every 8 weeks by subcutaneous injection. It has been found to be effective in patients with CAPS[41] and was approved by the FDA for this indication in June 2009.

In addition to treating the acute symptoms related to CAPS, such as fever, arthritis and rash, treatment with anti-IL-1 therapy may lead to stabilization of chronic symptoms such as deafness, vision loss and developmental delay.

Deficiency of Interleukin-1-Receptor Antagonist (DIRA)

Deficiency of interleukin-1-receptor antagonist (DIRA) is a very rare condition that was first reported in 2009.[42,43] Only 10 patients have been reported to date. These patients present in early infancy with fever, rash with pustulosis, thromboses and osteolytic lesions and share many clinical features with NOMID.

DIRA is an autosomal recessive condition, and is associated with the deletion or truncating mutations in a 175-kb of chromosome 2q13, which encompasses five IL-1 family members as well as the IL-1 receptor antagonist (ILRN). The IL1RN mutation appears to result in truncated proteins that are not secreted, leading to cells being hyperresponsive to IL-1α and IL-1β stimulation.

These patients respond well to treatment with corticosteroids and anti-IL-1 therapy (anakinra) with rapid response to therapy and full resolution of symptoms in the majority of patients.[42,43]

Blau Syndrome/Pediatric Granulomatous Arthritis

Blau syndrome is a systemic granulomatous condition which was first described in 1985 where 11 family members over four generations had granulomatous disease of the skin, eyes, and joints.[44] Recently it has been thought to include early onset sarcoidosis.[45] Blau syndrome typically presents at less than 5 years of age, and is characterized by a maculopapular rash, noncaseating granulomatous arthritis, uveitis, and lymphadenopathy. Fever may not be a prominent clinical symptom. It is distinguished from the autoimmune condition, sarcoidosis, based on its early age of onset and lack of lung and hilar lymph node involvement.

Blau syndrome is an autosomal dominant condition, involving chromosome 16q12, and over 90 mutations are described to date. Mutations in this region have also been associated with early-onset sarcoidosis. This gene encodes NOD2 (also known as CARD15), which is expressed primarily in myeloid cells, Paneth cells of the small intestine and activated intestinal epithelial cells, and is a member of the NLR protein family. NOD2, is made up of an N-terminal NOD/NACHT domain, an LRR region and two C-terminal CARD domains.

Similar to the cryopyrin, NOD2 appears to function as an intracellular pattern recognition receptor and recognizes pathogen-associated molecular patterns and is integral in IL-1β and NFκB activation. Bacterial cell wall peptidoglycans such as muramyl dipeptide, stimulate the NOD2 inflammasome, leading to the recruitment of RIP2 (also called RICK/CARDIAK) which then activates the IKK complex through IKKγ/NEMO and the release of NFκB and proinflammatory cytokines such as IL-1β and

IL-18.[46,47] Mutations in Blau syndrome appear to be a gain of function due to loss of auto-inhibition. However, patients with Blau syndrome, do not appear to have excess IL-1β activity, so the underlying mechanism for this condition remains under study.[48]

In contrast to Blau syndrome, in Crohn's disease (CD), another inflammatory granulomatous condition, mutations have been reported in the LRR region. These mutations may theoretically lead to diminished intracellular sensing of bacteria, thereby leading to diminished activity of the NOD2 inflammasome ('loss of function'). The exact role of these mutations in CD remains under investigation.

There are no case-controlled studies in the treatment of Blau syndrome, but anecdotal evidence supports the use of steroids, immunomodulation with TNF-α inhibitors and possibly other immunosuppressive therapies, such as methotrexate. There have been inconsistent results of clinical improvement with anti-IL-1 therapy.

Majeed Syndrome

Majeed syndrome is a very rare condition, first described in 1989 in a consanguineous Kuwaiti family, where three related children presented with congenital dyserythropoietic anemia, chronic recurrent multifocal osteomyelitis, and Sweet's syndrome. It has been found most commonly in Arabic populations.

These patients typically present at less than 2 years of age, with chronic recurrent episodes of sterile osteomyelitis and fever with associated destructive arthritis and deformities. Osteomyelitis more commonly involves the metaphyses. Fevers typically last 3 to 4 days, and occur about every 2 to 4 weeks, but symptoms have also been reported to be continuous. Rashes may include Sweet's syndrome and pustular lesions. Hepatosplenomegaly

and cholestatic jaundice are also reported. Patients may have transient neutropenia in infancy and chronic dyserythropoietic anemia may lead to transfusion dependence.

Majeed sydrome is an autosomal recessive disorder involving the LPIN2 gene on chromosome 18p.[49] Eight mutations have been described to date. The role that protein LPIN2 plays in Majeed syndrome is not clear. LPIN2 is similar to LPIN1, which plays a role in murine lipodystrophy but this has not helped to elucidate the role of LPIN2 mutations in Majeed syndrome. It may play a role in cellular response to oxidative stress.

Systemic corticosteroids and nonsteroidal antiinflammatory drugs appear to provide clinical improvement in patients. Data is limited with regard to disease-modifying antirheumatic agents or biologics.

Pyogenic Sterile Arthritis, Pyoderma Gangrenosum and Acne (PAPA)

Pyogenic sterile arthritis, pyoderma gangrenosum and acne (PAPA), first described in 1997,[50] is characterized by the clinical features described in its name. Typically, a very destructive arthritis is present, associated with pyoderma gangrenosum skin lesions and muscle inflammation.

PAPA is an autosomal dominant condition (chromosome 15q24-q25.1) and is associated with mutations in PSTPIP1, which is highly expressed in neutrophils and T cells. The genetic association was described in 2002,[51] and four mutations have been described to date. PSTPIP1 interacts with pyrin,[52] and the mutation implicated in PAPA, which leads to hyperphosphorylation, appears to increase the interaction of PSTPIP1 with pyrin, leading to a loss of function mutation, due to a reduction of pyrin's regulatory effect on the NALP3/cryopyrin inflammasome (Figure 21-1).

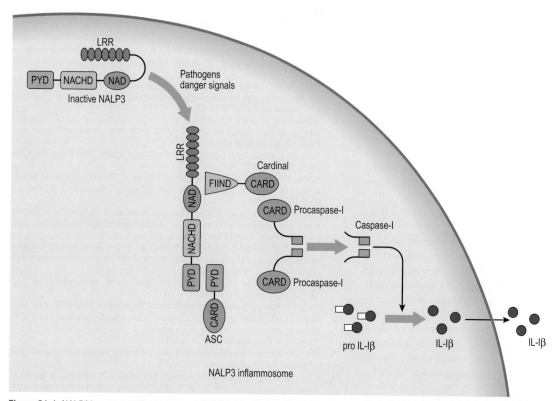

Figure 21-1 NALP3/cryopyrin inflammasome. NALP3 is usually found in an inactive state, and is activated by 'danger signals' such as peptidoglycans, ATP, uric acid crystals, bacterial RNA, etc, which leads to its unfolding and association with the remainder of the NALP3 inflammasome components FIIND (domain with function to find), CARDINAL, ASC and procaspase 1, via association between pyrin (*PYD*) and CARD domains. The NALP3 inflammasome induces the cleavage of procaspase-1 to caspase, leading to the activation of IL-1β from pro IL-1β.

PSTPIP1 is also known as CD2-binding protein (CDBP1) and interacts with CD2, Wiskott-Aldrich syndrome protein (WASP) and FasL, implicating its role in the adaptive immune system related to antigen recognition.

Limited anecdotal evidence suggests that steroids, anti-TNF therapy and anti IL-1 therapy may benefit these patients. Overall, anti-IL-1β therapy does not appear as effective in PAPA, compared to CAPS, suggesting that the mutations implicated in PAPA have additional effects beyond IL-1 over-expression.

Periodic Fevers, Apthous Stomatitis, Pharyngitis and Adenitis (PFAPA)

PFAPA is one of the periodic fever/autoinflammatory disorders with features described in the name, including periodic fevers with apthous stomatitis, pharyngitis and cervical adenitis. It was first described by Marshall in 1987,[53] followed by the publication of several other series.[54-57] PFAPA is clinically benign without any known long-term sequelae. It usually occurs in preschool age children with a male predominance. Regular intervals between episodes (usually every 4 weeks) as well as normal growth and development of the affected children are signature features of the syndrome, which help in diagnosis. Episodes usually last 4 to 6 days and frequently start with a sudden rise in temperature. Constitutional symptoms such as malaise, chills and headache may also be present, especially at the start of an episode. Less commonly, nausea, vomiting, and abdominal pain may occur. Oral ulcers usually are shallow and lymphadenopathy is often bilateral and tender. Parents are often able to predict fever episodes and the episodes usually end abruptly. Leukocytosis and mild elevation of the inflammatory markers are seen in most patients.[54-60]

Almost all of the patients with PFAPA respond to one or two doses of corticosteroids (0.5–2 mg/kg prednisone or prednisolone), especially when given before the onset of fever.[54-57] Corticosteroid therapy does not prevent subsequent episodes, and patients continue to respond on subsequent cycles. Unfortunately, in a subgroup of patients, the frequency of episodes increases with corticosteroid therapy. The dramatic response to a single oral dose of corticosteroids is classic for PFAPA, so steroid response has been suggested as a diagnostic criterion in patients with possible PFAPA[56,57] Two other effective treatments include tonsillectomy with or without adenoidectomy[61-64] and daily oral cimetidine use, both of which appear to induce remission in patients. Cimetidine treatment was first found to be beneficial in the early1990s,[65] though in later studies, the efficacy was shown to be modest (29%).

The etiology of PFAFA is still unknown. It is not clear if it is a primary infection or immune dysregulation. It certainly carries features supporting both. The rarity of PFAPA in older children and adults, as well as the predominance in boys, supports an infectious etiology. On the other hand, the lack of seasonal variation or geographical clustering make infection seem unlikely. The shortened intervals between febrile episodes after starting corticosteroids favor the infection model, and so does the remission of some children with tonsillectomy, after years of clockwork febrile episodes once an infected organ is removed. Conversely, one can hypothesize that tonsillectomy works because a tissue with localized aberrant immunologic response is removed.[60]

Though PFAPA shares several features with the known autoinflammatory disorders, it is considered nonhereditary to date, since no genetic base has been described. However, it is possible that PFAPA includes several different diseases with different etiologies causing a very similar phenotype, like those seen in common variable immunodeficiency. This may explain why various therapeutic modalities are effective in the treatment of the syndrome.

Conclusions

Discoveries in relatively rare conditions, that are well known clinically, such as FMF, can unveil the mechanisms of common, yet complicated homeostatic pathways of biologic systems, such as production of inflammation against nonself and danger signals. Autoinflammatory disorders were initially coined to describe the monogenic periodic fever syndromes when it was first proposed about 10 years ago. Today, it has become an encompassing term to include diverse conditions that involve not only the disorders of other aspects of innate immune system (hereditary angioedema [HAE], atypical hemolytic uremic syndrome [aHUS]) but also polygenic (Crohn's disease, Behcet's disease, systemic onset JIA), metabolic (gout, pseudogout) and storage (Gaucher's) disorders. In a relatively short time, our knowledge of the diverse roles of the innate immune system and its intimate cross-talk with the adaptive immune system has expanded exponentially. The significant role that innate immunity plays is becoming clearer in conditions previously thought to be solely related to abnormalities in the adaptive immune system, such as contact hypersensitivity and autoimmune conditions (RA and systemic lupus erythematosus). Finally, significant progress has also been achieved in understanding mechanisms of how environmental factors play a role in variable presentations of a particular condition. In short, the more we discover, the more the plot thickens, opening up new venues of exciting research and application to clinical practice.

References

1. McDermott MF, Aksentijevich I, Galon J, et al. Germline mutations in the extracellular domains of the 55 kDa TNF receptor, TNFR1, define a family of dominantly inherited autoinflammatory syndromes. Cell 1999;97:133–44.
2. Masters SL, Simon A, Aksentijevich I, et al. Horror autoinflammaticus: the molecular pathophysiology of autoinflammatory disease (*). Annu Rev Immunol 2009;27:621–68.
3. Milhavet F, Cuisset L, Hoffman HM, et al. The infevers autoinflammatory mutation online registry: update with new genes and functions. Hum Mutat 2008;29:803–8.
4. Touitou I, Kone-Paut I. Autoinflammatory diseases. Best Pract Res Clin Rheumatol 2008;22:811–29.
5. Bodar EJ, Drenth JP, van der Meer JW, et al. Dysregulation of innate immunity: hereditary periodic fever syndromes. Br J Haematol 2009;144:279–302.
6. Gattorno M, Sormani MP, D'Osualdo A, et al. A diagnostic score for molecular analysis of hereditary autoinflammatory syndromes with periodic fever in children. Arthritis Rheum 2008;58:1823–32.
7. Simon A, van der Meer JW, Vesely R, et al. Approach to genetic analysis in the diagnosis of hereditary autoinflammatory syndromes. Rheumatology (Oxford) 2006;45:269–73.
8. Ryan JG, Kastner DL. Fevers, genes, and innate immunity. Curr Top Microbiol Immunol 2008;321:169–84.
9. Siegal S. Benign paroxysmal peritonitis. Ann Intern Med 1945;23:1–22.
10. Janeway TC, Mosenthal HO. Unusual paroxysmal syndrome, probably allied to recurrent vomiting, with a study of nitrogen metabolism. Trans Assoc Am Physicians 1908;23:504–18.
11. Ozen S. Familial mediterranean fever: revisiting an ancient disease. Eur J Pediatr 2003;162:449–54.
12. Lachmann HJ, Sengul B, Yavuzsen TU, et al. Clinical and subclinical inflammation in patients with familial Mediterranean fever and in heterozygous carriers of MEFV mutations. Rheumatology (Oxford) 2006;45:746–50.
13. Pras E, Aksentijevich I, Gruberg L, et al. Mapping of a gene causing familial Mediterranean fever to the short arm of chromosome 16. N Engl J Med 1992;326:1509–13.

14. Ancient missense mutations in a new member of the RoRet gene family are likely to cause familial Mediterranean fever. The International FMF Consortium. Cell 1997;90:797–807.

15. A candidate gene for familial Mediterranean fever. Nat Genet 1997;17:25–31.

16. Chae JJ, Wood G, Masters SL, et al. The B30.2 domain of pyrin, the familial Mediterranean fever protein, interacts directly with caspase-1 to modulate IL-1beta production. Proc Natl Acad Sci U S A 2006;103:9982–7.

17. Brydges S, Kastner DL. The systemic autoinflammatory diseases: inborn errors of the innate immune system. Curr Top Microbiol Immunol 2006;305:127–60.

18. Booth DR, Lachmann HJ, Gillmore JD, et al. Prevalence and significance of the familial Mediterranean fever gene mutation encoding pyrin Q148. QJM 2001;94:527–31.

19. Bhat A, Naguwa SM, Gershwin ME. Genetics and new treatment modalities for familial Mediterranean fever. Ann N Y Acad Sci 2007;1110:201–8.

20. Tunca M, Akar S, Onen F, et al. Familial Mediterranean fever (FMF) in Turkey: results of a nationwide multicenter study. Medicine (Baltimore) 2005;84:1–11.

21. Lidar M, Livneh A. Familial Mediterranean fever: clinical, molecular and management advancements. Neth J Med 2007;65:318–24.

22. Matzner Y, Ayesh SK, Hochner-Celniker D, et al. Proposed mechanism of the inflammatory attacks in familial Mediterranean fever. Arch Intern Med 1990;150:1289–91.

23. Aral O, Ozdogan H, Yazici H. The other physician behind the use of colchicine for the treatment of familial Mediterranean fever. Clin Exp Rheumatol 2001;19:S13–14.

24. Williamson LM, Hull D, Mehta R, et al. Familial Hibernian fever. Q J Med 1982;51:469–80.

25. Stojanov S, McDermott MF. The tumour necrosis factor receptor-associated periodic syndrome: current concepts. Expert Rev Mol Med 2005;7:1–18.

26. van der Meer JW, Vossen JM, Radl J, et al. Hyperimmunoglobulinaemia D and periodic fever: a new syndrome. Lancet 1984;1:1087–90.

27. van der Hilst JC, Bodar EJ, Barron KS, et al. Long-term follow-up, clinical features, and quality of life in a series of 103 patients with hyperimmunoglobulinemia D syndrome. Medicine (Baltimore) 2008;87:301–10.

28. Houten SM, Kuis W, Duran M, et al. Mutations in MVK, encoding mevalonate kinase, cause hyperimmunoglobulinaemia D and periodic fever syndrome. Nat Genet 1999;22:175–7.

29. Drenth JP, Cuisset L, Grateau G, et al. Mutations in the gene encoding mevalonate kinase cause hyper-IgD and periodic fever syndrome. International Hyper-IgD Study Group. Nat Genet 1999;22:178–81.

30. Houten SM, Frenkel J, Waterham HR. Isoprenoid biosynthesis in hereditary periodic fever syndromes and inflammation. Cell Mol Life Sci 2003;60:1118–34.

31. Haas D, Hoffmann GF. Mevalonate kinase deficiencies: from mevalonic aciduria to hyperimmunoglobulinemia D syndrome. Orphanet J Rare Dis 2006;1:13.

32. Masters SL, Lobito AA, Chae J, et al. Recent advances in the molecular pathogenesis of hereditary recurrent fevers. Curr Opin Allergy Clin Immunol 2006;6:428–33.

33. Kile RL, Rusk RH. A case of cold urticaria with unusual family history. JAMA 1940;114:1067–8.

34. Muckle TJ, Wells M. Urticaria, deafness, and amyloidosis: a new heredofamilial syndrome. Q J Med 1962;31:235–48.

35. Ansell MB, Bywaters EG, Elderkin FM. Familial arthropathy with rash, uveitis and mental retardation. Proc R Soc Med 1975;68:584–5.

36. Jung M, Ross B, Wienker TF, et al. A locus for familial cold urticaria maps to distal chromosome 1q: familial cold urticaria and Muckle-Wells-syndrome are probably allelic. Am J Hum Genet 1996;A223.

37. Hoffman HM, Mueller JL, Broide DH, et al. Mutation of a new gene encoding a putative pyrin-like protein causes familial cold autoinflammatory syndrome and Muckle-Wells syndrome. Nat Genet 2001;29:301–5.

38. Shinkai K, McCalmont TH, Leslie KS. Cryopyrin-associated periodic syndromes and autoinflammation. Clin Exp Dermatol 2008;33:1–9.

39. Ramos E, Arostegui JI, Campuzano S, et al. Positive clinical and biochemical responses to anakinra in a 3-yr-old patient with cryopyrin-associated periodic syndrome (CAPS). Rheumatology (Oxford) 2005;44:1072–3.

40. Hoffman HM, Throne ML, Amar NJ, et al. Efficacy and safety of rilonacept (interleukin-1 Trap) in patients with cryopyrin-associated periodic syndromes: results from two sequential placebo-controlled studies. Arthritis Rheum 2008;58:2443–52.

41. Lachmann HJ, Kone-Paut I, Kuemmerle-Deschner JB, et al. Use of canakinumab in the cryopyrin-associated periodic syndrome. N Engl J Med 2009;360:2416–25.

42. Reddy S, Jia S, Geoffrey R, et al. An autoinflammatory disease due to homozygous deletion of the IL1RN locus. N Engl J Med 2009;360:2438–44.

43. Aksentijevich I, Masters SL, Ferguson PJ, et al. An autoinflammatory disease with deficiency of the interleukin-1-receptor antagonist. N Engl J Med 2009;360:2426–37.

44. Blau E. Familial granulomatous arthritis, uveitis and rash. J Pediatr 1985;107:689–93.

45. Rose CD, Doyle TM, McIlvain-Simpson G, et al. Blau syndrome mutation of CARD15/NOD2 in sporadic early onset granulomatous arthritis. J Rheumatol 2005;32:373–5.

46. Shaw MH, Reimer T, Kim YG, et al. NOD-like receptors (NLRs): bona fide intracellular microbial sensors. Curr Opin Immunol 2008;20:377–82.

47. Fritz JH, Ferrero RL, Philpott DJ, et al. Nod-like proteins in immunity, inflammation and disease. Nat Immunol 2006;7:1250–7.

48. Martin TM, Zhang Z, Kurz P, et al. The NOD2 defect in Blau syndrome does not result in excess interleukin-1 activity. Arthritis Rheum 2009;60:611–8.

49. Ferguson PJ, Chen S, Tayeh MK, et al. Homozygous mutations in LPIN2 are responsible for the syndrome of chronic recurrent multifocal osteomyelitis and congenital dyserythropoietic anaemia (Majeed syndrome). J Med Genet 2005;42:551–7.

50. Lindor NM, Arsenault TM, Solomon H, et al. A new autosomal dominant disorder of pyogenic sterile arthritis, pyoderma gangrenosum, and acne: PAPA syndrome. Mayo Clin Proc 1997;72:611–5.

51. Wise CA, Gillum JD, Seidman CE, et al. Mutations in CD2BP1 disrupt binding to PTP PEST and are responsible for PAPA syndrome, an autoinflammatory disorder. Hum Mol Genet 2002;11:961–9.

52. Shoham NG, Centola M, Mansfield E, et al. Pyrin binds the PSTPIP1/CD2BP1 protein, defining familial Mediterranean fever and PAPA syndrome as disorders in the same pathway. Proc Natl Acad Sci USA 2003;100:13501–6.

53. Marshall GS, Edwards KM, Butler J, et al. Syndrome of periodic fever, pharyngitis, and aphthous stomatitis. J Pediatr 1987;110:43–6.

54. Tasher D, Somekh E, Dalal I. PFAPA syndrome: new clinical aspects disclosed. Arch Dis Child 2006;91:981–4.

55. Feder HM Jr, Bialecki CA. Periodic fever associated with aphthous stomatitis, pharyngitis and cervical adenitis. Pediatr Infect Dis J 1989;8:186–7.

56. Thomas KT, Feder HM Jr, Lawton AR, et al. Periodic fever syndrome in children. J Pediatr 1999;135:15–21.

57. Padeh S, Brezniak N, Zemer D, et al. Periodic fever, aphthous stomatitis, pharyngitis, and adenopathy syndrome: clinical characteristics and outcome. J Pediatr 1999;135:98–101.

58. Pinto A, Lindemeyer RG, Sollecito TP. The PFAPA syndrome in oral medicine: differential diagnosis and treatment. Oral Surg Oral Med Oral Pathol Oral Radiol Endod 2006;102:35–9.

59. Matoussi N, M'Barek SB, Fitouri Z, et al. Periodic fever, aphthous stomatitis, pharyngitis, and adenitis (PFAPA) syndrome: a Tunisian report. Int J Pediatr Otorhinolaryngol Extra 2008;3:10–3.

60. Long SS. Syndrome of periodic fever, aphthous stomatitis, pharyngitis, and adenitis (PFAPA)–what it isn't. What is it? J Pediatr 1999;135:1–5.

61. Wong KK, Finlay JC, Moxham JP. Role of tonsillectomy in PFAPA syndrome. Arch Otolaryngol Head Neck Surg 2008;134:16–9.

62. Licameli G, Jeffrey J, Luz J, et al. Effect of adenotonsillectomy in PFAPA syndrome. Arch Otolaryngol Head Neck Surg 2008;134:136–40.

63. Renko M, Salo E, Putto-Laurila A, et al. A randomized, controlled trial of tonsillectomy in periodic fever, aphthous stomatitis, pharyngitis, and adenitis syndrome. J Pediatr 2007;151:289–92.

64. Garavello W, Romagnoli M, Gaini RM. Effectiveness of adenotonsillectomy in PFAPA syndrome: a randomized study. J Pediatr 2009;155:250–3.

65. Feder HM Jr. Cimetidine treatment for periodic fever associated with aphthous stomatitis, pharyngitis and cervical adenitis. Pediatr Infect Dis J 1992;11:318–21.

22

Laboratory Diagnosis and Management of Human Allergic Disease

Robert G. Hamilton

The diagnosis of human allergic disease begins and ends with the patient's clinical history and physical examination.[1] When the clinical history identifies allergic symptoms in temporal relationship with a definable and relevant allergen exposure, immunoglobulin E (IgE) antibody sensitization is then confirmed with in vivo skin tests (puncture/intradermal) or in vitro blood tests (allergen-specific IgE antibody serological assays). If there is a mismatch between the history and these primary diagnostic tests for sensitization, then a secondary provocation test (placebo-controlled food challenge, nasal challenge, bronchial challenge) may adjudicate the veracity of the history-driven diagnosis.[2] This chapter discusses analytes that serve as *diagnostic confirmatory tests* when there is high suspicion of allergic disease based on a clinical history, and provides quantification of the environmental allergen burden to permit *allergen exposure assessment and more effective management* of patients diagnosed with allergic disease.

Immediate (Type 1) Hypersensitivity Response

Prausnitz and Kustner first described the immediate-type hypersensitivity allergic reaction using an in vivo test when serum from Kustner, who was allergic to fish, was injected into the skin of Prausnitz.[3] An immediate wheal and flare reaction in the skin was then induced when fish antigen was injected into the same skin site. A serum factor or atopic reagin was later shown to be a novel immunoglobulin (IgE).[4,5]

Box 22-1 summarizes the immune system components that are involved in the induction of IgE antibody and elicitation of the effector mechanisms of type 1 hypersensitivity. Inhalation, skin or parenteral exposure to *allergens* are the initiating event, during which these foreign molecules are presented to antigen-presenting cells on mucosal surfaces. Antigen-presenting cells process present antigenic epitopes to *T helper cells* that secrete *cytokines* (IL-4, IL-10, IL-13) which induce *B cell* lymphocyte proliferation. Allergen-specific IgE antibody is produced and it circulates and binds onto FcεR1 receptors on *mast cells* and *basophils*. Upon re-exposure, allergen cross-links receptor bound IgE, causing an influx in calcium, which triggers pre-formed *mediator release (histamine, proteases)* and newly synthesized mediators (*leukotrienes, prostaglandins*). The pharmacological effects of these mediators on blood vessels and airways produce a spectrum of clinical symptoms including hay fever, asthma, eczema and anaphylaxis. Released *cytokines* (IL-4, IL-5, IL-6) from degranulating mast cells serve to enhance the inflammatory and IgE responses.

An investigation involving engineered antibodies and allergens showed that the concentration, specific activity (specific to total IgE ratio), affinity (tightness of binding) and clonality (epitope specificity) of the IgE antibody response each impact on effector cell activation.[6] The study concluded that higher levels of basophil activation occurred with higher overall total serum IgE levels, higher Derp2-specific IgE to total IgE ratios, broader clonality and higher IgE antibody affinities. Future designs of serological assays for IgE antibody need to quantify these four important humoral immune response parameters.[7]

Allergens

Allergens are mixtures of glycoproteins, lipoproteins or proteins that have been identified among the weeds, grasses, trees, animal danders, molds, house dust mites, parasites, insect venoms, occupational allergens, drugs and foods. Grass, for instance, has an estimated 9000 species that cover approximately 20% of the world surface. Cereals and forage plants reside in this family as well as grass mixtures for lawns. Extensive immunologic cross-reactivity exists within the grass genus *Festuceae* (Cocksfoot, Meadow Fescue, Rye, Meadow/Kentucky Blue/June and Timothy grass). In contrast, Bermuda grass (*Cynodon dactylon*) shows moderate cross-reactivity to Johnson and Bahia grass but not to the other distantly related grasses. A comprehensive compendium of these and other clinically important allergens with their scientific names, purified allergen components and identification codes is presented elsewhere.[8]

Natural rubber latex is another illustrative allergen group. Children who undergo multiple surgeries early in life are at an increased risk for becoming sensitized to natural rubber latex allergens. Frequent urologic, orthopedic and neurologic surgeries can result in repeated exposures to natural rubber latex gloves as well as rubber bladder catheters and nonsterile powdered examination gloves. A panel of potent latex allergens have been identified in latex-containing products (Table 22-1): *Hevea brasiliensis* (Hev-b) 1 and Hev-b 3 are proteins that envelop rubber particles and promote rubber chain formation. Hev-b 2, 6, 11, 12 and Hevamine are pathogenesis-related (PR) proteins in the central (C) serum or aqueous phase that serve to protect the plant against pathogenic microorganisms. Hev-b 2 (PR2) degrades fungal cell walls, Hev-b 11 (PR3) degrades chitin exoskeleton of insects and Hev-b 6 (PR3) is involved in plant would repair. Hev-b 6 comprises a separate group of allergens that are involved in modifying the latex coagulation process. Hevein or Hev-b 6.02

©2010 Elsevier Ltd, Inc, BV
DOI: 10.1016/B978-1-4377-0271-2.00022-5

Principal Immune System Components Involved in the Induction of IgE Antibody and Effector Mechanisms of Type I Hypersensitivity*

Antigen Presentation

Allergen (exposure, entry at mucosal surfaces or local lymph nodes)

Antigen presenting cells (processing and presentation)

T_H2 lymphocytes

Cytokines (promotors of IgE production: IL4, IL-10, IL-13 inhibitors of IgE production: IFγ)

B cell lymphocytes

IgE Production and Sensitization

IgE (allergen-specific IgE antibody)

Connective tissue fixed and mucosal mast cells with FcεRI receptors

Circulating basophils with FcεRI receptors

Mast Cell Activation and Mediator Release

Re-exposure to *allergen* induces calcium ion influx into mast cells

Mast cell releases preformed and newly synthesized mediators

Release of *trypase*

Exocytosis of preformed *histamine*

Synthesis of newly formed lipid mediators from arachidonic acid

Prostaglandin D_2

Leukotriene B_4, C_4, D_4

Humoral Immune Response

Chronic antigenic challenge (inadvertent or intentional [immunotherapy]) induces antigen-specific IgG and IgA antibodies in blood and secretions)

*Analytes in italics are routinely measured in the clinical diagnostic allergy laboratory and thus they are discussed in the text. Analytes that are underlined are considered research analytes and they are not routinely measured in the clinical immunology laboratory.

is a lectin-line protein that aids in latex coagulation by interacting with the n-acetyl d glucosamine and 22 kD glycoprotein receptor on the surface of the rubber particle. Hev-b 7 inhibits coagulation. Hev-b 4, 5, 8, 9, and 10 are structural proteins and housekeeping enzymes. The American Society for Testing Materials has standardized a new panel of analytical immunoassays to quantify Hev-b 1, 3, 5, and 6.02 in extracts of suspected natural rubber-containing products.[9]

In IgE antibody assays, there is an increasing trend toward the use of native and recombinant component allergens. Instead of measuring IgE antibody to crude cat dander extract, newer microarray assays are designed to measure IgE antibody specific to component allergens produced by cats, namely Fel-d 1 (uteroglobin), Fel-d 2 (cat albumin) and Fel-d 3 (cystatin), Fel-d 4 (lipocalin), Fel-d 5 (cat IgA), Fel-d 6 (cat IgM), and Fel-d 7 (cat IgG). Use of component allergens allows one to more effectively dissect the IgE antibody response into allergen families that share structural homologies that cross-react with each other.

Possibly the most well-studied example is the family of cross-reactive allergens called the PR-10 proteins or Bet-v 1 homologues. Group 1 allergen from birch tree pollen, Bet-v1, has a number of homologues. These include allergenic proteins from alder tree pollen (Aln g 1), hazelnut pollen (Cor-a 1), apple (Mal-d 1), peach (Pru-p 1), soybean (Gly-m 4), peanut (Ara-h 8), celery (Apr-g 1), carrot (Dau-c 1) and kiwi (Act-d 8). A primary sensitivity to Bet-v 1 may result in oral allergy symptoms after exposure to any of these structurally similar allergenic molecules. The chip-based microarray system discussed below is a comprehensive tool for identifying IgE antibodies in a given patient's serum that cross-react with components from among seemingly disparate allergen sources.

Diagnosis of Type 1 Hypersensitivity

The diagnostic algorithm for human allergic disease begins with a thorough clinical history and physical examination. A sugges-

Table 22-1 Natural Rubber Latex (*Hevea brasiliensis*) Allergens

Name	Description	MW kDa	Crossreactions and Plat Family	Allergen Group
Hev-b 1	Rubber elongation factor	58/14.6	Hevb3-rp	1
Hev-b 2	Beta 1/3 gluconase	34–36	PR-2	2
Hev-b 3	Prenyltransferase	24–27	Hevb1-rp	1
Hev-b 4	Microhelix	110/115		4
Hev-b 5	Acidic protein	16		4
Hev-b 6.02	Hevein protein	4.7	PR-3/foods	2, 3
Hev-b 7	Patatin homologue	43–35		2, 3
Hev-b 8	Hevea profilin	14–14.2	Pan-allergen	4
Hev-b 9	Hevea enolase	51	Molds	4
Hev-b 10	Superoxide dismutase	26	Molds	4
Hev-b 11	Class I chitinase	33	PR-3/foods	2
Hev-b 12	Lipid transfer protein	9.4	PR-14	4
Hev-b 13	Esterase	42		4

Allergen groups: 1, biosynthesis of polyisoprene polymer; 2, pathogenesis-related proteins; 3, latex coagulation-related proteins; 4, structural proteins and housekeeping enzymes. The plant families are pathogenesis-related-2 (PR-2), PR-3 and PR14.

BOX 22-2 Key concepts

Diagnosis

- Allergen-specific IgE antibody is the most important analyte measured in the clinical immunology laboratory for diagnosis of allergic disease. It is performed as a confirmatory test to support a clinical history that strongly suggests an allergic disorder.

- Allergen-specific IgE antibody is measured by nonisotopic autoanalyzers that employ the classical radioallergosorbent test or RAST assay design. The RAST is a two-stage noncompetitive immunoassay in which allergen-specific antibodies are bound to an allergosorbent and bound IgE antibodies are detected with radioiodinated antihuman IgE. A calibration curve analyzed is performed in each assay to allow interpolation of response data into dose estimates of allergen-specific IgE.

- Clinically used FDA-cleared allergen-specific IgE antibody immunoassays, which are patterned after the RAST, are more quantitative, reproducible, standardized, allergen-specific, rapid, automated and safer (nonisotopic). Quantitative IgE antibody results are reported in kUA/L, traceable to the World Health Organization IgE Standard (1 IU = 2.4 nanograms of IgE).

- The multi-allergen screen is a qualitative RAST-type assay that measures allergen-specific IgE antibody to multiple aeroallergens and/or food allergens, in a single test. The multi-allergen screening assay produces qualitative (positive or negative) results that lead to subsequent investigation of the patient's serum or skin for IgE antibodies specific for individual clinically defined allergen specificities.

- Competitive inhibition format of the RAST-type immunoassays is used to determine the relative potency of allergen extracts used in skin testing, to identify the extent of cross-reactivity of human IgE antibody for structurally similar allergens (e.g. Vespid vs Polistes Wasp venom allergens) and in *Hymenoptera* venom allergy, to select appropriate venoms for immunotherapy.

- Quantitative IgE antibody levels to selected foods (milk, egg, fish and peanut) if above a predefined IgE antibody threshold may eliminate the need for tedious and expensive double blind placebo-controlled food challenges (DBPCFC). However, food antigen-specific IgG and IgG4 antibody levels do not correlate with the diagnostic results of DBPCFCs.

BOX 22-3

Analytes Measured in the Clinical Immunology Laboratory

Diagnosis

Allergen-specific IgE

    Multi-allergen-specific IgE screen (adult and pediatric forms)

    Individual allergen specificities

Total serum IgE[1]

Precipitating antibodies specific for proteins in organic dusts

Tryptase (α, β) (mast cell protease and used as a marker for mast cell-mediated anaphylaxis)

Other tests: complete blood count (CBC), sputum examination for eosinophils and neutrophils

Management

Allergen-specific IgG (Hymenoptera)

Indoor aeroallergen quantitation in surface dust

    Der p 1/Der f 1 (Dust mite, *Dermatophagoides*)

    Fel d 1 (Cat, *Felis domesticus*)

    Can f 1 (Dog, *Canis familaris*)

    Bla g 1 / Bla g 2 (Cockroach: *Blattela germanica*)

    Mus m 1 (Mouse: *Mus musculus*)

    Rat n 1 (Rat: *Rattus norvegicus*)

Cotinine (metabolite of nicotine measured in serum, urine and sputum and used as a marker of smoke exposure)

Research Analytes

IgE specific autoantibodies

Eosinophil cationic protein

Mediators[2,3]

    Preformed biogenic amine: histamine

    Newly formed

        leukotriene C_4 (LTC_4)

        prostaglandin D_2 (PGD_2)

Proteoglycans[2]

    Heparin

    Chondroitin sulfate E

Proteases[2]

    Mast cell chymase

    Mast cell carboxypeptidase

    Cathepsin G

Fibroblast growth factor (bFGF)[2]

Cytokines

    Tumor necrosis factor (TNF)-alpha

    Interleukins (ILs) 4, 5, 6, 13[3]

[1]Total serum IgE is the only one of these tests listed that is regulated under the CLIA 88. [2]Primarily released from mast cells. [3]Primarily released from basophils.

tive history is followed by in vivo skin testing, in vitro serological assays and/or provocation challenge tests as confirmatory measures for the detection of IgE antibodies (BOX 22-3). The interrelationship between each of these components of the diagnostic plan is illustrated in this chapter using natural rubber latex as a model allergen system.

Clinical History

Latex allergy diagnosis begins with a comprehensive clinical history.[10] A child may present with complaints of hives, rhinoconjunctivitis, asthma or anaphylaxis that are temporally associated with exposure to a natural rubber product. The allergist probes the child's general atopic and specific latex allergy history using questions designed to identify predisposing risk factors, such as an atopic state (seasonal rhinitis, early onset asthma, ezcema, food allergy), the frequency, consistency and magnitude of latex exposure, the presence of concomitant food allergy and hand dermatitis.[11] Exposure to rubber-containing products

provide clues which strengthen the clinical suspicion of latex allergy. The rapid onset allergic symptoms around toy balloons, dental dams or other dipped rubber products (latex gloves, rubber toys) that contain high levels of allergen is supportive.[12] In contrast, respiratory or upper airway symptoms around latex paint that does not contain natural rubber, diminishes the likelihood of latex allergy. The type of exposure, time of onset, and duration and severity of the symptoms can help differentiate between immediate type 1 (protein-allergen induced) and delayed type 4 (rubber chemical induced) hypersensitivity.

Finally, a genetic predisposition for atopic disease or parental history of allergy, chronic infectious or acute viral illness, relative contribution of T_H1/T_H2 cells to the immune response and the nutritional status of the individual are other potential risk factors.

Diagnostic Laboratory Methods

Historically, total serum IgE was used as a diagnostic marker for allergic disease.[13] However, the wide overlap in the total serum IgE levels between atopic and nonatopic populations[14] caused it to be superseded by allergen-specific IgE as the single most important laboratory analyte in the diagnostic work-up for allergic disease. Since 2003, all patients receiving anti-IgE therapy (Xolair) must first have a total serum IgE to determine whether or not they are a candidate for the treatment. According to the Xolair indication, if the patient's total IgE falls between 30 and 700 kIU/L, (IU – international unit of IgE which is equivalent to approximately 2.4 nanograms of IgE) then the clinician can use the total serum IgE level to compute the starting Xolair dose using package insert criteria.

The radioallergosorbent test (RAST) was the first assay developed in 1968 for the detection of allergen-specific IgE antibodies in human serum.[15] The RAST is a noncompetitive, heterogeneous (separation step included), solid-phase immunoradiometric (radiolabeled antibody) assay in which allergen is covalently coupled to a solid phase (e.g. cellulose paper disc). In an initial incubation, human serum is added to the allergosorbent, during which time antibodies of all human isotypes, if present, bind to insolubilized antigens. Following a buffer wash, bound IgE is detected with ^{125}I-labeled antihuman IgE Fc. After a second buffer wash to remove unbound radiolabeled antihuman IgE, bound radioactivity is measured in a gamma counter. The counts per minute bound to the solid phase is proportional to the amount of allergen-specific IgE in the initial serum specimen.

The basic RAST chemistry has remained essentially unchanged over more than 35 years. The number and quality of allergen extracts used in preparing allergosorbents have increased as a result of extensive research with the use of new methods of extraction and quality control. While the paper disc is still employed in a clinically-used IgE antibody assay (Aligent-Hycor, IgE Turbo-MP), new matrix materials such as the cellulose sponge (Phadia ImmunoCAP) and the use of biotinylated allergens (Siemens Immulite) have enhanced the binding capacity and reduced the nonspecific binding properties of allergosorbents. Various polyclonal and monoclonal anti-IgE detection antibody combinations insure maximal assay sensitivity and specificity for human IgE. Automation has improved assay precision and reproducibility. Nonisotopic labels have increased the shelf-life of reagents and have made the assays more user-friendly. Calibration systems employ a common strategy[16] in which a (heterologous) total serum IgE curve is used to convert allergen-specific IgE assay response data into quantitative dose estimates of IgE antibody. All these modifications have resulted in assays with superior analytical sensitivity and specificity and are more quantitative, reproducible and automated than their earlier counterparts. These improvements have made the serological assay for IgE antibody more diagnostically competitive with its in vivo puncture skin test counterpart. The intradermal skin test still appears to possess an inherent advantage in terms of analytical sensitivity and disadvantage of a loss of diagnostic specificity.[1,17]

In 2009, a consensus guideline (I/LA20-A2) on allergen specific IgE assays was prepared by an international body of scientists in academia, industry and government regulatory agencies.[8] This effort has led to a more uniform strategy among the various assay manufacturers to report IgE antibody results in a common unitage (kUA/L) using a calibration system linked to the World Health Organization IgE standard (75/502). In spite of the use of a commonly calibration scheme, the clinically used assays measure different populations of IgE antibody.[18] This inter-assay difference stems from the use of extracts containing different compositions of allergens. The result, however, is that published IgE antibody data generated with one assay cannot be directly extrapolated to published predictive outcomes that are based on IgE antibody levels from a second assay method. Specific IgE antibody levels measured in different commercial assays are not interchangeable or equivalent.[8]

Until recently, all allergen preparations used in IgE antibody assays were mixtures of proteins from biological extracts that vary in their composition (molecular weight, charge [isoelectric point], relative content) and allergenic potency as a function of a number of factors. These factors include the season in which the raw material is collected, the degree of difficulty in identifying pure source of material, the presence of morphologically similar raw materials that may cross-contaminate and differences in the allergen extraction process. Allergen extracts undergo extensive quality control using isoelectrofocusing, SDS-polyacrylamide gel electrophoresis, crossed-immunoelectrophoresis, and immunoblotting methods. There are also issues of stability during storage, heterogeneity of the human IgE antibody containing quality control sera and different acceptance criteria for extract-based allergen-containing reagents. Thus, allergosorbents from different manufacturers should be expected to detect different populations of IgE antibodies for any given allergen specificity.

A trend has begun toward the supplementation of extract-based allergen-containing reagents with recombinant allergens that are either in low quantity or missing. For instance, the crude latex extract has been supplemented with recombinant Hev-b 5 which is labile and does not survive the extraction and coupling procedures. Addition of recombinant Hev-b 5 to the latex reagent increases the sensitivity of at least one IgE antibody assay by 10%, with no loss of specificity.[19] Problems can, however, occur when recombinant protein supplementation of extracts is performed without the knowledge of the end user. When hazelnut extract used on an allergosorbent was supplemented with recombinant Cor-a 1, it caused the enhanced detection of IgE anti-Bet-v 1.[20] This led to unusually high levels of IgE antihazelnut in patients with a concomitant birch pollen sensitivity which were difficult to interpret by the clinician.

In 2002, the microarray chip emerged.[21] Its current commercialized version, ImmunoCAP ISAC or immuno-solid phase allergen chip (VBC Genomics-Phadia), has 103 native/recombinant component allergens from 43 allergen sources that are dotted in triplicate onto glass slides. Twenty microliters of serum are pipetted onto the chip and antibodies specific for the allergens attached to the chip bind during a 2-hour incubation period. Following a buffer wash, bound IgE is detected with a fluorescently-labeled anti-IgE. The chip is read in a fluorometer and fluorescent signal units are interpolated into ISU or immuno-solid phase allergen chip (ISAC) units as semi-quantitative estimates of specific IgE antibody in the original serum. The analytical sensitivity of the ISAC varies as a function of the allergen specificity and is generally less than the ImmunoCAP system that employs the same allergen coupled to a sponge. The strength of the microarray system is its ability to identify cross-reactivity among structurally-similar allergens from different biological substances. The PR10-Bet-v 1 homologous family of allergens discussed earlier in this chapter is available on the ISAC chip.

They permit the assessment of cross-reactivity among this disparate allergen group. Other cross-reacting allergen families represented on the ISAC include the profilins (e.g. Bet-v 2-Birch, Ole-e 2-Olive, Hev-b 8-Latex, Phi-p 12-timothy grass), the lipid transfer proteins (e.g. Cor-a 9-hazelnut, Pru-p 3-peach, Art-v 3-mugwort and Par-j 2-Wall pellitory), the calcium binding proteins (e.g. Bet-v 4-birch, Phl-p 7-timothy grass), the tropomyosins (e.g. Pen-a 1-shrimp, Der-p 10-house dust mite, Bla-g 7-cockroach, Ani s 3-Anisakis), and the serum albumin family (e.g. Bos-d 6-bovine, Fel-d 2-cat, Can-f 3-dog, Equ-c 3-Horse and Gal-d 5-chicken). Knowledge of the extent of IgE cross-reactivity may provide useful information to the allergist as IgE serology is used to support a clinical history in the diagnostic process.

In addition to the chip-based microarray, another new trend in IgE antibody serology is the emergence of a point-of-care IgE test. A drop of blood from a finger prick is inserted into the sample well of a lateral-flow cassette. The current commercialized device (ImmunoCAP Rapid, Phadia) allows antibody to flow with the fluid front across a nitrocellulose strip that has been impregnated with lines of extract-based aeroallergens (cat dander, *D. farinae, D. pteronyssinus*, Bermuda grass, short ragweed, oak tree, *Alternaria*, timothy grass, elm tree and dog dander). If IgE antibody is bound, it is detected with anti-IgE-colloidal gold that subsequently migrates up the same nitrocellulose strip following the addition of developing solution to the appropriate well. This device is intended for use by primary care physicians who would then refer their IgE positive patient to an allergist for a comprehensive diagnostic work up.

Performance of IgE Antibody Confirmatory Tests using a Defined Positive Cut-Off Point

The practicing medical professional needs to know how well the available IgE antibody confirmatory assays perform analytically and diagnostically. The analytical performance of the available clinical assays is readily defined since the clinically used assays are all calibrated using the same WHO total serum IgE Standard (75/502). In general, available clinically used assays detect allergen-specific IgE antibody down to 0.1 kUa/L (≈0.24 ng of IgE) and false positive nonspecific binding typically occurs only with extremely high total IgE levels (e.g. >20 000 IU/mL). Analytical specificity is a function of the quality of the allergen-component and anti-IgE used in the assay.

Diagnostic sensitivity and specificity of IgE antibody assays are more difficult to determine because they require, first, differentiating individuals into those who have allergic disease from those who do not have allergic disease. There exists no perfect 'gold standard' method for defining the presence of human allergic disease. The diagnostic algorithm indicates, however, that the clinical history should be the primary decision criterion in making the final diagnosis. Unfortunately, a patient's history is not infallible.

Gendo and Larson propose three strategies for defining the presence of human allergic disease, with the expressed purpose of judging the performance of confirmatory IgE antibody tests.[22] The 'clinical criteria gold standard' correlates the patient's symptoms and signs with clinical criteria that have been established by expert opinion. It is easy to use, applicable to most patients but, unfortunately, it is prone to recall bias. Box 22-4 lists the principal patient and medical care professional factors that can influence the accuracy of the clinical criteria based gold standard approach. The 'composite gold standard' combines the clinical history and physical examination information with one or more IgE antibody confirmatory test results (skin tests or serological

tests). This approach is generally more robust than just using the history alone, however, it tends to overestimate the index test's diagnostic sensitivity and specificity if the index test is a part of the composite gold standard. Box 22-4 lists variables that influence the accuracy of skin test and serological test results. The third and possibly most rigorous strategy for defining the presence of allergic disease is the 'challenge gold standard'. Use of a challenge test to verify the presence of an allergic disease process on the surface sounds ideal. However, it too can be problematic

---

BOX 22-4

Variables that Influence the Accuracy of the Allergy Diagnosis

Patient Factors

Recognition of symptoms: recall bias related missing data, lack of knowledge or ability to accurately describe symptoms

Environment: rural, suburban, urban, pet ownership, smoking

Extent of allergen exposure: time between exposure and symptom recognition, exposure route (ingestion, inhalation, injection, adsorption)

Demographics: age (adult vs child-parent), gender, social economic status, language, race, family history of atopy

Prevalence of allergic disease in question in the population

Medical Care Professional Factors

Extent of education, training and experience

Physical examination skills

Questionnaire tools/skills: sensitivity and specificity

Differential interpretation of diagnostic test results

Skin Test Factors

Allergen extracts: potency, stability, standardization or characterization, concentration used, irritant in allergen extract, contaminant allergen in extract

Technique: puncture, intradermal, skin test device, number of skin tests, reporting scale [0 to 4+] vs mm of wheal/erythema, comparison to saline control or histamine control, skin test spacing application, insufficient penetration of the needle, testing in the week after anaphyaxis

Technologist and physician: education, training, experience in grading and interpretation of results

Quality control: negative control, positive control

Patient: dermagraphism, interfering premedication (antihistamines, tricyclic antidepressants, long-term oral steroids, topical steroids)

System factors: quality assurances practices, records, office procedures, level of documentation of results

Serological Test Factors

IgE antibody assay method: analytical sensitivity, degree of automation, method of standardization and quality control, reproducibility, linearity, units

Reagents: allergen containing reagent, anti-IgE detection reagent, buffers, protein matrix effects, recombinant allergen supplementation

Specimen/allergen specificity factors: specific to total IgE ratio, cross-reactive carbohydrate reactivity, high IgE nonspecific binding levels, allergen heterogeneity (analytical specificity)

Technical staff: education, training and experience

System factors: laboratory quality control practices, records, office procedures, level of documentation of results, laboratory certification

due to differences in threshold of organ sensitivity, a lack of standardization of methods and outcome measures, and the use of a higher allergen dose than is found in nature to elicit a clinically measurable response. Because skin and serological tests and provocation testing are analytical methods, they are inherently variable.[8,11,18,23] Thus, the validity of their results must always to be critiqued, especially if inconsistent with the history-based diagnosis.

A number of clinical studies have used one of these three gold standard approaches to define the presence of aeroallergen-related allergic disease.[24–26] With the cases defined, the investigators computed the diagnostic sensitivity and specificity of puncture skin tests and/or serological tests for IgE antibody to a limited number of aeroallergen specificities. Since the patient population studied, positive cut-off criteria and reagent sources used varied among the studies, generalized conclusions are not possible. Within the limits of these studies, the performance of the puncture skin test ranged from 55% to 98% (diagnostic sensitivity) and 70% to 90% (diagnostic specificity) using the clinical or composite gold standard to identify allergic disease. In the same studies, the performance of the serological tests for IgE antibody with the same allergen specificities ranged from 55% to 80% (diagnostic sensitivity) and 82% to 99% (diagnostic specificity) using the clinical or composite gold standard. Performance improved slightly for both the skin test and serology when a challenge-based gold standard was used to define the presence of clinical disease. Thus, as a general conclusion from these data, the diagnostic sensitivity and specificity of the puncture skin test and serology were shown to be comparable for aeroallergen related disease. Thus, the puncture skin test and serology are generally viewed today as equivalent for confirming a suggestive aeroallergen-related allergic history. However, if the confirmatory test result is inconsistent with the history-based diagnosis, it should be repeated with the same or an alternative confirmatory test for verification. Both skin and serological tests for IgE antibody are analytical methods with their inherent variability, and thus repetitive confirmation is often needed to minimize error associated with random or systematic bias.

Performance of IgE Antibody Confirmatory Tests using a Probability of Clinical Disease

Current assay technology produces quantitative estimates of IgE antibody in serum as international units per mL that are traceable to the WHO International Reference Preparation for human IgE. Rather than examine the dichotomize IgE antibody data as a positive or negative result based on a positive cut-off value, the alternative has been to examine the risk of clinical allergy associated with different IgE antibody levels as a series of probabilities. A 1997 study retrospectively investigated sera from 196 children and adolescents (mean age 5.2 years, 60% male) with atopic dermatitis who were evaluated for food allergy over a 10-year-period.[27] Levels of IgE antibodies specific for cow's milk, chicken egg, peanut, wheat, soy and fish were correlated with a diagnosis of food allergy as defined by positive double-blind, placebo-controlled food challenges or a convincing history of food-induced anaphylaxis. They were able to identify IgE antibody levels using the Phadia FEIA CAP system that could predict clinical reactivity (positive food challenges) with > 95% certainty for egg (6 kUa/L), milk (32 kUa/L), peanut (15 kUa/L), and fish (20 kUa/L). The significance of this report rests in the potential for eliminating double-blind placebo-controlled food challenges in children suspected of having IgE-mediated food allergy. In a 2001 report,[28] a prospective study was performed with sera from 100 children and adolescents (mean age: 3.8 years, 62% male) who had been referred for evaluation of food allergy. This prospective study verified the retrospective study based on 95% predictive decision points for egg, milk peanut and fish allergy. The study also confirmed that use of the positive criteria correctly diagnosed food allergy in >95% of children using the serum IgE antibody level. The study showed that quantitative food-specific IgE antibody measurements are useful in defining the probability of symptomatic allergies to egg, milk, peanut and fish in the pediatric population. The important conclusion of these studies is that judicious use of serological IgE antibody test results may eliminate the need for double-blind placebo-controlled food challenges in some children.

For inhalant allergies, quantitative cat allergen-specific IgE antibodies have been shown to be equivalent to puncture skin tests and superior in performance to intradermal skin tests in the diagnosis of clinical reactivity to cat allergen.[24] When compared to a positive cat inhalation challenge outcome, IgE antibody levels by the ImmunoCAP system displayed a diagnostic sensitivity of 69%, specificity of 100%, positive predictive value of 100% and negative predictive value of 73%. In the dust mite system, a significant correlation was observed between the concentration of dust mite specific IgE and the concentration of sensitizing mite allergen in the individual's mattress dust (p = 0.001).[29] They reported a 77% probability of being exposed to high dust mite allergen (>10 micrograms per gram of dust) when the serum IgE antimite levels were greater than 2kUa/L and vice-versa. Finally, using specific IgE as a continuous variable, the risk of current wheeze and reduced lung function in children increases significantly with increasing summed measurements of dust mite, cat and dog specific IgE antibody.[30] These data showed that quantitative estimates of serum IgE antibody can identify individuals who are not only sensitized but also who are in need of avoidance practices which they accomplish through environmental control measures. Other illustrations of the importance of quantitative allergen-specific IgE to respiratory allergy are reviewed elsewhere.[31] As a general rule for inhalant allergen specificities, the skin test and quantitative IgE antibody immunoassay can be viewed as interchangeable. One exception is in the monitoring of patients on immunotherapy where a decrease in the positivity of the puncture skin test titration alone was shown to predict continued remission after cessation of allergen immunotherapy.[32]

Multi-Allergen IgE Antibody Screening Assays

When a patient provides an equivocal history for allergic disease, it can be difficult to pinpoint with reasonable certainty the appropriate IgE antibody specificities for further diagnostic investigation. A multi-allergen screen is a single RAST-type test that has the highest negative predictive value for atopic disease of any laboratory test currently available. Multiple companies have multi-allergen screens which cover a broad number of specificities (e.g. 15 common indoor and outdoor aeroallergens that induce most upper and lower airway-related allergic disease). Other multi-allergen screens are specifically targeted at a limited number of specific allergens in a group such as the foods (e.g. chicken egg, cow's milk, peanut, soybean, wheat). A negative multi-allergen screen reduces the probability that allergic disease is the cause of the child's clinical problems. Multi-allergen screen results are particularly useful in the diagnosis of pediatric allergic diseases where there is a need to detect allergen-specific IgE antibody in serum as a marker for sensitization.

In one illustrative study,[33] 143 children and adolescent patients were assigned an allergy status (103 positive, 40 negative) based

Laboratory Diagnosis and Management of Human Allergic Disease on a combined history, skin prick test and specific IgE antibody (UniCAP, Phadia) to 6 common inhalants (mite, oak, ragweed, grass, dog, cat and *Alternaria*). The multi-allergen screen (Phadiatop, Phadia) run on these same sera correctly identified the allergy status of all subjects, verifying the diagnostic sensitivity and specificity of the Phadiatop in differentiating sensitized individuals from those who are not sensitized to common inhalant allergens.

Mast Cell Tryptase

Serum levels of tryptase can be useful as a marker of mast cell activation in making the definitive diagnosis of anaphylaxis. Tryptase is a 134 000 Da serine esterase with four subunits, each containing an enzymatically active site.[34] When tryptase becomes dissociated from heparin, it spontaneously degrades into enzymatically inactive monomeric subunits. It is released from activated mast cells in parallel with pre-stored histamine and other newly generated vasoactive mediators. The α tryptase concentration in blood is considered a measure of the mast cell number and it is estimated by subtracting the β tryptase from the total tryptase concentration. In contrast, β-tryptase levels in blood are considered a measure of mast cell activation.

An enzyme immunoassay is available to measure tryptase in human serum. It uses a capture monoclonal antibody that binds both α-protryptase and β-tryptase.[35] β-τryptase is measured with a solid phase noncompetitive immunoassay that uses a β-tryptase specific capture monoclonal antibody. Prior to analysis, both α- and β-forms of tryptase are converted into an enzymatically inactive form. Total serum tryptase concentrations in healthy (nondiseased) individuals range from 1 to 10 ng/mL (average 5 ng/mL). If baseline total serum tryptase levels exceed 20 ng/mL, systemic mastocytosis should be suspected. β-tryptase <1 ng/mL are observed in nondiseased individuals and β-tryptase levels >1 ng/mL indicate mast cell activation. For optimal results, blood samples should be collected from 0.5 to 4 hours following the initiation of a suspected mast cell-mediated systemic reaction.[36] A peak β-tryptase >10 ng/mL in a postmortem serum suggests systemic anaphylaxis as one probable cause of death. Systemic anaphylaxis induced by an insect sting can produce β-tryptase levels that peak at >5 ng/mL by 30 to 60 minutes after the sting and then decline with a biological half-life of ≈2 hours.[37]

Serum Markers of Hypersensitivity Pneumonitis

Extrinsic allergic alveolitis or hypersensitivity pneumonitis is an inflammatory reaction involving the lung interstitum and terminal bronchioles.[38] A heavy exposure to antigenic organic dusts (e.g molds, bird droppings) can induce chills, fever, malaise, cough and shortness of breath within hours of exposure. While histology of the lung lesions indicates that a cell-mediated pathology is involved in hypersensitivity pneumonitis, most individuals have high levels of IgG antibody in their serum to the offending antigen that is used as a marker of the disease. Precipitating IgG antibody specific for antigens in organic dusts has been measured in human serum to support the differential diagnosis of this condition. The classical double diffusion (Ouchterlony) analysis is routinely performed to detect precipitating antibodies in the diagnosis of this disease. In this assay, crude antigen extract and antibody (control or patient's serum) are delivered into closely spaced wells in a porous agarose gel. Visible white precipitin lines confirmed by lines of identity with known human antibody controls are considered a positive test. Precipitating antibodies or precipitins are detected in the serum

of nearly all ill patients in one study, but also in the serum of 50% of asymptomatic individuals exposed to the relevant organic dusts.[39] More recently, enzyme immunoassays for IgG antibody to selected organic dust antigens have been reported.[40] In many cases, however, the enzyme immunoassay appears to be too analytically sensitive and diagnostically nonspecific. Thus, the classical precipitin assays continue to be widely used for detecting IgG precipitins to antigens in pigeon serum, *Aureobasidium pullulans*, thermophillic actinomyces, *Aspergillus fumigatus,* and extractable proteins from fecal material produced by parakeets and a variety of exotic household birds.

Management of Type 1 Hypersensitivity

The management of individuals with allergic disease involves the combined use of pharmacotherapy, immunotherapy, anti-IgE therapy and avoidance therapy. A number of analytical measurements performed by the clinical immunology laboratory can aid the clinician in optimizing an immunotherapy regimen by monitoring the humoral (IgG antibody) immune responses in patients on venom immunotherapy. Anti-IgE therapy begins with a total serum IgE to determine proper dosing and subsequently, the clinical immunology laboratory may monitor free (non-anti-IgE bound) IgE. Finally, indoor aeroallergen levels may be measured in surface reservoir dust before remediation to document the need for allergen avoidance measures and after remediation to verify that the environment has been cleaned of allergen sources.

Optimizing Immunotherapy

When considering the medically important *Hymenoptera*, cross-reactivity has been known to exist between the vespid venoms (yellow jacket, white faced hornet and yellow hornet) and Polistes wasp venom (PWV) proteins. Results from a competitive inhibition format of the PWV-specific IgE antibody serology have allowed allergists to more effectively select the venom specificities and to minimize the number of venoms that must be admin-

---

BOX 22-5 Key concepts

Management

- Clinically successful aeroallergen immunotherapy is almost always accompanied by high (micrograms per mL) levels of allergen-specific IgG antibody in serum.

- Quantitative venom-specific IgG antibody levels can be useful in individualizing venom doses and injection frequencies for patients on maintenance venom immunotherapy for up to 4 years.

- Mast cell tryptase is a serine esterase that is used as a marker of mast cell activation during anaphylaxis. Immunoreactive tryptase levels in serum of healthy adults are typically <5 μg/L. Elevated levels (>10 μg/L) are detectable 1 to 4 hours after the onset of systemic anaphylaxis with hypotension.

- Indoor allergens from dust mites, animals (cat, dog, mouse, rat), cockroaches and a limited number of molds are quantified in processed house dust to investigate individual risk for allergic symptoms or sensitization and to monitor effects of environmental control.

istered during immunotherapy.[41] This targeted venom therapy is especially important for children where unnecessary administration of PWV may lead to denovo sensitization to Polistes allergens.

Monitoring Venom Immunotherapy

Allergen-specific IgG antibodies are not routinely measured in the clinical immunology laboratory. The one exception is *Hymenoptera* venom-related allergy. Some investigators use venom-specific IgG antibody measurements to assess the clinical and immunologic efficacy of venom immunotherapy, particularly in the early maintenance phase (3 to 6 months). Their measurement has also been used by some clinicians to periodically determine the efficacy of maintenance therapy doses and the frequency of injections and to evaluate adverse reactions and the relative need for increased venom immunotherapy doses.

Golden and colleagues[42] studied serum from 109 subjects who had a positive history of insect sting-induced systemic allergic reactions and positive intradermal skin tests with *Hymenoptera* venoms. A prospective discriminator of 3 μg/mL of IgG antivenom was able to define two groups who had been on similar maintenance venom immunotherapy for a minimum of 2 years. A total of 87 challenge stings were performed in 46 patients in the low venom-specific IgG group (<3 μg/mL) and 124 stings in 63 patients in the high group (venom-specific IgG >3 μg/mL). Systemic symptoms occurred in 1.6% of the subjects in the >3 μg/mL group, in 16% of those with <3 μg/mL and in 26% of subjects with low venom IgG who received less than 4 years of treatment. The venom-specific IgG level had no predictive value for subjects who received more than 4 year of therapy. Low venom-specific IgG levels are associated with an elevated risk of treatment failure during the first 4 years of immunotherapy with yellow jacket or mixed vespid venoms.

Monitoring Allergy Patients on Anti-IgE Therapy

Children with uncontrolled IgE-mediated asthma may be candidates for anti-IgE (Xolair) therapy. To compute the correct starting dose, a pre-Xolair total serum IgE is required. Once on Xolair, the total and allergen-specific IgE can be measured with one serological assay.[43] Moreover, the amount of free IgE unbound to Xolair can be computed[44] and used in some problematic cases to adjust the dosing regimen.

Aeroallergen Measurements of Indoor Environments to Facilitate Avoidance Therapy

Dust mite (*Dermatophagoides pteronyssinus*, *D. farinae*), cat epithelium/dander (*Felis domesticus*), dog epithelium/dander (*Canis familarias*), German cockroach (*Blatella germanica*), and mouse (*Mus muscularus*), rat (*Rattus norvegicus*) and molds are known sources of potent indoor aeroallergens.[45] Allergic proteins from each of these biosources are being used as 'indicator' allergens for relative levels in surface reservoir dust in the home, workplace or school (Box 22-3).

A surface dust specimen is collected from air ducts, floors or other horizontal surfaces (bed, upholstered furniture) using an inexpensive dust collector that is attached to a standard household vacuum cleaner. Crude dust is sent to a clinical immunology laboratory where it is sieved, extracted and quantified using a monoclonal antibody-based immunoenzymetric assays in plates (ELISA) or on fluorescent beads (BioPlex). A high level of one or more indoor aeroallergens identifies an allergen source that can sensitize or induce an allergic reaction in a sensitized individual. Levels of Der p1/f1 allergen > 2000 ng/G of fine dust have been associated with an increased risk for allergic symptoms in sensitized individuals. In contrast, cat allergen levels > 8000 ng/G of Fel-d1 in fine dust have been suggested as the threshold for sensitization. Comparable risk targets have also been used for dog (Can f1) allergen levels in indoor environments. For cockroach, mouse and/or rat urinary allergen, any detectable allergen in the indoor environment places cockroach, mouse or rat allergic individuals at risk for symptoms and further sensitization.[46]

Mold/Fungus Evaluation in Indoor Environments

Accurate quantitation of the mold content of an environment is a challenge. *Alternaria, Aspergillus, Cladosporium* and *Penicillium* comprise the majority of indoor molds.[46] The total spore counts (nonviable and viable) can be determined by collecting particulate from the air impactor or suction device and then assessing the spore's morphology for the purpose of speciating the mold. Viable fungal spores that grow when environmental conditions are favorable are considered by some allergists as more clinically important since they can colonize indoor environments and in some cases, the respiratory tract. In one clinical laboratory, a qualitative viable mold spore analysis is performed on 5 mg of fine dust that is distributed over a microbiological culture plate containing Sabouraud's dextrose agar. Visual inspection of the plate at 24 and 48 hours allows the total number of mold colonies to be quantified. The colony count at 24 hours is an estimate of the mold burden of the environment. Repetitive subculturing and morphological identification allows speciation of the predominant molds; however, this is infrequently performed. Rather, once a mold contamination has been identified, remediation by cleaning with bleach and reducing humidity is generally instituted.

There are no established mold spore contamination ranges that can be considered safe, partly because mold is ever present, different individuals have different relative sensitivities and the target airborne mold allergens are difficult to sample and verify. Thus, it is not possible to identify an environment that will place a mold-allergic person at risk for symptoms. Multiple variables associated with mold spore heterogeneity, differential growth based on nutrients and environmental conditions, the degree of aerosolization, and variable specificity of the patient's IgE antibody complicate the interpretation of a mold spore measurement when attempting to predict a clinical outcome from any environmental exposure. Sometimes the indoor mold levels are compared to the outdoor mold levels collected at the same time to judge if airborne mold spores are significantly higher and thus playing a more significant role in the allergy and asthma symptoms experienced indoors. Mold spore levels above 25 000 colonies per gram of fine dust have been identified in one study as a level that places a home in the 75th percentile for random homes monitored across the USA. When this proposed threshold level is exceeded, the allergic individual is encouraged to remediate their environment, which often involves replacing air duct filters, removing plants and decreasing indoor humidity.

Conclusions

The diagnostic allergy laboratory exists to provide serological testing that supports the clinician in the diagnosis and management of patients suspected of type 1 hypersensitivity reactions. To this end, the most important analyte measured in the clinical laboratory is allergen-specific IgE antibody. Selection of the laboratory and the IgE antibody assay methods and standards that it employs to insure quality are the ultimate responsibility of the referring physician.[47] Performance on national diagnostic allergy proficiency surveys and successful inspections leading to federal licensure under the Clinical Laboratory Improvement Act of 1988 are benchmarks that can be used by the healthcare professional to insure that the clinical laboratory provides quality diagnostic allergy testing.

References

1. Bernstein IL, Li JT, Bernstein DI, et al. Allergy diagnostic testing: an updated practice parameter. Ann Allergy Asthma Immunol 2008;100: S1–148.
2. Hamilton RG. Assessment of human allergic diseases. In: Rich RR, Fleisher TA, Shearer WT, Schroeder HW, Frew AJ, Weyand CM. Clinical immunology: principles and practice. 3rd ed. London: Mosby, Elsevier Ltd.; 2008. p. 1471–84.
3. Prausnitz C, Kustner H. Studien uber Uberempfindlicht. Centralb Baketerial 1 Abt Orog 1921;86:160–9. 1921. Originally published in English in Prausnitz C: In. Gell PGH, Coombs RRA, editors, Clinical aspects of immunology. Oxford: Blackwell, p 808–816, 1962.
4. Ishizaka K, Ishizaka T. Physiochemical properties of reaginic antibody. I. Association of reaginic activity with an immunoglobulin other than gamma A or gamma G globulin. J Allergy 1967;37:169–72.
5. Johansson SGO, Bennich H. Immunological studies of an atypical (myeloma) immunoglobulin. Immunology 1967;13:381–94.
6. Christensen LH, Holm J, Lund G, et al. Several distinct properties of the IgE repertoire determine effector cell degranulation in response to allergen challenge. J Allergy Clin Immunol 2008;122: 298–304.
7. Hamilton RG, Saito H. IgE antibody concentration, specific activity, clonality, and affinity measures from future diagnostic confirmatory tests. J Allergy Clin Immunol 2008;122:305–6.
8. Matsson PNJ, Hamilton RG, Homburger HA, et al. Analytical performance characteristics and clinical utility of immunological assays for human IgE antibodies of defined allergen specificities. 2nd ed. Wayne, PA: Clinical Laboratory Standards Institute; 2008 (Appendix A).
9. Hamilton RG, Palosuo T, the American Society for Testing Materials Working Group. Standard test method for immunological measurement of four principal allergenic proteins (Hev-b 1, 3, 5, and 6.02) in natural rubber and its products derived from latex. Report D7427. West Conshohocken, PA: American Society for Testing Materials International; 2008.
10. Hamilton RG. Diagnosis of natural rubber latex allergy. Methods 2002;27:22–31.
11. Hamilton RG, Peterson EL, Ownby DR. Clinical and laboratory based methods in the diagnosis of natural rubber latex allergy. J Allergy Clin Immunol 2002;110: S47–56.
12. Kostyal D, Horton K, Beezhold D, et al. Latex toy balloons and dental dams are a significant source of Hevea brasiliensis allergen exposure. Ann Allergy Clin Immunol (in press).
13. Hamilton RG. Human immunoglobulins. In: Donnenberg AD, O'Gorman M, editors. Handbook of human immunology. 2nd ed. Boca Raton: CRC Press; 2008. p. 63–106.
14. Barbee RA, Halomen M, Lebowitz M, et al. Distribution of IgE in a community population sample: correlations with age, sex and allergen skin tests reactivity. J Allergy Clin Immunol 1981;68: 106–14.
15. Wide L, Bennich H, Johansson SGO. Diagnosis by an in vitro test for allergen specific IgE antibodies. Lancet 1967;2:1105–9.
16. Butler JE, Hamilton RG. Quantification of specific antibodies: methods of expression, standards, solid phase considerations and specific applications. In: Butler JE, editor. Immunochemistry of solid phase immunoassays. Boca Raton: CRC Press; 1991. p. 173–98.
17. Wood RA, Phipatanakul W, Hamilton RG, et al. A comparison of skin prick tests, intradermal skin tests and RASTs in the diagnosis of cat allergy. J Allergy Clin Immunol 1999;102:773–9.
18. Wood RA, Segall N, Ahlstedt S, et al. Accuracy of IgE antibody laboratory results. Ann Allergy Asthma Immunol 2007;99:34–41.
19. Hamilton RG, Rossi CE, Yeang HY, et al. Latex-specific IgE assay sensitivity enhanced using Hev-b 5 enriched latex allergosorbent. J Allergy Clin Immunol 2003;111:S174 (A424).
20. Sicherer SH, Dhillon G, Laughery KA, et al. Caution: The Phadia hazelnut ImmunoCAP (f17) has been supplemented with recombinant Cor a 1 and now detects Bet v 1-specific IgE, which leads to elevated values for persons with birch pollen allergy. J Allergy Clin Immunol 2008;122: 413–4.
21. Hiller R, Laffer S, Harwanegg C, et al. Microarrayed allergen molecules: diagnostic gatekeepers for allergy treatment. FASEB J 2002;16: 414–6.
22. Gendo K, Larson EB. Evidence based diagnostic strategies for evaluating suspected allergic rhinitis. Ann Intern Med 2004;140:278–89.
23. McCann WA, Ownby DR. Reproducibility of the allergy skin test scoring and interpretation by board-certified/eligible allergists. Ann Allergy Asthma Immunol 2002;89:368–71.
24. Wood RA, Phipatanakul W, Hamilton RG, et al. A comparison of skin prick tests, intradermal skin tests, and RASTs in the diagnosis of cat allergy. J Allergy Clin Immunol 1999;103:773–9.
25. Petersson G, Dreborg S, Ingestad R. Clinical history, skin prick test and RAST in the diagnosis of birch and timothy pollinosis. Allergy 1986;41: 398–407.
26. Williams PB, Dolen WK, Koepke JW, et al. Comparison of skin testing and three in vitro assays for specific IgE in the clinical evaluation of immediate hypersensitivity. Ann Allergy 1992;68:34.
27. Sampson HA, Ho DG. Relationship between food-specific IgE concentrations and the risk of positive food challenges in children and adolescents. J Allergy Clin Immunol 1997;100:444–51.
28. Sampson HA. Utility of food-specific IgE concentrations in predicting food allergy. J Allergy Clin Immunol 2001;107:891–6.
29. De Lovinfosse S, Charpin D, Dornelas A, et al. Can mite specific IgE be used as a surrogate marker for mite exposure? Allergy 1994;49: 64–9.
30. Simpson A, Soderstrom L, Ahlstedt S, et al. IgE antibody quantification and the probability of wheeze in preschool children. J Allergy Clin Immunol 2005;116:744–9.
31. Yunginger JW, Ahlstedt S, Eggleston PA, et al. Quantitative IgE antibody assays in allergic diseases. (rostrum). J Allergy Clin Immunol 2000;105: 1077–84.
32. Des Roches A, Paradis L, Knani J, et al. Immunotherapy with a standardized Dermatophagoides pteronsynnisus extract. V. Duration of the efficacy of immunotherapy after it cessation. Allergy 1996;51:430–3.
33. Williams PB, Siegel C, Portnoy J. Efficacy of a single diagnostic test for sensitization to common inhalant allergens. Ann Allergy Asthma Immunol 2001;86:196–202.
34. Schwartz LB, Bradford TR. Regulation of tryptase from human lung mast cells by heparin. Stabilization of the active tetramer. J Biol Chem 1986;261:7372–9.
35. Enander I, Matsson P, Andesson AS, et al. A radioimmunoassay for human serum tryptase released during mast cell activation. J Allergy Clin Immunol 1990;85:154–9.
36. Schwartz LB, Yunginger JW, Miller J, et al. Time course of the appearance and disappearance of human mast cell tryptase in the circulation after anaphaylaxis. J Clin Invest 1989;83:1551–7.
37. Van der Linden PW, Hack CE, Poortman J, et al. Insect sting challenge in 138 patients: relation between clinical severity of anaphylaxis and mast cell activation. J Allergy Clin Immunol 1992;90: 110–8.
38. Zacharisen MC, Schuleter DP, Kurup VP, et al. The long-term outcome in acute, subacute and chronic forms of pigeon breeder's disease hypersensitivity pneumonitis. Ann Allergy Asthma Immunol 2002;88: 175–82.
39. Fan LL. Hypersensitivity pneumonitis in children. Curr Opin Pediatr 2002;14:323–6.
40. Mizobe T, Adachi S, Hamaoka A, et al. Evaluation of the enzyme-linked immunosorbent assay system for serodiagnosis of summer-type hypersensitivity pneumonitis. Arerugi 2002;51:20–3.
41. Hamilton RG, Wisenauer JA, Golden DB. Selection of Hymenoptera venoms for immunotherapy based on patient's IgE antibody cross-reactivity. J Allergy Clin Immunol 1993;92:651–9.
42. Golden DBK, Lawrence ID, Hamilton RG, et al. Clinical correlation of the venom specific IgG antibody level during maintenance venom immunotherapy. J Allergy Clin Immunol 1992;90:386–93.

43. Hamilton RG. Accuracy of Food and Drug Administration-cleared IgE antibody assays in the presence of anti-IgE (omalizumab). J Allergy Clin Immunol 2006;117:759–66.

44. Hamilton RG, Marcotte GV, Saini SS. Immunological methods for quantifying free and total serum IgE in asthma patients receiving omalizumab (Xolair) therapy. J Immunol Methods 2005;303:81–91.

45. Hamilton RG, Chapman MD, Platts-Mills TAE, et al. House dust aeroallergen measurements in clinical practice: a guide to allergen free home- and work- environments. Immunol Allergy Practice 1992;14: 96–112.

46. Hamilton RG, Eggleston PA. Environmental allergen analyses. Methods 1997;13:53–60.

47. Hamilton RG. Responsibility for quality IgE antibody results rests ultimately with the referring physician. (Invited Editorial). Ann Allergy Asthma Immunol 2001;86:353–5.

CHAPTER

23

In Vivo Testing for Immunoglobulin E-Mediated Sensitivity

Harold S. Nelson

Introduction

In the USA, in vivo testing for the diagnosis of allergy is virtually synonymous with skin testing. The preference for skin testing over allergen challenges to the conjunctiva, nose or lungs is attributable to skin testing being less time consuming and more comfortable for the patient. It provides an objective end-point, rather than the subjective end-points typical with conjunctival and nasal challenges. Finally, many allergens can be tested for in a single session, compared to the limitation to a single allergen with mucosal challenges. There is little to suggest that the information gained from mucosal testing is different from that obtained by skin testing. Results of nasal challenges have been shown to correlate closely with skin tests,[1] as do the results of bronchial challenges, when the additional factor of nonspecific airway responsiveness to histamine is included.[2] A joint committee of the American Academy of Allergy, Asthma and Immunology and the American College of Allergy Asthma and Immunology has developed a Practice Parameter for Allergy Diagnostic Testing which is comprehensive and based on the most current published literature on this topic.[3]

Prevalence of Positive Skin Tests

Reaction of the skin to extracts of environmental allergens is common, but not invariable, in patients with the so-called atopic diseases – perennial and seasonal rhinitis, bronchial asthma and atopic eczema. Of 656 asthmatic patients referred for an allergy evaluation in London, 544 (84%) had at least one positive immediate reaction to prick skin testing with 22 common allergens.[4] Skin test reactivity was more common in those with onset of asthma prior to 10 years of age, whereas those with onset after the age of 30 years were more commonly skin test negative. A similar percentage with positive skin tests has been reported in patients evaluated for rhinitis,[5] and eczema.[6]

Positive reactions on skin testing are also common in studies of unselected residents in westernized societies and there is a suggestion that the prevalence is increasing, including in the USA.[7] Allergy skin testing was administered in the 2nd and 3rd National Health and Nutrition Examination Survey (NHANES) from 1976 to 1980 and 1988 to 1994. In NHANES III, 10 allergens were tested in all subjects aged 6 to 19 years and a random half-sample of subjects aged 20 to 59 years. In NHANES III, 54.3% had a positive prick skin test to one or more allergens. Among those with positives, the median number was 3.0. For the six allergens common to NHANES II and III, prevalences were 2.1 to 5.5 times higher in NHANES III. Whether the higher prevalence observed in NHANES III reflected true changes in prevalence or methodological differences between the surveys cannot be determined with certainty.

It is clear that these positive reactions are not limited to persons with clinical allergy. A study was conducted in 200 young and middle-aged adults, employing a battery of 13 extracts (10 pollens, 2 mites and cat).[8] Three groups were recruited for prick skin testing. In those with a personal history of rhinitis or asthma, 90% had at least one positive prick skin test. In those with no personal history of rhinitis or asthma, but a close relative with one of these conditions, 46% had at least one positive prick skin test. Even in those who denied rhinitis or asthma personally, or in close relatives, 29% had at least one positive prick skin test.

Factors Affecting the Size and Prevalence of Positive Skin Tests

Age

Epidemiological studies in Tucson demonstrated the varying prevalence of positive immediate prick skin test reactions with age in their population.[9] When tested with a battery of five allergens or mixes, only 22% of those who were 3 and 4 years old had at least one positive test. The peak prevalence of reactivity was seen in the first half of the third decade, when 52% reacted to at least one test. The prevalence of a positive skin test then declined slowly until the age of 50 years, following which there was a more rapid fall-off, reaching a low of 16% in the subjects over 75 years of age. Further studies in this population related the presence of prick skin test reactivity to the reactivity of the skin to histamine and to the serum total immunoglobulin E (IgE) levels.[10] Dividing the population studied into four age groups, they found that total IgE was highest in those who were 9 to 19 years of age, and declined progressively in the other three groups (20 to 34, 35 to 50 and over 50 years). Histamine reactivity in the skin was lowest in the 9- to 19-year-old group, however, and was higher in the three older groups. The prevalence of positive skin tests, reflecting in part the interaction of specific IgE and

©2010 Elsevier Ltd, Inc, BV
DOI: 10.1016/B978-1-4377-0271-2.00023-7

reactivity of the skin to histamine, was highest in the 20- to 34-year-old group.

Supporting data for the above observations comes from separate studies of levels of specific IgE and cutaneous reactivity to histamine by age.[11,12] A retrospective review was conducted of results in 326 patients whose serum was analyzed for total and specific IgE.[11] The highest levels for grass and house dust mite-specific IgE were observed in those who were 10 to 15 years of age. A prospective study of cutaneous reactivity to histamine was conducted in 365 subjects from 1 to 85 years of age.[12] The size of the prick skin test to histamine increased progressively, peaking in those who were 1 to 30 years of age. There was then very little difference until the age of 50 years. Following this, there was a decline in the mean reaction size. Representative values with the 27 mg/mL concentration of histamine were: age 0 to 3 years, 3.8 mm; age 21 to 30 years, 6.2 mm, and age 61 to 70 years, 4.5 mm.

Reactivity of the skin to histamine and codeine was examined in children from infancy to the age of 2 years.[13] Prick skin tests with both histamine and codeine (a nonimmunologic mast cell degranulating agent) were particularly small up to the age of 6 months, although after 1 month of age there was usually some reactivity to both reagents. Due to the reduced reactivity to histamine in children under 2 years, adjustment of the interpretation for the size of the positive histamine control is important.

Varying reactivity to histamine can have a significant effect on skin test reactions, even in adults.[14] In an epidemiological study, 893 adult subjects were prick skin tested with 14 allergens and 10-fold dilutions of histamine, ranging from 1 mg/mL to 0.001 mg/mL. In those positive only to the highest concentration of histamine, 56% had all negative skin tests to allergens and only 15% had six or more positive skin tests. By comparison, of those responding to 0.01 and 0.001 mg/mL histamine concentrations, only 11% had all negative skin tests to allergens and 60% had six or more positive tests.

Physiologic Factors

The size of the reaction of the skin has been reported to vary with the time of day, the season of the year, the menstrual cycle, the subject's handedness and with the part of the body used for testing. Although it had been reported that there was a circadian pattern to skin reactivity, a study of 20 children and 20 adults did not find any significant variation during the normal clinic hours.[15] Subjects were tested in duplicate with serial dilutions of short ragweed and histamine at 8 a.m. and 4 p.m. No significant differences between the two sessions were observed at any dilution of either test material. The size of the skin reactions to histamine and allergens was examined over the course of a year.[16] It was found that reactions to both allergens and histamine were greater in October and February than in July and August.

Fifteen allergic women with seasonal rhinitis and/or asthma and 15 nonallergic female controls were skin tested three times during their menstrual cycle.[17] There were significantly greater reactions to histamine and morphine in both allergic and nonallergic women and to Parietaria extract in allergic women on days 12 to 16 of the cycle, corresponding to ovulation and peak estrogen levels. The size of the reaction to histamine on the forearms was compared with handedness in 176 subjects.[18] Significant differences between the size of the wheal and flare on the two forearms were observed. Subjects who were right-handed, with only right-handed relatives, had significantly larger reactions on the left arm. Subjects who were either left-handed or ambidextrous had significantly larger reactions on the right arm.

Reactivity of the Skin in Different Areas of the Body

The back is commonly used for percutaneous testing, since it provides a large surface that can accommodate many tests. Although it may be acceptable to consider the back as homogenous for clinical purposes, there is a significant gradient of reactivity, with the upper back being less reactive than the middle, which in turn is less reactive than the lower third. The wheal diameter with allergens was 30% less and with histamine 19% less on the upper compared with the lower back.[19] Often the forearm is employed as an alternative site for percutaneous testing, since there is no need for the patient to disrobe and testing may be done with the patient sitting in a chair, rather than lying down. It has been long recognized that the forearm is not as reactive as the back. In one study, allergen-induced wheal diameter was 27% smaller and flare diameter 14% smaller.[20] While the difference is not great, it is estimated that 2.3% of tests positive on the back would be negative if performed on the forearm.[20]

Viral Infections

Skin testing with inhalant allergens was performed in 16 adults before and up to 21 days following experimental inoculation with respiratory syncytial virus (RSV).[21] Even subjects with no measurable skin test reactions at baseline showed increased wheal-and-flare areas in response to histamine and allergen skin tests after RSV exposure. The altered skin test response persisted for up to 21 days after RSV inoculation. It was suggested that up-regulation of pathways relating to neurogenic inflammation may have played a role.

Medication

Since histamine is a major mediator of the immediate skin test, drugs that have antihistaminic properties suppress skin test reactions. Studies have assessed the duration of this suppression after the medication is discontinued, since this is often an important consideration for diagnostic allergy skin testing. Persisting suppression after multiple doses of first generation antihistamines was studied.[22] The mean time for skin reactivity to return to normal after stopping the drug was 3 days for chlorpheniramine and tripelennamine and 5 days for hydroxyzine. However, some patients remained suppressed for 6 to 8 days. After multiple doses of the second-generation antihistamine fexofenadine skin reactivity had returned to normal after 2 days.[23] Single 25 mg doses of the tricyclic antidepressants, desipramine and doxepin, produced suppression which lasted an average of 2 and 6 days respectively.[24] It was recommended that doxepin be withheld at least 7 days before skin testing. Multiple dosing of the H2 antagonist, ranitidine, produced significant suppression of both the wheal and flare of the histamine skin test.[25] Suppression was only 18% of the mean diameter, so withholding the drug on the day of testing should be adequate.

In 15 subjects, the leukotriene receptor antagonist, montelukast, significantly reduced the flare reaction to histamine, codeine and allergen.[26] There was a nonsignificant trend toward reduction in wheal size with all three agents. Other investigators found nonsignificant reductions in both wheal (9.6%) and flare (7.3%) following administration of montelukast.[27]

There is no consensus regarding the effect of corticosteroids on allergy skin tests. In a prospective study, topical application of corticosteroids for 4 weeks reduced the area of the allergen-induced wheal by 72% and the flare by 62%.[28] The reduction could at least, in part, be explained by an 85% reduction in the number of detectable skin mast cells in the treated skin. A prospective study of 1 week of oral corticosteroids, 24 mg daily of methylprednisolone, found no effect on reactivity to ragweed.[29] A retrospective analysis of 25 patients who had been on oral steroids for longer, but varying periods, suggested that they had diminished skin reactivity to codeine, a nonimmunologic mast cell degranulating agent.[30] However, a prospective study of 33 patients who received oral steroids for at least 1 year (median dose 20 mg of prednisone per day, median duration of 2 years) revealed no suppression of skin reactions to either codeine or allergen.[31]

The monoclonal antibody against IgE, omalizumab, has been reported to reduce skin test reactions.[32] In 19 subjects with perennial allergic rhinitis, 3 months of treatment with omalizumab 0.030 mg/kg/IU/mL reduced free IgE levels >98% and the cumulative wheaing response to titrated prick skin tests (150 to 10 000 AU/mL of house dust mite extract) by 78–83%.

Allergy immunotherapy has been observed to reduce the immediate reaction to allergen skin testing.[33] The reductions in the immediate skin test are accompanied by reductions in nasal and conjunctival sensitivity.[33] Allergen immunotherapy reduces the late cutaneous reaction even more than the immediate.[34]

Quantity and Quality of Extracts

The size of the reaction is a function of the patient's sensitivity and the amount of the relevant reagent injected. The relationship between dose and response is best expressed as a log:log relationship.[35] The slope is steeper when the size of the reaction is expressed as the log of the area, as opposed to the log of the diameter. When log-linear dose responses are calculated, the resulting curve is S-shaped, but linear in the midrange.[36] A 10-fold increase in the concentration of allergen or histamine will produce approximately a 1.5-fold increase in mean diameter[35] or a doubling of the area of the wheal.[35]

In the USA, standardized extracts are available for several grasses, ragweed, *Dermatophagoides pteronyssinus* and *farinae*, and cat. In general, other pollen extracts, although not standardized, are of good potency. Most extracts of dog dander,[37] probably most or all fungi[38] and all extracts of cockroach[39] are relatively weak. In the case of fungi and cockroach, proteases in the extracts may degrade susceptible proteins within the extract.[40] One exception to the low potency of most dog extracts is the acetone-precipitated dog extract manufactured by Holister-Steir (Spokane, WA). This extract contains 30 to 40 times as much major allergen as the other commercially available dog extracts. The increased allergen content has been shown to result in an increased number of positive prick skin tests in comparative skin testing.[37]

A unique problem appears to exist with extracts of some foods. Many patients with documented food sensitivity will fail to react to commercial extracts or in vitro tests prepared from these extracts but will react to testing with fresh extracts of the foods.[41,42] Reactions to fresh foods, but not commercial food extracts, have been reported with fruits and celery,[42,43] with shell fish and fish,[42,44] and even with peanuts and walnuts.[42] This report not withstanding, peanut extracts have been reported to be reliable in other studies.[43,45] In 76 children aged 5 months to 15 years, there were 31 positive blinded food challenges in 96 foods

which yielded positive prick skin tests.[45] All the positive challenges were to peanuts, eggs, milk or soy. There were no positive open feeding challenges to foods, which had not been positive on prick skin testing.

Methods of Skin Testing

Prick Versus Intradermal Testing

There are two approaches to allergen skin testing. One is performed by percutaneous introduction of the allergen through a break in the skin by pricking, puncturing or scratching.[46] In the latter, a linear scratch is made without drawing blood. The scratch may be performed first with the extract then dropped on the abraded skin, or the scratch may be made through a drop of extract. The scratch test has now largely been abandoned due to greater discomfort, poorer reproducibility, and the possibility of leaving multiple liner depigmented areas for some time afterwards.[47] The prick test is performed by introducing the tip of the device into the epidermis at approximately a 45-degree angle through a drop of extract; the tip is then lifted, creating a small, transient break in the epidermis. Prick testing can be performed with either solid needles or hollow hypodermic needles. Puncture testing is performed by pressing the tip of the device at a 90-degree angle to the skin. Usually the device employed has a sharp point approximately 1 mm long, with a widening above to limit penetration into the skin.

The alternative to percutaneous testing is intracutaneous testing. A hypodermic syringe and needle is employed. The needle is threaded into the dermis where, typically, 0.01 to 0.02 mL of extract is injected. Intradermal testing is more sensitive than prick/puncture. For equivalent reactions at threshold-sized reactions, the extract for prick/puncture testing must be 1000-fold more concentrated.[46] Also, direct comparisons indicate that intradermal testing is more reproducible than percutaneous testing.[46] Nevertheless, there are many arguments in favor of the percutaneous test as the routine for allergy testing. These include economy of time and patient comfort and safety. These apply to percutaneous versus intracutaneous, no matter what relative concentrations of extract are employed. If, in addition, the intradermal test is performed with a concentration greater than 1:1000 that of the percutaneous test, in order to increase its sensitivity, additional considerations arise as to whether this increased sensitivity is clinically necessary or useful.

Diagnostic Usefulness of the Percutaneous Test

The prick skin test has served well in epidemiological studies. Prick skin test reactivity to indoor allergens, but not pollens, has been shown to be a risk factor for asthma in children[48,49] and adolescents and adults.[50] Prick skin test reactivity in asymptomatic freshmen in college carried an increased risk for development of allergic rhinitis.[51,52] Three-year follow-up revealed that 18.2% of those with positive prick skin tests had developed allergic rhinitis compared to 1.8% of those with negative prick skin tests.[51] At 7-year follow-up, 31.9% of those with positive prick skin tests and 7.7% of those with negative skin tests had developed allergic rhinitis.[52] The larger the prick skin test as a freshman, the more likely the development of allergic rhinitis. Furthermore, after 7 years, new onset asthma had developed in 5% of the prick skin test positive group, versus 1.5% in the skin test negative group.[52]

Diagnostic Usefulness of the Intracutaneous Test

Although the intracutaneous test, at the strength customarily performed, is more sensitive, it may be questioned whether this increased sensitivity is clinically necessary. The prick test, performed with good quality extracts, is positive in many subjects who do not have personal, or even a family history of allergy.[8] A number of studies have addressed the clinical usefulness of intracutaneous testing. In the Tucson epidemiological study, 311 subjects representing a sample of the >3800 participants had prick skin testing followed, if negative, by intracutaneous testing with 1:1000 w/v extract to 14 common allergens.[53] Subjects were divided, by history, into allergic and nonallergic groups. Prick test reactivity correlated with the presence of allergy symptoms. Conversely, positive reactions to intracutaneous testing, which followed a negative prick test for that allergen, showed no correlation with either the patient's clinical allergic status or the level of total serum IgE. Studies in smaller groups of patients have supported this epidemiological data. Thirty-four subjects with perennial rhinitis who were prick skin test negative, but intracutaneous test positive, were compared to 19 who had positive prick skin tests and to 13 healthy controls.[54] Whereas, in the 19 prick skin test positive subjects, RAST was positive in 12, and leukocyte histamine release and nasal challenge were positive in 17 each, among those positive on intracutaneous testing there were no positive RASTs or leukocyte histamine release tests and only 1 of 34 had a positive nasal challenge. Similar results were reported in patients with a history of rhinoconjunctivitis.[55] Twenty nasal challenges were performed in 14 subjects with negative percutaneous and positive intradermal skin tests to cat, house dust mite, *Alternaria,* grass or ragweed extracts with results no different from the negative control group.

Two studies examined the intracutaneous test as a predictor of symptoms with natural exposure to the allergen.[56,57] In a study of the clinical usefulness of intradermal skin tests to grass, four groups were compared: three of the groups had a history of seasonal allergic rhinitis, one with positive prick skin tests to timothy, one with negative prick but a positive intradermal test to timothy, and one with both prick and intracutaneous tests to timothy negative. The fourth group was a nonallergic control.[56] On the basis of nasal challenge with timothy, grass pollen allergic reactions were present in 68% of those with positive prick skin tests to timothy and none of the nonallergic controls. In both the group with positive and those with negative intracutaneous tests to timothy, 11% were positive. Subjects were then followed through the grass pollen season. Their symptom scores, recorded in a diary, were examined for a correlation with grass pollen counts. A positive correlation was present in 64% of those with positive prick skin tests and none of the nonallergic controls. A positive correlation of symptoms and pollen count was present in 22% of those with a positive intracutaneous test and 21% of those with a negative intracutaneous test to timothy. Both criteria for allergy to timothy, a positive nasal challenge and a correlation between symptoms and grass pollen counts, were met in 46% of those with positive prick skin tests, but in none in the other three groups. Thus, under the conditions of this study, the presence of a positive intradermal skin test response to timothy in the presence of a negative skin prick test response to timothy did not indicate the presence of clinically significant sensitivity to timothy grass.[56]

In the second study, patients were challenged with cat exposure for 1 hour.[57] Both positive prick skin tests and RASTs to cat were highly predictive of development of symptoms on exposure to the cat room. Subjects with a negative skin prick test were just as likely to have a positive challenge result if they had a negative (31%) as if they had a positive intracutaneous skin test to cat (24%). The authors concluded that, at least with regard to cat allergy, these results strongly suggest that major therapeutic decisions, such as environmental control or immunotherapy should never be based on a positive intracutaneous skin test result alone.[57] It is clear from these studies that the intradermal skin test adds little to the diagnostic evaluation of allergy when allergy extracts of reasonable quality are available for skin testing. This probably includes almost all pollen extracts, house dust mite, cat and acetone-precipitated dog extracts. What of the extracts of poorer quality, particularly cockroach, fungi and some dander extracts? A study of the diagnosis of allergy to mouse extract is informative in this regard.[58] In this study, 49 workers reported symptoms on mouse exposure. The mouse extract contained only 2.37 μg of Mus m 1 per mL, about 6% the major allergen content in cat extract. Using a nasal challenge as the gold standard, sensitivity was only 47% for measurement of mouse IgE (mIgE), 67% for the prick skin test, and 100% for an intradermal test at a 1:100 dilution of the extract. On the other hand, specificity was 91% for mIgE, 94% for prick skin test, but only 65% for intradermal testing. The prick skin test performed best, but with this weak extract, intradermal testing was required to identify some clinically sensitized workers.

Expressing the Results of Skin Testing

The results of both percutaneous and intracutaneous skin tests are often reported in only semi-quantitative terms. Results may be recorded only as positive or negative, or graded 0 to 4+ without any indication of what size reactions these numbers represent.[59] At the very least, a record of skin testing should indicate certain information, which will allow another physician to interpret the results. In addition to the concentration of extract employed, the form should indicate whether the tests are percutaneous or intracutaneous, and if the former, which device was employed for testing, whether testing was performed on the back or the arm, and the size of the positive and negative reactions. Finally, if an arbitrary grading system is employed, the range of reaction for each grade should be clearly indicated on the form (see Table 23-1).

A superior method of expressing results is to measure and record actual size of the reaction. This need not be excessively time consuming. Although the area of the wheal is the most accurate, measurements of the product of the orthogonal diameters, the sum of the orthogonal diameters and even the longest diameter correlate very well with area, with r values greater than 0.9.[60]

The Scandinavian Society of Allergology recommended that skin test results be standardized in relation to the size of the reaction to histamine, employing 0.1 mg/mL of histamine for intradermal testing and 1 mg/mL of histamine for prick skin testing.[61] If the diameter of the reaction to allergen was the same size as the histamine reaction, the grade was 3+, if half that size 2+, and if twice as large 4+. A subsequent study suggested that the histamine control should be 10 mg/mL, because of the small reactions with high coefficient of variation with the 1 mg/mL histamine prick skin test.[62] Even the 20–30% coefficient of variation for reactions to 10 mg/mL raises questions regarding the desirability of basing grading on a histamine control, which if used for this purpose, should be performed at least in duplicate.[63]

The reliability of different means of expressing the results of prick skin testing was compared in patients sensitive to dogs.[64] A determination of sensitivity to dog was made in 202 children based on a composite score from history, RAST, and bronchial or conjunctival allergen challenges. The results with the three common means of expressing results (wheal diameter, wheal diameter compared to the histamine control and titrated prick skin tests) were compared for sensitivity, specificity and overall efficacy. Although the overall efficacy of the histamine reference was greatest in this study, most allergists would prefer to have the maximum sensitivity, which was provided by a wheal ≥3 mm diameter, in order not to miss any truly sensitive patients. Other methods, or clinical judgment, should then be used to distin-guish between those who are only sensitized and those who are clinically allergic.[64]

Devices for Percutaneous Skin Testing

Intracutaneous skin tests are performed using a hypodermic syringe and needle. Percutaneous tests are performed with an ever-increasing variety of devices.[19,65,66] These devices differ in whether they are used to prick or puncture (some being used both ways). Some have a single stylus with a single or several points and are used either to prick or puncture through a drop of extract or to carry a drop of extract from the extract bottle, so that application of extract and the puncture occur in one step. Increasingly, devices are being introduced which have multiple heads, so that up to 10 tests can be accomplished with one application (Figure 23-1). Generally the multiple-headed skin test devices are designed to first be dipped into the extract bottles, then applied to the skin so that testing is accomplished in one step. The devices for percutaneous testing vary in the degree of trauma that they impart to the skin. Therefore, they vary in the size of positive reactions and also in the likelihood of producing a reaction at the site of the negative control. Consequently, they require different criteria for what constitutes a positive reaction (see Table 23-2).

Placement of Adjacent Tests

There are two reports, both describing intracutaneous testing with hymenoptera venom, which indicate that false positive tests can result from an adjacent positive histamine controls.[67,68] The influence of large positive reactions to histamine or to inhalant allergen on adjacent prick skin tests was prospectively studied.[20] There was no evidence of falsely positive skin prick tests attributable to the large adjacent reactions, even when the test sites were only separated by 2 cm. Thus, it appears that the augmentation which has been observed may be limited to intracutaneous testing, and perhaps also to the active constituents in the hymenoptera venom.

Special Considerations

Safety of Skin Testing

Deaths have been reported with skin testing.[69,70] For the most part these were reactions to testing with horse serum or other potent allergens and, almost without exception, they were associated with intradermal testing.[69] Severe reactions can occur, however, even with prick skin testing in very sensitive patients

Table 23-1 Semiquantitative Reporting of Skin Test Results

Criteria to Read Prick/Puncture Skin Tests

Negative	0	No reaction or no different from control
One plus	+	Erythema < a nickel in diameter
Two plus	++	Erythema > a nickel in diameter
Three plus	+++	Wheal with surrounding erythema
Four plus	++++	Wheal with pseudopods and surrounding erythema

Criteria to Read Intracutaneous Tests When Control ≥2 mm

Negative	0	No different from control
One plus	+	Wheal 11/2 to 2 times control or definite erythema > a nickel in size
Two plus	++	Wheal 2–3 times control
Three plus	+++	Wheal >3 times control
Four plus	++++	Wheal with pseudopods

Criteria to Read Intracutaneous Tests When Control <2 mm

Negative	0	No difference from control
One plus	+	3–4 mm wheal with erythema or erythema > a nickel in size.
Two plus	++	4–8 mm wheal without pseudopods
Three plus	+++	>8 mm wheal without pseudopods
Four plus	++++	Wheal with pseudopods and erythema

From Esch RG. Role of proteases on the stability of allergic extracts. In: Klein R, ed. Regulatory control and standardization of allergic extracts. Stuttgart: Gustav Fischer; 1990:171–177.

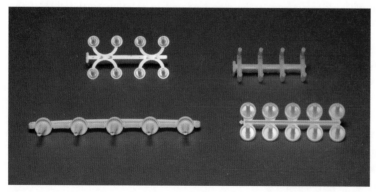

Figure 23-1 Four multiple-pronged skin test devices. Left upper: Quick-Test (Penatrex Inc, Placentia, CA), Right upper: Multi-Test (Lincoln Diagnostics, Decatur, IL), Left lower: Quintest (Hollister-Stier Laboratories, Spokane, WA), Right lower: Omni (Greer laboratories, Lenoir, NC)

Table 23-2 Size of Wheals on the Back That are Larger Than 99% of the Wheals with Saline Using the Same Device by the Same Operator

Devices for Which a 3-mm Wheal Would be Significant		Devices for Which a >3-mm Wheal Should be Used as Significant	
Device	0.99 Quantile of Reactions at the Negative Control Sites	Device	0.99 Quantile of Reactions at the Negative Control Sites
Quintest(HS) multiple puncture	0 mm	DermaPIK (Greer) single Prick	3.25 mm
Smallpox needle (HS) single prick	0 mm	DuoTip (Lincoln) single twist	3.5 mm
DuoTip (Lincoln) single prick	1.5 mm	Greer tract (Greer) multiple puncture	4.0 mm
Lancet (HS) single puncture	2.0 mm	Bifurcated needle (ALO) single prick	4.0 mm
Lancet (ALK) single puncture	3.0 mm	MultiTest II (Lincoln) multiple puncture	4.0 mm
		Quick test (Panatrex) multiple puncture	4.0 mm
		Bifurcated needle (ALO) single puncture	4.5 mm
DermaPik (HS) multiple puncture	0 mm	DermaPIK (Greer) single twist	5.0 mm

Data from:
Kalogeromitros D, Katsarou A, Armenaka M, et al. Clin Exp Allergy 1995;25:461–466.
Nelson HS, Oppenheimer JJ, Buchmeier A, et al. J Allergy Clin Immunol 1996;97:1193–1201.
HS: Hollister Steir; *Greer*: Greer laboratories; *Lincoln*: Lincoln Diagnostics; *ALK*: ALK America; *ALO*: Allergy Labs of Ohio

treated with undiluted commercial or fresh food extracts.[71] A fatal reaction was reported in a young woman with moderate asthma, probably poorly controlled, following application of 90 food allergens employing the Dermapik (Greer Laboratories, Lenoir, NC) skin testing device.[70] In a private practice, 10 400 patients were skin tested first by prick, followed, if negative, by intradermal testing.[72] Two systemic reactions occurred, both with intradermal testing. One was in a patient who had had a negative prick skin test, and the other a patient who did not have preliminary prick skin testing. The experience with allergy skin testing at the Mayo clinic between 1992 and 1997 was reviewed.[69] Puncture skin testing was performed in 16 505 patients, while 1806 received puncture tests followed by intracutaneous tests for selected allergens (hymenoptera venom, penicillin, and other drugs). Five patients experienced systemic reactions following puncture tests, while one patient experienced a systemic reaction to an intracutaneous test following a negative puncture test. Two of the five patients who experienced systemic reactions to puncture testing had positive reactions to latex. One patient reacted to both latex and aeroallergens, while two reacted only to aeroallergens. Thus, for prick/puncture testing to aeroallergens systemic reactions, none of which were life threatening, occurred with an incidence of about 15 to 23 per 100 000 tests.

Local Allergy

Patients sometimes present with what sounds like a convincing clinical history for an allergic respiratory condition, but they have negative skin tests to the suspected and sometimes to all allergens. There are several studies that suggest that patients may be sensitive to an allergen and have IgE antibodies to that allergen in their nasal secretions, even though prick skin tests and serum in vitro tests for that same allergen are negative. A group of patients with perennial rhinitis were reported to have nasal challenges to house dust mite extract and have a positive RAST for house dust mites performed on their nasal secretions, even though prick skin tests and RAST on peripheral

blood were negative.[73] Nine children, with a mean age of 2 years and 5 months, and with rhinitis or asthma, had both negative prick skin tests and serum RASTS for house dust mites. Mast cells from the nasal secretions from 7 out of 9 of the children bound house dust mite allergen on their surface.[74] The investigators were able to block the binding by anti-IgE, indicating the mast cells were sensitized with house dust mite specific IgE. Fifty adult subjects with persistent rhinitis who had negative prick skin tests and no specific IgE for perennial allergens and who had negative intradermal skin tests for house dust mites (PNAR) were compared to 30 subjects with persistent allergic rhinitis (PAR) and 30 nonallergic controls.[75] Subjects with PNAR and PAR did not differ in symptoms or nasal cytology. All of the PAR, 54% of the PNAR and none of the normal control had a positive nasal challenge with house dust mite allergen *Dermatophygoides pteronyssinus* (DP). Nasal DP-specific IgE was found in 23/30 with PAR and 6/50 with PNAR, all of whom had positive nasal challenges with DP. The data support the concept that some patients with PNAR have local IgE production which contributes to their disease.

Delayed Reactions to Skin Tests

Immediate skin reactions to histamine typically peak at 8 minutes, while those to allergen peak at 15 minutes. Large allergen induced immediate skin tests may be followed by a late cutaneous reaction. Progressive erythema and induration occur at the site of the immediate reaction, peaking at 4 to 6 hours. These reactions can be triggered by mast cell mediators released by a variety of mechanisms including allergens, anti-IgE and nonimmunologic mast cell degranulating agents, but not by histamine alone.[76] There appears to be a threshold size of the immediate reaction below which the late phase reaction does not occur. Beyond that size, there is a rough correlation between the size of the immediate reaction and the size of the resulting late phase reaction in the same individual[76] and in unselected patients.[77] The IgE-mediated late cutaneous reaction has not been described in the absence of the immediate reaction. The late phase cutaneous reaction is not suppressed by antihistamines, but is reduced by corticosteroids. Furthermore, it is marked reduced by allergen immunotherapy, more so than the immediate reactions.[34]

Isolated, delayed reactions to allergy skin testing have been described.[68–70] Furthermore, when looked for, they appear to fairly commonly follow intracutaneous testing.[78,79] Two hundred and ninety two adult patients who had received a total of 2700 intracutaneous tests were examined after 20 minutes for immediate reactions and again after 48 hours for evidence of delayed reactions.[78] Immediate reactions were observed in 17% of the skin tests in allergic and 5% of the skin tests in nonallergic patients. At 48 hours, delayed reactions were present at 7% of the skin test sites in the allergic and 5% in the nonallergic patients. Delayed reactions were over twice as common at sites of positive immediate as negative immediate skin reactions. Those occurring at the site of negative immediate skin tests had the histology of a delayed-type hypersensitive reaction. There was no suggestion that the late or delayed cutaneous reactions had clinical relevance.

Relation of Skin Tests to In Vitro Measurements of Specific IgE

For most aeroallergens, the RAST tests and its enzyme-employing variations are somewhat less sensitive than percutaneous tests, and both are much less sensitive than intracutaneous tests at the concentrations of allergen extracts that are commonly employed. Even though they are less sensitive than the intracutaneous test, the prick/puncture and RAST tests still are often positive in patients without clinical symptoms. This has led to attempts to increase the diagnostic precision of these tests by defining cut-offs that enhance specificity without too great a loss in sensitivity. An ambitious study recruited 267 patients who were prick skin test positive and had a clear history of respiratory symptoms in relation to the allergen producing the positive skin test.[79] They were compared to 232 subjects with similar positive prick skin tests but negative histories of respiratory symptoms caused by the aeroallergens producing the positive prick skin tests. Finally, there were 243 nonallergic controls. Patients also had RASTs testing for the allergens that produced the positive prick skin tests. The investigators constructed receiver operating characteristic curves for sensitivity versus specificity for both RAST and prick skin tests. They found maximum diagnostic accuracy at cut-offs of 11.7 KU/L in the Pharmacia CAP system (where threshold for sensitivity is 0.35 KU/L). The cut-off for prick skin testing was a wheal area of 32.2 mm (roughly 6 mm diameter). They also reported the diagnostic accuracy of the RAST exceeded that of the prick skin test. This conclusion may have been biased, however, by the inclusion criteria that all subjects have positive prick skin tests.

Despite similar sensitivity and performances by the in vitro and percutaneous tests, the quantitative relationship between them in individuals is relatively weak. Reactivity on intracutaneous skin testing and RAST was measured in 43 patients with rhinitis and/or asthma employing five purified major allergens.[80] The overall correlation for skin testing versus serum IgE was only 0.68. For the same level of specific IgE, the amount of the allergen required in different subjects for a positive skin test varied by as much as 100-fold. Skin reactivity was adversely affected by total IgE. Skin testing correlated better than RAST with histamine release, suggesting that 'releasability' might account for part of the residual variation in

the correlation between skin test results and levels of IgE antibodies.

An additional factor may be the affinity for IgE-allergen binding.[81] Reactions on prick skin testing to ragweed and *Dermatophagoides pteronyssinus* were compared to serum Amb a 1- and Der p 1-specific IgE levels in 165 members from families with histories of clinical atopy. Those donors with positive skin test reactions tended to have higher concentrations of specific IgE than those donors with negative skin tests. However, there was considerable overlap between the skin test positive and skin test negative groups, without a clear demarcation between them. Mean values between skin prick test-positive and skin prick test-negative groups were not statistically significant. Donors with positive skin test reactions had, on average, higher binding affinities than those with negative skin test results. These values differed significantly for the two groups (p < 0.001). The product of affinity and concentration, termed the antibody capacity, provided a much clearer demarcation between donors who were skin test positive and those who were skin test negative.

Relation of Skin Tests to Nasal Allergen Challenge and In Vitro Assessment of Specific IgE

Nasal allergen challenges with 3-fold increasing numbers of grass pollen grains, prick skin tests with 3-fold increasing concentrations of grass pollen extract and RASTs utilizing the same grass pollen extract were compared in 44 subjects with rhinitis and 10 nonallergic controls during the grass pollen season.[1] The nasal challenge method, which employs a total symptom score of 5 as an end-point, has been validated by demonstration of release of PGD_2 into nasal secretion at end-point and by correlation of threshold scores with symptoms on seasonal exposure to grass pollen. Nasal challenges were positive in 41 of 43 patients and 0 of 10 controls. There was a significant correlation ($R_s = 0.54$, p < 0.005) between threshold for nasal challenge and threshold for prick skin testing. There was no significant correlation between nasal threshold and levels of specific IgE, suggesting that releasability of mast cells and basophils may be an important parameter in determining symptoms. In a related study, the correlation between threshold for nasal allergen challenge and titrated prick skin test was confirmed and both were shown to correlate with symptoms during natural pollen exposure.[82]

Relation of Skin Tests to Bronchial Allergen Challenge

There is a relatively poor correlation between the results of allergen skin testing and bronchial allergen challenge. The reason is the presence of a second variable, nonspecific bronchial hyperresponsiveness as measured by histamine or methacholine inhalation challenge. It was observed that positive bronchial allergen challenges occurred almost exclusively in subjects with positive prick skin tests,[83] but that the correlation between skin testing and bronchial allergen challenge could be improved considerably by incorporating the threshold of nonspecific bronchial responsiveness.[84,85] A prospective study confirmed these retrospective observations.[2] The early bronchoconstrictor response to allergen challenge could be predicted within an 8-fold range by a formula employing skin test reactivity and bronchial sensitivity to histamine. It was pointed out that this degree of prediction was better than the reproducibility of bronchial allergen challenge achieved by some investigators.

References

1. Bousquet J, Lebel B, Dhlvert H, et al. Nasal challenge with pollen grains, skin-prick tests and specific IgE in patients with grass pollen allergy. Clin Allergy 1987;17:529–36.

2. Cockcroft DW, Murdock KY, Kirby J, et al. Prediction of airway responsiveness to histamine. Am Rev Respir Dis 1987;135:264–7.

3. Bernstein IL, Li JT, Bernstein DI, et al. Allergy diagnostic testing: an updated practice parameter. Ann Allergy, Asthma Immunol 2008; 100(no 3, Supplement 3): S1–148.

4. Hendrick DJ, Davies RJ, D'Souza MF, et al. An analysis of skin prick test reactions in 656 asthmatic patients. Thorax 1975;30:2–8.

5. Viner AS, Jackman N. Retrospective study of 1271 patients diagnosed as perennial rhinitis. Clin Allergy 1976;6:251–9.

6. Rajka G. Prurigo Besnier (atopic dermatitis) with special reference to the role of allergy factors. II. The evaluation of the results of skin reactions. Acta Dermato-Venereol 1961;41:1–39.

7. Arbes SJ Jr, Gergen PJ, Elliott L, et al. Prevalences of positive skin test responses to 10 common allergens in the US population: results from the Third National Health and Nutrition Examination Survey. JACI 2005;116:377–83.

8. Adinoff AD, Rosloniec DM, McCall LL, et al. Immediate skin test reactivity to Food and Drug Administration-approved standardized extracts. J Allergy Clin Immunol 1990;86:766–74.

9. Barbee RA, Lebowitz MD, Thompson HC, et al. Immediate skin test reactivity in a general population sample. Ann Intern med 1976;84: 129–33.

10. Barbee RA, Brown WG, Kaltenborn W, et al. Allergen skin-test reactivity in a community population sample: correlation with age, histamine skin reactions, and total serum immunoglobulin E. J Allergy Clin Immunol 1981;68:15–9.

11. Hanneuse Y, Delespesse G, Hudson D, et al. Influence of ageing on IgE-mediated reactions in allergic patients. Clin Allergy 1978;8:165–74.

12. Skassa-Brociek W, Manderscheid J-C, Michel F-B, et al. Skin test reactivity to histamine from infancy to old age. J Allergy Clin Immunol 1987;80:711–6.

13. Menardo JL, Bousquet J, Rodiere M, et al. Skin test reactivity in infancy. J Allergy Clin Immunol 1985;75:646–51.

14. Stuckey MS, Witt CS, Schmitt LH, et al. Histamine sensitivity influences reactivity to allergens. J Allergy Clin Immunol 1985;75:373–6.

15. Vichyanond P, Nelson HS. Circadian variation of skin reactivity and allergy skin tests. J Allergy Clin Immunol 1989;83:1101–6.

16. Oppenheimer JJ, Nelson HS. Seasonal variation in immediate skin test reactions. Ann Allergy 1993;71:227–9.

17. Kalogeromitros D, Katsarou A, Armenaka M, et al. Influence of the menstrual cycle on skin-prick test reactions to histamine, morphine and allergen. Clin Exp Allergy 1995;25:461–6.

18. Wise SL, Meador KJ, Thompson WO, et al. Cerebral lateralization and histamine skin test asymmetries in humans. Ann Allergy 1993;70: 328–32.

19. Nelson HS, Rosloniec DM, McCall LL, et al. Comparative performance of five commercial skin test devices. J Allergy Clin Immunol 1993;92:750–6.

20. Nelson HS, Knoetzer J, Bucher B. Effect of distance between sites and region of the body on results of skin prick tests. J Allergy Clin Immunol 1996;97:596–601.

21. Skoner DP, Gentile DA, Angelini B, et al. Allergy skin test responses during experimental infection with respiratory syncytial virus. Ann Allergy Asthma Immunol 2006;96:834–9.

22. Cook TJ, MacQueen DM, Wittig HJ, et al. Degree and duration of skin test suppression and side effects with antihistamines. J Allergy Clin Immunol 1973;51:71–7.

23. Dockhorn RJ, Hill EK, Hafner KB, et al. The duration of inhibition of skin prick test reactions after bid administration to steady-state of the non-sedating antihistamine Allegra (abst). J Allergy Clin Immunol 1997;99(1 Part 2):S446.

24. Rao KS, Menon PK, Hillman BC, et al. Duration of the suppressive effect of tricyclic antidepressants on histamine-induced wheal-and-flare reactions in human skin. J Allergy Clin Immunol 1988;82:752–7.

25. Miller J, Nelson HS. Suppression of immediate skin tests by ranitidine. J Allergy Clin Immunol 1989;84:895–99.

26. Kupczyk M, Kuprys I, Gorski P, et al. The effect of montelukast (10 mg daily) and loratadine (10 mg daily) on wheal, flare and itching reactions in skin prick tests. Pulm Pharmacol Therapeut 2006;20:85–9.

27. While M, Rothrock S, Meeves S, et al. Comparative effects of fexofenadine and montelukast on allergen-induced wheal and flare. Allergy Asthma Proc 2005;26:221–8.

28. Pipkorn U, Hammarlund A, Enerback L. Prolonged treatment with topical glucocorticoids results in an inhibition of the allergen-induced weal-and-flare response and a reduction in skin mast cell numbers and histamine content. Clin Exp Allergy 1989;19:19–25.

29. Slott RI, Zweiman B. A controlled study of the effect of corticosteroids on immediate skin test reactivity. J Allergy Clin Immunol 1974;554: 229–34.

30. Olson R, Karpink MH, Shelanski S, et al. Skin reactivity to codeine and histamine during prolonged corticosteroid therapy. J Allergy Clin Immunol 1990;86:153–9.

31. Des Roches A, Paradis L, Bougeard Y-H, et al. Long-term oral corticosteroid therapy does not alter the results of immediate allergy skin prick tests. J Allergy Clin Immunol 1996;98:522–7.

32. Corren J, Shapiro G, Reimann J, et al. Allergen skin tests and free IgE levels during reduction and cessation of omalizumab therapy. J Allergy Clin Immunol 2008;121:506–11.

33. Dantzler BS, Tipton WR, Nelson HS, et al. Tissue threshold changes during the first months of immunotherapy. Ann Allergy 1980;45: 213–6.

34. Nish WA, Charlesworth EN, Davis TL, et al. The effect of immunotherapy on the cutaneous late phase reaction to allergen. J Allergy Clin Immunol 1994;93:484–93.

35. Dreborg S, Holgersson M, Nilsson G, et al. The dose response relationship of allergen, histamine, and histamine releasers in skin prick test and the precision of the skin prick test method. Allergy 1987;42:117–25.

36. Harris RI, Stern MA, Watson HK. Dose response curve of allergen and histamine in skin prick tests. Allergy 1989;43:565–72.

37. Meiser JP, Nelson HS. Comparing conventional and acetone-precipitated dog allergen extract skin testing. J Allergy Clin Immunol 2001;107: 744–5.

38. Esch RE. Manufacturing and standardizing fungal allergen products. J Allergy Clin Immunol 2004;113:210–5.

39. Patterson ML, Slater JE. Characterization and comparison of commercially available German and American cockroach allergen extracts. Clin Exp Allergy 2002 May;32:721–7.

40. Esch RG. Role of proteases on the stability of allergic extracts. In: Klein R, editor. Regulatory control and standardization of allergic extracts. Stuttgart: Gustav Fischer Verlag 1990, p. 171–7.

41. Dreborg S, Foucard T. Prick-prick skin test with fresh foods. Allergy 1983;38:167–71.

42. Rosen JP, Selcow JE, Mendelson ML, et al. Skin testing with natural foods in patients suspected of having food allergies: is it a necessity? J Allergy Clin Immunol 1994;93:1068–70.

43. Ortolani C, Ispano M, Pastorello EA, et al. Comparison of results of skin prick tests (with fresh foods and commercial food extracts) and RAST in 100 patients with oral allergy syndrome. J Allergy Clin Immunol 1989;83:683–90.

44. Ancona GR, Schumacher IC. The use of raw foods as skin testing material in allergic disorders. California Med 1950;73:473–5.

45. Bock SA, Lee W-Y, Remigio L, et al. An appraisal of skin tests with food extracts for diagnosis of food hypersensitivity. Clin Allergy 1978;8:559–64.

46. Indrajana T, Spieksma F, Th M, et al. Comparative study of the intracutaneous, scratch and prick tests in allergy. Ann Allergy 1971;29:639–50.

47. Vanselow NA. Skin testing and other diagnostic procedures. In: Sheldon JM, Lovell RG, Mathews KP, editors. A manual of clinical allergy. 2nd ed. Chapter 4. Philadelphia: WB Saunders Company; 1967.

48. Sears MR, Herbison GP, Holdaway MD, et al. The relative risks of sensitivity to grass pollen, house dust mite and cat dander in the development of childhood asthma. Clin Exp Allergy 1989;19:419–24.

49. Henderson FW, Stewart PW, Burchinal MR, et al. Respiratory allergy and the relationship between early childhood lower respiratory illness and subsequent lung function. Am Rev Respir Dis 1992;145:283–90.

50. Gergen PJ, Turkeltaub PC. The association of individual allergen reactivity with respiratory disease in a national sample: data from the second National Health and Nutrition Examination Survey, 1976–80 (NHANNES II). J Allergy Clin Immunol 1992;90:579–88.

51. Hagy GW, Settipane GA. Prognosis of positive allergy skin tests in an asymptomatic population: a three year followup of college students. J Allergy 48:200–11, 1971.

52. Hagy GW, Settipane GA. Risk factors for developing asthma and allergic rhinitis: a 7-year follow-up of college students. J Allergy Clin Immunol 1976;58:330–6.

53. Brown WG, Hhalonen MJ, Kaltenborn WT, et al. The relationship of respiratory allergy, skin test reactivity, and serum IgE in a community population sample. J Allergy Clin Immunol 1979;63:328–35.

54. Reddy PM, Nagaya H, Pascual HC, et al. Reappraisal of intracutaneous tests in the diagnosis of reaginic allergy. J Allergy Clin Immunol 1978;61:36–41.

55. Schwindt CD, Hutcheson PS, Leu SY, et al. Role of intradermal skin tests in the evaluation of clinically relevant respiratory allergy assessed using patient history and nasal challenges. Ann Allergy Asthma Immunol 2005;94:627–33.

56. Nelson HS, Oppenheimer JJ, Buchmeier A, et al. An assessment of the role of intradermal skin testing in the diagnosis of clinically relevant allergy to timothy grass. J Allergy Clin Immunol 1996;97:1193–1201.

57. Wood RA, Phipatanakul W, Hamilton RG, et al. A comparison of skin prick tests, intradermal skin tests, and RASTs in the diagnosis of cat allergy. J Allergy Clin Immunol 1999;103:773–9.

58. Sharma HP, Wood RA, Bravo AR, et al. A comparison of skin prick tests, intradermal skin tests, and specific IgE in the diagnosis of mouse allergy. J Allergy Clin Immunol 2008;121:933–9.

59. Oppenheimer J, Nelson HS. Skin testing: a survey of allergists. Ann Allergy Asthma Immunol 2006;96:19–23.

60. Ownby DR. Computerized measurement of allergen-induced skin reactions. J Allergy Clin Immunol 1982;69:536–8.

61. Scandinavian Society of Allergology. Standardization of diagnostic work in allergy. Acta Allergologica 1974;29:239–40.

62. Taudorf E, Malling H-J, Laursen LC, et al. Reproducibility of histamine skin prick test. Allergy 1985;40:344–9.

63. Dreborg S. Skin testing: the safety of skin tests and information obtained from using different methods and concentrations of allergens. Allergy 1993;48:473–8.

64. Vanto T. Efficacy of different t skin prick testing methods in the diagnosis of allergy to dog. Ann Allergy 1983;50:340–3.

65. Nelson HS, Lahr J, Buchmeier BA, et al. Evaluation of devices for prick skin testing. J Allergy Clin Immunol 1998;101:153–6.

66. Nelson HS, Kolehmainen C, Lahr J, et al. A comparison of multiheaded devices for allergy skin testing. J Allergy Clin Immunol 2004;113:1218–9.

67. Tipton WR. Influence of histamine controls on skin tests with hymenoptera venom. Ann Allergy 1980;44:204–5.

68. Koller DY, Pirker C, Jarisch R, et al. Influence of the histamine control on skin reactivity in skin testing. Allergy 1992;47:58–9.

69. Valyaseui MA, Maddox DE, Li JTC. Systemic reactions to allergy skin tests. Ann Allergy 1999;83:132–6.

70. Bernstein DI, Wanner M, Boorish L, et al. Twelve-year survey of fatal reactions to allergen injections and skin testing: 1990–2001. J Allergy Clin Immunol 2004;113:1129–36.

71. Novembre E, Bernardini R, Bertini G, et al. Skin-prick-test-induced anaphylaxis. Allergy 1995;50:511–3.

72. Lin MS, Tanner E, Lynn J, et al. Non-fatal systemic allergic reactions induced by skin testing and immunotherapy. Ann Allergy 1993;71:557–62.

73. Huggins KG, Brostoff J. Local production of specific IgE antibodies in allergic rhinitis patients with negative skin tests. Lancet 1975;ii:148–50.

74. Shimojo N, Hirano K, Saito K, et al. Detection of house dust mite (HDM)-specific IgE antibodies on nasal mast cells from asthmatic patients whose skin prick test and RAST are negative for HDM. Int Arch Allergy Immunol 1992;98:135–9.

75. Rondon C, Romero JJ, Lopez S, et al. Local IgE production and positive nasal provocation test in patients with persistent nonallergic rhinitis. J Allergy Clin Immunol 2007;119:899–905.

76. DeShazo RD, Levinson AI, Dvorak HF, et al. The late phase skin reaction: evidence for activation of the coagulation system in an IgE-dependent reaction in man. J Immunol 1979;122:692–8.

77. Agarwal K, Zetterstrom O. Diagnostic significance of late cutaneous allergic responses and their correlation with radioallergosorbent test. Clin Allergy 1982;12:489–97.

78. Green GR, Zweiman B, Beerman H, et al. Delayed skin reactions to inhalant antigens. J Allergy 1967;40:224–36.

79. Pastorello EA, Incorvaia C, Ortolani C, et al. Studies on the relationship between the level of specific IgE antibodies and the clinical expression of allergy. I. Definition of levels distinguishing patients with symptomatic from patients with asymptomatic allergy to common aeroallergens. J Allergy Clin Immunol 1995;96:580–7.

80. Witteman AM, Stapel SSO, Perdok GJ, et al. The relationship between RAST and skin test results in patients with asthma or rhinitis: a quantitative study with purified major allergens. J Allergy Clin Immunol 1996;97:16–25.

81. Pierson-Mullany LK, Jackola DR, Blumenthal MN, et al. Evidence of an affinity threshold for IgE-allergen binding in the percutaneous skin test reaction. Clin Exp Allergy 2002;32:107–16.

82. Bousquet J, Maasch H, Martinot B, et al. Double-blind, placebo-controlled immunotherapy with mixed grass-pollen allergoids. II. Comparison between parameters assessing the efficacy of immunotherapy. J Allergy Clin Immunol 1988;82:439–46.

83. Bryant DH, Burns MW, Lazarus L. The correlation between skin tests, bronchial provocation tests and the serum level of IgE specific for common allergens in patients with asthma. Clin Allergy 1975;5:145–57.

84. Killian D, Cockcroft DW, Hargreave FE, et al. Factors in allergen-induced asthma: relevance of the intensity of the airways allergen reaction and nonspecific bronchial reactivity. Clin Allergy 1976;6:219–25.

85. Bryant DH, Burns WM. Bronchial histamine reactivity: its relationship to the reactivity of the bronchi to allergens. Clin Allergy 1976;6:523–32.

Outdoor Allergens

Richard W. Weber

Aerobiology is the science of airborne emanations of an organic or biologic origin. Allergists are generally concerned with only a portion of that discipline, namely, the impact of airborne allergens. Such aeroallergens may be dispersed through the air on a variety of particle sizes and come from a variety of sources and settings (see Table 24-1).[1] The originating source may be: microscopic, such as bacteria or protozoa; at the limits of visual detection, such as dust mites; or easily seen, such as mushrooms, bracket fungi, or animals such as cats, dogs, or horses. The airborne particle may be: a cell, intact pollen grain or cytoplasmic component thereof, fungal spore or mycelial fragment, protein adhering to epidermal scales or dust particles, or protein dissolved in water droplets. Outdoor sources are more likely to be of plant origin, while animal allergens are usually a greater problem indoors; however, there are exceptions, for example, fungal spores may be troublesome both inside and outdoors. Once entrained into airstreams, aeroallergens may be deposited on conjunctival membranes to induce allergic conjunctivitis, on nasal membranes to induce allergic rhinitis, or fragments can be inhaled into the lungs to induce allergic asthma.

General Principles of Allergen Aerobiology

Pollen

Vascular plants propagate through extension via trunk or root shoots, rhizomes or stolons, or by seed. Sexual reproduction is accomplished by transport of the male gamete, the pollen or spore, to the female gamete, the ovary. Pollen dispersal mechanisms make use of the wind, anemophily, or a vector such as an insect, entomophily. Insect-pollinated plants are seldom inducers of hay fever, although there are exceptions. Some amphiphilous plants utilize both mechanisms: although primarily insect-pollinated, sufficient pollen is produced to become airborne.

Fungi

Fungi comprise one of seven kingdoms of living organisms, more closely related to the animal kingdom than to the plant kingdom. Where plants can be looked on as producers, and animals as consumers, fungi fulfill an ecologic role of decomposers and recyclers. Fungi are eukaryotic organisms with chromosomes within membrane-bound nuclei, dividing through mitosis. Fungi have chitin-containing cell walls, a polysaccharide found also in insect exoskeletons. Fungi may be unicellular, syncitial

(many nuclei not divided into separate cells), and multi-cellular (nuclei separated by septa). Life cycles can be very complex, with multiple life stages, with both sexual and asexual reproduction. 'Holomorph' refers to the whole fungus, which is comprised of the 'anamorph' (asexual reproductive stage) plus the 'teleomorph' (sexual reproductive stage). In some cases, only the anamorph or the teleomorph is identified, and the alternate life stage is not known. Anamorphs without a known teleomorph stage are frequently classified as Deuteromycota, also known as Fungi Imperfecta. This is an artificial taxon, a paraphyletic group united only in asexual propagation.[2]

Animal

While animal sources are primarily indoors, some may be significant outdoor allergens as well. Heavy hatches of caddis flies or mayflies, or miller moth infestations have been reported to induce allergic symptoms.[3] Occupational exposures to tussock moths in pine trees may bother lumberjacks, and sewer flies, municipal sanitation workers.[4] Horse dander allergen can be sampled down-stream of stables.[5]

Submicronic Allergenic Particles

The observation that ragweed hay fever symptoms might persist for days after intact pollen is no longer collectable from the air spurred studies that demonstrated airborne allergens in submicronic particles.[6,7] The assumption was that such particles represented fragmented pollen grains. Airborne birch antigenic activity has also been demonstrated on particles smaller than 2.4 microns. Starch granules are prominent in the cytoplasm of certain pollens such as the grasses (Poaceae) and docks (Rumex, Polygonaceae).[8] It has been discovered that grass starch granules have heavy concentrations of groups 1, 5 and 13 allergens.[9–11] It is suggested that the force of storm-driven raindrops disrupts grass pollen grains, releasing large amounts of respirable allergen-laden starch granules.[12] Schäppi and colleagues have demonstrated that a moisture-drying cycle of grass pollen will result in starch granules emanating through the aperture.[9]

Characteristics of Wind-Pollinated Plants

Although wind-pollination may appear to be a simpler process than vector-facilitated pollination, it is felt to be a later evolutionary mechanism than the latter. Characteristics are summarized in Box 24-1. Anemophilous plants have incomplete flowers, that

DOI: 10.1016/B978-1-4377-0271-2.00024-9

Table 24-1 Aeroallergen Sources and Types

Allergen Source	Particle Type
Bacteria	Cells, fragments, metabolites
Thermophilic actinomycetes	Spores, metabolites
Algae	Cells, fragments, metabolites
Protozoa	Metabolites
Fungi	Spores, mycelial fragments, metabolites
Ferns and mosses	Spores
Grasses, weeds and trees	Pollens, cytoplasmic particles
Arthropods	Feces, saliva, body parts
Birds	Feces, serum proteins, epidermal debris
Mammals	Dander, saliva, urine

Modified from Burge HA. Ann Allergy 1992;69:9–18.

BOX 24-1

Characteristics of Wind-Pollinated Plants

- Incomplete flowers (spatially separate male and female)
- Male flowers exposed to wind
- Petals and sepals insignificant or absent
- Absent attractants (color, aroma, nectar)
- Pollen grains small and dry, reduced ornamentation

BOX 24-2

Thommen's Postulates

- Pollen must contain excitant of hay fever
- Pollen must be anemophilous
- Pollen must be produced in sufficiently large amounts
- Pollen must be buoyant to carry long distances
- Plant must be widely and abundantly distributed

From Thommen AA. Which plants cause hayfever? In: Asthma and hay fever in theory and practice. Springfield, IL: Charles C Thomas; 1931:546–554.

is, male and female functions are found on separate structures. The male, or pollen-producing flowers, are exposed to the wind. On trees, this is usually on dangling structures called catkins, frequently having hundreds of small individual flowers. On weeds or grasses the inflorescences are thrust up into the air on the higher portions of the plant. Female flowers may be lower, often at axils of leaves, or at stem junctions. Petals and sepals, rather than being showy, are insignificant or absent. Attractants such as color, fragrance, or nectar are absent. The pollen grains themselves tend to be small and dry, with reduced ornamentation to minimize turbulence, and with little sticky resin.

Wind-pollinated trees produce extraordinary amounts of pollen. Each catkin may have more than 200 individual tiny flowers. Erdtman reported that a single birch catkin produced about 6 million pollen grains, and an alder catkin 4.5 million. An English oak catkin released 1.25 million grains.[13] Erdtman tabulated the number of catkins on such trees, and calculated the amount of pollen produced in a single year. A birch tree released over 5.5 billion grains over a single year, alder 7.2 billion, and an oak 0.6 billion grains. Spruce, like birch, produced about 5.5 billion grains in a year. Cereal rye grass produced 4.25 million pollen grains per inflorescence.[13]

Almost 80 years ago, August Thommen set out five principles that he felt were necessary for a plant to be an important inducer of pollinosis (Box 24-2). These are now referred to as Thommen's Postulates, and they have generally remained correct, although there are some caveats.[14] That the pollen must contain an excitant of hay fever appears self-evident, and such excitants are either proteins or glycoproteins easily elutable on contact with a moist surface, or are coated on the surface of expelled cytoplasmic particles that are of a respirable size. While the majority of pollinosis inducers are wind-pollinated, some primarily insect-pollinated plants will release sufficient airborne pollen to cause

sensitization in the proper setting. Such a setting may be a tree or shrub situated at a bedroom window, and a single point source could lead to sensitization. Although most pollen grains come to rest within meters of the source, grains may be transported for hundreds of miles.[13]

Floristic Zones

The distribution of individual plant species is dependent on a multitude of factors. Foremost are conditions that constitute 'climate': average high and low temperatures, ambient humidity and average precipitation. Soil factors, such as mineral content, pH, and density, will also impact on plant adaptation and selection.[15] Certain plants are cosmopolitan, adapting to diverse circumstances, while others are limited to a niche, adapting to extremes of moisture or temperature. The range of native indigenous species may be limited by niche selectivity. The extent to which an introduced plant has spread will be determined by its adaptability, and by its aggressiveness and the length of time from the point of introduction. Which plants may be found in different locations may be induced from several sources. Numerous gardening texts contain 'hardiness zone' maps defined by the United States Department of Agriculture (USDA).[16] There are 10 climatic zones in the North American continent based on the average annual minimum temperature: beginning with zone 1 at −50°F, and progressing by about 10° increments to zone 10 at 30–40°F. These isotherms generally define northern limits of species, due to their inability to survive the cold of the winter. Exceptions may occur in protected sites with extraneous sources of heat. The USDA map does not take into consideration other factors such as rainfall or maximum temperature. A more exact classification system has been developed for the western half of the USA. Twenty-four climate zones have been described, determined by the interplay of six factors: latitude, elevation, Pacific Ocean influence, continental air mass influence, mountains and hills, and local terrain.[17] This is helpful to define the likely vegetation in any given region of the western states. However, 24 zones are cumbersome to consider. Solomon has popularized 10 floristic zones which are a cross between the USDA hardiness zones and factors like those considered in the western system, and which offer a useful compromise.[18,19] While the borders of the zones are purposely ill-defined, they are perhaps more descriptive of the territory encompassed. The zones are: Northern Forest, Eastern Agricultural, Southeastern Coastal Plain, Florida Subtropical, Central Plains, Rocky Mountain, Arid Southwest, Great Basin, Northwest Coastal, and California Lowland. A useful reference source is *Airborne and Allergenic Pollen of North America*[20] which has distribution maps of many native allergenic plants. However, numbers of introduced major allergenic plants do not have distribution maps.

Characterized Allergens

Numerous allergens from plant, fungal, and animal sources have now been fully or partially characterized. A list of those that have been sequenced is maintained and updated on-line by the International Union of Immunological Societies (IUIS).[21] Allergen nomenclature, by convention, is the first three letters of the genus followed by the first letter of the species, followed by a number. An example would be the major allergen of short ragweed, Amb a 1, initially known as Antigen E. A lower number may signify either importance or chronology of discovery, but not invariably. Occasionally, allergens are renamed to conform to the function of another numbered allergen from a related source. Variations in the molecular weight or charge of an allergen due to amino acid substitutions or glycosylation are called isoallergens and are designated by a decimal point followed by four digits (e.g. Phl p 5.0102 and Phl p 5.0201).

Aeroallergen Sampling

In order to assess the type and intensity of the aeroallergen exposure in different settings, it is necessary to monitor the environment. Table 24.2 lists the types of samplers that can be used to assess both outdoor and indoor air. The earliest samplers were crude devices that relied on gravity to deposit particles on sticky surfaces. The Durham sampler is a greased microscope slide mounted horizontally on a stand, with a roof, or rain shield, above. Petrie dishes with the appropriate agar medium have been used indoors for mold studies, with the advantage of the growth medium allowing identification of viable spores by distinctive colony characteristics. Disadvantages of gravimetric samplers are that they can only be quantified in terms of surface area (cm^2) and do not give an estimate of particle burden in a volume of air. Also, capture is skewed to larger particles, and smaller particles such as smaller mold spores are underrepresented as air currents may carry them over the top of the surface. Gravimetric samplers are no longer considered adequate for meaningful study.

Volumetric devices sample volumes of air over a given time interval and results are reported in particles/cubic meter/24 hr (Table 24-2). The Rotorod seen in Figure 24-1A is a rotary impaction device that spins two small plastic rods at fixed time intervals, usually adjusted at 1 minute out of every 10 (or a total of 144 minutes in 24 hours). The rods are lowered into the ambient air from the spinning armature by centripetal force. The leading side

of the rod is greased with silicone. It has a fixed surface area (length and width) that sweeps a given length of air (circumference of the circle) for a given length of time. The advantages are that it is not affected by wind direction. The disadvantages are that it loses capture efficiency as the surface becomes loaded with impacted particles, explaining the necessity of not running continually over 24 hours. Suction devices use vacuum pumps to move air through an aperture to impact on tape on a rotating drum (with the Burkard) or an advancing microscope slide (Kramer-Collins). The Burkard (Figure 24-1B) can be configured for a 24-hour or 7-day sample. Capture efficacy is best when the aperture is facing into the wind, and when the wind velocity matches the intake flow. The Burkard has a large weather vane to orient the aperture into the wind. Another suction device, used either indoors or outside, is the Andersen cascade impactor, which can segregate particles by size through several stages. Figure 24-1C and D show the Andersen intact and disassembled revealing the individual stages. The use of agar plates can be used to identify fungi by culture characteristics. Small personal-sized samplers have been developed which can be worn or carried, and with stationary samplers have been useful in risk assessment, especially, but not exclusively, in indoor occupational settings. High-volume suction devices are fitted with fiberglass filters that can be scanned microscopically, or eluted and stained with specific monoclonal antibodies. The subtleties of outdoor sampling and interpretation, as well as the importance of pauci-micronic particles carrying allergen, has been well described.[22] Immunochemical techniques to measure such outdoor allergen loads have come into vogue.[23,24] Unfortunately, the number of pollen or fungal related allergens contributing to the aeroallergen atmospheric burden exceeds, by several orders of magnitude, the number of characterized allergens that can be used as the basis of monoclonal specific immunochemical assays.

Outdoor aeroallergen sampling has for the most part been based on microscopic examination with identification based on morphologic pattern recognition, which is labor intensive and requires an experienced counter.[25] The National Allergy Bureau is the AAAAI-sponsored pollen-and-mold counting stations primarily scattered around the contiguous USA (with additional stations in Alaska, Hawaii, Puerto Rico, Canada, and Argentina). The stations number over 85, and the majority of stations have only a single qualified counter; therefore, the prospect of automated systems is highly tantalizing. Automated counters evaluated by Delaunay and associates are elegant in their concept, but have significant drawbacks.[26] The inability to discern ice particles from pollen by one sampler was a major problem, but the major difficulty was the relatively high particle detection threshold, which was above that necessary to induce symptoms in the majority of patients. Therefore, more work is needed before automated counters can be used for common monitoring.

Representative Pollens

Grasses

The grass family, Poaceae, is a huge botanical group with several subfamilies and numerous tribes. The fescue subfamily, including the temperate climate pasture grasses and most cereal grains, is the most prominent in pollinosis. These grasses have a wide range throughout the USA. With only minor exceptions, members of the fescue subfamily have strongly cross-reactive major allergens.[27] Representative members include Kentucky bluegrass, timothy, cereal rye, and foxtail barley (Figure 24-2A). Bermuda (*Cynodon dactylon*) is the most important southern grass,

Table 24-2 Types of Aeroallergen Samplers

Type	Example	Comment
Gravimetric	Durham	Large particles overrepresented
	Petrie dish	Particles per surface area (p/cm^2)
Volumetric		Particles per air volume (p/m^3)
Impaction		
intermittent rotary	Rotorod	Easily overloaded
suction drum	Burkard	Wind orientation necessary
cascade	Anderson	Indoor or outdoor use
Filtration	Accu-Vol	Microscopic or immunoassay
Personal sampler		Clinically relevant exposure
Automatic counter	NTT-Shinyei	Misreading likely
	KH300	Lack of sensitivity

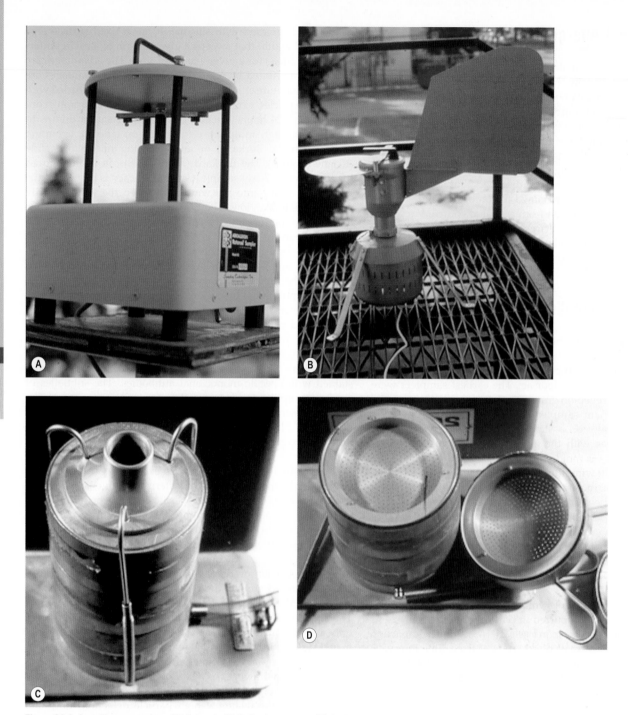

Figure 24-1 Aeroallergen samplers. **(A)** Rotorod; **(B)** Burkard spore trap; **(C)** Andersen cascade impactor; **(D)** Andersen sampler showing inner layers.

generally found south of the 38° parallel, with extension further north along the coasts. Johnson (*Sorghum halepense*) is primarily a southern grass, but is found throughout the Eastern Agricultural zone and across the Arid Southwest. Buffalo grass and grama grass are two native prairie grasses related to Bermuda grass. Included within the superorder containing the grasses are the rush, sedge, and cattail families, and while producing airborne pollen, they are not considered significant inducers of pollinosis.

Conifers

The most important member of the order Coniferales is the cedar family (Cupressaceae), containing cedars, junipers (*Juniperus spp*, *Thuja spp*), and cypresses (*Cupressus spp*). Exposure is not only

from forest stands, but also from the ubiquitous use of junipers in home landscaping. In Texas and parts of Oklahoma, mountain cedar (*Juniperus ashei*) counts may be > 20 000 grains/m³. Members of this family are strongly cross-reactive.[27] A subfamily includes bald cypress, redwoods, sequoias, and the foremost producer of pollinosis in Japan, Japanese cedar, (*Cryptomeria japonica*). The pine family consists of pines (*Pinus spp*), spruces (*Picea spp*), hemlocks (*Tsuga spp*), and firs (*Abies spp, Pseudotsuga*). The pollens of this family are produced in copious amounts, but they are weak allergens, and induce little hay fever.

Other Trees

Deciduous trees are scattered throughout a great number of botanical orders and families, some of which contain perennial

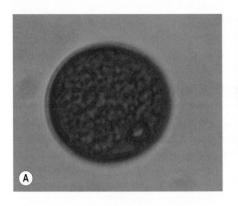

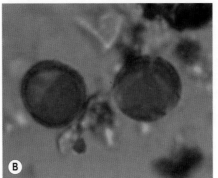

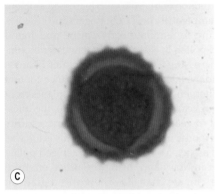

Figure 24-2 Representative pollens. **(A)** grass; **(B)** maple; **(C)** ragweed.

shrubs and weeds as well. With only a few exceptions, there is little cross-reactivity between these diverse plants. Cottonwoods, aspens, poplars, and willows are within the same family. Aspens are prevalent in the Rocky Mountains and throughout the Northern Forest. Poplars and cottonwoods are common throughout the eastern states and Great Plains. Willows, although primarily insect-pollinated, may release significant amounts of airborne pollen. Several birch species (*Betula*) and alder (*Alnus*) are found throughout the Northern Forest, Northwest Coastal, California Lowlands, and Great Basin zones. Alder is especially prevalent in the Northern Forest and Pacific Northwest zones. Red and white oaks (*Quercus spp*) have a wide range from the entire east through the Central Plains. Live oaks are evergreen, and found throughout the Southern Tier. American elm (*Ulmus americana*), with a wide range, has been decimated by disease. Siberian and Chinese elms (*U. pumila* and *U. parvifolia*) are now more common, with a similar range. Numerous maples (*Acer spp*) are found across the USA, with box elder (*A. negundo*) having a wide range in the Eastern zones, Central Plains, Rocky Mountain, Southwest, and California Lowlands (Figure 24-2B). Box elder is entirely wind-pollinated, and a prodigious pollen producer, while other maples are amphiphilous, both insect and wind pollinated. Ash trees are found across the continent, and have strong cross-reactivity with the European olive. Linden, or basswood (*Tilia spp.*), is another amphiphilous tree, which will produce large amounts of airborne pollen in summer, and is associated with significant sensitization. Russian olive, *Elaeagnus angustifolia*, has been widely planted across the Great Plains as a drought-resistant windbreak. It is also both wind and insect pollinated.

Weeds

Numerous annual or perennial weeds are significant inducers of hay fever. The sorrels and docks pollinate earlier than many weeds, coinciding with the grass pollen season. Sheep sorrel, (*Rumex acetosella*) is considered a moderate hay fever inducer, while curly or yellow dock (*R. crispus*), though a lower pollen producer, is a common plant. Nettle (*Urtica spp*) is common across the floristic zones with the exception of Florida and the Southeast Coastal zone; pellitory (*Parietaria spp*) is found throughout the zones. Nettle produces large amounts of small, pale pollen, and is under-appreciated as a source of hay fever. Pellitory is a major inducer of pollinosis in the Mediterranean basin. The closely related chenopod and amaranth weeds of Amaranthaceae are major inducers of hay fever in the later summer. Their pollen grains are very similar, and difficult to identify by species on counters. Pigweeds such as *Amaranthus retroflexus* are ubiquitous. The two major tumbleweeds found in the Central Plains, Russian thistle (*Salsola kali*) and burning bush (*Kochia scoparia*), are introduced and have expanded throughout the central states to the gulf and California coasts. *Kochia* is now even found in the northeastern states. Lamb's quarter (*Chenopodium album*), although a modest pollen producer, has a worldwide distribution. Plantains (*Plantago* spp.) are common weeds, which, while moderate pollen producers, have a long season, stretching from spring into fall.

Short (*Ambrosia artemisiifolia*) and giant (*A. trifida*) ragweed predominate in the eastern states through the Central Plains, with false (*A. acanthicarpa*) and western (*A. psilotachya*) ragweed common in the Rocky Mountain, Great Basin, Arid Southwest, and California Lowlands (Figure 24-2C). These four major ragweed plants strongly cross-react.[27] Cocklebur (*Xanthium commune*) and the marshelders (*Iva spp*) are within the same botanical tribe as the ragweeds, but are of lesser significance due to moderate pollen production. Mugwort (*Artemisia vulgaris*) in the east and a number of western sages (*Artemisia spp*) are important pollen producers in the late summer, rivaling the importance of ragweed in the western states. Goldenrod, *Solidago spp.*, is a showy, late summer blooming flower which has, historically, been blamed for much of the misery caused by the less conspicuous ragweed. Although goldenrod and sunflower are primarily insect pollinated, they can produce moderate amounts of pollen, which may persist in higher levels as ragweed pollen is waning.

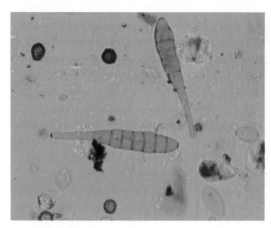

Figure 24-3 Alternaria. Two club-shaped *Alternaria*; four clear cigar-shaped *Cladosporium* in lower right quadrant; two pairs of dark brown Basidiomycete smut spores in upper and lower left quadrants.

Representative Fungi

A landmark paper by Long and Kramer demonstrated that airborne fungal spora should be classified as two types: those facilitated by dry windy conditions and those with greater spore release with increased humidity or precipitation.[28] In the Central Plains, fungi such as *Alternaria*, *Cladosporium*, and *Epicoccum* grow on grasses and grains, and spores are released through wind turbulence. These mold spores are generally in greatest concentrations on dry windy afternoons (Figure 24-3). On the other hand, many Basidomycetes and Ascomycetes have spore release dependent on increased humidity, and puffballs release spores when hit by raindrops. Such fungi will then be in greatest concentrations during or after rainfall and during the damper hours of darkness.[28] Although *Alternaria* is recovered on samplers to a much lesser degree than for *Cladosporium*, it is a more potent allergenic source, and has been incriminated in the severity of asthma and life-threatening events.[29,30] *Epicoccum* and Basidiospores have also been linked with decreases in pulmonary function and asthma admissions.[31,32]

Meteorological Variables

While prevalent weather helps define climate, individual factors such as rain, humidity, wind speed and direction, temperature, or amount of sunshine may all have effects on bioaerosols.[33] Effects may be direct or indirect, immediate or cumulative. Precipitation and humidity will decrease particle air burden acutely, while sufficient moisture preseasonally is necessary to assure proper growth of flower buds on perennials and trees, and growth of annuals in general. Ambient temperature rise is necessary for pollen anthesis in many plants, and cumulative heat above a threshold value has been linked to onset and intensity of pollination in grasses, weeds, and trees.

Wind direction only impacts if there is lack of uniformity in pollen sources surrounding sampling sites. Wind speed may factor in re-entrainment of settled particles, or act to scour the air. Thunderstorms provide a unique sum of factors that may greatly increase aeroallergen burden due to outflows from storm cells as well as disruption of pollen grains with increase in airborne submicronic particles.[34,35]

As discussed above, dispersal of mold spores is intimately linked to precipitation and humidity, but effects may be diametrically opposed, depending on the type of fungi. Certain ascospores and basidiospores require active rainfall for release of spores, while other Deuteromycetes will be suppressed by precipitation.

Impact of Climate Change on Aeroallergens

Periods of pollen anthesis have been used as a monitor of global warming, and specifically anthropogenic climate change. Not only can outdoor aeroallergen sampling be used as a marker, but conversely, climate change can also affect quantity of airborne allergens. Ziska and Caulfield in 2000, and Wayne and associates in 2002, reported increased short ragweed (*A. artemisiifolia*) biomass and pollen production of 61–90% with increased ambient CO_2.[36,37] Manipulating temperature and CO_2, Rogers and coworkers increased temperature to simulate early spring and found more inflorescences and pollen in earlier rather than later blooming ragweed plants.[38] Increasing CO_2 resulted in greater biomass and pollen production in the later growing cohorts. Since content of the ragweed major allergen Amb a 1 will vary in plants from site to site and even from year to year at the same site, the question was raised whether increased pollen production necessarily implies an increase in airborne allergenic load.[39,40] This issue was addressed by Ziska and associates who collected ragweed pollen along an urban transect in Maryland, using the urban environment as a surrogate for climate change.[41] There was a gradient of both air temperature and CO_2 level through four sites: urban, suburban, semi-rural, and rural. The urban site averaged 2°C higher and a 30% higher CO_2 level than the rural site. As expected, the urban ragweed grew faster with a greater above-ground biomass, flowered earlier, and produced more pollen than the rural site. There was about a 2-fold greater concentration of Amb a 1 per microgram of protein in the rural versus the other sites. However, there was a greater than 7-fold production of pollen from the urban sites compared to the rural site, supporting the premise that there was indeed an increased airborne allergenic burden.

There is now a wealth of evidence that climate change has had, and will have further impact on a variety of allergenic plants.[42,43] Increased CO_2 increases plant biomass and pollen production. It is conceivable that increases in airborne pollen numbers will increase the efficiency of wind-borne pollination, thereby increasing propagation of such plants. The expectation then is that there will be increasing amounts of robust allergenic plants and an increasing aeroallergen burden for inhalant allergy sufferers.

References

1. Burge HA. Monitoring for airborne allergens. Ann Allergy 1992;69: 9–18.
2. Kendrick B. The fifth kingdom. Waterloo, Ontario, Canada: Mycologue Publications; 1985.
3. Kraut A, Sloan J, Silviu-Dan F, et al. Occupational allergy after exposure to caddis flies at a hydroelectric power plant. Occup Environ Med 1994;51:408–13.
4. Smith TS, Hogan MB, Welch JE, et al. Modern prevalence of insect sensitization in rural asthma and allergic rhinitis. Allergy Asthma Proc 2005;26:356–60.
5. Elfman L, Brannstrom J, Smedje G. Detection of horse allergen around a stable. Int Arch Allergy Immunol 2008;145:269–76.
6. Busse W, Reed C, Hoehne J. Where is the allergic reaction in ragweed asthma? II. Demonstration of ragweed antigen in airborne particles smaller than pollen. J Allergy Clin Immunol 1972;50:289–93.
7. Habenicht HA, Burge HA, Muilenberg ML, et al. Allergen carriage by atmospheric aerosol. II. Ragweed-pollen determinants in submicronic atmospheric fractions. J Allergy Clin Immunol 1984;74:64–7.
8. Weber RW. Pollen identification. Ann Allergy Asthma Immunol 1998;80:141–7.

9. Schäppi GF, Taylor PE, Pain MCF, et al. Concentrations of major grass group 5 allergens in pollen grains and atmospheric particles: implications for hay fever and allergic asthma sufferers sensitized to grass pollen allergens. Clin Exp Allergy 1999;29:633–41.

10. Grote M, Vrtala S, Niederberger V, et al. Expulsion of allergen-containing materials from hydrated ryegrass (*Lolium perenne*) pollen revealed using immunogold field emission scanning and transmission electron microscopy. J Allergy Clin Immunol 2000;105:1140–5.

11. Grote M, Swoboda I, Valenta R, et al. Group 13 allergens as environmental and immunological markers for grass pollen allergy: studies by immunogold field emission scanning and transmission electron microscopy. Int Arch Allergy Immunol 2005;136:303–10.

12. Suphioglu C, Singh MB, Taylor PE, et al. Mechanism of grass-pollen-induced asthma. Lancet 1992;399:569–72.

13. Erdtman G. Output and dissemination of pollen. In: An introduction to pollen analysis. Waltham, MA: Chronica Botanica Co.; 1954, p. 175–85.

14. Thommen AA. Which plants cause hayfever? In: Asthma and hay fever in theory and practice. Springfield, IL, Charles C: Thomas Publisher; 1931, p. 546–54.

15. Weber RW. Floristic zones and aeroallergen diversity. Immunol Allergy Clin N Amer 2003;23:357–69.

16. Clausen RR, Ekstrom NH. Perennials for American gardens. New York: Random House; 1989, p. xi–xv.

17. Williamson JF. Sunset New Western garden book. 4th ed. Menlo Park, CA: Lane Publishing Co.; 1979, p. 8–29.

18. Solomon WR. Pollens and fungi. In: Aerobiology and inhalant allergens. In: Middleton E Jr, Reed CE, Ellis EF, Adkinson NF Jr, Yunginger JW, Busse WW, editors. Allergy principles and practice. 4th ed. St Louis: Mosby-Year Book, Inc.; 1993, p. 469–514

19. Solomon WR. Common pollen and fungus allergens. In: Bierman CW, Pearlman DS, editors. Allergic diseases from infancy to adulthood. 2nd ed. Philadelphia: WB Saunders Co.; 1988, p. 141–64.

20. Lewis WH, Vinay P, Zenger VE. Airborne and allergenic pollen of North America. Baltimore: Johns Hopkins University Press; 1983.

21. Allergen nomenclature. International Union of Immunological Societies Allergen Nomenclature Subcommittee, http://www.allergen.org/Allergen.aspx, updated 02-03-2009.

22. Solomon WR. How ill the wind? Issues in aeroallergen sampling. J Allergy Clin Immunol 2003;112:3–8.

23. Johnson CR, Weeke ER, Nielsen J, et al. Aeroallergen analyses and their clinical relevance. II. Sampling by high-volume air sampler with immunochemical quantification versus Burkard pollen trap sampling with morphologic quantification. Allergy 1992;47:510–16.

24. Razmovski V, O'Meara TJ, Taylor DJM, et al. A new method for simultaneous immunodetection and morphologic identification of individual sources of pollen allergens. J Allergy Clin Immunol 2000;105:725–31.

25. Weber RW. Outdoor aeroallergen sampling: not all that simple. Ann Allergy Asthma Immunol 2007;98:505–6.

26. Delauney J-J, Sasajima H, Okamoto Y, et al. Side-by-side comparison of automatic pollen counters for use in pollen information systems. Ann Allergy Asthma Immunol 2007;98:553–8.

27. Weber RW. Guidelines for using pollen cross-reactivity in formulating allergen immunotherapy. J Allergy Clin Immunol 2008;122:219–21.

28. Long DL, Kramer CL. Air spora of two contrasting ecological sites in Kansas. J Allergy Clin Immunol 1972;49:255–66.

29. Zureik M, Neukirch C, Leynaert B, et al. Sensitisation to airborne moulds and severity of asthma: cross sectional study from European Community respiratory health survey. Br Med J 2002;325:411–7.

30. O'Halloran MT, Yuninger JW, Offord KP, et al. Exposure to an aeroallergen as a possible precipitating factor in respiratory arrest in young patients with asthma. N Engl J Med 1991;324:359–63.

31. Salvaggio J, Seabury J, Schoenhardt FA. New Orleans asthma. V. Relationship between Charity Hospital asthma admission rates, semiquantitative pollen and fungal spore counts, and total particulate aerometric sampling data. J Allergy Clin Immunol 1971;48:96–114.

32. Atkinson RW, Strachan DP, Anderson HR, et al. Temporal associations between daily counts of fungal spores and asthma exacerbations. Occup Environ Med 2006;63:580–90.

33. Weber RW. Meteorological variables in aerobiology. Immunol Allergy Clin N Amer 2003;23:411–22.

34. Marks GB, Colquhoun JR, Girgis ST, et al. Thunderstorm outflows preceding epidemics of asthma during spring and summer. Thorax 2001;56:468–71.

35. Newsom R, Strachan D, Archibald E, et al. Effect of thunderstorms and airborne grass pollen on the incidence of acute asthma in England, 1990–94. Thorax 1997;52:680–5.

36. Ziska LH, Caulfied F. Rising CO_2 and pollen production of common ragweed (*Ambrosia artemisiifolia*), a known allergy-inducing species: implications for public health. Aust J Plant Physiol 2000;27:893–8.

37. Wayne P, Foster S, Connelly J, et al. Production of allergenic pollen by ragweed (*Ambrosia artemisiifolia* L.) is increased in CO_2-enriched atmospheres. Ann Allergy Asthma Immunol 2002;88:279–82.

38. Rogers CA, Wayne PM, Macklin EA, et al. Interaction of the onset of spring and elevated atmospheric CO_2 on ragweed (*Ambrosia artemisiifolia* L.) pollen production. Environ Health Perspect 2006;114:865–9.

39. Lee YS, Dickinson DB, Schlager D, et al. Antigen E content of pollen from individual plants of short ragweed (*Ambrosia artemisiifolia*). J Allergy Clin Immunol 1979;63:336–9.

40. Weber RW. Mother Nature strikes back: global warming, homeostasis, and the implications for allergy. Ann Allergy Asthma Immunol 2002;88:251–2.

41. Ziska LH, Gebhard DE, Frenz DA, et al. Cities as harbingers of climate change: common ragweed, urbanization, and public health. J Allergy Clin Immunol 2003;111:290–5.

42. Beggs PJ. Impacts of climate change on aeroallergens: past and future. Clin Exp Allergy 2004;34:1507–13.

43. Shea KM, Truckner RT, Weber RW, et al. Climate change and allergic disease. J Allergy Clin Immunol 2008;122:443–53.

25

Indoor Allergens

Martin D. Chapman

Allergens found in house dust have been associated with asthma since the 1920s, when Kern[1] and Cooke[2] independently reported a high prevalence of immediate skin tests to house dust extracts among patients with asthma. Van Leeuven[3] showed that asthmatics who were admitted to a modified hospital room free of 'climate allergens' (thought to be bacteria and molds) showed clinical improvement: these were the first experiments that used allergen avoidance for asthma management. Allergists sought to explain how a heterogenous material such as house dust could contain a potent allergen that appeared to be ubiquitous. The prevailing theory was that a chemical reaction occurred in dust resulting in synthesis of the 'house dust allergen'.[4] Researchers extracted house dust with organic solvents to identify allergenically active compounds. The puzzle was finally resolved in 1967, when Voorhorst and Spieksma[5] showed that the origin of house dust allergen was biologic rather than chemical. The allergenic potency of Dutch house dust extracts correlated with the numbers of house dust mites (Acari, Pyroglyphidae: *Dermatophagoides pteronyssinus* and *D. farinae*) in the samples. Extracts of mite cultures gave positive skin tests at dilutions of 10^{-6}, and asthma symptoms correlated with seasonal variation in mite numbers. Exposure to 100 mites per gram of dust was associated with sensitization, and 500 mites per gram was associated with symptom exacerbation.

The prevalence of asthma has increased during the past 40 years. Current data suggest that approximately 10% of US children have asthma. Sensitization and exposure to indoor allergens, principally dust mites, cat, dog, mouse, cockroach (CR), and fungi, are among the most important risk factors.[6,7] The two principal mite species, *D. pteronyssinus* and *D. farinae,* account for more than 90% of the mite fauna in US house dust samples. Other allergenic mites include *Euroglyphus maynei* and *Blomia tropicalis* (found in subtropical regions such as Florida, southern California, Texas, and Puerto Rico). Storage mites, such as *Lepidoglyphus destructor, Tyrophagus putrescentiae,* and *Acarus siro,* cause occupational asthma among farmers, farm workers and grain handlers. Childhood asthma is also strongly associated with sensitization to animal allergens, CR, and, to a lesser extent, mold allergens. Cat allergen (Fel d 1) has a ubiquitous distribution in the environment and can be found at clinically significant levels in houses that do not contain cats (similarly for dog allergen).[8–10] Rodent urinary proteins have long been associated with occupational asthma among laboratory animal handlers. A high prevalence of sensitization and exposure to mouse allergen is a risk factor for asthma among inner-city children.[11,12] Children living in urban areas are also at risk of developing CR allergy. Cockroach infestation of housing results in the accumulation of potent allergens that are associated with increased asthma mortality and morbidity among US children, particularly African-American and Hispanic children, living in inner cities.[6,13,14] Cockroach allergens appear to be particularly potent. Atopic individuals develop immunoglobulin E (IgE) responses after exposure to 10-fold to a 100-fold lower levels of CR allergens than to dust mite or cat.[15]

Investigation of the role of indoor allergens in asthma has involved the identification of the most important allergens and the development of techniques to accurately monitor allergen exposure. This chapter reviews the structure and biologic function of indoor allergens, methods for assessing environmental exposure and the clinical significance of indoor allergens.

Allergen Structure and Function

Allergens are proteins or glycoproteins of 10 to 50 kDa that are readily soluble and able to penetrate the nasal and respiratory mucosae. A systematic allergen nomenclature has been developed by the International Union of Immunological Societies' (IUIS) Allergen Nomenclature Subcommittee: the first three letters of the source genus followed by a single letter for the species and a number denoting the chronologic order of allergen identification. Thus the abbreviated nomenclature for *Dermatophagoides pteronyssinus* allergen 1 is Der p 1 (see http://www.allergen.org). To be included in the IUIS nomenclature, the allergen must have been purified to homogeneity and/or cloned, and the prevalence of IgE antibody (ab) must have been established in an appropriate allergic population by skin testing or in vitro IgE ab assays.[16] Molecular cloning has determined the primary amino acid sequences of more than 500 allergens and most common allergens can be manufactured as recombinant proteins. There are over 50 three-dimensional structures of allergens in the Protein Database (PDB) and allergens are found in ≈180 protein families in the Pfam protein family database (http://www.sanger.ac.uk/software/Pfam) (Figure 25-1).[16–19] It has been argued that this is a small number of protein families, given that there are over 10 000 protein families in Pfam, and that this implies that only a limited group of proteins (with certain structural features) have the potential to become allergens.[17,20] However, detailed structural analyses have not revealed any common features or motifs that are associated with the induction of IgE responses. Recent studies have resolved the crystal structure of Bla g 2/mAb complexes. Mutagenesis of surface residues is being used to identify IgE epitopes and generate hypoallergenic variants for vaccine development.[18]

©2010 Elsevier Ltd, Inc, BV
DOI: 10.1016/B978-1-4377-0271-2.00025-0

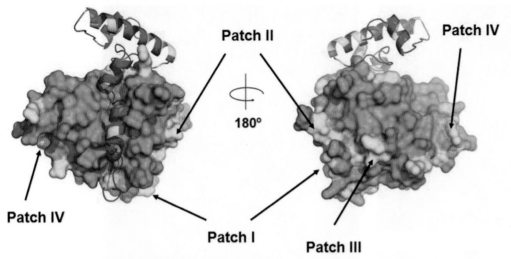

Figure 25-1 X-ray crystal structures of the mite cysteine protease allergens, Der p 1 and Der f 1. Residues that differ between the two allergens are shown in yellow and labeled as patches I, II, III, and IV. The conserved Cys35 active site residue is shown in orange. (From Chruszcz M, Chapman M, Vailes L et al. J Mol Biol 2009; 386:520–530.)

BOX 25-1 Key concepts

Indoor Allergens: Structure and Function

- Allergens are soluble proteins or glycoproteins of molecular weights of 10 to 50 kDa.
- More than 500 allergen sequences are deposited in protein databases (GenBank, PDB), and about 50 tertiary structures have been resolved by X-ray crystallography.
- Allergens have diverse biologic functions and may be enzymes, enzyme inhibitors, lipid-binding proteins, lipocalins, or regulatory or structural proteins.
- Allergens promote T cells to differentiate along the Th2 pathway to produce IL-4 and IL-13 and to initiate iso-type switching to IgE.
- Biologic functions of allergens, such as proteolytic enzyme activity or other adjuvant-like effects, can enhance IgE responses, damage lung epithelium and cause allergic inflammation.

Allergens belong to protein families with diverse biologic functions: they may be enzymes, enzyme inhibitors, lipid-binding proteins, ligand-binding proteins, structural or regulatory proteins (Box 25-1, Figure 25-2).[16] Some dust mite allergens are digestive enzymes excreted with the feces, such as Der p 1 (cysteine protease), Der p 3 (serine protease), and Der p 6 (chymotrypsin). Enzymatic activity of mite allergens promotes IgE synthesis and local inflammatory responses via cleavage of CD23 and CD25 receptors on B cells and by causing the release of proinflammatory cytokines (interleukin [IL]-8, IL-6, monocyte chemotactic protein-1 [MCP-1], and granulocyte-monocyte colony-stimulating factor [GM-CSF]) from bronchial epithelial cells.[21] Mite protease allergens cause detachment of bronchial epithelial cells in vitro and disrupt intercellular tight junctions. Activation of mite proteases could damage lung epithelia and allow access of other nonenzymatic allergens, such as Der p 2, to antigen-presenting cells. Der p 2 has structural homology to MD-2, the lipopolysaccharide (LPS) binding component of the Toll-like receptor 4 (TLR4) complex. Recent studies have shown that Der p 2 can drive signaling of the TLR4 complex and may enhance the expression of TLR4 on the airway epithelium and have intrinsic adjuvant activity.[22] Mite feces contain other elements, including endotoxin, bacterial DNA, mite DNA, and chitin that could also influence IgE responses and inflammation.[23,24]

With the exception of cat allergen Fel d 1, most animal allergens are ligand-binding proteins (lipocalins) or albumins. Lipocalins are 20- to 25-kDa proteins with a conserved, eight-stranded, antiparallel β-barrel structure that bind and transport small hydrophobic chemicals. In contrast, Fel d 1 is a calcium-binding, steroid-inducible, uteroglobin-like molecule – a tetrameric 35-kDa glycoprotein, comprising two subunits which are heterodimers of two chains comprising eight α-helices.[25] Fel d 1 has two amphipathic water-filled cavities which may bind biologically important ligands. Rat and mouse urinary allergens are pheromone- or odorant-binding proteins. The CR allergen Bla g 4 is a lipocalin that is produced in utricles and conglobate glands of male CRs and may have a reproductive function. Other important CR allergens include: Bla g 1, a gut-associated allergen; Bla g 2, an inactive aspartic proteinase; Bla g 5 (glutathione transferase family); and the Group 7 tropomyosin allergens (Figure 25-2).[26] Fungal allergens have been cloned from *Alternaria, Aspergillus, Cladosporium, Penicillium,* and *Trichophyton* spp., and they include proteolytic enzymes, heat shock proteins, or ribonucleases.

Evaluation of Allergen Exposure

Environmental Assessments

Counting Critters

Biologists and pest management companies have counted dust mites in dust samples and trapped CRs to assess infestation and allergen exposure. These methods are useful in studying population dynamics, seasonal variation, and the effect of physical and chemical methods for reducing mite and CR populations. However, they are time-consuming and unsuitable for routine measurements of allergen exposure. Allergen levels may remain high when mite or CR levels have been reduced, and simply enumerating mites/CRs may not be a reliable indicator of allergen exposure. Similarly, several epidemiologic studies on cat allergen exposure have relied on questionnaires and direct

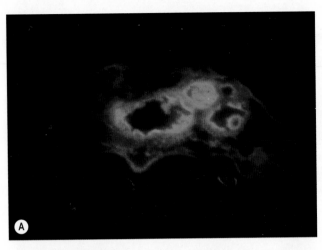

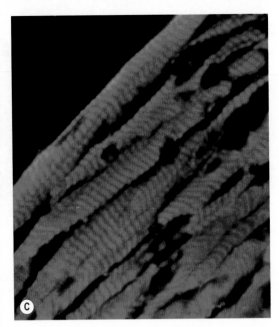

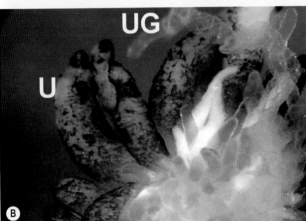

Figure 25-2 Biologic functions of indoor allergens. **(A)** Localization of Der p 1 in the mite digestive tract by immunofluorescence (courtesy of Dr. Euan Tovey, University of Sydney, Australia.). **(B)** In situ hybridization showing Bla g 4 in the uricose gland (UG) and utricles (U) of male cockroach (from Fan Y, Gore C, Redding K et al. Insect Mol Biol 2005;14:45–53). **(C)** Immunofluorsecence of tropomyosin (Per a 7) in cockroach muscle tissue (from Arruda LK, Vailes L, Ferriani V et al. J Allergy Clin Immunol 2001;107:419–428.)

observations of the numbers of cats in children's homes as a measure of exposure. The amount of cat allergen that accumulates in homes is dependent on furnishings (especially carpets) and air exchange rates, so the number of animals is not a sufficient measure of exposure.

Enzyme-Linked Immunosorbent Assays (ELISA) for Major Allergens

Since the mid-1980s, quantitative assessments of allergen exposure have been made by measuring major allergens in reservoir dust samples (bed, carpet, soft furnishings) using monoclonal antibody (mAb)-based ELISA. ELISA methods have defined specificity, high sensitivity (≈1 ng/mL), and provide accurate and reproducible measurements.[6,27] The ELISA use either pairs of mAbs directed against nonoverlapping epitopes on the allergen molecule or capture mAb and polyclonal rabbit antibody for detection. Robust ELISA tests require high-affinity mAb of defined specificity and standards with known allergen content. ELISA has been the gold standard for indoor allergen exposure assessment for 25 years. A growing number of academic and commercial laboratories in the USA and in Europe offer ELISA testing services. While ELISA provides reliable quantitative exposure assessment, it does require a separate test for each allergen. The associated time and cost involved is an impediment for large studies of exposure assessment and especially for studies involving multiple allergens.

Multiplex Array for Indoor Allergens (MARIA)

Recently, innovative fluorescent multiplex array technology has been developed that allows the most common indoor allergens to be detected at once in a single test.[28] The multiplex array for indoor allergens (MARIA) uses mAb that are covalently bound to polystyrene beads containing different ratios of orange-red fluorescent dyes. Up to 100 dye combinations are available to create different bead sets. Beads coupled with mAb directed against different allergens are incubated with the dust samples and bound allergen is detected using a cocktail of biotinylated detector mAb and streptavidin phycoeryhthrin. Fluorescent intensity is measured using a two channel laser flow cytometer: a red laser identifies beads by their internal color as bearing a specific allergen; a green laser quantifies the intensity of the bound streptavidin-conjugated fluorophore, and measures the amount of allergen bound. In most cases, the same combinations of mAb used in ELISA can be used in MARIA and there is an excellent quantitative correlation between the results for MARIA and ELISA (Table 25-1).[28] The multiplex test occurs within a single microtiter well and the assay conditions are the same for each allergen, resulting in improved standardization and reproducibility. Other advantages of MARIA compared to ELISA are the time savings achieved by analyzing multiple allergens at once, as well as improved sensitivity, accuracy and greater inter-laboratory reproducibility. For allergen exposure assessment, nine indoor allergens can be measured by MARIA: Der p 1, Der f 1,

Table 25-1 Antibody Combinations and xMAP Bead Sets Used in MARIA*

Allergen	Capture Monoclonal Antibody	Biotinylated Antibody	xMAP Bead Set
Der p 1	10B9	5H8	33
Der f 1	6A8	4C1	51
Mite Group 2	1D8	7A1	53
Fel d 1	6F9	3E4	58
Can f 1	10D4	6E9	20
Rat n 1	RUP-6	RUP-1	69
Mus m 1*	Rabbit anti-Mus m 1	Ra anti-Mus m 1	62
Bla g 2	1F3	4C3	47
Alt a 1	121G	121G	28

*The Mus m 1 bead set uses polyclonal antibodies.

mite group 2, Fel d 1, Can f 1, Mus m 1, Rat n 1, Bla g 2, and Alt a 1 (Table 25-1).

Allergen standards are an integral component for calibration of both ELISA and MARIA and enable allergen measurements made by different laboratories to be directly compared.[29,30] In the past, ELISA standards were allergen extracts (not purified allergens) that were calibrated to contain a known amount of allergen by reference to national or international standards, where available. For example, Der p 1 measurements were standardized using the WHO/IUIS international *D. pteronyssinus* reference (NIBSC 82/518) which was estimated to contain 12.5 μg Der p 1 per ampoule.[6] In 2000, the WHO/IUIS Allergen Standardization Committee initiated a project to produce international standards of purified allergens with verifiable allergen content. The project was funded through the European Union as the Certified Reference Materials for Allergenic Products (CREATE) study. The aim was to develop recombinant allergen standards for mite group 1 and group 2 allergens, as well as birch, rye grass, and olive pollen allergens. Purified natural and recombinant allergens were rigorously compared for protein content, structure, allergenic activity and ability to serve as primary standards for immunoassays.[31] Two of the allergens developed in CREATE, Bet v 1 and Phl p 5, are currently being evaluated by the European Directorate for the Quality of Medicines as biological reference materials for inclusion in the European Pharmacopoeia.[31,32] It is anticipated that other allergen standards will be developed through a similar mechanism. The principles of CREATE were used to formulate a single standard of purified natural allergens that could be used for calibration of both ELISA and MARIA.[28,32] The single 'universal' allergen standard contained eight purified allergens whose protein content was determined by amino acid analysis. The standard was compared with previous ELISA standards and conversion factors were developed to enable previous ELISA results to be compared with the current single standard.[32]

'Point-of-Care' Tests

Simple qualitative or semiquantitative tests that can be used in allergy clinics or physicians' offices or by consumers have been developed. The aim of these 'point of care' tests is to provide patients with tests that can be used to monitor allergen levels in their homes and to reinforce education about the role of allergens in causing asthma. The first such test was Acarex, a dipstick that

measures guanine in house dust (a surrogate for dust mites). Lateral flow technology has been used to develop rapid tests that can measure specific allergens in 10 minutes. These tests are analogous to pregnancy or drug tests and are designed for use by patients and other consumers. The mite allergen test uses the same mAb as the mite group 2 ELISA and can detect both *D. pteronyssinus* and *D. farinae*. The test includes a simple dust collection and extraction device that allows dust to be collected and extracted within 2 minutes. The rapid test has indicator lines that provide patients with estimates of high, medium, and low allergen levels and which broadly correlate with group 2 levels determined by ELISA.[33]

Allergen Sampling in Dust and Air

Allergens are typically measured on dust samples that are collected by vacuuming an area of 1 m² for 2 minutes and extracting 100 mg of fine dust in 2 mL of buffer. Samples are usually collected from three or four sites in the home, including mattresses, bedding, bedroom or living room carpet, soft furnishings, or kitchen floors. The results are expressed as nanograms or micrograms of allergen per gram of dust. Measurements of group 1 allergens in bedding provide the best index of mite exposure and show a good correlation between results expressed as micrograms of allergen per gram of dust or per unit area ($\mu g/m^2$).[34] Cat and dog allergens are widely distributed throughout the house and accumulate at clinically significant levels in houses that do not contain pets. Not surprisingly, the highest concentrations of CR allergens are usually found in kitchens, although in heavily infested homes allergen accumulates on flooring and in bedding.

Measurement of allergen levels in dust provides a valid index of exposure but cannot be used to monitor personal exposure. The aerodynamic properties of mite, cat, dog, and CR allergens have been studied using particle sizing devices such as the Cascade impactor and Andersen sampler.[9,35,36] Mite and CR allergens occur on large particles of 10 to 40 μm in diameter and cannot be detected in rooms under undisturbed conditions. After a disturbance, such as using a vacuum cleaner without a filter, these particles remain airborne for about 20 to 40 minutes. In contrast, cat and dog allergens can be easily detected in air samples under undisturbed conditions and persist in the air for several hours.[37] Animal dander particles (skin flakes) are less dense than mite feces, and approximately 25% of animal allergen occurs on smaller particles, 5 μm in diameter, that remain airborne.[9,37]

Clinical Significance of Indoor Allergens

Measurement of indoor allergen levels in reservoir dust and air samples has played a key role in determining risk levels for allergen exposure. Previous International Workshop reports recommended that allergen exposure be expressed as μg allergen/gram dust (or ng/m^3 for air samples).[6] Exposure data collected in epidemiologic studies, population surveys and birth cohort studies has strengthened the association between indoor allergen exposure and allergic respiratory diseases. Prominent studies include the National Inner-City Asthma Studies (ICAS)[13,14] and the National Survey of Lead and Allergens in Housing (NSLAH) in the USA;[38,39] the European Community Respiratory Health Survey (ECRHS);[40,41] and a series of birth cohort studies in the USA, Europe, Australia and New Zealand.[42-46] Childhood asthma is more closely linked to allergic sensitization and allergen exposure than adult asthma. Studies in both inner-city and suburban children with asthma indicated that >80% of school-age children with asthma are sensitized to at least one indoor allergen and that allergic sensitization is a strong predictor of disease persistence in later life.[44,47,48] In the ICAS, 94% of the study population of severe asthmatics was sensitized to at least one allergen and the number of sensitivities correlated with asthma severity.[14] Equally compelling is the recently confirmed observation in the German MAAS cohort that high-level allergen exposure in early life is associated with chronic asthma in children.[44,44,48]

Epidemiologic studies have allowed risks for allergic sensitization to be attributed to certain levels of allergen exposure among different populations of atopic individuals (Table 25-2). Mite allergen levels at high altitude or in 'allergen-free' rooms are generally <0.3 µg/g and <10% of atopic individuals are likely to become sensitized at this low level of mite exposure. Persistent exposure of atopic individuals to ≈2 µg of mite allergen is likely to result in sensitization in a majority of atopic individuals and will increase as mite allergen levels exceed 2 µg/g. Adjusted odds ratios (ORs) for sensitization and exposure to 2 µg/g mite group 1 allergen range from 3 to 6, and in many parts of the world sensitization to mites is the strongest independent risk factor for asthma. A survey of 1054 middle school children in Virginia showed that dust mite sensitization was independently associated with asthma (OR 6.6, $P < 0.0001$) and that dust from 81% of homes contained more than 2 µg/g mite group 1 allergen.[49] A prospective study of 939 German schoolchildren, which followed them up to the age of 7 years, showed a 7-fold difference in sensitization to mites between children exposed to less than 0.03 µg/g mite group 1 (first quartile) compared to those exposed to 1 to 240 µg/g (fourth quartile).[50] This data is consistent with a dose response relationship between exposure and sensitization for mite allergens. Mite allergen exposure levels above 10 µg/g are considered high risk for sensitization and results of NSLAH indicate that these levels are found in ≈23% of US homes (22 million housing units).[39]

Data on cat and dog allergen exposure in relation to sensitization are more difficult to interpret. Exposure to Fel d 1 of <0.5 µg/g is considered to be low and is a low risk for sensitization (Table 25-2).[15] Paradoxically, the prevalence of sensitization can be reduced among atopic individuals who keep cats from birth and are continuously exposed to Fel d 1 levels of >20 µg/g.[51-53] This level of exposure appears to reduce the prevalence of sensitization by ≈50%. High exposure to Fel d 1 (>20 µg/g) gives rise to a modified Th2 response – a form of tolerance that results in a lower prevalence of IgE antibody responses. In contrast, low-dose exposure to Fel d 1 (1 to 8 µg/g) is most strongly associated with the development of IgE antibody. The dose-response studies may explain why, in population surveys, sensitization to cats is often lower than that to dust mites. In countries such as New Zealand, where 78% of the population owns cats and high levels of allergen occur in houses, the prevalence of sensitization to cat is only 10% and cat is not as important a cause of asthma as dust mites.[46]

Most houses that contain cats or dogs have Fel d 1 or Can f 1 levels of greater than 10 µg/g, whereas homes that do not contain these pets may contain 1 to 10 µg/g animal allergen.[8-10] What distinguishes animal allergen exposure from other indoor allergens is the wide range of exposure levels (from <0.5 to >3000 µg/g) and the ubiquitous allergen distribution. Cat and dog allergens occur in schools, offices, workplaces, and public buildings, where they are passively transported by their owners, and they can cause both sensitization and symptoms in these environments. An atopic child who lives at home without a cat can become sensitized by visiting homes or attending schools where cat allergen is present. A Swedish study showed a 9-fold increased risk of asthma exacerbations at school among 6- to 12-year-old children who attended classes with other children who kept cats compared with those in classes with fewer than 18% cat owners.[54] Thus passive exposure of schoolchildren to animal allergens can exacerbate asthma, even among children who are being treated with asthma medications.

CR allergen exposure has been assessed by measuring Bla g 1 and Bla g 2, which cause sensitization in 30% and 60% of CR-allergic patients, respectively.[55] Most dust samples from CR-infested homes contain both allergens, although there is only a modest quantitative correlation between levels of the two allergens. Analysis of Bla g 1 and Bla g 2 levels in the homes of asthma patients admitted to the emergency departments in Atlanta, Georgia, and Wilmington, Delaware, showed that homes with visible evidence of CRs contained more than 8 U/g Bla g 1 and more than 2 U/g (approximately 0.1 µg/g) Bla g 2.[56] In inner-city Baltimore, the proportion of asthmatic children (aged 4 to 9 years) with positive skin tests to CR increased from 32% among children exposed to 1 to 2 U/g Bla g 1 to 45% among children exposed to more than 4 U/g.[47] Multicenter case-control studies carried out among 12- to 13-year-old schoolchildren in Charlottesville, Virginia, and Los Alamos, New Mexico, showed that a 4-fold increase in Bla g 2 exposure (from 0.08 to 0.33 µg/g) was associated with highly significant increases in wheal size of CR skin tests.[15] These studies provide evidence for a dose-response relationship between CR allergen exposure and sensitization. The reported CR allergen levels are several-fold lower than those for either mite or animal allergens, suggesting that CR may be more potent in stimulating IgE responses. The National Cooperative Inner City Asthma Study (NCICAS) showed that sensitization and exposure to CRs (>8 U/g Bla g 1) was associated with increased asthma morbidity. Among inner-city children from

Table 25-2 Allergen Exposure Thresholds for Sensitization

	Allergen Level in Dust Sample				
Risk for Sensitization*	Mite Group 1 (µg/g)	Fel d 1 (µg/g)	Can f 1 (µg/g)	Bla g 1 (U/g)	Bla g 2 (µg/g)
High	>10	1–8	1–8	>8	>1
Medium	2–10	8–20	8–20	1–8	0.08–0.4
Low	<0.3†	<0.5	<0.5	<0.6	<<0.08
		>20	>20?		

*For atopic children.
†Levels found in 'allergen-free' hospital rooms or in houses/apartments maintained for at least 6 months are less than 45% relative humidity.

eight US cities enrolled in the study, 37% were allergic to CRs, and hospitalizations, unscheduled medical visits, and days lost from school due to wheezing or asthma were strongly associated with CR allergen exposure.[13,47] These data have been confirmed in the ICAS study which showed similar correlations between sensitization, CR exposure and asthma morbidity in Bronx, New York and in Dallas.[14] In the USA, high CR allergen levels are associated with lower socioeconomic status, living in inner cities, and race (African-American or Hispanic). Cockroach allergy is not an entirely urban problem. Suburban and rural homes, including trailer homes, that harbor high levels of CRs, cause sensitization and respiratory disease in these populations.

Monitoring Allergen Exposure as Part of Asthma Management

The most recent National Asthma Education and Prevention Program (NAEPP) Expert Panel Report 3 (EPR-3) significantly strengthened guidelines recommending allergen avoidance as an important goal of asthma management (Box 25-2). Targeted interventions in the homes of allergic individuals can significantly improve health and should be part of the management of children with asthma. Studies of inner-city asthma demonstrated that reduction of indoor allergen exposure leads to improvement of asthma symptoms, associated with a reduced use of medication and also a reduction in lost work or school time due to asthma.[57] The guidelines recommend using patient histories and allergic sensitization as evidence of allergen exposure but do not include any environmental assessment. There are several flaws with this approach. Allergen levels in homes vary widely across the USA, depending on climate, geographic location, housing type and condition, and socioeconomic status. The NSLAH publications illustrate that high indoor allergen levels are a potential problem in many homes.[39,58] Conversely, many US homes have low or undetectable allergen levels. For example, Der f 1 levels in Boston, Massachusetts, were 10-fold to 100-fold higher in single-family homes than in centrally heated apartments.[59] Thus marked variations in allergen exposure were demonstrated in a single US city and are related to changes in relative humidity.[59–61] Other observations show that inner-city homes located on the East Coast have lower mite allergen levels than those reported in the urban South.[47,62] Clinically relevant levels of cat allergen are found in homes that do not contain cats and in some schools.

Finally, CR allergen is found in about 20% of homes that have no visible evidence of CR infestation.[56] The significance of these studies is that allergen exposure should not be assumed and that knowledge of allergen levels in the home is needed to provide objective advice about exposure and avoidance.

Allergen measurements have been used to validate the efficacy of a variety of physical and chemical control procedures and devices, including mattress encasings, vacuum cleaner filters, acaricides, protein denaturants, detergents and carpet cleaners, steam cleaning, humidity control and air filtration systems.[63] It is important that products and devices be tested for their effects on specific allergens so that allergists can verify claims made by manufacturers and make evidence-based recommendations.

Despite over 20 years of study supporting a role for allergen avoidance in the treatment of asthma, a recent review from the Nordic Cochrane Centre concluded that extensive US and EU expert panel reports on allergen avoidance were misleading and that reducing dust mite allergen levels was 'ineffective' as a treatment strategy.[64] Earlier meta-analyses by the Cochrane Center were criticized because they included studies that used avoidance protocols that did not result in reduction of allergen levels. In a rebuttal of the most recent Cochrane review, Platts-Mills argued that meta-analysis was compromised in avoidance studies because of the variability in the studies that have been performed and because the Cochrane review was selective about which studies were included in the meta-analysis.[65] Successive Cochrane reviews have failed to take into account that patients are rarely sensitized only to dust mite allergens and one of the most clinically effective avoidance studies involved tailored approaches to allergen control together with comprehensive patient education.[57]

The availability of point-of-care tests for indoor allergens will educate patients about the role of allergens in causing allergic disease. The importance of educating patients so that they can play a leading role in controlling their disease has been emphasized.[63] The objectives of making exposure measurements are to show that in addition to having IgE reactivity to an allergen, the patient may be exposed to the relevant allergen at home. This information is expected to reinforce the link among allergen sensitization, exposure, and disease activity; enable informed decisions to be made about treatment options, and encourage implementation and compliance with intervention procedures.

Conclusions

Indoor allergens are a risk factor for the development of asthma as well as other allergic diseases. The most important indoor allergens have been cloned, sequenced and expressed and over 50 three-dimensional structures of allergens have been resolved. Indoor allergens have diverse biologic functions and may be enzymes, lipid-binding proteins, ligand-binding proteins, structural or regulatory proteins. The biologic function of allergens may enhance IgE responses and play a direct role in causing allergic inflammation. The level of environmental exposure to allergen as well as the atopic predisposition of the individual also influences the development of IgE responses and Th2 responses. Measurement of allergen in reservoir dust samples provides the best index of allergen exposure and can be accurately measured by ELISA for major allergens. A new generation of tests (MARIA) uses fluorescent multiplex array technology and enables multiple allergens to be tested simultaneously in dust or air samples. The MARIA technology is especially suited to large population studies or cohort studies and for routine allergen exposure assessment. The NAEPP-EPR 3 guidelines for the management

---

BOX 25-2 Therapeutic principles

Control of Environmental Factors that Affect Asthma (NAEPP EPR-3)

- For patients who have persistent asthma, the clinician should evaluate the potential role of indoor allergens.
- Use the patient's medical history, skin testing or in vitro testing to identify allergen exposures that may worsen the patient's asthma.
- Patients who have asthma at any level of severity should reduce, if possible, exposure to allergens to which the patient is sensitized and exposed.
- Know that effective allergen avoidance requires a multifaceted, comprehensive approach.
- Consider allergen immunotherapy when there is clear evidence of a relationship between symptoms and exposure to an allergen to which the patient is sensitive.

of asthma recommend that for any patient with persistent asthma, the clinician should (1) identify allergen exposures; (2) use skin testing or in vitro testing to assess specific sensitivities to indoor allergens; and (3) implement environmental controls to reduce exposure to relevant allergens. Avoidance procedures that can help to reduce exposure to indoor allergens have been developed and can reduce symptoms and medication requirements. The combination of improved allergen-monitoring techniques and validated allergen-avoidance procedures should improve asthma management and reduce the public health problems associated with sensitization to indoor allergens.

Acknowledgements

This chapter is dedicated to the memory of Dr Richard Sporik, pediatric allergist and friend, whose premature death in 2008 was a great loss. Richard's seminal studies of the role of indoor allergens in the etiology of childhood asthma are a lasting legacy.

Our work on indoor allergens has been supported by Small Business Innovation Research awards from the National Institute for Environmental Health Sciences (ES011920 and ES55545).

References

1. Kern RA. Dust sensitization in bronchial asthma. Med Clin North Am 1921;5:751–8.
2. Cooke RA. Studies in specific hypersensitiveness. IV. New aetiologic factors in bronchial asthma. J Immunol 1922;7:147–62.
3. van Leeuwen SW. Asthma and tuberculosis in realtion to 'climate allergens'. Br Med J 1927;2:344–7.
4. Berrens L, Young E. Preparation and properties of purified house dust allergen. Nature 1961;190:536–7.
5. Voorhorst R, Spieksma FThM, Leupen MJ. The house dust mite (*Dermatophagoides pteronyssins*) and the allergens it produces. Identity with the house dust allergen. J Allergy 1967;39:325–39.
6. Platts-Mills TA, Vervloet D, Thomas WR, et al. Indoor allergens and asthma: report of the Third International Workshop. J Allergy Clin Immunol 1997;100(6 Pt 1):S2–24.
7. Sporik R, Chapman MD, Platts-Mills TA. House dust mite exposure as a cause of asthma. Clin Exp Allergy 1992;22:897–906.
8. Bollinger ME, Eggleston PA, Flanagan E, et al. Cat antigen in homes with and without cats may induce allergic symptoms. J Allergy Clin Immunol 1996;97:907–14.
9. Custovic A, Green R, Fletcher A, et al. Aerodynamic properties of the major dog allergen Can f 1: distribution in homes, concentration, and particle size of allergen in the air. Am J Respir Crit Care Med 1997;155:94–8.
10. Ingram JM, Sporik R, Rose G, et al. Quantitative assessment of exposure to dog (Can f 1) and cat (Fel d 1) allergens: relation to sensitization and asthma among children living in Los Alamos, New Mexico. J Allergy Clin Immunol 1995;96:449–56.
11. Phipatanakul W, Eggleston PA, Wright EC, et al. Mouse allergen. II. The relationship of mouse allergen exposure to mouse sensitization and asthma morbidity in inner-city children with asthma. J Allergy Clin Immunol 2000;106:1075–80.
12. Matsui EC, Simons E, Rand C, et al. Airborne mouse allergen in the homes of inner-city children with asthma. J Allergy Clin Immunol 2005;115:358–63.
13. Rosenstreich DL, Eggleston P, Kattan M, et al. The role of cockroach allergy and exposure to cockroach allergen in causing morbidity among inner-city children with asthma. N Engl J Med 1997;336:1356–63.
14. Gruchalla RS, Pongracic J, Plaut M, et al. Inner City Asthma Study: relationships among sensitivity, allergen exposure, and asthma morbidity. J Allergy Clin Immunol 2005;115:478–85.
15. Sporik R, Squillace SP, Ingram JM, et al. Mite, cat, and cockroach exposure, allergen sensitisation, and asthma in children: a case-control study of three schools. Thorax 1999;54:675–80.
16. Chapman MD, Pomes A, Breiteneder H, et al. Nomenclature and structural biology of allergens. J Allergy Clin Immunol 2007;119:414–20.
17. Radauer C, Breiteneder H. Pollen allergens are restricted to few protein families and show distinct patterns of species distribution. J Allergy Clin Immunol 2006;117:141–7.
18. Li M, Gustchina A, Alexandratos J, et al. Crystal structure of a dimerized cockroach allergen Bla g 2 complexed with a monoclonal antibody. J Biol Chem 2008;283:22806–14.
19. Chruszcz M, Chapman MD, Vailes LD, et al. Crystal structures of mite allergens Der f 1 and Der p 1 reveal differences in surface-exposed residues that may influence antibody binding. J Mol Biol 2009;386:520–30.
20. Radauer C, Bublin M, Wagner S, et al. Allergens are distributed into few protein families and possess a restricted number of biochemical functions. J Allergy Clin Immunol 2008;121:847–52.
21. Shakib F, Ghaemmaghami AM, Sewell HF. The molecular basis of allergenicity. Trends Immunol 2008;29:633–42.
22. Trompette A, Divanovic S, Visintin A, et al. Allergenicity resulting from functional mimicry of a Toll-like receptor complex protein. Nature 2009;457:585–8.
23. Platts-Mills TA. The role of indoor allergens in chronic allergic disease. J Allergy Clin Immunol 2007;119:297–302.
24. Dickey BF. Exoskeletons and exhalation. N Engl J Med 2007;357:2082–4.
25. Kaiser L, Velickovic TC, Badia-Martinez D, et al. Structural characterization of the tetrameric form of the major cat allergen Fel d 1. J Mol Biol 2007;370:714–27.
26. Gore JC, Schal C. Cockroach allergen biology and mitigation in the indoor environment. Annu Rev Entomol 2007;52:439–63.
27. Chapman MD, Tsay A, Vailes LD. Home allergen monitoring and control–improving clinical practice and patient benefits. Allergy 2001;56:604–10.
28. Earle CD, King EM, Tsay A, et al. High-throughput fluorescent multiplex array for indoor allergen exposure assessment. J Allergy Clin Immunol 2007;119:428–33.
29. Becker WM, Vogel L, Vieths S. Standardization of allergen extracts for immunotherapy: where do we stand? Curr Opin Allergy Clin Immunol 2006;6:470–5.
30. van RR. Indoor allergens: relevance of major allergen measurements and standardization. J Allergy Clin Immunol 2007;119:270–7.
31. van RR, Chapman MD, Ferreira F, et al. The CREATE project: development of certified reference materials for allergenic products and validation of methods for their quantification. Allergy 2008;63:310–26.
32. Chapman MD, Ferreira F, Villalba M, et al. The European Union CREATE Project: a model for international standardization of allergy diagnostics and vaccines. J Allergy Clin Immunol 2008;122:882–889.
33. Tsay A, Williams L, Mitchell EB, et al. A rapid test for detection of mite allergens in homes. Clin Exp Allergy 2002;32:1596–601.
34. Custovic A, Taggart SC, Niven RM, et al. Evaluating exposure to mite allergens. J Allergy Clin Immunol 1995;96:134–5.
35. Luczynska CM, Li Y, Chapman MD, et al. Airborne concentrations and particle size distribution of allergen derived from domestic cats (*Felis domesticus*): measurements using cascade impactor, liquid impinger, and a two-site monoclonal antibody assay for Fel d I. Am Rev Respir Dis 1990;141:361–7.
36. de Blay F, Heymann PW, Chapman MD, et al. Airborne dust mite allergens: comparison of group II allergens with group I mite allergen and cat-allergen Fel d I. J Allergy Clin Immunol 1991;88:919–26.
37. de Blay F, Chapman MD, Platts-Mills TA. Airborne cat allergen (Fel d I). Environmental control with the cat in situ. Am Rev Respir Dis 1991;143:1334–9.
38. Cohn RD, Arbes SJ Jr, Jaramillo R, et al. National prevalence and exposure risk for cockroach allergen in U.S. households. Environ Health Perspect 2006;114:522–6.
39. Arbes SJ Jr, Cohn RD, Yin M, et al. House dust mite allergen in US beds: results from the First National Survey of Lead and Allergens in Housing. J Allergy Clin Immunol 2003;111:408–14.
40. Zock JP, Heinrich J, Jarvis D, et al. Distribution and determinants of house dust mite allergens in Europe: the European Community Respiratory Health Survey II. J Allergy Clin Immunol 2006;118:682–90.
41. Heinrich J, Bedada GB, Zock JP, et al. Cat allergen level: its determinants and relationship to specific IgE to cat across European centers. J Allergy Clin Immunol 2006;118:674–81.
42. Celedon JC, Litonjua AA, Ryan L, et al. Exposure to cat allergen, maternal history of asthma, and wheezing in first 5 years of life. Lancet 2002;360:781–2.
43. Woodcock A, Lowe LA, Murray CS, et al. Early life environmental control: effect on symptoms, sensitization, and lung function at age 3 years. Am J Respir Crit Care Med 2004;170:433–9.
44. Illi S, von ME, Lau S, et al. Perennial allergen sensitisation early in life and chronic asthma in children: a birth cohort study. Lancet 2006;368:763–70.
45. Almqvist C, Egmar AC, Hedlin G, et al. Direct and indirect exposure to pets–risk of sensitization and asthma at 4 years in a birth cohort. Clin Exp Allergy 2003;33:1190–7.
46. Sears MR, Greene JM, Willan AR, et al. A longitudinal, population-based, cohort study of childhood asthma followed to adulthood. N Engl J Med 2003;349:1414–22.
47. Eggleston PA, Rosenstreich D, Lynn H, et al. Relationship of indoor allergen exposure to skin test sensitivity in inner-city children with asthma. J Allergy Clin Immunol 1998;102(4 Pt 1):563–70.

48. Sporik R, Holgate ST, Platts-Mills TA, et al. Exposure to house-dust mite allergen (Der p I) and the development of asthma in childhood. A prospective study. N Engl J Med 1990;323:502–7.

49. Squillace SP, Sporik RB, Rakes G, et al. Sensitization to dust mites as a dominant risk factor for asthma among adolescents living in central Virginia: multiple regression analysis of a population-based study. Am J Respir Crit Care Med 1997;156:1760–4.

50. Lau S, Illi S, Sommerfeld C, et al. Early exposure to house-dust mite and cat allergens and development of childhood asthma: a cohort study. Multicentre Allergy Study Group. Lancet 2000;356:1392–7.

51. Platts-Mills T, Vaughan J, Squillace S, et al. Sensitisation, asthma, and a modified Th2 response in children exposed to cat allergen: a population-based cross-sectional study. Lancet 2001;357:752–6.

52. Ownby DR, Johnson CC, Peterson EL. Exposure to dogs and cats in the first year of life and risk of allergic sensitization at 6 to 7 years of age. JAMA 2002;288:963–72.

53. Custovic A, Hallam CL, Simpson BM, et al. Decreased prevalence of sensitization to cats with high exposure to cat allergen. J Allergy Clin Immunol 2001;108:537–9.

54. Almqvist C, Wickman M, Perfetti L, et al. Worsening of asthma in children allergic to cats, after indirect exposure to cat at school. Am J Respir Crit Care Med 2001;163(3 Pt 1):694–8.

55. Satinover SM, Reefer AJ, Pomes A, et al. Specific IgE and IgG antibody-binding patterns to recombinant cockroach allergens. J Allergy Clin Immunol 2005;115:803–9.

56. Gelber LE, Seltzer LH, Bouzoukis JK, et al. Sensitization and exposure to indoor allergens as risk factors for asthma among patients presenting to hospital. Am Rev Respir Dis 1993;147:573–8.

57. Morgan WJ, Crain EF, Gruchalla RS, et al. Results of a home-based environmental intervention among urban children with asthma. N Engl J Med 2004;351:1068–80.

58. Salo PM, Arbes SJ Jr, Crockett PW, et al. Exposure to multiple indoor allergens in US homes and its relationship to asthma. J Allergy Clin Immunol 2008;121:678–84.

59. Chew GL, Higgins KM, Gold DR, et al. Monthly measurements of indoor allergens and the influence of housing type in a northeastern US city. Allergy 1999;54:1058–66.

60. Chew FT, Yi FC, Chua KY, et al. Allergenic differences between the domestic mites *Blomia tropicalis* and *Dermatophagoides pteronyssinus*. Clin Exp Allergy 1999;29:982–8.

61. Arlian LG, Neal JS, Morgan MS, et al. Reducing relative humidity is a practical way to control dust mites and their allergens in homes in temperate climates. J Allergy Clin Immunol 2001;107:99–104.

62. Miller RL, Chew GL, Bell CA, et al. Prenatal exposure, maternal sensitization, and sensitization in utero to indoor allergens in an inner-city cohort. Am J Respir Crit Care Med 2001;164:995–1001.

63. Platts-Mills TA. Allergen avoidance. J Allergy Clin Immunol 2004;113:388–91.

64. Gotzsche PC, Johansen HK. House dust mite control measures for asthma: systematic review. Allergy 2008;63:646–59.

65. Platts-Mills TA. Allergen avoidance in the treatment of asthma: problems with the meta-analyses. J Allergy Clin Immunol 2008;122:694–6.

26

Environmental Control

Robert A. Wood

There is no doubt that aeroallergens play a major role in the pathogenesis of allergic disease, including asthma, allergic rhinitis, and atopic dermatitis. Among these, the indoor allergens are of particular importance. These principally include the allergens of house dust mites, domestic pets, molds, and pests such as cockroaches and rodents. The relative importance of these different allergens varies in different environments depending on a variety of geographic, climatic, and socioeconomic factors. All studies agree, however, that children with asthma have a high likelihood of becoming sensitized to whichever of these allergens are prominent in their local environments. This chapter focuses on the possible role that allergen avoidance may play in the management of allergic disease.

As a general concept, it is important to recognize that allergen avoidance should be based on knowledge of the patient's specific allergic sensitivities as well as their environemental exposures. Based on this information, it is important to recommend a comprehensive strategy to reduce exposure to as many relevant allergens as possible. In fact, most of the studies in which environmental control has been proven effective are those that utilize a multi-faceted approach tailored to the patient's sensitivities and enviroronment,[1,2] which requires both thoughtful consideration and detailed patient education.

Dust Mites

Dust mites are arachnids that live in the dust that accumulates in most homes, particularly the dust contained within fabrics. Favorite habitats include carpets, upholstered furniture, mattresses, pillows, and bedding materials. Their major food source is shed human skin scales, which are present in high numbers in most of these items. The major dust mite species known to be associated with allergic disease are *Dermatophagoides pteronyssinus* and *Dermatophagoides farinae*.[3-5] Other mites, including *Euroglyphus maynei* and *Blomia tropicalis* are also important in some areas, although their distribution is considerably more limited. Dust mites grow optimally in areas that are both warm and humid, and they grow very poorly when the relative humidity remains below 40%.[6] Dust mites grow from eggs to adults over the course of about 4 weeks and adult dust mites live for about 6 weeks, during which time females produce 40 to 80 eggs.[7]

Assessment of dust mite exposure has been accomplished largely through the analysis of settled dust samples. Although some studies have not been able to show a relationship between dust mite levels and allergic sensitization or disease activity,

there is now general agreement that dust mite levels of greater than 2 μg of group 1 allergen per gram of dust should be considered a risk factor for sensitization and that levels greater than 10 μg/g of dust are a risk factor for acute asthma.[5,7-11] Airborne sampling for dust mite allergen has proven difficult or impossible.[12]

The prevalence of dust mite sensitivity in asthmatic patients varies considerably from one geographic area to another. For example, studies have demonstrated prevalence rates ranging from 5% in asthmatic children in Los Alamos, New Mexico, to 66% in Atlanta, Georgia, to 91% in Papua, New Guinea.[13,14] These differences are roughly proportional to differences in mite exposure in these areas of the world.

At least as significant as the relationship between mite exposure and mite sensitization is the evidence that mite exposure contributes not just to sensitization but to the asthmatic state itself. In a prospective trial, Sporik and colleagues[10] demonstrated a significant increase in asthma, as well as mite sensitivity, in 11-year-old children who had experienced high mite exposure during infancy. Other studies have demonstrated a striking association between asthma development and mite sensitivity,[13,15-17] although these studies lacked a prospective evaluation of mite exposure. While these studies suggest that allergen avoidance early in life could prevent the development of asthma in some patients, studies of prevention have yielded inconsistent results.[18,19]

Extensive evidence also exists to support a relationship between ongoing mite exposure and disease activity.[20-23] With regard to chronic symptoms, Vervloet and colleagues[22] demonstrated a significant correlation between medication requirements and current mite exposure in a group of mite-sensitive adult asthma patients. Custovic and colleagues[20] also demonstrated a relationship between mite exposure and asthma severity as evidenced by bronchial hyperreactivity (BHR), peak expiratory flow rate variability, and forced expiratory volume in 1 second (FEV$_1$). Several studies have also demonstrated mite exposure to be a risk factor for acute asthma and emergency room visits.[11,23] In a study by Call and colleagues,[11] inner-city children in Atlanta were evaluated after presentation to the emergency room with acute asthma. Of these children, 72% were found to be allergic to either dust mite alone or both dust mite and cockroach allergen. The combination of mite exposure and mite sensitization was highly associated with the development of acute asthma.

The most compelling evidence for the role of dust mites in asthma comes from studies of allergen avoidance, either through

©2010 Elsevier Ltd, Inc, BV
DOI: 10.1016/B978-1-4377-0271-2.00026-2

environmental control in the home or the removal of mite-allergic patients from their homes. Two classic studies from the early 1980s provided dramatic evidence for the potential benefits of dust mite avoidance. Platts-Mills and colleagues[24] investigated the effects of mite avoidance by placing nine young adults with mite-induced asthma in a hospital setting for a minimum of 2 months. All patients experienced reduced symptoms, seven patients had reduced medication requirements, and five patients showed at least an 8-fold reduction in bronchial reactivity as measured by the concentration of histamine required to induce a 30% fall in FEV_1. In the second study Murray and Ferguson[25] studied 20 mite-allergic asthmatic children in a controlled trial of mite avoidance in the patients' homes. They found significant reductions in asthma symptoms, days on which wheezing was observed, days with low peak flow rates, and BHR in the group using active mite control measures.

Most subsequent trials of mite avoidance have yielded similar results.[26-30] Ehnert and colleagues[28] studied 24 children with asthma and mite sensitivity in a 1-year trial of mite avoidance. The patients were divided into three groups. The first had their mattresses, pillows, and comforters covered with impermeable encasements; the second had their mattresses and carpets treated with an acaricide (benzyl benzoate); and the third had their mattresses and carpets treated with placebo. Significant reductions in dust mite allergen levels were found only in the group with mattress and pillow encasements. Similarly, a highly significant reduction in BHR was noted in that group compared with the other two. In another study, Peroni and colleagues[30] performed an extensive clinical study of mite avoidance by moving asthmatic children to a high-altitude environment and demonstrated significant reductions in total immunoglobulin E (IgE) levels, dust mite-specific IgE levels, methacholine reactivity, and response to dust mite bronchoprovocation.

However, it is also important to recognize that there have also been several important negative studies of mite avoidance, especially when using single intervention such as bedding encasements.[31-33] In one, Woodcock and colleagues studied the efficacy of impermeable bed covers in over 1100 adults with asthma and dust mite sensitivity.[32] While the impermeable covers resulted in significant decreases in mite allergen in mattress dust, asthma symptoms were not significantly reduced. These studies again point to the need for a comprehensive allergen reduction plan rather than relying on single interventions.

Dust Mite Control Measures

A variety of approaches to dust mite control have been utilized and there is, in fact, still some controversy as to the specific measures that are necessary to sufficiently reduce mite exposure to control disease. This controversy arises for three major reasons. First, some environmental control measures have not been adequately studied to make any firm conclusions. Second, for some measures, studies of their efficacy have yielded conflicting results. Third, in many studies a combination of environmental control measures was used, making it difficult to determine which measures actually led to the benefit that was observed. Specific environmental control measures will therefore be reviewed individually and then summarized in Box 26-1.

It is very clear that allergen-proof encasements for mattresses and pillows significantly reduce dust mite exposure.[28,34-36] In the study by Ehnert and colleagues,[28] polyurethane mattress encasements produced a 91% decrease in mite allergen by day 14 of treatment, which rose to 98% by month 12 of the study. Encasements of the mattress, pillows, and box springs should therefore

---

BOX 26-1

Environmental Control of House Dust Mites

First Line (Necessary and Cost Effective)

Replace mattress and pillow encasements

Wash bed linen every 1 to 2 weeks, preferably in hot water

Remove stuffed toys

Regularly vacuum carpeted surfaces

Regularly dust hard surfaces

Reduce indoor relative humidity (dehumidify and do not add humidity)

Second Line (Helpful but More Expensive)

Remove carpets, especially in the bedroom

Remove upholstered furniture

Avoid living in basements

Third Line (Limited or Unproven Benefit)

Acaricides

Tannic acid

Air cleaners

---

be recommended for all patients with mite sensitivity. In addition, although encasements had been constructed of impermeable plastic or vinyl materials that were very uncomfortable, they are now also available in tightly woven fabrics that are considerably more comfortable.[36]

The effects of vacuum cleaning on mite exposure have been studied. Live mites are difficult to remove from carpeting, and it is clear that vacuum cleaning in the absence of other measures will provide only limited benefit. However, regular vacuum cleaning does remove significant amounts of dust from carpets, which will at least help to reduce the allergen reservoir. Patients should also be warned that vacuuming creates considerable disturbance, with transient increases in airborne mite levels. Vacuum cleaners equipped with special bags or HEPA filters help prevent this problem and may be of some added benefit.[37] There is some evidence that wet vacuum cleaning or steam cleaning may provide additional benefit,[38,39] although one study showed that wet vacuum cleaning led to a subsequent increase in mite numbers.[40]

A variety of carpet treatments have also been developed in an effort to control dust mite allergen exposure. At this time, one acaricide, benzyl benzoate, and one denaturing agent, tannic acid, are available in the USA. Although there is little doubt that benzyl benzoate is effective in killing dust mites, studies regarding the efficacy of this compound in home environments have provided only modest, short-lived effects.[27,41,42]

Tannic acid is designed to reduce allergen levels by denaturing allergenic proteins but it does not affect dust mite growth or allergen production. It has also been shown in the laboratory to be highly effective but its efficacy in home environments not convincing.[43] Because of the limitations of both vacuuming and chemically treating carpets, carpet removal is always best when feasible, especially from the bedroom of the allergic person. Bed linens, stuffed animals, and other soft furnishings also provide excellent environments for dust mite growth. Objects such as stuffed animals should be removed whenever possible. The mite content of bedding materials and other objects that cannot be removed can be reduced by washing. Washing in hot water (greater than 55°C) is ideal in that it both removes allergen and kills dust mites.[44] These water temperatures, however, may not be available in many homes due to safety concerns. It is important to note, therefore, that washing in cooler water does not kill mites but does remove most live mites as well as mite allergens very effectively. Weekly washing of all bed linens in a hot cycle is therefore recommended for all mite-allergic patients. Dry cleaning also kills dust mites,[44,45] as does tumble drying at temperatures greater than 55°C for at least 20 minutes.[34]

Dust mites are susceptible to the effects of low as well as high temperatures. Freezing in a typical household freezer for 24 hours will kill most dust mites, although the mite allergen in the object will not necessarily be reduced.[46] Exposing carpets to direct sunlight for several hours will also kill dust mites because of the high temperature, the low humidity, or both.[47] It has also been shown that electric blankets will reduce mite growth.[48] None of these methods have been established in clinical trials.

Because of the reliance of dust mites on humidity for growth, it has been suggested that methods capable of reducing relative humidity would be useful in the control of mite exposure. Korsgaard and Iversen[49] demonstrated that dust mite growth could be significantly reduced by keeping indoor humidity below 7 g/kg by ventilation, whereas Arlian[50] demonstrated that mite growth could be prevented by maintaining relative humidity below 35% for at least 22 hours a day. Air conditioning and dehumidification may also help to deter mite growth and should be used whenever possible, and humidifiers should be avoided.[51] It is clear, however, that achieving low humidity will be difficult or impossible in very humid environments. A prime example of this fact is the difficulty in eliminating dust mites from carpets over cement slab floors in basements.

Finally, air filtration devices are frequently purchased by patients for the control of their dust mite allergies; however, there is little evidence to support their use.[52-55] One would logically not anticipate much effect because of the fact that dust mite allergens do not remain airborne for extended periods and would therefore not be available for filtration in most instances.

In summary, effective dust mite control can be accomplished in most homes with a combination of mattress and pillow covers, hot washing of bed linens, removal of stuffed animals and other soft furnishings, and carpet removal. In the absence of carpet removal, intense vacuum cleaning and the use of acaricides and denaturing agents may have some benefit. Because of the convincing benefits provided through dust mite avoidance in mite-sensitive asthmatic patients, these measures should be routinely recommended, and compliance with these recommendations should be reassessed at each subsequent visit.

Animal Allergens

Animal allergens are also potent causes of both acute and chronic asthma symptoms.[56] Cat and dog allergens are the most important, although significant exposure to a wide variety of other furred animals is not uncommon. Sensitivity to cat and dog allergens has been shown to occur in up to 67% of asthmatic children, and in some settings these are clearly the dominant indoor allergens.[14,57,58] This fact was best demonstrated in a study conducted in Los Alamos, New Mexico.[14] In this environment, where cat and dog allergens are common but exposure to dust mite and cockroach allergens is rare, IgE antibody to cat and dog allergens was detected in 62% and 67% of asthmatic children, respectively. The presence of this IgE antibody was highly associated with

asthma, whereas sensitivity to mite or cockroach allergen was not associated with asthma.

A number of studies have investigated the distribution of cat and dog allergens in the home and other environments.[14,58-61] Using settled dust analysis, it has been shown that levels of cat and dog allergens are clearly highest in homes housing these animals. However, it is also clear from a number of studies that the vast majority of homes contain cat and dog allergen even if a pet has never lived there. This widespread distribution of cat and dog allergens has also been documented in a variety of other settings, including office buildings and schools. Whereas most of the environments with no animals have relatively low allergen levels compared to those with a cat or dog, it is not uncommon to find rather high levels in some of these homes. This widespread distribution is presumed to occur primarily through passive transfer of allergen from one environment to another. The particles carrying animal allergens appear to be very sticky and, unlike dust mite allergens, can be found in high levels on walls and other surfaces within homes.[62]

The characteristics of airborne cat allergen have also been extensively studied. Cat allergen has been shown to be carried on particles that range from less than 1 μ to greater than 20 μ in mean aerodynamic diameter.[63,64] Although estimates have varied, studies agree that at least 15% of airborne cat allergen is carried on particles less than 5 μ. Less information is available for dog allergen, but evidence to date suggests that it is distributed very much like cat allergen, with about 20% of airborne dog allergen being carried on particles less than 5 μ in diameter.[65]

Cat allergen can also be detected in air samples from all homes with cats and from many homes without cats.[66] In an attempt to determine the clinical significance of this unsuspected cat exposure, patients were challenged in an experimental cat exposure facility to varying levels of cat allergen. It was found that allergen levels of less than 100 ng/m^3 were capable of inducing upper and lower respiratory symptoms as well as significant pulmonary function changes. These levels are similar to those found in homes with cats as well as a subset of homes without cats, suggesting that even patients without known cat exposure may be exposed to clinically significant concentrations of airborne cat allergen on a regular basis.

Control of Animal Allergens

At the present time much less is known about the control of animal allergens than about the control of dust mite allergens.[56] In particular, there are still no convincing studies on the clinical benefit of environmental control measures for animal allergens. Although it is assumed that removing an animal from the home will lead to clinical improvement in patients who have disease related to their pets, this has not been proven. Even less data is available regarding the potential benefits of methods that might be used in lieu of animal removal. Cat allergen will be specifically discussed here because the most information is available regarding this important allergen. Most of the information should be applicable to other allergens, and the overall approach to the control of animal allergens is summarized in Box 26-2.

To begin, it should be stated that in any asthmatic patient who is known to be cat or dog sensitive and whose asthma is believed to be related to a significant degree to the pet, the most appropriate recommendation is to remove the pet from the home. This is clearly the correct advice from a medical standpoint, and it should be recommended strenuously. A number of potential alternative measures will also be discussed, however, because of the high proportion of patients who are either reluctant or completely unwilling to remove a household pet.

Once a cat has been removed from the home, it is important to recognize that the clinical benefit may not be seen for a period of at least several months because allergen levels fall quite slowly after cat removal.[61] In most homes, levels in settled dust will have fallen to those seen in homes without cats within 4 to 6 months of cat removal. Levels may fall much more quickly if extensive environmental control measures are undertaken, such as removal of carpets, upholstered furniture, and other reservoirs from the home, whereas in other homes the process may be considerably slower. This information points to the fact that thorough and repeated cleaning will be required once the animal has been removed. It has also been shown that cat allergen may persist in mattresses for years after a cat has been removed from a home,[67] so new bedding or impermeable encasements must therefore also be recommended.

A number of studies have investigated other measures that might help to reduce cat allergen exposure without removing the animal from the home. De Blay and colleagues[68] demonstrated significant reductions in airborne Fel d 1 with a combination of air filtration, cat washing, vacuum cleaning, and removal of furnishings, although these results were based on a small sample size and did not include any measure of clinical effect. When cat washing was evaluated separately in that study, dramatic reductions in airborne Fel d 1 were seen afterward. Subsequent studies, however, have presented conflicting results. Klucka and colleagues[69] studied both cat washing and Allerpet/c (Allerpet, Inc., New York, New York) and found no benefit from either treatment. More recently, Avner and colleagues[70] studied three different methods of cat washing and found transient reductions in airborne cat allergens after each. There was no sustained benefit, however, with levels returning to baseline within 1 week of washing.

Information is very limited as to the clinical benefits of these environmental control measures if one or more cats is allowed to remain in the home. Four studies have evaluated different combinations of control measures, and although all have shown reductions in allergen levels, clinical effect was less consistent.[71-74] Two studies showed a clear benefit, one showed benefit only in the group in which environmental control was done along with intranasal steroid treatment, and the fourth showed

no clinical benefit whatsoever. It therefore still remains to be seen whether allergen exposure can be sufficiently reduced to produce a clinical effect in the absence of animal removal.

In families who insist on keeping their pets, the following should be recommended pending more definitive studies.[56] The animals should be restricted to one area of the home and certainly kept out of the patient's bedroom. HEPA or electrostatic air cleaners should be used, especially in the patient's bedroom. Carpets and other reservoirs for allergen collection should be removed whenever possible, again focusing on the patient's bedroom. Finally, mattress and pillow covers should be routinely used. Although tannic acid has been shown to reduce cat allergen levels, the effects are modest and short-lived when a cat is present, so this treatment should not be routinely recommended. Similarly, cat washing appears to be of such transient benefit that it is only likely to add significantly to the other avoidance measures if it is done at least twice a week.

Cockroach Allergen

The importance of cockroach allergen in asthma and allergy has been recognized only over the past 30 years. It is now clear that cockroach allergens play a major role in asthma, particularly in urban areas.[75] Significant cockroach exposure has been demonstrated in a number of cities, and the prevalence of cockroach sensitivity in urban patients with asthma has been shown to range from 23 to 60%.[9,76,77] In addition, cockroach exposure has been associated with higher rates of sensitization.[78] The combination of cockroach exposure and cockroach sensitization has been shown to be a risk factor for increased asthma morbidity and acute asthma exacerbations.[11,23,59]

In the first comprehensive study on the problem of asthma in inner-city children, 1528 children with asthma from eight major inner-city areas were extensively investigated with regard to the factors, both allergic and otherwise, that contributed to their disease.[59] Although sensitivity to cockroaches, dust mites, and cats were all common (36.8%, 36.9%, and 22.7%, respectively), exposure to cockroach allergen was much more common than exposure to either dust mite or cat (50.2%, 9.7%, and 12.8%, respectively). The combination of cockroach sensitivity and high cockroach exposure was associated with significantly more hospitalizations, unscheduled medical visits for asthma, days of wheezing, missed days from school, and nights with sleep loss because of asthma. Such a correlation was not seen for dust mite or cat allergens. These data argue persuasively that cockroach allergen is a major factor, if not *the* major factor, in the high degree of morbidity seen in this patient population.

Although there are at least 50 cockroach species in the USA, only four or five are domiciliary.[75] Two species, the German cockroach (*Blatella germanica*), and the American cockroach (*Periplaneta americana*), are the most common causes of both household infestation and allergic sensitization. Several allergens from each species have been identified and characterized.[79,80] The most important among these are Bla g 1, Bla g 2, and Per a 1. There is significant cross reactivity between *B. germanica* and *P. americana*, although most patients in the USA are primarily sensitized to *B. germanica*. The source of the major cockroach allergens is still not completely clear, although they do appear to be secreted or excreted, suggesting that they may also be digestive proteins.

The distribution of cockroach allergens has been studied in a number of settings. The highest levels tend to be found in kitchens, although the allergen is widely distributed through the home, including the bedroom.[59,77,80] In fact, in the inner-city asthma study noted above, the 50.2% exposure rate was found in bedroom dust samples.[59] It has been suggested that cockroach allergen levels of greater than 2 units per gram are associated with sensitization and levels greater than 8 units per gram are associated with disease activity.[59] Cockroach allergen has also been detected at significant concentrations in schools in urban Baltimore.[81] Finally, studies have shown that cockroach allergen is very much like dust mite allergen, with little or no measurable airborne allergen in the absence of significant disturbance.[75]

Cockroach Allergen Control

Extensive study has been performed on the chemical control of cockroach infestation, and a variety of pesticides and traps are readily available. These include chlorpyrifos, diazanon, boric acid powder, and bait stations that contain hydranethylon. All of these agents, with the exception of boric acid, can reduce cockroach numbers by 90% or more, whereas boric acid reduces numbers by 40% to 50%. Several studies have shown that cockroach extermination is possible in most homes and that a combination of extermination and thorough cleaning can reduce cockroach allergen levels by 80% to 90%,[82-84] although studies to date have not convincingly demonstrated that cockroach eradication alone is capable of significantly reducing disease activity.[85-87]

Other measures that should help to reduce cockroach infestation include eliminating food sources and hiding and entry points (Box 26-3). All foods should be stored in sealed containers and the kitchen should be cleaned regularly. Finally, extensive cleaning should be performed after extermination to remove the cockroach debris as completely as possible. Even with the most aggressive measures, however, it may be difficult to adequately reduce cockroach exposure in some environments. This is particularly true of the older, multiple dwelling units that house a preponderance of inner-city residents. It may be necessary to exterminate in the homes or apartments surrounding the patient's home to obtain maximum effect, and some patients may need to find new housing altogether.

A more encouraging study related to inner-city asthma did demonstrate a convincing benefit from a multifaceted, allergen specific environmental control program in asthmatic children living in urban areas.[1] In that study, cockroach extermination was part of a global environmental treatment that also included education, a HEPA filtered vacuum cleaner, allergen-proof bedding encasings, and a HEPA filter in the child's bedroom.

Bla g 1 in floor dust was reduced by 53% compared to 19% in the control group but more importantly, symptoms were also significantly reduced in the treated group. This trial once again supports the concept that global environmental avoidance strategies have the highest likelihood of produce beneficial clinical effects.

Rodent Allergens

Mice and rats produce allergens, which are primarily urinary proteins, that have been shown to cause sensitization and disease in both occupational and home environments.[88-91] The widespread distribution of mouse allergen in home environments and its potential importance in asthma, especially in those living in inner cities, has recently been demonstrated in a number of studies. In fact, mouse allergens are measurable in nearly all inner-city homes and as many as 75% of suburban homes.[91-93] However, the levels in the inner-city homes are far higher, in fact, 100 to 1000-fold higher in comparison to suburban homes.[94] With regard to effects on disease, mouse exposure in infancy has been associated with the development of asthma[95] and in older children with increased sensitization, poorer asthma control, and increased health-care utilization.[90,96,97] Even in adults, sensitization to mouse allergens has been shown to be associated with asthma and asthma morbidity.[98]

To date, there has been relatively little study of environmental control for the mouse, although Phipatanakul and colleagues did demonstrate reduced allergen exposure using an integrated pest management strategy.[99] Based on this study, and general information about pest management, recommendations for mouse allergen control include professional extermination, thorough cleaning after extermination, keeping food and trash in covered containers, cleaning food scraps from the floor and countertops, and sealing cracks in the walls, doors, and floors (Box 26-4).[100]

Mold Allergens

A wide variety of mold species can be present in both indoor and outdoor environments. *Aspergillus* and *Penicillium* species are generally regarded as the most numerous indoor molds,[60,101] whereas *Alternaria* is important in both indoor and outdoor environments. Several mold allergens, including Alt n 1 and Asp f 1, have been identified and characterized. Mold exposure has been associated with chronic asthma symptoms and as well as with asthma exacerbations.[101-103]

Molds tend to grow best in warm, moist environments and mold exposure is therefore roughly correlated with these conditions. Basements, window sills, shower stalls, and bathroom carpets are common sites of mold infestation. Air conditioners and humidifiers have also been shown to be sources of significant mold exposure.[104,105] The assessment of mold exposure

---

BOX 26-3

Environmental Control of Cockroach Allergen

Regular and thorough extermination

Thorough cleaning after extermination

Extermination of neighboring dwellings

Roach traps

Repair leaky faucets and pipes

Repair holes in walls and other entry points

Behavioral changes to reduce food sources

    Clean immediately after cooking

    Clean dirty dishes immediately

    Avoid open food containers

    Avoid uncovered trash cans

BOX 26-4

Environmental Control of Rodent Allergens

Regular and thorough extermination

Thorough cleaning after extermination

Keep food and trash in covered containers

Seal cracks in walls, door, and floors

has been improved by the development of immunoassays to measure major allergens, although for most molds one must still rely on culture and microscopic examination of air or dust samples. Airborne mold allergens have been shown to be carried on particles ranging in size from less than 2 μ to greater than 100 μ.[101]

The control of mold allergens requires a concerted approach combining fungicides, measures to reduce humidity, and the removal of mold-infested items whenever possible[101] (Box 26-5). With more severe infestation such as after flooding has occurred, professional remediation may be required.[106] A variety of fungicides are commercially available that are highly effective as long as the sites of mold growth are carefully investigated. Any measures that can then be taken to reduce humidity should be recommended, including dehumidification, air-conditioning, increased ventilation, and a ban on the use of humidifiers and vaporizers. Moldy items, such as a basement carpet that has suffered water damage, should be removed altogether. Although no specific data are available, air filtration devices may also assist in reducing mold exposure; no clinical studies on the efficacy of mold avoidance measures have been undertaken.

Indoor Air Pollution

Although a detailed discussion of indoor air pollution is beyond the scope of this chapter, it should be emphasized that effective environmental control cannot be achieved without attention to a variety nonspecific irritants. The deleterious effects of passive cigarette smoke on pediatric asthma have been well documented in a number of studies.[107,108] No studies to date have assessed the clinical benefit of removal from a smoke-containing environment, but one would predict that this would have highly beneficial effects. In addition to passive cigarette smoke, a variety of other indoor pollutants, such as nitrous oxide, have been documented to exacerbate pediatric asthma, especially in inner-city environments.[109,110] All patients must therefore be queried about these exposures and counseled about their control. Parents who are smokers and who have asthmatic children need to be reminded at each visit about the ongoing damage that they are causing.

Outdoor Allergens

There is far less ability to control exposure to outdoor allergens than indoor allergens. Source control is rarely an option because the airborne pollens and molds travel so widely. Local mold control may be accomplished by ensuring good drainage, removing leaves and other debris as they accumulate, and limiting the use of mulch and other ground cover that might support mold growth. Otherwise, exposure may be reduced by staying indoors when pollen and mold counts are high, as long as windows and doors are kept closed. An air filter may help to reduce exposure, especially if windows are being left open; some activities, such as lawn mowing or plowing, may need to be avoided altogether. After being outside, it is important that allergic individuals wash their hands and faces immediately and that they wash their hair daily. When outside, masks and goggles can be very effective but there are very few children and adolescents willing to wear them.

Conclusions

Indoor allergens are of tremendous importance to pediatric allergic disease (Box 26-6). Exposure is a risk factor for the development of asthma as well as for more severe disease. Thankfully, there are measures that can help to reduce exposure to most allergens, which can significantly reduce symptoms and medication requirements. The guidelines for the management of asthma that were originally published in 1997 and most recently revised in 2007[111] have consistently stressed the importance of indoor allergens and environmental control, stating that for any patient with persistent asthma, the clinician should (1) identify allergen exposures; (2) use skin testing or in vitro testing to assess specific sensitivities to indoor allergens; and (3) implement environmental controls to reduce exposure to relevant allergens. With all the time, effort, and money put forth for the use of medications and immunotherapy for asthma and allergic rhinitis, it is very important that we do not lose sight of this logical and important recommendation.

Helpful Websites

Allergy & Asthma Network Mothers of Asthmatics (www.breatherville.org)

The American Academy of Allergy, Asthma and Immunology website (www.aaaai.org/)

The American College of Allergy, Asthma and Immunology website (www.acaai.org/)

The Asthma and Allergy Foundation of America website (www.aafa.org/)

American Lung Association (www.lungusa.org)

Association of Asthma Educators (www.asthmaeducators.org)

Asthma and Allergy Foundation of America (www.aafa.org)

Centers for Disease Control and Prevention (www.cdc.gov)

National Heart, Lung, and Blood Institute Information Center (www.nhlbi.nih.gov)

U.S. Environmental Protection Agency National Center for Environmental Publications (www.airnow.gov)

References

1. Morgan WJ, Crain EF, Gruchalla RS, et al. Results of a home-based environmental intervention among urban children with asthma. N Engl J Med. 2004;351:1068–73.

2. van Schayck OC, Maas T, Kaper J, et al. Is there any role for allergen avoidance in the primary prevention of childhood asthma? J Allergy Clin Immunol. 2007;119:1323–30.

3. Platts-Mills TAE, De Weck A. Dust mite allergens and asthma—a worldwide problem. Bull WHO. 1989;66:769–80.

4. Platts-Mills TAE, Thomas WR, Aalberse RC, et al. Dust mite allergens and asthma: report of a second international workshop. J Allergy Clin Immunol. 1992;89:1046–60.

5. Arlian LG, Platts-Mills TAE. The biology of dust mites and the remediation of mite allergens in allergic disease. J Allergy Clin Immunol. 2001;107: S406-13.

6. Arlian LG. Biology and ecology of house dust mites Dermatophagoides spp. and Euroglyphus spp. Immunol Allergy Clin North Am. 1989;9:339–56.

7. Kueher J, Frischer J, Meiner R, et al. Mite exposure is a risk factor for the incidence of specific sensitization. J Allergy Clin Immunol. 1994;94:44–52.

8. Lau S, Falkenhorst G, Weber A, et al. High mite-allergen exposure increases the risk of sensitization in atopic children and young adults. J Allergy Clin Immunol. 1989;84:718–25.

9. Peat JK, Tovey E, Mellis CM, et al. Importance of house dust mite and Alternaria allergens in childhood asthma: an epidemiological study in two climatic regions of Australia. Clin Exp Allergy. 1993;23: 812–20.

10. Sporik R, Holgate ST, Platts-Mills TAE, et al. Exposure to house-dust mite allergen (Der p I) and the development of asthma in childhood: a prospective study. N Engl J Med. 1990;323:502–7.

11. Call RS, Smith TF, Morris E, et al. Risk factors for asthma in inner-city children. J Pediatr. 1992;121:862–6.

12. Platts-Mills TAE, Heymann PW, Longbottom JL, et al. Airborne allergens associated with asthma: particle sizes carrying dust mite and rat allergens measured with a cascade impactor. J Allergy Clin Immunol. 1986;77:850–7.

13. Dowse GK, Turner KJ, Stewart GA, et al. The association between Dermatophagoides mites and the increasing prevalence of asthma in village communities within the Papua New Guinea highlands. J Allergy Clin Immunol. 1985;75:75–83.

14. Ingram JM, Sporik R, Rose G, et al. Quantitative assessment of exposure to dog (Can f 1) and cat (Fel d 1) allergens: relationship to sensitization and asthma among children living in Los Alamos, New Mexico. J Allergy Clin Immunol. 1995;96:449–56.

15. Burrows B, Sears MR, Flannery EM, et al. Relations of bronchial responsiveness to allergy skin test reactivity, lung function, respiratory symptoms and diagnoses in thirteen-year-old New Zealand children. J Allergy Clin Immunol. 1995;95:548–56.

16. Peat JK, Tovey ER, Toelle BG, et al. House-dust mite allergens: a major risk factor for childhood asthma in Australia. Am J Respir Crit Care Med. 1996;153:141–6.

17. Sears MR, Herbison GP, Holdaway MD, et al. The relative risk of sensitivity to grass pollen, house dust mite, and cat dander in the development of childhood asthma. Clin Exp Allergy. 1989;19: 419–24.

18. Hide DW, Matthews S, Tariq S, et al. Allergen avoidance in infancy and allergy at 4 years of age. Allergy. 1996;51:89–93.

19. Marinho S, Simpson A, Custovic A. Allergen avoidance in the secondary and tertiary prevention of allergic diseases: does it work? Prim Care Respir J. 2006;15:152–8.

20. Custovic A, Taggart SCO, Francis HC, et al. Exposure to house dust mite allergens and the clinical activity of asthma. J Allergy Clin Immunol. 1996;98:64–72.

21. Kivity S, Solomon A, Soferman R, et al. Mite asthma in childhood: a study of the relationship between exposure to house dust mites and disease activity. J Allergy Clin Immunol. 1993;91:844–9.

22. Vervloet D, Charpin D, Haddi E, et al. Medication requirements and house dust mite exposure in mite-sensitive asthmatics. Allergy. 1991;46:554–8.

23. Pollart SM, Chapman MD, Fiocco GP, et al. Epidemiology of acute asthma: IgE antibodies to common inhalant allergens as a risk factor for emergency room visits. J Allergy Clin Immunol. 1989;83: 875–82.

24. Platts-Mills TAE, Tovey ER, Mitchell EB, et al. Reduction of bronchial hyperreactivity following prolonged allergen avoidance. Lancet. 1982;ii: 675–8.

25. Murray AB, Ferguson AC. Dust-free bedrooms in the treatment of asthmatic children with house dust or house dust mite allergy. Pediatrics. 1983;71:418–22.

26. Carswell F, Birmingham K, Weeks J, et al. The respiratory effects of reduction of mite allergen in bedrooms of asthmatic children: a double-blind controlled trial. Clin Exp Allergy. 1996;26:386–96.

27. Dietemann A, Bessot JC, Hoyet C, et al. A double-blind, placebo-controlled trial of solidified benzyl benzoate applied in dwellings of asthmatic patients sensitive to mites: clinical efficacy and effect on mite allergens. J Allergy Clin Immunol. 1993;91:738–46.

28. Ehnert B, Lau-Schadendorf S, Weber A, et al. Reducing domestic exposure to dust mite allergen reduces bronchial hyperreactivity in sensitive children with asthma. J Allergy Clin Immunol. 1992;90: 135–8.

29. Gillies DRN, Littlewood JM, Sarsfield JK. Controlled trial of house dust mite avoidance in children with mild to moderate asthma. Clin Allergy. 1987;105–11.

30. Peroni DG, Boner AL, Vallone G, et al. Effective allergen avoidance at high-altitude reduced allergen-induced bronchial hyerresponsiveness. Am J Resp Crit Care Med. 1994;149:1442–6.

31. de Vries MP, van den Bemt L, Aretz K, et al. House dust mite allergen avoidance and self-management in allergic patients with asthma: randomised controlled trial. Br J Gen Pract. 2007;57:184–89.

32. Woodcock A, Forster L, Matthews E, et al. Control of exposure to mite allergen and allergen-impermeable bed covers for adults with asthma. N Engl J Med. 2003;349:225–30.

33. Terreehorst I, Hak E, Oosting AJ, et al. Evaluation of impermeable covers for bedding in patients with allergic rhinitis. N Engl J Med. 2003;349: 237–41.

34. Owen S, Morganstern M, Hepworth J, et al. Control of house dust mite antigen in bedding. Lancet. 1990;335:396–7.

35. Tovey E, Marks G, Shearer M, et al. Allergens and occlusive bed covers. Lancet. 1993;342:126.

36. Miller JD, Naccara L, Satinover S, et al. Nonwoven in contrast to woven mattress encasings accumulate mite and cat allergen. J Allergy Clin Immunol. 2007;120:977–82.

37. Kalra S, Owen SJ, Hepworth J, et al. Airborne house dust mite antigen after vacuum cleaning. Lancet. 1990;336:449.

38. de Bohr R. The control of house dust mite allergens in rugs. J Allergy Clin Immunol. 1990;86:808–14.

39. Htut T, Higenbottam TW, Gill GW, et al. Eradication of house dust mite from homes of atopic asthmatic subjects: a double-blind trial. J Allergy Clin Immunol. 2001;107:55–60.

40. Wassenaar DP. Effectiveness of vacuum cleaning and wet cleaning in reducing house-dust mites, fungi and mite allergen in a cotton carpet: a case study. Exp Appl Acarol. 1988;4:53–62.

41. Lau-Schadendorf S, Rusche AF, Weber AK, et al. Short-term effect of solidified benzyl benzoate on mite-allergen concentrations in house dust. J Allergy Clin Immunol. 1991;87:41–7.

42. Woodfolk JA, Hayden ML, Couture N, et al. Chemical treatment of carpets to remove allergen. J Allergy Clin Immunol. 1996;96:325–33.

43. Woodfolk J, Hayden M, Miller J, et al. Chemical treatment of carpets to reduce allergen: a detailed study of the effects of tannic acid on indoor allergens. J Allergy Clin Immunol. 1994;94:19–26.

44. McDonald LG, Tovey ER. The role of water temperature and laundry procedures in reducing house dust mite populations and allergen content of bedding. J Allergy Clin Immunol. 1992;90:599–608.

45. Vendenhove T, Soler M, Birnbaum J, et al. Effect of dry cleaning on the mite allergen levels in blankets. Allergy. 1993;48:264–6.

46. Dodin A, Rak H. Influence of low temperature on the different stages of the human allergy mite Dermatophagoides pteronyssinus. J Med Entomol. 1993;30:810–1.

47. Tovey E, Woolcock A. Direct exposure of carpets to sunlight can kill all mites. J Allergy Clin Immunol. 1993;93:1072–4.

48. Mosbech H, Korsgaard J, Lind P. Control of house dust mites by electrical heating blankets. J Allergy Clin Immunol. 1988;81:706–10.

49. Korsgaard J, Iversen M. Epidemiology of house dust mite allergy. Allergy. 1991;46:14–8.

50. Arlian LG, Neal JS, Vyszenski-Moher HL. Reducing humidity to control the house dust mite Dermatophagoides farinae. J Allergy Clin Immunol. 1999;104:852–6.

51. Custovic A, Taggart S, Kennaugh J, et al. Portable dehumidifiers in the control of house dust mites and mite allergens. Clin Exp Allergy. 1995;25:312–6.

52. Antonicelli L, Bilo MB, Pucci S, et al. Efficacy of an air-cleaning device equipped with a high-efficiency particulate air filter in house dust mite respiratory allergy. Allergy. 1991;46:594–600.

53. Nelson HS, Roger Hirsch S, Ohman JL Jr, et al. Recommendations for the use of residential air-cleaning devices in the treatment of respiratory diseases. J Allergy Clin Immunol. 1988;82:661–9.

54. Reisman R, Mauriello P, Davis G, et al. A double-blind study of the effectiveness of a high-efficiency particulate air (HEPA) filter in the treatment of patients with perennial allergic rhinitis and asthma. J Allergy Clin Immunol. 1990;85:1050–9.

55. Warner JA, Marchant JL, Warner JO. Double-blind trial of ionisers in children with asthma sensitive to the house dust mite. Thorax. 1993;48:330–3.

56. Chapman MD, Wood RA. The role and remediation of animal allergens in allergic diseases. J Allergy Clin Immunol. 2001;107:S414-21.

57. Sporik R, Ingram JM, Price W, et al. Association of asthma with serum IgE and skin test reactivity to allergens among children living at high altitude: tickling the dragon's breath. Am J Respir Crit Care Med. 1995;151:1388–92.

58. Munir AKM, Bjorksten B, Einarsson R, et al. Cat (Fel d I), dog (Can f 1) and cockroach allergens in homes of asthmatic children from three climatic zones in Sweden. Allergy. 1994;49:508–16.

59. Rosenstreich DL, Eggleston P, Kattan M, et al. The role of cockroach allergy and exposure to cockroach allergen in causing morbidity among inner-city children with asthma. N Engl J Med. 1997;336:1356–63.

60. Wood RA, Eggleston PA, Ingemann L, et al. Antigenic analysis of household dust samples. Am Rev Resp Dis. 1988;137:358–63.

61. Wood RA, Chapman MD, Adkinson NF, et al. The effect of cat removal on allergen content in household dust samples. J Allergy Clin Immunol. 1989;83:730–4.

62. Wood RA, Mudd KE, Eggleston PA. The distribution of cat and dust mite allergens on wall surfaces. J Allergy Clin Immunol. 1992;89:126–30.

63. Wood RA, Laheri AN, Eggleston PA. The aerodynamic characteristics of cat allergen. Clin Exp Allergy. 1993;23:733–9.

64. Luczynska CM, Li Y, Chapman MD, et al. Airborne concentrations and particle size distribution of allergen derived from domestic cats (Felis domesticus). Am Rev Respir Dis. 1990;141:361–7.

65. Custovic A, Green R, Pickering CAC, et al. Major dog allergen Can f 1: distribution in homes, airborne levels, and particle sizing (abstract). J Allergy Clin Immunol. 1996;97:302.

66. Bollinger ME, Eggleston PA, Wood RA. Cat antigen in homes with and without cats may induce allergic symptoms. J Allergy Clin Immunol. 1996;97:907–14.

67. Van der Brempt X, Charpin D, Haddi E, et al. Cat removal and Fel d 1 levels in mattresses. J Allergy Clin Immunol. 1991;87:595–6.

68. De Blay F, Chapman MD, Platts-Mills TAE. Airborne cat allergen (Fel d 1): environmental control with the cat in situ. Am Rev Respir Dis. 1991;143:1334–9.

69. Klucka CV, Ownby DR, Green J, et al. Cat shedding of Fel d 1 is not reduced by washings, Allerpet-C spray, or acepromazine. J Allergy Clin Immunol. 1995;95:1164–71.

70. Avner DB, Perzanowski MS, Platts-Mills TAE, et al. Evaluation of different techniques for washing cats: quantitation of allergen removed from the cat and effect on airborne Fel d 1. J Allergy Clin Immunol. 1997;100:357–62.

71. Bjornsdottir US, Jakobinudottir S, Runarsdottir V, et al. Environmental control with cat in situ reduces cat allergen in house dust samples but does it alter clinical symptoms? J Allergy Clin Immunol. 1997;99:S389.

72. Soldatov D, De Blay F, Greiss P, et al. Effects of environmental control measures on patient status and airborne Fel d 1 levels with a cat in sit. J Allergy Clin Immunol. 1995;95:263.

73. Wood RA, Johnson EF, Van Natta ML, et al. A placebo-controlled trial of a HEPA air cleaner in the treatment of cat allergy. Am J Resp Crit Care Med. 1998;158:115–20.

74. Van der Heide S, van Aalderen WMC, Kaufmann HF, et al. Clinical effects of air cleaners in homes of allergic children sensitized to pet allergens. J Allergy Clin Immunol. 1999;104:447–51.

75. Eggleston PA, Arruda LK. Ecology and elimination of cockroaches and allergens in the home. J Allergy Clin Immunol. 2001;107:S422–9.

76. Kang BC, Johnson J, Veres-Thorner C. Atopic profile of inner-city asthma with a comparative analysis on the cockroach-sensitive and ragweed-sensitive subgroups. J Allergy Clin Immunol. 1993;92:802–11.

77. Sarpong SB, Hamilton RG, Eggleston PA, et al. Socioeconomic status and race as risk factors for cockroach allergen exposure and sensitization in children with asthma. J Allergy Clin Immunol. 1996;97:1393–401.

78. Gruchalla RS, Pongracic J, Plaut M, et al. Inner city asthma study: relationships among sensitivity, allergen exposure and asthma morbidity. J Allergy Clin Immunol. 2005;115:478–85.

79. Arruda LK, Vailes LD, Mann BJ, et al. Molecular cloning of a major cockroach (Blattella germanica) allergen, Bla g 2. J Biol Chem. 1995;270:19563–8.

80. Pollart S, Smith TF, Morris EC, et al. Environmental exposure to cockroach allergens: analysis with monoclonal antibody-based enzyme immunoassays. J Allergy Clin Immunol. 1995;87:505–10.

81. Sarpong S, Wood RA, Karrison T, et al. Cockroach allergen (Bla g 1) in school dust. J Allergy Clin Immunol. 1997;99:486–92.

82. Sarpong SB, Wood RA, Eggleston PA. Short-term effects of extermination and cleaning on cockroach allergen Bla g 2 in settled dust. Ann Allergy Asthma Immunol. 1996;76:257–60.

83. Eggleston PA, Wood RA, Rand C, et al. Removal of cockroach allergen from inner-city homes. J Allergy Clin Immunol. 1999;104:842–6.

84. Wood RA, Eggleston PA, Rand C, et al. Cockroach allergen abatement with sodium hypochlorite in inner-city homes. Annals Allergy. 2001;87:60–4.

85. Sever ML, Arbes SJ Jr, Gore JC, et al. Cockroach allergen reduction by cockroach control alone in low-income urban homes: a randomized control trial. J Allergy Clin Immunol. 2007;120:849–55.

86. Gergen PJ, Mortimer KM, Eggleston PA, et al. Results of the National Cooperative Inner-City Asthma Study (NCICAS) environmental intervention to reduce cockroach allergen exposure in inner-city homes. J Allergy Clin Immunol. 1999;103:501–7.

87. Carter MC, Perzanowski MS, Raymond A, et al. Home intervention in the treatment of asthma among inner-city children. J Allergy Clin Immunol. 2001;108:732–37.

88. Matsui EC, Diette GB, Krop EJ, et al. Mouse allergen-specific immunoglobulin G4 and risk of mouse skin test sensitivity. Clin Exp Allergy. 2006;36:1097–103.

89. Eggleston PA, Ansari AA, Ziemann B, et al. Occupational challenge studies with laboratory workers allergic to rats. J Allergy Clin Immunol. 1990;86:63–70.

90. Phipatanakul W, Eggleston PA, Wright EC, et al. Mouse allergen. II. The relationship of mouse allergen exposure to mouse sensitization and asthma morbidity in inner-city children with asthma. J Allergy Clin Immunol. 2000;106:1075–80.

91. Matsui EC, Simons E, Rand C, et al. Airborne mouse allergen in the homes of inner-city children with asthma. J Allergy Clin Immunol. 2005;115:358–63.

92. Matsui EC, Eggleston PA, Breysse P, et al. Mouse allergen levels vary over time in inner-city homes. J Allergy Clin Immunol. 2007;120:956–9.

93. Chew GL, Perzanowski MS, Miller RL, et al. Distribution and determinants of mouse allergen exposure in low-income New York City apartments. Environ Health Perspect. 2003;111:1348–52.

94. Simons E, Curtin-Brosnan J, Buckley T, et al. Indoor environmental differences between inner city and suburban homes of children with asthma. J Urban Health. 2007;84:577–90.

95. Phipatanakul W, Celedon JC, Sredl DL, et al. Mouse exposure and wheeze in the first year of life. Ann Allergy Asthma Immunol. 2005;94:593–7.

96. Matsui EC, Eggleston PA, Buckley TJ, et al. Household mouse allergen exposure and asthma morbidity in inner-city preschool children. Ann Allergy Asthma Immunol. 2006;97:514–18.

97. Matsui EC, Eggleston PA, Breysse PN, et al. Mouse allergen-specific antibody responses in inner-city children with asthma. J Allergy Clin Immunol. 2007;119:910–5.

98. Phipatanakul W, Litonjua AA, Platts-Mills TA, et al. Sensitization to mouse allergen and asthma and asthma morbidity among women in Boston. J Allergy Clin Immunol. 2007;120:954–8.

99. Phipatanakul W, Cronin B, Wood RA, et al. Effect of environmental intervention on mouse allergen levels in homes of inner-city Boston children with asthma. Ann Allergy Asthma Immunol. 2004;92:420–4.

100. Sharma HP, Hansel NN, Matsui E, et al. Indoor environmental influences on children's asthma. Pediatr Clin North Am. 2007;54:103–20.

101. Bush RK, Portnoy JM. The role and abatement of fungal allergens in allergic diseases. J Allergy Clin Immunol. 2001;107:S430-40.

102. Halonen M, Stern D, Wright AL, et al. Alternaria as a major allergen for asthma in children raised in a desert environment. Am J Respir Crit Care Med. 1997;155:1356–61.

103. Bush RK, Portnoy JM, Saxon A, et al. The medical effects of mold exposure. J Allergy Clin Immunol. 2006;117:326–33.

104. Burge HA, Solomon W, Boise JR. Microbial prevalence in domestic humidifiers. Appl Environ Microbiol. 1980;39:840–4.

105. Kumar P, Lopez M, Fan W, et al. Mold contamination of automobile air conditioner systems. Annals Allergy. 1990;64:174–7.

106. Barnes CS, Dowling P, Van Osdol T, et al. Comparison of indoor fungal spore levels before and after professional home remediation. Ann Allergy Asthma Immunol. 2007;98:262–8.

107. Chilmonczyk BA, Salmun LM, Megathlin KN, et al. Association between exposure to environmental tobacco smoke and exacerbations of asthma in children. N Engl J Med. 1993;328:1665–9.

108. Cook DG, Strachan DP. Health effects of passive smoking. Thorax. 1999;54:357–66.

109. Matsui EC, Hansel NN, McCormack MC, et al. Asthma in the inner city and the indoor environment. Immunol Allergy Clin North Am. 2008;28:665–8.

110. Hansel NN, Breysse PN, McCormack MC, et al. A longitudinal study of indoor nitrogen dioxide levels and respiratory symptoms in inner-city children with asthma. Environ Health Perspect. 2008;116:1428–32.

111. National Asthma Education and Prevention Program. Expert panel report III: Guidelines for the diagnosis and management of asthma. Bethesda, MD: National Heart, Lung, and Blood Institute, 2007. (NIH publication no. 08–4051). Full text available online: www.nhlbi.nih.gov/guidelines/asthma/asthgdln.htm.

Immunotherapy for Allergic Disease

Elizabeth C. Matsui • Peyton A. Eggleston

In 1911, Noon[1] found that by administering increasing doses of grass pollen extract, he could induce a marked decrease in conjunctival sensitivity to grass pollen. It was this observation that eventually led to the widespread use of immunotherapy for the treatment of allergic disease.[1] *Immunotherapy* is the term used to describe a prolonged process of repeated administration of extracts of pollens or other allergen sources to patients with diseases with a demonstrable allergic etiology for the purpose of reducing symptoms. It has also been called *desensitization* or *allergy injection therapy.* It is recommended in most discussions of the treatment of allergic airway disease, along with allergen avoidance and symptomatic drug therapy.

Principles of Immunotherapy

In allergic rhinitis (AR), the effectiveness of immunotherapy has been demonstrated in many carefully conducted placebo-controlled trials. The results of a typical clinical trial are shown in Figure 27-1.[2] Three groups of patients matched on the basis of their allergic sensitivity to ragweed allergen were treated with injections of whole ragweed pollen extracts, purified Antigen E (Amb a 1) or placebo. Although everyone became symptomatic during the ragweed pollen season, it is obvious that those receiving placebo injections were more symptomatic than those receiving pollen extracts. These trials have been reviewed in detail elsewhere[3,4] and are addressed here only to review the principles learned for the safe and effective use of immunotherapy.

The first principle is that clinical effectiveness is dose dependent; that is, a certain minimal dose of allergen extract must be administered to produce effective symptomatic control.[5] These extracts are prepared by suspending source material (pollen, fungal cultures, dust mites, or animal pelts) in buffers to extract the water-soluble components into the buffer, and they are now available commercially under license by the Food and Drug Administration. Extracts are complex mixtures of dozens of proteins, of which only a few are major allergens. Clinical trials that compare treatment with purified allergens or with partially purified extracts containing high concentrations of allergens with treatment with currently available crude extracts have shown them to be equally effective. For instance, symptoms are reduced to a similar extent with immunotherapy with purified ragweed allergen Amb a 1 and with whole ragweed extract in the study illustrated in Figure 27-1.

Another lesson from these studies is that therapeutic effectiveness increases with time. Significant improvement is generally not seen before 3 months or more of therapy.[6] It is not clear why

such a long time is needed, but in part it reflects the time required to increase the injected dose from the very small dose that can be tolerated initially to the 10000-fold higher dose that produces immunologic and clinical effects. Clinical benefit increases for several years after the maximal doses of antigens are achieved. Although the reason for the delayed effect of immunotherapy is not clear, it is important to discuss with patients so that their expectations will be realistic.

In clinical trials when symptom scores are compared with those in untreated patients, a placebo effect is seen consistently. This placebo effect is especially easy to see in the asthma trials in which most placebo-treated patients improve and 25–30% improve significantly.[6] For clinical investigators, this fact has made it absolutely essential to include a placebo group in any immunotherapy trial. For clinicians, it is important to recognize that there is a significant and powerful placebo effect associated with the repeated injections and frequent visits with sympathetic physicians and nurses. Only by administering concentrated antigen preparations to carefully selected patients are the benefits greater than those seen with sympathetic support.

For most patients, symptomatic improvement is partial and immunotherapy serves to decrease the severity of symptoms without totally eliminating them. In addition, a significant number of allergic patients, perhaps as many as 25% do not benefit from immunotherapy regardless of the potency of the antigen or the length of therapy. The reasons why certain patients are 'nonresponders' are unclear, but the point is an important one to bear in mind when discussing immunotherapy with patients.

In clinical trials, systemic anaphylactic reactions are common. Although these are usually mild and not life threatening, they may require epinephrine therapy and may be fatal. Such reactions are not surprising because patients are selected who are clearly allergic on the basis of skin tests and/or specific immunoglobulin E (IgE) tests and history of severe symptoms on allergen exposure. Although the patient population in clinical trials is more highly sensitive than that encountered in most clinical practices, even in a large clinical series, 7% of patients experienced at least one systemic reaction, most of which were mild and responded to a single injection of epinephrine.[7] Therapy with newer, modified antigens is associated with fewer systemic reactions, but they still occur.

Research in immunotherapy continues in several directions. Standardization of allergen extracts to make available products with consistent potency has dramatically increased the reliability of commercially available extracts. Studies have demonstrated the safety and efficacy of shortening the dose escalation phase

©2010 Elsevier Ltd, Inc, BV
DOI: 10.1016/B978-1-4377-0271-2.00027-4

with schedules for rush and ultrarush immunotherapy.[4] Investigators have also been studying adjuvants to improve efficacy of immunotherapy as well as modified allergens to reduce the risk of serious reactions to immunotherapy. Other routes of administering allergen extracts are also being studied, as well as the use of immunotherapy for other allergic diseases such as food allergy. Finally, therapies targeted at immune mediators are currently in clinical trials; these include agents such as anti-IgE and anticytokine therapies. All of these new directions are addressed in further detail in this chapter.

Mechanisms of Action

Many observations about patients' immunologic and cellular responses to immunotherapy have been made, but the precise

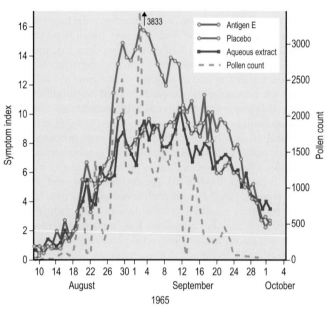

FIGURE 27-1 Typical result of an immunotherapy trial in patients allergic to ragweed pollen. (From Norman PS, Winkenwerder WL, Lichtenstein LM, et al: J Allergy Clin Immunol 1968;42:93–108.)

mechanism of action of immunotherapy remains unknown. What is generally recognized is that skin test sensitivity decreases and allergen-specific IgG increases with immunotherapy.[8] It is not until after several years of immunotherapy that allergen-specific IgE decreases.[9] There has also been much speculation that immunotherapy acts on the T helper cell type 1 (Th1)/Th2 axis to shift the T cell phenotype away from the allergic Th2 phenotype. More recently, some evidence has emerged to suggest that immunotherapy may promote regulatory T cells which may play a role in attenuating allergic symptoms.[10]

Antibody Response and Immunotherapy

Studies have consistently demonstrated an increase in allergen-specific IgG and IgE within months of starting immunotherapy. One trial of ragweed immunotherapy in adults that examined allergen-specific antibody responses can be seen in Figure 27-2. Within months of starting immunotherapy, subjects demonstrated significant dose-dependent increases in ragweed-specific IgG long before symptom relief was seen. Ragweed-specific IgE initially increased and did not decrease until years into therapy.[9] Similar observations have been made by other investigators for both venom immunotherapy and inhalant allergen immunotherapy. It has been suggested that allergen-specific IgG acts as blocking antibody either by blocking antigen binding by IgE or by preventing aggregation of the high-affinity IgE receptor (FcERI) at the cell surface. To further confound the issue, the allergen-specific IgG response does not correlate with clinical efficacy, leaving many questions unanswered about its role in the clinical effectiveness of immunotherapy.[10,11]

Effects on T Cells

Because a Th2 phenotype has been associated with allergic disease and a Th1 phenotype with protection against allergic disease, it has been hypothesized that immunotherapy exerts its effects through modulation of the T helper phenotype. This modulation may result in either a shift from the Th2 to Th1 phenotype or through induction of CD8[+] suppressor activity. Indeed, evidence has been published in support of both of these hypotheses. Rocklin and colleagues[12] demonstrated the genera-

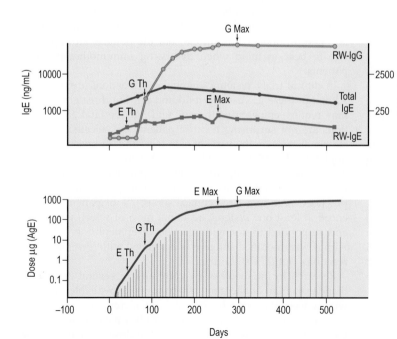

FIGURE 27-2 A profile of a typical patient receiving ragweed immunotherapy. (**Top**) Ragweed-specific IgE (*RW-IgE*), IgG (*RW-IgG*), and total IgE responses during ragweed immunotherapy plotted against time expressed in days. E Th: Threshold dose for ragweed-specific IgE response; G Th: Threshold dose for ragweed-specific IgG response; E Max: maximum ragweed-specific IgE; G Max: maximum ragweed-specific IgE. (**Bottom**) Cumulative dose (*curve*) and single doses (*lines*) plotted against time expressed in days. (From Creticos PS, Van Metre TE, Mardiney MR, et al. J Allergy Clin Immunol 1984;73:94–104.)

tion of allergen-specific suppressor cells during immunotherapy and provided evidence that the suppressor cells decrease IgE synthesis. Other studies have examined the cytokine profile of peripheral blood Th2 cells and demonstrated decreases in interleukin (IL)-4 production and, in some cases, concomitant increases in interferon (IFN)-γ production,[13] suggesting a modulation of the T helper phenotype from Th2 to Th1. The mechanism of these changes has recently advanced with the recognition of CD4+CD25+ regulatory T cells that are capable of directing the Th1:Th2 balance and are activated by effective immunotherapy.[10]

Effects on Inflammatory Cells

There also is evidence that immunotherapy affects mast cells, basophils, and eosinophils. One study demonstrated a significant decrease in metachromatic cells (mast cells and basophils) in nasal scrapings after dust mite immunotherapy.[14] Ragweed immunotherapy has also been demonstrated to decrease peripheral blood basophil histamine release.[13] In addition, successful immunotherapy has been associated with a decrease in the numbers of eosinophils from nasal and bronchial specimens.[15-17]

Specific Disease Indications

Although immunotherapy has been demonstrated to be effective for stinging insect hypersensitivity, AR, and allergic asthma, appropriate patient selection is imperative. In the case of stinging insect hypersensitivity, children with a history of a life-threatening reaction combined with evidence of venom-specific IgE warrant treatment with immunotherapy. Immunotherapy should be considered for the treatment of AR in those patients with evidence of clinically relevant allergen-specific IgE, significant symptoms despite reasonable avoidance measures (e.g., dust mite allergen-proof mattress and pillow covers), and maximal medical therapy. Although similar criteria apply to patients with asthma, poorly controlled asthma is a contraindication for immunotherapy because of the risk of severe systemic reactions for these patients.

Allergic Rhinitis

Immunotherapy has been demonstrated to be quite effective in both seasonal and perennial AR. Many well-designed studies have examined the efficacy of immunotherapy for pollen-allergic patients with seasonal AR.[18-20] These randomized, controlled trials have recently been the subject of a meta-analysis which demonstrated significant symptom relief and reduction of medication requirements.[21] Immunotherapy has also been shown to be effective for mite-induced perennial AR[22] and may also be effective in mold-induced rhinitis.[23] The duration of treatment is generally 3 to 5 years, and symptomatic improvement continues for years after discontinuation.

Asthma

Many studies in the past decade have examined the efficacy of immunotherapy for allergic asthma.[8,24-26] Certainly, allergic sensitization and subsequent allergen exposure contribute significantly to asthma morbidity in children, making immunotherapy an appealing option for children with allergic asthma. However, IgE-mediated mechanisms are only part of the underlying pathophysiology of asthma, making the rationale for immunotherapy as a treatment option in allergic asthma less straightforward.

Results of clinical trials examining the efficacy of immunotherapy in allergic asthma have been conflicting. To complicate matters further, many studies have not included placebo arms, making it difficult to draw any conclusions about efficacy from those studies. Abramson and colleagues[27] conducted a meta-analysis of randomized, controlled trials for immunotherapy in asthma. Twenty trials met inclusion criteria of being double blind, randomized, and placebo-controlled. After analysis of the combined results from these trials, immunotherapy was found to reduce bronchial hyperreactivity and medication use and to improve asthma symptoms. The results were similar when the dust mite trials were analyzed separately. The effects of immunotherapy on pulmonary function were less pronounced.

A comprehensive review also concluded that immunotherapy is effective in the treatment of asthma but in carefully selected circumstances.[28] The authors concluded that immunotherapy is effective in grass pollen asthma but that results from studies for ragweed asthma were inconclusive. In addition, mite immunotherapy with standardized extracts was effective in reducing symptoms and increasing the threshold dose of mite extract needed to induce bronchial obstruction in bronchial challenges. The authors also make the point that children receiving mite immunotherapy benefited to a greater extent than adults.

Immunotherapy for animal-induced asthma has been more controversial. Some proponents of immunotherapy believe that there is a role for animal immunotherapy in the treatment of asthmatic patients who live with pets, but consensus statements from respected international organizations maintain that allergen avoidance is first-line therapy for these patients.[3] There have been carefully conducted, placebo-controlled trials demonstrating the efficacy of specific immunotherapy for cat asthma.[25] Studies have demonstrated a decrease in the quantitative airway responsiveness to cat allergen and decreased skin test reactivity in those treated with cat immunotherapy, but studies examining improvement in clinical symptoms have been inconclusive.

Clinical trials evaluating mold immunotherapy for asthma have been published for *Alternaria* and *Cladosporium*. One of the *Cladosporium* trials was conducted in children and demonstrated a decrease in allergen sensitivity on inhalation challenge, but did not provide good evidence of a decrease in symptoms or medication use.[23] Some studies evaluating *Alternaria* immunotherapy have demonstrated an improvement in asthma symptoms and a decrease in medication use. Although there is evidence to support the addition of certain mold extracts to an immunotherapy prescription, more data are needed before any firm conclusions can be made about immunotherapy in mold asthma.

Although many studies support a role for immunotherapy in the treatment of allergic asthma, there have been some studies that have not demonstrated the efficacy of immunotherapy for asthma. One of these was a well-conducted, placebo-controlled trial of immunotherapy for children with allergic asthma, and the investigators found little evidence to support the efficacy of immunotherapy.[8] One hundred and twenty-one children with moderate to severe asthma were randomly assigned to receive either polyvalent immunotherapy (i.e. a mixture of extracts of various allergens) or placebo. Both groups demonstrated statistically significant improvements in medication use and PD_{20} FEV_1. The improvement seen in the treatment group was not statistically significantly better than that seen in the placebo group. Despite the negative results of this well-conducted study, many other published studies have demonstrated the efficacy of immunotherapy for allergic asthma. One of the major differences in this trial is that multiple allergen extracts were included in the injections. Although this is the usual approach to immunotherapy for allergic asthma in the USA, European standards require therapy with a single allergen extract (e.g. dust mite, cat, *Alternaria*), and this trial is the only one dealing with polyvalent immunotherapy. It is possible that this approach differs in some important way from immunotherapy with single-allergen extracts.

Stinging Insect

Immunotherapy for venom allergy is highly efficacious, affording protection for more than 95% of individuals undergoing treatment.[29] Although venom immunotherapy is indicated in adults with evidence of IgE to Hymenoptera venom and a history of a systemic reaction to Hymenoptera, the indications in children are somewhat different. Studies of the natural history of venom allergy in children indicate that the risk of a serious reaction from a subsequent sting for a child with a history of a cutaneous systemic reaction is small. There is an approximately 10% incidence of subsequent systemic reactions in this patient population and a 0.4% incidence of more severe reactions involving the respiratory and cardiovascular systems.[30] In light of these findings, venom immunotherapy has been reserved for those children who have had 'life-threatening' reactions to Hymenoptera as well as evidence of IgE to Hymenoptera venom[31] (see also Chapter 60).

Food

Although immunotherapy is not a recommended treatment for food allergy, this treatment option is being actively investigated. One randomized trial of subcutaneous immunotherapy for peanut allergy demonstrated increased tolerance to peanut allergen, but the incidence of systemic reactions to the peanut immunotherapy was substantial.[32] The six patients receiving immunotherapy experienced a mean of 34.7 systemic reactions and required a mean of 9.8 epinephrine injections. A recent clinical trial of oral immunotherapy in cow's milk allergy was encouraging.[33] Over 4 months of therapy, 12 children randomized to active treatment were able to tolerate 2 to 8 grams of milk protein compared to 0.04 grams in controls. Almost half of the oral immunotherapy doses induced reactions, but these were usually mild and local.

Practical Considerations

Patient Selection

Allergic Rhinitis

Immunotherapy should be considered for patients with clear evidence of IgE-mediated symptoms who have not been adequately controlled with first-line medical therapy, including antihistamines, nasal corticosteroids, and ocular antihistamines or antiinflammatory medications. Other aspects of the patient's history should be taken into consideration. For example, successful immunotherapy requires that a patient be able to visit a physician's office weekly and spend a minimum of 30 minutes there. Certain medications, such as beta blockers, put a patient at higher risk for systemic reactions to immunotherapy.

Asthma

Although some of the same principles of patient selection apply, immunotherapy for asthma deserves separate commentary. Like

AR, patients must have demonstrable IgE to allergens to which they are exposed and the clinical history should be consistent with exacerbation of asthma symptoms with exposure to the allergens. A patient's ability to visit a medical facility weekly, as well as his or her medications and age, should be taken into consideration. Immunotherapy may be appropriate for treating asthma that has been difficult to control, but it should not be prescribed for patients with unstable asthma and an FEV_1 less than 70% of predicted, so it may be least appropriate for patients who continue to have clinical symptoms of asthma despite maximal medical therapy. It should be emphasized that every clinical situation is unique and guidelines cannot replace clinical judgment.

Allergen Extracts

Allergen Extracts for Immunotherapy

Allergen extracts are prepared by extracting bulk source materials (e.g. pollens, mite cultures, fungal cultures) in aqueous buffers; typically the potency of these extracts is expressed in a ratio of the weight of source material extracted to the extraction volume, such as 1:10 wt/v. Variations in the bulk sources and in the manufacturing process have led to vast differences in the quantity of active allergens in these extracts.[34] A second approach to labeling is based on the total protein content of the extract and is expressed in protein nitrogen units (PNUs); this method has little relationship to allergenic potency but is still commonly used in the USA. Efforts to standardize extracts in Europe and the USA have produced fundamentally different approaches. One approach measures the content of the major allergen or allergens in the mixture using crossed immunoelectrophoresis, immunodiffusion, RAST inhibition, or enzyme-linked immunosorbent assay. Another approach compares the biologic activity of the material with the diameter of a control intradermal injection of histamine and expresses this as a BU (biologic unit). The US Food and Drug Administration uses a slightly different approach to establish a BU, in which the flare diameter of reference extract in a select group of allergic volunteers is compared with a reference extract and expresses the result in allergen units (AU) or bioequivalent allergen units (BAU). The results are somewhat confusing, and most commercially available extracts are labeled with more than one method to try to simplify administration of the materials. Studies that have established guidelines for effective maintenance doses for particular allergens report these doses in micrograms of major allergen, but translating wt/v, PNU, BU, AU, or BAU into microgram doses can be difficult. Fortunately, some products have also been standardized by the major allergen concentration expressed as micrograms per milliliter (μg/mL). There are also some data translating allergen content into micrograms of major allergen; this information may be helpful in guiding dosing decisions. Table 27-1 is adapted from a recent comparison of labeling methods.[35] Where they are available, standardized extracts should always be used for therapy.

Storage

Some loss of potency is usual over time; therefore, manufactured extracts are supplied with expiration dates. These expiration dates are based on the assumption that the extracts will be refrigerated because loss of activity is more rapid at temperatures above 5°C. Loss of potency is faster in more diluted solutions, but it can be decreased by the addition of 50% glycerol or 0.03% human serum albumin; because glycerol is irritating, most allergen solutions are diluted in albumin-containing buffers. Fungal,

Table 27-1 Major Allergen Content of Extracts

Source	Label	Allergen	N	Mean (µg)	Maximum (µg)	Minimum (µg)
Orchard grass	100 000 BAU/mL	Dac g 5	14	918	2414	294
Short ragweed	1:10 wt/v	Amb a 1	13	268	458	87
D. farinae	10 000 AU/mL	Der f 1	18	44	72	30
Cat hair	10 000 BAU/ml	Fel d 1	12	40	52	26
Dog hair	1:10 wt/v	Can f 1	4	5.4	7.2	2.7

Modified from Nelson HS. J Allergy Clin Immunol 2000;106:41–45.

dust mite, and cockroach extracts have been found to have significant protease activity[36] and therefore may accelerate the deterioration of allergen solutions. Some experts recommend that when making up immunotherapy solutions, dust mite, cockroach, and fungal extracts should be placed in vials separate from other allergen extracts that do not contain protease activity.

Injection Regimens

A prescription for immunotherapy should reflect the patient's demonstrated specific IgE-mediated sensitization, as well as the clinical history of symptoms on exposure and other medical illnesses. The decision is a complex one and should be made by a trained allergist rather than a manufacturer or testing service. Typically, a prescription is written for a treatment set, with one vial containing a 1:10 dilution of concentrated material from a manufacturer and three or four other vials containing 10-fold dilutions (i.e. 1:100, 1:1000, etc.). Each vial of the set should be clearly labeled with the patient's name, the allergens contained in the vial, the dilution, and an expiration date.

Administration and Dosing

Dosing instructions are shown in Table 27-2, modified from Nelson.[4] The principle is that a dose is administered that is 10-fold smaller than the dose that will induce a positive skin test; then increasing doses are administered weekly until a dose 1000 to 10 000 times greater is tolerated (Table 27-2). Once the maximum dose is reached (0.5 mL of the 1:10 dilution in Table 27-2), the patient continues to receive this dose every other week for the first year. Generally, it takes 6 months of weekly doses to reach the maintenance dose. Alternative dosing schedules have been proposed in which the build-up doses are administered every 20 to 30 minutes (rush immunotherapy) or 2 or 3 times a week (cluster immunotherapy). All of these regimens allow a patient to reach the maintenance dose in a shorter period of time, but each has a greater risk of allergic reactions to the injections.

Duration of Immunotherapy

Once maintenance doses have been reached, these are generally continued for 3 years or longer. If a patient is able to tolerate two sequential pollen seasons with minimal symptoms or none at all, they are able to stop immunotherapy without a relapse for up to 3 years. Although this has been shown in adult clinical trials,[20] it is likely to be true for children as well. Duration of treatment for asthma is less clear.

Reactions to Immunotherapy

The risks of immunotherapy are not trivial. Clinical surveys report 3% to 7% of patients experience systemic reactions and

TABLE 27-2 Allergen Extract Prescription

Begin with vial A and progress to vial D, which is the most concentrated, or 'maintenance', solution. Injections should be administered subcutaneously every week until the highest maintenance dose is administered, 0.5 mL of vial D. Then repeat this dose every other week for the next year. After the first year, maintenance doses can be given every 3 to 4 weeks.

- Call the center before resuming treatment if the treatment has lapsed by 4 weeks or more.
- During the build-up phase, repeat a dose if the last dose produced local swelling of more than 3 cm in diameter (the size of a silver dollar) or if treatment lapses for 1 to 2 weeks.
- Drop back 2-fold (i.e. from 0.4 to 0.2 mL) if the previous dose has produced local swelling of 5 cm or more in diameter, if a mild systemic reaction occurs, or if treatment lapses for more than 2 weeks.
- Drop back 4-fold (i.e. from 0.4 to 0.1 mL) if a systemic reaction occurs.
- The patient should remain for observation for 30 minutes after each injection.

Vial A (1:10 000)	Vial B (1:1000)	Vial C (1:100)	Vial D (1:10)
0.05 mL	0.05 mL	0.05 mL	0.05 mL
0.10 mL	0.10 mL	0.10 mL	0.07 mL
0.20 mL	0.20 mL	0.20 mL	0.10 mL
0.40 mL	0.40 mL	0.40 mL	0.15 mL
			0.20 mL
			0.30 mL
			0.50 mL

Modified from Nelson HS: Immunotherapy for inhalant allergens. In: Adkinson NF Jr, Busse WW, Bochner BS, eds. Middleton's allergy: principles and practice. 7th edn. St Louis: Mosby; 2008.

that one reaction occurs for every 250 to 1600 injections.[7] Reactions may be limited to urticaria, but 40% to 73% include respiratory reactions and almost 10% include hypotension; fatal reactions occur in 1 per 2 to 3 million injections.[37] From 70% to 90% of reactions begin within the first 30 minutes of an injection. The risk of reactions is greater during the build-up phase, but about half of the reactions occur during maintenance therapy. Reactions are more common in adolescents and young adults and during pollen or mold seasons. Other risk factors for serious systemic reactions include severe asthma, age of less than 5 years, and use of a beta blocker.[38] For these reasons, injections should be given in a medical facility and by personnel who know how to recognize and treat a local and systemic reaction to allergenic extract and who are trained in basic cardiopulmonary resuscitation.[39] Resuscitation equipment should be available (minimal equipment is summarized in Box 27-1. Patients should remain in the facility for 30 minutes after an injection and should report immediately if a reaction begins. Injections should not be administered at home.

Future Directions

Allergoids and Adjuvants

Allergoids are produced by chemically modifying or denaturing native allergens. The goal is to retain the ability of the allergen to elicit an immunologic response (specifically a T cell response) while decreasing the risk of anaphylaxis (the IgE-mediated response). Various chemical agents have been used, including urea, glutaraldehyde, and polyethylene glycol. Although some of these agents have appeared promising, the inability to standardize the process of chemical modification has made this approach impractical. Adjuvants are used with the allergen extract to boost immunologic response to immunotherapy in hopes of increasing its efficacy. Substances such as alum, tyrosine absorbate, and Freund's adjuvant have been used with the rationale that they have the ability to boost Th1-type immune responses.[40] It remains unclear whether adjuvants improve the efficacy of immunotherapy.

Peptides and Recombinant Allergens

As more is discovered about T cell epitopes, peptides of major allergens can be produced and used as a means of decreasing the risk of IgE-mediated reactions while retaining immunologic potency. In fact, fragments of both the dust mite allergens Der p 1 and Der f 1 and the cat allergen Fel d 1 were found to contain epitopes that were capable of inducing tolerance in mice.[41] This led to clinical trials that showed that injections of mixtures of small synthetic peptides containing the Fel d 1 epitope modified T cell responsiveness in allergic patients and decreased symptoms on exposure to cats.[42] The effects were modest, and it is not clear whether this will be a clinically useful therapy.

Immunostimulatory DNA

Immunostimulatory sequences (ISSs) are short base-pair segments of DNA that are thought to enhance a Th1 immune response by inducing IL-12 production. In preclinical studies, the activity of ragweed protein-linked ISSs was studied in peripheral blood mononuclear cultures from subjects with ragweed allergy. The ISS-tagged ragweed protein resulted in an IFN-γ-predominant cytokine profile, whereas Amb a 1 alone promoted a Th2 profile with increased IL-4 and IL-5 production.[43] A randomized controlled clinical trial demonstrated that 6 injections at weekly intervals significantly reduced rhinitis symptoms, not only in the season immediately following, but in the next year as well. No systemic reactions were seen and local reactions were similar to those seen with placebo injections.[44] With further study, the addition of ISS may prove to be an effective strategy to enhance the efficacy and reduce the risk of immunotherapy.

Immune Modulators

Many immunomodulators are being actively investigated as therapeutic strategies for allergic disease; these include treatment strategies aimed at IgE as well as those aimed at cytokines. Two such therapies that have made it to human trials are an anti-IgE humanized monoclonal antibody and a humanized monoclonal antibody to IL-5. Anti-IgE has been evaluated as a treatment for allergic asthma and AR. Milgrom and colleagues[45] conducted a randomized, placebo-controlled trial of anti-IgE in adolescent and adult patients with moderate to severe allergic asthma. Symptom scores in the active treatment groups were improved compared with the placebo arm, but perhaps the most striking result was the steroid-sparing effect of anti-IgE. Anti-IgE has also been shown to be effective in reducing the symptoms of seasonal AR in adolescents and adults with ragweed allergy.[46] One randomized, double-blinded study in children and adolescents examined its therapeutic value in seasonal AR when added to immunotherapy. Those subjects receiving anti-IgE in addition to specific immunotherapy had significant reduction in symptoms compared with those receiving immunotherapy alone.[47]

Monoclonal anti-IL-5 has been demonstrated in a placebo-controlled trial to significantly reduce peripheral and sputum eosinophilia without affecting the early- or late-phase responses with inhaled allergen challenges.[48] Despite serious methodologic concerns regarding this study,[49] it has tempered enthusiasm for anti-IL-5 therapy. Recent studies in a rare form of adult-onset asthma characterized by persistent eosinophilia, despite systemic corticosteroid therapy, have demonstrated significant benefit in terms of reduced exacerbations and steroid requirement.[50] Antagonists to IL-4 and IL-13 are also in development. Other cytokines, such as IL-12 and IL-10, are 'anti-allergic' in nature and may play a role in the treatment of allergic disease.[51]

Alternative Routes of Administration

Interest in sublingual swallow immunotherapy or SLIT began in Europe as a method to reduce the risk of serious allergic reactions to therapy. Since then, many clinical trials have examined efficacy and safety, and the results of these trials have been examined in recent meta-analyses. In adults with allergic rhinitis, 22 high quality randomized clinical trials were identified and demonstrated a significant reduction in symptoms (p = 0.002) and medication requirements (p = 0.00003).[52] In children with asthma, 9 high quality trials were examined and the reduction in symptoms and medication requirements was significant, although less consistent than that seen in adults.[53] Dose requirements of relevant aeroallergens are now better defined and an order of magnitude larger than those used for injection immunotherapy.

Successful studies using these doses produce symptomatic changes and immunologic changes similar to those seen with injection immunotherapy.[54] Systemic reactions are uncommon, but local (oral and gastrointestinal) reactions are common. Allergen extracts are not yet approved by the FDA for use in SLIT, but several phase II trials are underway, and phase III trials, including one in children with asthma, are planned. Because SLIT is still being studied, at this point in time, it is advisable that SLIT only be carried out in an allergist's office, particularly because appropriate patient selection and dosing are still being defined.

Immunotherapy as Prevention

Immunotherapy has traditionally been used as a therapeutic intervention rather than a preventive one. However, some evidence suggests that specific immunotherapy may have a future role in the secondary prevention of allergic diseases. The Preventative Allergy Treatment Study is a European multicenter, randomized trial of specific immunotherapy for seasonal AR. Among those children without asthma, those who had received 3 years of immunotherapy had significantly fewer asthma symptoms than those in the open control group.[55] The children who had received immunotherapy continued to be at lower risk for asthma 10 years after initiation of treatment.[56] In addition, a study evaluating dust mite immunotherapy in monosensitized children demonstrated a decreased risk of the development of additional sensitizations in the active treatment group compared with the control group.[57] The evidence is preliminary, but there is a suggestion that immunologic intervention at an early stage of immune development may alter the natural progression of the allergic phenotype.

Conclusions

Immunotherapy is an effective treatment option for pediatric patients with stinging insect hypersensitivity and AR (Box 27-2). It is also effective in selected patients with asthma. There is a small but definite risk of systemic allergic reactions; therefore facilities administering immunotherapy should be adequately prepared to handle such an event and patients should remain in the medical facility for 30 minutes after receiving the injection (Box 27-3).

Immunotherapy may act to suppress allergic symptoms through modification of antibody responses, lymphocyte responses, or target cell responses to allergen. Studies are under way to determine whether modifications of immunotherapy reagents or dosing route will improve its efficacy or reduce side-effects. Immunotherapy is also being pursued as a treatment option for food allergy, and there is some evidence to suggest

that immunotherapy may alter the natural progression of sensitization.

References

1. Noon L. Prophylactic inoculation for hay fever. Lancet. 1911;1:1572.
2. Norman PS, Winkenwerder WL, Lichtenstein LM. Immunotherapy of hay fever with ragweed antigen E: comparisons with whole pollen extract and placebos. J Allergy Clin Immunol. 1968;42:93–108.
3. Thompson R, Bousquet J, Cohen S, et al. The current status of allergen immunotherapy (hyposensitization). Report of WHO/IUIS Working Group. Lancet. 1989;1:259–61.
4. Nelson HS. Immunotherapy for inhalant allergens. In: Adkinson NF Jr, Bochner BS, Busse WW, Holgate ST, Lemanske RF, Simons FER, editors. Middleton's allergy: principles and practice. 7th edn. St Louis: Mosby; 2009.
5. Johnstone DE. Study of the role of antigen dosage in the treatment of pollenosis and pollen asthma. Am J Dis Child. 1957;94:1.
6. Warner JO, Price JF, Southill JF, et al. Controlled trial of hyposensitization to *Dermatophagoides pteronyssinus* in children with asthma. Lancet. 1978;2:912.
7. Greenberg MA, Kaufman CR, Gonzalez GE, et al. Late and immediate systemic allergic reactions to inhalant allergen immunotherapy. J Allergy Clin Immunol. 1986;77:865.
8. Adkinson NF, Eggleston PA, Eney D, et al. A controlled trial of immunotherapy for asthma in allergic children. N Engl J Med. 1997;336:324–31.
9. Creticos PS, Van Metre TE, Mardiney MR, et al. Dose response of IgE and IgG antibodies during ragweed immunotherapy. J Allergy Clin Immunol. 1984;73:94–104.
10. James LK, Durham SR. Update on mechanisms of allergen injection immunotherapy. Clin Exp Allergy. 2008;38:1074–88.
11. Gleich GJ, Jacob GL, Yunginger JW, et al. Measurement of the absolute levels of IgE antibodies in patients with ragweed hay fever: effect of immunotherapy on seasonal changes and relationship to IgG antibodies. J Allergy Clin Immunol. 1977;60:188–98.
12. Rocklin RE, Sheffer AL, Greineder DK, et al. Generation of antigen-specific suppressor cells during allergy sensitization. N Engl J Med. 1980;302:1213–9.
13. Durham SR, Ying S, Varney VA, et al. Grass pollen immunotherapy inhibits allergen-induced infiltration of CD4+ T lymphocytes and eosinophils in the nasal mucosa and increase the number of cells expressing messenger RNA for interferon-gamma. J Allergy Clin Immunol. 1996;97:1356–65.
14. Otsuka H, Mezawa A, Ohnishi M, et al. Changes in nasal metachromatic cells during allergen immunotherapy. Clin Exp Allergy. 1991;21:115–9.
15. Creticos PS, Adkinson NF, Kagey-Sobotka A, et al. Nasal challenge with ragweed pollen in hay fever patients: effect of immunotherapy. J Clin Invest. 1985;76:2247–53.
16. Furin MJ, Norman PS, Creticos PS, et al. Immunotherapy decreases antigen-induced eosinophil cell migration into the nasal cavity. J Allergy Clin Immunol. 1991;88:27–32.
17. Rak S, Lowhagen O, Venge P. The effect of immunotherapy on bronchial hyperresponsiveness and eosinophil cationic protein in pollen-allergic patients. J Allergy Clin Immunol. 1988;82:470–80.

18. Varney VA, Gaga M, Frew AJ, et al. Usefulness of immunotherapy in patients with severe summer hay fever uncontrolled by antiallergic drugs. Br Med J. 1991;302:265–9.

19. Lowell FC, Franklin W. A double-blind study of the effectiveness and specificity of injection therapy in ragweed hay fever. N Engl J Med. 1965;273:675–9.

20. Durham SR, Walker SM, Varga EM, et al. Long-term efficacy of grass pollen immunotherapy. N Engl J Med. 1999;341:468–75.

21. Calderon MA, Alves B, Jacobson M, et al. Allergen injection immunotherapy for seasonal allergic rhinitis, *Cochrane Database of Systematic Reviews* 2007, Issue 1. Art. No.: CD001936. DOI: 10.1002/14651858. CD001936.pub2. accessed March, 2009.

22. Bousquet J, Hejjaoui A, Clauzel AM, et al. Specific immunotherapy with standardized *Dermatophagoides pteronyssinus* extract. J Allergy Clin Immunol. 1988;82:971–7.

23. Dreborg S, Agrell B, Foucard T, et al. A double-blind, multicenter immunotherapy trial in children using a purified and standardized *Cladosporium herbarum* preparation. I. Clinical results. Allergy. 1986;41:131–40.

24. Ohman JL Jr. Allergen immunotherapy in asthma: evidence for efficacy. J Allergy Clin Immunol. 1989;84:133–40.

25. Van Metre TE, Marsh DG, Adkinson NF, et al. Immunotherapy for cat asthma. J Allergy Clin Immunol. 1988;82:1055–68.

26. Bousquet J, Maasch A, Hejjaoui W, et al. Double blind placebo controlled immunotherapy with mixed grass pollen allergoids. III. Efficacy and safety of unfractionated and high molecular weight preparations in rhinoconjunctivitis and asthma. J Allergy Clin Immunol. 1989;84:546–56.

27. Abramson MJ, Puy RM, Weiner JM. Is allergen immunotherapy effective in asthma? Am J Respir Crit Care Med. 1995;151:969–74.

28. Bousquet J, Hejjaoui A, Michel FB. Specific immunotherapy in asthma. J Allergy Clin Immunol. 1990;86:292–305.

29. Hunt KJ, Valentine MD, Kagey-Sobotka A, et al. A controlled trial of immunotherapy in insect sting hypersensitivity. N Engl J Med. 1978; 299:157.

30. Valentine MD, Schuberth KC, Kagey-Sobotka A, et al. The value of immunotherapy with venom in children with allergy to insect stings. N Engl J Med. 1990;323:1601.

31. Golden DBK. Stinging insect vaccines: patient selection and administration of Hymenoptera venom immunotherapy. Immunol Allergy Clin North Am. 2000;20:553–70.

32. Nelson HS, Lahr J, Rule R, et al. Treatment of anaphylactic sensitivity to peanuts by immunotherapy with injections of aqueous peanut extract. J Allergy Clin Immunol. 1997;99:744–51.

33. Skripak JM, Nash SD, Rowley H, et al. A randomized, double-blind, placebo-controlled study of milk oral immunotherapy for cow's milk allergy. J Allergy Clin Immunol. 2008;122:1154–60.

34. Chapman MD, Ferriera F, Villalba M, et al. The European Union CREATE project: a model for international standardization of allergy diagnostics and vaccines. J Allergy Clin Immunol. 2008;122:882–9.

35. Nelson HS. The use of standardized extracts in allergen immunotherapy. J Allergy Clin Immunol. 2000;106:41–5.

36. Stewart GA, Thompson PS, McWilliam AS. Biochemical properties of aeroallergens: contributory factors in allergic sensitization? Pediatr Allergy Immunol. 1993;4:163–72.

37. Tinkelman DG, Cole WQ III, Tunno J. Immunotherapy: a one-year prospective study to evaluate risk factors of systemic reactions. J Allergy Clin Immunol. 1995;95:8–14.

38. Reid MJ, Lockey RF, Turkeltaub PC, et al. Survey of fatalities from skin testing and immunotherapy 1985–1989. J Allergy Clin Immunol. 1993;92:6–13.

39. Executive Committee, American Academy of Allergy and Immunology. Personnel and equipment for allergenic extracts. J Allergy Clin Immunol. 1986;77:271–3.

40. Platts-Mills TAE, Mueller GA, Wheatley LM. Future directions for allergen immunotherapy. J Allergy Clin Immunol. 1998;102:335–43.

41. Briner TJM, Kuo M-C, Keating KM, et al. Peripheral T tolerance induced in naive and primed mice by subcutaneous injection of peptides from the major cat allergen Fel d 1. Proc Natl Acad Sci USA. 1993;90: 7608–12.

42. Norman PS, Ohman JL Jr, Long AA, et al. Treatment of cat allergy with T cell reactive peptides. Am J Respir Crit Care Med. 1996;154:1623–8.

43. Marshall JD, Abtahi S, Eiden JJ, et al. Immunostimulatory sequence DNA linked to the Amb a 1 allergen promotes T(H)1 cytokine expression while downregulating T(H)2 cytokine expression in PBMCs from human patients with ragweed allergy. J Allergy Clin Immunol. 2001;108: 191–7.

44. Creticos PS, Schroeder JT, Hamilton RG, et al. Immunotherapy with a ragweed-toll-like receptor agonist vaccine for allergic rhinitis. N Engl J Med. 2006;355:1445–55.

45. Milgrom H, Fick RB Jr, Su JQ. Treatment of allergic asthma with monoclonal anti-IgE antibody. rhuMAb-E25 Study Group. N Engl J Med. 1999;341:1966–73.

46. Casale TB, Condemi J, LaForce C, et al. Effect of omalizumab on symptoms of seasonal allergic rhinitis: a randomized controlled trial. JAMA. 2001;286:2956–67.

47. Kuehr J, Brauburger J, Zielen S, et al. Efficacy of combination treatment with anti-IgE plus specific immunotherapy in polysensitized children and adolescents with seasonal allergic rhinitis. J Allergy Clin Immunol. 2002;109:274–80.

48. Leckie MJ, ten Brinke A, Khan J, et al. Effect of an interleukin-5 blocking monoclonal antibody on eosinophils, airway hyper-responsiveness, and the late asthmatic response. Lancet. 2000;356:2144–8.

49. O'Byrne PM, Inman MD, Parameswaran K. The trials and tribulations of IL-5, eosinophils, and allergic asthma (editorial). J Allergy Clin Immunol. 2001;108:503–8.

50. Nair P, Pizzichini MM, Kjarsgaard M, et al. Mepolizumab for prednisone-dependent asthma with sputum eosinophilia. N Engl J Med. 2009;360:985–93.

51. Barnes PJ. Cytokine-directed therapies for asthma. J Allergy Clin Immunol. 2001;108:S72–6.

52. Wilson DR, Torres Lima M, Durham SR. Sublingual immunotherapy for allergic rhinitis: systematic review and meta-analysis. Allergy. 2005;60: 4–12.

53. Penagos M, Pasalacqua G, Compaliti E, et al. Meta analysis of the efficacy of sublingual immunotherapy in the treatment of allergic asthma in pediatric patients 3 to 18 years of age. Chest. 2008;133:599–609.

54. O'Hehir RE, Sandrini A, Anderson GP, et al. Sublingual allergen immunotherapy: immunologic mechanisms and prospects for refined vaccine preparations; Curr Med Chem. 2007;14:2335–44.

55. Moller C, Dreborg S, Ferdousi HA, et al. Pollen immunotherapy reduces the development of asthma in children with seasonal rhinoconjunctivitis (the PAT-study). J Allergy Clin Immunol. 2002;109:251–6.

56. Jacobsen L, Niggemann B, Dreborg S, et al. Specific immunotherapy has long-term preventive effect of seasonal and perennial asthma: 10-year follow-up on the PAT study. Allergy. 2007;62:943–8.

57. Pajno GB, Barberio G, De Luca F, et al. Prevention of new sensitizations in asthmatic children monosensitized to house dust mite by specific immunotherapy: a six-year follow-up study. Clin Exp Allergy. 2001;31:1392–7.

28

Allergic Rhinitis

Deborah A. Gentile • David P. Skoner

Rhinitis is defined as inflammation of the membranes lining the nose and is characterized by one or more of the following nasal symptoms: sneezing, itching, rhinorrhea, and nasal congestion. Rhinitis is frequently accompanied by symptoms that involve the eyes, ears, and throat.[1,2]

There are many different causes of rhinitis in children. Approximately 50% of all cases of rhinitis are caused by allergy. In allergic rhinitis, symptoms arise as a result of inflammation induced by an immunoglobulin E (IgE)-mediated immune response to specific allergens such as pollen, mold, animal dander, and dust mites. The immune response involves the release of inflammatory mediators and the activation and recruitment of cells to the nasal mucosa.[1,2]

A careful history and physical examination are the most effective diagnostic maneuvers for the identification of allergic rhinitis in children. Because allergic rhinitis and nonallergic rhinitis are frequently indistinguishable based on symptoms and because they require different management strategies and pharmacologic treatments, the value of an accurate differential diagnosis cannot be underestimated. Clinicians should pursue specific diagnostic testing when indicated. Management options for allergic rhinitis include treatment with pharmacologic agents and preventative measures such as environmental control and immunotherapy.

Epidemiology

Although allergic rhinitis reportedly occurs very frequently, data regarding the true underlying causes of rhinitis are difficult to interpret. Most population surveys rely on physician-diagnosed rhinitis for their data, possibly underestimating the actual frequency with which rhinitis occurs. Some population studies have been conducted by means of questionnaires administered to subjects, followed by telephone interviews to attempt to make a specific diagnosis of rhinitis. Results of such studies reflect a more accurate prevalence of rhinitis but are likely to continue to underreport this disease.[2-12]

Most epidemiologic studies have been directed toward the identification of seasonal allergic rhinitis because of the easy identification of the rapid and reproducible onset and offset of symptoms in association with pollen exposure. Perennial allergic rhinitis is more difficult to identify because its symptom complex often overlaps with chronic sinusitis, recurrent upper respiratory tract infections, and vasomotor rhinitis.

The reported prevalence of rhinitis in epidemiologic studies, conducted in various countries, ranges from 3% to 19%. Studies that have included the most information suggest that seasonal allergic rhinitis is found in approximately 10% of the general population and perennial rhinitis is found in 10–20% of the population.[2-12] Overall, allergic rhinitis affects 20 to 40 million people in the USA.[11,12]

The frequency of allergic rhinitis in the general population has risen in parallel with that of all IgE-mediated diseases during the past decade. Swedish army studies have shown that the prevalence of seasonal allergic rhinitis has increased from 4% to 8% in the 10-year period from 1971 to 1981.[13] In addition, atopic skin test reactivity increased from 39% to 50% in Tucson, Arizona, during an 8-year period of testing.[5,12]

The prevalence of allergic rhinitis in the pediatric population also appears to be rising. One study showed a prevalence of physician-diagnosed allergic rhinitis in 42% of 6-year-old children.[5] Another study conducted in Finland reported a near tripling of the prevalence from 1977 to 1991.[14] Currently, allergic rhinitis is the most common atopic disease and one of the leading chronic conditions in children younger than 18 years.[15] These figures relate to industrialized nations; there is generally less atopic disease in underdeveloped countries for reasons that are not entirely clear but involve genetic and environmental interactions.

Sex

In childhood, boys with allergic rhinitis outnumber girls, but, in general, equal numbers are affected during adulthood.

Age

Symptoms of allergic rhinitis develop before the age of 20 years in 80% of cases. Children in families with a bilateral family history of allergy generally have symptoms before puberty; those with a unilateral family history tend to have symptoms later in life or not at all.[5-7] Symptoms of allergic rhinitis develop in 1 of 5 children by 2 to 3 years of age and in approximately 40% by the age of 6 years. Approximately 30% develop symptoms during adolescence.

Risk Factors

Studies have shown that the frequency of allergic rhinitis increases with age and that positive allergy skin tests are significant risk factors for the development of new symptoms of allergic rhinitis. There appears to be a higher prevalence of rhinitis in higher socioeconomic classes, in nonwhites, in some polluted areas, in individuals with a family history of allergy, and in individuals born during the pollen season. Also, allergic rhinitis is more likely to occur in firstborn children. Studies in children in the first years of life have shown that the risk of rhinitis was higher in those with early introduction of foods or formula, heavy maternal cigarette smoking in the first year of life, exposure to indoor allergens such as animal dander and dust mites, higher serum IgE levels (>100 IU/mL before the age of 6 years), the presence of positive allergen skin-prick tests, and parental allergic disorders.[5] Recent studies have demonstrated associations between obesity, nutrition and atopy.[16-18]

Socioeconomic Impact

Because of the high prevalence of allergic rhinitis, impaired quality of life, costs of treatment, and the presence of comorbidities such as asthma, sinusitis, and otitis media, allergic rhinitis has a tremendous impact on society.[19] The severity of allergic rhinitis ranges from mild to seriously debilitating. The cost of treating allergic rhinitis and indirect costs related to loss of workplace productivity resulting from the disease are significant and substantial. The estimated cost of allergic rhinitis, based on direct and indirect costs, was $2–5 billion for 2004, exclusive of costs for associated medical problems such as sinusitis and asthma.[20] In children with allergic rhinitis, the quality of life of both the parents and the child, including the ability to learn, may be affected.[20,21]

Pathophysiology

Under normal conditions, the nasal mucosa quite efficiently humidifies and cleans inspired air. This is the result of orchestrated interactions of local and humoral mediators of defense.[22] In allergic rhinitis, these mechanisms do not function appropriately and contribute to signs and symptoms of the disorder.[23]

Components of the Allergic Response

The allergic sensitization that characterizes allergic rhinitis has a strong genetic component. The tendency to develop IgE, mast cell, and T helper cell type 2 (Th2) lymphocyte immune responses is inherited by atopic individuals. Exposure to threshold concentrations of dust mite fecal proteins; cockroach allergen; dog, cat, and other danders; pollen grains; or other allergens for prolonged periods of time leads to the presentation of the allergen by antigen-presenting cells to CD4$^+$ T lymphocytes, which then release interleukin (IL)-3, -4, and -5 and other Th2 cytokines. These cytokines drive proinflammatory processes, such as IgE production, against these allergens through the mucosal infiltration and actions of plasma cells, mast cells, and eosinophils.

Once the patient has become sensitized to allergens, subsequent exposures trigger a cascade of events that result in the symptoms of allergic rhinitis. The response in allergic rhinitis can be divided into two phases: the immediate-, or early-, phase response and the late-phase response.

Early Phase

During periods of continuous allergen exposure, increasing numbers of IgE-coated mast cells traverse the epithelium, recognize the mucosally deposited allergen, and degranulate.[24] Products of this degranulation include preformed mediators such as histamine, tryptase (mast cell-specific marker), chymase (connective tissue mast cells only), kininogenase (generates bradykinin), heparin, and other enzymes. In addition, mast cells secrete several inflammatory mediators de novo (i.e. not preformed and stored in mast cell granules), including prostaglandin D$_2$ and sulfidopeptidyl leukotriene (LT) C$_4$, LTD$_4$, and LTE$_4$. These mediators cause blood vessels to leak and produce the mucosal edema and watery rhinorrhea that are characteristic of allergic rhinitis. Glands secrete mucoglycoconjugates and antimicrobial compounds and dilate blood vessels to cause sinusoidal filling and thus occlusion and congestion of nasal air passages. These mediators also stimulate sensory nerves, which convey the sensation of nasal itch and congestion, and recruit systemic reflexes such as sneezing. These responses develop within minutes of allergen exposure and thus constitute the early-phase, or 'immediate', allergic response.[25] Sneezing, itching, and copious, clear rhinorrhea are characteristic symptoms during early-phase allergic responses, although some degree of nasal congestion can also occur.

Late Phase

The mast cell-derived mediators released during early-phase responses are hypothesized to act on postcapillary endothelial cells to promote the expression of vascular adhesion molecule and E-selectin, which facilitate the adhesion of circulating leukocytes to the endothelial cells. Chemoattractant cytokines such as IL-5 promote the infiltration of the mucosa with eosinophils, neutrophils, and basophils; T lymphocytes; and macrophages.[26,27] During the 4- to 8-hour period after allergen exposure, these cells become activated and release inflammatory mediators, which in turn reactivate many of the proinflammatory reactions of the immediate response. This cellular-driven, late inflammatory reaction is termed the *late-phase response*. This reaction may be clinically indistinguishable from the immediate reaction, but congestion tends to predominate.[28] Eosinophil-derived mediators such as major basic protein, eosinophil cationic protein, and leukotrienes have been shown to damage the epithelium, leading ultimately to the clinical and histologic pictures of chronic allergic disease.

Subsets of the T helper lymphocytes are the likely orchestrators of the chronic inflammatory response to allergens. Th2 lymphocytes promote the allergic response by releasing IL-3, IL-4, IL-5, and other cytokines that promote IgE production, eosinophil chemoattraction and survival in tissues, and mast cell recruitment.[29] Cytokines released from Th2 lymphocytes and other cells may circulate to the hypothalamus and result in fatigue, malaise, irritability, and neurocognitive deficits that are commonly noted in patients with allergic rhinitis. Cytokines produced during late phase allergic responses can be reduced by glucocorticoids.[30]

When subjects are challenged intranasally with allergen repeatedly, the amount of allergen required to produce an immediate response decreases.[31] This effect is termed 'priming' and is hypothesized to be a result of the influx of inflammatory cells that occurs during late-phase allergic responses. The response is clinically significant because exposure to an allergen may promote an exaggerated response to other allergens. Priming represents an increase in airway reactivity and highlights the importance of fully defining the spectrum of allergens for a given patient and the need to prevent this process by initiating preseasonal, prophylactic, antiinflammatory therapy.

Classification

On the basis of timing and duration of allergen exposure, and thus the allergen pathogenesis, allergic rhinitis is classified as seasonal or perennial. Overall, approximately 20% of all cases are strictly seasonal, 40% are perennial, and 40% are mixed (perennial with seasonal exacerbation).

Seasonal Allergic Rhinitis

Tree, grass, and weed pollens and outdoor mold spores are common seasonal allergens. The symptoms typically appear during a defined season in which aeroallergens are abundant in the outdoor air. The length of seasonal exposure to these allergens is dependent on geographic location. Therefore, familiarity with the pollinating season of the major trees, grasses, and weeds of the locale makes the syndrome easier to diagnose.[32] Certain outdoor mold spores also display seasonal variation with the highest levels in the summer and fall months.[33]

Typical symptoms during pollen exposure include the explosive onset of profuse, watery rhinorrhea; itching; and sneezing; along with frequent allergic symptoms of the eye. Congestion also occurs but usually is not the most troubling symptom. The onset and offset of symptoms usually track the seasonal pollen counts. However, hyperresponsiveness to irritant triggers, which develops from the inflammatory reaction of the late phase and priming responses, often persists after cessation of the pollen season. Such triggers include tobacco smoke, noxious odors, changes in temperature, and exercise.

Perennial Allergic Rhinitis

Year-round exposure to dust mites, cockroaches, indoor molds, and cat, dog, and other danders leads to persistent tissue edema and infiltration with eosinophils, mast cells, Th2 lymphocytes, and macrophages.[34] Perennial allergic rhinitis can also be caused by pollen in areas where pollen is prevalent perennially.

A universally accepted definition of perennial rhinitis does not exist. Most often, it is defined as a disease that persists for longer than 9 months each year and produces two or more of the following symptoms: serous or seromucus hypersecretion, nasal blockage caused by a swollen nasal mucosa, and sneezing paroxysms. Nasal congestion and mucous production (postnasal drip) symptoms predominate in most patients, and sneezing, itching, and watery rhinorrhea may be minimal.[2] Because late-phase reactivity is commonly ongoing, it becomes difficult to sort out early- from late-phase reactions; therefore the history of trigger factor exposure is often difficult to decipher.

Perennial Allergic Rhinitis with Seasonal Exacerbation

Symptoms of allergic rhinitis may also be perennial with seasonal exacerbation, depending on the spectrum of allergen sensitivities.

Differential Diagnosis

The causes of rhinitis are summarized in Box 28-1.[2] The most common form of nonallergic rhinitis in children is infectious rhinitis. Infectious rhinitis may be acute or chronic. Acute infectious rhinitis, such as the common cold, is usually caused by one of a large number of viruses, but secondary bacterial infection with sinus involvement may be a complication. Symptoms of chronic infectious rhinosinusitis include mucopurulent nasal discharge, facial pain and pressure, olfactory disturbance, and postnasal drainage with cough.

The symptoms of allergic rhinitis are frequently confused with those of infectious rhinitis when patients complain of a constant

BOX 28-1

Causes of Rhinitis

Allergic rhinitis
  Seasonal
  Perennial
  Perennial with seasonal exacerbation
Nonallergic rhinitis
  Structural/mechanical factors
    Deviated septum/septal wall anomalies
    Hypertrophic turbinates
    Adenoidal hypertrophy
    Foreign bodies
    Nasal tumors
      Benign
      Malignant
    Choanal atresia
  Infectious
    Acute
    Chronic
  Inflammatory/immunologic
    Wegener granulomatosis
    Sarcoidosis
    Midline granuloma
    Systemic lupus erythematosus
    Sjögren's syndrome
    Nasal polyposis
  Physiologic
    Ciliary dyskinesia syndrome
    Atrophic rhinitis
    Hormonally induced
      Hypothyroidism
      Pregnancy
      Oral contraceptives
      Menstrual cycle
      Exercise
      Atrophic
  Drug induced
    Rhinitis medicamentosa
    Oral contraceptives
    Antihypertensive therapy
    Aspirin
    Nonsteroidal antiinflammatory drugs
  Reflex induced
    Gustatory rhinitis
    Chemical or irritant induced
    Posture reflexes
    Nasal cycle
  Environmental factors
    Odors
    Temperature
    Weather/barometric pressure
    Occupational
Nonallergic rhinitis with eosinophilia syndrome
Perennial nonallergic rhinitis (vasomotor rhinitis)
Emotional factors

From Skoner DP. J Allergy Clin Immunol 2001;108:S2–S8.

cold. Symptoms persisting longer than 2 weeks should prompt a search for a cause other than infection. If tests for atopy or airway disease (e.g. asthma) are negative, foreign body rhinitis should be considered in the differential diagnosis. In such cases, symptoms may be acute or chronic and unilateral or bilateral, and the nasal discharge may be bloodstained or foul smelling.

Exacerbation of rhinitis symptoms with predominant, clear rhinorrhea in patients with a known history of allergic rhinitis may be difficult to diagnose. The difference between active infection and allergy should be noted. When the history or physical examination is not diagnostic, a nasal smear should be obtained to aid in differentiation. The presence of more than 5% eosinophils suggests allergic disease, whereas a preponderance of neutrophils suggests infection.

Allergy, mucociliary disturbance, and immune deficiency may predispose certain individuals to the development of chronic infection.[35,36] Mucociliary abnormalities may be congenital, as in primary ciliary dyskinesia, Young syndrome, or cystic fibrosis, or they may be secondary to infection.[37,38] Similarly, immune deficiency may be congenital or acquired.

Tumors or nasal polyps (Figure 28-1) as well as other conditions (e.g. nasal septal deviation, adenoidal hypertrophy, hypertrophy of the nasal turbinates) can produce nasal airway obstruction.[39,40] Nasal polyps are common in children with cystic fibrosis but not in children with allergic rhinitis. Tumors as a cause of rhinitis are very uncommon in children; other anatomic anomalies are more common in children. Nasal septal deviation and nasal turbinate or adenoidal hypertrophy may block the flow of nasal secretions, leading to rhinorrhea or postnasal drip as well as causing nasal blockage. The most common acquired anatomic cause of nasal obstruction in infants and children is adenoidal hypertrophy.

Children with rhinitis should also be assessed for congenital and acquired anatomic causes of nasal obstruction. Reduced airflow through the nasal passages in infants may be caused by congenital choanal atresia.

Refractory, clear rhinorrhea may be caused by cerebrospinal fluid leak, even in the absence of trauma or recent surgery. Any case of suspected tumor should be promptly referred to an otolaryngologist for a complete examination of the upper respiratory tract.

Evaluation and Management

History and Physical Examination

A careful history and physical examination are the most effective diagnostic maneuvers for the identification of allergic rhinitis in children.[2] The key to accurate and timely diagnosis in children is a heightened awareness of the condition and its potential comorbidities. Allergic rhinitis in children is often undiagnosed or misdiagnosed as other disorders such as recurrent colds. When cough is predominant, especially at night, allergic rhinitis may be misdiagnosed as 'cough-variant asthma'. To make a correct diagnosis with appropriate accuracy and timeliness, the clinician must be knowledgeable of and attentive to the symptoms and signs of rhinitis, ask specific questions directed at the presence and cause of rhinitis symptoms at each well-child visit, and understand the differential diagnosis of allergic rhinitis in children[2,41] (see Box 28-1). One must be aware of the comorbidities of allergic rhinitis (asthma, sinusitis, otitis media), pursue specific diagnostic tests when indicated, and often administer therapeutic trials of antiinflammatory medications.[42,43]

Parents must also be aware of signs and symptoms and report them to physicians because the more subtle case presentations

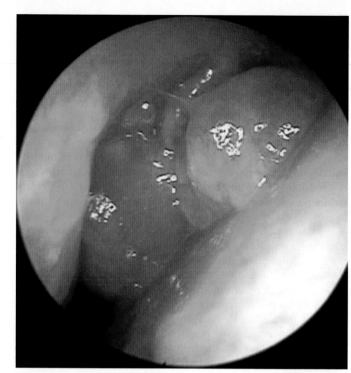

Figure 28-1 Appearance of nasal polyps on rhinoscopy. (Courtesy of Dr. Sylvan Stool, Department of Otolaryngology, Children's Hospital, Denver, Colo.)

BOX 28-2

Signs and Symptoms of Allergic Rhinitis

Itching of the nose, ears, palate, or throat

Sneezing episodes

Thin, clear rhinorrhea

Nasal congestion

Sinus headache

Eustachian tube dysfunction

Mouth breathing or snoring

Chronic postnasal drip

Chronic, nonproductive cough

Frequent throat clearing

Sleep disturbance

Daytime fatigue

---

may otherwise go undiagnosed. Such underdiagnosis may be responsible for substantial morbidity in children, who often do not report their symptoms. Unfortunately, children who live with allergic symptoms on a daily basis for prolonged periods of time may mistakenly assume that their altered state is normal.

The signs and symptoms of allergic rhinitis are summarized in Box 28-2. Typical symptoms of allergic rhinitis include sneezing, itching, clear rhinorrhea, and congestion. Congestion may be bilateral or unilateral and may alternate from side to side. It is generally more pronounced at night. With nasal obstruction, the patient is likely to be a mouth breather, and snoring can be a nocturnal symptom. As such, sleep disturbances may indicate the presence of an allergic disorder. With chronic disease, abnormalities of facial development, dental malocclusion, and the allergic facies may ensue, with an open mouth and gaping habitus.

Older children blow their noses frequently, whereas younger children do not. Instead, they sniff, snort, and repetitively clear their throats. Their voices may be abnormally hyponasal. Nasal pruritis may stimulate grimacing and twitching and picking of the nose. The latter may result in epistaxis. Children often have the allergic salute, an upward rubbing of the nose with the palm of the hand. This often produces an allergic nasal crease, which is an accentuated, horizontal skin fold over the lower third of the nose. Children with allergic rhinitis may also have recurrent sinusitis or otitis media, eczema, or asthma.

Patients may also complain of red, itchy eyes, along with itchy throat and ears. They may also lose their senses of smell and taste. Increased symptoms are frequently noted with increased exposure to the responsible allergen, such as after grass is cut.

With development of the allergic reaction, clear nasal secretions will be evident, and the nasal mucous membranes will become edematous without much erythema. The mucosa appears boggy and blue-gray. With continued exposure to the allergen, the turbinates will appear swollen and can obstruct the nasal airway. Conjunctival edema, itching, tearing, and hyperemia are frequent findings in patients with associated allergic conjunctivitis. Allergic rhinitis patients, particularly children with significant nasal obstruction and venous congestion, may also demonstrate edema and darkening of the tissues beneath the eyes. These 'shiners' are not pathognomonic for allergic rhinitis because they can also be seen in patients with chronic rhinitis and/or sinusitis.

In severe cases, especially during the peak pollen season, mucous membranes of the eyes, eustachian tube, middle ear, and paranasal sinuses may be involved. This produces conjunctival irritation (itchy, watery eyes), redness and tearing, ear fullness and popping, itchy throat, and pressure over the cheeks and forehead. Malaise, weakness, and fatigue may also be present. The coincidence of other allergic syndromes, such as atopic eczema or asthma, and a positive family history of atopy point toward an allergic pathology. Approximately 20% of cases are accompanied by symptoms of asthma.[4]

When a clear relation between onset of pollination and the typical rhinitis symptoms is present, the diagnosis of allergic rhinitis is relatively simple. However, when all of the typical rhinitis symptoms are not expressed, the diagnosis is more difficult. Chronic nasal obstruction alone may be the major symptom of perennial allergic rhinitis as a result of ongoing inflammation and late-phase allergic reactions.[28]

Distinct temporal patterns of symptom production may aid in the diagnosis. Symptoms of rhinitis, which occur each time the patient is exposed to a furry pet, suggest IgE-mediated sensitivity to that pet. Furthermore, patients who are sensitive to animal proteins may develop symptoms of rhinitis and asthma when entering a house, even though the animal was removed several hours earlier. Exposure to airborne allergens in the school or work environment may produce symptoms only during the week, with a symptom-free period during weekends. Likewise, vacations may be notably symptom free.

Several processes and anomalies in presentation may complicate the diagnosis of allergic rhinitis. For example, the symptoms on any particular day of pollen exposure will be influenced by exposure on that day but also on previous days because of the *priming phenomenon*. As a consequence, at the end of the pollen season, the decline of symptoms usually takes place more slowly than the decline of pollen counts.[44] In cases of perennial rhinitis, the symptoms are chronic and persistent, and patients may have secondary complaints of mouth breathing, snoring sinusitis, otitis media, or a 'permanent cold'.[45]

Diagnostic Tests

Laboratory confirmation of the presence of IgE antibodies to specific allergens such as dust mites, pollens, and animal dander is helpful in establishing a specific allergic diagnosis, especially if the history of specific allergen exposure is not clear cut. In many patients, it is necessary to test for specific allergens to convince the family and patient of an allergic diagnosis and to reinforce the importance of environmental control measures.

Although skin testing can be performed on any child of any age, children younger than 1 year may not display a positive reaction. Often the child with seasonal respiratory allergy will not have a positive test until after two seasons of exposure. Clinicians should be selective in the use of allergens for skin testing and should use only common allergens of potential clinical importance. The most useful allergens for testing in the child with perennial inhalant allergy are dust mite, animal dander, and fungi. Allergens important in the diagnosis of seasonal allergic rhinitis are weed, grass, and tree pollen. Because there is a significant geographic specificity with regard to pollens, the importance of these seasonal allergens varies not only by season of the year but also by geographic distribution. Therefore allergens used for skin testing must be individualized and should be selected on the basis of prevalence in the patient's geographic area of the country and the home and school environment in which they live and play.

There are two methods for specific IgE antibody testing: in vivo skin testing and in vitro serum testing. Each has advantages and disadvantages[46] (Table 28-1). At the present time, properly performed skin tests are the best available method for detecting the presence of allergen-specific IgE. The skin prick, which is also called the *puncture* or *epicutaneous skin test*, is the preferred method of IgE antibody testing. Scratch testing has been abandoned as too traumatic. If skin prick test results are negative and allergy is highly suspected, then intradermal testing, which is more sensitive but less specific, may be used if indicated.

In vitro tests are acceptable substitutes for skin tests in the following circumstances: (1) the patient has abnormal skin conditions such as dermatographism or extensive dermatitis, (2) the patient cannot or did not discontinue antihistamines or other interfering medications, (3) the patient is very allergic by history and anaphylaxis is a possible risk, and (4) the patient is noncompliant for skin testing.

To avoid false-negative tests, most antihistamine medications should be withheld for 72 hours because antihistamines suppress the skin results. Longer-acting antihistamines, such as astemi-

Table 28-1 Comparison of In Vivo Skin Tests and In Vitro Serum IgE Antibody Immunoassay in Allergic Diagnosis

Skin Test	Serum Immunoassay
Less expensive	No patient risk
Greater sensitivity	Patient-doctor convenience
Wide allergen selection	Not suppressed by antihistamines
Results available immediately	Results are quantitative
	Preferable to skin testing in: Dermatographism Widespread dermatitis Uncooperative children

From Skoner DP. J Allergy Clin Immunol 2001;108:S2–S8.

zole, should be withheld for 4 to 6 weeks before skin tests are performed.

Physicians must remember that positive tests for allergen-specific IgE themselves are not sufficient for a diagnosis of allergic disease. These tests only indicate the presence of IgE molecules with a particular immunologic specificity. A decision of whether the specific IgE antibodies are responsible for clinically apparent disease must be based on the physician's assessment of the entire clinical picture. The ultimate standard for the diagnosis of allergic disease remains the combination of (1) positive history, (2) the presence of specific IgE antibodies, and (3) demonstration that the symptoms are the result of IgE-mediated inflammation.

Blood eosinophilia and total serum IgE levels have been proposed as screening tests for allergies, but they have relatively low sensitivity and should not be used routinely for the diagnosis of allergic rhinitis. The nasal secretions or sputum of patients with respiratory allergy contains increased numbers of eosinophils, which form the basis of a useful nonspecific test (nasal smear for eosinophils) but one that will not identify any specific allergen etiology. Nasal smears for eosinophil/neutrophil counts can be useful in the differential diagnosis when the diagnosis is unclear.

Guidelines for Diagnosis and Management

Recently, evolving evaluation and management trends were delineated in an updated algorithm proposed by the Joint Task Force on Practice Parameters in Allergy, Asthma and Immunology[1] (Figure 28-2). As outlined, the initial evaluation of a patient with rhinitis symptoms (e.g. rhinorrhea, nasal congestion, sneezing, nasal pruritus, postnasal drainage, and conjunctivitis) should be performed by a primary care physician. The primary care physician should pay particular attention to the nature and history of the symptoms, the presence of complications and comorbid conditions, the identification and timing of factors that trigger symptoms, the effect on rhinitis symptoms of medications taken for rhinitis and for other conditions, and the effects of

rhinitis symptoms on the patient's ability to function and have a good quality of life. The primary care physician should institute an appropriate therapeutic trial. Upon follow-up, the primary care physician should determine if the patient has responded to treatment and/or meets the criteria for consultation with an allergist. Routine assessment of response to therapy includes evaluation of improvements in nasal symptoms, functional ability, quality of life, and comorbid conditions. Routine follow-up of patients is important when treatment is successful to ensure continued control of symptoms, absence of side-effects, and maintenance of improved quality of life.

The indications for referral to an allergist are summarized in Box 28-3. One of the primary purposes of a consultation with an allergist is the differential diagnosis of allergic rhinitis based on the combined results of a detailed medical history, physical examination of the airway, and ancillary tests, particularly skin tests. Effective management of allergic rhinitis may require a combination of aggressive avoidance measures, patient education regarding allergen avoidance and the administration of pharmacologic therapy, allergen immunotherapy, management of coexisting conditions, and adjustments in pharmacologic therapy. Cooperative follow-up is an essential part of the successful management of allergic rhinitis and ideally includes the patient, the family, and all health-care providers (e.g. primary care provider, allergist, and otolaryngologist). With the common goal of reducing symptoms and improving functional ability, all involved would cooperatively manage exacerbations and complications through the optimal use of environmental avoidance measures, medications, and immunotherapy in appropriately selected patients. Periodic assessments and continued patient education should also be included in the follow-up protocol.

Management

Specific treatment options include environmental control for allergen avoidance, pharmacotherapy, and immunotherapy. In all cases, the primary goal of treatment is to control the symptoms and to improve the quality of life without altering the patient's ability to function. A second but equally important goal is to prevent the development of sequelae of allergic rhinitis, including sinusitis and otitis media.[1,43]

Environmental Control for Allergen Avoidance

Educating families about avoiding exposure to allergens is an essential part of the treatment of allergic rhinitis (Table 28-2). Unfortunately, the specific measures are often highly impractical; moreover, they may have negative psychosocial ramifica-

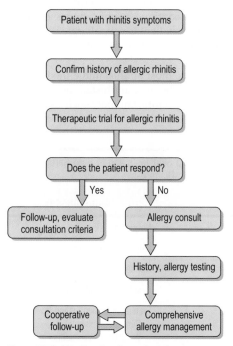

Figure 28-2 Algorithm for diagnosis and management of rhinitis. (Modified from Wallace DV, Dykewicz MS, Bernstein DI, et al. J Allergy Clin Immunol 2008;122:S1–S84.)

BOX 28-3
Indications for Referral to an Allergist/Immunologist
Prolonged history of rhinitis
Presence of complications or comorbid conditions including asthma, otitis media, sinusitis and/or nasal polyposis
Prior systemic corticosteroid for the treatment of rhinitis
Treatment that is either ineffective or produces adverse events
Symptoms that significantly interfere with the patient's functional ability or reduce the quality of life
Diagnosis of rhinitis medicamentosa
Need to further define allergic/environmental triggers of rhinitis
Need for more education

Table 28-2 Environmental Control of Allergen Exposure

Allergens	Control Measures
Dust mites	Encase bedding in airtight covers Wash bedding in water at temperatures >130°F Remove wall-to-wall carpeting Remove upholstered furniture
Animal dander	Avoid furred pets Keep animals out of patient's bedroom
Cockroaches	Control available food supply Keep kitchen/bathroom surfaces dry and free of standing water Professionally exterminate
Mold	Destroy moisture-prone areas Avoid high humidity in patient's bedroom Repair water leaks Check basements, attics, and crawl spaces for standing water and mold
Pollen	Keep automobile and house windows closed Control timing of outdoor exposure Restrict camping, hiking, and raking leaves Drive in air-conditioned automobile Air-condition the home Install portable, high-efficiency particulate air filters

Table 28-3 Second- and Third-Generation Antihistamines

Medication	Formulations	Recommended Dosage
Azelastine	Nasal spray	≥12 yr: 2 sprays per nostril bid 5–11 yr: 1 spray per nostril bid
Cetirizine	Tablets 5, 10 mg Syrup 5 mg/5 mL	≥12 yr: 10 mg qd 6–11 yr: 5–10 mg qd 6 mo–5 yr: 5 mg qd
Desloratadine	Tablets 5 mg Syrup 2.5 mg/5 mL	≥12 yr: 5 mg qd 6–11 yr: 2.5 mg qd 1–5 yr: 1.25 mg qd 6–11 mo: 1 mg qd
Fexofenadine	Capsules/tablets 30, 60, 180 mg Syrup 30 mg/5 mL	≥12 yr: 60 mg bid or 180 mg qd 2–11 yr: 30 mg bid
Levocetirizine	Tablets 5 mg Syrup 2.5 mg/5 mL	≥12 yr: 5 mg qd 6–11 yr: 2.5 mg qd
Loratadine	Tablets 10 mg Syrup 5 mg/5 mL	≥12 yr: 10 mg qd 6–11 yr: 5–10 mg qd 2–5 yr: 5 mg qd
Olopatadine	Nasal spray	≥12 yr: 2 sprays per nostril bid

tions for children that should not be ignored. Avoiding outdoor sports in the springtime and banishing furred pets from the home, for example, may have adverse effects on children that range beyond allergen control. Nevertheless, families should be taught about the importance of environmental control measures and advised to adhere to them to the extent possible.[1]

Oral Antihistamines

The Joint Task Force on Practice Parameters in Allergy, Asthma and Immunology recently updated published guidelines on the diagnosis and management of allergic rhinitis.[1] These guidelines review the considerations in selecting an antihistamine for the treatment of allergic rhinitis. As with any medication, the choice of an antihistamine should be considered in the context of an individual patient's needs and response to a given agent regarding the benefit obtained versus the risk of adverse effects. Adherence issues are also important because treatment is usually administered chronically.

Three generations of antihistamines are available: the first-generation (sedating) antihistamines, which are available without prescription; the second-generation (hypose-dating or non-sedating) agents, most of which require a prescription; and the third-generation (nonsedating metabolites of second-generation agents), all of which require a prescription in the USA at this time (Table 28-3). Antihistamines act primarily by blocking the H_1-histamine receptor, but several of the newer agents have also been shown to have mild antiinflammatory properties. The problems of sedation and frequent dosing that limited treatment with the first-generation antihistamines have been in large part eliminated by the second- and third-generation agents. The second- and third-generation agents have several advantages over the first-generation agents, including preferential binding to peripheral H_1-receptors, which results in minimal penetration of the central nervous system; minimal antiserotinergic, anticholinergic, and α-adrenergic blocking activities; and minimal sedative and performance-impairing effects.[47–49]

As a general rule, antihistamines reduce symptoms of sneezing, pruritis, and rhinorrhea but have little or no effect on nasal congestion. Consequently, a topical or oral decongestant may have to be added. Many antihistamine/decongestant formulations are available. The major advantage of these combinations is their convenience. Disadvantages are intolerance of the fixed dose of decongestant in certain patients and an inability to titrate each agent independently.[48,49]

Patients should be educated about the appropriate use of antihistamines. For optimal results, antihistamines should be administered prophylactically (2 to 5 hours before allergen exposure) or on a regular basis if needed chronically. Although antihistamines are effective on an as-needed basis, these agents work best when they are administered in a maintenance fashion.[48,49]

Decongestants

Decongestants produce vasoconstriction within the nasal mucosa through α-adrenergic receptor activation and therefore are effective in relieving the symptoms of nasal obstruction. However, these agents have no effect on other symptoms such as rhinorrhea, pruritis, or sneezing and may be most effective when used in combination with other agents, such as antihistamines.[48,49]

A number of decongestants are available for oral use, but the most commonly used decongestant is pseudoephedrine. The most common side-effects of oral decongestants are central nervous system (nervousness, insomnia, irritability, headache) and cardiovascular (palpitations, tachycardia) effects. In addition, these drugs may elevate blood pressure, raise intraocular pressure, and aggravate urinary obstruction.[48,49]

Topical intranasal decongestants are sometimes used by patients with allergic rhinitis. However, when these agents are used for longer than 3 to 5 days, many patients experience rebound congestion after withdrawal of the drug. If patients continue to use these medications over several months, a form of rhinitis, rhinitis medicamentosa, will develop, which can be difficult to treat effectively.[48,49]

Intranasal Corticosteroids

Topical intranasal corticosteroids represent the most efficacious agents for the treatment of allergic rhinitis and are useful in relieving symptoms of nasal pruritus, rhinorrhea, sneezing, and congestion. These drugs exert their effects through multiple mechanisms, including vasoconstriction and reduction of edema, suppression of cytokine production, and inhibition of inflammatory cell influx. Physiologically, prophylactic treatment before nasal allergen challenge reduces both the early and late phase allergic responses.[50]

These agents work best when taken regularly on a daily basis or prophylactically in anticipation of an imminent pollen season. However, because of their rapid onset of action (within 12 to 24 hours for many agents), there is increasing evidence that they may also be effective when used intermittently. A number of glucocorticoid compounds are available for intranasal use in both aerosol and aqueous formulations (Table 28-4). Although the topical potency of these agents varies widely, clinical trials have been unable to demonstrate significant differences in efficacy.[51,52]

The most important pharmacologic characteristic differentiating these agents is systemic bioavailability. After intranasal administration, the majority of the dose is swallowed. Most of the available compounds, including beclomethasone dipropionate, budesonide, flunisolide, and triamcinolone acetonide, are absorbed readily from the gastrointestinal tract into the systemic circulation and subsequently undergo significant first-pass hepatic metabolism. The resulting bioavailabilities can be as high as 50%. However, neither fluticasone propionate nor mometasone furoate is well absorbed through the gastrointestinal tract, and the small amount of drug that reaches the portal circulation is rapidly and thoroughly metabolized. The newest agent, ciclesonide, is administered as a prodrug and metabolized to a bioactive metabolite by esterases in the nasal mucosa. Ciclesonide has low oral bioavailability due to low gastrointestinal absorption and high first-pass metabolism. The lower systemic availabilities of these newer agents may be most important in growing children and in patients who are already using inhaled corticosteroids for asthma. Nevertheless, there are no studies to document the comparative effects of nasal corticosteroids on growth and development at this time.[53-56]

Patients who use intranasal corticosteroids experience dryness and irritation of the nasal mucous membranes in 5% to 10% of mild cases and mild epistaxis in approximately 5%. For mild symptoms, the dose of intranasal corticosteroid may be reduced if tolerated, and/or saline nasal spray should be instilled before the drug is sprayed.

Mast Cell Stabilizers

Mast cell stabilizers, such as cromolyn sodium, can be useful in relieving nasal pruritus, rhinorrhea, and sneezing; however, they have minimal effects on congestion. Cromolyn sodium is generally well tolerated and is most efficacious when taken prophylactically, well in advance of allergen exposure. In addition, because of its short duration of action, it should be taken 4 times a day; as a result, compliance is difficult for many patients.[1]

Ipratropium Bromide

Topical intranasal ipratropium bromide 0.03% and 0.06% solution reduces the volume of watery secretions but has little or no effect on other symptoms. Therefore this agent is most helpful in allergic rhinitis, when rhinorrhea is refractory to topical intranasal corticosteroids and/or antihistamines. The most common side-effects include nasal irritation, crusting, and mild epistaxis. This drug can be helpful for blocking reflex-mediated rhinitis, which occurs in people with profuse rhinorrhea after the ingestion of spicy foods or in those with cold-air exposure.[1]

Leukotriene Receptor Antagonists

These agents are effective in the treatment of seasonal and perennial allergic rhinitis.[57-60] Because allergic rhinitis often coexists with asthma and montelukast is approved for both of these diagnoses, montelukast may be considered in such patients. It should also be considered in patients who are unresponsive or noncompliant with intranasal corticosteroids. Montelukast has an excellent safety profile and is approved down to 6 months of age. An attractive attribute of this drug is that it is available as a once daily oral formulation. Dosing is one 10 mg tablet daily for patients ≥14 years, one 5 mg chewable tablet daily for patients aged 6 to 13 years, and 4 mg daily (chewable tablet or granules) for children of 6 months to 5 years of age. Adverse effects are rare, with the most common complaints being headache or stomachache shortly after dosing.

Omalizumab

Omalizumab is a monoclonal antibody against IgE and is currently approved for the treatment of severe persistent allergic asthma that is refractory to all other available treatment options. Studies have shown efficacy in both seasonal and perennial allergic rhinitis; however, the high cost of this treatment precludes its use for allergic rhinitis without concomitant asthma.[61]

Saline

Isotonic and hypertonic saline are of modest benefit in reducing symptoms and improving quality of life in patients with allergic rhinitis.[62] Various mechanisms of action, including improvement in mucociliary clearance, removal of allergen and inflammatory mediators and a protective effect on nasal mucosa, have been proposed but not confirmed. Side-effects are minimal and include

Table 28-4 Intranasal Corticosteroid Sprays

Corticosteroid	Dose per Actuation (μg)	Recommended Dosage
Beclomethasone	42	≥6 yr: 168–336 μg/day bid
Budesonide	32	≥12 yr: 64–256 μg/day qd 6–11 yr: 64–128 μg/day qd
Ciclesonide	50	≥6 yr: 200 μg/day qd
Flunisolide	25	≥14 yr: 200–400 μg/day bid 6–14 yr: 100–200 μg/day bid
Fluticasone furoate	27.5	>12 yr: 110 μg/day qd 2–11 yr: 55 ug/day qd
Fluticasone propionate	50	≥4 yr: 100–200 μg/day qd
Mometasone furoate	50	≥12 yr: 100–200 μg/day qd 2–11 yr: 100 μg/day qd
Triamcinolone acetonide	55	≥12 yr: 110–220 μg/day qd 6–11 yr: 110 μg/day qd

local burning and irritation as well as nausea. Optimal delivery techniques, volumes, concentrations and dose frequency have not been established.

Allergen Immunotherapy

Specific-allergen immunotherapy continues to be a useful and important treatment for many patients with severe allergic rhinitis.[63,64] Research performed during the past decade has demonstrated that allergen immunotherapy induces a state of allergen-specific T lymphocyte tolerance with a subsequent reduction in mediator release and tissue inflammation. When administered to appropriately selected patients, immunotherapy is effective in most cases. In addition to short-term benefits, recently published data suggest that the improvement in rhinitis symptoms persists for several years after the treatment is discontinued. Immunotherapy should be considered in patients who (1) do not respond to a combination of environmental control measures and medications, (2) experience substantial side-effects with medications, (3) have symptoms for a significant portion of the year that require daily therapy, or (4) prefer long-term modulation of their allergic symptoms. In making the decision to prescribe this therapy, the clinician should consider the positive and potentially negative effects of regular office visits for the administration of injections. If the decision is made to prescribe immunotherapy, it must be administered by a physician who is experienced in its use and whose office is set up to deal with the management of adverse allergic reactions, including anaphylaxis should this rare, untoward event occur.

Sublingual immunotherapy is an evolving treatment option for allergic rhinitis.[65,66] It has been approved for use in European countries for several years and is currently being tested in the USA. Preliminary results demonstrate efficacy that is somewhat less than injected immunotherapy. Potential advantages of sublingual immunotherapy include ease of administration, decreased adverse reactions and the potential to initiate treatment in very young children.

Conclusions

Despite the high prevalence of allergic rhinitis in the pediatric population, this disease is often overlooked or undertreated. Untreated allergic rhinitis impairs the quality of life of the child and his or her parents. Accurate and timely diagnosis of allergic rhinitis in children relies on awareness of the symptoms and signs of the disease and its comorbidities, including asthma, sinusitis, and otitis media. Clinicians should understand the differential diagnosis of allergic rhinitis in children and pursue specific diagnostic testing when indicated. Treatment options include environmental controls and the use of intranasal corticosteroids, nonsedating antihistamines, and immunotherapy. The key concepts of allergic rhinitis in children are summarized in Box 28-4.

Helpful Websites

The American Academy of Allergy, Asthma, and Immunology website (www.aaaai.org)

The American College of Allergy, Asthma and Immunology website (www.allergy.mcg.edu)

The Journal of Allergy and Clinical Immunology website (www.jaci@aaaai.org)

The Annals of Allergy, Asthma and Immunology website (www.annallergy.org)

> **BOX 28-4   Key concepts**
>
> **Allergic Rhinitis**
>
> - Allergic rhinitis is one of the most common chronic disorders of childhood.
> - Allergic rhinitis in children is an inflammatory airway disease.
> - The distinction between allergic and nonallergic forms of rhinitis is important in children.
> - Treatment should be individualized, aggressive, and targeted toward decreasing inflammation.
> - Attention should be given to decreasing environmental exposures (e.g. allergens, tobacco smoke) and the use of intranasal corticosteroids and nonsedating antihistamines.
> - Intranasal steroids constitute very effective therapy for allergic rhinitis and are safe despite a potential small drug-specific effect on growth rates.
> - Allergic rhinitis in children may predispose to the development of otitis media, sinusitis, and asthma.

References

1. Wallace DV, Dykewicz MS, Bernstein DI, et al. The diagnosis and management of rhinitis: an updated practice parameter. J Allergy Clin Immunol 2008;122:S1–84.
2. Blaiss MS. Pediatric allergic rhinitis: physical and mental complications. Allergy Asthma Proc 2008;29:1–6.
3. Nathan RA, Meltzer EO, Derebery J, et al. The prevalence of nasal symptoms attributed to allergies in the United States: findings from the burden of rhinitis in an American Survey. Allergy Asthma Proc 2008;29: 600–8.
4. Tang EA, Matsui E, Wiesch DG, et al. Epidemiology of asthma and allergic diseases. In: Adkinson Jr NF, Bochner BS, Busse WW, et al, editors. Middleton's allergy: principles and practice. 7th ed. St Louis: Mosby; 2009.
5. Wright AL, Holberg CJ, Martinez FD, et al. Epidemiology of physician diagnosed allergic rhinitis in childhood. Pediatrics 1994;94:895–901.
6. Aberg N, Engstrom I. Natural history of allergic diseases in children. Acta Paediatr Scand 1990;79:206–11.
7. Tang RB, Tsai LC, Hwang HM, et al. The prevalence of allergic disease and IgE antibodies to house dust mite in schoolchildren in Taiwan. Clin Exp Allergy 1990;20:33–8.
8. Schachter J, Higgins MW. Median age at onset of asthma and allergic rhinitis in Tecumseh, Michigan. J Allergy Clin Immunol 1976;57: 342–51.
9. Aberg N. Familial occurrence of atopic disease: genetic vs environmental factors. Clin Exp Allergy 1993;23:829–43.
10. Gerrard JW, Vickers P, Gerrard CD. The familial incidence of allergic disease. Ann Allergy 1976;36:10–15.
11. Fineman S. Rhinitis. In: Lieberman PL, Blaiss MS, editors. Atlas of allergic diseases. Philadelphia: Current Medicine Inc; 2002.
12. Meltzer EO. The prevalence and medical and economic impact of allergic rhinitis in the United States. J Allergy Clin Immunol 1997;99:S805–28.
13. Aberg N. Asthma and allergic rhinitis in Swedish conscripts. Clin Exp Allergy 1989;19:59–63.
14. Rimpela AH, Savonius B, Rimpela MK, et al. Asthma and allergic rhinitis among Finnish adolescents in 1977–1991. Scand J Soc Med 1995;23: 60–5.
15. Newacheck PW, Stoddard JJ. Prevalence and impact of multiple childhood chronic illnesses. J Pediatr 1994;124:40–8.
16. Visness CM, London SJ, Daniels JL. Association of obesity with IgE levels and allergy symptoms in children and adolescents: results from the National Health and Nutrition Examination Survey 2005–2006. J Allergy Clin Immunol 2009;123:1163–69.
17. Brehm JM, Celedon JC, Soto-Quiros ME, et al. Serum vitamin D levels and markers of severity of childhood asthma in Costa Rica. Am J Respir Crit Care Med 2009;179:765–1.
18. Pesonen M, Ranki A, Siimes MA, et al. Serum cholesterol level in infancy is inversely associated with subsequent allergy in children and adolescents: a 20-year follow-up study. Clin Exp Allergy 2008;38:178–84.
19. Fineman SM. The burden of allergic rhinitis: beyond dollars and cents. Ann Allergy Asthma Immunol 2002;88:2–7.

20. Reed SD, Lee TA, McCrory DC. The economic burden of allergic rhinitis: a critical evaluation of the literature. Pharmacoeconomics 2004;22:345–61.

21. Vuurman EF, van Vaggel LM, Uiterwijk MM, et al. Seasonal allergic rhinitis and antihistamine effects on children's learning. Ann Allergy 1993;71: 121–6.

22. Raphael GD, Baraniuk JN, Kaliner MA. How and why the nose runs. J Allergy Clin Immunol 1991;87:457–67.

23. Baraniuk J, Kaliner M. Functional activity of upper airway nerves. In: Busse W, Holgate S, editors. Mechanisms in asthma and rhinitis: implications for diagnosis and treatment. London: Blackwell Scientific; 1995.

24. Naclerio RM. Allergic rhinitis. N Engl J Med 1991;325:860–9.

25. Mygind N, Naclerio R. Allergic and nonallergic rhinitis. Philadelphia: WB Saunders; 1993.

26. Naclerio RM, Proud D, Togias AG, et al. Inflammatory mediators in late antigen-induced rhinitis. N Engl J Med 1985;313:65–70.

27. Bascom R, Pipkorn U, Lichtenstein LM, et al. The influx of inflammatory cells into nasal washings during the late response to antigen challenge: effect of systemic steroid pretreatment. Am Rev Respir Dis 1988;138:406–12.

28. Skoner D, Doyle W, Boehm S, et al. Late phase eustachian tube and nasal allergic responses associated with inflammatory mediator elaboration. Am J Rhinol 1988;2:155–61.

29. Durham SR, Ying S, Varney VA, et al. Cytokine messenger RNA expression for IL-3, IL-4, IL-5, and granulocyte/macrophage-colony-stimulating factor in the nasal mucosa after local allergen provocation: relationship to tissue eosinophilia. J Immunol 1992;148:2390–4.

30. Sim TC, Reece LM, Hilsmeier KA, et al. Secretion of chemokines and other cytokines in allergen-induced nasal responses: inhibition by topical steroid treatment. Am J Respir Crit Care Med 1995;152:927–33.

31. Connell JT. Quantitative intranasal pollen challenges. III. The priming effect in allergic rhinitis. J Allergy 1969;43:33–44.

32. Jelks M. Allergy plants that cause sneezing and wheezing. London: Worldwide Publications; 1986.

33. Platts-Mills TA, Hayden ML, Chapman MD, et al. Seasonal variation in dust mite and grass-pollen allergens in dust from the houses of patients with asthma. J Allergy Clin Immunol 1987;79:781–91.

34. Bradding P, Feather IH, Wilson S, et al. Immunolocalization of cytokines in the nasal mucosa of normal and perennial rhinitic subjects: the mast cell as a source of IL-4, IL-5, and IL-6 in human allergic mucosal inflammation. J Immunol 1993;151:3853–65.

35. MacKay I, Cole P. Rhinitis, sinusitis, and associated chest disease. In: MacKay I, Null T, editors. Scott-Brown's otolaryngology. London: Butterworths; 1987.

36. Lund VJ, Scadding GK. Immunologic aspects of chronic sinusitis. J Otolaryngol 1991;20:379–81.

37. Afzelius BA. A human syndrome caused by immotile cilia. Science 1976;193:317–9.

38. Young D. Surgical treatment of male infertility. J Reprod Fertil 1970;23:541–2.

39. Skoner D, Casselbrant M. Diseases of the ear. In: Bierman C, et al, editors. Allergy, asthma, and immunology from infancy to adulthood. 3rd ed. Philadelphia: WB Saunders; 1996.

40. Gentile DA, Michaels MG, Skoner DP. Pediatric allergy and immunology. In: Davis H, Zitelli B, editors. Atlas of pediatric physical diagnosis. 4th ed. St Louis: Mosby; 2002.

41. Settipane RA, Lieberman P. Update on nonallergic rhinitis. Ann Allergy Asthma Immunol 2001;86:494–508.

42. Lack G. Pediatric allergic rhinitis and comorbid conditions. J Allergy Clin Immunol 2001;108:9–15.

43. Skoner DP. Complications of allergic rhinitis. J Allergy Clin Immunol 2000;105:S605–9.

44. Brostrom G, Moller C. A new method to relate symptom scores with pollen counts: a dynamic model for comparison of treatments of allergy. Grana 1990;28:123–8.

45. Lucente FE. Rhinitis and nasal obstruction. Otolaryngol Clin North Am 1989;22:307–18.

46. Bernstein IL, Storms WW. Practice parameters for allergy diagnostic testing: Joint Task Force on Practice Parameters for the Diagnosis and Treatment of Asthma. The American Academy of Allergy, Asthma and Immunology and the American College of Allergy, Asthma and Immunology. Ann Allergy Asthma Immunol 1995;75:543–625.

47. Berger WE. Treatment update: allergic rhinitis. Allergy Asthma Proc 2001;22:191–8.

48. Gentile DA, Friday GA, Skoner DP. Management of allergic rhinitis: antihistamines and decongestants. Immunol Allergy Clin North Am 2000;20:355–68.

49. Schad CA, Skoner DP. Antihistamines in the pediatric population: achieving optimal outcomes when treating seasonal allergic rhinitis and chronic urticaria. Allergy Asthma Proc 2008;29:7–13.

50. Mygind N, Nielsen LP, Hoffman HJ, et al. Mode of action of intranasal corticosteroids. J Allergy Clin Immunol 2001;108:S16–25.

51. Szefler SJ. Pharmacokinetics of intranasal corticosteroids. J Allergy Clin Immunol 2001;108:S26–31.

52. Scadding GK. Corticosteroids in the treatment of pediatric allergic rhinitis. J Allergy Clin Immunol 2001;108:S26–31.

53. Schenkel EJ, Skoner DP, Bronsky EA, et al. Absence of growth retardation in children with perennial allergic rhinitis following 1 year of treatment with mometasone furoate aqueous nasal spray. Pediatrics 2000;105:E22.

54. Skoner JD, Schaffner TJ, Schad CA, et al. Addressing steroid pobia: improving the risk-benefit ratio with new agents. Allergy Asthma Proc 2008;29:358–68.

55. Skoner DP, Rachelefsky GS, Meltzer EO, et al. Detection of growth suppression in children during treatment with intranasal beclomethasone dipropionate. Pediatrics 2000;105:E23.

56. Pederson S. Assessing the effect of intranasal steroids on growth. J Allergy Clin Immunol 2001;108:S26–31.

57. Meltzer EO, Malmstrom K, Lu S, et al. Concomitant montelukast and loratadine as treatment for seasonal allergic rhinitis: a randomized, placebo-controlled clinical trial. J Allergy Clin Immunol 2000;105:917–22.

58. Chervinsky P, Philip G, Malice MP, et al. Montelukast for treating fall allergic rhinitis: effect of pollen exposure in three studies. Ann Allergy Asthma Immunol 2004;92:367–73.

59. Metlzer EO, Philip G, Weinstein SF, et al. Montelukast effectively treats the nighttime impact of seasonal allergic rhinitis. Am J Rhinol 2005;19:591–8.

60. Patel P, Philip G, Yang W, et al. Randomized, double-blind, placebo-controlled study of montelukast for treating perennial allergic rhinitis. Ann Allergy Asthma Immunol 2005;95:551–7.

61. Casale TB, Bernstein IL, Busse WW, et al. Use of an anti-IgE humanized antibody in ragweed-induced allergic rhinitis. J Allergy Clin Immunol 1997;100:110–21.

62. Harvey R, Hannan SA, Badia L, et al. Nasal saline irrigations for the symptoms of chronic rhinosinusitis. Cochrane Database Syst Rev 2007:CD006394.

63. DuBuske L. Appropriate and inappropriate use of immunotherapy. Ann Allergy Asthma Immunol 2001;87:56–67.

64. Bousquet J, Demoly P, Michel FB. Specific immunotherapy in rhinitis and asthma. Ann Allergy Asthma Immunol 2001;87:38–42.

65. Larenas-Linnemann D. Sublingual immunotherapy in children: complete and updated review supporting evidence of effect. Curr Opin Allergy Clin Immunol 2009;9:168–76.

66. Compalati E, Penagos M, Tarantini F, et al. Specific immunotherapy for respiratory allergy: stare of the art according to current meta-analyses. Ann Allergy Asthma Immunol 2009;102:22–8.

29

Otitis Media

Lauren Segal • Bruce Mazer

Introduction

Acute otitis media (AOM), with the potential resultant otitis media with effusion (OME), is the most common disease requiring pediatric care in the first decade of life, except for viral upper respiratory infections. The costs of primary and specialty care, as well as the indirect costs incurred by the family in providing care for these patients, are enormous. In 1998, the direct cost of treating otitis media in the USA totalled $ 5.3 billion, not including indirect costs. Toddlers with otitis media account for about 40% of this expenditure.[1] Some authors estimate that indirect costs incurred by families (such as hours of work lost, transportation, etc.) equal the direct costs, doubling the financial burden.[2] Even though there have been significant advances in the past 30 years in understanding the pathogenesis, pathophysiology, and immunopathology of otitis media (OM), there has not been a significant decrease in the incidence of this illness. The possibility that allergy contributes to OM is not a new concept, and its role has been debated for many years.[3] This chapter provides a review of the epidemiology, pathogenesis, Eustachian tube (ET) physiology, and immunology of OM as well as medical and surgical therapies employed to treat it.

Definitions

OM is characterized by acute or chronic inflammation of the middle ear (ME).[4] AOM is typically preceded by or associated with a viral upper respiratory tract infection (URTI); up to 37% of viral URTIs may be complicated by OM.[5] Persistent OM is defined as the persistence of symptoms and signs of ME infection despite antimicrobial therapy (i.e. treatment failure) and/or a relapse of AOM within 1 month of completion of antibiotic therapy. When two episodes of OM occur within 1 month, it may be difficult to distinguish recurrence of AOM (new episode) from persistent otitis media (relapse). Recurrent AOM is defined as having 3 or more episodes of AOM in 6 months or 4 episodes in 12 months.[6] (Box 29-1)

The inflammation of AOM often evolves into OME, a chronic middle ear effusion (MEE) without signs or symptoms of an acute infection. Two weeks after an episode of AOM, 60–70% of children have OME, decreasing to 40% at 1 month and 10–25% at 3 months post AOM.[7] When the duration exceeds 12 weeks without resolution, the process is termed *chronic OME*. Children with certain sensory, physical, cognitive and behavioral conditions are particularly vulnerable to the hearing loss, speech, language and learning problems associated with OME.[8]

Epidemiology

The peak incidence for AOM occurs during the first 2 years of life, and most cases occur between 6 and 12 months of age.[9] By 1 year of age almost 50% of children have had a least one episode of AOM,[10] and two thirds by 3 years. Three or more episodes of OM occur in 10% of children by 1 year of age and in 33% by 3 years of age. Tos and colleagues reported a point prevalence of OME of 13% during the first 2 years of life. In 4- to 6-year-old children, point prevalence decreased to 7% and then further decreased to 2–4% in 8- to 10-year-old children.[11–13] Population-based studies in the USA and Finland suggest that the incidence of recurrent otitis media (ROM) has increased 44–68% during the last 3 decades.[14,15] We must interpret these large increases with caution, because changes in health-care systems, access to care, patterns of using services and awareness of OM may be partially responsible for the increase.[16]

Multiple factors appear to increase the risk of OM in children. The best-defined risk factor in the development of AOM is a preceding viral URTI. A prospective cohort study by Wald and colleagues reported that 25% to 40% of URTIs in children from birth to 3 years of age were accompanied by an episode of AOM,[17] most commonly in children under the age of 1 year. Although not all of these episodes of AOM were confirmed by physical examination and no cultures or laboratory studies were performed, the extensive nature of follow-up (phone calls every 2 weeks) gave the data considerable power.

Universally, males are affected more than females. Populations, such as North American Indians, native Canadians, and Polynesian children have a much higher incidence than white children.[18] Compared with bottle-feeding, breast-feeding for at least 6 months is associated with a decreased risk of acute otitis or recurrent otitis during the first year of life.[19] This protective effect on both the frequency of URTIs and the resultant AOM may not be seen with shorter durations of breast-feeding.[20–22] Cigarette smoking by the parents, especially the mother, is a significant risk factor for AOM during the first year of life.[23] Children whose parents or siblings have had a history of chronic otitis have a higher incidence than those with no family history.[10] A cohort study of 2512 children in Finland concluded that, while family size, low socioeconomic status and cigarette smoking were all individually correlated with an increased risk of recurrent AOM, they were all interdependent variables. The authors also concluded that the association of these factors with AOM was best accounted for by the strong correlation with attendance at large (about 20 children) daycare centers as well as short duration of breast-feeding.[24] A prospective study that followed 175

DOI: 10.1016/B978-1-4377-0271-2.00029-8

BOX 29-1

Classification of Otitis Media

Acute otitis media

Recurrent acute otitis media

Persistent acute otitis media

Otitis media with effusion

Chronic otitis media with effusion

BOX 29-2

Risk Factors for Otitis Media

Environmental Factors

Viral upper respiratory tract infection

Day care attendance

Cigarette smoke (passive)

Socioeconomic status

Environmental pollution

Host Factors

Male gender

Genetic predisposition

Premature birth

Not breast-fed

Supine bottle feeding

Immune deficiency (primary and secondary)

Craniofacial abnormalities

Eustachian tube dysfunction

Cilia dysfunction

Allergic rhinitis

sets of twins and triplets from birth documented a genetic component to susceptibility to AOM. The estimate of discordance of AOM in monozygotic twins was 0.04 compared with 0.49 in dizygotic twins ($P < 0.005$).[25] Numerous studies confirm an augmented risk of AOM, ROM and OME as the number of children in the childcare setting increases.[26] Other factors, such as preterm birth and greater number of siblings in the household also increased a child's risk of AOM.[27] Several specific conditions, such as Down's syndrome, craniofacial anomalies,[28,29] ciliary dysfunction syndromes, and primary and secondary immune deficiency syndromes,[30,31] have been associated with an increased risk of AOM. (Box 29-2)

Several authors have investigated the point prevalence of MEEs in healthy children in daycare and school settings. Using tympanometry, Mandel and Casselbrandt found that asymptomatic OME is relatively frequent, especially in the winter months. Repeated evaluations indicated that many resolved spontaneously without therapy and could persist for up to 6 months without overt symptoms.[32]

Whether allergy predisposes children to AOM and OME is an area of much controversy. Several large Scandinavian and US studies have shown that, during the first 3 years of life, there is no association between AOM and allergic disease. This finding is fairly consistent throughout the literature, with very few studies conclusively proving a link.[33] Allergy is cited as an epidemiologic risk factor for OME, especially in studies of children

necessitating surgical intervention.[34] Unfortunately, significant methodological limitations abound in many of the approximately 70 clinical studies in this area. For example, one study of children with chronic OM referred for the placement of ventilation tubes found that approximately half of these children had positive allergy skin tests or increased serum immunoglobulin E (IgE) antibodies to specific allergens.[35] However, there was no comparison to normal controls, nor is it clear whether these children had clinical allergies or simply asymptomatic sensitization.[36] Japanese investigators reported that allergic rhinitis was found in 50% of 259 patients (mean age of 6 years) who were being treated for OME. Conversely, OME was found in 21% of 605 patients being treated for allergic rhinitis. Surgical intervention may be more frequently required in subjects with untreated allergic rhinitis.[37] A controlled trial from Italy compared 172 children with OME (mean age of 6 years) with 200 controls. The children were defined as having atopic disease if they had both positive skin prick tests to aeroallergens and allergic symptoms as determined by history. About a third of both children with OME and controls were sensitized to aeroallergens. However, children with OME were 2.6 times more likely to have clinical allergic rhinitis. These children also had a 2.6 fold risk of having eczema.[38] Several in vitro studies also substantiate a pathophysiological link between allergy and OME.[39]

No association between OM and food ingestion has been conclusively proven, although a large unblinded trial did show some efficacy of elimination diets in OME.[40] One study showed a link between true IgE-mediated cow's milk allergy and recurrent otitis media, however, the effect could be completely accounted for by the presence of respiratory allergies in these children.[41]

Pathophysiology

Structure and Function

OM should be considered a disease of the upper respiratory tract. Ventilation of the ME is accomplished via the ET from the posterior nasopharynx. Middle ear effusions in children are most often related to abnormal functioning of the ET. The ET provides an anatomic communication between the nasopharynx and the ME. Like mucosa elsewhere in the respiratory tract, the mucosa lining the ET contains mucus-producing cells, ciliated cells, plasma cells, and mast cells.[42] Unlike the bronchial tree, the ET is usually collapsed and thus closed to the nasopharynx and its contents. In this regard the ET, like the bronchial airway, serves several physiologic functions. The ET protects the ME from nasopharyngeal secretions, drains secretions produced within the ME into the nasopharynx, ventilates the ME to equilibrate pressures and replenishes oxygen in the ME that has been absorbed. In normal tubal function, intermittent opening of the ET maintains near-ambient pressure in the ME cavity. It is suspected that in cases in which active swallowing is inadequate to overcome tubal resistance, the tube remains persistently collapsed, resulting in progressively negative ME pressure. This type of ventilation appears to be common in children. While normal children may have negative ME pressures, periodic or persistently high negative pressure may be pathologic and have been associated with abnormal function of the ET and may lead to AOM. If effective ventilation does not occur because of persistent ET obstruction, transudation of sterile ME effusion in the tympanum can result as a consequence of the constant absorption of oxygen by the ME epithelium.

Types of Eustachian Tube Obstruction

Mechanical obstruction
  Intrinsic
    Infectious inflammation
    Allergic inflammation
  Extrinsic (peritubular)
    Adenoidal hypertrophy
    Nasopharyngeal tumor
Functional obstruction
  Poor tensor veli palatini muscle function
  Increased tubal compliance

Eustachian Tube Obstruction

Two types of ET obstruction, mechanical and functional, could result in acute or chronic OME (Box 29-3). Intrinsic mechanical obstruction may result from the inflammation of infection or allergy, whereas extrinsic obstruction may result from enlarged adenoids or, in rare instances, nasopharyngeal tumors. Experimentally, allergic rhinitis provoked in patients with a history of allergy has been associated with the development of ET obstruction.[43] A persistent collapse of the ET during swallowing may result in functional obstruction, which appears to be related to increased tubal compliance; an inefficient, active opening mechanism by the tensor veli palatine muscle; or both. The angulation of the craniofacial base changes with age, which renders the tensor veli palatine muscle less efficient before puberty. Another factor that may contribute to the frequency of functional ET obstruction in infants and younger children may be because the cartilaginous support of the ET is less robust.[18,44]

Pathogenesis

A role for ET dysfunction in the pathogenesis of AOM during a viral URI is supported by the results of a variety of clinical and experimental studies. Studies reported tubal dysfunction in children and adults with natural viral URI,[45] experimental infection,[46] and animals models.[47]

Research involving experimental virus infection of adult volunteers showed that rhinovirus infection results in significant increases in nasal inflammation, impaired tubal function in a majority of subjects, abnormal ME pressures in more than 40% of subjects, and asymptomatic OM in approximately 2% of subjects.[46] These events occurred sequentially and in descending frequency, supporting a causal pathway. This pattern was generalizable in infection with rhinovirus, influenza A virus, and coxsackievirus A.[48] Similar studies with influenza virus caused significant nasal symptoms, ET dysfunction, and ME underpressures in the majority of subjects and OM in approximately 20%.[49] In the majority of cases, the OM episode was asymptomatic and the recovered effusion was negative by culture for viruses and bacteria but positive for genomic sequences of Influenza-A and *Streptococcus pneumoniae* by PCR.[50] These results indicate that the various components of OM pathogenesis are indeed realized during a viral URI, which may also potentiate the allergic inflammatory response.

The inflammatory response to acute infection is a key part of the pathophysiology of the disease. Animal models have contributed to understanding the inflammatory changes and the infiltrate in the ME following acute infection. Using a murine model of ME and *H. influenzae* infection, Ryan and colleagues documented that ME mucosa undergoes rapid hypertrophy and within 24 hours exhibits edema, mucosal thickening, and a lymphocytic infiltrate.[51] This progressed over a 5- to 7-day period and resolved. Similar pathology was noted in larger animal models of AOM, including rats, guinea pigs and chinchillas.[47] Middle ear effusions are accompanied by an influx of inflammatory cytokines, including TNF-α, IL-1, IL-8, IL-10 and IL-6, which diminish over 48 to 72 hours.[52,53] The inflammatory infiltrate is potentiated by a wide variety of chemokines that are also produced as a response to the infectious process. What is lacking in the animal models of acute OM is a combined inflammatory profile that mimics both the early viral infection, and the subsequent bacterial superinfection that is characteristic in humans. Most models induce OM primarily via introduction of bacteria to the ME via the tympanic membrane (TM) or the bulla (i.e. the ME in mice). While this certainly duplicates the pathogens that are found within ME fluid in AOM, this does not completely mimic AOM pathogenesis. A small number of models have employed co-exposure to viruses and bacteria, primarily to assess therapeutic approaches.

A novel, potentially highly important contribution of animal models is the discovery of genes that may predispose to OM. Recent genetic work in mice has identified the key role of innate immunity in the inflammatory response of the ME. It is well recognized in human studies that, in addition to humoral immune defects, children with more subtle defects in mucosal immunity such as mannose-binding ligand defects are more susceptible to OM. Using murine models, a crucial role for proteins in the Toll receptor pathways has been identified.[54-57] MyD-88 signaling may also be crucial for the defence against bacterial pathogens in AOM.[54] Indeed, defects in chemokines such as IL-8, MCP-1 and CCL3, normally play integral roles in promoting early neutrophillic inflammation[58-60] and can predispose animals to AOM.[61]

The role of mast cells and innate immune responses in AOM has been the subject of multiple studies. Mast cells, as primarily mucosal leucocytes, are the most common hematopoetic cells found in normal ME, including the lining of the ME, ET and the TM. This has led to a focus on allergy in the pathogenesis of otitis. However, it is unlikely that the primary role of the mast cell in OM is via its ability to bind IgE on Fc epsilon R1, but rather its role in innate immunity and the ability to bind IgG via the Fc gamma receptors. In cKit knock-out mice, which are unable to produce mast cells, infection induced into the ME did not cause the inflammation, mucosal changes or remodeling that was found in mast cell sufficient mice or cKit knock out mice that had received infusions of normal mast cells.[62] ME fluid has been found to harbour mast cell mediators in both acute and chronic models of OM, further underlining the role of mast cells in the normal host response against bacterial pathogens.

Another major advantage of the expanding role of murine models is the ability to detect potential new genes that predispose to OM. Examples of potential defects that can affect the development of the ET and ME include mutations in the transcription factor EVI1 and the Eyes Absent Homologue Eya1.[63-65] A mouse model of deafness that is known to develop chronic suppurative OM, known as Jeff, carries a mutation in an F-box gene, Fbxo11, which predisposes to the development of cleft palate.[66,67] Even well-known genetic syndromes such as DiGeorge/Velocardiofacial syndrome have been advanced in the study of OM pathogenesis by murine models.[64-68]

Table 29-1 Bacteria Cultured from Middle Ear Effusion Tympanocentesis of Acute Otitis Media

Bacteria	Percentage
Haemophilus influenzae	51
Streptococcus pneumoniae	38
Moraxella catarrhalis	12
Staphylococcus aureus	5
Two pathogens	12
No growth	30

Etiology

Acute Otitis Media and Otitis Media with Effusion

Bacteria are found in approximately 60–70% children with AOM who are treated with tympanocentesis.[69] Historically, *Streptococcus pneumoniae*, *Moraxella catarrhalis*, and nontypeable *H. influenzae* have been the predominant causative bacterial pathogens in AOM. Group A β-hemolytic *Streptococcus*, *Staphylococcus aureus* and even more rarely, anaerobes, account for the minority of cases of AOM. Viruses, alone, are recovered from ME fluid in about 15% of cases.[70] Since the routine institution of the heptavalent pneumococcal conjugate vaccine (PCV7), the microbiology of AOM has changed as illustrated in Table 29-1. About 50% of children in one case series of children requiring myringotomy for AOM refractory to second-line antimicrobial treatment had positive cultures, most growing organisms such as *S. pneumoniae*, *Staph. aureus* and coagulase negative *Staphylococcus*.[71] Finnish and US trials have demonstrated that PCV7 has resulted in a 6% overall reduction in the clinical incidence of AOM.[72] It may also diminish ROM and reduce the need for tympanostomy tube placement.[73,74]

Antimicrobial resistance is an increasingly troublesome problem worldwide. Penicillin-resistant *S. pneumoniae* is a significant clinical problem and is found in up to two thirds of pneumococcal isolates.[75] Approximately 50% of *H. Influenzae* and 90% of *M. catarrhalis* strains produce β-lactamase, making them resistant to amoxicillin. These increases in resistance have an important impact on the choice and dosing of antibiotic therapy.

Previously it had been assumed, incorrectly, that chronic MEF effusions were sterile. In several studies, about 50% of the chronic, persistent ME effusions had positive cultures for bacteria whose microbiology was similar to that found in acute otitis.

Mediators of Allergy and Otitis Media with Effusion

Recent work has focused on analysis of the inflammatory infiltrate found in MEEs from individuals with OME. There is no uniform infiltrate; both Th1 and Th2 inflammation have been found in analyses of ME fluid.[76] MEE with infiltrates characteristic of allergic inflammation have been studied in detail and whether or not there is a correlation between allergic disease and the pattern of inflammation found in MEE has been explored. Eosinophilia and proteins derived from eosinophil degranulation are unique features of ME disease in allergic patients.[77]

Statistically significant differences in major basic protein and IL-5 mRNA were found in ME biopsy specimens, suggesting both eosinophil recruitment and degranulation in the ME. Elevated levels of IL-4, mast cell-derived tryptase, eosinophilic cationic protein and RANTES (regulated upon activation normal T cell-expressed and secreted) were all found in higher concentration in children with atopic backgrounds compared with nonatopic children.[39]

Using a cohort of 75 children who were skin tested prior to surgery for OME, Sobol and colleagues[78] and Nguyen and colleagues[79,80] studied the cellular components and cytokine expression in the MEEs of patients undergoing tympanostomy tube insertion. The incidence of atopy in these 3 studies was 24–30%. Children with positive skin testing to at least one of 12 common substances were considered to be atopic. Atopic children had significantly higher levels of eosinophils, T lymphocytes, and IL-4+ and IL-5+ cells on immunohistochemistry compared with the nonatopic cohort, as well as a trend toward higher mast cell and basophil counts in atopic children. Nonatopics had higher levels of IFNγ+ cells.[78] Th2 cells and cytokines were found in the ME fluid in atopic children and in biopsy specimens from adenoid tissue as well as the torus tubaris, demonstrating a strong correlation between allergic inflammation in MEE and in the upper airway.[79,80] A UK study with an incidence of atopy of 7% defined four groups of children with OME based on their MEE infiltrate and cytokine profiles.[76,81] Two groups were predominantly Th1 (subacute and chronic), one had Th1–Th2 overlap, and one was strongly Th2. In addition, a strong correlation between mucin production and the Th2 cytokines IL-4 and IL-13 was observed.

Diagnosis of Otitis Media

Acute Otitis Media

The American Academy of Pediatrics (AAP) and American Association of Family Physicians recently put out a clinical practice guideline outlining the diagnosis of AOM. The guidelines stipulate three criteria that must be fulfilled. There must be acute, often abrupt onset of signs and symptoms of AOM such as otalgia, otorrhea, irritability and fever. There must be a documented MEE. One can document this on examination of the ME by noting one of the following: a bulging TM, an air fluid level behind the TM, otorrhea, or limited TM mobility on tympanometry, pneumatic otoscopy or acoustic reflectometry. The patient must also have signs or symptoms of inflammation in the ME, such as distinct erythema of the TM. However, crying and/or fever can both result in an erythematous TM.[27,82] The diagnosis of AOM is often difficult in infants who are too young to clearly express themselves. They often have coexisting viral upper respiratory tract infections, and it is often a challenge to clear the external ear canal of cerumen. The ultimate management of the infant or child will differ depending on the physician's degree of certainty of the diagnosis of AOM.

Chronic Otitis Media with Effusion

The AAP, American Academy of Family Physicians, and American Academy of Otolaryngology and Head and Neck Surgery recently developed clinical practice guidelines describing the diagnosis and management of OME in children.[82] According to these evidence-based guidelines, during follow-up of all children with OME, it is important to document the laterality, duration of

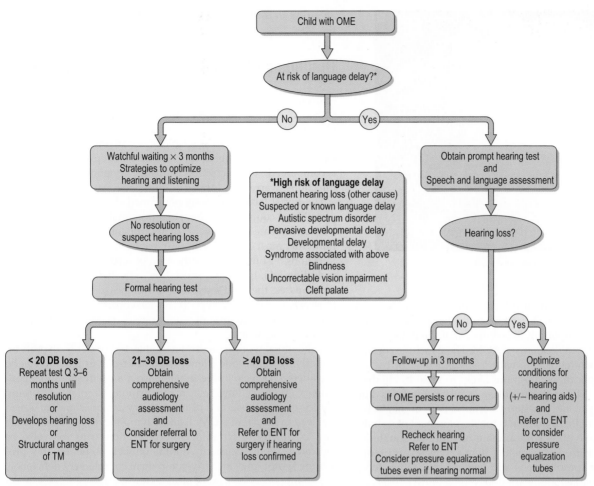

Figure 29-1 Algorithm for management of otitis media with effusion. (Modified from Mandel EM, Casselbrant ML. Acute otitis media in decision making. In: Alper CM, Myers EN, Eibling DE, eds. Ear, nose, and throat disorders. Philadelphia: WB Saunders; 2001.)

effusion, and presence and severity of any associated symptoms at each clinical assessment. The presence of OME can be confirmed by a combination of visual inspection, tympanometry and pneumatic otoscopy. Children at 'high risk' for the development of speech, language, or learning problems as a result of an MEE causing hearing loss should be promptly evaluated and may need more timely surgical intervention than low-risk children. A low-risk child with OME can be managed with watchful waiting for 3 months from the onset of the effusion (if known), or from the date of diagnosis. All children with OME lasting > 3 months should have a hearing test and be reexamined at 3- to 6-month intervals until the effusion is no longer present, significant hearing loss is identified, or structural abnormalities of the eardrum or ME are suspected.[8] (Figure 29-1)

Chronic Otitis Media and Allergy

Some children presenting with OM have associated rhinitis. It is important to decide whether this rhinitis is infectious or allergic in nature. A prolonged, perennial or recurrent seasonal rhinitis with itching and sneezing would suggest an allergic basis, as would coexistent allergic rhinoconjunctivitis. A family history of allergy, a personal history of atopic dermatitis, allergic asthma and food allergies also raise clinical suspicion of allergic rhinitis.

It is advisable that children with persistent OME be screened for allergic rhinitis by taking a clinical history looking for allergic rhinitis. If this is suspected, these children should be referred to a specialist in allergy for further evaluation and investigations.[39] Skin prick testing is preferred to serologic anti-IgE antibody tests for the detection of IgE antibodies to specific allergens because of the increased clinical sensitivity and lower cost of these tests. For either test result to be considered clinically relevant there must be a correlation between exposure to a particular allergen and clinical symptoms. Total serum IgE levels are usually not especially useful, as it does not assist in defining specific allergen sensitivity and only a third of allergic individuals have elevated total serum IgE.

Diagnostic Techniques

Physical Findings

Otoscopic inspection requires visualization of the TM. The normal TM is thin, translucent, neutrally positioned and mobile. The bony ossicles, particularly the malleus, are generally visible through the TM. Adequate assessment requires that the physician take note of the TM's thickness, degree of translucency, position and its mobility to applied pressure. A bulging eardrum and air bubbles or air-fluid levels both indicate the presence of excessive ME fluid and document effusion. While hyperemia suggests acute inflammation, erythema can be seen in 5% of OME, and thus should not be used as the only indicator of acute inflammation.[83] The ear canal may be filled with pus which, when removed, will usually reveal an inflamed TM with perforation. (Figure 29-2)

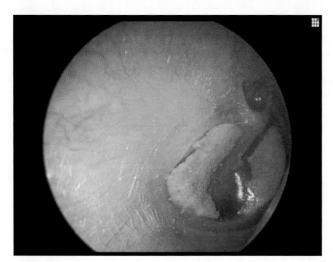

Figure 29-2 Demonstration of acute otitis media with effusion.

Children with AOM may also have coexistent sinusitis as a complication of a viral URTI, which should be considered and addressed. It is also important to be mindful of the potential for more severe, acute complications of AOM. These include coexistent mastoiditis, meningitis, brain abscess, sepsis and/or bacteremia. These complications are more likely to arise in children with underlying ME malformations, cochlear implants and immunodeficiency. One long-term complication of neglected otitis with recurrent inflammation is the development of a cholesteatoma, a cyst-like mass with a lining of stratified squamous epithelium filled with desquamating debris, which can predispose to infectious complications and hearing loss. Other long-term complications include hearing loss, tympanosclerosis and vestibular problems.[84]

Pneumatic Otoscopy

Clinicians should use pneumatic otoscopy as the primary diagnostic method for OME.[8] A meta-analysis showed that when done by trained observers, pneumatic otoscopy has a sensitivity of 87% and specificity of 74%.[85] Both choosing the correct size of speculum to fit the patient's ear canal, and obtaining a good pneumatic seal during an otoscopic examination, help to ascertain the motility of the tympanic membrane. The loss of normal movement of the eardrum during the gentle application of air pressure via a hand-held bulb indicates a loss of compliance of the eardrum. This may be seen with either an ME effusion or increased stiffness from scarring or thickening of an inflamed eardrum.

Tympanometry

When otoscopic findings are unclear or otoscopy is difficult to perform, tympanometry can be very useful in evaluating children older than 4 months.[86] This instrument, which measures the compliance of the eardrum as well as ME pressure, is also helpful in clinical practice in confirming the diagnosis of OME. Unlike pneumatic otoscopy, which requires clinicians to be specifically trained in order for it to be an accurate tool, tympanometry is easy and seems to have better diagnostic accuracy.[8]

Audiogram

An audiogram to evaluate for a conductive hearing deficit is necessary for the management of recurrent and chronic OME. OME is most often associated with a conductive hearing loss of about 25 to 30 dB, directly attributable to the effects of fluid in the ME.[87,88]

Diagnosis of Immunodeficiency Syndromes

The possibility of an immune deficiency syndrome should be considered if the child has an undue susceptibility to infections. One consensus statement suggests eight or more diagnosed episodes of AOM should raise suspicion for an underlying immunodeficiency. The combination of multiple episodes of AOM, accompanied by recurrent sinusitis, pneumonia, or other infections, warrants a formal immunologic assessment.

The initial laboratory tests performed should include a complete blood count and leukocyte differential to ensure that there is no underlying lymphopenia or neutropenia. Defects of humoral immunity most often present with recurrent oto-sino-pulmonary infections.[89] Thus, the quantification of serum immunoglobulins including IgG, IgA, IgM, and IgE is indicated. It is also mandatory to assess the child's response to vaccines (diphtheria, tetanus, *Haemophilus influenzae* type B, *Pneumococcus*) to determine the child's capacity to mount an immune response and sustain immunologic memory.[90,91]

If the initial workup is unremarkable, but one still suspects an underlying immunodeficiency, second-line investigations can be considered. Defects in the innate barrier system should be considered, such as inner ear malformations, implanted foreign bodies, cystic fibrosis and primary ciliary dyskinesia, all of which can lead to recurrent AOM. B and T lymphocyte enumeration by flow cytometry or lymphocyte proliferation assay may also be indicated. While recurrent AOM is unlikely to be the only presenting symptom of an early-component complement deficiency, depending on associated clinical features, levels of C3, C4, mannose-binding ligand and total hemolytic complement can be measured.[92] Less common conditions that can also predispose to recurrent oto-sino-pulmonary infections include specific polysaccharide antibody deficiency[90] and IRAK-4 deficiency (a defect in signaling through Toll-like receptors).[93,94] Defects in cell-mediated immunity, both primary and secondary (such as HIV) can also predispose patients to have recurrent AOM.

Treatment

Acute Otitis Media

The therapy for acute OM is outlined in Figure 29-3. If there are no potential or documented complications, the initial management consists of treating associated pain and deciding if antibiotics are indicated. Several meta-analyses have found that OM resolves without antibiotics in 80% of children over 2 years old and in 30% of children younger than 2 years of age.[95,96] The AAP subcommittee review recommended that selected patients can be managed with 'observation only' providing pain control without antibacterial treatment for 48 to 72 hours, as long as follow-up is ensured. This is not an option in patients with known or suspected immunodeficiencies, infants under 6 months of age and children presenting with severe disease (moderate-severe otalgia or fever > 39°C). This option can be considered for children aged 6 to 24 months with an uncertain diagnosis of AOM *and* nonsevere disease, or children older than 2 years of age without severe disease *or* uncertain diagnosis. If symptoms worsen on follow-up, the patient should then be treated with antibiotics. A randomized controlled trial in the UK found that 86% of a group treated immediately with antibiotics was better at 3 days, as was

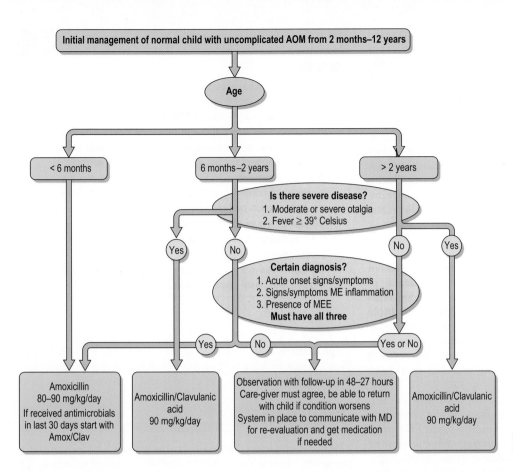

Initial management of normal child with uncomplicated AOM from 2 months–12 years

Age

< 6 months | 6 months–2 years | > 2 years

Is there severe disease?
1. Moderate or severe otalgia
2. Fever ≥ 39° Celsius

Yes | No | No | Yes

Certain diagnosis?
1. Acute onset signs/symptoms
2. Signs/symptoms ME inflammation
3. Presence of MEE
Must have all three

Yes | No | Yes or No

Amoxicillin
80–90 mg/kg/day
If received antimicrobials in last 30 days start with Amox/Clav

Amoxicillin/Clavulanic acid
90 mg/kg/day

Observation with follow-up in 48–27 hours
Care-giver must agree, be able to return with child if condition worsens
System in place to communicate with MD for re-evaluation and get medication if needed

Amoxicillin/Clavulanic acid
90 mg/kg/day

Figure 29-3 Algorithm for management of acute otitis media.

70% of the group randomized to observation only. The groups did not differ with respect to pain or distress scores or school absence. The immediate treatment group had a 1-day shorter clinical course and consumed half a teaspoon less acetaminophen per day.[97] A recent meta-analysis found that if a child is younger than 2 years of age with bilateral acute OM, they are more likely to 'fail' the 'observation only' option and eventually require antibiotics. In this trial 55% of children in the 'observation only' group versus 30% of children treated initially with antibiotics still had pain, fever, or both on days 3 to 7 after diagnosis.[98] There does not appear to be an increase in severe complications such as mastoiditis, bacteremia or meningitis with this approach.

According to treatment guidelines, the majority of children with AOM who require antibiotics should receive amoxicillin 80 to 90 mg/kg/day. Amoxicillin is considered first-line therapy because it covers strains of *S. pneumoniae* that are both sensitive and intermediately resistant to penicillin and it has a narrow microbiologic spectrum. High-dose amoxicillin-clavulanate (80–90 mg/kg/day) is preferred for severe illness (moderate to severe otalgia and/or fever > 39°C) in order to cover β-lactamase-producing *H. influenzae* and *M. catarrhali*. In penicillin-allergic patients, azithromycin, clarithromycin or trimethoprim-sulfamethoxazole are potential alternatives. Antimicrobials should be prescribed for 10 days in children < 6 years and for 5 to 7 days in children over 6 years of age.[27]

In the event of no clinical improvement within 48 to 72 hours, the child should be reevaluated. The physician should ensure that the patient does not present signs of complications of AOM and reassess if the patient still meets the diagnostic criteria for AOM. If the diagnosis of AOM is maintained, and the patient was initially observed, antibiotics should be prescribed. A patient initially treated with amoxicillin, should be switched to amoxicillin-clavulanate. If the patient fails to respond to second-line

antibiotics, 3 daily doses of parenteral ceftriaxone may be given. If this too fails, therapeutic and diagnostic tympanocentesis should be done. A culture of the ME fluid can help tailor antimicrobial therapy. In the case of penicillin-allergic patients, clindamycin is the optimal second-line therapy. When a patient has had an episode of AOM in the previous 30 days, a second-line antibiotic should be prescribed initially because the causative organism is more likely to be penicillin-resistant. When symptoms of the acute infection improve, the patient should be scheduled for follow-up in 4 to 6 weeks to determine if OME persists. If OME is present at follow-up, the clinician should consider follow-up, audiology testing, and, if necessary, tympanostomy on a case-by-case basis (see Figure 29-2).

Antimicrobial prophylaxis for recurrent acute OM, usually with trimethoprim-sulfamethoxazole, has demonstrated efficacy, but because of the problem of increased bacterial resistance, this therapy should be limited to selected cases.[89] Data from a recent Cochrane review do not support the use of decongestant treatment in children with AOM, given the lack of benefit and increased risk of side-effects.[99]

Otitis Media with Effusion

OME may be a complication of AOM or it may be detected as an occult condition without previous signs or symptoms of an infection. OME is frequently asymptomatic but may cause a hearing loss or balance disturbance.[100] If the patient is identified as not at 'high risk' of suffering language or developmental delay as a result of hearing loss secondary to OME and the OME has been present for less than 3 months, and the patient is asymptomatic, then the patient should be reexamined at 4 to 6 weeks to determine whether the effusion has resolved. An effusion that persists

CHAPTER **29**

Otitis Media

for longer than 3 months should prompt a hearing evaluation with audiometry. A normal audiogram for at least one ear is reassuring and the patient can then be rechecked periodically. This watchful waiting strategy is employed because up to 90% of OME will resolve spontaneously after 3 months.[82] Children should have scheduled pediatric follow-up every 3 to 6 months, verifying if hearing is normal and the tympanic membrane examination free of pathology such as retraction pockets, atelectasis or cholesteatoma. Children with moderate (> 40 dB) hearing loss should be referred for consideration of surgery, whereas low-risk children with mild hearing loss can continue to be observed with close follow-up and strategies to optimize hearing, such as minimizing background noise and standing close to the child when speaking.[8]

In all patients with OME in whom persistent nasal inflammation is documented, allergy should be considered. If allergic rhinitis is documented in association with OME, management should include intranasal corticosteroids and avoidance of offending allergens. Antihistamine therapy and decongestants alone have been proven to be ineffective for OME in multiple meta-analyses,[99] as have antibiotics for treatment of asymptomatic OME.[101] Oral steroids are not recommended for the management of chronic OME or recurrent OM and the risks of systemic steroids largely outweighed any potential short-term benefits.[102]

There are no placebo-controlled trials that document the efficacy of immunotherapy for reducing the frequency or promoting the resolution of OME. Recently, a community-based ENT practice examined the effect of treating patients who warranted pressure equalixation (PE) tubes for OME with immunotherapy. Although this study strongly supported the use of immunotherapy in the treatment of subjects with OME, there were methodological problems with the evaluation and treatment of the subjects.[103] Similar methodological issues were found in an older pediatric otolaryngologic study.[104]

In some cases of OME, surgical management is indicated. The surgical management of OME includes the insertion of tympanostomy tubes, also known as ventilation tubes or pressure equalization (PE) tubes to promote drainage of persistent unresolved effusions and improve hearing. According to the AAP guidelines on management of OME, the indications for consultation with an otolaryngologist to consider insertion of tympanostomy tubes include children with OME lasting 4 months or longer with persistent hearing loss, recurrent or persistent OME in high-risk children regardless of hearing status and OME associated with structural damage to the TM or ME. The decision of whether or not to proceed to surgery should be individualized. Children with OME of any duration who are at 'high risk' of language delay are candidates for earlier surgery.[8] Other plausible indications for referral include the following: (1) appropriate medical management has not been successful in alleviating the OME, (2) recurrent OME (three or more episodes in the preceding 6 months), (3) OME has persisted for more than 6 months, (4) documented persistent conductive hearing loss.

There continues to be a great deal of controversy regarding the indications for PE tube placement in children with OME. One must weigh the benefits of PE tube placement with the risks of surgery, including mortality with anesthesia and TM perforation. While PE tubes decrease number of days per year that children have OME by about half, hearing improves only minimally (about 10 dB).[104] Also a third of children have relapse of OME after their PE tubes fall out, and later require repeated PE tube placement. Furthermore, low-risk children with long-standing OME and hearing loss, derived no benefit from the insertion of PE tubes,[87,88] and only one RCT has shown minimal

improvement with PET placement in children with OME and hearing loss which resulting in disruptions of speech, language, learning or behavior.

> **BOX 29-4** Key concepts
>
> **Otitis Media**
>
> - Acute otitis media, a frequent multifactorial illness of early childhood, can evolve into a chronic otitis media with effusion associated with obstruction of the Eustachian tube.
> - Viral upper respiratory infection often precedes acute otitis media with bacteria cultured in 70% of patients with acute otitis media and 50% of patient with otitis media with effusion.
> - Chronic otitis media with effusion of more than 3 months' duration promotes a conductive hearing deficit with potential resultant speech pathology.
> - Increased frequency of bacterial resistance to antibiotics requires judicious selection of antibiotics without excessive use.
> - Epidemiologic and experimental studies suggest a role for allergic rhinitis in the patient with chronic otitis media with effusion and nasal obstruction but not in acute otitis media.

Conclusions

OM is a multifactorial illness that affects many children as either an acute, chronic or recurrent disease. Roles of infection, ET obstruction, allergy, and host defense defects have been delineated and discussed. Infection and ET obstruction are the principal contributing factors in acute OM. However, in a child who has clinically significant allergic rhinitis, the role of allergy in the child with chronic or recurrent OM cannot be ignored. Clinicians should be diligent about using the available tools and most recent evidence-based techniques when diagnosing AOM and OME, and not hesitate to involve consultants such as allergist-immunologists, otolaryngologist and audiologists when clinically indicated. In treating patients with OM, being mindful of indications for treatment, considering the adverse effects of various therapies, treating associated co-morbidities, and identifying children at risk for language delays reduce the health-care costs, as well as increase the well-being of these children. (Box 29-4)

Acknowledgements

We would like to thank Dr Phillip Fireman for allowing us to incorporate portions of his excellent original chapter on otitis media into this work.

We would like to thank Dr Sam Daniel, Otorhinolaryngologist at the McGill University Health Care Center for his expertise and help with this chapter.

References

1. Bondy J, Berman S, Glazner J, et al. Direct expenditures related to otitis media diagnoses: extrapolations from a pediatric medicaid cohort. Pediatrics 2000;105:E72.
2. Capra AM, Lieu TA, Black SB, et al. Costs of otitis media in a managed care population. Pediatr Infect Dis J 2000;19:354–5.
3. Fireman P. Otitis media and its relation to allergic rhinitis. Allergy Asthma Proc 1997;18:135–43.
4. Revai K, Dobbs LA, Nair S, et al. Incidence of acute otitis media and sinusitis complicating upper respiratory tract infection: the effect of age. Pediatrics 2007;119:e1408–12.

5. Winther B, Doyle WJ, Alper CM. A high prevalence of new onset otitis media during parent diagnosed common colds. Int J Pediatr Otorhinolaryngol 2006;70:1725–30.

6. Pichichero ME. Recurrent and persistent otitis media. Pediatr Infect Dis J 2000;19:911–6.

7. Rosenfeld RM, Kay D. Natural history of untreated otitis media. Laryngoscope 2003;113:1645–57.

8. Rosenfeld RM, Culpepper L, Doyle KJ, et al. Clinical practice guideline: otitis media with effusion. Otolaryngol Head Neck Surg 2004;130: S95–118.

9. Cober MP, Johnson CE. Otitis media: review of the 2004 treatment guidelines. Ann Pharmacother 2005;39:1879–87.

10. Teele DW, Klein JO, Rosner B. Epidemiology of otitis media during the first seven years of life in children in greater Boston: a prospective, cohort study. J Infect Dis 1989;160:83–94.

11. Stangerup SE, Tos M. Epidemiology of acute suppurative otitis media. Am J Otolaryngol 1986;7:47–54.

12. Stangerup SE, Tos M, Arnesen R, et al. A cohort study of point prevalence of eardrum pathology in children and teenagers from age 5 to age 16. Eur Arch Otorhinolaryngol 1994;251:399–403.

13. Tos M. Epidemiology and natural history of secretory otitis. Am J Otol 1984;5:459–62.

14. Lanphear BP, Byrd RS, Auinger P, et al. Increasing prevalence of recurrent otitis media among children in the United States. Pediatrics 1997;99:E1.

15. Joki-Erkkila VP, Laippala P, Pukander J. Increase in paediatric acute otitis media diagnosed by primary care in two Finnish municipalities–1994–5 versus 1978–9. Epidemiol Infect 1998;121:529–34.

16. Rovers MM, Schilder AG, Zielhuis GA, et al. Otitis media. Lancet 2004;363:465–73.

17. Wald ER, Guerra N, Byers C. Upper respiratory tract infections in young children: duration of and frequency of complications. Pediatrics 1991;87:129–33.

18. Bluestone CD, Hebda PA, Alper CM, et al. Recent advances in otitis media. 2. Eustachian tube, middle ear, and mastoid anatomy; physiology, pathophysiology, and pathogenesis. Ann Otol Rhinol Laryngol Suppl 2005;194:16–30.

19. Teele DW, Klein JO, Rosner BA. Epidemiology of otitis media in children. Ann Otol Rhinol Laryngol Suppl 1980;89:5–6.

20. Chantry CJ, Howard CR, Auinger P. Full breastfeeding duration and associated decrease in respiratory tract infection in US children. Pediatrics 2006;117:425–32.

21. Kramer MS, Chalmers B, Hodnett ED, et al. Promotion of Breastfeeding Intervention Trial (PROBIT): a randomized trial in the Republic of Belarus. JAMA 2001;285:413–20.

22. Kuiper S, Muris JW, Dompeling E, et al. Interactive effect of family history and environmental factors on respiratory tract-related morbidity in infancy. J Allergy Clin Immunol 2007;120:388–95.

23. Jacoby PA, Coates HL, Arumugaswamy A, et al. The effect of passive smoking on the risk of otitis media in Aboriginal and non-Aboriginal children in the Kalgoorlie-Boulder region of Western Australia. Med J Aust 2008;188:599–603.

24. Alho OP, Koivu M, Sorri M, et al. Risk factors for recurrent acute otitis media and respiratory infection in infancy. Int J Pediatr Otorhinolaryngol 1990;19:151–61.

25. Casselbrant ML, Mandel EM, Fall PA, et al. The heritability of otitis media: a twin and triplet study. JAMA 1999;282:2125–30.

26. Daly KA, Casselbrant ML, Hoffman HJ, et al. Recent advances in otitis media. 2. Epidemiology, natural history, and risk factors. Ann Otol Rhinol Laryngol Suppl 2002;188:19–25.

27. Pediatrics AAO. Diagnosis and management of acute otitis media. Pediatrics 2004;113:1451–65.

28. Bluestone CD. Studies in otitis media: Children's Hospital of Pittsburgh-University of Pittsburgh progress report–2004. Laryngoscope 2004;114:1–26.

29. Clarke RW. Ear, nose and throat problems in children with Down syndrome. Br J Hosp Med (Lond) 2005;66:504–6.

30. Boyle RJ, Le C, Balloch A, et al. The clinical syndrome of specific antibody deficiency in children. Clin Exp Immunol 2006;146:486–92.

31. Wilson NW, Hogan MB. Otitis media as a presenting complaint in childhood immunodeficiency diseases. Curr Allergy Asthma Rep 2008;8:519–24.

32. Mandel EM, Casselbrant ML. Recent developments in the treatment of otitis media with effusion. Drugs 2006;66:1565–76.

33. Bentdal YE, Nafstad P, Karevold G, et al. Acute otitis media in schoolchildren: allergic diseases and skin prick test positivity. Acta Otolaryngol 2007;127:480–5.

34. Bernstein JM. The role of IgE-mediated hypersensitivity in the development of otitis media with effusion: a review. Otolaryngol Head Neck Surg 1993;109:611–20.

35. Bernstein JM, Lee J, Conboy K, et al. Further observations on the role of IgE-mediated hypersensitivity in recurrent otitis media with effusion. Otolaryngol Head Neck Surg 1985;93:611–5.

36. Arbes SJ Jr, Gergen PJ, Vaughn B, et al. Asthma cases attributable to atopy: results from the Third National Health and Nutrition Examination Survey. J Allergy Clin Immunol 2007;120:1139–45.

37. Tomonaga K, Kurono Y, Mogi G. The role of nasal allergy in otitis media with effusion: a clinical study. Acta Otolaryngol Suppl 1988;458: 41–7.

38. Caffarelli C, Savini E, Giordano S, et al. Atopy in children with otitis media with effusion. Clin Exp Allergy 1998;28:591–6.

39. Tewfik TL, Mazer B. The links between allergy and otitis media with effusion. Curr Opin Otolaryngol Head Neck Surg 2006;14:187–90.

40. Nsouli TM, Nsouli SM, Linde RE, et al. Role of food allergy in serous otitis media. Ann Allergy 1994;73:215–9.

41. Juntti H, Tikkanen S, Kokkonen J, et al. Cow's milk allergy is associated with recurrent otitis media during childhood. Acta Otolaryngol 1999;119:867–73.

42. Ishii T, Toriyama M, Suzuki JI. Histopathological study of otitis media with effusion. Ann Otol Rhinol Laryngol Suppl 1980;89:83–6.

43. Friedman RA, Doyle WJ, Casselbrant ML, et al. Immunologic-mediated eustachian tube obstruction: a double-blind crossover study. J Allergy Clin Immunol 1983;71:442–7.

44. Bluestone CD. Impact of evolution on the eustachian tube. Laryngoscope 2008;118:522–7.

45. Bylander A. Upper respiratory tract infection and eustachian tube function in children. Acta Otolaryngol 1984;97:343–9.

46. McBride TP, Derkay CS, Cunningham MJ, et al. Evaluation of noninvasive eustachian tube function tests in normal adults. Laryngoscope 1988;98:655–8.

47. Giebink GS. Otitis media: the chinchilla model. Microb Drug Resist 1999;5:57–72.

48. Reuman PD, Swarts JD, Maddern BD, et al. The effects of influenza A H3N2, rhinovirus 39 and coxsackie A 21 infection on nasal and middle ear function in adult subjects. In: Proceedings of the 5th International Symposium on Recent Advances in Otitis Media. Toronto: BC Decker; 1993.

49. Doyle WJ, Skoner DP, Hayden F, et al. Nasal and otologic effects of experimental influenza A virus infection. Ann Otol Rhinol Laryngol 1994;103:59–69.

50. Post JC, Aul JJ, White GJ, et al. PCR-based detection of bacterial DNA after antimicrobial treatment is indicative of persistent, viable bacteria in the chinchilla model of otitis media. Am J Otolaryngol 1996;17:106–11.

51. Ryan AF, Ebmeyer J, Furukawa M, et al. Mouse models of induced otitis media. Brain Res 2006;1091:3–8.

52. Tong HH, Chen Y, Liu X, et al. Differential expression of cytokine genes and iNOS induced by nonviable nontypeable Haemophilus influenzae or its LOS mutants during acute otitis media in the rat. Int J Pediatr Otorhinolaryngol 2008;72:1183–91.

53. Chen A, Li HS, Hebda PA, et al. Gene expression profiles of early pneumococcal otitis media in the rat. Int J Pediatr Otorhinolaryngol 2005;69:1383–93.

54. Hernandez M, Leichtle A, Pak K, et al. Myeloid differentiation primary response gene 88 is required for the resolution of otitis media. J Infect Dis 2008;198:1862–9.

55. Lee HY, Takeshita T, Shimada J, et al. Induction of beta defensin 2 by NTHi requires TLR2 mediated MyD88 and IRAK-TRAF6-p38MAPK signaling pathway in human middle ear epithelial cells. BMC Infect Dis 2008;8:87.

56. McCoy SL, Kurtz SE, Macarthur CJ, et al. Identification of a peptide derived from vaccinia virus A52R protein that inhibits cytokine secretion in response to TLR-dependent signaling and reduces in vivo bacterial-induced inflammation. J Immunol 2005;174:3006–14.

57. Moon SK, Woo JI, Lee HY, et al. Toll-like receptor 2-dependent NF-kappaB activation is involved in nontypeable Haemophilus influenzae-induced monocyte chemotactic protein 1 up-regulation in the spiral ligament fibrocytes of the inner ear. Infect Immun 2007;75:3361–72.

58. Tong HH, Chen Y, James M, et al. Expression of cytokine and chemokine genes by human middle ear epithelial cells induced by formalin-killed Haemophilus influenzae or its lipooligosaccharide htrB and rfaD mutants. Infect Immun 2001;69:3678–84.

59. Tong HH, Long JP, Shannon PA, et al. Expression of cytokine and chemokine genes by human middle ear epithelial cells induced by influenza A virus and Streptococcus pneumoniae opacity variants. Infect Immun 2003;71:4289–96.

60. Tsuchiya K, Toyama K, Tsuprun V, et al. Pneumococcal peptidoglycan-polysaccharides induce the expression of interleukin-8 in airway epithelial cells by way of nuclear factor-kappaB, nuclear factor interleukin-6, or activation protein-1 dependent mechanisms. Laryngoscope 2007;117:86–91.

61. Wasserman SI, Leichtle A, Hernandez M, et al. CCL3 restores bacterial clearance in nontypeable Haemophilus influenzae (NTHi)-induced otitis media in TNF−/− mice. J Allergy Clin Immunol 2009;123:S257.

62. Ebmeyer J, Furukawa M, Pak K, et al. Role of mast cells in otitis media. J Allergy Clin Immunol 2005;116:1129–35.

63. Parkinson N, Hardisty-Hughes RE, Tateossian H, et al. Mutation at the Evi1 locus in Junbo mice causes susceptibility to otitis media. PLoS Genet 2006;2:e149.

64. Depreux FF, Darrow K, Conner DA, et al. Eya4-deficient mice are a model for heritable otitis media. J Clin Invest 2008;118:651–8.

65. Lazaridis E, Saunders JC. Can you hear me now? A genetic model of otitis media with effusion. J Clin Invest 2008;118:471–4.

66. Hardisty RE, Erven A, Logan K, et al. The deaf mouse mutant Jeff (Jf) is a single gene model of otitis media. J Assoc Res Otolaryngol 2003;4:130–8.

67. Hardisty-Hughes RE, Tateossian H, Morse SA, et al. A mutation in the F-box gene, Fbxo11, causes otitis media in the Jeff mouse. Hum Mol Genet 2006;15:3273–9.

68. Liao J, Kochilas L, Nowotschin S, et al. Full spectrum of malformations in velo-cardio-facial syndrome/DiGeorge syndrome mouse models by altering Tbx1 dosage. Hum Mol Genet 2004;13:1577–85.

69. Fletcher MA, Fritzell B. Brief review of the clinical effectiveness of PRE-VENAR against otitis media. Vaccine 2007;25:2507–12.

70. Heikkinen T, Thint M, Chonmaitree T. Prevalence of various respiratory viruses in the middle ear during acute otitis media. N Engl J Med 1999;340:260–4.

71. Shiao AS, Guo YC, Hsieh ST, et al. Bacteriology of medically refractory acute otitis media in children: a 9-year retrospective study. Int J Pediatr Otorhinolaryngol 2004;68:759–65.

72. Jacobs MR. Prevention of otitis media: role of pneumococcal conjugate vaccines in reducing incidence and antibiotic resistance. J Pediatr 2002;141:287–93.

73. Fireman B, Black SB, Shinefield HR, et al. Impact of the pneumococcal conjugate vaccine on otitis media. Pediatr Infect Dis J 2003;22:10–6.

74. Poehling KA, Szilagyi PG, Grijalva CG, et al. Reduction of frequent otitis media and pressure-equalizing tube insertions in children after introduction of pneumococcal conjugate vaccine. Pediatrics 2007;119:707–15.

75. Pichichero ME, Casey JR, Hoberman A, et al. Pathogens causing recurrent and difficult-to-treat acute otitis media, 2003–2006. Clin Pediatr (Phila) 2008;47:901–6.

76. Smirnova MG, Birchall JP, Pearson JP. Evidence of T-helper cell 2 cytokine regulation of chronic otitis media with effusion. Acta Otolaryngol 2005;125:1043–50.

77. Wright ED, Hurst D, Miotto D, et al. Increased expression of major basic protein (MBP) and interleukin-5(IL-5) in middle ear biopsy specimens from atopic patients with persistent otitis media with effusion. Otolaryngol Head Neck Surg 2000;123:533–8.

78. Sobol SE, Taha R, Schloss MD, et al. T(H)2 cytokine expression in atopic children with otitis media with effusion. J Allergy Clin Immunol 2002;110:125–30.

79. Nguyen LH, Manoukian JJ, Sobol SE, et al. Similar allergic inflammation in the middle ear and the upper airway: evidence linking otitis media with effusion to the united airways concept. J Allergy Clin Immunol 2004;114:1110–5.

80. Nguyen LH, Manoukian JJ, Tewfik TL, et al. Evidence of allergic inflammation in the middle ear and nasopharynx in atopic children with otitis media with effusion. J Otolaryngol 2004;33:345–51.

81. Smirnova MG, Birchall JP, Pearson JP. The immunoregulatory and allergy-associated cytokines in the aetiology of the otitis media with effusion. Mediators Inflamm 2004;13:75–88.

82. American Family Physicians, American Academy of Academy of Otolaryngology-Head and Neck Surgery, American Academy of Pediatrics. Otitis media with effusion. Pediatrics 2004;113:1412–29.

83. Karma PH, Penttila MA, Sipila MM, et al. Otoscopic diagnosis of middle ear effusion in acute and non-acute otitis media. I. The value of different otoscopic findings. Int J Pediatr Otorhinolaryngol 1989;17:37–49.

84. Bluestone CD. Clinical course, complications and sequelae of acute otitis media. Pediatr Infect Dis J 2000;19:S37–46.

85. Kaleida PH, Stool SE. Assessment of otoscopists' accuracy regarding middle-ear effusion. Otoscopic validation. Am J Dis Child 1992;146:433–5.

86. Palmu A, Puhakka H, Rahko T, et al. Predicting the development and outcome of otitis media by tympanometry. Int J Pediatr Otorhinolaryngol 2002;62:135–42.

87. Lous J. Which children would benefit most from tympanostomy tubes (grommets)? A personal evidence-based review. Int J Pediatr Otorhinolaryngol 2008;72:731–6.

88. Lous J, Burton MJ, Felding JU, et al. Grommets (ventilation tubes) for hearing loss associated with otitis media with effusion in children. Cochrane Database Syst Rev 2005;:CD001801.

89. Bonilla FA, Bernstein IL, Khan DA, et al. Practice parameter for the diagnosis and management of primary immunodeficiency. Ann Allergy Asthma Immunol 2005;94:S1–63.

90. Paris K, Sorensen RU. Assessment and clinical interpretation of polysaccharide antibody responses. Ann Allergy Asthma Immunol 2007;99:462–4.

91. Orange JS, Hossny EM, Weiler CR, et al. Use of intravenous immunoglobulin in human disease: a review of evidence by members of the Primary Immunodeficiency Committee of the American Academy of Allergy, Asthma and Immunology. J Allergy Clin Immunol 2006;117:S525–553.

92. Wiertsema SP, Herpers BL, Veenhoven RH, et al. Functional polymorphisms in the mannan-binding lectin 2 gene: effect on MBL levels and otitis media. J Allergy Clin Immunol 2006;117:1344–50.

93. Picard C, von Bernuth H, Ku CL, et al. Inherited human IRAK-4 deficiency: an update. Immunol Res 2007;38:347–52.

94. Ku CL, von Bernuth H, Picard C, et al. Selective predisposition to bacterial infections in IRAK-4-deficient children: IRAK-4-dependent TLRs are otherwise redundant in protective immunity. J Exp Med 2007;204:2407–22.

95. Fischer TF, Singer AJ, Gulla J, et al. Reaction toward a new treatment paradigm for acute otitis media. Pediatr Emerg Care 2005;21:170–2.

96. Rovers MM, Zielhuis GA. Otitis media meta-analysis. Pediatrics 2004;114:508–9; author reply 508–9.

97. Little P, Gould C, Williamson I, et al. Pragmatic randomised controlled trial of two prescribing strategies for childhood acute otitis media. BMJ 2001;322:336–42.

98. Rovers MM, Glasziou P, Appelman CL, et al. Antibiotics for acute otitis media: a meta-analysis with individual patient data. Lancet 2006;368:1429–35.

99. Coleman C, Moore M. Decongestants and antihistamines for acute otitis media in children. Cochrane Database Syst Rev 2008:CD001727.

100. Casselbrant ML, Villardo RJ, Mandel EM. Balance and otitis media with effusion. Int J Audiol 2008;47:584–9.

101. Koopman L, Hoes AW, Glasziou PP, et al. Antibiotic therapy to prevent the development of asymptomatic middle ear effusion in children with acute otitis media: a meta-analysis of individual patient data. Arch Otolaryngol Head Neck Surg 2008;134:128–32.

102. Thomas CL, Simpson S, Butler CC, et al. Oral or topical nasal steroids for hearing loss associated with otitis media with effusion in children. Cochrane Database Syst Rev 2006;3:CD001935.

103. Hurst DS. Efficacy of allergy immunotherapy as a treatment for patients with chronic otitis media with effusion. Int J Pediatr Otorhinolaryngol 2008;72:1215–23.

104. McMahan JT, Calenoff E, Croft DJ, et al. Chronic otitis media with effusion and allergy: modified RAST analysis of 119 cases. Otolaryngol Head Neck Surg 1981;89:427–31.

30
Sinusitis

Kenny H. Chan • Mark J. Abzug • Andrew H. Liu

This chapter on sinusitis in children will provide a current overview of the pathogenesis and management of acute and chronic sinus disease. The goals of sinusitis treatment are to relieve sinusitis symptoms and signs and to prevent complications. Although acute sinusitis has been substantially investigated, relatively little is known about chronic sinusitis in children.

Sinus Development in Childhood

There are four pairs of paranasal sinuses in humans: maxillary, ethmoid, frontal, and sphenoid. The maxillary and ethmoid sinuses are present at birth and invaginate to become radiographically visible in the first 1 to 2 years of life (Figure 30-1). In comparison, frontal and sphenoid sinuses begin to develop in the first few years of life and gradually become pneumatized and radiographically visible between 7 and 15 years of age. The maxillary, anterior ethmoid, and frontal sinus ostia enter the nasal cavity through the middle meatus, under the middle turbinate (i.e. osteomeatal complex; see Figure 30-1). The sphenoid and posterior ethmoid ostia join the nasal cavity through the superior meatus, above the middle turbinate.

Clinical Definitions of Sinusitis

Several descriptive modifiers for sinusitis are commonly used, although the pathogenic and therapeutic relevance of the differences between subgroups has not been well clarified. In terms of sinusitis duration, (1) *acute* sinusitis refers to sinus symptoms of 10 to 30 days, with complete resolution of symptoms,[1] (2) *subacute* sinusitis refers to symptoms that last 30 to 90 to 120 days, and (3) *chronic* sinusitis is used for symptoms that last more than 90 to 120 days. *Recurrent* sinusitis occurs in patients who improve with sinus therapy but experience multiple episodes. *Refractory* sinusitis refers to patients who do not respond to conventional therapy for sinusitis.

The uses of the term *sinusitis* and *rhinosinusitis* have been debated; *sinusitis* implies that the disease is the manifestation of an infectious process of the sinuses.[2] In comparison, the term *rhinosinusitis* implies that the nasal and sinus mucosae are involved in similar and concurrent pathogenic (e.g. inflammatory) processes.[1] In this chapter the two terms will be used interchangeably, although the bias of the authors is that sinusitis is both pathogenically and clinically linked to rhinitis.

Epidemiology

Sinusitis is a common problem in childhood, but only a few epidemiologic studies have assessed its prevalence and natural history in childhood. In a study of 1- to 5-year-old children seen in pediatric practices, 9.3% met the clinical criteria of sinusitis (i.e. ≥10 days of symptoms).[3] In a large birth cohort study primarily intended to study the natural history of childhood asthma (Children's Respiratory Study, Tucson, Arizona), 13% of 8-year-old children reported physician-diagnosed sinusitis within the past year.[4] Of children with sinusitis, 50%, 18%, and 11% had sinusitis diagnosed for the first time at ages 6 years, 3 years, and 2 years, respectively. The main risk factors for sinusitis were current allergic rhinitis and grass pollen hypersensitivity.

The National Center for Health Statistics in the USA reported that from 1980 to 1992, sinusitis was the fifth leading diagnosis for which antibiotics was prescribed.[5] The annual outpatient visit rates for sinusitis increased about 3-fold over this period and the use of amoxicillin and cephalosporin antibiotics for sinusitis also increased significantly. Antibiotic resistance of bacterial pathogens from the sinuses of children with acute sinusitis[6] and chronic sinusitis[7] is currently common. Severe alterations in quality of life can result from chronic recurrent sinusitis in children. Using a standardized child health questionnaire, children with chronic sinusitis and their parents reported more bodily pain and greater limitation in their physical activity than those typically reported by children with asthma or juvenile rheumatoid arthritis.[8] Complications of sinusitis, such as intracranial or intraorbital extension of bacterial infection from the sinuses, are medical emergencies that are life-threatening and carry a high risk of morbidity and mortality.

Etiology

A combination of anatomic, mucosal, microbial, and immune pathogenic processes is believed to underlie sinusitis in children. Children with congenital mucosal diseases (e.g. cystic fibrosis, ciliary dyskinesias) and lymphocyte immune deficiencies (congenital and acquired) typically have chronic recurrent sinus disease. Also, allergic airway diseases in children have both epidemiologic and pathogenic links to sinusitis.

©2010 Elsevier Ltd, Inc, BV
DOI: 10.1016/B978-1-4377-0271-2.00030-4

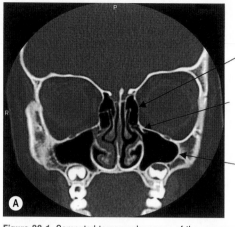 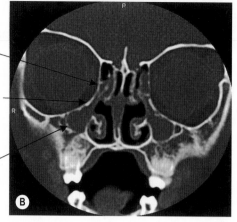

Figure 30-1 Computed tomography scans of the paranasal sinuses. Coronal views of a 4-year-old child with **(A)** normal maxillary and ethmoid sinuses and patent osteomeatal complex and **(B)** opacified maxillary and ethmoid sinuses consistent with sinusitis. *E*, Ethmoid sinus; *M*, maxillary sinus; *OMC*, osteomeatal complex.

Anatomic Pathogenesis

Anatomic obstructions of the sinus ostia in the nasopharynx have long been suspected causes of sinusitis. The pathophysiology of osteomeatal obstruction leading to sinusitis is believed to be similar to that of otitis media.[9] For the middle ear space, animal model studies reveal that a lack of ventilation (i.e. oxygenation) of the middle ear results in negative pressure in the closed space, leading to mucosal vascular leakage, edema, inflammation, and middle ear fluid accumulation.[10,11] Both anatomic obstructive lesions and mucosal disorders such as mucosal injury from viral upper respiratory tract infections (URTIs), inhalant allergies, cystic fibrosis, and ciliary dyskinesias may begin this cascade of pathogenic events. Anatomic variations associated with sinusitis in children in uncontrolled studies include concha bullosa (10%), paradoxical turbinates (4% to 8%), lateralized uncinate process with hypoplastic maxillary sinus (7% to 17%); Haller cell (5% to 10%), and septal deviation (10%).[12,13] Recent studies have failed to establish a relationship between anatomic variations and the severity and extent of chronic sinusitis in children.[14,15] Adenoid hypertrophy has also been implicated as a possible predisposing factor to sinusitis in children by serving as a mechanical obstruction to nasal drainage; however, an etiologic role has not been established.[16,17] Therefore, it is not prudent to base surgical intervention on anatomic variations alone.

Microbial Pathogenesis

Both viral and bacterial infections have integral roles in the pathogenesis of sinusitis. Viral URTIs commonly cause sinus mucosal injury and swelling, resulting in osteomeatal obstruction, loss of ciliary activity, and mucous hypersecretion. Indeed, radiologic sinus imaging studies of adults with common colds revealed that sinus mucosal abnormalities are the norm, and even air-fluid levels in the maxillary sinuses and opacification of the maxillary sinuses are common.[18,19] Specifically, coronal sinus computed tomography (CT) scans of adults with URTIs revealed that 87% had abnormalities of one or both maxillary sinuses, 77% had obstruction of the ethmoid infundibulum, 65% had abnormal ethmoid sinuses, 32% had abnormal frontal sinuses, and 39% had abnormal sphenoid sinuses.[19]

Sneezing and nose blowing are thought to introduce nasal flora into the sinuses. Chronically infected adenoids, which may be colonized by bacterial biofilms, and intracellular bacteria (in particular, *Staphylococcus aureus*) in the nasopharynx have been proposed as nasopharyngeal reservoirs of pathogens that may be introduced into the sinuses.[17,20] Normal nasopharyngeal flora such as alpha streptococci and anaerobes may elaborate bacteriocins and other inhibitory compounds that interfere with colonization and infection by pathogenic bacteria.[21] Bacterial growth conditions are favorable in obstructed sinuses, reflected by bacterial concentrations of up to 10^7 bacterial colony-forming units (cfu)/mL in sinus aspirates. Additionally, bacterial biofilms have been demonstrated in sinus mucosal specimens obtained from 45–80% of children and adults with chronic sinusitis[22,23] White blood cell counts in excess of 10 000 cells/mL in sinus aspirates are evidence of a robust inflammatory response to infection. The combination of infection, biofilm formation, and inflammation can be directly destructive, resulting in intense epithelial damage and transmucosal injury.[24,25]

Microbiology of Acute and Subacute Sinusitis

The gold standard for microbiologic diagnosis of bacterial sinusitis has been the recovery of $\geq 10^4$ cfu/mL of pathogenic bacteria from a sinus aspirate.[1,26] Studies employing sinus aspirates indicate that the pathogens responsible for acute and subacute sinusitis are similar to each other and mirror those responsible for acute otitis media[26–31] (Table 30-1). *Streptococcus pneumoniae* is recovered in approximately 30% of cases, nontypable *Haemophilus influenzae* in approximately 20%, and *Moraxella catarrhalis* in approximately 20%. Similar to observations for acute otitis media, a modest reduction in the proportion due to *S. pneumoniae* and a corresponding increase in the proportion due to *H. influenzae* is suggested in populations with routine pneumococcal conjugate vaccination of young children.[21] A significant proportion of *S. pneumoniae* isolates have intermediate or high-level resistance to penicillin due to alterations in penicillin-binding proteins (15–50%). *H. influenzae* and *M. catarrhalis* isolates are frequently β-lactamase positive (25–50% and 90–100%, respectively), and a minority of *H. influenzae* are ampicillin-resistant due to altered penicillin-binding proteins and/or an efflux pump.[21,32] Actual resistance rates vary with time period, geographic region, and the prevalence of risk factors for resistance (e.g. age <2 years, daycare attendance, recent antibiotic exposure). *Streptococcus pyogenes* and other streptococcal species are generally recovered in only a small number of cases, although several series have highlighted a frequent association between recovery of *Streptococcus milleri* and other streptococcal species with acute sinusitis leading to intraorbital and/or intracranial

Table 30-1 Microbiology of Acute, Subacute, and Chronic Sinusitis

Microorganism	Frequency		
	Common	Occasional	Uncommon
Streptococcus pneumoniae	A*, C†		
Haemophilus influenzae, nontypable	A, C		
Moraxella catarrhalis	A, C		
Streptococcus pyogenes		A, C	
Other streptococcal species (including *Streptococcus milleri*)		A, C	
Staphylococcus aureus (including methicillin-resistant *S. aureus*)		C	A
Diphtheroids		C	
Coagulase-negative staphylococci		C	
Other Gram-negatives, moraxella, neisseria		C	A
Anaerobes		C	A
Respiratory viruses		A, C	
Fungi (aspergillus, alternaria, other dematiaceous fungi, zygomycetes)‡		C	A
Acanthamoeba§			A

*Acute and subacute sinusitis.
†Chronic sinusitis.
‡Primarily in immunocompromised hosts or associated with allergic fungal sinusitis.
§Primarily in immunocompromised hosts.

complications in children and adults.[33,34] *Staphylococcus aureus* and anaerobes are uncommon causes of acute and subacute pediatric sinusitis; however, they are more frequently identified in severe, complicated disease, or, in the case of anaerobes, associated with dental disease.[35] Less commonly recovered bacteria include Gram-negative organisms such as *Eikenella corrodens* and other *Moraxella* and *Neisseria* species. Fungi are uncommonly recovered in acute sinusitis except in immunocompromised patients.[27] The protozoan *Acanthamoeba* has also been identified as a rare cause of sinusitis in severely immunosuppressed hosts.[36,37] Sinus aspirates are sterile in approximately 30% to 35% of children with clinically and/or radiographically diagnosed sinusitis.[1,26,30,38] Respiratory viruses are recovered from approximately 10% of sinus aspirates; whether or not they play a direct pathogenic role in the sinus is poorly understood, but it is clear that viral rhinosinusitis and bacterial sinusitis may have overlapping clinical (and radiographic) features that make clinical diagnosis of the latter entity challenging.[32]

Microbiology of Chronic Sinusitis

Infection is a key component in most cases of pediatric chronic sinusitis, although concomitant factors may be an important contributor to the chronic inflammatory process.[39] In numerous studies, 65% to 100% of children with chronic sinusitis have positive cultures of sinus aspirates.[7,40-44] Rates of recovery of specific organisms vary among studies; this variability is likely to be

explained by differences in patient populations, sinuses evaluated, specimen collection methods, and microbiologic culture techniques. Despite these differences, certain general observations can be made. *S. pneumoniae*, *H. influenzae*, and *M. catarrhalis* are frequently isolated from children with chronic sinusitis and mirror common pathogens in acute and subacute sinusitis[7,41,45] (see Table 30-1). With increasing chronicity, other organisms may also be recovered, including *S. aureus*, *S. pyogenes*, alpha streptococci (including *Streptococcus milleri*), group D streptococci, diphtheroids, coagulase-negative staphylococci, neisseria species, Gram-negative aerobic rods (including *Pseudomonas aeruginosa*), and anaerobes; infection is frequently polymicrobial.[40,42-44] *S. aureus* and anaerobes tend to be disproportionately associated with protracted, severe, or complicated disease.[46-49] In concert with the overall increase in community-acquired methicillin-resistant *S. aureus* (MRSA) infections, an increased frequency of MRSA-associated sinus infections has been observed.[50] Recovery of anaerobes (e.g. peptococcus, peptostreptococcus, *Propionibacterium acnes*, prevotella, veillonella, fusobacterium, bacteroides, and actinomyces) has varied widely from less than 5% to more than 90%, depending on the populations and sinuses evaluated and microbiologic methods employed.[40-44,51,52] Many anaerobic isolates are β-lactamase producing.[35,53] Fungi, including Aspergillus, Alternaria, and other dematiaceous species (e.g., Bipolaris and Curvularia), and zygomycetes are occasionally isolated, although invasive disease is uncommon except in immunocompromised children.[43] Respiratory viruses are occasionally identified in sinus mucosal or lavage specimens.[54,55] Interestingly, bilateral cultures of the sinuses are often discordant.[7,44]

Antibiotic resistance has emerged as an important factor in the microbiology of chronic sinusitis. For example, in a 4-year retrospective review of maxillary sinus aspirates from children with sinusitis for more than 8 weeks, rates of nonsusceptibility of *S. pneumoniae* (recovered in 19% of cultures) were 64% for penicillin, 40% for cefotaxime, and 18% for clindamycin.[7] Of *H. influenzae* isolates (recovered in 24%), 44% were nonsusceptible to ampicillin, and all *M. catarrhalis* isolates (recovered in 17%) were β-lactamase positive.

Immune Pathogenesis

There are few studies in the literature on the immunopathology of sinusitis in children. Most of our knowledge is derived from studies conducted on adults with chronic hyperplastic sinusitis and nasal polyposis (CHS/NP). In adults, chronic sinusitis is characterized by mucosal thickening, goblet cell hyperplasia, subepithelial fibrosis, and persistent inflammation[57] (Figure 30-2). Although not fully understood, these fibrotic changes are thought to be driven by activated eosinophils and their products, including the profibrotic transforming growth factor-β,[58] GM-CSF,[59,60] and interleukin (IL)-11.[61] Tissue fibroblasts are stimulated to increase the synthesis and deposition of collagen and matrix products, resulting in thickening of the sub-basement membrane layer.

Current views associate sensitivity to aeroallergens as a primary pathologic mechanism in the development of chronic sinusitis in both adults[62,63] and children.[64] Many studies have shown that the composition of the inflammatory substrate in chronic sinusitis is similar to that seen in allergic rhinitis and the late-phase response to antigen challenge.[62,65]

Th2-Mediated Eosinophilic Inflammation

Although many immune cell types are involved in the pathogenesis of chronic sinusitis, a specific subclass of T lymphocytes (i.e.

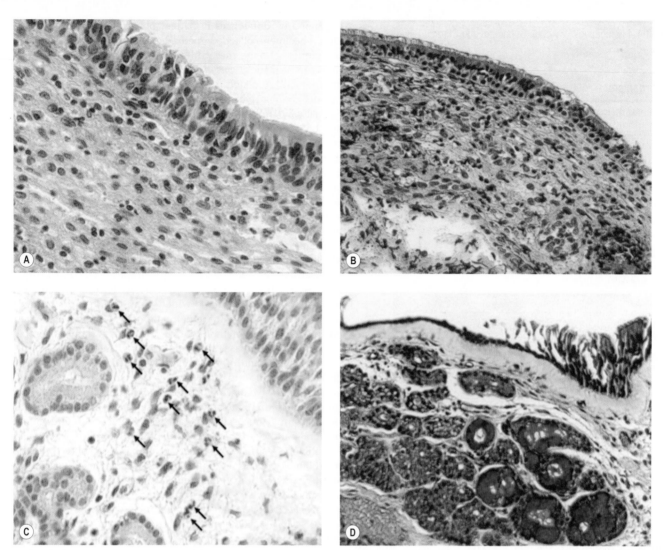

Figure 30-2 Chronic sinusitis: sinus mucosal biopsies from children (A and B) and adults (C and D). **(A)** and **(C)**: Hematoxylin and eosin stained (original magnification ×400). Arrows on the adult photo (C) point to some of the eosinophils in this image. There is a relative abundance of lymphocytes and scarcity of eosinophils in the pediatric specimen (A) compared with adult tissue (C). **(B)** and **(D)**: Pentachrome stained (original magnification ×200). Arrows on the adult photo (D) point to thickened basement membrane. Basement membrane thickening, mucous gland hyperplasia and hypertrophy, and loss of columnar epithelium in the adult sample (D) are not seen in the pediatric sample (B).

T helper cell type 2 [Th2] lymphocytes) and eosinophils appear to have a central role. The orchestration of cellular recruitment and activation of the inflammatory infiltrate in CHS/NP have been largely attributed to the Th2 cells and their cytokines (i.e. IL-3, IL-4, IL-5, IL-9, IL-13, GM-CSF). Among immune cell types, eosinophils are the most characteristic and are found in 80% to 90% of nasal polyps.[66] A histopathologic study has investigated the inflammatory cells in pediatric chronic sinusitis and reported similar findings: the numbers of eosinophils, and to a much lesser extent mast cells and T lymphocytes, are significantly increased in children with chronic sinusitis compared to control subjects[67] (see Figure 30-2). In these studies, the degree of tissue eosinophilia was not affected by the allergic status of patients. This is in agreement with published studies on chronic sinusitis in the adult population where the level of eosinophilic infiltration was found to be similar between allergic and nonallergic patients with either chronic sinusitis without nasal polyps[68,69] or CHS/NP.[70,71] Levels of neutrophils are also increased in the sinus lavage fluid of adults with chronic sinusitis, particularly in nonallergic patients.[72]

Allergic fungal sinusitis (AFS), an uncommon condition due to an intense and chronic allergic reaction to fungi growing in aller-

gic mucin within the sinus cavities, is believed to be pathogenically similar to allergic bronchopulmonary mycoses.[73,74] Mostly dematiaceous fungi (e.g. *Aspergillus, Alternaria, Curvularia, Bipolaris*) have been cultured from affected sinuses. Nasal polyposis, facial deformity, bony erosion of the sinuses, proptosis, and fungal hyphae in allergic mucin filling the sinuses are common in children with AFS.[75-77] Because of its destructive nature, AFS is managed aggressively, with topical and oral corticosteroids after surgical debridement.[73,77] Antifungal therapy (e.g. itraconazole) has been associated with clinical improvement, oral steroid reduction, and resolution of disease.[56,78] A randomized, controlled trial with antifungal therapy has not yet been performed.

Chronic rhinosinusitis in young children differs pathologically from the common phenotypes in older children and adults. Sinus mucosal biopsies from younger children (median age 3.9 years; range 1.4–8.2) with chronic rhinosinusitis (i.e. despite at least two courses of antibiotics, one with a second-line agent), when compared with adult sinusitis controls, had significantly less eosinophils, less basement membrane thickness, less submucosal mucous glands, and less epithelial injury.[79] These young children had more CD8+ (cytotoxic T lymphocytes), CD20+ (B lymphocytes), myeloperoxidase-positive (neutrophils), and CD68[+] (monocytes, macrophages) cells in sinus epithelium and/or submucosal tissues.[80] Those whose sinus cultures grew a bacterial pathogen (55%) had significantly more submucosal neutrophils. This pan-immune histopathology might indicate inadequate and/or dysregulated immune responses to bacterial biofilms and/or common respiratory viruses.

It seems, therefore, that the immunopathologic mechanisms underlying the development of some forms of chronic sinusitis, especially CHS/NP and allergic fungal sinusitis, are largely related to the effects of Th2 cytokines and their receptors, such that the final pathologic profile of intense eosinophilic infiltration is a common finding of chronic sinusitis in both atopic and nonatopic patients. In young children, the common pathology differs from CHS/NP, indicating different immunopathologic mechanisms.

Asthma and Allergy Risk Factors

Along with histologic evidence that the immune pathologic processes of chronic sinusitis and asthma can be similar, radiographic and clinical studies also link sinusitis with asthma. Using plain radiography of the sinuses, the prevalence of radiographic sinus abnormalities was significantly higher in asthmatic children (31%) than nonasthmatic controls (0%).[81] In asthmatic children who were hospitalized for an acute exacerbation, significant radiographic abnormalities of the sinuses were revealed in 87% of the patients.[82] A study of patients undergoing surgery for chronic sinusitis found that sinus CT evidence of extensive disease was associated with asthma, allergen sensitization, and peripheral blood eosinophilia.[83] Of those with eosinophilia, 87% had extensive sinus disease.

Allergic rhinitis and inhalant allergen sensitization have also been associated with sinusitis in children. In a large birth cohort study (Children's Respiratory Study, Tucson, Arizona), both allergic rhinitis and grass pollen sensitization were significant and independent risk factors for sinusitis in childhood (i.e. age 8 years).[4] Experimentally, in allergic rhinitis subjects, nasal provocation with allergen induced sinus radiographic changes (i.e. mucosal thickening, sinus opacification) and symptoms of headache and pressure in the maxillary sinuses.[84]

Genetic Risk Factors

Association studies between chronic sinusitis and genetic markers in a few candidate genes have been reported. Chronic rhinosinusitis, and sometimes nasal polyposis, are hallmark features of cystic fibrosis (CF) and primary ciliary dyskinesia, two autosomal recessive inherited disorders. In some chronic sinusitis patients without CF, mutations in the cystic fibrosis transmembrane regulator (CFTR) gene have been recently observed. In a cohort of 147 white adults with chronic sinusitis, the proportion of chronic sinusitis patients who were found to have a CFTR mutation (7%) was significantly higher than in nonsinusitis controls (2%).[85] Furthermore, 9 of the 10 CF carriers also had the CFTR polymorphism M470V. M470V homozygotes were also overrepresented in the remaining sinusitis patients. A similar study in children with chronic sinusitis found that 12% were carrying CFTR mutations compared with the expected 3% to 4% in the nonsinusitis control group.[86] However, if a CFTR mutation carrier is susceptible to chronic sinusitis, then one would expect the siblings of CF patients to have a higher incidence of chronic sinusitis. A questionnaire survey failed to detect a difference in the prevalence of rhinosinusitis between 261 obligate CF heterozygotes and 201 control subjects.[87]

Modest to marginally significant linkages of promoter region polymorphisms in other candidate genes with specific phenotypes of chronic rhinosinusitis have been reported, including TNF-α (CHS/NP),[88] LTC4 synthase (chronic hyperplastic eosinophilic sinusitis),[89] TGF-β1 (chronic rhinosinusitis with aspirin-intolerant asthma),[90] TNF-β2 (chronic sinusitis),[91] and the major histocompatilbility B54 haplotype (chronic sinusitis).[92] Replicated observations for these genetic linkages have not yet been reported. One genome-wide screen suggested that a locus in chromosome 7q31.1-7q32.1 was linked to chronic rhinosinusitis.[93] This locus includes the CFTR gene, although genotyping 38 CFTR mutations did not reveal CFTR variation accounting for this linkage.

Other Risk Factors

Medical conditions that render children susceptible to acute and chronic sinus disease include immune deficiencies (especially T and B lymphocyte defects and acquired immune deficiencies, such as AIDS, and patients receiving immunosuppressive medications) and primary ciliary dyskinesias. The association of gastroesophageal reflux disease (GERD) with chronic sinusitis has also received attention. GERD, diagnosed by pH-monitored nasopharyngeal acid reflux[94] or esophageal biopsy,[95] was associated with rhinosinusitis in children. Phipps and colleagues[96] also reported significantly increased nasopharyngeal reflux in children with chronic sinusitis when compared with a historical control group. Antireflux treatment of their GERD-positive cohort resulted in a 79% improvement in chronic sinusitis symptoms. However, a randomized, controlled trial demonstrating posttreatment improvement in sinus disease by radiographic imaging and resolution of GERD by pH studies is currently lacking.

Sinusitis Management

Overview

Medical histories and physical examinations can help to distinguish sinusitis in children from URTIs and other masqueraders and to identify complications from sinusitis and underlying risk factors for chronic recurrent disease. Radiographic imaging studies are particularly helpful in evaluating children with chronic, recurrent, or complicated sinusitis. Sinus washings for bacterial culture and targeted antimicrobial therapy, while ideal, are surgical procedures (e.g. antral irrigation) that require general anesthesia in children. Therefore, their use is generally reserved for (1) children with chronic sinusitis that does not adequately improve with multiple courses of antibiotics, (2) sinusitis with complications, and (3) sinusitis in immunocompromised hosts. Differential diagnostic considerations are provided in Box 30.1.

Consensus-based guidelines on the management of sinusitis in children have been published,[1,97,98] including a report from a subcommittee of the American Academy of Pediatrics in conjunction with the American Academy of Allergy, Asthma and Immunology, the American Academy of Otolaryngology–Head and Neck Surgery, and the American College of Emergency Physicians. These consensus guidelines, along with randomized controlled trials, systematic reviews and meta-analyses of specific management topics, when reported, have been considered in the following discussion.

BOX 30-1

Differential Diagnosis and Risk Factors for Acute and Chronic Sinusitis in Children

Acute Sinusitis

Prolonged viral upper respiratory tract infection

Foreign body in the nose

Acute exacerbation of inhalant allergies

Acute adenoiditis or adenotonsillitis

Chronic Sinusitis

Rhinitis, allergic and nonallergic

Anatomic causes of nasopharyngeal obstruction

    Turbinate hypertrophy

    Adenoid hypertrophy

    Nasal polyps

    Severe septal deviation

    Choanal atresia

    Asthma

Neoplasms of the nose and nasopharynx

    Juvenile angiofibroma

    Rhabdomyosarcoma

    Lymphoma

    Dermoid cyst

Cystic fibrosis

Lymphocyte immune deficiencies

    B lymphocytes – antibody deficiencies

    T lymphocyte deficiencies – congenital and acquired

Primary ciliary dyskinesias

Wegener's granulomatosis

Churg-Strauss vasculitis

Dental caries/abscess

Gastroesophageal reflux disease with nasopharyngeal reflux

History and Physical Examination

Acute Sinusitis

Nasal discharge (77%) and cough (80%) lasting longer than 10 to 14 days are the common symptoms of sinusitis in children.[26] Nasal discharge can be of any quality, and cough can be daytime, nighttime, or both. Fever may accompany the illness. Although headaches and sinus tenderness are generally believed to be the hallmarks of sinusitis, a study of 200 sinusitis patients did not find a significant correlation of facial pain or headache with abnormal findings on sinus CT.[99] Additionally, the reported regions of facial pain did not correlate with radiographically identified sinus abnormalities. The nasal cavity is usually filled with discharge and the nasal muscosa and turbinates are generally edematous. Following decongestion of the nasal cavity, purulent drainage coming from the middle meatus can sometimes be observed in older children. Tenderness over the frontal sinus in older children may indicate frontal sinus disease, but tenderness, in general, is rare in children with acute disease. Transillumination, considered by some to be a useful tool in adults, is unreliable in children.

Chronic Sinusitis

The most common symptoms associated with chronic sinusitis in children are nasal discharge (59%), facial pain/discomfort (33%), nasal congestion (30%), cough (19%), and wheezing (19%).[97]

Nasal discharge can be of any quality, but purulent discharge is the most common. Daytime mouth-breathing and snoring are common complaints. Examination of the nasal cavity may or may not reveal nasal discharge. The nasal turbinates are generally enlarged and can be edematous or erythematous. Although facial pain or discomfort may be a common complaint, tenderness over the sinuses is an uncommon finding in children.

Radiographic Imaging

A consensus report provided by the American College of Radiology[100] provided appropriateness criteria of various radiographic imaging modalities in assessing pediatric sinus disease. Currently, coronal CT is the recommended examination for imaging persistent or chronic sinusitis in patients of any age. Plain sinus radiographs (Waters and Caldwell projections), although widely available, can both underdiagnose and overdiagnose sinus soft tissue changes. Magnetic resonance imaging provides superlative soft tissue delineation; however, it is expensive, has limited availability, and does not provide bony details of the osteomeatal complex. Conventional tomography, nuclear medicine studies, and ultrasound have significant limitations for imaging the sinuses.

It is tempting to consider sinus mucosal abnormalities and associated anatomic variations seen in imaging studies in symptomatic patients as clear indications for sinusitis therapy (e.g. antimicrobial therapy and sinus surgery). However, the clinical importance of such findings is challenged by studies that have revealed a high prevalence of such soft tissue findings in people without sinusitis symptoms or with URTIs.[18,19] In these studies, URTI symptoms and associated radiographic sinus abnormalities have improved without specific sinusitis therapy (i.e. no antibiotics or surgery for sinusitis).

The American College of Radiology consensus report has the following recommendations: (1) the diagnoses of acute and chronic sinusitis should be made clinically and not on the basis of imaging findings alone; (2) no imaging studies are indicated for acute sinusitis except for cases where complications are suspected or cases that are not responding to therapy; and (3) if imaging information in patients with chronic sinusitis is desired, coronal sinus CT is recommended. The use of plain radiographs of the sinuses (i.e. Waters and Caldwell views) is generally discouraged in this report, except in children younger than 4 years of age. The use of Waters view radiographs in children is supported by a study in which the sensitivity and specificity of a Waters view radiograph to diagnose chronic sinusitis in children were 76% and 81%, respectively.[101] In the same study, limited coronal CT scans were better than sinus X-rays and nearly as good as full sinus CT evaluations.

Sinusitis Complications

Complications of sinusitis (Table 30-2) are generally believed to be acute events that result from a combination of outflow obstruction and pathogenic bacteria in the sinuses. Intracranial extension of infection is by direct erosion, thrombophlebitis, or extension through preformed pathways (e.g. fracture lines). The incidence of intracranial complications in children hospitalized for sinusitis was 3%.[102]

Orbital complications from sinusitis are primarily the result of acute ethmoid disease but could occasionally be extensions of frontal disease.[103] A classic description of the progression of sinusitis to orbital complications is as follows: inflammatory edema, orbital cellulitis, subperiosteal abscess, orbital abscess, and cavernous sinus thrombosis.[104] The most common presentations of orbital complications include eyelid edema, orbital pain,

Table 30-2 Sinusitis Complications (by Sinus Involvement)

Complication	Maxillary Sinus	Ethmoid Sinus	Frontal Sinus	Sphenoid Sinus
Osteomyelitis	+		+ +	
Mucocele	+ +	++	++	+
Preseptal cellulitis		+++		
Orbital cellulitis		+++	+	
Subperiosteal abscess		+++		
Orbital abscess	+			
Meningitis			++	
Epidural abscess			++	
Subdural abscess			+	
Brain abscess			+	

+++, Frequent; ++, less frequent; +, least frequent.

diplopia, proptosis, and chemosis, as well as fever, nasal discharge, and headache.[105] In a cohort of children with orbital complications from sinusitis, 72% of hospitalized children had a history of a URTI, and 24% had received oral antibiotic therapy prior to their presentation with orbital complications.[105] It can be difficult to differentiate between preseptal cellulitis and orbital cellulitis on clinical parameters alone (i.e. based on lid edema and pain without an imaging study). In orbital cellulitis, proptosis progresses and leads to chemosis and ophthalmoplegia. Fortunately, orbital abscesses and cavernous sinus thrombosis caused by sinusitis are rarely seen today.

Intracranial complications from sinusitis are primarily the result of frontal sinus disease.[102] There are many similarities between the pathogenesis of intracranial extension of frontal sinusitis and that of otitis media. The classic presentations of the progression from meningitis to the various intracranial abscesses will not be discussed here. Intracranial complications in the pre-antibiotic era were devastating, with mortality rates of up to 75%. Current mortality rates for these complications are between 10% to 20%. Cavernous sinus thrombosis is a unique intracranial complication of ethmoid and sphenoid sinusitis by direct extension. This complication is characterized by a toxic-appearing patient with infectious/inflammatory involvement of cranial nerves III, IV and VI, resulting in ophthalmoplegia. Progressive disease within the cavernous sinus can lead to carotid artery thrombosis and mycotic aneurysm formation, resulting in neurologic sequelae and death.

Complications of maxillary sinusitis are rare. Mucoceles in the maxillary sinus are occasionally encountered in children with cystic fibrosis, but they are unusual in the general pediatric population. Osteomyelitis of the maxillary sinus was more prevalent in the preantibiotic era and in adults with dental disease. This appears to be a rare complication today – there have been no reported cases in the literature since the 1950s.

Sinusitis Treatment

Antimicrobial Therapy

Acute and Subacute Sinusitis

The goals of therapy for acute and subacute sinusitis are to hasten clinical improvement, prevent intracranial and orbital complica-

---

BOX 30-2 Key concepts

Use of Antimicrobials in Sinusitis

- For acute and subacute sinusitis, target therapy toward the same pathogens responsible for acute otitis media: *Streptococcus pneumoniae, Haemophilus influenzae,* and *Moraxella catarrhalis.*

- Broad-spectrum antibiotics targeting β-lactamase-producing organisms and resistant *S. pneumoniae* should be used when there is:

  Poor response to first-line antibiotics

  Moderate–severe, chronic, or recurrent disease

  Complicated or potentially complicated disease (including frontal or sphenoidal involvement)

  High risk for first-line antibiotic-resistant organisms: antibiotic therapy within the preceding 30–90 days, daycare attendance, age <2 years

- Treat until asymptomatic plus an additional 7 days (at least 10 days).

- Consider sinus aspiration for microbiologic identification and targeted antimicrobial therapy if disease is:

  Severe

  Associated with orbital or intracranial complications

  Unresponsive to multiple antibiotic courses

  In immunocompromised patients

---

tions, and prevent mucosal damage that may predispose to chronic sinus disease[27,28] (Box 30.2). The actual benefit of antibiotics in achieving these goals has not been conclusively proven. A pivotal randomized trial showed that antibiotic therapy (amoxicillin or amoxicillin-clavulanic acid) for acute sinusitis, defined by clinical and plain radiograph criteria, was associated with symptom resolution in 66% of children at 10 days, significantly greater than the 43% rate of resolution among placebo-treated subjects.[106] Two more recent randomized trials call into question the benefit of antibiotic treatment. One compared amoxicillin, amoxicillin-clavulanate, and placebo in children with clinically diagnosed acute sinusitis and found no differences among groups in symptom improvement at 14 days (79% to 81% in each) nor in relapse and recurrence rates.[107] The other compared cefuroxime and placebo in children with nonimproving respiratory symptoms and abnormal maxillary sinus ultrasonography; no difference in rates of clinical cure (57–63%) or in rates of improvement or cure (84–91%)at 14 days were observed.[108] A meta-analysis of six randomized, controlled (comparison to placebo or symptomatic therapies) pediatric trials, four of which were limited to acute sinusitis and two of which included chronic sinusitis, suggested the benefit of antibiotics in reducing persistence of symptoms. Benefit was modest, however, with approximately eight children requiring therapy for one additional child with cure or improvement.[109] As in children, meta-analyses of studies in adults with acute sinusitis suggest a benefit of antibiotic therapy, but note that these benefits are small to modest.[110–114] Because studies suggest that about two thirds of adults with acute sinusitis improve without antibiotic treatment,[110] the need for antibiotic treatment in adults with acute sinusitis, except in moderate to severe disease, has been questioned.[112,114–117]

Despite lack of definitive proof of efficacy, antibiotic treatment is recommended for most children with acute and subacute sinusitis because bacterial pathogens are recoverable from the majority of affected sinuses,[1,17] and preventing sinusitis complications is a major concern. There is a paucity of trial data in children to indicate which antibiotics may be superior, although studies performed in adults suggest comparable clinical efficacy of commonly used agents.[21] Antibiotic selection is frequently directed by typical susceptibility profiles of frequently isolated bacteria and pharmacokinetic properties of candidate antibiotics[27,28] (Table 30-3). Because their microbiology is similar, the approach to antibiotic selection for acute and subacute sinusitis is similar. Amoxicillin is commonly recommended for previously untreated, mild, and uncomplicated acute sinusitis based on its excellent tolerability, low cost, narrow spectrum, and track record for both sinusitis and otitis media.[1,116,118] This parallels recommendations for adults, in whom meta-analyses of randomized trials support the efficacy of amoxicillin (and penicillin) for acute sinusitis.[110,119,120] However, a 5% to 20% failure rate can be expected with amoxicillin because of resistant *S. pneumoniae*, *H. influenzae*, and *M. catarrhalis*.[1,31] High-dose amoxicillin (80 to 90 mg/kg/day) can be used to improve eradication of potentially resistant *S. pneumoniae* in children with risk factors for antibiotic resistance (e.g. antibiotic therapy within the preceding 30 to 90 days, daycare attendance, and/or age <2 years).[1,27] Initial therapy with a broader antibiotic targeting β-lactamase-producing organisms and resistant *S. pneumoniae* should be considered in the following circumstances: a history of poor response to amoxicillin; moderate-severe, complicated, or potentially complicated disease (including frontal or sphenoidal involvement); protracted or recurrent disease; and high risk for antibiotic resistance.[31,118] Options include amoxicillin-clavulanic acid (80 to 90 mg/kg/day of amoxicillin component if risk factors for resistance are present), cefuroxime, and oral third-generation cephalosporins (especially cefpodoxime and cefdinir). Macrolides such as clarithromycin and azithromycin are less useful because of increasing resistance of *S. pneumoniae* and marginal in vivo activity versus *H. influenzae* unless other options are limited by the patient being allergic to β-lactams.[1,27,118] The role of trimethoprim-sulfamethoxazole has been reduced by increasing resistance of both *S. pneumoniae* and *H. influenzae*; it remains an option in patients with beta-lactam allergy or known infection with methicillin-resistant *Staphylococcus aureus*.[1,27,28,118] Clindamycin can be useful if there is a known or suspected Gram-positive (e.g. *S. pneumoniae* or *S. aureus*, including many methicillin-susceptible and methicillin-resistant *S. aureus*) and/or anaerobic pathogen, but it offers no activity against *H. influenzae* or *M. catarrhalis*. Newer quinolones (e.g. levofloxacin, moxifloxacin, gatifloxacin) are active against the most frequent pathogens and have excellent sinus penetration and demonstrated efficacy in adults; however, evaluation of their safety and efficacy in children is needed.[27,121,122] In some cases, combinations of antimicrobial agents targeting Gram-positive and Gram-negative organisms may be appropriate.[28]

If amoxicillin is chosen for initial therapy, lack of clinical response within 48 to 72 hours should prompt a change to a broader agent if sinusitis is still considered the correct diagnosis.[28,31] If the disease becomes severe, protracted, associated with orbital or intracranial complications, or unresponsive to multiple antibiotic trials, sinus lavage for microbiologic diagnosis and/or intravenous antibiotics (e.g. cefotaxime, ceftriaxone, vancomycin, clindamycin) can be considered.[1,19,118] In immunocompromised hosts, sinus lavage should be considered earlier because of their increased risk for atypical and resistant organisms and their impaired immune response to them.[31,118]

There has been no systematic evaluation of the optimal duration of antibiotic therapy for acute sinusitis in children. Data obtained in adults suggest that treatment for 10 days affords microbiologic cure rates in excess of 90%, whereas 7-day courses are associated with microbiologic failure in 20%. However, treatment courses as short as 1 to 5 days in children have had encouraging clinical results in a limited number of trials.[123–125] In general, a 10- to 14-day treatment course is recommended for the majority of children, tailored to a patient's response (e.g. treat until asymptomatic plus an additional 7 days).[1,31,118,126] Longer courses (e.g. 3 to 4 weeks) should be considered for severe disease or if resolution is unusually slow.[27,32,118,126]

Table 30-3 Selected Antibiotics for Acute, Subacute, and Chronic Sinusitis

Antibiotic	Comments
Penicillins	
Amoxicillin	Untreated, mild, uncomplicated disease; high dose targets resistant *Streptococcus pneumoniae*
Amoxicillin-clavulanate	Poor response to amoxicillin; moderate–severe, complicated, or protracted disease; or high risk for antibiotic resistance
	High dose of amoxicillin component targets resistant *S. pneumoniae*
Cephalosporins Cefuroxime Cefpodoxime Cefdinir Cefotaxime Ceftriaxone	Poor response to amoxicillin; moderate–severe, complicated, or protracted disease; or high risk for antibiotic resistance. Intravenous agents for severe or complicated disease or disease unresponsive to oral antibiotics
Macrolides Clarithromycin Azithromycin	Option if significant β-lactam allergy; increasing resistance of *S. pneumoniae* and marginal activity against *Haemophilus influenzae*
Trimethoprim-sulfamethoxazole	Option if significant β-lactam allergy or if known methicillin-resistant *Staphylococcus aureus*; increasing resistance of *S. pneumoniae* and *H. influenzae*
Clindamycin	Activity against Gram-positive aerobes (including many *S. pneumoniae*, many methicillin-susceptible and methicillin-resistant *S. aureus*, and streptococci) and anaerobes; option if significant β-lactam allergy
Vancomycin	Intravenous; severe or complicated disease or disease unresponsive to oral antibiotics

Chronic Sinusitis

Few studies of the efficacy of antibiotics in hastening clinical improvement from and preventing complications of chronic sinusitis have been reported, and have inconsistent findings. In atopic children with chronic sinusitis, amoxicillin and trimetho-prim-sulfamethoxazole were associated with higher response rates than either erythromycin or an oral antihistamine/decongestant without antibiotic.[127] However, in other studies of subacute or chronic sinusitis, response rates with antibiotic therapy plus decongestant were not greater than those with decongestant plus nasal saline[128] or with placebo or drainage procedures.[45]

Despite lack of firm evidence of efficacy, antibiotics are generally prescribed for chronic sinusitis because pathogenic bacteria in the sinuses have been well documented. Broad-spectrum antibiotics are chosen for empirical therapy, with the choice dependent on previous treatments and anticipated resistance patterns of pathogens such as *S. pneumoniae, H. influenzae, M. catarrhalis, and S. aureus* (see Table 30-3). Favorable options include amoxicillin-clavulanic acid, cefuroxime, and third-generation cephalosporins such as cefpodoxime and cefdinir. If these agents are unsuccessful, a trial of clindamycin to target β-lactam-resistant *S. pneumoniae,* methicillin-susceptible and methicillin-resistant *S. aureus,* and anaerobes is reasonable.[27,129,130] Trimethoprim-sulfamethoxazole may be helpful for a patient with known infection with methicillin-resistant *S. aureus* resistant to clindamycin. The roles of oxazolidinones (e.g. linezolid) and newer quinolones for pediatric chronic sinusitis are yet to be determined. After multiple failed antibiotic courses, concern for resistant organisms increases, and sinus lavage for culture and susceptibilities should be considered to facilitate targeted antibiotic treatment.[7,31,41,118,131] Nasal swabs have insufficient positive predictive value to accurately guide antibiotic therapy.[38,44,54,132] Middle meatus swabs may have better, although still imperfect, correlation with sinus cultures.[44,54,133] Patients with very resistant isolates and/or extremely refractory disease may benefit from intravenous therapy with agents such as cefotaxime, ceftriaxone, cefuroxime, ampicillin-sulbactam, ticarcillin-clavulanate, piperacillin-tazobactam, vancomycin, or clindamycin.[41,118,131,134] For invasive fungal sinusitis, surgical debridement and systemic antifungal therapy are indicated.[135]

The optimal duration of therapy is unknown. A minimum of 14 days is generally recommended if there is a prompt response. Longer courses (e.g. 3 to 6 weeks) can be considered for slower responses, and treatment for 7 days beyond the patient becoming symptom-free has been suggested.[32,118,126] It has been suggested that prolonged courses of intravenous antibiotics may be effective for treating bacteria in sinus-containing biofilms; however, this concept remains to be proven.[17]

Antibiotic prophylaxis with agents such as amoxicillin or sulfonamides was previously used for children with recurrent sinusitis by analogy with recurrent otitis media.[31,97] An alternative approach was short-term, preemptive prophylaxis with the onset of a URTI in children who have frequently recurrent sinusitis triggered by URTIs, a strategy that was beneficial for recurrent otitis media.[136] However, increasing rates of antibiotic resistance and resulting impetus to reduce antibiotic exposure has restricted prophylactic antibiotic strategies in recent years.[1,32,137]

Sinus Surgery

Acute Sinusitis

The indications to perform sinus surgery on a child with acute and uncomplicated sinusitis are limited. Acute sinusitis symptoms are generally relieved by medical therapy consisting of antibiotics and adjunctive medical therapy. However, acute frontal or sphenoidal sinusitis in an adolescent may benefit from emergent surgical drainage for pain relief. In immunocompromised hosts, sinus irrigations to obtain specimens for microbial staining and culturing may be needed to identify potentially unusual, opportunistic pathogens.

Chronic Sinusitis

Endoscopic sinus surgery (ESS) was popularized after sinus surgery using endoscopes was imported from Europe by American surgeons in the 1980s. The safety and efficacy of this procedure in pediatric sinusitis cases have been reported, based primarily on satisfaction questionnaires.[138-140] A meta-analysis using data from eight published studies and personal data on the outcomes of pediatric ESS concluded that ESS is a safe and effective treatment of chronic sinusitis in children.[141] However, it is important to note that all the studies included in this analysis lack an untreated control group, and all except one of the nine data sources used were retrospective chart reviews.

Others have reported symptomatic and clinical improvements following ESS in special populations such as children with severe asthma[142] and cystic fibrosis.[143] Opposing this trend have been sporadic commentaries challenging the impression that pediatric sinusitis is a surgical disease.[137,144] Indeed, in a cohort of children who have undergone ESS at an early age, a markedly higher rate of revision surgeries (50%) was required (e.g. for postsurgical osteomeatal scarring), in comparison with a control group of young, chronic sinusitis patients who had not had prior sinus surgery (9%).[145]

Despite its unproven clinical efficacy and uncertain indications, ESS has safety attributes that surpass those of its predecessors. ESS with pediatric instrumentation can provide sinus drainage and sinus ablation. Specifically, the ostium of the maxillary sinuses can be widened by endoscopic antrostomy. By performing endoscopic ethmoidectomy, the ethmoid cells and polypoid tissue can be removed, frontal duct drainage can be enhanced, and the sphenoid sinus can be entered and drained.

Surgery for Sinusitis Complications

The type of sinusitis complication dictates whether an otolaryngologist will need the additional expertise of an ophthalmologist or a neurosurgeon. Generally, the participation of a pediatrician or an infectious disease consultant in the care of a child with sinusitis complications is beneficial.

Subperiosteal and orbital abscesses can be drained through either an external or endoscopic approach. Small epidural abscesses may be treated medically. Other intracranial abscesses are usually drained by a neurosurgeon. Complicated frontal sinusitis (e.g. mucocele, osteomyelitis of the frontal bone) is treated through an external approach, with the intent to achieve drainage and debridement. Severe cases in which long-term antimicrobial therapy has failed may need sinus obliteration, cranialization, and/or other reconstructive procedures. Mucoceles of the ethmoid and sphenoid sinuses can be drained endoscopically. Children with toxic shock syndrome from sinusitis should undergo sinus irrigation for culture and drainage. Neurosurgical drainage is sometimes indicated.

Adjunctive Surgical Procedures

Adenoid hypertrophy as a cause of chronic sinusitis and the benefits of adenoidectomy for chronic sinusitis have been suggested by earlier uncontrolled studies.[146,147] A meta-analysis of 10 trials (6 cohort and 4 case series) showed significant reduction of postoperative sinusitis symptoms.[148] The basis for improvement of adenoidectomy is unknown. No correlation between maxillary sinus and adenoid cultures in patients with chronic rhinosinusitis was found by Tuncer.[16] The authors suggested that the adenoids may act as a barrier for mechanical obstruction. However, the potential role of biofilm on the adenoids was raised by Coticchia and colleagues,[149] who found an abundance of biofilm coating the surface of adenoid surgical specimens in patients with chronic rhinosinusitis as compared to patients with obstructive sleep apnea. Chronic sinusitis patients with nasal obstruction from adenoid hypertrophy are likely to have some symptomatic benefit from an adenoidectomy regardless of effects on the sinuses.

Some children with chronic sinusitis have inferior turbinate hypertrophy causing nasal obstruction. There are no published reports on the efficacy of inferior turbinate cauterization or reduction in the treatment of chronic sinusitis. In subjects in whom intranasal corticosteroid therapy for nasal obstructive symptoms associated with inferior turbinate hypertrophy has failed, a turbinate reduction procedure for symptomatic relief may be considered.

Adjunctive Medical Therapy

Clinicians have used an assortment of agents in conjunction with oral antibiotics for the treatment of both acute and chronic sinusitis in children, including: nasal saline (isotonic and hypertonic) washes, topical and oral decongestants, topical and oral antihistamines, topical anticholinergic agents, leukotriene receptor antagonists, antiinfectives, and corticosteroids (intranasal and oral). The use of these agents is largely based on their theoretical benefits of improving associated rhinitis and rhinorrhea by decreasing mucosal inflammation, edema, and mucous production, and increasing mucociliary transport, thereby improving nasal patency and presumably ostial drainage. Two Cochrane Reviews addressed the efficacy of intranasal saline washes[150] and intranasal corticosteroids[151] for the symptoms of chronic rhinosinusitis in adults. Symptom scores were significantly improved by saline washes as a monotherapy and in combination with intranasal corticosteroids. There was limited support for the use of intranasal corticosteroids as monotherapy, or in combination with oral antibiotics to resolve or reduce the symptoms of sinusitis.[152] The efficacy/safety of these adjunctive medical therapies for sinusitis in children have not been reported.

Conclusions

Sinusitis in children is a common problem of widely varying duration. Unfortunately, symptoms, physical examination, and radiographic findings of sinusitis are blurred with those of common URTIs, without clearly distinguishing features. Sinusitis rarely leads to severe, life-threatening complications, which are usually the result of direct extension of bacterial infection from the sinuses.

Management of uncomplicated sinusitis consists of antimicrobial and medical adjunctive treatment aiming for symptom relief and prevention of complications and recurrence. Radiographic imaging studies may be helpful in chronic and/or recurrent sinusitis. In uncomplicated cases, limited coronal sinus CT scans are generally preferred. In complicated cases, complete coronal sinus CT series are recommended. Antral irrigation can provide sinus specimens for bacterial culture and targeted antimicrobial therapy in patients with chronic, refractory, and complicated disease. Sinus surgery in uncomplicated sinusitis, especially in young children, should generally be avoided. Great reductions in mortality caused by sinusitis complications coincide with improvements in antimicrobial and surgical therapy.

References

1. American Academy of Pediatrics. Clinical practice guideline: management of sinusitis. Pediatrics 2001;108:798–808.
2. Clement PA, Gordts F. Epidemiology and prevalence of aspecific chronic sinusitis. Int J Pediatr Otorhinolaryngol 1999;49:S101–3.
3. Aitken M, Taylor JA. Prevalence of clinical sinusitis in young children followed up by primary care pediatricians. Arch Pediatr Adolesc Med 1998;152:244–8.
4. Lombardi E, Stein RT, Wright AL, et al. The relation between physician-diagnosed sinusitis, asthma, and skin test reactivity to allergens in 8-year-old children. Pediatr Pulmonol 1996;22:141–6.
5. McCaig LF, Hughes JM. Trends in antimicrobial drug prescribing among office-based physicians in the United States. JAMA 1995;273:214–9.
6. Doern GV, Brueggemann AB, Huynh H, et al. Antimicrobial resistance with Streptococcus pneumoniae in the United States, 1997–1998. Emerg Infect Dis 1999;5:757–65.
7. Slack CL, Dahn KA, Abzug MJ, et al. Antibiotic-resistant bacteria in pediatric chronic sinusitis. Pediatr Infect Dis J 2001;20:247–50.
8. Cunningham JM, Chiu EJ, Landgraf JM, et al. The health impact of chronic recurrent rhinosinusitis in children. Arch Otolaryngol Head Neck Surg 2000;126:1363–8.
9. Parsons DS, Wald ER. Otitis media and sinusitis: similar diseases, Otolaryngol Clin North Am 1996;29:11–25.
10. Swarts JD, Alper CM, Seroky JT, et al. In vivo observation with magnetic resonance imaging of middle ear effusion in response to experimental underpressures, Ann Otol Rhinol Laryngol 1995;104:522–8.
11. Piltcher OB, Swarts JD, Magnuson K, et al. A rat model of otitis media with effusion caused by eustachian tube obstruction with and without Streptococcus pneumoniae infection: methods and disease course. Otolaryngol Head Neck Surg 2002;126:490–8.
12. Milczuk HA, Dalley HA, Wessbacher RW, et al. Nasal and paranasal sinus anomalies in children with chronic sinusitis. Laryngoscope 1993;103:247–52.
13. Lusk RP, McAlister B, el Fouley A. Anatomic variation in pediatric chronic sinusitis: a CT study. Otolaryngol Clin North Am 1996;29:75–91.
14. Al-Qudah M. The relationship between anatomical variations of the sinonasal region and chronic sinusitis extension in children. Int J Pediatr Otorhinolaryngol 2008;72:817–21.
15. Kim HJ, Jung Cho M, Tae Kim Y, et al. The relationship between anatomic variations of paranasal sinuses and chronic sinusitis in children. Acta Otolaryngol 2006;126:1067–72.
16. Tuncer U, Aydogan B, Soylu L, et al. Chronic rhinosinusitis and adenoid hypertrophy in children. Am J Otolaryngol 2004;25:5–10.
17. Novembre E, Mori F, Pucci N, et al. Systemic treatment of rhinosinusitis in children. Pediatr Allergy Immunol 2007;18(Suppl 18):56–61.
18. Puhakka T, Makela MJ, Alanen A, et al. Sinusitis in the common cold. J Allergy Clin Immunol 1998;102:403–8.
19. Gwaltney JMJ, Phillips CD, Miller RD, et al. Computed tomographic study of the common cold. N Engl J Med 1994;330:25–30.
20. Plouin-Gaudon I, Clement S, Huggler E, et al. Intracellular residency is frequently associated with recurrent Staphylococcus aureus rhinosinusitis. Rhinology 2006;44:249–54.
21. Brook I. Current issues in the management of acute bacterial sinusitis in children. Int J Pediatr Otorhinol 2007;71:1653–61.
22. Sanclement JA, Webster P, Thomas J, et al. Bacterial biofilms in surgical specimens of patients with chronic rhinosinusitis. Laryngoscope 2005;115:578–82.
23. Harvey RJ, Lund VJ. Biofilms and chronic rhinosinusitis: systematic review of evidence, current concepts and directions for research. Rhinology 2007;45(1):3–13.
24. Bolger WE, Leonard D, Dick JEJ, et al. Gram negative sinusitis: a bacteriologic and histologic study in rabbits. Am J Rhinol 1997;11:15–25.
25. Gwaltney JM. Principles and practice of infectious diseases. Philadelphia: Churchill Livingstone; 2000.
26. Wald ER, Milmoe GJ, Bowen A, et al. Acute maxillary sinusitis in children. N Engl J Med 1981;304:749–54.

27. Brook I, Gooch WM, Jenkins S, et al. Medical management of acute bacterial sinusitis. Ann Otol Rhinol Laryngol 2000;109:S2–20.
28. Sinus and Allergy Health Partnership. Antimicrobial treatment guidelines for acute bacterial rhinosinusitis. Otolaryngol-Head Neck Surg 2000;123:S1–32.
29. Tinkleman DG, Silk HJ. Clinical and bacteriologic features of chronic sinusitis in children. Am J Dis Child 1989;143:938–41.
30. Wald ER, Byers C, Guerra N, et al. Subacute sinusitis in children. J Pediatr 1989;115:28–32.
31. Wald ER. Sinusitis. Pediatr Ann 1998;27:811–8.
32. Principi N, Esposito S. New insights into pediatric rhinosinusitis. Pediatr Allergy Immunol 2007;18(Suppl 18):7–9.
33. Rankhethoa NM, Prescott CA. Significance of *Streptococcus milleri* in acute rhinosinusitis with complications. J Laryngol Otol 2008;122:810–3.
34. Hwang SY, Tan KK. *Streptococcus viridans* has a leading role in rhinosinusitis complications. Ann Otol Rhinol Laryngol 2007;116:381–5.
35. Brook I, Frazier EH, Gher ME. Microbiology of periapical accesses and associated maxillary sinusitis. J Periodontol 1996;67:608–10.
36. Kim SY, Syms MJ, Holtel MR, et al. Acanthamoeba sinusitis with subsequent dissemination in an AIDS patient. Ear Nose Throat J 2000;79:168–74.
37. Teknos TN, Poulin MD, Laruentano AM, et al. Acanthamoeba rhinosinusitis: characterization, diagnosis, and treatment. Am J Rhinol 2000;14:387391.
38. Arruda LK, Mimica IM, Sole D, et al. Abnormal maxillary sinus radiographs in children: do they represent bacterial infection? Pediatrics 1990;85:553–8.
39. Steele RW. Chronic sinusitis in children. Clin Pediatr 2005;44:465–71.
40. Brook I. Bacteriologic features of chronic sinusitis in children. JAMA 1981;246:967–9.
41. Don DM, Yellon RF, Casselbrant ML, et al. Efficacy of a stepwise protocol that includes intravenous antibiotic therapy for the management of chronic sinusitis in children and adolescents. Arch Otolaryngol Head Neck Surg 2001;127:1093–8.
42. Erkan M, Ozcan M, Arslan S, et al. Bacteriology of antrum in children with chronic maxillary sinusitis. Scand J Infect Dis 1996;28:283–5.
43. Muntz HR, Lusk RP. Bacteriology of the ethmoid bullae in children with chronic sinusitis. Arch Otolaryngol Head Neck Surg 1991;117:179–81.
44. Orobellow PW, Park RI, Belcher LJ, et al. Microbiology of chronic sinusitis in children. Arch Otolaryngol Head Neck Surg 1991;117:980–3.
45. Otten FWA, Grote JJ. Treatment of chronic maxillary sinusitis in children. Int J Pediatr Otorhinolaryngol 1988;15:269–78.
46. Brook I, Frazier EH, Foote PA. Microbiology of the transition from acute to chronic maxillary sinusitis. J Med Microbiol 1996;45:372–5.
47. Brook I, Yocum P, Frazier EH. Bacteriology and beta-lactamase activity in acute and chronic maxillary sinusitis. Arch Otolaryngol Head Neck Surg 1996;122:418–23.
48. Brook I, Frazier EH. Microbiology of subperiosteal orbital abscess and associated maxillary sinusitis. Laryngoscope 1996;106:1010–3.
49. Frederick J, Braude A. Anaerobic infection of the paranasal sinuses. N Engl J Med 1974;290:135–7.
50. Brook I, Foote PA, Hausefeld JN. Increase in the frequency of recovery of methicillin-resistant *Staphylococcus aureus* in acute and chronic maxillary sinusitis. J Med Microbiol 2008;57:1015–7.
51. Brook I. Bacteriology of chronic maxillary sinusitis in adults. Ann Otol Rhinol Laryngol 1989;98:426–8.
52. Erkan M, Aslan T, Ozcan M, et al. Bacteriology of antrum in adults with chronic maxillary sinusitis. Laryngoscope 1994;104:321–4.
53. Brook I. Chronic sinusitis in children and adults: role of bacteria and antimicrobial management. Curr Allergy Asthma Rep 2005;5:482–90.
54. Chan KH, Liu A, Abzug MJ, et al. Unpublished data.
55. Ramadan HH, Farr RW, Wetmore SJ. Adenovirus and respiratory syncytial virus in chronic sinusitis using polymerase chain reaction. Laryngoscope 1977;107:923–5.
56. Andes D, Proctor R, Bush RK, et al. Report of successful prolonged antifungal therapy for refractory allergic fungal sinusitis. Clin Infect Dis 2000;31:202–4.
57. Van Nostrand AWP, Goodman WS. Pathologic aspects of mucosal lesions of the maxillary sinus. Otolaryngol Clin North Am 1976;9:21–7.
58. Rochester CL, Ackerman SJ, Zheng T, et al. Eosinophil-fibroblast interactions: granule major basic protein interacts with IL-1 and transforming growth factor-beta in the stimulation of lung fibroblast IL-6-type cytokine production. J Immunol 1996;156:4449–56.
59. Broide DH, Paine MM, Firestein GS. Eosinophils express interleukin 5 and granulocyte macrophage-colony-stimulating factor mRNA at sites of allergic inflammation in asthmatics. J Clin Invest 1992;90:1414–24.
60. Kita H, Ohnishi T, Okubo Y, et al. Granulocyte/macrophage colony-stimulating factor and interleukin 3 release from human peripheral blood eosinophils and neutrophils. J Exp Med 1991;174:745–8.
61. Minshall E, Chakir J, Laviolette M, et al. IL-11 expression is increased in severe asthma: association with epithelial cells and eosinophils. J Allergy Clin Immunol 2000;105:232–8.
62. Durham SR, Ying S, Varney VA, et al. Cytokine messenger RNA expression for IL-3, IL-4, IL-5 and granulocyte/macrophage-colony-stimulating factor in the nasal mucosa after local allergen provocation: relationship to tissue eosinophilia. J Immunol 1992;148:2390–4.
63. Hamilos DL, Leung DYM, Wood R, et al. Evidence for distinct cytokine expression in allergic versus nonallergic chronic sinusitis. J Allergy Clin Immunol 1995;96:537–4.
64. Rachelefsky GS. Chronic sinusitis: a disease of all ages. Am J Dis Child 1989;143:886–8.
65. Varney VA, Jacobson MR, Sudderick RM, et al. Immunohistology of the nasal mucosa following allergen-induced rhinitis: identification of activated T lymphocytes, eosinophils and neutrophils. Am Rev Respir Dis 1992;146:170–6.
66. Settipane GA. Epidemiology of nasal polyps. Allergy Asthma Proc 1996;17:231–6.
67. Baroody FM, Hughes T, McDowell PR, et al. Eosinophilia in chronic childhood sinusitis. Arch Otolaryngol Head Neck Surg 1995;121:1396–02.
68. Demoly P, Crampette L, Mondain M, et al. Assessment of inflammation in noninfectious chronic maxillary sinusitis. J Allergy Clin Immunol 1994;94:95–108.
69. Wright ED, Frenkiel S, Al-Ghamdi K, et al. Interleukin-4, interleukin-5, and granulocyte-macrophage colony-stimulating factor receptor expression in chronic sinusitis and response to topical steroids. Otolaryngol Head Neck Surg 1998;118:490–5.
70. Hamilos DL, Leung DYM, Wood R, et al. Chronic hyperplastic sinusitis: association of tissue eosinophilia with mRNA expression of granulocyte-macrophage colony-stimulating factor and interleukin-3. J Allergy Clin Immunol 1993;92:39–48.
71. Hamilos DL. Chronic sinusitis. J Allergy Clin Immunol 2000;106:213–27.
72. Demoly P, Crampette L, Mondain M, et al. Myeloperoxidase and interleukin-8 levels in chronic sinusitis. Clin Exp Allergy 1997;27:672–5.
73. Schubert MS, Goetz DW. Evaluation and treatment of allergic fungal sinusitis. II. Treatment and follow-up. J Allergy Clin Immunol 1998;102:395402.
74. Schubert MS, Goetz DW. Evaluation and treatment of allergic fungal sinusitis. I. Demographics and diagnosis. J Allergy Clin Immunol 1998;102:387394.
75. Manning SC, Vuitch F, Weinberg AG, et al. Allergic aspergillosis: a newly recognized form of sinusitis in the pediatric population. Laryngoscope 1989;99:681–5.
76. Kupferberg SB, Bent JP. Allergic fungal sinusitis in the pediatric population. Arch Otolaryngol Head Neck Surg 1996;122:1381–4.
77. Campbell JM, Graham M, Gray HC, et al. Allergic fungal sinusitis in children. Ann Allergy Asthma Immunol 2006;96:286–90.
78. Seiberling K, Wormald PJ. The role of itraconazole in recalcitrant fungal sinusitis. Am J Rhinol Allergy. 2009;23:303–6.
79. Chan KH, Abzug MJ, Coffinet L, et al. Chronic rhinosinusitis in young children differs from adults: a histopathology study. J Pediatr 2004;144(2):206–12.
80. Coffinet L, Chan KH, Abzug MJ, et al. Immunopathology of chronic rhinosinusitis in young children. J Pediatr 2009;154(5):754–8.
81. Zimmerman B, Stinger D, Feanny S, et al. Prevalence of abnormalities found by sinus X-rays in childhood asthma: lack of relation to severity of asthma. J Allergy Clin Immunol 1987;80:268–73.
82. Rossi OVJ, Pirila T, Laitinen J, et al. Sinus aspirates and radiographic abnormalities in severe attacks of asthma. Int Arch Allergy Immunol 1994;103:209–13.
83. Newman LJ, Platts-Mills TAE, Phillips CD, et al. Chronic sinusitis: relationship of computed tomographic findings to allergy, asthma, and eosinophilia. JAMA 1994;271:363–7.
84. Pelikan Z, Pelikan-Filipek M. Role of nasal allergy in chronic maxillary sinusitis-diagnostic value of nasal challenge with allergen. J Allergy Clin Immunol 1990;86:484–91.
85. Wang X, Moylan B, Leopold DA, et al. Mutation in the gene responsible for cystic fibrosis and predisposition to chronic rhinosinusitis in the general population. JAMA 2000;284:1814–9.
86. Raman V, Clary R, Siegrist KL, et al. Increased prevalence of mutations in the cystic fibrosis transmembrane conductance regulator in children with chronic rhinosinusitis. Pediatrics 2002;E13.
87. Castellani C, Quinzii C, Altieri S, et al. A pilot survey of cystic fibrosis clinical manifestations in CFTR mutation heterozygotes. Genet Test 2001;5:249–54.
88. Bernstein J, Anon JB, Rontal M, et al. Genetic polymorphisms in chronic hyperplastic sinusitis with nasal polyposis. Laryngoscope 2009;119:1258–64.

89. de Alarcon A, Steinke JW, Caughey R, et al. Expression of leukotriene C4 synthase and plasminogen activator inhibitor 1 gene promoter polymorphisms in sinusitis. Am J Rhinol 2006;20:545–9.

90. Kim SH, Park HS, Holloway JW, et al. Association between a THFbeta1 promoter polymorphism and rhinosinusitis in aspirin-intolerant asthmatic patients. Respir Med 2007;101:490–5.

91. Takeuchi K, Majima Y, Shimizu T. Tumor necrosis factor gene polymorphism in chronic sinusitis. Laryngoscope 2000;110:1711–4.

92. Takeuchi K, Majima Y, Shimizu T, et al. Analysis of HLA antigens in Japanese patients with chronic sinusitis, Laryngoscope 1999;109:275–8.

93. Pinto JM, Hayes MG, Schneider D, et al. A genomewide screen for chronic rhinosinusitis genes identifies a locus on chromosome 7q. Laryngoscope 2008;118:2067–72.

94. Contencin P, Narcy P. Nasopharyngeal pH monitoring in infants and children with chronic rhinopharyngitis. Int J Pediatr Otorhinolaryngol 1991;22:249–56.

95. Yellon RF, Coticchia J, Dixit S. Esophageal biopsy for the diagnosis of gastroesophageal reflux-associated otolaryngologic problems in children. Am J Med 2000;108:131S–8S.

96. Phipps CD, Wood WE, Gibson WS, et al. Gastroesophageal reflux contributing to chronic sinus disease in children: a prospective analysis, Arch Otolaryngol Head Neck Surg 2000;126:831–6.

97. Chan KH, Winslow CP, Levin MJ, et al. Clinical practice guidelines for the management of chronic sinusitis in children. Otolaryngol Head Neck Surg 1999;120:328–34.

98. Slavin RG, Spector SL, Bernstein IL, et al. The diagnosis and management of sinusitis: a practice parameter update. J Allergy Clin Immunol 2005;116(6 Suppl):S13–47.

99. Mudgil SP, Wise SW, Hopper KD, et al. Correlation between presumed sinusitis-induced pain and paranasal sinus computed tomographic findings. Ann Allergy Asthma Immunol 2002;88:223–6.

100. McAlister WH, Parker BR, Kushner DC, et al. Sinusitis in the pediatric population: American College of Radiology. ACR appropriateness criteria. Radiology 2000;215(suppl):811–8.

101. Garcia DP, Corbett ML, Eberly SM, et al. Radiographic imaging studies in pediatric chronic sinusitis. J Allergy Clin Immunol 1994;94:523–30.

102. Lerner DN, Zalzal GH, Choi SS, et al. Intracranial complications of sinusitis in childhood. Ann Otol Rhinol Laryngol 1995;104:288–93.

103. Garcia CE, Cunningham MJ, Clary RA, et al. The etiologic role of frontal sinusitis in pediatric orbital abscesses. Am J Otolaryngol 1993;14:449–52.

104. Chandler JR, Lanenbrunner DJ, Steven ER. The pathogenesis of orbital complications in acute sinusitis. Laryngoscope 1970;141:1414–28.

105. Samad I, Riding K. Orbital complications of ethmoiditis: B.C. Children's Hospital experience. J Otolaryngol 1991;20:400–3.

106. Wald ER, Chiponis D, Ledesma-Medina J. Comparative effectiveness of amoxicillin and amoxicillin-clavulanate potassium in acute paranasal sinus infections in children: a double-blind, placebo-controlled trial. Pediatrics 1986;77:795–800.

107. Garbutt JM, Goldstein M, Gellman E, et al. A randomized, placebo-controlled trial of antimicrobial treatment for children with clinically diagnosed acute sinusitis. Pediatrics 2001;107:619–25.

108. Kristo A, Uhari M, Luotonen J, et al. Cefuroxime axetil versus placebo for children with acute respiratory infection and imaging evidence of sinusitis: a randomized, controlled trial. Acta Paediatrica 2005;94:1208–13.

109. Morris P, Leach A. Antibiotics for persistent nasal discharge (rhinosinusitis) in children (review). Cochrane database of systematic reviews 2002;Issue 4, Art. No.:CD001094. DOI: 10.1002/14651858.CD001094.

110. Benninger MS, Sedory Holzer SE, Lau J. Diagnosis and treatment of uncomplicated acute bacterial rhinosinusitis: summary of the Agency for Health Care Policy and Research evidence-based report. Otolaryngol Head and Neck Surg 2000;122:1–7.

111. Ahuvoo-Saloranta A, Borisenko OV, Kovanen N, et al. Antibiotics for acute maxillary sinusitis. Cochrane Database Syst Rev 2008;CD000243.

112. Young J, De Sutter A, Merenstein D, et al. Antibiotics for adults with clinically diagnosed acute rhinosinusitis: a meta-analysis of individual patient data. Lancet 2008;371:908–14.

113. de Ferranti SD, Ioannidis JP, Lau J, et al. Are amoxicillin and folate inhibitors as effective as other antibiotics for acute sinusitis? A meta-analysis. Br Med J 1998;317:632–7.

114. Falagas ME, Giannopoulou KP, Vardakas KZ, et al. Comparison of antibiotics with placebo for treatment of acute sinusitis: a meta-analysis of randomized controlled trials. Lancet Infect Dis 2008;8:543–52.

115. Hickner JM, Bartlett JG, Besser RE, et al. Principles of appropriate antibiotic use for acute rhinosinusitis in adults: background. Ann Intern Med 2001;134:498–505.

116. Piccirillo JF, Mager DE, Frisse ME, et al. Impact of first-line vs. second-line antibiotics for the treatment of acute uncomplicated sinusitis, JAMA 2001;286:1849–56.

117. Snow V, Mottur-Pilson C, Hickner JM. Principles of appropriate antibiotic use for acute sinusitis in adults. Ann Intern Med 2001;134:495–7.

118. Clement PAR, Bluestone CD, Gordts F, et al. Management of rhinosinusitis in children. Arch Otolaryngol Head Neck Surg 1998;124:31–4.

119. Williams JWJ, Aguilar C, Makela M, et al. Antibiotics for acute maxillary sinusitis. Cochrane Database Syst Rev 2000;2:CD000243.

120. Williams JW Jr, Aguilar C, Makela M. Which antibiotics lead to higher clinical cure rates in adults with acute maxillary sinusitis? West J Med 2000;173:42.

121. Rakkar S, Roberts K, Towe BF, et al. Moxifloxacin versus amoxicillin clavulanate in the treatment of acute maxillary sinusitis: a primary care experience. Int J Clin Pract 2001;55:309–15.

122. Siegert R, Gehanno P, Nikolaidis P, et al. A comparison of the safety and efficacy of moxifloxacin (BAY 12–8039) and cefuroxime axetil in the treatment of acute bacterial sinusitis in adults: the sinusitis study group. Respir Med 2000;94:337–44.

123. Ng DK, Chow PY, Leung I, et al. A randomized controlled trial of azithromycin and amoxicillin/clavulanate in the management of sub-acute rhinosinusitis. J Paediatr Child Health 2000;36:378–81.

124. Pichichero M. Short course antibiotic therapy for respiratory infections: a review of the evidence. Pediatr Infect Dis J 2000;19:929–37.

125. Alagic-Smailbegovic J, Saracevic E, Sutalo K. Azythromycin versus amoxicillin-clavulanate in the treatment of acute sinusitis in children. Bosn J Basic Med Sci 2006;6:76–8.

126. Zacharisen MC, Kelly KJ. Allergic and infectious pediatric sinusitis. Pediatr Ann 1998;27:759–66.

127. Rachelefsky GS. Chronic sinusitis in children with respiratory allergy: the role of antimicrobials. J Allergy Clin Immunol 1982;69:382–7.

128. Dohlman AW, Hemstreet MP, Odrezin GT, et al. Subacute sinusitis: are antimicrobials necessary? J Allergy Clin Immunol 1993;91:1015–23.

129. Brook I, Yocum P. Antimicrobial management of chronic sinusitis in children. J Laryngol Otol 1995;109:1159–62.

130. Bussey MF. Acute sinusitis. Pediatr Rev 1999;20:142.

131. Buchman CA, Yellon RF, Bluestone CD. Alternative to endoscopic sinus surgery in the management of pediatric chronic rhinosinusitis refractory to oral antimicrobial therapy. Otolaryngol-Head Neck Surg 1999;120:219–24.

132. Sener B, Hascelik G, Onerci M, et al. Evaluation of the microbiology of chronic sinusitis. J Laryngol Otol 1996;110:547–50.

133. Vogan JC, Bolger WE, Keyes AS. Endoscopically guided sinonasal cultures: a direct comparison with maxillary sinus aspirate cultures. Otolaryngol Head Neck Surg 2000;122:370–3.

134. Adappa ND, Coticchia JM. Management of refractory chronic rhinosinusitis in children. Am J Otolaryngol 2006;27:384–9.

135. Rizk SS, Kraus DH, Gerresheim G, et al. Aggressive combination treatment for invasive fungal sinusitis in immunocompromised patients. Ear Nose Throat J 2000;79:278–80, 282, 284–5.

136. Prellner K, Fogle-Hansson M, Jorgensen F. Prevention of recurrent acute otitis media in otitis-prone children by intermittent prophylaxis with penicillin. Acta Otolaryngol 1994;114:182–7.

137. Baroody FM. Pediatric sinusitis. Arch Otolaryngol Head Neck Surg 2001;127:1099–101.

138. Parsons DS, Phillips SE. Functional endoscopic surgery in children: a retrospective analysis of results. Laryngoscope 1993;103:899–903.

139. Lazar RH, Younis RT, Long TE. Functional endonasal sinus surgery in adults and children. Laryngoscope 1993;103:1–5.

140. Gross CW, Gurucharri MJ, Lazar RH, et al. Functional endonasal sinus surgery (FESS) in the pediatric age group. Laryngoscope 1989;99:272–5.

141. Hebert RL, Bent JP III. Meta-analysis of outcomes of pediatric functional endoscopic sinus surgery. Laryngoscope 1998;108:796–9.

142. Manning SC, Wasserman RL, Silver R, et al. Results of endoscopic sinus surgery in pediatric patients with chronic sinusitis and asthma. Arch Otolaryngol Head Neck Surg 1994;120:1142–5.

143. Rosbe KW, Jones DT, Rahbar R, et al. Endoscopic sinus surgery in cystic fibrosis: do patients benefit from surgery? Int J Pediatr Otorhinolaryngol 2001;61:113–9.

144. Poole MD. Pediatric sinusitis is not a surgical disease. Ear Nose Throat J 1992;71:622–3.

145. Chan KH, Winslow CP, Abzug MJ. Persistent rhinosinusitis in children following endoscopic sinus surgery. Otolaryngol Head Neck Surg 1999;121:577–80.

146. Vandenberg SJ, Heatley DG. Efficacy of adenoidectomy in relieving symptoms of chronic sinusitis in children. Arch Otolaryngol Head Neck Surg 1997;123:675–8.

147. Rosenfeld RM. Pilot study of outcomes in pediatric rhinosinusitis. Arch Otolaryngol Head Neck Surg 1995;121:729–36.

148. Brietzke SE, Brigger MT. Adenoidectomy outcomes in pediatric rhinosinusitis: a meta-analysis. Int J Pediatr Otorhinolaryngol. 2008;72(10):1541–5.

149. Coticchia J, Zuliani G, Coleman C, et al. Biofilm surface area in the pediatric nasopharynx: chronic rhinosinusitis vs obstructive sleep apnea. Arch Otolaryngol Head Neck Surg 2007;133:110–4.

150. Harvey R, Hannan SA, Badia L, et al. Nasal saline irrigations for the symptoms of chronic rhinosinusitis. Cochrane Database of Systematic Reviews 2007, Issue 3.

151. Zalmanovici A, Yaphe J. Steroids for acute sinusitis. Cochrane Database of Systematic Reviews 2007, Issue 2.

152. Dolor RJ, Witsell DL, Hellkamp AS, et al. Comparison of cefuroxime with or without intranasal fluticasone for the treatment of rhinosinusitis. The CAF trial: a randomized controlled trial. JAMA 2001;286:3097–105.

31

Chronic Cough

Henry Milgrom

Introduction

Cough is a pervasive sign and symptom of diseases ranging from simple respiratory tract infections to serious illnesses affecting several organ systems. It is a source of discomfort for the young patient and emotional distress for the parents.[1,2] In the years 1995–1996, 24 million annual physician visits for cough took place in the USA, the largest number documented for a single symptom.[3] Nearly half the patients were under 15 years. In this young cohort, cough accounted for 8.5% of all medical appointments, exceeded only by well-baby visits.[3] Pediatric texts generally describe chronic cough as a condition that persists for more than 3 weeks. This definition leads to the observation that chronic cough is likely to improve in time without treatment.[4] A better-founded classification by Irwin and colleagues divides cough into three categories: acute, lasting less than 3 weeks; subacute, lasting 3 to 8 weeks; and chronic, lasting more than 8 weeks.[5] Irwin's definition of chronic cough excludes a greater proportion of self-limiting cases. A chronic cough by his criteria often lasts much longer than 8 weeks and requires medical attention.

Viral infections of the upper respiratory tract are the most common causes of acute cough. Typically, the symptoms resolve within 10 to 14 days. Patients with subacute cough most often have a history of recent upper respiratory tract infection or seasonal allergic rhinitis. Consider postinfectious cough, bacterial sinusitis, and asthma. Children with chronic or recurrent episodes of dry, nonproductive cough that lasts for months, require careful and systematic evaluation for the presence of specific diagnostic indicators.[6] They pose a perplexing problem in pediatric practice. Their coughs, the subject of this chapter, calls for a careful evaluation. It is often an exhausting process that contributes to the child's morbidity and adversely affects both the patient and the family. It may be a manifestation of an underlying disorder that must be identified and treated. Many children with chronic cough have experienced repeated treatment failure, and the families have come to regard the condition as permanent and untreatable. Fortunately, in most cases, this perception is incorrect. However, a systematic approach to the diagnosis is necessary, and therapy, to be effective, may have to be directed simultaneously at several involved cough mechanisms.

Differential Diagnosis (Figure 31-1)

The differential diagnosis of cough in childhood varies with the age of the patient, the duration, character and time of occurrence of the cough, associated signs and symptoms, and the patient's exposure history. In the neonatal period, congenital abnormalities, especially pulmonary or cardiac, must be considered. Prematurity, especially in a patient who had required mechanical ventilation, may lead to bronchopulmonary dysplasia or the development of tracheal or bronchial stenosis. Vomiting and regurgitation may be the presenting signs and symptoms of gastroesophageal reflux or a tracheoesophageal fistula. Recurrent choking or cough associated with difficulty in sucking or swallowing suggests aspiration. Cough may occur in the course or following resolution of a respiratory infection. Attendance in daycare increases the risk of upper respiratory symptoms and infections in young children. In the toddler, foreign body aspiration and cystic fibrosis is added to the list of causes. A history of fever and/or presentation in winter suggests a viral etiology; seasonal occurrence suggests asthma or seasonal allergic rhinitis; year-round symptoms suggest perennial allergic rhinitis, with maternal smoking, in particular, appearing to influence the development of respiratory symptoms in young children.[7] In the older child, immune deficiency, tuberculosis and psychogenic cough enter into the differential diagnosis. Sinusitis, postnasal drip and gastroesophageal reflux may contribute to cough at any age, most commonly in adolescence. Cigarette smoking and psychogenic causes also require consideration in this age group.[8] An important recent publication questions the importance of upper airway disease and gastroesophageal reflux in the etiology of chronic cough (defined by the authors as cough lasting longer than 3 weeks) of young children.[9] We agree that these conditions are more important in older children, but they also rise in significance in the younger child whose cough has been present for over 8 weeks. Further, we agree with the salient comments of Boren and colleagues who stress the importance of early evaluation and treatment of children with recurrent cough, sinusitis, potential foreign-body aspiration, or gastroesophageal reflux to prevent bronchiectasis, which is even more important now that infectious causes of this complication have been largely eliminated in developed countries through the use of vaccines and antibiotics.[10]

How often do normal children cough? Accurate answers come from studies that used cough recorders. Cough frequency over 24 hours was 11.3, with a range of 1 to 34 in 41 children free from respiratory infection for at least 1 month. Only two children coughed at night.[11] In children with chronic cough the frequency was 65/day and in normal controls 10/day.[12] Unfortunately, most studies rely on parents to report their children's cough, a method that has been shown to provide inaccurate information.[13,14] When questionnaires administered to parents about

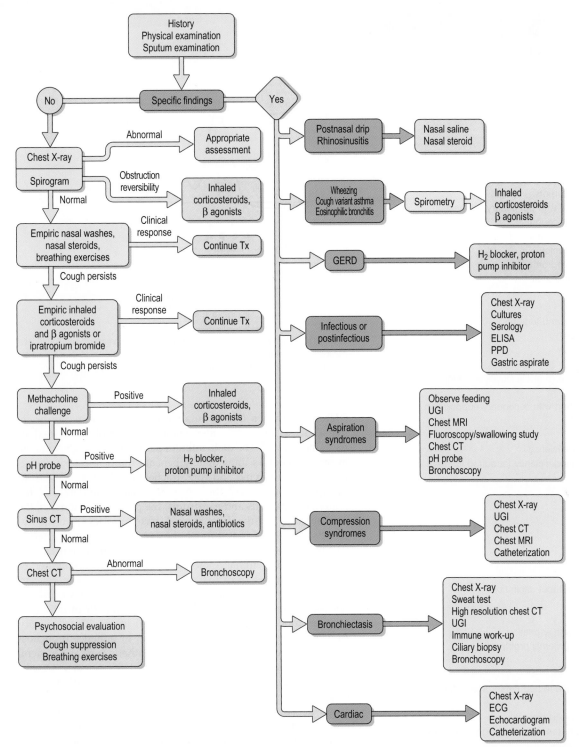

Figure 31-1 Algorithm for the evaluation and treatment of chronic cough in childhood. *CT,* Computed tomography; *Tx,* therapy; *GERD,* gastroesophageal reflux disease; *ELISA,* enzyme-linked immunosorbent assay; *PPD,* purified protein derivative; *UGI,* upper gastrointestinal series; *MRI,* magnetic resonance imaging; *ECG,* electrocardiogram.

their children's coughing were compared to overnight recordings performed in 145 homes the agreement was low, with kappa statistics ranging from 0.02 to 0.10.[15]

Pathophysiology (Figures 31-2 and 31-3)

Cough serves as a protective mechanism to clear the respiratory tract and to defend it against the aspiration of noxious materials.

While mechanical barriers limit the exposure of the respiratory tract to inhaled pathogens, the mucociliary apparatus and cough act to expel any organisms that may have bypassed the primary defenses. Two associated processes, bronchoconstriction and mucus secretion, add to its effectiveness. Recurrent partial collapse or incomplete inflation of the lungs and pneumonia associated with ineffective cough attest to its importance.[16]

Cough is executed as a complex reflex, an automatic or involuntary response to a stimulus, completed by the afferent and

BOX 31-1

Differential Diagnosis of Chronic Cough

Congenital anomalies
  Connection of the airway to the esophagus
    Laryngeal cleft
    Tracheoesophageal fistula
  Laryngotracheomalacia
    Primary laryngotracheomalacia
    Laryngotracheomalacia secondary to vascular or other compression
  Bronchopulmonary foregut malformation
  Congenital mediastinal tumors
  Congenital heart disease with pulmonary congestion
Infectious or postinfectious cough
  Recurrent viral infection (infants and toddlers)
  Chlamydial infection (infants)
  Whooping cough-like syndrome
    Bordetella pertussis infection
    Chlamydial infection
    Mycoplasma infection
    Cystic fibrosis (infants and toddlers)
  Granulomatous infection
    Mycobacterial infection
    Fungal infection
  Suppurative lung disease (bronchiectasis and lung abscess)
    Cystic fibrosis
    Foreign body aspiration with secondary suppuration
    Ciliary dysfunction
    Immunodeficiency
      Primary immunodeficiency
      Secondary immunodeficiency (acquired immune deficiency syndrome)
  Paranasal sinus infection
  Cough-variant asthma
Rhinitis related
  Allergic rhinitis
  Rhinosinusitis
  Vasomotor rhinitis
  Postnasal drip
Gastroesophageal reflux without aspiration
Vocal cord dysfunction
Aspiration (fluid material)
  Dyskinetic swallowing with aspiration
    General neurodevelopmental problems
    Möbius' syndrome
    Chiari malformations
  Bottle-propping and bottle in bed (infant and toddlers)
  Gastroesophageal reflux
Foreign body aspiration (solid material)
  Upper airway aspiration (tonsillar, pharyngeal, laryngeal)
  Tracheobronchial aspiration
    Esophageal foreign body with an obstruction or aspiration resulting from dysphagia
Physical and chemical irritation
  Smoke from tobacco products (active and passive)
  Wood smoke from stoves and fireplaces
  Dry, dusty environment (hobbies and employment)
  Volatile chemicals (hobbies and employment)
  Dampness
  Mold
Psychogenic cough
Habit cough

Modified from Brown MA, Morgan WJ. Clinical assessment and diagnostic approach to common problems. In: Taussig LM, Landau LI, eds: Pediatric respiratory medicine. St Louis: Mosby; 1999.

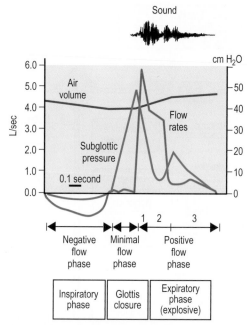

Figure 31-2 Changes in flow rate, air volume, subglottic pressure, and sound level generated during the act of coughing. (From Bianco S, Robuschi M. Mechanics of cough. In: Braga PC, Allegra L, eds. Cough. New York: Raven; 1989.)

efferent pathways and a putative cough center in the brain, but at least, in part, under voluntary control intensified or restrained at will. The main afferent pathways of cough originate in nerve receptors immediately beneath the respiratory epithelium in the larynx and the tracheobronchial tree, and in extrapulmonary sites: the nose, the paranasal sinuses, the pharynx, ear canals and ear drums, the pleura, the stomach, the pericardium, and the diaphragm. Nerve impulses from the tracheobronchial tree pass through the vagus, the principal afferent pathway. Cough may result from direct stimulation of this nerve.[17] The trigeminal, glossopharyngeal, and phrenic nerves conduct impulses from extrapulmonary sites.[18] Axon reflexes traveling through branches of sensory end-organs may cause the release of neuropeptides and subsequent smooth muscle contraction, mucus secretion, and epithelial injury. Thus, sensory signals taking part in cough may trigger or enhance bronchospasm. Reflexes regulate the parasympathetic nervous system, and chronic cough lowers the threshold for sensory signals. Efferent impulses of the cough reflex are transmitted to the respiratory musculature through the phrenic and other spinal motor nerves and to the larynx through the recurrent laryngeal branches of the vagus. The vagus also provides efferent innervation to the tracheobronchial tree where its branches mediate bronchoconstriction.

Cough and Bronchospasm

Cough and bronchospasm are two closely related reflexes that enhance one another, but neither depends on the other for its action.[19] Cough clears the airways effectively only at high lung volumes; sufficient air velocity to shear mucus from bronchial walls can be achieved only down to the sixth or seventh generation of airway branching.[20] Coexisting bronchoconstriction adds to the effectiveness of cough by extending peripherally the region of rapid and turbulent airflow. Challenge with either methacholine or histamine provokes both cough and bronchoconstriction.[21] However, the receptors for both reflexes are functionally

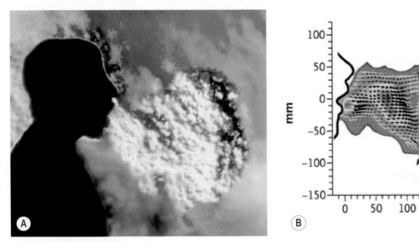

Figure 31-3 When a healthy volunteer coughs, he expels a turbulent jet of air with density changes that distort a projected schlieren light beam (**A**). A velocity map early in the cough (**B**) was obtained from image analysis. (From Tang J, Settles G. N Engl J Med 2008;359:e19.)

distinct, and either response can arise independently. Challenge with hyperosmolar solutions causes both cough and bronchoconstriction, but hypoosmolar solutions tend to bring about cough alone.[22] Pretreatment sets apart induced cough and bronchoconstriction.[23] When aerosolized water serves as a provoking agent, inhaled lidocaine blocks cough but not bronchoconstriction, while the opposite is true for cromolyn. When inhaled capsaicin is used, opiates administered systemically suppress cough while the same agents administered by inhalation suppress bronchoconstriction.[23] Bronchoconstriction, but not the urge to cough, can be blocked by pretreatment with intravenous atropine, consistent with the role of cholinergic pathways in the efferent limb of reflex bronchoconstriction. The mechanisms that trigger cough and bronchospasm following exercise or exposure to cold air appear to be different. Cough results mainly from excessive water loss while bronchoconstriction follows airway rewarming.[24] Cold, air-induced bronchoconstriction can be blocked by β-adrenergic agents, but cough cannot. Cough most often results from excitation of receptors concentrated in the larynx and proximal airways, while bronchoconstriction can be triggered from the lower airways as well. And finally, inflammatory changes in the airways may result in cough without simultaneously giving rise to bronchospasm.[25]

Cough-Variant Asthma

Childhood asthma is a syndrome of inflammation in medium and small airways that gives rise to hyperresponsiveness and constriction of the bronchial smooth muscle, edema and disruption of the mucosa, and obstruction of the airway lumen.[26] Inflammation may lead to airway remodeling with proliferation of smooth muscle and deposition of matrix proteins. Cough-variant asthma is associated with the same disordered physiological processes and presenting signs, but overt wheezing is absent, and cough is the most evident clinical manifestation. However, substantial evidence shows that the awareness of symptoms by children with asthma is poor,[27] and both the children and their parents may be more conscious of cough than of other symptoms that may be present as well.

Unconsidered diagnosis of asthma on the basis of cough alone accounts for the profusion of unsustainable cases of cough-variant asthma.[28] In 1991, 10% of children with cough as the only symptom were diagnosed as having asthma; 2 years later, the figure had increased to 22.6%.[28] Whereas, in the past, cough may have been underrecognized as a sign of asthma, at present the opposite appears to be true.[29,30] This is borne out by reports in which children with persistent nocturnal cough improved after 2 weeks of placebo therapy and received only modest additional benefit from a course of high-dose inhaled corticosteroids.[31] Inhaled albuterol and beclomethasone in children with cough, but without wheezing, were no more effective than placebo in reducing cough frequency.[32] Surprisingly, even the documentation of airway hyperreactivity did not predict a child's response to these asthma medications. A study of nocturnal cough showed that in the absence of wheeze, shortness of breath, or tightness of the chest, cough did not indicate hidden or atypical asthma in most children.[33] Children under 4 years of age with frequent recurrent wheeze and a stringent index for the prediction of asthma at school age showed significantly higher median fractional exhaled NO levels (11.7 [11.85]) than children with recurrent cough but no history of wheeze (6.5 [5.5]; P < 0.001) and those with early recurrent wheeze and a loose index for the prediction of asthma at school age (6.4 [6.5]; P < 0.001). No difference in FeNO levels was found between children from the latter two groups (P = 0.91).[34] A prospective study of infants followed up to age 11 years, showed that recurrent cough present early in life resolved in the majority of children. Children with recurrent cough but without wheeze did not have airway hyperresponsiveness or atopy, and significantly differed from those with classical asthma, with or without cough.[35] Brooke and colleagues reassessed, during the early school years, a cohort of children identified as having recurrent cough in the preschool period. Seventy of 125 (56.0% [95% CI 47.3–64.5%]) were symptom-free at follow-up, 46 (36.8% [28.7–45.5%]) continued to have recurrent cough in the absence of colds, and only 9 (7.2% [3.6–12.8%]) reported recent wheezing. The authors concluded that there are children with long-term recurrent cough consistent with the diagnosis of cough-variant asthma, but that few progress to develop asthma characterized by wheeze.[36]

Isolated cough is rarely due to asthma and often fails to respond to asthma medications.[37] On the other hand, patients with a prolonged history of cough who respond to treatment with asthma medications or show evidence of bronchospasm or hyperresponsiveness without concurrent wheezing may be considered to have cough-variant asthma. Patients may be free of bronchoconstriction at the time of their evaluation. Their history of respiratory disease may be difficult to assess while physical findings and routine pulmonary function tests may disclose no evidence of airway obstruction. In such cases, evaluation of airway function by bronchial provocation with methacholine, histamine or exercise is recommended. In children too young to perform pulmonary function testing, the diagnosis of cough-variant asthma may be confirmed by the patient developing unequivocal evidence of reversible airways obstruction later in the clinical course and by the patient's response to asthma therapy.

Cough During and After Respiratory Infection

Children have an average of six to eight respiratory infections per year, and the number may be higher in those with siblings or in daycare. Repeated infections common in winter months may result in a chronic cough. Acute bronchitis usually follows the symptoms of upper respiratory illness. Mucus gland activity increases and desquamation of ciliated epithelium becomes prominent. Infiltration of polymorphonuclear leukocytes into the lumen and in the airway walls contributes to purulent appearance of the secretions that does not necessarily indicate a bacterial infection. Cough associated with infection with *respiratory syncytial virus* (RSV), other respiratory viruses and cytomegalovirus; *Mycoplasma pneumoniae, Chlamydia trachomatis, Ureoplasma urealyticum,* and *Pneumocystis carinii; Corynebacterium diphtheriae,* and *Bordetella pertussis* often lasts beyond the acute stage. Measles causes a cough with coryza, conjunctivitis, and fever. In the immunized patient, atypical measles is more likely to cause cough or pneumonia than the characteristic rash.

The pathogenesis of postinfectious cough is not known. Children with persistent postinfectious cough do not have airway eosinophilia typical of untreated asthma, but some manifest increased reactivity of the airways. These observations suggest that postinfectious cough has different pathophysiologic features than asthma.[38] The infection causing the cough, in most cases, remains unidentified. The diagnosis is clinical and one of exclusion. It should be considered in patients with normal chest X-rays who cough only after respiratory tract infections. Postinfectious cough generally regresses over time, but it often recurs. Its resolution may be accelerated by the administration of corticosteroids or ipratropium bromide.[39]

Acute Viral Bronchiolitis

Bronchiolitis occurs in epidemics during the winter months in temperate regions and during the hottest months and the rainy season in tropical climates. Cough set off by microorganisms contributes to their spread and survival. RSV is the leading cause of epidemic bronchiolitis, accounting for over 40% of cases. Influenza, parainfluenza type 3, and adenovirus are responsible for many of the remaining cases. New isolation techniques have led to the discovery of previously unrecognized viruses, including the human metapneumovirus and bocavirus, which also play a significant role.[40] The risk of RSV illness in the first year is over 60%, and it infects nearly all children by the age of 2 years.[41] RSV lower respiratory tract infections lead to 125 000 hospital admissions per year in the USA. Eighty percent occur in infants with peak incidence at 2 to 8 months.[42] RSV accounts for 25% of all acute hospitalizations in children younger than 5 years with chronic lung disease. Between 0.5% and 3.2% of children with RSV infection require hospitalization, and there are approximately 4500 deaths per year. Environmental risk factors for severe RSV infection include poverty, crowding, exposure to tobacco smoke, and malnutrition. Older children and adults develop antibodies to RSV, but the immunity is incomplete, and reinfection may occur at any age. In these older patients infection with RSV usually takes the form of an upper respiratory illness often with bronchitis.

There is a general consensus that following even mild RSV bronchiolitis, children are at increased risk for repeated bouts of respiratory symptoms during the first 3 years of life.[43] Stein and colleagues reported a relationship to recurrent respiratory symptoms up to 6 years of age but not to asthma after the of age 13 years.[44] However, more recent evidence points to an association between severe RSV infection early in life and increased incidence of asthma and eczema later.[45]

Mycoplasma pneumoniae

Most infections with *Mycoplasma pneumoniae* in infants and young children are asymptomatic or are associated only with upper respiratory symptoms.[46] However, it is the most frequent cause of pneumonia in children between 5 and 15 years of age,[47] and a cause of bronchiolitis in all age groups. *Mycoplasma pneumoniae* pneumonia presents with a gradual onset of malaise, fever, and headache. Cough begins several days after the onset of the illness and often persists for weeks. It may be productive of white or blood-tinged sputum. Physical findings include crackles, rhonchi, and bronchial breath sounds. The incidence of wheezing with the acute infection has been reported to be 40%. X-ray findings, though not diagnostic, frequently show unilateral lower lobe involvement. Initially the pattern is reticular and interstitial. Later, patchy segmental consolidation is seen. Hilar adenopathy and pleural effusions may be present. Ten percent of the children develop an exanthem, and 36% have elevated hepatic transaminases. The diagnosis can be made by measuring specific IgM antibody. A rise in IgG antibody takes between 1 and 2 weeks. Cold agglutinins are positive in about 40% to 60% of patients; however, the results are not specific. There is little evidence that treatment with antibiotics is helpful during the acute illness; however, macrolide antibiotics may shorten the duration of fever and respiratory symptoms.

Infection with mycoplasma may produce a long-term impairment in lung function even in asymptomatic children. Clinical reports, throat culture and serological studies, and animal models suggest a role for mycoplasma in airway hyperresponsiveness. In nonasthmatic subjects, significant response to bronchodilators has been noted 1 month after infection. More significantly, abnormal FEV_1 and forced expiratory flow after 50% of the expired vital capacity have been noted as long as 3 years after initial infection.[48]

Bordetella pertussis

Whooping cough, a highly communicable respiratory disease, caused serious morbidity and mortality among infants and children before the introduction of whole-cell pertussis vaccine. Regrettably, reported pertussis cases increased from a historic low of 1010 in 1976 to 11 647 cases in 2003 with substantial increase among adolescents, who become susceptible to pertussis approximately 6 to 10 years after childhood vaccination.[49] While in the prevaccine era pertussis was primarily a childhood disease, today with widespread vaccination, there has been a shift in the incidence of disease to adolescents and adults.[50,51] As many as 90% of nonimmune household contacts acquire the disease. Infection in immunized children and older persons is often mild.[52] Whooping cough continues to be the main cause of postinfectious bronchiectasis in underdeveloped countries. The widespread use of this vaccine in combination with diphtheria and tetanus toxoids (DTP), starting in the USA in the late 1940s, led to a historic low point of 1010 cases of pertussis in 1976. However, since the early 1980s, cases of pertussis have increased with cyclical peaks every 3 to 4 years. In 1996, the US Centers for Disease Control and Prevention reported 7796 cases of pertussis, almost half among individuals aged 10 years or older. In the same year, acellular pertussis vaccines were licensed and recommended for routine immunization of infants.[53] The effectiveness of the complete vaccination series is 80% (95% CI 66 to 88). Having received less than three doses constitutes a significant risk factor (relative risk, 5.1; 95% CI, 3 to 8.6).[54] More recently, acellular vaccines and a genetically inactivated mutant pertussis toxoid appear to be safer and more immunogenic than the current chemically inactivated pertussis toxin.[55,56] The burden of disease assessed by rates of complications and death remains greatest in the youngest patients, but there has been a recent resurgence of pertussis in adolescents and adults. These groups constitute a major source of disease transmission to younger children. Increased exposure to pertussis in the community, delay in identification and treatment, and high contact rates among children attending school or daycare contribute to the spread of the disease.

In the unimmunized child, infection with *Bordatella. pertussis* leads to a catarrhal phase with rhinitis, conjunctivitis, low-grade fever and cough. *B. pertussis* infection causes infiltration of airway mucosa by lymphocytes and polymorphonuclear leukocytes, necrosis of the midzonal layers of the mucosa and injury to the ciliated epithelium of the respiratory tract. A stage of tracheobronchitis ensues with episodes of paroxysmal cough that increase in number and severity. Repetitive forceful coughs during a single expiration are followed by an abrupt inspiration that produces the characteristic whoop. Many children experience posttussive emesis. Fever is absent or minimal. The duration of classic pertussis is 6 to 10 weeks. Pertussis is more severe in the first year of life. A clinical case is defined as an acute cough illness lasting a minimum of 14 days in a person with at least one pertussis-associated symptom (i.e. paroxysmal cough, posttussive vomiting, or inspiratory whoop) or 14 days of cough during an established outbreak. A confirmed case is a cough illness of any duration in a person from whom *Bordetella pertussis* has been isolated, or a case that meets the clinical definition and is confirmed by polymerase chain reaction or by an epidemiologic connection to a laboratory-confirmed case.[53] Although *B. pertussis* infection should be suspected in children with paroxysmal cough, other organisms, most notably adenovirus, parainfluenza viruses, respiratory syncytial virus, and mycoplasma have been implicated.[37]

There is growing evidence that *B. pertussis* is an important cause of persistent cough in adolescents and adults. Pertussis has been implicated in 16% of cases of chronic cough of adults in Denmark. Susceptibility to infection with *B. pertussis* recurs several years after vaccination. Moreover, cases of laboratory proven reinfection have been reported.[57] *B. pertussis* should be considered in patients with symptoms of typical or atypical whooping cough, irrespective of their vaccination status or past history of the disease.[57] By demonstrating *B. pertussis* in an adult, one can reassure the patient that the symptoms will subside without the need for extensive evaluation and treatment, and recommend measures to protect others, especially unvaccinated infants.[58] Droplet precautions are recommended for 5 days after initiation of effective therapy or until 3 weeks after the onset of paroxysms if appropriate antimicrobial therapy has not been given. Erythromycin or clarithromycin eliminates pertussis from the nasopharynx in 3 to 4 days, decreasing the spread of the disease.[59] Given within 14 days of onset, these antibiotics may abort pertussis. Once paroxysms of cough develop, antibiotics have little effect on the course of illness. An association between erythromycin and idiopathic hypertrophic pyloric stenosis has been reported in infants.[60] There are no such reports for clarithromycin.[61]

In addition to maintaining high vaccination rates among preschool children, effort must be directed at identification and treatment of pertussis cases to prevent further spread of the disease. Erythromycin (40–50 mg/kg per day orally in four divided doses, maximum 2 g/day) for 14 days is recommended for all close contacts irrespective of age or immunization status. Exposure of infants to children and adults with cough illnesses should be minimized. A major public health challenge at present is to address the illness in adolescents and adults. A rational strategy might be a universal booster vaccination for adolescents and a program targeted at those adults most likely to have contact with infants.

Chlamydia trachomatis

Infants with *Chlamydia trachomatis* infection present with a high-pitched, staccato, nonproductive cough and tachypnea without fever that begin around 4 weeks of age and last for several weeks, even after therapy with erythromycin.[62] Concomitant conjunctivitis is a frequent finding.

Mycobacterium tuberculosis

Pediatric pulmonary tuberculosis remains a major cause of morbidity and mortality worldwide.[63] From 1985 to 1992, the number of cases of childhood TB increased; however, between 1992 and 1998, the numbers declined substantially in all age groups.[64] The incidence of TB among children is lower than among adults, and most of the pediatric morbidity and mortality occur in children less than 5 years of age. In the USA the groups with the highest rates include immigrants from Asia, Africa and Latin America, the homeless and residents of correctional facilities.[64]

Children contract TB from adults and adolescents; disease transmission among youngsters is most uncommon. When the tuberculin skin test converts to positive, most infections with *M. tuberculosis* in children are asymptomatic. The radiographs at that time are usually negative, and the primary infection progresses slowly. Infection with *Mycobacterium tuberculosis* that becomes symptomatic usually involves the hilar and mediastinal lymph nodes as well as lung parenchyma. Early manifestations become evident 1 to 6 months after initial infection. They include fever, weight loss, cough, night sweats, and chills. Chest X-rays may show lymphadenopathy of the hilar and mediastinal nodes, involvement of a lung segment or lobe with atelectasis or infiltrate, cavitary lesions, and military disease. Tuberculous meningitis may be an early finding. Later extrapulmonary manifestations may involve the middle ear, the mastoid, bones, joints, skin, and kidneys.[64]

The recommended treatment regimen for TB disease consists of an initial 2-month phase of four drugs: isoniazid, rifampin, pyrazinamide, and ethambutol followed by a 4-month continuation phase of isoniazid and rifampin. Ethambutol is generally not used for young children whose visual acuity cannot be monitored. Streptomycin may be substituted for ethambutol, but must be given by injection. Ethambutol (or streptomycin) can be discontinued when drug susceptibility results show the infecting organism to be fully drug-susceptible.[53]

Children from Asia or Africa where tuberculosis is endemic may have cough, often with hemoptysis, and without fever, as a result of an infestation with a fluke of the genus *Paragonimus* acquired by eating undercooked freshwater crab or crayfish.

Cough Associated with Allergic Rhinitis, Rhinosinusitis, and/or Postnasal Drip

Allergic rhinitis and rhinosinusitis, (both described elsewhere in this text), are associated with cough that results from postnasal drip and irritation of the larynx.[65] Chronic sinusitis may be an early manifestation of immunodeficiency or ciliary dysfunction. Irwin and colleagues have identified postnasal drip as the most common cause of chronic cough among their patients.[5] The diagnosis can be established by history. Mucoperiosteal changes on X-ray or sinus CT of an atopic child in the absence of opacification or air-fluid levels and acute symptoms do not constitute an indication for treatment with antibiotics or sinus surgery. A most effective treatment is once or twice daily nasal irrigation with normal saline buffered by bicarbonate, followed by the instillation of a nasal corticosteroid spray.

Cough Associated with Compression Syndromes

Tracheobronchomalacia

Tracheo- or bronchomalacia is characterized by flaccidity or congenital absence of the cartilaginous rings supporting the trachea and/or the bronchi. Although most infants are asymptomatic, some present with cough, often described as brassy,[37] paroxysmal dyspnea, wheezing, and stridor. Chest X-rays frequently show recurrent 'pneumonia' that results from the collapse of segments of the airway during expiration. Increased secretions associated with respiratory infections precipitate symptoms. The caliber of the airways on chest X-ray varies from normal to markedly reduced depending on the phase of respiration. The appearance of pneumonia is most often caused by atelectasis, but secondary infection of the collapsed lung may occur. Prolongation of the expiratory phase and suprasternal and intercostal retractions are common. The diagnosis is established by observation of the collapse of tracheal or bronchial walls on fluoroscopy or bronchoscopy. Intrinsic airway stenosis or extrinsic compression exaggerates the manifestation of tracheomalacia. These complications must be considered during endoscopy. If associated bronchospasm is present, it must be treated aggressively. Although the symptoms usually subside by 12 to 18 months of age some infants may require a trial of continuous positive airway pressure or mechanical ventilation.[8]

Vascular Rings

The trachea can become partially obstructed by a vascular abnormality involving a right aortic arch with left ligamentum arteriosum or persistent ductus arteriosus, double aortic arch, anomalous innominate, or left carotid artery. These abnormalities are generally referred to as vascular rings. Typical symptoms include inspiratory stridor, expiratory wheezing, and a barking cough. Respiratory distress may be present, especially during feeding or when infection intervenes. Feeding difficulties may be present in the first few weeks of life. There may be recurrent pneumonia and atelectasis.

The presence of vascular rings must be considered in any infant with stridor. The chest X-ray may show a right or an indeterminate aortic arch. Tracheal compression by an anomalous innominate artery causes a curvilinear indentation of the anterior trachea. While barium esophagrams may show characteristic indentations from various anomalies of the aortic arch, magnetic resonance imaging (MRI) with its multiplanar images has become the procedure of choice at many institutions. Laryngotracheobronchoscopy is useful in excluding upper airway obstruction. Tracheal compression viewed endoscopically may be recognizable as a pulsatile, extrinsic mass. Vascular rings may be life-threatening, but with prompt recognition and surgical treatment, they are usually completely correctable.[8,66]

Mediastinal Masses

Mediastinal masses may be present at birth. Children under 2 years are likely to present with respiratory symptoms including dyspnea, cough, stridor, and chest pain. Additional signs and symptoms may include cyanosis, atelectasis, superior vena cava syndrome, Horner's syndrome, dysphagia, spinal cord compression, intercostal nerve neuralgia, and cervical lymphadenopathy. These masses may be categorized as congenital or neoplastic. Most neoplastic tumors are malignant, and prompt diagnosis and treatment are required. In a large number of older children, the masses are asymptomatic, and are recognized coincidentally on chest X-rays. The asymptomatic masses are often benign. Chest X-rays provide information about location, size, and presence or absence of calcifications. The barium swallow may be helpful in defining the anatomy. Computed tomography (CT) and MRI provide the most useful information for further diagnosis and treatment. Other helpful tests include percutaneous biopsy, bone marrow aspiration, urinary catecholamines, and skeletal survey. Monoclonal antibodies have been used for the diagnosis, assessment of response to therapy, and monitoring for relapse.[66]

Bronchial Stenosis

Bronchial stenosis is a fixed narrowing of the bronchus, usually not associated with other congenital malformations, although coexisting segmental bronchomalacia, most commonly of the left main bronchus has been reported. In the past, tuberculosis was a common cause of bronchial stenosis. It can occur at any level along the bronchial tree although it most commonly involves a main bronchus, just distal to the carina. The degree of stenosis is variable. Wheezing, both inspiratory and expiratory, is a typical presenting symptom. It may be associated with cough, dyspnea, and stridor. Chest X-rays reveal recurrent atelectasis that may become secondarily infected. Hyperinflation is usually noted on the X-rays of patients with stenosis of the main bronchus. In patients with segmental bronchomalacia, the involved lung is usually hyperlucent. If the orifices of the upper lobes or right middle lobe are involved there may be an associated collapse. Recurrent consolidation or persistent collapse is a common radiologic finding of stenosis of a lobar bronchus. Diagnosis is accomplished by endoscopy. Treatment varies with the severity of obstruction. In some cases, the administration of bronchodilators and chest physical therapy is sufficient; more severe cases may require positive pressure ventilation or surgery to remove the stenotic segment. Lobar resection may be necessary to control persistent infection.[67]

Tracheal Stenosis

Signs and symptoms of congenital tracheal stenosis include persistent cough and respiratory distress in the newborn period.

Patients may have expiratory stridor and wheezing. History of feeding difficulties is common. Chest X-rays and fluoroscopy may reveal a missing segment of the trachea. Highly penetrated films of the neck may show tracheal narrowing. In congenital tracheal stenosis there is intrinsic narrowing of the tracheal lumen caused by complete cartilaginous rings. The size of the lumen can be assessed by CT or MRI. The definitive diagnosis is made by endoscopy. The differential diagnosis includes extrinsic compression of the trachea by vascular rings or mediastinal masses. Tracheotomy may be necessary to maintain a patent airway. Endoscopic procedures can be used to treat thin tracheal webs and unilateral lesions. Conservative management of patients with mild symptoms should be attempted. Dilation of tracheal stenosis may provide a temporary solution until definitive surgical repair can be accomplished. Surgical treatment is associated with significant morbidity and mortality.[66]

Cough Associated with Aspiration Syndromes

Aspiration pneumonia is a common disorder frequently mistaken for nonspecific respiratory infection while aspiration bronchitis is mistaken for asthma. In infants, these conditions are most commonly associated with the inhalation of milk as a result of one of three disorders: impairment of sucking or swallowing likely to be neurogenic in origin, gastroesophageal reflux, or tracheoesophageal fistula. These are conditions that must not be overlooked.

The initial step in diagnosis is to observe the child, while nursing, for difficulty with sucking or swallowing or for associated cough or choking. Gross structural abnormalities of the mouth, jaw, or palate can be noted. Placing a finger in the baby's mouth can assess the act of the sucking. X-rays of children with aspiration bronchitis typically show perihilar thickening and increased bronchovascular markings, while those of children with aspiration pneumonia show patchy areas of uniform opacity that may have a segmental or lobar distribution. In infants, the posterior parts of the upper and lower lobes are most commonly involved with the right side predominating. Fluoroscopy is used to evaluate the anatomy of the upper airway and esophagus and the swallowing function. Esophageal pH probe or impedance probe monitoring establishes the presence of reflux.[68] Bronchoscopy and microscopic examination for lipid-laden macrophages substantiate the diagnosis of aspiration.

Tracheoesophageal fistulas require prompt surgical repair. The management of a child with a swallowing disorder requires the assistance of a clinic that specializes in this problem.

Gastroesophageal Reflux

Gastroesophageal reflux (GER) is a common cause of chronic cough in individuals of all ages and of apnea in infants, even without coexisting aspiration. Its most likely mode of action is through vagal stimulation, although aspiration must be considered. GER has been documented in about half of the adults with chronic cough, and it commonly occurs in children.[69] The respiratory manifestations of GER – cough, wheezing, sore throat, hoarseness, throat clearing, choking, and throat irritation – often persist in the absence of more familiar symptoms such as heartburn and regurgitation.[70] Proton pump inhibitors or H-2 blockers effectively reduce the respiratory complications of GER. However, higher than standard doses may be necessary and therapy may need to be continued for several months before a therapeutic effect is achieved. Laparoscopic fundoplication has been performed safely, even in high-risk children.[71]

Foreign Body

A foreign body may lodge in the hypopharynx, larynx, trachea, bronchus, or esophagus. Aspiration of a foreign body into the airway typically causes stridor. It is a pediatric emergency requiring immediate management by a specialist, even though unsuspected bronchial foreign bodies may be present for a long time and lead to chronic bronchitis and bronchiectasis. Unrecognized esophageal foreign bodies resulting in tracheal compression have caused recurrent wheezing or cough without dysphagia for as long as a year. Cough, wheezing, or dyspnea may date from the time of aspiration or may begin later, after edema and inflammation have set in and reflex bronchospasm has resulted. The majority of aspirated foreign bodies are foods such as peanuts or sunflower seeds, but a remarkable variety of objects has been removed at bronchoscopy. It is of note that peanuts release oils that are irritating to the bronchial mucosa, causing inflammation and edema. Other organic solids, such as beans, peas, corn, or seeds, can absorb water and increase considerably in size.

In one third of patients with foreign body aspiration, the actual event goes unobserved by caretakers.[72] The diagnosis may be suspected on the basis of history and physical findings. Classical signs are wheezing, coughing, and decreased breath sounds. Use of a differential stethoscope may be helpful in detecting localized airway obstruction. The diagnosis is established by radiographic findings, and ultimately by bronchoscopy. Chest X-rays show atelectasis in cases of complete obstruction of a bronchus. In cases of partial obstruction, the foreign body may act as a valve that allows air entry but impedes exhalation from a portion of a lung. Comparison of inspiratory and expiratory films shows a hyperinflated obstructed portion in comparison to the unaffected lung following expiration. On decubitus films and fluoroscopy the dependent lung should show less inflation unless obstructive hyperinflation from the valve-like mechanism is present. Bronchoscopy provides decisive evidence for diagnosis and treatment. Rigid bronchoscopy is preferred because it allows for the removal of the foreign body at the time of diagnosis. Treatment with bronchodilators, postural drainage and chest physical therapy as an alternative to bronchoscopic removal of the foreign body is no longer recommended.

Cystic Fibrosis

Cystic fibrosis is diagnosed with increasing frequency during neonatal screening. The presenting symptoms of this disease are cough, poor weight gain, and abnormal stools. The earliest symptom is usually a loose cough. Most patients experience recurrent lower respiratory infection before 12 months, but the age of onset is variable. Purulent bronchitis may be associated with wheezing and cough, and the diagnosis of asthma is often made in error. Purulent chronic cough in children must always be regarded as a pathologic finding.[37]

Allergic Bronchopulmonary Aspergillosis

Timely diagnosis of allergic bronchopulmonary aspergillosis (ABPA) is important because untreated ABPA results in progressive, irreversible lung damage. ABPA is a disease differentiated by recurrent infiltrates on chest X-ray, markedly elevated serum immunoglobulin E (IgE), eosinophilia, and underlying asthma.

Clinically it is characterized by afebrile episodes of cough, sputum production, dyspnea, and wheezing.

Hypersensitivity Lung Disease

Hypersensitivity pneumonitis or extrinsic allergic alveolitis is a syndrome that results from sensitization to inhaled organic dusts, which in children are most often avian antigens. Bird fancier's disease has been reported to occur in families. During acute attacks patients suffer from both respiratory and systemic symptoms including cough, dyspnea, temperature as high as 40°C, chills, and myalgia.

Vocal Cord Dysfunction

Vocal cord dysfunction (VCD) is a condition characterized by a paradoxical adduction of the vocal cords on inspiration that causes shortness of breath, cough, and stridor.[73] VCD in children commonly occurs during exertion and must be differentiated from exercise-induced bronchospasm (EIB). VCD has been documented in adolescents, usually female athletes.[74] Among these patients, perfectionism, depression, and anxiety are common.

The chest X-rays in uncomplicated VCD are normal. Spirometry shows blunting or truncation of the inspiratory portion of the flow-volume curve. Because of the episodic nature of VCD, the flow rate patterns may vary, and during asymptomatic periods, normal flow-volume curves are likely to be found. It is possible to replicate symptoms and spirometric findings of VCD by exercise or inhalation challenge, but negative results do not rule out the diagnosis. Observation of the vocal cords of a patient experiencing either spontaneous or induced symptoms by flexible fiberoptic rhinolaryngoscopy documents the presence of VCD.[73] The examination can be videotaped or photographed for the medical record. Complications are rare and discomfort is minimal. In VCD, the vocal cords adduct anteriorly from the vocal process, and the posterior glottic chink remains open. The adduction occurs during inspiration or in both the inspiratory and expiratory phases. The adduction of vocal cords with an open glottic chink in a symptomatic patient unequivocally establishes the diagnosis of VCD.

In the author's experience, the most successful treatment of VCD is derived from breathing exercises used for hyperfunctional voice disorders to decrease the laryngeal muscle tone.[75] These techniques are likely to desensitize the cough pathways.[76] In some extreme cases, hypnosis, biofeedback, and psychotherapy have been used successfully. An approach reserved for acute attacks is the administration of a mixture of helium and oxygen. More aggressive therapies under study for patients with intractable, recurrent symptoms include injection of botulinum toxin directly into one vocal cord or sectioning of the laryngeal nerve.[73,76]

Psychogenic Cough

Although it has been suggested that psychogenic cough typically ceases at night and has a barking or honking character, in actual fact, there are no distinguishing clinical features, and the diagnosis should be considered only after other possibilities have been excluded.[39] In some cases, a complete evaluation may require an assessment of the psychosocial factors that influence the origin, progression, persistence and/or exacerbation of chronic cough. Some children derive secondary gain in the form

of greater attention or emotional support from their parents. In others, trauma such as physical abuse or school phobia may cause a conversion syndrome. A psychological evaluation may be necessary to focus on specific detrimental effects of the cough, a disruptive process that may affect negatively a broad spectrum of social and interpersonal experiences. This may range from distress at school to exclusion from play, social functions, or participation in sports. As in other chronic medical conditions, emotional responses to the symptom may need to be addressed. Depression and frustration are the most common adjustment reactions, but negative responses may range over the entire affective spectrum.

Patients with psychogenic cough often believe that they have a serious chest problem. The diagnosis has been made in 3% to 10% of children with cough of unknown etiology that persists for more than 1 month. In 17 published reports, 149 of 153 patients were under 18 years of age.[39] While wholly psychogenic cough is rare, children and/or parents may exaggerate some or all aspects of the cough. Occasionally it is difficult to reconcile the parents' or children's accounts with clinical findings. The parents may demand inappropriate treatment and may instill in the child the belief that he or she is physically disabled. When clinical findings differ from the history, confirmation of the cough by the use of a recording device and/or admission to the hospital for observation may be invaluable. The circumstances call for sympathy and understanding, and the doctor's responsibility to the child must take precedence over the doctor-parent relationship.

Habit cough, a diagnosis of exclusion, results from the lowering of the threshold for sensory signals in chronic nonproductive cough that may become self-perpetuating and persist even after the initial inciting reason is no longer present.

Evaluation

Information about the history of onset, character of the cough (harsh, dry, productive, paroxysmal), triggers, the time of occurrence and accompanying symptoms or sensations may offer clues about its etiology. A detailed health history must be obtained with attention to the neonatal period; feeding problems; congenital malformations affecting the heart, great vessels, nasopharynx and upper respiratory tract, and gastrointestinal tract; respiratory infections; signs and symptoms of chronic illness; respiratory symptoms including those relating to the upper airway such as postnasal drip or irritation and lower respiratory tract such as wheezing, dyspnea and exercise tolerance; heartburn; nocturnal symptoms; and environmental exposures including cigarette smoke at home, at school, at daycare, and at the homes of close playmates. The social history provides information about family or school problems that may contribute to psychogenic cough.

The physical examination focuses on the head and neck and the respiratory and cardiovascular systems. We seek out signs of allergic rhinitis, stridor, tachypnea, hyperinflation, wheezes, crackles, rhonchi (with special attention paid to unilateral or asymmetric findings), heart murmurs, gallops, and congestive heart failure.

Eosinophils on the nasal smear suggest allergic rhinitis and neutrophils infectious sinusitis. Eosinophils in the sputum suggest asthma. Pulmonary function testing should be used in any child capable of performing the necessary maneuvers. Generally, useful data include a complete blood count with differential, serum IgE, allergy skin tests, an examination of the vocal cords, chest and sinus X-rays and/or CT, bronchial challenge, and esophageal pH or impedance monitoring.[77] Exhaled NO may help to identify toddlers with recurrent cough who will go on to develop asthma. Other laboratory tests based on clinical findings comprise specific studies recommended for the conditions discussed in the sections above. They include sputum culture, immunoglobulins, PPD, sweat test, and ciliary biopsy. Bronchoscopy is rarely indicated. For dynamic evaluation of compression syndromes, flexible bronchoscopy provides the best detail, but if a foreign body aspiration is likely, rigid bronchoscopy should be used. Cough with hemoptysis is an indication for a chest X-ray, chest CT and bronchoscopy.

Environment

It is important to obtain an environmental history of children with chronic cough because it may be possible to make improvements in their surroundings. Environmental history for chronic cough should include exposure to cigarette smoke in all children, to aeroallergens, especially indoor, in older children, and dietary history in infants and toddlers. In utero exposure to mainstream smoke from the mother and even to environmental tobacco smoke changes fetal lung development and causes airflow obstruction and airway hyperresponsiveness. Children exposed to environmental tobacco smoke postnatally have more symptoms of cough, wheeze, respiratory illnesses, decreases in lung function, and increases in airway responsiveness.[78] A survey of respiratory symptoms in children aged 12 to 14 years was conducted throughout Great Britain as part of the International Study of Asthma and Allergies in Childhood (ISAAC). The response rate was 79.3%, and 25 393 children in 93 schools participated.[79] Cough and phlegm were associated with active and passive smoking. Gas cooking was significantly associated with dry night cough. The prevalence of cough and phlegm tended to be higher in metropolitan areas; the opposite applied to asthma. Exposure to any passive smoking raised the odds ratio (OR) for night cough (OR = 1.8), snoring (OR = 1.4), and respiratory infections during the first 2 years of life (OR = 1.3). Respiratory problems were more prevalent in homes with reported molds or dampness with adjusted OR ranging from 1.32 (95% confidence interval 1.06–1.39) for bronchitis to 1.89 (95% confidence interval 1.58–2.26) for cough.[80] There is an association between coal fires and nocturnal cough.[81]

Treatment

The goal of clinical evaluation of chronic cough is to identify its causes and to prescribe specific remedies such as modification of the child's environment and treatment of postnasal drip or gastroesophageal reflux. Antiasthma drugs are not reliably effective in patients with chronic dry cough, nevertheless a 2- to 4-week course of a potent inhaled corticosteroid should be administered to children with prolonged cough without wheeze who have not already received such therapy, especially if they have obstructive pulmonary function tests or positive bronchial challenge results. Inhaled corticosteroids should be discontinued in children who have received an adequate trial and are continuing to cough, and whose pulmonary function tests are normal. Failure to improve after 4 weeks of inhaled corticosteroids and/or normal pulmonary function tests call for consideration of alternative diagnoses and for proceeding with the clinical evaluation described above. New treatment should be directed at all conditions identified that may be responsible for the patient's cough and should include breathing exercises.[75]

Parents have access to a great deal of information, some of questionable value, and they are exposed to a barrage of advertising. Health information available on the Internet relating to treatment of cough is generally unreliable. A review of websites identified more incorrect than correct information, and only 1 of 19 received a high score.[82] Parents may hold unrealistic expectations and may demand needless medications. In such cases, it is best to acknowledge the child's discomfort, to give a realistic time course for resolution of symptoms and to promote active management with nonpharmacologic treatments. Patient education fills an important role in the management of chronic cough. The patient and family who understand how individual mechanisms contribute to the cough and where each type of treatment fits, carry out their regimen with greater adherence and reduced anxiety. They cope more effectively with the symptoms, especially during periods of exacerbation. On rare occasions, it may be necessary to enlist the help of a psychotherapist to help the family accept the diagnosis and to adhere to therapy.

Over-the-counter pediatric cough and cold medications are widely marketed and used despite lack of evidence of efficacy and numerous recent reports challenging their safety. Serious adverse effects have been associated with accidental overdose, inadvertent misuse, and drug–drug or drug–host interactions in children given standard doses.[83] An estimated 7091 children under 12 years are treated annually in the USA in emergency departments for adverse drug events attributable to cough and cold medications. Most visits (64%). are for children aged 2 to 5 years. Unsupervised ingestions account for 66% of estimated emergency department visits.[84] Data obtained from 4267 children enrolled from 1999 to 2006 in the Slone Survey, a random-digit-dial telephone survey of medication use by the US population, disclosed that in a given week, 10.1% of US children use a cough and cold medication. Exposure is highest to decongestants (6.3%; mostly pseudoephedrine) and first-generation antihistamines (6.3%; most common were chlorpheniramine, diphenhydramine, and brompheniramine), followed by antitussives (4.1%; mostly dextromethorphan) and expectorants (1.5%; almost exclusively guaifenesin). Multiple-ingredient products accounted for 64.2% of all cough and cold medications used. Exposure to antitussives, decongestants, and first-generation antihistamines was highest among 2- to 5-year-olds (7.0%, 9.9%, and 10.1%, respectively) followed by children who were younger than 2 years (5.9%, 9.4%, and 7.6%, respectively).[85] During 2004 to 2005, an estimated 1519 children under 2 years of age were treated in US emergency departments for adverse events associated with cough and cold medications. A review by the Food and Drug Administration (FDA) covering several decades identified 123 deaths related to the use of such products in children under 6 years.[83,86] The infants ranged in age from 17 days to 10 months. Postmortem testing showed evidence of recent administration of pseudoephedrine, antihistamine, dextromethorphan, and/or other cold-medication ingredients.[87] On a positive note, pseudoephedrine use by children appears to be declining since the institution of the 2005 Combat Methamphetamine Epidemic Act.[88] In the Slone survey conducted from 1999 to 2006, use in 2006 (2.9%) was significantly lower than in 1999–2005 (5.2%)

Conclusions

As the ability to perform pulmonary function tests in infants and toddlers expands and surrogate markers of disease become identified, prospective longitudinal studies starting at a very young age will become feasible, and it will become possible to assess both immediate and long-term consequences of cough and its

BOX 31-2 Key concepts

Evaluation of Chronic Cough

- Cough is a common manifestation of disease in childhood.

- Cough is an important defense mechanism.

- Cough functions as a complex neurologic reflex.

- Cough may be classified as acute (lasting < 3 weeks), subacute (lasting 3 to 8 weeks), or chronic (lasting > 8 weeks).

- The cause of chronic cough can be determined in most patients; specific therapy based on a systematic evaluation is usually successful.

- A chest radiograph should be obtained in children with chronic cough to rule out lower respiratory tract and cardiac pathology.

- Postnasal drip, acting alone or with other conditions, is the most common cause of chronic cough.

- Asthma is very often associated with chronic cough, but few children with chronic cough develop asthma.

- Cough-variant asthma is suggested by (1) airway obstruction and reversibility, (2) airway hyperresponsiveness, and/or (3) clinical improvement after treatment with asthma medications.

- Gastroesophageal reflux may cause or intensify chronic cough through a vagal reflex or as a result of aspiration of stomach contents.

- Postinfectious cough resolves over time; the use of oral or inhaled corticosteroids or ipratropium bromide may shorten its duration.

- Congenital anomalies and aspiration are relatively uncommon causes of chronic cough in children.

- Bronchiectasis is a rare cause of chronic cough in children.

- Psychogenic cough and habit cough are diagnoses of exclusion.

treatment. The ultimate goals are not merely to find effective therapies for chronic cough but also to identify and eliminate factors that predispose children to this troublesome complaint. In the meantime, let us strive to limit children's exposure to tobacco smoke and the families' reliance on over-the-counter medications.

References

1. Marchant JM, Newcombe PA, Juniper EF, et al. What is the burden of chronic cough for families? Chest 2008;134:303–9.
2. Newcombe PA, Sheffield JK, Juniper EF, et al. Development of a parent-proxy quality-of-life chronic cough-specific questionnaire: clinical impact vs psychometric evaluations. Chest 2008;133:386–95.
3. Vital and Health Statistics: National Ambulatory Medical Care Survey: 1995–96 summary. Series 13: data from the National Health Care Survey No. 142, Hyattsville, MD, 1999, U.S. Department of Health and Human Services, Centers for Disease Control and Prevention, National Center for Health Statistics.
4. Powell CV, Primhak RA. Stability of respiratory symptoms in unlabelled wheezy illness and nocturnal cough. Arch Dis Child 1996;75:385–91.
5. Irwin RS, Madison JM. The diagnosis and treatment of cough. N Engl J Med 2000;343:1715–21.
6. Irwin RS, Baumann MH, Bolser DC, et al. Diagnosis and management of cough executive summary: ACCP evidence-based clinical practice guidelines. Chest 2006;129:1S–23S.
7. Lister SM, Jorm LR. Parental smoking and respiratory illnesses in Australian children aged 0–4 years: ABS 1989–90 National Health Survey results. Aust N Z J Public Health 1998;22:781–6.
8. Milgrom H, Wood RI, Ingram D. Respiratory conditions that mimic asthma. Immunol Allergy Clin N Amer 1998;18:113–32.
9. Marchant JM, Masters IB, Taylor SM, et al. Evaluation and outcome of young children with chronic cough. Chest 2006;129:1132–41.
10. Boren EJ, Teuber SS, Gershwin ME. A review of non-cystic fibrosis pediatric bronchiectasis. Clin Rev Allergy Immunol 2008;34:260–73.
11. Munyard P, Bush A. How much coughing is normal? Arch Dis Child 1996;74:531–4.
12. Chang AB, Asher MI. A review of cough in children. J Asthma 2001;38:299–309.
13. Falconer A, Oldman C, Helms P. Poor agreement between reported and recorded nocturnal cough in asthma. Pediatr Pulmonol 1993;15:209–11.
14. Shann F. How often do children cough? Lancet 1996;348:699–700.
15. Dales RE, White J, Bhumgara C, et al. Parental reporting of children's coughing is biased. Eur J Epidemiol 1997;13:541–5.
16. Chang AB. Cough, cough receptors, and asthma in children. Pediatr Pulmonol 1999;28:59–70.
17. Helmers SL, Wheless JW, Frost M, et al. Vagus nerve stimulation therapy in pediatric patients with refractory epilepsy: retrospective study. J Child Neurol 2001;16:843–8.
18. Irwin RS, Rosen MJ, Braman SS. Cough: a comprehensive review. Arch Intern Med 1977;137:1186–91.
19. Cough and wheeze in asthma: are they interdependent? Lancet 1988;1:447–8.
20. Leith DE. Cough. Phys Ther 1968;48:439–47.
21. Chausow AM, Banner AS. Comparison of the tussive effects of histamine and methacholine in humans. J Appl Physiol 1983;55:541–6.
22. Eschenbacher WL, Boushey HA, Sheppard D. Alteration in osmolarity of inhaled aerosols cause bronchoconstriction and cough, but absence of a permeant anion causes cough alone. Am Rev Respir Dis 1984;129:211–5.
23. Fuller RW, Karlsson JA, Choudry NB, et al. Effect of inhaled and systemic opiates on responses to inhaled capsaicin in humans. J Appl Physiol 1988;65:1125–30.
24. McFadden ER, Jr., Nelson JA, Skowronski ME, et al. Thermally induced asthma and airway drying. Am J Respir Crit Care Med 1999;160:221–6.
25. Chang AB, Harrhy VA, Simpson J, et al. Cough, airway inflammation, and mild asthma exacerbation. Arch Dis Child 2002;86:270–5.
26. Lemanske RF, Jr. Inflammation in childhood asthma and other wheezing disorders. Pediatrics 2002;109:368–72.
27. Baker RR, Mishoe SC, Zaitoun FH, et al. Poor perception of airway obstruction in children with asthma. J Asthma 2000;37:613–24.
28. Kelly YJ, Brabin BJ, Milligan PJ, et al. Clinical significance of cough and wheeze in the diagnosis of asthma. Arch Dis Child 1996;75:489–93.
29. McKenzie S. Cough – but is it asthma? Arch Dis Child 1994;70:1–2.
30. Chang AB. Isolated cough: probably not asthma. Arch Dis Child 1999;80:211–3.
31. Davies MJ, Fuller P, Picciotto A, et al. Persistent nocturnal cough: randomised controlled trial of high dose inhaled corticosteroid. Arch Dis Child 1999;81:38–44.
32. Chang AB, Powell CV. Non-specific cough in children: diagnosis and treatment. Hosp Med 1998;59:680–4.
33. Ninan TK, Macdonald L, Russell G. Persistent nocturnal cough in childhood: a population based study. Arch Dis Child 1995;73:403–7.
34. Moeller A, Diefenbacher C, Lehmann A, et al. Exhaled nitric oxide distinguishes between subgroups of preschool children with respiratory symptoms. J Allergy Clin Immunol 2008;121:705–9.
35. Wright AL, Holberg CJ, Morgan WJ, et al. Recurrent cough in childhood and its relation to asthma. Am J Respir Crit Care Med 1996;153:1259–65.
36. Brooke AM, Lambert PC, Burton PR, et al. Recurrent cough: natural history and significance in infancy and early childhood. Pediatr Pulmonol 1998;26:256–61.
37. Chang AB. Cough. Pediatr Clin North Am 2009;56:19–31.
38. Zimmerman B, Silverman FS, Tarlo SM, et al. Induced sputum: comparison of postinfectious cough with allergic asthma in children. J Allergy Clin Immunol 2000;105:495–9.
39. French CL, Irwin RS, Curley FJ, et al. Impact of chronic cough on quality of life. Arch Intern Med 1998;158:1657–61.
40. Yanney M, Vyas H. The treatment of bronchiolitis. Arch Dis Child 2008;93:793–8.
41. Law BJ, Carbonell-Estrany X, Simoes EA. An update on respiratory syncytial virus epidemiology: a developed country perspective. Respir Med 2002;96(Suppl B):S1–7.
42. Schlesinger C, Koss MN. Bronchiolitis: update 2001. Curr Opin Pulm Med 2002;8:112–6.
43. McBride JT, McConnochie KM. RSV, recurrent wheezing, and ribavirin. Pediatr Pulmonol 1998;25:145–6.
44. Stein MT, Harper G, Chen J. Persistent cough in an adolescent. J Dev Behav Pediatr 1999;20:434–6; discussion 6–8.
45. Castro M, Schweiger T, Yin-Declue H, et al. Cytokine response after severe respiratory syncytial virus bronchiolitis in early life. J Allergy Clin Immunol 2008;122:726–33 e3.

46. Fernald GW, Collier AM, Clyde WA, Jr. Respiratory infections due to *Mycoplasma pneumoniae* in infants and children. Pediatrics 1975;55: 327–35.

47. Murphy TF, Henderson FW, Clyde WA, Jr., et al. Pneumonia: an eleven-year study in a pediatric practice. Am J Epidemiol 1981;113:12–21.

48. Sabato AR, Martin AJ, Marmion BP, et al. *Mycoplasma pneumoniae*: acute illness, antibiotics, and subsequent pulmonary function. Arch Dis Child 1984;59:1034–7.

49. Centers for Disease Control and Prevention. Pertussis–United States, 2001–2003. MMWR Morb Mortal Wkly Rep 2005;54:1283–6.

50. Bamberger ES, Srugo I. What is new in pertussis? Eur J Pediatr 2008;167:133–9.

51. Sotir MJ, Cappozzo DL, Warshauer DM, et al. A countywide outbreak of pertussis: initial transmission in a high school weight room with subsequent substantial impact on adolescents and adults. Arch Pediatr Adolesc Med 2008;162:79–85.

52. American Academy of Pediatrics. Report of the Committee on Infectious Diseases. Pertussis. Elk Grove Village, Ill; 2003.

53. Centers for Disease Control and Prevention. Pertussis–United States, 1997–2000. JAMA 2002;287:977–9.

54. Khetsuriani N, Bisgard K, Prevots DR, et al. Pertussis outbreak in an elementary school with high vaccination coverage. Pediatr Infect Dis J 2001;20:1108–12.

55. Pichichero ME, Casey JR. Acellular pertussis vaccines for adolescents. Pediatr Infect Dis J 2005;24:S117–26.

56. Robbins JB, Schneerson R, Keith JM, et al. Pertussis vaccine: a critique. Pediatr Infect Dis J 2009;28:237–41.

57. Versteegh FG, Schellekens JF, Nagelkerke AF, et al. Laboratory-confirmed reinfections with *Bordetella pertussis*. Acta Paediatr 2002;91: 95–7.

58. Birkebaek NH, Kristiansen M, Seefeldt T, et al. *Bordetella pertussis* and chronic cough in adults. Clin Infect Dis 1999;29:1239–42.

59. Lebel MH, Mehra S. Efficacy and safety of clarithromycin versus erythromycin for the treatment of pertussis: a prospective, randomized, single blind trial. Pediatr Infect Dis J 2001;20:1149–54.

60. Cooper WO, Griffin MR, Arbogast P, et al. Very early exposure to erythromycin and infantile hypertrophic pyloric stenosis. Arch Pediatr Adolesc Med 2002;156:647–50.

61. Goldstein LH, Berlin M, Tsur L, et al. The safety of macrolides during lactation. Breastfeed Med 2009.

62. Chen CJ, Wu KG, Tang RB, et al. Characteristics of *Chlamydia trachomatis* infection in hospitalized infants with lower respiratory tract infection. J Microbiol Immunol Infect 2007;40:255–9.

63. Eamranond P, Jaramillo E. Tuberculosis in children: reassessing the need for improved diagnosis in global control strategies. Int J Tuberc Lung Dis 2001;5:594–603.

64. American Academy of Pediatrics. Report of the Committee on Infectious Diseases. Tuberculosis. Elk Grove Village, Ill; 2003.

65. Lack G. Pediatric allergic rhinitis and comorbid disorders. J Allergy Clin Immunol 2001;108:S9–15.

66. Andrews T, Myer C, Bailey W. Intrathoracic lesions involving the tracheobronchial tree. Philadelphia: JB Lippincott; 1995.

67. Oermann CM, Moore RH. Foolers: things that look like pneumonia in children. Semin Respir Infect 1996;11:204–13.

68. Condino AA, Sondheimer J, Pan Z, et al. Evaluation of gastroesophageal reflux in pediatric patients with asthma using impedance-pH monitoring. J Pediatr 2006;149:216–9.

69. McGeady S. GERD and airways disease in children and adolescents. In Stein M, editor. Gastroesophageal reflux disease and airway disease. New York: Marcel Dekker; 1999.

70. Block BB, Brodsky L. Hoarseness in children: the role of laryngopharyngeal reflux. Int J Pediatr Otorhinolaryngol 2007;71:1361–9.

71. Rothenberg SS, Bratton D, Larsen G, et al. Laparoscopic fundoplication to enhance pulmonary function in children with severe reactive airway disease and gastroesophageal reflux disease. Surg Endosc 1997;11: 1088–90.

72. Cohen SR, Herbert WI, Lewis GB, Jr., et al. Foreign bodies in the airway. Five-year retrospective study with special reference to management. Ann Otol Rhinol Laryngol 1980;89:437–42.

73. Wood RP 2nd, Milgrom H. Vocal cord dysfunction. J Allergy Clin Immunol 1996;98:481–5.

74. Landwehr LP, Wood RP 2nd, Blager FB, et al. Vocal cord dysfunction mimicking exercise-induced bronchospasm in adolescents. Pediatrics 1996;98:971–4.

75. Blager FB, Gay ML, Wood RP. Voice therapy techniques adapted to treatment of habit cough: a pilot study. J Commun Disord 1988;21: 393–400.

76. Chung KF, Pavord ID. Prevalence, pathogenesis, and causes of chronic cough. Lancet 2008;371:1364–74.

77. Pattenden S, Antova T, Neuberger M, et al. Parental smoking and children's respiratory health: independent effects of prenatal and postnatal exposure. Tob Control 2006;15:294–301.

78. Joad JP. Smoking and pediatric respiratory health. Clin Chest Med 2000;21:37–46.

79. Burr ML, Anderson HR, Austin JB, et al. Respiratory symptoms and home environment in children: a national survey. Thorax 1999;54: 27–32.

80. Dales RE, Zwanenburg H, Burnett R, et al. Respiratory health effects of home dampness and molds among Canadian children. Am J Epidemiol 1991;134:196–203.

81. Strachan DP, Elton RA. Relationship between respiratory morbidity in children and the home environment. Fam Pract 1986;3:137–42.

82. Pandolfini C, Impicciatore P, Bonati M. Parents on the web: risks for quality management of cough in children. Pediatrics 2000; 105:e1.

83. Sharfstein JM, North M, Serwint JR. Over the counter but no longer under the radar: pediatric cough and cold medications. N Engl J Med 2007;357:2321–4.

84. Schaefer MK, Shehab N, Cohen AL, et al. Adverse events from cough and cold medications in children. Pediatrics 2008;121:783–7.

85. Vernacchio L, Kelly JP, Kaufman DW, et al. Cough and cold medication use by US children, 1999–2006: results from the Slone Survey. Pediatrics 2008;122:e323–9.

86. Food and Drug Administration. Division of Drug Risk Evaluation. Nonprescription Drug Advisory Committee meeting: cold, cough, allergy, bronchodilator, antiasthmatic drug products for over-the-counter human use. 2007:29. memorandum. http://www.fda.gov/ohrms/dockets/ac/07/briefing/2007-4323b1-02-FDA.pdf accessed 4/22/09

87. Rimsza ME, Newberry S. Unexpected infant deaths associated with use of cough and cold medications. Pediatrics 2008;122: e318–22.

88. Vernacchio L, Kelly JP, Kaufman DW, et al. Pseudoephedrine use among US children, 1999–2006: results from the Slone Survey. Pediatrics 2008;122:1299–304.

CHAPTER

32

Immunology of the Asthmatic Response

Philippe Stock • Claudia Macaubas • Rosemarie H. Dekruyff • Dale T. Umetsu

Asthma is an immunologic disease in which adaptive and innate immunity play major roles. Asthma, as a complex trait, develops after environmental exposures, such as to innocuous allergens, infectious agents, and air pollutants, in genetically susceptible individuals.[1] These events generally induce an immune response associated with a specific type of inflammation in the lungs that causes asthma, and characterized by the presence of T helper cell type 2 (Th2) lymphocytes, eosinophils, and basophils. This Th2-biased immune response results in increased mucus production, mucosal edema, reversible airway obstruction, bronchial hyper-responsiveness (BHR), airway remodeling, and in the symptoms of asthma. In addition, the inflammatory response in asthma is associated with sensitization to indoor and outdoor allergens,[2,3] and with elevated serum IgE levels,[4] which have been shown to be major risk factors for the development of asthma and persistent wheezing in children.

Components of the Allergic Inflammatory Response

The Th2-biased inflammatory response that results in asthma is complex and involves a number of cell types producing a large number of cytokines and chemokines (Figure 32-1). Together, these cell types and mediators are responsible for the *immediate-phase response* (IPR), as well as the *late-phase response* (LPR). The IPR occurs within minutes after allergen challenge due to binding of allergen to IgE on the surface of mast cells, resulting in mast cell degranulation and causing increased vascular permeability, extravasation of fluid into the tissues and smooth muscle contraction. The LPR occurs 6 to 12 hours later as a result of the accumulation of eosinophils, basophils, and activated T cells that typify the allergic inflammatory response. The LPR and its accompanying inflammation are associated with BHR, a cardinal feature of asthma.

Th2 Cells and Th2 Cytokines

CD4[+] T lymphocytes producing Th2 cytokines play a prominent role in asthma and are present in lung biopsy specimens and bronchoalveolar lavage (BAL) fluid from patients with asthma.[5] Several studies showed a correlation between the presence of CD4[+] Th2 cells and Th2 cytokine levels with the severity of asthma.[6] Although several cell types produce Th2 cytokines, including mast cells, basophils, and natural killer T (NKT) cells, Th2 lymphocytes are considered fundamental in asthma, because

in animal models, CD4[+] T cell depletion prevents the development of asthma. In fact, B cell-, IgE-, and mast cell-deficient mice can still develop asthma, whereas CD4[-], STAT-6-, and interleukin (IL)-13-deficient mice cannot. The signature Th2 cytokine, IL-4, plays an important initiator role. *IL-4* is essential for the differentiation of Th2 lymphocytes, and in the absence of IL-4, Th2 cell differentiation is severely impaired. IL-4 is critical for the induction of IgE synthesis and for the up-regulation of IgE receptor expression on B cells (low affinity IgE receptor, CD23), mast cells, and basophils (high affinity IgE receptor, FcεRI). Inhalation of recombinant IL-4 leads to BHR and eosinophil recruitment in asthmatic people.[7] IL-4 also increases the production of cysteinyl leukotrienes from IgE-primed mast cells[8] and induces expression of adhesion molecules, such as vascular cell adhesion molecule-1 (VCAM-1) on pulmonary endothelium, which is involved in the recruitment of eosinophils, basophils, and lymphocytes. IL-4 induces expression of eotaxin by lung cells, although IL-13, another Th2 cytokine, is more potent in this regard. In addition, IL-4 increases mucus production and may have direct effects on smooth muscle cells, but the exact role of IL-4 in causing BHR and mucus production is complex and overlaps with that of IL-13 (see below).

IL-5 is another central Th2 cytokine that is coordinately produced with IL-4. IL-5, together with IL-3 and granulocyte-macrophage colony-stimulating factor (GM-CSF), promotes the differentiation and maturation of eosinophil progenitors (CD34[+] cells) in the bone marrow and induces the release of mature eosinophils from the bone marrow into the circulation. Although IL-3 and GM-CSF also promote the differentiation of multiple cell lineages, IL-5 promotes only the terminal differentiation of eosinophils. IL-5 has also been shown to be important for the survival of eosinophils once in the tissues and for priming eosinophils for response to several stimuli. Clinically, the presence of eosinophils in the airways (and in the circulation) is associated with the presence of asthma, suggesting that eosinophil-induced damage to the pulmonary epithelium causes BHR and asthma. However, studies have shown that the depletion of eosinophils in patients with asthma through neutralization of IL-5 with anti-IL-5 monoclonal antibody does not reduce BHR,[9] except in a small fraction of patients, who have very large numbers of airway eosinophils.[10,11] Eosinophils produce cysteinyl leukotrienes, and may enhance the production of IL-13[12] which can directly induce BHR (see below).

Another Th2 cytokine, *IL-13*, has been shown to play a critical role in asthma. IL-13 has 30% homology with IL-4, and the receptors for both cytokines share one receptor chain, the IL-4Rα, involved in signal transduction. Accordingly, IL-4 and IL-13

©2010 Elsevier Ltd, Inc, BV
DOI: 10.1016/B978-1-4377-0271-2.00032-8

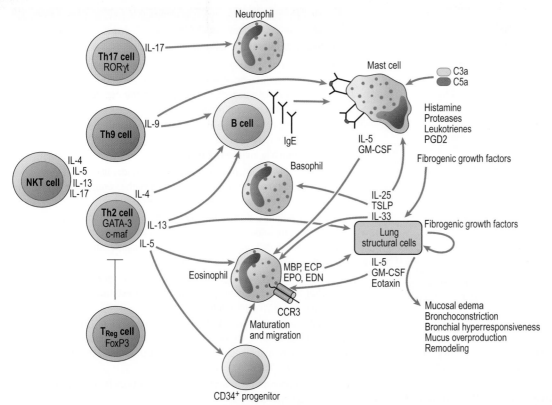

Figure 32-1 Schematic representation of the effector phase in asthma. Cytokines derived from CD4$^+$ Th2 T cells, NKT, Th9, Th17 cells and B cells producing IgE orchestrate the asthmatic response. Innate cells such as neutrophils, basophils, eosinophils, mast cells, as well as airway structural/epithelial cells participate in the response. CD4$^+$ T regulatory cells (T_{Reg}) down-modulate Th2 cells, Th17 cells and other inflammatory cells.

share several functions, including the promotion of IgE switch, and use the same transduction pathways (STAT-6). However, IL-13 is not able to induce Th2 differentiation because of the absence of the IL-13 receptor on the surface of T lymphocytes. Nevertheless, IL-13 directly increases mucus production by epithelial cells in the lung and directly causes BHR by binding to IL-13 receptors on airway smooth muscle cells.[13,14] High IL-13 levels are observed in bronchial biopsy samples from patients with asthma and in BAL fluid and serum of atopic asthmatic subjects. IL-13-deficient mice fail to develop BHR, even though they develop pulmonary eosinophilia.[15] Selective overexpression of IL-13 in the lungs results in pulmonary inflammation, airway epithelial and goblet cell hyperplasia with increased mucus production, increased collagen deposition, an increase in eotaxin, and an increase in BHR in response to methacholine. These findings indicate that IL-13 is a critical cytokine required for the development of asthma. It should be noted, however, that an IL-4 mutant protein that binds to IL-4Rα, blocking the binding of both IL-4 and IL-13, was unable in clinical trials to reduce BHR, although it reduced the severity of the LPR.[16] This suggests that other factors, in addition to IL-13/IL-4, function to induce BHR in patients with asthma.

Th2 Cell Development

The production of Th2 cytokines and the development of polarized T cells are regulated by specific transcription factors, which are induced by antigenic stimulation in the presence of a specific set of cytokines.[17] Th2 cell differentiation is enhanced by the presence of IL-4, which binds to IL-4R, composed of the IL-4Rα and the common β chain (also part of the receptors for IL-2, IL-7, IL-9, and IL-15). Binding of IL-4 to its surface receptor

activates STAT-6. The binding of IL-13 to its receptors, which consist of IL-13Rα1 and IL-13Rα2 and the IL-4Rα chain, also results in phosphorylation of STAT-6. Increased expression of STAT-6 in bronchial mucosa of asthmatic patients has been observed.[18] STAT-6 may directly translocate to the nucleus and bind to STAT-6 transcriptional elements or interact with additional Th2-associated transcription factors such as GATA-3. In contrast to STAT-6, GATA-3 is selectively expressed in Th2 cells and is critical for Th2 cytokine expression. GATA-3 is expressed in higher levels in the bronchial mucosa of asthmatic individuals.[19]

Costimulatory Requirements for the Development of Sensitization

Dendritic cells (DCs, see below) present allergen to naïve T cells in a process that requires costimulation (Figure 32-2). The best characterized costimulatory molecule expressed on T cells is CD28, which binds to CD80 (B7-1) and CD86 (B7-2) expressed on antigen-presenting cells (APCs).[20] Human studies with isolated peripheral blood mononuclear cells indicate that blockage of CD28-B7 interactions with CTLA-4-Ig inhibits allergen-induced proliferation and production of IL-5 and IL-13.[21]

Another more recently described member of the CD28 family, called inducible T cell costimulator (ICOS), is expressed by activated T cells and germinal center T cells[20] and appears to be important for both the development and effector function of Th2 cells. ICOS binds to the B7-related protein ICOS ligand (ICOSL) or B7RP-1, expressed on DCs, monocytes, B cells, and endothelial cells. ICOS is expressed by naïve T cells on activation but is preferentially expressed on Th2 but not Th1 cells. Inhibition of

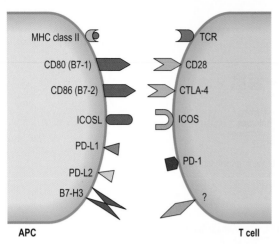

Figure 32-2 Antigen presentation and costimulation. Major histocompatibility complex (MHC) class II molecules on the surfaces of antigen-presenting cells present processed allergen to the T cell receptor. Costimulatory signals are also necessary to modulate the T cell response. Known members of the best characterized costimulatory family, the B7/CD28, are represented in the figure.

ICOS signaling decreases Th2 effector activity but not Th1 responses and blocks both the development and expression of experimental asthma.[22]

Other costimulatory pathways for T cells include CTLA-4-B7, which induces T cell inhibitory signals. Consistent with this, treatment with a neutralizing anti-CTLA-4 monoclonal antibody increased IgE production, eosinophilic inflammation and BHR, and Th2 cytokine production but decreased transforming growth factor (TGF)-β production in mice.[23] Another member of the CD28 family is the PD-1 (programmed death) receptor, which interacts with the B7 family members PD-L1 and PD-L2.[24] PD-1 expression is up-regulated in T, B, and myeloid cells on activation. Binding of PD-1 to both PD-L1 and PD-L2 has been associated mainly with inhibition of T cell function in both CD4+ and CD8+ T cells, although some studies reported T cell stimulation, especially production of IL-10. Finally, the latest identified member of the B7 family is B7-H3.[20] B7-H3 expression is induced on DCs and monocytes by proinflammatory cytokines. The receptor for B7-H3 is still unknown and is distinct from CD28, CTLA-4, ICOS, and PD-1. B7-H3 costimulation induces proliferation in both CD4+ and CD8+ T cells, induces cytotoxic activity, and selectively increases expression of interferon (IFN)-γ[25] (Box 32-1).

Th1/Th2 Paradigm

As part of the *Th1/Th2 paradigm*, Th1 cells were thought to balance Th2 responses and protect against allergic disease by dampening the activity of Th2 responses, as has been shown in models of infection with intracellular bacteria. In support of this idea, infants having greater quantities of IFN-γ in their cord blood have been shown to be less likely to develop atopy.[26] Furthermore, expression of T-bet, the transcription factor that greatly increases IFN-γ production and directs Th1 cell commitment, is decreased in the airways of patients with asthma,[27] and in the absence of T-bet, enhanced airway inflammation and BHR occurs. Moreover, IL-12 production, which greatly enhances Th1 cell development, has been reported to be decreased in patients with asthma and allergy,[28] and expression of the receptor for IL-12, IL-12Rβ2, may be decreased in patients with atopic asthma.[29]

Updating the Th2 Paradigm

Although the Th2 paradigm of asthma explains many features of asthma, particularly in allergic and mild asthma, many other observations cannot be explained by this paradigm. For example, non-Th2 factors such as IFN-γ, neutrophils and IL-17 are present in the airways of many patients with asthma, particularly patients with severe asthma and corticosteroid resistant asthma. This suggests that IFN-γ is a proinflammatory cytokine, and that Th1 cells are not necessarily the polarized opposite of Th2 cells. This idea is supported by the observations that Th1-mediated autoimmune diseases such as type 1 diabetes and inflammatory bowel disease, like atopic diseases, have increased in prevalence in westernized cultures during the past three decades. This suggests that the environmental changes that have occurred in westernized cultures have affected immunity in a way that has enhanced the development of both Th2- and Th1-mediated diseases.

Another observation that cannot be explained by the Th2 paradigm of asthma is that patients with severe asthma and with steroid-resistant asthma often have few Th2 cells in their airways.[16] Additionally, many nonallergic factors, such as viral infection, exercise and air pollution, induce symptoms of asthma.

Also, allergen sensitization does not automatically presage the development of asthma, as only 30–40% of patients with allergic rhinitis develop asthma, suggesting that Th2 cells by themselves are not sufficient for the development of asthma. Finally, therapies targeting Th2 factors in clinical trials have not been as effective as predicted,[30] suggesting that distinct subtypes of asthma exist, of which only some involve Th2 cells.[31] Thus, other inflammatory pathways must be considered beyond what was proposed by the Th1/Th2 paradigm to explain the development of asthma, and to understand the heterogeneity of asthmatic phenotypes and the variability of treatment responses.

New T Cell Subsets

Recently, additional subsets of CD4+ T cells have been described, including Th17 cells, regulatory T (T_{Reg}) cells and Th9 cells. These stubsets have potential roles in asthma, requiring modification of the Th1/Th2 paradigm.

Th17 Cells

Recently, a new T cell lineage, called *Th17 cells*, has been identified secreting large quantities of *IL-17A*, also known as IL-17.[32,33] Production of IL-17A has been found in the inflamed tissues of patients with psoriasis, Crohn's disease and rheumatoid arthritis, and mouse models suggest a causal role for Th17 cells, rather than Th1 cells, in mouse models of diabetes, inflammatory bowel disease and multiple sclerosis. Moreover, IL-17, which is a potent neutrophil chemotactic factor, is found in high amounts in sputum and BAL fluid of some asthmatic subjects,[34,35] particularly in patients with nonallergic asthma,[36] in association with neutrophils. Recent studies in mice and in humans suggest that Th17 cells, as well as IL-17 producing NKT cells and γδT cells may play important roles in asthma associated with neutrophils, since IL-17 potently attracts neutrophils.[37]

Th17 cells are normally thought to be involved in clearance of bacterial and fungal infections. APCs producing IL-6 and TGF-β induce the development of Th17 cells, which express the transcription factor, retinoid-related orphan receptor (ROR)γt. Low levels of TGF-β (with IL-6) induce Th17 cells, whereas higher levels of TGF-β in the absence of IL-6 result in the development of FoxP3+ T_{Reg} cells. Thus, Th17 cells and T_{Reg} cells have a reciprocal relationship (see below). IL-23 is necessary for the maintenance of murine Th17 cells, as it fixes the phenotype of these cells. In humans, TGF-β with IL-1β and IL-6, IL-21 or IL-23 are able to induce development of Th17 cells.[38] Th17 cells are absent in patients with autosomal dominant hyper-IgE syndrome (having hypomorphic mutations in Stat3).[38,39]

Regulatory T Cells and Tolerance

Cells that can down-modulate the function of Th2 cells (and Th1 cells) are now known as T_{Reg} cells. There are several subsets of T_{Reg} cells, including natural T_{Reg} cells, which develop in the thymus and prevent autoimmunity, adaptive T_{Reg} cells, which are antigen-specific and develop on exposure to antigen, as well as T_r1 cells, which are also antigen-specific but develop on exposure to IL-10. In humans, the induction of T_{Reg} cells is related to degree of allergen exposure. Lower doses of allergen appear to induce greater numbers of T_{Reg} cells, and higher doses may induce a greater deletion of antigen-specific cells.[40] Allergen-specific CD4 T_{Reg} cells may mediate T cell tolerance by inhibiting effector Th2 cells, thereby inhibiting airway inflammation and BHR.[41] In addition, the development of the tolerance process and the function of the T_{Reg} cells depend on ICOS-ICOSL pathways,

on CD28-B7-2 pathways, IL-10, CTLA-4 and direct cell-to-cell contact.[42] TGF-β production by T_{Reg} cells may also inhibit the development of BHR.[43] Natural and adaptive T_{Reg} cells express the transcription factor, Forkhead box p3 (Foxp3), which is essential for the development and function of T_{Reg} cells, since mutations in Foxp3 results in a multi-organ inflammatory disease, both in mice (scurfy) and in humans (x-linked immune dysregulation, polyendocrinopathy, and enterophathy syndrome, IPEX).[44] Allergic manifestations such as dermatitis and elevated IgE are part of this disease,[45] indicating that T_{Reg} cells are critically important in preventing allergic symptoms. Allergic and asthmatic individuals are thought to have a deficiency in the frequency of T_{Reg} cells, and allergen immunotherapy increases the number of allergen specific T_{Reg} cells.[46]

Th9 Cells

Recently, it has been shown that TGF-β is also able to reprogram Th2 cells to become selective producers of IL-9 (Th9), or, in combination with IL-4, to induce the direct development of 'Th9' cells.[47,48] IL-9 has a role in hematopoiesis, participates in mast cell maturation, and potentiates IgE production elicited by IL-4.[49] No specific transcription factor has been yet ascribed to this subpopulation. The expression of IL-9 and IL-9 receptor is increased in bronchial tissue of atopic asthmatic subjects,[50] and constitutive overexpression of IL-9 is associated with several manifestations of experimental asthma, such as BHR, inflammation, mucus production, and increased number of tissue mast cells.[51]

Innate Inflammatory Pathways to Asthma

The contribution of innate immune inflammatory pathways may have been underestimated in the past in asthma, in both allergic asthma and nonallergic forms of asthma. The innate inflammatory systems involve any response that does not involve memory, which is a characteristic of the adaptive immune system. Innate cells participate in the asthmatic response from the initial allergen presentation, to the effector phase of asthma. Compared to adaptive immunity, innate immunity is less sensitive to corticosteroids,[52] which may explain why nonallergic asthma and severe asthma tend to be steroid resistant. The innate pathways may involve pattern recognition receptors (PRRs) recognizing molecular patterns released from pathogens (pathogen-associated molecular patterns, PAMPs) or from damaged tissues (damage associated molecular patterns, DAMPs). These pathways involve cells intrinsic to the lungs, such as epithelial cells, other airway cells, as well as neutrophils, eosinophils, dendritic cells, NK cells and NKT cells.[30] For example, exposure to cigarette smoke may directly damage respiratory tissues, activating damage PRRs, or respiratory viruses may activate toll-like receptor (TLR)3, TLR7 or TLR8, inducing inflammation, and both together, may greatly exacerbate lung inflammation.[53,54] Other innate pathways include lung epithelial cells, which produce many mediators, including chemokines (RANTES/CCL5, eotaxin/CCL11, and MCP-1/CCL2), growth factors (platelet-derived growth factor, fibroblast growth factor, and endothelins), nitric oxide that increase airway inflammation,[55] as well as cytokines such as IL-25, IL-33 and TSLP (see below), which may activate innate cells, including mast cells, basophils and NKT cells, and independent of Th2 cells.

IL-25, also known as IL-17E, a newly identified cytokine and a member of the IL-17 cytokine family, is produced by Th2 cells and epithelial cells.[56,57] IL-25 may play an important role in asthma by promoting increases in IgE synthesis, increases in Th2 cytokine production, and increases in blood eosinophils, epithelial hypertrophy, and mucus production. IL-25 mediates its effects through the induction of Th2 cytokine production (IL-4, IL-5, and IL-13) in non-B/non-T (NBNT) c-kit+FcεRI− cells in mesenteric lymph nodes, and in a subset of natural killer T (NKT) cells.[58] The IL-25 receptor IL-17RB has been shown to be expressed by a subset of CD4+ NKT cells, which when stimulated with IL-25 greatly enhance BHR.[58,59] In murine models, IL-25 was sufficient to induce allergic diseases of the airways, and neutralization of IL-25 prevented BHR[60] This indicates that IL-25 amplifies allergic-type inflammatory responses by effects on several different cell types, although there is still some debate regarding the cell types that respond to IL-25.

IL-33, also expressed by bronchial epithelial cells (and by fibroblasts and smooth muscle cells), plays a significant role in the regulation of mucosal immune responses of the airways.[61] IL-33 potently activates human eosinophils and induces production and release of inflammatory mediators by binding to its receptor, ST2, expressed on Th2 cells, mast cells and some NKT cells.[62] IL-33 is increased in the serum during anaphylaxis and in the skin of patients with atopic dermatitis, and mediates direct degranulation of mast cells in the absence of allergen.[63] In mice, IL-33 induces IL-5-producing T cells, thereby promoting airway inflammation, independent of IL-4.[64] Finally, a genome-wide association scan for sequence variants affecting eosinophil counts identified IL-33 as an important determinant associated with atopic asthma.[65] Together, these data indicate that IL-33 may have significant effects on mast cell function and the induction of eosinophilic inflammation of the airways, and that IL-33 might provide a future target for the treatment of eosinophilic inflammations like asthma.

Human epithelial cells in the lung and skin produce another cytokine, thymic stromal lymphopoietin (*TSLP*), which triggers dendritic cells (DCs) to induce T cell production of IL-4, IL-5, and IL-13 while down-regulating IL-10 and interferon (IFN)-γ.[66,67] Basophils also produce TSLP, and may produce TSLP, not only when activated through their IgE receptors (FcεR1), but also after sensing protease activity of some allergens.[68] TSLP activates DCs to induce Th2 cytokine production and to produce the Th2-attracting chemokines thymus and activation-regulated chemokine (TARC) and monocyte-derived chemokine (MDC). These functions of TSLP may help localize allergic inflammatory responses to the respiratory mucosa and skin of atopic individuals.[45,69] TSLP expression is increased in asthmatic airways (and in the skin of individuals with atopic dermatitis), and correlates with the expression of Th2 attracting chemokines and with disease severity, indicating that TSLP is crucially involved in the pathogenesis of human asthma.[70]

Antigen-Presenting Cells

Environmental allergens are taken up by specialized antigen-presenting cells (APCs), processed, and presented to cells in the adaptive immune system. DCs, B cells, basophils and macrophages are all able to present antigen to T cells, but DCs, which line the mucous membranes of the airways,[71] are the most potent stimulators of naïve T cells. In contrast, alveolar macrophages, which are abundant in the lung, phagocytize antigen but appear normally to actively tolerize CD4+ T cells.[72] Alveolar macrophages fail to up-regulate expression of CD80 (B7.1) and CD86 (B7.2) costimulatory antigens and consequently are not competent in inducing T cell-mediated immune responses in the pulmonary compartment. On the other hand, DCs, which are derived from bone marrow progenitors, populate most peripheral tissues, including the lung in small numbers, but are extremely effective in activating T cells. DCs in the periphery and in the lung survey the environment by constantly sampling and capturing antigens. These tissue DCs are considered 'immature' because they lack expression of costimulatory molecules and cannot stimulate T cells well. However, these immature DCs migrate to regional lymph nodes, and in the process, they mature and express chemotactic receptors as well as costimulatory molecules, such as MHC class II, CD80, and CD86. The maturation and migration of DCs are greatly enhanced by the presence in the lungs or tissue of necrotic cells or pathogens. After reaching the regional lymph nodes, the mature DCs encounter T and B cells, which they efficiently activate (Figure 32-3).

Based on the expression of distinct cell surface markers, cell culture requirements, and functional differences, DCs have been classified into distinct subsets.[73] In humans, one subset, called DC1, derives from blood monocytes, whereas another subset, called DC2, appears as plasmacytoid cells and expresses high levels of CD123 (IL-3 receptor α chain). DC1 cells induce naive CD4+ T cells to produce large quantities of IFN-γ but few Th2 cytokines, such as IL-4 and IL-5, whereas DC2 induce CD4+ T cells to produce large amounts of Th2 cytokines but not IFN-γ. It is not clear whether DC1 and DC2 cells are of different lineages or represent different maturation/differentiation steps of a single lineage. Plasmacytoid pre DC2s express Toll-like receptors (TLRs) 7 and 9 and respond to microbial TLR9 ligand CpG-oligodeoxynucleotides (ODNs containing unmethylated CpG motifs) by producing large quantities of IFN-α. In contrast, pre-DC1 express TLR1, 2, 4, 5, and 8 and respond to microbial ligands for TLR2 (peptidoglycan, lipoteichoic acid) and TLR4 (lipopolysaccharide [LPS]) by producing TNF-α and IL-6. The expression of distinct sets of TLRs and the difference in reactivity to microbial molecules support the concept that DC1s and DC2s developed through distinct evolutionary pathways to recognize different microbial antigens.[74] In the respiratory tract, DCs are recruited to the airway epithelium after the administration of infectious agents or challenge with soluble protein allergens. DC2s are thought to be preferentially recruited to the respiratory mucosa during allergic-type responses.[75]

Other Innate Cell Types that Affect Asthma

Mast Cells and Neutrophils

The IPR is IgE dependent and mediated by mast cells, which migrate from the bone marrow as precursors to the tissues where they mature locally in response to stem cell factor. The number of mast cells infiltrating smooth muscle cells in the airways in asthmatic compared with nonasthmatic individuals is increased, suggesting that mast cells contribute to the development of BHR via direct effects on smooth muscle cells.[76] The LPR is characterized by an inflammatory infiltrate that includes mainly eosinophils but also basophils, neutrophils, and activated T cells. Recent work has suggested that neutrophilic infiltration is an important feature of severe asthma, and that the number of neutrophils (and not eosinophils) in lungs and IL-17, a potent neutrophil chemotactic agent, correlates with disease severity.[77] The LPR is dependent on the IPR and is thought to be responsible for the development of BHR and the chronic symptoms of asthma.

Basophils

Recently, basophils have been shown to express class II MHC molecules and to directly activate naïve CD4+ T cells to differentiate into Th2 cells.[78,79] Basophils produce large quantities of IL-4,

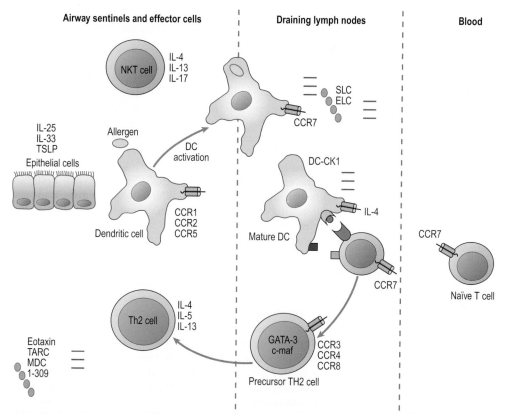

Figure 32-3 Cell trafficking and the initiation of allergic response. Immature dendritic cells (*DCs*) survey the airways and capture allergen. Allergen-loaded DCs (as well as basophils) migrate from the lungs to draining regional lymph nodes in response to chemokines such as secondary lymphoid tissue chemokine (*SLC, CCL21*) and EBL-1–ligand chemokine (*ELC, CCL19*). In the lymph nodes DCs and basophils activate naïve T cells from the peripheral blood. NKT cells in the airways, as well as airway epithelial cells also function as sentinels for environmental pathogens and antigens, and can be rapidly activated to produce cytokines such as IL-4, IL-13 and IL-17, or IL-25, IL-33 and TSLP, respectively, which can then amplify adaptive immune responses. Other chemoattractants produced by alveolar macrophages such as DC-CK1 (CCL18), attract Th2 cells and basophils to the airways. Activated Th2 cells express distinct chemokine receptors that bind to Th2-associated chemokines such as eotaxin (CCL11), TARC (CCL17), MDC (CCL22), and I-309, expressed in sites of allergic inflammation.

IL-13 and TSLP,[80] and are as effective as DCs in stimulating the differentiation of naïve T cells into Th2 cells, although they cannot induce IFN-γ production in naïve T cells. Therefore, basophils not only enhance the IPR, but can also enhance adaptive immunity and Th2 responses.

Natural Killer T Cells

Another lymphocyte subset, called *natural killer T (NKT) cells*, appears to play an important role in asthma. These cells express characteristics of NK cells as well T cells. A large fraction of NKT cells express an invariant or conserved T cell receptor (TCR), and as such, these cells are thought to be part of the innate immune system. Moreover, activation of NKT cells results in the rapid (within minutes to hours of stimulation) production of cytokines, which can then amplify adaptive immune responses. Furthermore, recent studies have indicated that NKT cells may play a critical role in the development of BHR. These studies have shown that in different models of asthma, different subsets of NKT cells are required. For example, in a model of allergic asthma, NKT cells producing IL-4 and IL-13 were required for the developmenmt of BHR,[81] but in a model of air pollution associated asthma induced with ozone and associated with airway neutrophils, NKT cells producing IL-17 were required.[37] In another model of virus induced BHR, CD4⁻ NKT cells were required.[82] Of note, in the ozone-induced and virus-induced BHR, NKT cells caused BHR in the absence of Th2 cells and adaptive immunity, which may explain some forms of nonallergic asthma. The frequency of NKT cells in the lungs of asthma patients appears to be highly variable,[83,84] although the number of pulmonary NKT cells in the lungs of asthma patients may be loosely related to asthma severity and symptom control.[85] These studies suggest that while Th2 cells are necessary for responses to allergens, the development of BHR may also require the presence of NKT cells.

Natural Killer Cells

NK cells, which are lymphocytes that do not express CD3, CD4, or CD8, are important in controlling certain microbial infections and killing virus-infected cells and tumors. Subsets of NK cells (CD56^bright CD16^dull) rapidly produce cytokines on activation, including IFN-γ, tumor necrosis factor (TNF)-α, TGF-β, IL-5, IL-10 and IL-22. Depletion of NK cells in a murine model resulted in a reduction in pulmonary eosinophilia, suggesting that NK cells normally exacerbate airway inflammation and increase Th2 cytokine production.[86] However, the activation of NK cells, such as that with CpG oligonucleotides, greatly increases NK cell production of IFN-γ, which may protect against the development of asthma.[87] Production of IL-22 by NK cells enhances epithelial cell integrity and the production of antimicrobial peptides.

γδ Cells

T cells expressing γδ T cell receptors (γδ T cells) have been shown to promote allergic sensitization in models of systemic sensitization.[88] These cells, which are found in high numbers in mucosal tissue, are thought to be involved in the initiation of immune response to bacterial antigens in mucosal epithelium. It is thought that subsets of γδ T cells producing Th2-type cytokines develop after allergen challenge.[89] Increased γδ T cell numbers have been reported in BAL fluid from patients with asthma,[90] suggesting that these cells exacerbate asthma symptoms. However, the precise role of γδ T cells in asthma is controversial, and other studies show that atopic asthmatics have decreased numbers of peripheral blood γδ cells.[91]

CD8⁺ T Cells

CD8⁺ T cells producing IL-4 and IL-5 (type 2 CD8⁺ cells) in the lungs and blood of asthmatic individuals may contribute to asthma pathogenesis.[92] CD8⁺ cells producing IFN-γ (type 1 CD8⁺ cells) may also contribute to asthma symptoms and to asthma exacerbation,[93] although they may protect against asthma, by eliminating allergen-specific Th2 cells. The precise role of CD8⁺ cells in asthma is not clear and may depend on the relative number of type 1 versus type 2 CD8 T⁺ cells present. Allergen-specific CD8⁺ cells respond to exogenous allergens cross-presented through class I pathways. In addition, virus-specific CD8⁺ cells producing type 2 cytokines may develop during certain viral infections, suggesting a mechanism for virus-induced asthma exacerbation.[94] (Box 32-2)

BOX 32-2 Key concepts

Allergic Inflammatory Response

- Allergic inflammation is mediated by Th2 and Th9 lymphocytes and their products, IgE and mast cells, eosinophils, basophils and epithelial cells. Innate immunity, involving epithelial cells producing IL-25, IL-33 and TSLP as well as NKT cells producing Th2 cytokines may contribute to this inflammation.

- Nonallergic asthma, associated with neutrophils, Th17 cells and NKT cells may be associated with more severe airways disease and corticosteroid resistance.

- The Th1/Th2 paradigm requires modification. Other CD4⁺ T helper cell types, such as Th17, Th9 T$_{Reg}$ cells must be added to the paradigm, and all of these cells interact with a large number of innate immune cells.

- CD8⁺ T cells, natural killer (NK), γδ T cells, and the complement components C3a and C5a may also contribute to asthma pathology.

- CD4⁺ T$_{Reg}$ can down-modulate the function of pro-inflammatory cells.

- Airway inflammation is associated with an increase in mucus production, mucosal edema, reversible obstruction, bronchial hyperresponsiveness, and remodeling of the airways.

- Bronchial hyperresponsiveness can be induced independent of eosinophilic inflammation through IL-13 or IL-33.

Clinical Relevance

- Neutralization of some components of the inflammatory response is being investigated as therapy for asthma (e.g. anti-IgE monoclonal antibody, anti-IL-5 monoclonal antibody, or IL-13 antagonists).

- Severe asthma, associated with airway neutrophils, NKT cells and corticosteroid resistance may not respond to therapies focused on neutralizing Th2 cytokines and mediators.

- Strategies to increase the number of allergen-specific T$_{Reg}$ cells may be beneficial in asthma.

Epithelial-Mesenchymal Trophic Unit and Airway Remodeling

A factor intrinsic to the lung that may contribute to the development of asthma involves epithelial and mesenchymal cell interactions and the epithelial cell response to injury. Under normal circumstances, the pulmonary epithelium and underlying mesenchymal cells communicate with each other through cytokines and growth factors (TGF-β and epithelial growth factor [EGF]) and coordinate growth and the response to damage after injury from the environment in this epithelial-mesenchymal unit.[95] In asthma, the mesenchymal cells differentiate into myofibroblasts that deposit interstitial collagens, resulting in thickening of the subepithelial basement membrane (lamina reticularis). These structural remodeling changes are only partially reversible and account for a portion of the deterioration in lung function associated with persistent disease.[96] The alterations observed in the airways include thickening of the bronchial wall, subepithelial fibrosis, mucus hypersecretion, hyperplasia and hypertrophy of the smooth muscle layer, and neovascularization.[97] Genetic polymorphisms in asthma susceptibility genes may affect all of these pathways and result in the development of asthma. Recently, the ADAM33 gene was identified through positional cloning as a major asthma susceptibility gene.[96] This gene codes for a metalloprotease, which may regulate the response of the respiratory epithelium to damage and stress, and asthma-inducing alleles of ADAM33 may amplify repair mechanisms, leading to greater inflammation, airway remodeling, and the development of asthma (Box 32-1). In addition, recent reports indicate a strong association of atopic dermatitis and asthma with null mutations in the gene encoding for **filaggrin** (FLG), a member of the epidermal differentiation complex on chromosome 1q21.[98-100] It is thought that disruption of barrier function in the skin and possibly the lung, may allow enhanced allergen sensitization through the skin and possibly the lung, which ultimately results in allergic asthma.

The Role of Cell Trafficking in Pulmonary Inflammation

The development of asthma and lung inflammation also involves the homing of the inflammatory cells to the lung (see Figure 32-3). This cell trafficking process involves several families of proteins, including cytokines, chemokines, adhesion molecules, and matrix metalloproteinases (MMPs), in processes that are complex and redundant.

The first cells to be recruited to the lungs during allergic inflammation are basophils (expressing the chemokine receptors CCR2, 3, and 4) by chemokines MCP-1/CCL2, MCP-2/CCL8, and eotaxin/CCL11, which are produced by several cells in the lung. Eosinophils (expressing CCR3, CXCR4, and α4β1/VLA-4 and α4β7/LPAM-1 integrins) are also recruited into the lung by chemokines MCP-3/CCL7, MCP-4/CCL13, and VCAM-1 and MadCAM-1.[101] Expression of CCR3 and eotaxin/CCL11 is increased in atopic asthma, demonstrating the importance of these chemokines.[102] Th2 cells express CCR4 and CCR8 and are recruited into the lungs by MDC/CCL22, TARC/CL17, and I-309/CCL1 and by specific antigen. Expression of the CCR4 ligands MDC and TARC is up-regulated in epithelial cells after allergen challenge but not of the CCR8 ligand I-309/CCL1.

After recruitment to the lungs, migration of cells into the tissues requires integrin-mediated, firm adhesion. Chemokine-mediated activation of lymphocytes, which increases expression of and activates integrins, assists in this process. Chemokines and cytokines are also involved in lymphocyte extravasation/diapedesis by regulating the expression of proteinases such as MMPs, matrix-degrading enzymes that allow the leukocytes to penetrate through the basement membrane and into the tissue stroma. Recent studies showed that MMPs, especially MMP2 and possibly MMP9, are important in airway inflammation. MMP2 and MMP9 are increased in BAL fluid after allergen challenge in experimental asthma.[103] If MMP2 inhibitor TIMP-2 was administered, egression of eosinophils out of the lungs into airway lumen would be blocked, causing greater airway inflammation. These results were extended in an MMP2-deficient mouse model, in which allergen challenge resulted in severe airway inflammation and death of mice by asphyxia.[104]

Biological and Environmental Factors in Asthma

During the past several decades in industrialized countries, atopic diseases, including asthma, have increased dramatically in both prevalence and severity. Because the environment in westernized cultures has also changed significantly, particularly in terms of the prevalence of infectious diseases, it is thought that infections may affect the immune system in ways that protect against the development of asthma (hygiene hypothesis). However, the specific infectious pathogens that can protect against asthma have not been identified, and thus the link between asthma pathogenesis and infections remains nebulous.

Respiratory Viruses

A link between infection with specific respiratory viruses and asthma has been recognized for decades, in which respiratory viruses precipitate acute airway obstruction and wheezing in patients with asthma. Although reduced asthma prevalence in children who enter daycare early or in those who have older siblings suggests otherwise, frequent respiratory viral infections may exacerbate rather than prevent the development of asthma.

Rhinovirus

The common cold virus, rhinovirus, has emerged as the most frequent illness associated with exacerbations and other aspects of asthma. The mechanisms by which rhinovirus influences asthma are not fully understood. Infection of epithelial cells generates a variety of proinflammatory mediators to attract inflammatory cells to the airway with a subsequent worsening of underlying disease. It has been shown, that rhinovirus infection of bronchial endothelial cells induces the secretion of IL-1, IL-6, IL-8, GM-CSF, eotaxins and RANTES.[105-107] At the same time, Th2 might be augmented during the course of human rhinovirus (HRV) infection, while Th1 polarization or IL-10 secretion by T cells are impaired.[108] Additionally, virus-specific CD8$^+$ cells producing type 2 cytokines may develop during viral infections.[94]

Respiratory Syncytial Virus (RSV)

During the first 3 years of life, acute viral bonchilolitis is often caused by infections with the respiratory syncicial virus (RSV). RSV-induced lower respiratory tract illnesses in early life are associated with the subsequent development of recurrent wheezing.[109,110] On the other hand, patients with atopic diseases and asthma have an increased risk of lower respiratory tract infection

and RSV hospitalization, and early wheezing is a strong risk factor for subsequent RSV hospitalization.[111,112] Recent in vitro studies have shown that lung epithelial cells have the capacity to inhibit T cell activation in healthy airway mucosa and that they induce T$_{Reg}$ cells, which suppress unwanted adaptive immune responses. Upon respiratory viral infection with RSV, the inhibitory capacity of lung epithelial cells was compromised, allowing local activation of T cell responses in the respiratory mucosa and consequently airway inflammation.[113] Also, recent data suggests that RSV infection may induce airway remodeling and thus prime the lung epithelium to become susceptible to subsequent allergic responses to inhaled allergens.[114] Consequently, ribavirin treatment of children hospitalized with RSV bronchiolitis was shown to decrease the risk of subsequent allergic sensitization and development of asthma.[115] In this line, prevention of RSV bronchiolitis with palivizumab was able to reduce subsequent recurrent wheezing in premature infants.[116]

Endotoxins

In contrast to respiratory viral infection, gastrointestinal exposure to bacteria and bacterial products may have a significant effect on the maturation of the immune system and indeed protect against the development of asthma. Recent studies have shown that increased incidence of allergy is associated with reduced colonization of the gastrointestinal tract in children with *Bifidobacteria* and *Lactobacillus* strains, two Gram-positive commensal bacteria.[117] Furthermore, exposure of infants to *Lactobacillus* in the neonatal period appears to protect against the development of atopy.[118] The effect of gastrointestinal bacteria on the developing immune system may be mediated through TLRs, which may inhibit the development of Th2-biased immune responses. 'Improved' hygiene may eliminate exposure and the protective effects of these commensal gastrointestinal bacteria. The specific TLRs that may protect against asthma are not clear, although several investigators suggest that, based on epidemiologic studies of farm environments, TLR4 and exposure to bacterial LPS may be protective against asthma.[119]

The Hygiene Hypothesis

It thus appears that the natural environment in the past (before widespread industrialization) maintained the respiratory and gastrointestinal mucosal systems in a state that favored the development of T cell tolerance to nonreplicating antigens encountered on mucosal surfaces, such as in food and in inhaled material. The establishment of these tolerance mechanisms at mucosal surfaces may require the presence of commensal bacteria in the gastrointestinal and upper respiratory tracts because immune tolerance induced by mucosal exposure to antigen does not occur in germ-free animals.[120] Commensal bacteria may enhance the production of IL-10 through mechanisms involving the innate immune system and receptors such as nucleotide-binding oligomerization domain 2 (NOD2). NOD2 is a member of the NOD family of proteins involved in the regulation of programmed cell death and host defense against pathogens.[121] Infection with high levels of helminths may also favor the development of tolerance to nonreplicating environmental antigens by enhancing IL-10 production.[122] Therefore, some microorganisms may diminish inflammation at mucosal surfaces, and changes in the environment in westernized societies limit exposure to these types of organisms and thereby diminish the normal tolerance-inducing state of mucosal surfaces, resulting in enhanced mucosal inflammation. These changes prevent the development of allergen-specific T_{Reg} cells in some individuals, resulting in an aberrant form of T_{Reg} cells developing in atopic individuals (i.e. Th2 cells) that induces the development of allergy. The responsible environmental changes may include frequent use of antibiotics or changes in diet,[123] which alter the normal gastrointestinal flora, resulting in reduced IL-10 and TGF-β production by epithelial cells, DCs, and B cells in the mucosa, causing increased development of Th2 cells and allergy.

Hepatitis A Virus and the *TIM1* Gene

In addition to gastrointestinal bacteria, several other gastrointestinal pathogens appear to have potent effects in the protection against the development of asthma. For example, evidence of infection with hepatitis A virus (HAV) is strongly associated with protection against the development of asthma.[124] Infection with other gastrointestinal pathogens such as *Helicobacter pylori* and *Toxoplasma gondii* may also protect against the development of asthma.[125] However, because HAV, *H. pylori*, and *T. gondii* are not respiratory pathogens and because HAV is transmitted via fecal-oral routes, clinical investigators have assumed that infections with these agents are merely markers of poor hygiene and that other infectious pathogens, possibly involving the respiratory tract, are more directly involved in protecting against asthma. The mechanisms by which HAV infection prevents the development of asthma may be more direct than previously suspected, since *TIM1*, which codes for the cellular receptor for HAV and functions as a receptor for apoptotic cells,[126] has been shown to be an atopy susceptibility gene.[127] This suggests that HAV binds to its receptor, TIM-1, preferentially expressed on Th2 cells,[126] thereby preventing the development of atopic diseases. Together, these observations with HAV, *H. pylori*, and *T. gondii* suggest that the microbiota in the intestinal tract have important effects on innate immunity and determining whether atopic diseases develop.

How Can Asthma be Treated to Induce Protective Immunity?

Most available treatments for asthma are effective at controlling symptoms, but none so far are curative. If the increase in asthma could be ascribed to alterations in tolerance, then procedures to induce tolerance to environmental allergens could be used to better treat asthma. Several strategies are possible. Conventional immunotherapy, although efficient in controlling symptoms and even reversing established disease,[128] is burdensome to administer. Strategies to increase the efficiency of conventional immunotherapy are being developed. This approach is antigen-specific, can change the course of the disease, and can provide long-lasting remission. For example, allergens used in conventional immunotherapy might be modified by conjugating the allergen with CpG oligonucleotide motifs. CpG motifs bind to TLR9; induce the production of IL-12, IFN-γ, and IL-10; and have been shown to inhibit development of several asthmatic features, including BHR and eosinophil infiltration in a model of asthma and to reduce symptoms in patients with allergic rhinitis.[129] Another possible strategy is the induction of T_{Reg} cells, either by DC manipulation or by administration of other agents[130] or by use of allergen peptides.[131] Oral immunotherapy through the oral administration of allergens could be used to stimulate the mucosal mechanisms of tolerance. Oral tolerance has been shown to be able to prevent development of experimental asthma.

Finally, because intestinal flora has been shown to be essential for the establishment of tolerance in animal models,[120] the administration of probiotics such as *Lactobacillus* may also be helpful in altering the immune system and inducing protective immunity[118] (Box 32-3). The effect of intestinal flora may be mediated by activation of the innate immune system, which might have broader, prolonged effects than therapies focused on the adaptive immunity.

Conclusions

Our understanding of the immunology of asthma has progressed rapidly during the past decade and is radically changing the focus of therapy for this disease. Although past therapies were based on relieving airway obstruction in asthma, current therapy focuses on reducing airway inflammation and neutralizing the effects of mast cell mediators. As even more is learned about the underlying immunologic mechanisms that enhance and prolong airway inflammation and the immunologic processes that prevent and reverse airways disease, therapies will become more specific and effective. Thus knowledge of critical mediators involved in the Th2-biased asthmatic immune response (e.g. IL-4, IL-13, IL-25, IL-33, TSLP, chemokines, and integrins) and in airway remodeling (e.g. metalloproteases [ADAM33] and EGF) has spurred the development of strategies to limit the activity of these mediators as therapies for asthma. Furthermore, as our understanding of innate immunity and other specific mechanisms involved in regulating and reversing Th2-driven response becomes more complete (e.g. of microbial exposure, HAV infection, and the *TIM1* gene), additional preventive, and potentially curative, immunotherapies are likely to develop in the near future, bringing about a new era in asthma management.

References

1. Holt PG, Macaubas C, Stumbles PA, et al. The role of allergy in the development of asthma. Nature 1999;402:B12–17.

2. Martinez FD, Wright AL, Taussig LM, et al. Asthma and wheezing in the first six years of life. N Engl J Med 1995;332:133–8.

3. O'Hollaren MT, Yunginger JW, Offord KP, et al. Exposure to an aeroallergen as a possible precipitating factor in respiratory arrest in young patients with asthma. N Engl J Med 1991;324:359–63.

4. Sears MR, Burrows B, Flannery EM, et al. Relation between airway responsiveness and serum IgE in children with asthma and in apparently normal children. N Engl J Med 1991;325:1067–71.

5. Robinson DS, Hamid Q, Ying S, et al. Predominant Th2-like bronchoalveolar T lymphocyte population in atopic asthma. N. Engl J Med 1992;326:298–304.

6. Robinson DS, Ying S, Bentley AM, et al. Relationships among numbers of bronchoalveolar lavage cells expressing messenger ribonucleic acid for cytokines, asthma symptoms, and airway methacholine responsiveness in atopic asthma. J Allergy Clin Immunol 1993;92:397–403.

7. Shi HZ, Deng JM, Xu H, et al. Effect of inhaled interleukin-4 on airway hyperreactivity in asthmatics. Am J Respir Crit Care Med 1998;157:1818–21.

8. Hsieh FH, Lam BK, Penrose JF, et al. T helper cell type 2 cytokines coordinately regulate immunoglobulin E-dependent cysteinyl leukotriene production by human cord blood-derived mast cells: profound induction of leukotriene C(4) synthase expression by interleukin 4. J Exp Med 2001;193:123–33.

9. Leckie M, ten Brinke A, Khan J, et al. Effects of an interleukin-5 blocking monoclonal antibody on eosinophils, airway hyper-responsiveness, and the late asthmatic response. Lancet 2000;356:2144–8.

10. Nair P, Pizzichini MM, Kjarsgaard M, et al. Mepolizumab for prednisone-dependent asthma with sputum eosinophilia. N Engl J Med 2009;360:985–93.

11. Haldar P, Brightling CE, Hargadon B, et al. Mepolizumab and exacerbations of refractory eosinophilic asthma. N Engl J Med 2009;360:973–84.

12. Mattes J, Yang M, Mahalingam S, et al. Intrinsic defect in T cell production of interleukin (IL)-13 in the absence of both IL-5 and eotaxin precludes the development of eosinophilia and airways hyperreactivity in experimental asthma. J Exp Med 2002;195:1433–44.

13. Wills-Karp M, Luyimbazi J, Xu X, et al. Interleukin-13: central mediator of allergic asthma. Science 1998;282:2258–61.

14. Grunig G, Warnock M, Wakil AE, et al. Requirement for IL-13 independently of IL-4 in experimental asthma. Science 1998;282:2261–3.

15. Walter D, McIntire J, Berry G, et al. Critical role for IL-13 in the development of allergen-induced airway hyperreactivity. J Immunol 2001;167:4668–75.

16. Wenzel S, Wilbraham D, Fuller R, et al. Effect of an interleukin-4 variant on late phase asthmatic response to allergen challenge in asthmatic patients: results of two phase 2a studies. Lancet 2007;370:1422–31.

17. Murphy KM, Ouyang W, Farrar JD, et al. Signaling and transcription in T helper development. Annu Rev Immunol 2000;18:451–94.

18. Mullings RE, Wilson SJ, Puddicombe SM, et al. Signal transducer and activator of transcription 6 (STAT-6) expression and function in asthmatic bronchial epithelium. J Allergy Clin Immunol 2001;108:832–8.

19. Nakamura Y, Ghaffar O, Olivenstein R, et al. Gene expression of the GATA-3 transcription factor is increased in atopic asthma. J Allergy Clin Immunol 1999;103:215–22.

20. Sharpe AH, Freeman GJ. The B7-CD28 superfamily. Nat Rev Immunol 2002;2:116–26.

21. Larche M, Till SJ, Haselden BM, et al. Costimulation through CD86 is involved in airway antigen-presenting cell and T cell responses to allergen in atopic asthmatics. J Immunol 1998;161:6375–82.

22. Gonzalo JA, Tian J, Delaney T, et al. ICOS is critical for T helper cell-mediated lung mucosal inflammatory responses. Nat Immunol 2001;2:597–604.

23. Hellings P, Vandenberghe P, Kasran A, et al. Blockade of CTLA-4 enhances allergic sensitization and eosinophilic airway inflammation in genetically predisposed mice. Eur J Immunol 2002;32:585–94.

24. Freeman GJ, Long AJ, Iwai Y, et al. Engagement of the PD-1 immunoinhibitory receptor by a novel B7 family member leads to negative regulation of lymphocyte activation. J Exp Med 2000;192:1027–34.

25. Chapoval AI, Ni J, Lau JS, et al. B7-H3: a costimulatory molecule for T cell activation and IFN-gamma production. Nat Immunol 2001;2:269–74.

26. Katamura K, Tabata Y, Oshima Y, et al. Selective induction of IL-4 and IFN-γ producing T cells from cord blood naive T cells: effects of costimulatory signaling through CD28. Intern Arch Allerg Immunol 1995;106:101–6.

27. Finotto S, Neurath M, Glickman J, et al. Development of spontaneous airway changes consistent with human asthma in mice lacking T-bet. Science 2002;295:336–8.

28. Tang L, Benjaponpitak S, DeKruyff RH, et al. Reduced prevalence of allergic disease in patients with multiple sclerosis is associated with enhanced IL-12 production. J Aller Clin Immunol 1998;102:428–35.

29. Rogge L, Papi A, Presky DH, et al. Antibodies to the IL-12 receptor beta 2 chain mark human Th1 but not Th2 cells in vitro and in vivo. J Immunol 1999;162:3926–32.

30. Anderson GP. Endotyping asthma: new insights into key pathogenic mechanisms in a complex, heterogeneous disease. Lancet 2008;372:1107–19.

31. MacDonald C, Sternberg A, Hunter PR. A systematic review and meta-analysis of interventions used to reduce exposure to house dust and their effect on the development and severity of asthma. Environ Health Perspect 2007;115:1691–5.

32. Park H, Li Z, Yang XO, et al. A distinct lineage of CD4 T cells regulates tissue inflammation by producing interleukin 17. Nat Immunol 2005;6:1133–41.

33. Harrington LE, Hatton RD, Mangan PR, et al. Interleukin 17-producing CD4+ effector T cells develop via a lineage distinct from the T helper type 1 and 2 lineages. Nat Immunol 2005;6:1123–32.

34. Molet S, Hamid Q, Davoine F, et al. IL-17 is increased in asthmatic airways and induces human bronchial fibroblasts to produce cytokines. J Allergy Clin Immunol 2001;108:430–8.

35. Kolls JK, Linden A. Interleukin-17 family members and inflammation. Immunity 2004;21:467–76.

36. Pene J, Chevalier S, Preisser L, et al. Chronically inflamed human tissues are infiltrated by highly differentiated Th17 lymphocytes. J Immunol 2008;180:7423–30.

37. Pichavant M, Goya S, Meyer EH, et al. Ozone exposure in a mouse model induces airway hyperreactivity that requires the presence of natural killer T cells and IL-17. J Exp Med 2008;205:385–93.

38. Boniface K, Blom B, Liu YJ, et al. From interleukin-23 to T-helper 17 cells: human T-helper cell differentiation revisited. Immunol Rev 2008;226:132–46.

39. Milner JD, Brenchley JM, Laurence A, et al. Impaired T(H)17 cell differentiation in subjects with autosomal dominant hyper-IgE syndrome. Nature 2008;452:773–6.

40. Platts-Mills T, Vaughan J, Squillace S, et al. Sensitisation, asthma, and a modified Th2 response in children exposed to cat allergen: a population-based cross-sectional study. Lancet 2001;357:752–6.

41. Akbari O, Freeman GJ, Meyer EH, et al. Antigen-specific regulatory T cells develop via the ICOS-ICOS-Ligand pathway and inhibit allergen-induced airway hyperreactivity. Nature Medicine 2002;8:1024–32.

42. Bacchetta R, Gambineri E, Roncarolo MG. Role of regulatory T cells and FOXP3 in human diseases. J Allergy Clin Immunol 2007;120:227–35; quiz 236–227.

43. Hansen G, McIntire JJ, Yeung VP, et al. CD4(+) T cells engineered to produce latent TGF-beta1 reverse allergen-induced airway reactivity and inflammation. J Clin Invest 2000;105:61–70.

44. Hill JA, Feuerer M, Tash K, et al. Foxp3 transcription-factor-dependent and -independent regulation of the regulatory T cell transcriptional signature. Immunity 2007;27:786–800.

45. Ziegler SF, Liu YJ. Thymic stromal lymphopoietin in normal and pathogenic T cell development and function. Nat Immunol 2006;7:709–14.

46. Stock P, DeKruyff RH, Umetsu DT. Inhibition of the allergic response by regulatory T cells. Curr Opin Allergy Clin Immunol 2006;6:12–6.

47. Veldhoen M, Uyttenhove C, van Snick J, et al. Transforming growth factor-beta 'reprograms' the differentiation of T helper 2 cells and promotes an interleukin 9-producing subset. Nat Immunol 2008;9:1341–6.

48. Dardalhon V, Awasthi A, Kwon H, et al. IL-4 inhibits TGF-beta-induced Foxp3+ T cells and, together with TGF-beta, generates IL-9+ IL-10+ Foxp3(-) effector T cells. Nat Immunol 2008;9:1347–55.

49. Demoulin JB, Renauld JC. Interleukin 9 and its receptor: an overview of structure and function. Int Rev Immunol 1998;16:345–64.

50. Shimbara A, Christodoulopoulos P, Soussi-Gounni A, et al. IL-9 and its receptor in allergic and nonallergic lung disease: increased expression in asthma. J Allergy Clin Immunol 2000;105:108–15.

51. Temann UA, Geba GP, Rankin JA, et al. Expression of interleukin 9 in the lungs of transgenic mice causes airway inflammation, mast cell hyperplasia, and bronchial hyperresponsiveness. J Exp Med 1998;188:1307–20.

52. Zhang N, Truong-Tran QA, Tancowny B, et al. Glucocorticoids enhance or spare innate immunity: effects in airway epithelium are mediated by CCAAT/enhancer binding proteins. J Immunol 2007;179:578–89.

53. Kang MJ, Lee CG, Lee JY, et al. Cigarette smoke selectively enhances viral PAMP- and virus-induced pulmonary innate immune and remodeling responses in mice. J Clin Invest 2008;118:2771–84.

54. Gualano RC, Hansen MJ, Vlahos R, et al. Cigarette smoke worsens lung inflammation and impairs resolution of influenza infection in mice. Respir Res 2008;9:53.

55. Holgate ST, Lackie P, Wilson S, et al. Bronchial epithelium as a key regulator of airway allergen sensitization and remodeling in asthma. Am J Respir Crit Care Med 2000;162:S113–117.

345

56. Fort MM, Cheung J, Yen D, et al. IL-25 induces IL-4, IL-5, and IL-13 and Th2-associated pathologies in vivo. Immunity 2001;15:985–95.

57. Fallon PG, Ballantyne SJ, Mangan NE, et al. Identification of an interleukin (IL)-25-dependent cell population that provides IL-4, IL-5, and IL-13 at the onset of helminth expulsion. J Exp Med 2006;203:1105–16.

58. Terashima A, Watarai H, Inoue S, et al. A novel subset of mouse NKT cells bearing the IL-17 receptor B responds to IL-25 and contributes to airway hyperreactivity. J Exp Med 2008;205:2727–33.

59. Stock P, Lombardi V, Kohlrautz V, et al. Induction of airway hyperreactivity by IL-25 is dependent on a subset of invariant NKT cells expressing IL-17RB. J Immunol 2009;182:5116–22.

60. Ballantyne SJ, Barlow JL, Jolin HE, et al. Blocking IL-25 prevents airway hyperresponsiveness in allergic asthma. J Allergy Clin Immunol 2007;120:1324–31.

61. Schmitz J, Owyang A, Oldham E, et al. IL-33, an interleukin-1-like cytokine that signals via the IL-1 receptor-related protein ST2 and induces T helper type 2-associated cytokines. Immunity 2005;23:479–90.

62. Cherry WB, Yoon J, Bartemes KR, et al. A novel IL-1 family cytokine, IL-33, potently activates human eosinophils. J Allergy Clin Immunol 2008;121:1484–90.

63. Pushparaj PN, Tay HK, H'ng SC, et al. The cytokine interleukin-33 mediates anaphylactic shock. Proc Natl Acad Sci U S A 2009;106:9773–8.

64. Kurowska-Stolarska M, Kewin P, Murphy G, et al. IL-33 induces antigen-specific IL-5+ T cells and promotes allergic-induced airway inflammation independent of IL-4. J Immunol 2008;181:4780–90.

65. Gudbjartsson DF, Bjornsdottir US, Halapi E, et al. Sequence variants affecting eosinophil numbers associate with asthma and myocardial infarction. Nat Genet 2009;41:342–7.

66. Ito T, Wang YH, Duramad O, et al. TSLP-activated dendritic cells induce an inflammatory T helper type 2 cell response through OX40 ligand. J Exp Med 2005;202:1213–23.

67. Wang YH, Ito T, Wang YH, et al. Maintenance and polarization of human TH2 central memory T cells by thymic stromal lymphopoietin-activated dendritic cells. Immunity 2006;24:827–38.

68. Sokol CL, Barton GM, Farr AG, et al. A mechanism for the initiation of allergen-induced T helper type 2 responses. Nat Immunol 2007;9:310–8.

69. Soumelis V, Reche PA, Kanzler H, et al. Human epithelial cells trigger dendritic cell mediated allergic inflammation by producing TSLP. Nat Immunol 2002;3:673–80.

70. Holgate ST. Pathogenesis of asthma. Clin Exp Allergy 2008;38:872–97.

71. McWilliam AS, Holt PG. Immunobiology of dendritic cells in the respiratory tract: steady-state and inflammatory sentinels? Toxicology letters 1998;102–3:323–9.

72. Blumenthal R, Campbell D, Hwang P, et al. Human alveolar macrophages induce functional inactivation of antigen-specific CD4+ T cells. J Aller Clin Immunol 2001;107:258–64.

73. Shortman K, Liu YJ. Mouse and human dendritic cell subtypes. Nat Rev Immunol 2002;2:151–61.

74. Kadowaki N, Ho S, Antonenko S, et al. Subsets of human dendritic cell precursors express different toll-like receptors and respond to different microbial antigens. J Exp Med 2001;194:863–9.

75. Jahnsen FL, Lund-Johansen F, Dunne JF, et al. Experimentally induced recruitment of plasmacytoid (CD123high) dendritic cells in human nasal allergy. J Immunol 2000;165:4062–8.

76. Brightling CE, Bradding P, Symon FA, et al. Mast-cell infiltration of airway smooth muscle in asthma. N Engl J Med 2002;346:1699–705.

77. Ordonez CL, Shaughnessy TE, Matthay MA, et al. Increased neutrophil numbers and IL-8 levels in airway secretions in acute severe asthma: Clinical and biologic significance. Am J Respir Crit Care Med 2000;161:1185–90.

78. Perrigoue JG, Saenz SA, Siracusa MC, et al. MHC class II-dependent basophil-CD4+ T cell interactions promote T(H)2 cytokine-dependent immunity. Nat Immunol 2009;10:697–705.

79. Yoshimoto T, Yasuda K, Tanaka H, et al. Basophils contribute to T(H)2-IgE responses in vivo via IL-4 production and presentation of peptide-MHC class II complexes to CD4+ T cells. Nat Immunol 2009;10:706–12.

80. Schroeder JT, Lichtenstein LM, Roche EM, et al. IL-4 production by human basophils found in the lung following segmental allergen challenge. J Allergy Clin Immunol 2001;107:265–71.

81. Akbari O, Stock P, Meyer E, et al. Essential role of NKT cells producing IL-4 and IL-13 in the development of allergen-induced airway hyperreactivity. Nat Med 2003;9:582–8.

82. Kim EY, Battaile JT, Patel AC, et al. Persistent activation of an innate immune response translates respiratory viral infection into chronic lung disease. Nat Med 2008;14:633–40.

83. Akbari O, Faul JL, Hoyte EG, et al. CD4+ invariant T cell-receptor+ natural killer T cells in bronchial asthma. N Engl J Med 2006;354:1117–29.

84. Vijayanand P, Seumois G, Pickard C, et al. Invariant natural killer T cells in asthma and chronic obstructive pulmonary disease. N Engl J Med 2007;356:1410–22.

85. Matangkasombut P, Marigowda G, Ervine A, et al. Natural killer T cells in the lungs of patients with asthma. J Allergy Clin Immunol 2009;123:1181–5.

86. Korsgren M, Persson CG, Sundler F, et al. Natural killer cells determine development of allergen-induced eosinophilic airway inflammation in mice. J Exp Med 1999;189:553–62.

87. Broide D, Schwarze J, Tighe H, et al. Immunostimulatory DNA sequences inhibit IL-5, eosinophililc inflammation, and airway hyperresponsiveness in mice. J Immunol 1998;161:7054–62.

88. Schramm CM, Puddington L, Yiamouyiannis CA, et al. Proinflammatory roles of T cell receptor (TCR)gammadelta and TCRalphabeta lymphocytes in a murine model of asthma. Am J Respir Cell Mol Biol 2000;22:218–25.

89. Krug N, Erpenbeck VJ, Balke K, et al. Cytokine profile of bronchoalveolar lavage-derived CD4(+), CD8(+), and gammadelta T cells in people with asthma after segmental allergen challenge. Am J Respir Cell Mol Biol 2001;25:125–31.

90. Spinozzi F, Agea E, Bistoni O, et al. Increased allergen-specific, steroid-sensitive gamma delta T cells in bronchoalveolar lavage fluid from patients with asthma. Ann Intern Med 1996;124:223–7.

91. Chen KS, Miller KH, Hengehold D. Diminution of T cells with gamma delta receptor in the peripheral blood of allergic asthmatic individuals. Clin Exp Allergy 1996;26:295–302.

92. Stanciu LA, Shute J, Promwong C, et al. Increased levels of IL-4 in CD8+ T cells in atopic asthma. J Allergy Clin Immunol 1997;100:373–8.

93. Magnan AO, Mely LG, Camilla CA, et al. Assessment of the Th1/Th2 paradigm in whole blood in atopy and asthma. Increased IFN-gamma-producing CD8(+) T cells in asthma. Am J Respir Crit Care Med 2000;161:1790–6.

94. O'Sullivan S, Cormican L, Faul JL, et al. Activated, cytotoxic CD8(+) T lymphocytes contribute to the pathology of asthma death. Am J Respir Crit Care Med 2001;164:560–4.

95. Holgate S, Davies D, Lackie P, et al. Epithelial-mesenchymal interactions in the pathogenesis of asthma. J Allergy Clin Immunol 2000;105:193–204.

96. Van Eerdewegh P, Little RD, Dupuis J, et al. Association of the ADAM33 gene with asthma and bronchial hyperresponsiveness. Nature 2002;418:426–30.

97. Elias JA, Zhu Z, Chupp G, et al. Airway remodeling in asthma. J Clin Invest 1999;104:1001–6.

98. Palmer CN, Irvine AD, Terron-Kwiatkowski A, et al. Common loss-of-function variants of the epidermal barrier protein filaggrin are a major predisposing factor for atopic dermatitis. Nat Genet 2006;38:441–6.

99. Marenholz I, Nickel R, Rüschendorf F, et al. Filaggrin loss-of-function mutations predispose to phenotypes involved in the atopic march. J Allergy Clin Immunol 2006;118:866–71.

100. Palmer CN, Ismail T, Lee SP, et al. Filaggrin null mutations are associated with increased asthma severity in children and young adults. J Allergy Clin Immunol 2007;120:64–8.

101. Kunkel EJ, Butcher EC. Chemokines and the tissue-specific migration of lymphocytes. Immunity 2002;16:1–4.

102. Lamkhioued B, Renzi PM, Abi-Younes S, et al. Increased expression of eotaxin in bronchoalveolar lavage and airways of asthmatics contributes to the chemotaxis of eosinophils to the site of inflammation. J Immunol 1997;159:4593–601.

103. Kumagai K, Ohno I, Okada S, et al. Inhibition of matrix metalloproteinases prevents allergen-induced airway inflammation in a murine model of asthma. J Immunol 1999;162:4212–9.

104. Corry DB, Rishi K, Kanellis J, et al. Decreased allergic lung inflammatory cell egression and increased susceptibility to asphyxiation in MMP2-deficiency. Nat Immunol 2002;3:347–53.

105. Papadopoulos NG, Papi A, Meyer J, et al. Rhinovirus infection up-regulates eotaxin and eotaxin-2 expression in bronchial epithelial cells. Clin Exp Allergy 2001;31:1060–6.

106. Terajima M, Yamaya M, Sekizawa K, et al. Rhinovirus infection of primary cultures of human tracheal epithelium: role of ICAM-1 and IL-1beta. Am J Physiol 1997;273:L749–759.

107. Zhu Z, Tang W, Gwaltney JM, et al. Rhinovirus stimulation of interleukin-8 in vivo and in vitro: role of NF-kappaB. Am J Physiol 1997;273:L814–824.

108. Message SD, Laza-Stanca V, Mallia P, et al. Rhinovirus-induced lower respiratory illness is increased in asthma and related to virus load and Th1/2 cytokine and IL-10 production. Proc Natl Acad Sci U S A 2008;105:13562–7.

109. Stein RT, Sherrill D, Morgan WJ, et al. Respiratory syncytial virus in early life and risk of wheeze and allergy by age 13 years. Lancet 1999;354:541–5.

110. Kusel MM, de Klerk NH, Kebadze T, et al. Early-life respiratory viral infections, atopic sensitization, and risk of subsequent development of persistent asthma. J Allergy Clin Immunol 2007;119:1105–10.

111. Goetghebuer T, Kwiatkowski D, Thomson A, et al. Familial susceptibility to severe respiratory infection in early life. Pediatr Pulmonol 2004;38:321–8.

112. Stensballe LG, Kristensen K, Simoes EA, et al. Atopic disposition, wheezing, and subsequent respiratory syncytial virus hospitalization in Danish children younger than 18 months: a nested case-control study. Pediatrics 2006;118:e1360–1368.

113. Wang H, Su Z, Schwarze J. Healthy, but not RSV-infected, lung epithelial cells profoundly inhibit T cell activation. Thorax 2008;64(4):283–90.

114. Tourdot S, Mathie S, Hussell T, et al. Respiratory syncytial virus infection provokes airway remodelling in allergen-exposed mice in absence of prior allergen sensitization. Clin Exp Allergy 2008;38:1016–24.

115. Chen CH, Lin YT, Yang YH, et al. Ribavirin for respiratory syncytial virus bronchiolitis reduced the risk of asthma and allergen sensitization. Pediatr Allergy Immunol 2008;19:166–72.

116. Simoes EA, Groothuis JR, Carbonell-Estrany X, et al. Palivizumab prophylaxis, respiratory syncytial virus, and subsequent recurrent wheezing. J Pediatr 2007;151:34–42, 42.e31.

117. Bjorksten B, Naaber P, Sepp E, et al. The intestinal microflora in allergic Estonian and Swedish 2-year-old children. Clin Exp Allergy 1999;29:342–6.

118. Kalliomaki M, Salminen S, Arvilommi H, et al. Probiotics in primary prevention of atopic disease: a randomised placebo-controlled trial. Lancet 2001;357:1076–9.

119. Gehring U, Bolte G, Borte M, et al. Exposure to endotoxin decreases the risk of atopic eczema in infancy: a cohort study. J Allergy Clin Immunol 2001;108:847–54.

120. Sudo N, Sawamura S, Tanaka K, et al. The requirement of intestinal bacterial flora for the development of an IgE production system fully susceptible to oral tolerance induction. J Immunol 1997;159:1739–45.

121. Ogura Y, Inohara N, Benito A, et al. Nod2, a Nod1/Apaf-1 family member that is restricted to monocytes and activates NF-kappaB. J Biol Chem 2001;276:4812–8.

122. Yazdanbakhsh M, Kremsner PG, van Ree R. Allergy, parasites, and the hygiene hypothesis. Science 2002;296:490–4.

123. Diez-Gonzalez F, Callaway TR, Kizoulis MG, et al. Grain feeding and the dissemination of acid-resistant Escherichia coli from cattle. Science 1998;281:1666–8.

124. Matricardi PM, Rosmini F, Ferrigno L, et al. Cross sectional retrospective study of prevalence of atopy among Italian military students with antibodies against hepatitis A virus. Br Med J 1997;314:999–1003.

125. Matricardi P, Rosmini F, Riondino S, et al. Exposure to foodborne and orofecal microbes versus airborne viruses in relation to atopy and allergic asthma: epidemiological study. Br Med J 2000;320:412–7.

126. McIntire JJ, Umetsu SE, Akbari O, et al. Identification of Tapr (an airway hyperreactivity regulatory locus) and the linked Tim gene family. Nat Immunol 2001;2:1109–16.

127. McIntire J, Umetsu S, Macaubas C, et al. Immunology: hepatitis A virus link to atopic disease. Nature 2003;425:576.

128. Moller C, Dreborg S, Ferdousi HA, et al. Pollen immunotherapy reduces the development of asthma in children with seasonal rhinoconjunctivitis (the PAT-study). J Allergy Clin Immunol 2002;109:251–6.

129. Creticos PS, Schroeder JT, Hamilton RG, et al. Immunotherapy with a ragweed-toll-like receptor 9 agonist vaccine for allergic rhinitis. N Engl J Med 2006;355:1445–55.

130. Zuany-Amorim C, Sawicka E, Manlius C, et al. Suppression of airway eosinophilia by killed Mycobacterium vaccae-induced allergen-specific regulatory T cells. Nat Med 2002;8:8625–9.

131. Oldfield W, Larche M, Kay A. Effect of T cell peptides derived from Fel d 1 on allergic reactions and cytokine production in patients sensitive to cats: a randomised controlled trial. Lancet 2002;360:47–53.

CHAPTER
33

Guidelines for the Treatment of Childhood Asthma: Gains and Opportunities

Stanley J. Szefler

Over the past 30 years, we have witnessed the evolution of guidelines for the management of many common diseases, including asthma. As indicated in the excellent summary by John Warner in the previous edition of this book,[1] there has been a transition of guidelines from a consensus approach to one that is based on a backbone of evidence. Many authorities argue that the guidelines have not been thoroughly tested and theoretically have little impact on the clinician. Some may even argue that asthma guidelines have had little impact on asthma management.[2] However, if anything, the early asthma guidelines exposed the weaknesses in the literature on childhood asthma as compared to the volume of information that was available on the management of adult asthma and thus directed attention to new research in this area.

The guidelines have also served to consolidate a wealth of information and carefully assimilated it into recommendations for clinical management. While the guidelines were initially based on consensus opinion with available literature support, that consensus opinion has been gradually replaced with landmark studies supported by industry and government sources. Whether or not this area of advance in asthma care is related to the introduction of guidelines, we have witnessed a reduction in asthma mortality and also morbidity as measured by asthma hospitalizations.[3] However, there are still populations at risk for a higher rate of asthma mortality and morbidity, especially the African American population.[4] Now there is the distinct opportunity for healthcare systems to address these issues and embrace the principles of the guidelines, apply new techniques in managing the disease, identify poor responders to conventional treatment, and to pave the way for the application of personalized medicine.

This review will focus on the current status of the asthma guidelines as they pertain to children. The National Heart, Lung and Blood Institute, National Asthma Education and Prevention Program Expert Panel Report-3, Guidelines for the Diagnosis and Management of Asthma will serve as the base for discussion.[3,5] The key message in the recently revised guidelines is that the current version, Expert Panel-3 Report, is an evolution in asthma management rather than a revolution. Therefore, this review will focus on the key messages within the guidelines that pertain particularly to the management of childhood asthma and the new terminology that was introduced to help evaluate and monitor asthma control. This chapter will conclude with a brief discussion of opportunities to improve future asthma management in children. More details on this topic can be found in the chapter on new directions in childhood asthma (Chapter 43).

Why Guidelines?

The driving force for the development of guidelines began in the 1980s in New Zealand as a reaction to a documented pattern of increasing and potentially preventable asthma deaths. There was a strong feeling that corticosteroid therapy was underutilized and that a concerted effort to educate physicians on the principles of asthma management could improve overall outcomes and thus reduce asthma mortality. While the goals of this effort have been achieved with a recognized stabilization and even reduction of asthma deaths and hospitalizations in the USA, one should not be satisfied with this accomplishment.

As previously mentioned, initial guidelines were primarily opinion-based and lacked specific information on pediatric asthma.[1] As a result, opinions differed nationally and even regionally on the key messages and separate guidelines were developed among countries. This was largely related to cultural and financial reasons for choices in management. Although specific country guidelines still exist, there is a movement to develop global guidelines in order to harmonize the principles of management.[6]

Individual guidelines by country take into account availability of specific medications and approval by the respective governing bodies, such as the Food and Drug Administration (FDA) in the USA.[3] For example, in most of the world, there is regulatory approval for the use of combination inhaled corticosteroid (ICS) therapy and long-acting β-adrenergic agonist (LABA) to be used as needed along with maintenance therapy. However, that principal of management will likely never receive approval in the USA based on concerns expressed by the FDA regarding an increased risk of asthma deaths associated with the use of LABA.[7,8] For this reason, there is some good reason to have country-specific guidelines. However, it is still good to solidify the central themes around some unifying principles. Some of these unifying principles include the assessment for the correct diagnosis, monitoring to achieve asthma control, importance of patient education, therapeutic intervention and the management of exacerbations. How these principles are applied differ somewhat among countries, especially regarding medication selection. Amazingly, another area that is very susceptible to variation among and within countries, even within

©2010 Elsevier Ltd, Inc, BV
DOI: 10.1016/B978-1-4377-0271-2.00033-X

geographic areas, is the precise specifications for an asthma action plan.

The introduction of asthma guidelines, along with the advances in development of more effective medications, has resulted in a plateau in asthma deaths and hospitalizations in most countries. Some countries have actually witnessed a trend downwards for these outcomes and that probably speaks for the benefits of organized healthcare and easy access to medications.

Changing Concepts

There are several new areas included in the recent version of the asthma guidelines that merit attention.[3,5,9] First, the recent revision reflects a total review of all areas in the asthma guidelines. There is every attempt possible to support major conclusions and each change from previous versions with evidence consistent with an evidence-based approach. Grading of the evidence for these conclusions can be found on the full website version.[3] In addition, evidence tables are provided for conclusions that involve multiple studies, for example inhaled corticosteroids (ICS) as preferred long-term control therapy, step-care decisions for addition of supplementary therapy to ICS, etc.

Second, consideration is directed towards the needs of three different age groups regarding assessment, treatment steps and monitoring. The three age groups include: 12 years and older, 5 to 11 years of age, and less than 5 years of age. Each of these three populations differ in the amount of information available for decisions on treatment steps, age-limited ability to apply assessment techniques, such as spirometry, and the presentation of the disease in the various age groups, for example, young children usually present with severe exacerbations rather than evidence of persistent symptoms.

Third, some new terminology was introduced to better characterize asthma severity and asthma control. Several key terms were introduced with the new NAEPP asthma guidelines, including severity, control, responsiveness, impairment and risk.[3,5,9] Severity is defined as the intrinsic intensity of the disease process and can be measured most readily and directly in patients who are not receiving long-term controller therapy. Control is the degree to which the manifestations of asthma (symptoms, functional impairment, and risks of untoward events) are minimized and the goals of therapy are achieved. Responsiveness is the ease with which control is achieved by therapy.

Asthma severity and asthma control are both divided into two domains: impairment and risk. Impairment is the assessment of the frequency and intensity of symptoms, as well as the functional limitations that the patient is experiencing now or in the past because of his or her asthma. Risk is the estimate of the likelihood of an asthma exacerbation, progressive loss of pulmonary function over time caused by asthma, or an adverse event from medication or even death. The assessment of severity and control provide guidance on the direction to take in stepping up or stepping down medications.

In a recent theme issue on asthma in *The Lancet*, McIvor and Chapman[2] provide an overview of the past 20 years of asthma guidelines by pointing out some of the challenges in addressing the appropriate target audience and assuring application of these principles to improve outcomes. They point to the many ways that clinicians have ignored key messages in these reports and support the new direction in making guidelines practical and implementable. There are ways to do this but it will require cooperation from all stakeholders including patients, healthcare providers, and clinicians, to name a few.

Fourth, the asthma guidelines emphasize the importance of a step-wise approach to asthma management, and the importance of early diagnosis and intervention.[3,5] The core principles remain as assessment and monitoring, education for a partnership in care, control of environmental factors and comorbid conditions that affect asthma, and medications.

Assessing Asthma Severity in Children

Asthma severity is best assessed in the absence of treatment since severity reflects the intrinsic intensity of the disease. Once treatment is started, then symptoms, pulmonary function and other parameters of disease presentation are altered. Figure 33-1 is a summary of the components of asthma severity for the age groups 0 to 4 years and 5 to 11 years. The two domains include impairment and risk. Impairment includes symptoms, nighttime awakenings, short-acting β-agonist use for symptom control, interference with activity, and lung function. With this revision of the guidelines, parameters were included to assess severity based on two measures of lung function, FEV_1 % predicted and FEV_1/FVC ratio. It is recognized that pulmonary function can be measured in children 5 and above and cannot be measured reliably in children less than 5 years of age. In children between 5 and 11 years of age, the FEV_1/FVC ratio may be more helpful since FEV_1% predicted is often within the normal range. This may be a reflection of the early development of the disease and impact on specific lung function parameters.

The risk category is primarily defined by the assessment of exacerbations requiring oral systemic corticosteroids in the past year. In assessing the use of corticosteroids the severity of the exacerbation and the interval since the last exacerbation should be considered.

For less severe asthma that is considered intermittent, treatment can be limited to rescue short-acting β-agonist use for mild symptoms and prevention of exercise-induced asthma and systemic corticosteroids for managing more severe exacerbations. However, when asthma is deemed persistent, the additional treatment should be considered, specifically long-term control therapy, as discussed in the treatment section.

For severity in regards to impairment, the main differentiation between intermittent and persistent asthma in children up to 12 years of age includes either symptoms or use of short-acting β agonists more than 2 days per week, or minor limitation in activity due to asthma symptoms. Young children less than 5 years of age are considered persistent if they have nighttime awakenings due to asthma 1 to 2 times per month or more. For children 5 to 11 years, nighttime awakenings 3 to 4 times per month or more places them in a category of persistent. Regarding pulmonary function in children 5 to 11 years of age, an FEV_1 % predicted or FEV_1/FVC less than 80% places them in the moderate persistent category.

For the risk domain, the differentiation between intermittent and persistent asthma in children less than 5 years of age occurs at the level of 2 or more exacerbations within 6 months requiring systemic corticosteroids, or 4 or more wheezing episodes per year lasting more than 1 day along with risk factors for persistent asthma. The risk factors are associated with the Asthma Predictive Index and consist of either (1) one of the following: parental history of asthma, a physician diagnosis of atopic dermatitis, or evidence of sensitization to aeroallergens, or (2) two of the following: evidence of sensitization to foods, ≥4% peripheral blood eosinophilia, or wheezing apart from colds.[3,10] For children between the ages of 5 to 11 years, persistent asthma is defined by two or more exacerbations and should therefore prompt a

Components of Severity		Classifying Asthma Severity and Initiating Therapy in Children							
		Intermittent		Persistent					
				Mild		Moderate		Severe	
		Ages 0–4	Ages 5–11	Ages 0–4	Ages 5–11	Ages 0–4	Ages 5–11	Ages 0–4	Ages 5–11
Impairment	Symptoms	≤ 2 days/week		< 2 days/week but not daily		Daily		Throughout the day	
	Nighttime awakenings	0	≤ 2x/ month	1–2x/month	≤ 2x/ month	3–4x/ month	> 1x/week but not nightly	> 1x/ week	Often 7x/week
	Short-acting β₂-agonists use of symptom control	≤ 2 days/week		> 2 days/week but not daily		Daily		Several times per day	
	Interference with normal activity	None		Minor limitations		Some limitation		Extremely limited	
	Lung function • FEV₁ (predicted) or peak flow (personal best) • FEV₁/FVC	N/A	Normal FEV₁ between exacerbations >80% >85%	N/A	>80% >80%	N/A	60–80% 75–80%	N/A	< 60% 75%
Risk	Exacerbations requiring oral systemic corticosteroids (consider severity and interval since last exacerbation)	0–1/year (see notes)		≥ 2 exacerbations in 6 months requiring oral systemic conticosteroids, or ≥ 4 wheezing episodes/1 year lasting > 1 day AND risk factors for persistent asthma	≥ 2x/year (see notes) Relative annual risk may be related to FEV₁				
Recommended Step for Initiating Therapy (See "Stepwise Approach for Managing Asthma" for treatment steps) The stepwise approach is meant to assist, not replace, the clinical decisionmaking required to meet individual patient needs.		Step 1 (for both age groups)		Step 2 (for both age groups)		Step 3 and consider short course of oral systemic cortico-steroids	Step 3: medium dose ICS option and consider short course of oral systemic cortico-steroids	Step 3 and consider short course of oral systemic cortico-steroids	Step 3: medium dose ICS option OR step 4 and consider short course of oral systemic cortico-steroids

In 2–6 weeks, depending on severity, evaluate level of asthma control that is achieved.
• Children 0–4 years old: If no clear benefit is observed in 4–6 weeks, stop treatment and consider alternative diagnoses or adjusting therapy.
• Children 5–11 years old: Adjust therapy accordingly.

Figure 33-1 Classifying asthma severity and initiating therapy in children. (Adapted from Expert Panel Report 3 (EPR-3). J Allergy Clin Immunol 2007;120:S94–138.)

careful evaluation of the impairment domain as well as a consideration for long-term control therapy.

In the absence of treatment, the assessment of severity into intermittent, mild, moderate or severe will direct treatment according to the six-step treatment algorithm described in the following section.

Asthma Treatment Steps for Children

In the past, once severity was assessed, there was a matching level of preferred and alternative treatments. With the revision of the national asthma guidelines, six treatment steps have been created to reflect a pattern of beginning long-term control therapy at Step 2 with low-dose inhaled corticosteroid therapy to either an alternative long-term control therapy at Step 2 or increasing doses of ICS or addition of supplemental long-term controllers at Step 3 and above. Information regarding appropriate choices has been derived from key studies that have been conducted over the last 15 years to define choices based on age and level of severity and this information, based on available evidence, is summarized in the full document.[3]

Figure 33-2 summarizes the treatment steps for children less than 12 years of age by the two categories of 0 to 4 years and 5 to 11 years of age. For children between the ages of 0 and 4 years,

there are only a few medications that have been labeled by the FDA for use in young children as long-term control therapies, namely an ICS in the form of nebulized budesonide and a leukotriene receptor antagonist (LTRA), montelukast. All other currently used long-term control medications for asthma remain to be studied for this age group. Thus, there is currently no long-acting β agonist approved for use in children less than 5 years of age. A close evaluation of the treatment steps for children less than 5 years of age shows the relative paucity of treatment choices due to either the absence of studies or the approval of medications for this age group. Also, to date, there is no preferred delivery method for inhaled corticosteroids although there is only one ICS approved for use in young children, namely nebulized budesonide. Studies are needed to directly compare the relative effectiveness and safety of inhaled corticosteroids administered via the nebulizer/face mask and metered-dose inhaler with spacer/face-mask in young children.

For children between the ages of 5 and 11 years, the treatment steps are relatively similar to those defined for those 12 years and above. However, noteworthy is the absence of omalizumab as a treatment option at Steps 5 and 6 due to the absence of product information and FDA approval for children less than 12 years of age. Also, for children of 5 to 11 years of age, medium-dose ICS is an alternative preferred option in Step 3 to low-dose ICS plus long-acting β-adrenergic agonist (LABA). This is largely due to

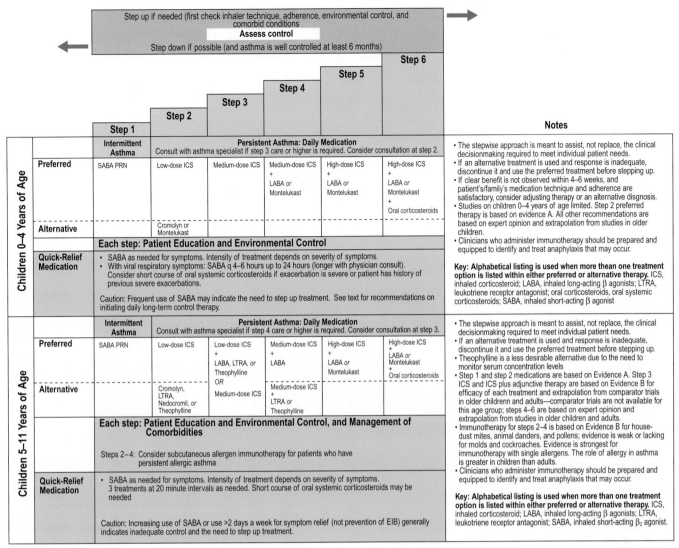

Figure 33-2 Step-wise approach for managing asthma long-term in children 0 to 4 years of age and 5 to 11 years of age. *PRN*, as necessary; *q*, every. (Adapted from Expert Panel Report 3 (EPR-3). J Allergy Clin Immunol 2007;120:S94–138.)

the absence of comparative studies of medium-dose ICS to low-dose ICS/LABA in this age group. The study of these two treatment options plus a third option of low-dose ICS/LTRA is currently being conducted in the NHLBI Childhood Asthma Research and Education Network and should soon be available. This study will not only compare the three treatment options but will also define patient features that might be associated with a favorable response to one treatment option versus the others.

Monitoring Asthma Control in Children

A new direction in the current revision of the asthma guidelines is the focus on asthma control as a goal of management. An assessment of asthma control begins once treatment is initiated. There are three defined levels of control, including well controlled, not well controlled and very poorly controlled as summarized in Figure 33-3. These three levels prompt different decisions to reduce, maintain or advance treatment. In particular, those with very poorly controlled asthma should be considered for treatment with a short course of systemic corticosteroids and stepping up treatment. Those with asthma that is considered not well controlled should be evaluated for an increase in treatment by at least one step. One note of caution is to reassess the diag-

nosis of asthma and adherence to the current treatment regimen before advancing treatment steps. Also, for those patients who are not well controlled, information is provided on the frequency of evaluations that should occur until the patient is well controlled.

In those patients who are considered well controlled, a consideration should be given to stepping down therapy, especially if they have been well controlled for at least 3 months. One note of caution is not to consider a reduction in treatment prior to the time of the year when there is increased risk of an exacerbation based on past history, for example the past history of an exacerbation in the fall, shortly after starting the school year.[11]

For the assessment of control, the two domains of impairment and risk should be evaluated. In addition to the parameters indicated in the assessment of severity, two additional parameters are added to the risk category, including assessment of reduction in lung function as an indication of asthma progression, as well as treatment-related adverse effects. The latter parameters require long-term follow-up and serial measures of lung function and other measures, such as linear growth and weight in children.

For the impairment domain, children less than 12 years of age are considered not well controlled when the symptoms or short-acting β-agonist use occurs more than two times per week or

Components of Control		Assessing Asthma Control and Adjusting Therapy in Children					
		Well Controlled		Not Well Controlled		Very Poorly Controlled	
		Ages 0–4	Ages 5–11	Ages 0–4	Ages 5–11	Ages 0–4	Ages 5–11
Impairment	Symptoms	≤ 2 days/week but not more than once on each day		>2 days/week or multiple times on ≥ 2 days/week		Throughout the day	
	Nighttime awakenings	<1x/month		>1x/month	≥ 2x/month	>1x/week	≥ 2x/week
	Interference with normal activity	None		Some limitation		Extremely limited	
	Short-acting β_2 agonists use of symptom control (not prevention of EIB)	≤ 2 days/week		>2 days/week		Several times per day	
	Lung function • FEV_1 (predicted) or peak flow (personal best)	N/A	>80%	N/A	60–80%	N/A	<60%
	• FEV_1/FVC		>80%		75–80%		<75%
Risk	Exacerbations requiring oral systemic corticosteroids	0–1x/year		2–3x/year	≥ 2x/year	> 3x/year	≥ 2x/year
	Reduction in lung growth	N/A	Requires long-term follow-up	N/A		N/A	
	Treatment-related adverse effects	Medication side effects can vary in intensity from none to very troublesome and worrisome. The level of intensity does not correlate to specific levels of control but should be considered in the overall assessment of risk.					

Recommended Action for Treatment

(See "Stepwise Approach for Managing Asthma" for treatment steps)

The stepwise approach is meant to assist, not replace, the clinical decisionmaking required to meet individual patient needs.

- Maintain current step
- Regular followup every 1–6 months
- Consider step down if well controlled for at least 3 months

Step up 1 step | Step up at least 1 step

- Consider short course of oral systemic corticosteroids
- Step up 1–2 steps

- **Before step up:**
  Review adherence to medication, inhaler technique, and environmental control.
  If alternative treatment was used, discontinue it and use preferred treatment for that step.
- **Reevaluate the level of asthma control in 2–6 weeks to achieve control; every 1–6 months to maintain control.**
  Children 0–4 years old: If no clear benefit is observed in 4–6 weeks, consider alternative diagnoses or adjusting therapy.
  Children 5–11 years old: Adjust therapy accordingly.
- **For side effects,** consider alternative treatment options.

EIB, exercise-induced bronchospasm; *FEV₁*, forced expiratory volume in 1 second; *FVC*, forced vital capacity; *ICU*, intensive care unit; *N/A*, not applicable

Notes;

- The level of control is based on the most severe impairment or risk category. Assess impairment domain by patient's or care-giver's recall of previous 2–4 weeks. Symptom assessment for long periods should reflect a global assessment, such as whether the patient's asthma is better or worse since the last visit.
- At present there are inadequate data to correspond frequencies of exacerbations with different levels of asthma control. In general, more frequent and intense exacerbations (e.g., requiring urgent, unscheduled care, hospitalization, or ICU admission) indicate poorer disease control.

Figure 33-3 Assessing asthma control and adjusting therapy in children. (Adapted from Expert Panel Report 3 (EPR-3). J Allergy Clin Immunol 2007;120:S94–138.)

multiple times on 2 or more days. For nocturnal exacerbations, not well controlled is defined by awakenings due to asthma more than once per month for children 5 to 11 years and one or more per month for those less than 5 years. Also for children of 5 to 11 years, an FEV_1 % predicted or FEV_1/FVC less than 80% is an indication that asthma is not well controlled. For that age group, an FEV_1 % predicted less than 60% or FEV_1/FVC less than 75% is considered very poorly controlled. For the risk domain, exacerbations two or more times per year indicate the asthma is not well controlled. This number can be adjusted based on the last change in treatment.

Application of Guidelines to Clinical Practice

In the past, clinicians appreciated the availability of the guidelines as a resource of information but did not necessarily apply them to day-to-day management of their patients. However, advances in electronic medical records, web-based communication systems, and disease management programs should facilitate the implementation of the principles established in the asthma guidelines. In addition, monitoring by providers will also enhance awareness of the established principles of management and reinforce a standard level of care.

Clearly, there are areas that need to be advanced to assure optimal care for all patients. These areas include access to healthcare including specialists when needed, affordability of medications, education regarding proper self-care, and programs for individualizing therapy. For example, asthma exacerbations are often unpredictable and difficult to manage and thus require urgent care and hospitalization. While it is assumed that better overall management will reduce exacerbations, they do not abolish them. Therefore, advances are needed in identifying the patient at risk for an exacerbation and appropriate preventive therapy. Also, the introduction of biomarkers and genetics offer the promise of tools that could assist in advancing or personalizing management to either identify those at risk for developing asthma or to select treatments that offer the greatest likelihood of success and the lowest risk of adverse effects.

Overall, the message should be that we have advanced asthma care considerably over the past 20 years with new medications and new directions in management. However, we should not rest assured with a stabilization of mortality and hospitalization rate but should direct our attention to continued reduction in mortality and morbidity by identifying those who are at risk for treatment failure and who are not responding to conventional management plans and available therapy. This path should direct us to even better methods to manage the disease and to discover more effective treatment modalities.

Acknowledgement

Dr Szefler would like to thank Gretchen Hugen for assistance with preparation of this chapter.

This chapter has been supported in part by Public Health Services Research Grants HR-16048, HL64288, HL 51834, AI-25496, HL081335, HL075416, the General Clinical Research Center Grant 5 MO1 RR00051 and the Colorado Cancer, Cardiovascular and Pulmonary Disease Program.

References

1. Warner JO. Guidelines for the treatment of asthma. In: Leung DYM, Sampson HA, Geha RS, Szefler SJ, editors. Pediatric allergy: principles and practice. St. Louis: Mosby, 2003, p. 350-6.
2. McIvor RA, Chapman KR. The coming of age of asthma guidelines. Lancet 2008;372:1021-2.
3. National Institutes of Health. National Heart, Lung, and Blood Institute. National Asthma Education and Prevention Program. Expert Panel Report 3: Guidelines for the Diagnosis and Management of Asthma. August 2007. NIH Publication No. 07-4051, http://www.nhlbi.nih.gov/guidelines/asthma/index.htm.
4. Moorman JE, Rudd RA, Johnson CA, et al. National surveillance for asthma - United States, 1980-2004, MMWR 2007;56:1-54.
5. Expert Panel Report 3 (EPR-3). Guidelines for the Diagnosis and Management of Asthma - Summary Report 2007. J Allergy Clin Immunol 2007;120:S94-138.
6. Global Initiative for Asthma. Global strategy for asthma management and prevention. 2008. [Accessed may 2009]. Available from www.ginasthma.com.
7. Kramer JM. Balancing the benefits and risks of inhaled long-acting beta-agonists: the influence of values. N Engl J Med 2009;360:1592-5.
8. Drazen JM, O'Byrne PM. Risks of long-acting beta-agonists in achieving asthma control. N Engl J Med 2009;360:1671-2.
9. Busse WW, Lemanske RF. Expert Panel Report 3: Moving forward to improve asthma care. J Allergy Clin Immunol 2007;120:1012-4.
10. Castro-Rodriguez JA, Holberg CJ, Wright AL, et al. A clinical index to define risk of asthma in young children with recurrent wheezing. Am J Respir Crit Care Med 2000;162(4 Pt 1):1403-6.
11. Sears MR. Epidemiology of asthma exacerbations. J Allergy Clin Immunol 2008;122:662-68.

CHAPTER 34

Functional Assessment of Asthma

Gary L. Larsen • David P. Nichols

Asthma is characterized in part by intermittent airway obstruction, which commonly manifests as shortness of breath, cough, wheezing, and chest tightness. However, even moderate degrees of obstruction may not be clinically apparent. Airflow limitation varies greatly in asthmatic subjects, from mild and self-limited to life threatening. Between these extremes are gradations of obstruction that should be quantified if the patient is to be optimally assessed and managed. This chapter deals with functional assessments of asthma in the pediatric patient, with an emphasis on tests that reflect airway and lung function. Although the primary focus is on studies that can be easily performed in an office or a clinic setting, tests that require more sophisticated equipment than usually found in these locations are also noted. Furthermore, because asthma often first presents in preschool children, tests of lung function that may be performed in the youngest patients are also mentioned. Many of the latter studies are not usually available within the scope of general clinical practice, but they may be performed in centers with expertise in pediatric pulmonary medicine. In addition, knowledge of airway function close to the onset of disease is an important subject of ongoing investigations into the pathogenesis of the disorder.

Because structural changes within airways may relate to the functional assessments, this chapter initially addresses the pathology of asthma. This is relevant for several reasons. For example, an understanding of the pathologic findings in severe asthma identifies components contributing to obstruction that are poorly responsive to acute treatment and take time to resolve. This will be reflected in tests of airway function. At the other end of the clinical spectrum of disease activity, tests that define airway responsiveness may also correlate with lung pathology in subjects in whom the disease is clinically quiescent. Thus this chapter first focuses on a brief review of asthma pathology and then on physiologic correlates before a discussion of functional assessments of the disease. The use of tests of lung function to identify diseases that may mimic asthma is then presented. The ways in which pulmonary function tests may be helpful in guiding therapy in both acute and chronic settings are also considered. Studies involving infants, children, and adolescents are cited whenever possible because of the focus of this text and chapter on childhood asthma. Investigations into structural and functional assessments of the disease in adults are cited when they provide additional insight into the process.

The Pathology of Asthma

Fatal asthma is typified by marked airway inflammation with mucus and cellular debris, epithelial desquamation, subepithelial collagen deposition, and airway wall thickening resulting in luminal obstruction.[1-3] Airway wall thickening occurs as a result of a combination of factors, including smooth muscle hypertrophy, edema, goblet cell hyperplasia, and infiltration of inflammatory cells into airway walls. These features have been noted in autopsy material, not only from adults, but also from pediatric patients of varying ages.[4] We also know that severe asthma can be characterized by similar pathologic findings. For example, Cutz and colleagues[5] found that lower airway biopsy samples obtained from children with severe but clinically stable asthma had features that were also found when the disease led to death. This observation is especially important to keep in mind when considering the length of time it may take for the functional assessment of airway mechanics to return to an acceptable level after an acute episode of the disease.

With the more recent use of bronchoalveolar lavage (BAL) and endobronchial biopsies to address asthma pathogenesis, it is apparent that even clinically mild asthma is also characterized by airway inflammation.[6,7] Common features of this inflammation include infiltration of airways by eosinophils, activation of T cells within airways, an increase in mast cell numbers, and desquamation of airway epithelium.[8] These invasive studies have been performed primarily in adults, with a loose correlation found between indices of inflammation and the level of airway responsiveness to agents such as histamine and methacholine (see later). Although information on pediatric patients is more limited, work using BAL in older children and adolescents suggests that pathologic findings are similar to some of the abnormalities described in adults.[9,10] For example, Ferguson and colleagues[10] reported an association between the level of airway responsiveness to histamine and both eosinophil numbers and mast cell tryptase within BAL fluid of 6- to 16-year-old children. The characteristics of the inflammation present in lungs of preschool children with wheezing are not as clearly defined. However, this is an area being addressed through research involving analysis of lavage fluid.[11,12] Wheezing phenotypes have been characterized physiologically in infants and small children,[13] but the association between pulmonary inflammation and objective measures of airway function in this group of subjects remains to be addressed in more detail.

The Physiology of Asthma

Asthma is defined by physiologic abnormalities. As noted earlier, these abnormalities include increased responsiveness of airways, variable airflow limitation, and reversible airway obstruction. Given these features, asthma is a disease that is best quantified

©2010 Elsevier Ltd, Inc, BV
DOI: 10.1016/B978-1-4377-0271-2.00034-1

by tests of lung function. Several measures of lung mechanics have been used to describe asthma during both symptomatic and asymptomatic phases of the disease.[14] These measures include lung volumes, the pressure-volume characteristics of the lung, resistance to airflow, and flow rates. A discussion of each of these measures in severe childhood asthma is presented.[15] This discussion focuses on measures commonly used by practicing physicians to assess asthma of varying severity in children. Therefore, the emphasis is primarily on flow rates and lung volumes. These considerations follow a general discussion of airway hyperresponsiveness, a fundamental feature of this disease.[16,17] This chapter also includes a review of the changes that occur in arterial blood gases as the severity of obstruction increases.

Heightened Airway Responsiveness

Airway responsiveness is commonly defined as the ease with which airways narrow in response to various nonallergic and nonsensitizing stimuli, including inhaled pharmacologic agents (e.g. histamine, methacholine) as well as natural physical stimuli (e.g. exercise, exposure to cold air). Heightened airway responsiveness to several stimuli is a hallmark of asthma.[16,17] Even when conventional assessments of lung function are normal in children with chronic stable asthma, the airways often exhibit this heightened responsiveness. The most common method of quantifying airway responsiveness is to assess lung function (usually forced expiratory volume in 1 second [FEV_1]) before and after inhaling increasing concentrations of methacholine. The test is concluded when a defined decrease in lung function has been achieved; for the FEV_1, this is usually a 20% decrease from baseline values. The more responsive the airways, the less methacholine is needed to decrease lung function.

The level of airway responsiveness to pharmacologic agents has been noted to roughly correlate with the severity of disease in both adults[16] and children.[18,19] Thus asthmatic subjects who are the most responsive are generally the most symptomatic (wheeze, cough, chest tightness) and require the most medications to control their disease. Although there can be great variability in responsiveness within groups of patients classified by disease severity,[20] the concept that the level of responsiveness correlates with disease severity is important when considering factors that lead to loss of control of the disease. In this respect, the level of airway responsiveness is not static in either normal individuals or asthmatic subjects but may increase or decrease in response to various stimuli. When responsiveness increases, control of the disease is often lost in that this is when asthmatic subjects develop signs and symptoms of their disease. In general, stimuli that increase responsiveness are found in our environment and induce or exacerbate airway inflammation. For children, these stimuli commonly include various viral respiratory infections, air pollutants (including cigarette smoke), and allergens.[21]

A viral respiratory infection is a common antecedent to acute episodes of asthma in children.[22] This has been documented for several respiratory viruses, including respiratory syncytial virus[23] and rhinovirus.[24] In terms of air pollutants, both nitrogen dioxide[25] and ozone[26] have been shown to enhance airway responsiveness. Cigarette smoke is arguably the most serious environmental air pollutant in terms of the respiratory health of children and has been implicated in the onset as well as the perpetuation of the disease.[27-29] In addition, exposure of atopic individuals to relevant allergens can lead to significant increases in airway responsiveness that persist for days to months.[30,31] These classes of disease precipitants are often considered separately, but they assuredly have combined effects in an asthmatic subject's airways which contribute to disease instability.[24]

Just as airway responsiveness will increase in response to certain stimuli that lead to airway inflammation, the level of responsiveness will also decrease if measures are taken to decrease inflammation within airways.[21] These measures include use of medications with antiinflammatory properties (e.g. inhaled corticosteroids) and the avoidance of relevant allergens (atopic asthmatic subjects) and cigarette smoke.[17]

Flow Rates

The usual method of measuring the degree of airflow limitation is to assess lung function during a maximal forced exhalation.[32] The subject exhales forcibly from total lung capacity (TLC) to residual volume (RV) into either a spirometer or through a flow meter by which flow is integrated to give volume. The results are usually expressed as either a time-based recording of expired volume (spirogram) or a plot of instantaneous airflow against lung volume (maximal expiratory flow-volume [MEFV] curve). The tests of lung function derived from a spirogram are the forced vital capacity (FVC), the FEV_1, and the forced expiratory flow from 25% to 75% of the FVC (FEF $_{25-75}$). From the flow-volume curve, the maximal expiratory flow rate (MEFR) achieved approximates the peak expiratory flow rate (PEFR) obtained from a flow meter. Flow rates at and below 50% of the vital capacity (VC) are also obtained as part of this maneuver. Because airflow is related to lung volume, plethysmography combined with the MEFV maneuver plotted as a flow-volume curve or loop allows assessment of the relationship between airflow and absolute lung volumes (Figure 34-1). Measurement of flow rates in this manner may be informative when an isovolumetric shift occurs (discussed later).

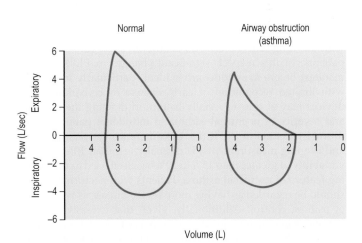

Figure 34-1 Maximal inspiratory and expiratory curves that together constitute a flow-volume loop are shown in a patient with asthma when the disease is under control (*left loop*) and when control is lost (*right loop*). Flow is shown on the y-axis, whereas absolute lung volume is displayed on the x-axis. The point of maximal inspiration (TLC) is the point of zero flow on the left side of the loops while the point of maximal expiration (RV) is at the point of zero flow at the right side of the loops. When asthma control is lost, hyperinflation is noted, with an increase in RV. In addition, expiratory flow rates decrease, as demonstrated in the maximal expiratory portion of the curve, which becomes concave. With milder instability, as shown in this example, the inspiratory portion of the loop is fairly well preserved. With more severe obstruction, inspiratory flows will be more compromised. (From Wenzel SE, Larsen GL, Assessment of lung function: pulmonary function testing. In: Bierman CW, Pearlman DS, Shapiro GS, et al, eds: Allergy, asthma, and immunology from infancy to adulthood. 3rd edn. Philadelphia: WB Saunders; 1996.)

In subjects with asthma, the expected pattern of altered flow rates during an exacerbation has been described. On spirometry, both the FEV1 and FEF$_{25-75}$ are diminished, although the former is more preserved as a percent of predicted than the latter. On the MEFV curve, the expiratory portion of the loop typically becomes concave, or 'scooped out' at the distal portion of the loop (see Figure 34-1) due to a greater impairment in flows at low lung volumes. These flows are the first to decrease and the last to return to normal. The MEFR, like its counterpart, the FEV$_1$, is more preserved during acute attacks and is quicker to normalize.

In a minority of episodes of asthma, the spirogram or MEFV curve alone will not reflect significant airway obstruction. However, if subjects are studied with both an MEFV maneuver and plethysmography to assess lung volumes, they will have a displacement of the flow-volume curve to a higher lung volume without a change in the configuration of the curve itself.[33] Thus if flow is measured as a percent of the VC, no change in flow is appreciated. However, when the same curve is plotted as a function of the absolute lung volumes present before and after onset of symptoms, substantial changes in flow become apparent at the same lung volume, that is, at an isovolume. This represents an isovolumetric shift to a higher lung volume. The factors responsible for isovolumetric shifts are poorly defined but may include closure of some airways with loss of the contribution of these more-obstructed units to the flow-volume pattern.

In acute asthma, loss of symptoms and signs of asthma do not mean that lung function has returned to normal. Classic studies by McFadden and colleagues[34] demonstrated that when patients with severe, acute asthma became asymptomatic, the overall mechanical function of their lungs in terms of the FEV$_1$ was still only 40% to 50% of predicted normal values. Thus loss of clinical signs of airway obstruction does not mean there has been physiologic recovery.

The use of peak flow meters within the home is an inexpensive method of monitoring a flow rate to assess asthma stability.[35] Although there are limitations in that the PEFR may be normal while other spirometric indices are abnormal,[36] home monitoring with this lung function can still contribute to the care of selected patients. In this respect, significant changes in PEFR may be manifest before symptoms are evident, particularly in patients with limited recognition of early disease exacerbation. These devices may also be especially helpful in defining the presence and severity of nocturnal asthma in individual patients.[37] The diurnal variation of PEFR (i.e. the difference between morning and evening measurements) is normally less than 10%. A PEFR variability of greater than 15% to 20% has been used as one defining feature of nocturnal asthma. Patients with nocturnal asthma should be regarded as having more severe disease as well as loss of asthma control. Additionally, given that excessive diurnal variations in lung function during recovery from status asthmaticus have been associated with an increased risk of sudden death,[38] this vulnerable period of time may warrant close monitoring both in the hospital and home environment. Therefore, in more severe patients or those with limited recognition of signs and symptoms of exacerbation, monitoring the PEFR as part of their daily routine may allow for earlier recognition of loss of control with more timely intervention.

Lung Volumes

During an exacerbation of asthma, all of the various capacities and volumes of gas contained in the lung may be altered to some extent. The RV, functional residual capacity (FRC), and TLC are usually increased (RV > FRC >TLC), whereas the VC and its subdivisions are decreased (see Figure 34-1). These alterations have been described during natural exacerbation of asthma in adults[39] and children.[40] Although laboratory-induced changes in lung volumes (exercise, histamine challenge) may be immediately normalized with inhalation of a bronchodilator, it may take weeks after an episode of severe, acute asthma for the RV to return to a normal range.[14] The mechanisms responsible for the increases in RV, FRC (hyperinflation), and TLC (overdistension) are not completely understood. However, several factors have been identified that may contribute, including a generalized decrease in the elastic properties of the lung, a ball-valve phenomenon caused by swollen and mucus-plugged airways, and tonic activity in the intercostal muscles and diaphragm during episodes of obstruction.[14]

Arterial Blood Gases

The primary function of the lung is to provide for gas exchange such that oxygen is taken up and delivered to the body while carbon dioxide is eliminated. This function may be altered when control of asthma is lost. Several studies of acute asthma have correlated arterial blood gases with the level of airway obstruction. One of the classic descriptions is the work of McFadden and Lyons.[41] These authors studied a large population (101 subjects) who, because of age (14 to 45 years) and medical history, were unlikely to have their asthma complicated by bronchitis and emphysema. This study and others (cited later) provide an important description of the expected abnormalities in gas exchange as a function of the degree of airway obstruction.

Oxygen Tension

McFadden and Lyons[41] found that the characteristic blood gas pattern in patients who were experiencing acute asthma was hypoxemia associated with respiratory alkalosis. The hypoxemia was the most consistent abnormality found in their study. A near linear correlation was found between values of FEV$_1$ and arterial oxygen tension (Figure 34-2, top). Patients with an FEV$_1$ of 50% to 85% of their predicted normal values were arbitrarily classified as having mild airway obstruction; those with values of 26% to 50%, moderate obstruction; and those with values of less than 25%, severe obstruction. The mean values of arterial oxygen tension (in mm Hg as measured at sea level) ranked by disease severity were 82.8, 71.3, and 63.1, respectively. Thus there was almost a 20-mm Hg difference in arterial oxygen tensions between the mild and severe groups. Just as important, it was also noted that some degree of hypoxemia was encountered at all levels of airway obstruction. In terms of studies in children, Weng and colleagues[42] noted similar findings in asthmatic subjects who were 14 months to 14 years old. The study found that all symptomatic asthma patients were hypoxemic, with the level of hypoxemia correlating with the degree of airflow obstruction.

Several mechanisms are likely to contribute to the hypoxemia just described. The primary mechanism is thought to be an alteration in ventilation-perfusion ratios.[41,42] In severely obstructed subjects, in whom atelectatic alveoli are still being perfused, transitory anatomic shunts may also contribute to the hypoxemia. In the most severely obstructed subjects, alveolar hypoventilation is also likely to be important.

The normal response of the body to a decrease in arterial oxygen is to increase ventilation. A reduced chemosensitivity to hypoxia coupled with a blunted perception of dyspnea may predispose patients to fatal asthma attacks. Kikuchi and colleagues[43] found that adult patients with a history of near-fatal asthma had

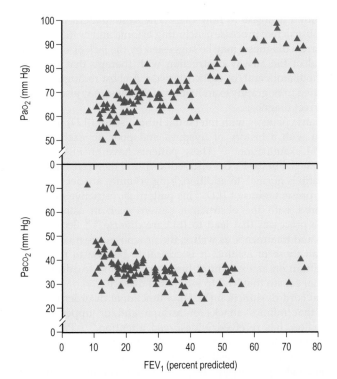

Figure 34-2 The relationship between arterial oxygen (mm Hg) and degree of airway obstruction (FEV₁ as a percent of predicted) **(top)** and the relationship between arterial carbon dioxide (mm Hg) and FEV₁ **(bottom)**. Although the level of hypoxemia correlates with the level of airway obstruction, an elevation in carbon dioxide levels is seen only when the FEV₁ is markedly compromised. (Data from McFadden ER Jr, Lyons HA. N Engl J Med 1968;278:1027–1032.)

respiratory responses to hypoxia that were significantly lower than responses in normal subjects and in asthmatic subjects without near-fatal attacks. The lower hypoxic response was seen in conjunction with a blunted perception of dyspnea. These abnormalities could occur because of preexisting genetic factors as well as adaptation of the body to recurrent hypoxia. The relative importance of these and other factors is unknown. Children with poor perception of airway obstruction may be at risk for fatal or near-fatal asthma.[44]

Carbon Dioxide Tension

McFadden and Lyons[41] demonstrated that respiratory alkalosis often accompanies hypoxemia in asthmatic subjects experiencing exacerbations. In terms of carbon dioxide tensions, their study suggested that most attacks were associated with alveolar hyperventilation and that hypercapnia was not likely to occur until extreme degrees of obstruction were reached. Plotting airway obstruction (percent predicted FEV₁) against the carbon dioxide tension indicated that hypercapnia was not seen until the FEV₁ fell to less than 20% of its predicted value (see Figure 34-2, *bottom*). Thus a 'normal' or elevated $PaCO_2$ in a patient with acute asthma is cause for concern.

Arterial Values of pH

Arterial pH values in acute asthma typically reflect this respiratory alkalosis. In the study of McFadden and Lyons,[41] 73 of the 101 subjects had a respiratory alkalosis (mean pH 7.46); 21, normal pH; and 7, respiratory acidosis (mean pH 7.32). Weng and colleagues[42] reported similar results in children. A metabolic acidosis may also be seen in acute asthma. Although this is not commonly seen in adults, it has been noted in combination with a respiratory acidosis in children with severe asthma.[42,45] This

acid-base imbalance is usually associated with very severe airway obstruction.[46] Although the mechanisms responsible for the metabolic acidosis remain to be clarified, we know that these subjects are in imminent danger of respiratory failure.[42]

Functional Assessments of Asthma in Infants and Small Children

Assessment of lung function in a quantitative manner in infants and small children is very challenging. Noninvasively assessing arterial oxygenation and gas exchange may be relatively straightforward (see later), but measuring pulmonary mechanics, including airflow and lung volumes, is more problematic. Foremost among the problems encountered in working with young subjects is that many are unable to cooperate in the performance of conventional respiratory maneuvers. There has been progress in addressing spirometric lung function in healthy preschool children,[47] but limits remain related to the age and developmental level of the child. Thus many assessments must be done while the youngest subjects are sedated and asleep. In this respect, methods exist for assessing lung function in infants using spirometric techniques in which the patient is passive and forced exhaled flows are generated from near TLC to RV through rapid compression of the chest.[48] When this is accomplished, functional measures similar to those that can be performed in older children and adults may also be obtained in young subjects. Although it is beyond the scope of this chapter to discuss in detail the methods that are used for these studies, it is important to point out that insight into normal maturation of airway function has been gained by this and similar approaches. For example, the highest flow rates corrected for lung size are found in newborns and healthy premature infants, with size-corrected flows decreasing to values found in older children and adults by the end of the first year of life.[49] In addition, studies have demonstrated that normal infants bronchoconstrict when exposed to low concentrations of bronchoreactive agents such as methacholine[50] and histamine[51] as well as to the physical stimulus of cold, dry air.[52] Goldstein and colleagues[53] also found that the response in infants to the inhaled bronchodilator albuterol as assessed by forced expiratory flows was greatest in the youngest subjects. These observations have led to speculation that the level of responsiveness is normally quite high and decreases with postnatal maturation. Although there is an age-dependent variability in the levels of airway responsiveness in normal individuals,[54] higher levels of responsiveness in infants may also reflect technical factors inherent in the administration of a bronchoconstricting stimulus to a small airway. Nevertheless, there is information suggesting that an insult to an airway at a young age may interfere with this normal age-related decrease in responsiveness.[55,56] In this respect, the cross-sectional and longitudinal data of Montgomery and Tepper[57] demonstrate that normal infants and young children have a decrease in airway responsiveness to methacholine as they become older.

The onset of asthma is commonly during the early years of life. This has been noted in several studies, including work from Europe[58] as well as the USA.[59,60] Investigations of asthma are beginning to focus on disease pathogenesis closer to the time of onset. One practical consequence of this is that younger subjects must be assessed, given that the onset of disease is often in preschool children. In terms of quantitative assessments that help categorize disease severity as well as the effects of any intervention, measurements of lung function become essential. However, conventional methods are neither technically feasible nor practical when considering multicenter studies involving large numbers of infants and preschool children. These conventional measures are likewise impractical in the day-to-day care of young asthmatic subjects within many clinical settings. Thankfully, newer techniques offer promise when the assessment must be done in a time-effective manner in subjects with limited ability to cooperate.

Forced oscillation is one of several new techniques that have been used to obtain lung function measures in young subjects.[49,61,62] This method involves the application of sine waves to the airway opening via a mouthpiece while the child breathes normally (tidal breathing). Several variables can be assessed, including resistance, reactance, and resonant frequency of the respiratory system. Although use of this technique has not been applied to large populations of children, results from a published study demonstrate a reasonable agreement with more traditional measures of lung function.[63] There are reports of the use of this technique in young children with acute asthma.[64] This technique has also been used to quantify the response to bronchoconstrictor agents, including methacholine,[63,64] in young asthmatic subjects when clinically stable. In addition, the bronchodilator response in healthy and stable asthmatic children has been addressed.[65] Use of this approach is also feasible when assessing lung function reponses to chronic therapy in very young[66] as well as older children with asthma (below). Therefore, forced oscillation may prove useful in following the course of the disease.

Uses of Assessments of Lung Function

The preceding paragraphs have provided an overview of the tests of lung function that are commonly used to provide a functional assessment of asthma. Reference has been made to pathologic and physiologic correlates in the disease. This section is provided to address practical ways in which these functional assessments are commonly used. In this respect, we concentrate on lung function in diseases that may masquerade as asthma and therefore must be considered in the differential diagnosis of children with wheezing and other nonspecific pulmonary symptoms. We also address how these tests may be used to assess and follow asthma once that diagnosis has been established. In terms of the latter, the value of functional assessments during both acute and chronic phases of the disease is considered.

Functional Assessments of Diseases that Masquerade as Asthma

Shortness of breath, cough, wheezing, and chest tightness are not specific for asthma. Thus children who present in this manner may have medical problems other than asthma. The differential diagnosis of wheezing and dyspnea in pediatric subjects is influenced by the age of the patient. The younger the child, the more one has to consider congenital problems involving the airways. This is especially true for infants and toddlers. In terms of older children and adolescents, the confounding conditions will be more analogous to the problems seen in adults. When considering the differential diagnosis, an assessment of lung function will often help arrive at the correct diagnosis.

Children with bronchiolitis obliterans have experienced insults to their lungs (e.g. adenovirus infection, Stevens-Johnson syndrome with pulmonary involvement) that have led to scarring within small airways and severe airway obstruction.[67] They may present with dyspnea and/or wheezing, leading to the impression that they have asthma. On assessment of lung function, they demonstrate an obstructive pattern with evidence of hyperinfla-

tion with a decrease in flow rates. The same pattern is seen in other obstructive processes, including asthma and cystic fibrosis. The correct diagnosis may be suggested by the lack of significant reversal of the airway obstruction with therapy that includes bronchodilators and/or corticosteroids. A chest radiograph and computed tomography examination of the chest may also suggest the correct diagnosis.

Pediatric patients with interstitial lung disease (ILD) may also present with a history of dyspnea and poor air exchange on physical examination.[68,69] These patients have an FEV_1 that is diminished, but the FVC is also reduced, and therefore the FEV_1/FVC ratio is normal. In addition, lung volumes are decreased in classic presentations of ILD. This pattern is restrictive in nature compared with the obstructive pattern seen in asthma. The disease processes that lead to ILD are diverse.[68,69] Because the causes and treatments, as well as the prognosis, are much different than those of asthma, it is critical to be able to recognize this pattern on assessment of lung function and to address the potential causes that lead to interstitial disease.

Vocal cord dysfunction (VCD), a functional disorder of vocal cords that mimics attacks of asthma and/or upper airway obstruction, has received widespread attention.[70,71] Paroxysms of wheezing and dyspnea seen with VCD are refractory to standard therapy for asthma. During symptomatic episodes, the maximal expiratory and inspiratory flow-volume loop resembles a variable extrathoracic obstruction (Figure 34-3). The diagnosis is confirmed by laryngoscopy results, which demonstrate that the wheezing and/or stridor is associated with paradoxic adduction of the vocal cords during inspiration and sometimes during the entire respiratory cycle. Both the flow-volume loops and the laryngoscopic findings are completely normal when the subjects are asymptomatic. In the vast majority of patients, VCD is subconscious and may be associated with stress. In pediatric patients as young as 4 years, underlying factors such as stress related to athletic or academic performance may be found.[72-74] It must be noted that VCD and asthma frequently coexist in children.[73] Truncation of the inspiratory portion of the flow-volume loop together with a concave shape of the expiratory curve may then be found. Treatment of VCD is primarily accomplished through speech therapy together with psychotherapy in selected patients.[71] Although rarely needed, breathing a mixture of 70% helium/30% oxygen can relieve dyspnea and abort acute attacks.

Just as flow-volume loops may be helpful in making a diagnosis of VCD, they can also aid in the diagnosis of other types of obstructive lesions in the proximal airways (larynx and trachea) that may present with wheezing. For example, with a lesion that is circumferential, preventing either compression or dilation of the airway with respiratory efforts, a 'fixed' pattern is seen (see Figure 34-3) with truncation of both the inspiratory and expiratory curves. Subglottic stenosis and vascular rings that surround an airway might present with such a pattern. If a lesion permits compression or dilation with respiration, the pattern will depend on the location of the lesion (intrathoracic or extrathoracic). With an extrathoracic problem, a picture like that noted previously regarding VCD is seen. With an intrathoracic lesion, greater impairment of expiratory flow rates will be found.[32] One example of such an intrathoracic lesion is tracheomalacia.

Functional Assessment of Acute Asthma

The severity of acute asthma may be gauged by findings on physical examination, tests of lung function, and the adequacy of oxygenation and ventilation (oximetry, arterial blood gases).

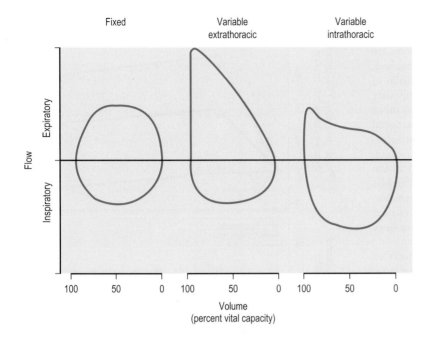

Fixed   Variable   Variable
extrathoracic   intrathoracic

Figure 34-3 Flow-volume loops are displayed for various types of obstructive lesions in the proximal airways (larynx and trachea) that may present with wheezing. For comparison, the normal contour of a flow-volume loop is shown (see left side of Figure 34-1). With a lesion that is circumferential, preventing either compression or dilation of the airway with respiratory efforts, a 'fixed' pattern is seen with truncation of both the inspiratory and expiratory curves. Subglottic stenosis and vascular rings that surround an airway might present with such a pattern. If a lesion permits compression or dilation with respiration, the pattern will depend on whether the lesion is intrathoracic or extrathoracic. With extrathoracic lesions (vocal cord dysfunction) *(middle)*, the inspiratory curve is more affected. An intrathoracic lesion (mass that compresses only part of the airway, tracheomalacia) *(right)* will have more of an effect on expiratory flow rates. (From Wenzel SE, Larsen GL. Assessment of lung function: pulmonary function testing. In: Bierman CW, Pearlman DS, Shapiro GS, et al, eds. Allergy, asthma, and immunology from infancy to adulthood. 3rd edn. Philadelphia: WB Saunders; 1996.)

Pertinent findings on physical examination include use of the accessory muscles of respiration, particularly the sternocleidomastoid muscle, which is an indication of significant airflow obstruction.[75] The presence of a pulsus paradoxus of greater than 20 mm Hg is also a useful indicator of severe airflow limitation in children with acute asthma.[76,77] The finding of a 'quiet chest' in an anxious patient struggling to breathe is an ominous finding.

Although it is critical to recognize and appreciate the importance of these physical findings, quantitative assessments are also of great value in the patient with acute asthma. In asthmatic subjects who are extremely breathless, tests of lung mechanics, although highly desirable, may be difficult or impossible to obtain. Repeated spirometry alone may lead to greater airway obstruction in some children with moderate to severe acute asthma, precluding this manner of assessing the subject. When tests can be performed, assessments commonly include PEFR and FEV$_1$. Flow rates on presentation are important to record, but a lack of improvement in lung function after initial treatment may be a better predictor of the need for hospitalization than the pretreatment value.[78]

In critically ill children, arterial blood gases may need to be performed at presentation and then serially as dictated by abnormalities in gas exchange and clinical status. The expected abnormalities in terms of arterial oxygen and carbon dioxide levels as a function of the level of obstruction (FEV$_1$) were discussed earlier and are displayed in Figure 34-2. In most clinical settings, advances made in noninvasive monitoring allow for relatively quick assessments in patients with acute asthma regardless of age or degree of obstruction; these methods include pulse oximetry and transcutaneous measurements of oxygen and/or carbon dioxide. The latter has been applied primarily to infants and young children, but it has also been used in older pediatric patients.[79] Oximetry has become the most widely applied and clinically useful tool for assessing oxygenation in emergent situations. Oximeters offer a rapid and reliable noninvasive method of assessing the most vital physiologic consequence of obstructed breathing. Physical signs of hypoxemia, such as irritability, pallor, and cyanosis, are variable and may not be present at mild-to-moderate levels of oxygen desaturation. In children, oximetry provides a gauge of the acuity of their asthma and may be helpful in decision-making regarding the need for hospitalization. In a

study from Australia, Geelhoed and colleagues[80] found that the initial arterial oxygen saturation was highly predictive of outcome in pediatric asthma patients in an emergency department. A saturation of 91% was found to discriminate between favorable and unfavorable outcomes as defined in part by the need for subsequent care after the initial visit. In addition, continuous measurements of oxygen saturation during therapy allow care providers to quickly address fluctuations in oxygenation that may be the consequence of both the disease and the therapy provided to the patient. In terms of the latter, lung mechanics may improve after inhalation of a bronchodilator while oxygenation deteriorates.[81] This phenomenon has been attributed in part to the vasodilatory effect of the drugs on the pulmonary vessels, counteracting local vasoconstrictive factors in the lung. Both oximetry and electrodes that assess transcutaneous oxygen provide a noninvasive approach that allows quick responses to fluctuating oxygen needs.

In instances when the episode is mild and the therapy is initiated early within the home environment, administration of one respiratory treatment via metered-dose inhaler (two actuations) or by nebulization may lead to substantial and prolonged bronchodilation. A good response is commonly defined as a return of the PEFR to greater than 80% of that predicted or personal best, with the response sustained for 4 hours.[35] Children who improve with home bronchodilator therapy may then safely repeat this treatment as frequently as every 4 hours. Serial measurements of peak flow before and after therapy are useful not only to assess the severity of acute asthma but also to monitor the response to treatment. A lack of response or an incomplete response to inhalation of a β_2-adrenergic agonist in a patient with asthma should always be a concern and is reason for evaluation and treatment by a physician.

Functional Assessment of Chronic Asthma

As noted earlier, airway obstruction may be present in children with asthma who are asymptomatic. In a subset of subjects who deny symptoms, the degree of obstruction can be quite remarkable. When this is encountered on a child's initial evaluation, the significance of the findings is difficult to assess. Therefore serial tests of lung function in subjects with chronic asthma will be helpful in several respects. First, when several determinations are made over time, the child's personal best lung functions are defined and serve as a point of reference for that child. Second, serial tests of lung function will help support the diagnosis of asthma if fluctuations in PEFR or FEV$_1$ are noted spontaneously or as a result of therapy. When this lability is not seen, other diagnoses may need to be considered. Third, the functional response to therapy (or lack thereof) provides important information on the degree of reversibility in the individual child. When little or no reversibility of lung function is found in the face of significant obstruction, a disease such as bronchiolitis obliterans may be present. Fourth, simple tests of lung function may help identify subjects with increased risk of future asthma attacks[82] or those at greater risk for the persistence of respiratory symptoms.[83]

Serial tests of lung function also help define the effects of various approaches to therapy. This was demonstrated in a long-term study that compared three controller regimens.[84] Children aged 6 to 14 years with mild-to-moderate persistent asthma were characterized with both impulse oscillometry and spirometry before entry into a clinical trial and then serially during 48 weeks of therapy with either an inhaled corticosteroid, a combination inhaled corticosteroid with a long-acting β agonist, or a leukotriene receptor antagonist. The spirometric parameters FEV$_1$, FEV$_1$/FVC, and FEF$_{25-75}$ all demonstrated significant improvement during the first 12 weeks of therapy in the groups receiving corticosteroid and combination therapy. However, improvement appeared to plateau at that time with improvement maintained but not increasing during the latter part of therapy (12 to 48 weeks). Conversely, reactance area (XA), a measurement obtained with oscillometry that reflects both reactance and resonant frequency, demonstrated improvement during the latter part of the study in the corticosteroid treatment arm of the trial. These changes with treatment over time are shown in Figure 34-4. Studies such as this demonstrate not only the time course and magnitude of effects that may be expected with different approaches to therapy, but also suggest that information from oscillometry may complement information obtained with spirometry.

Conclusions

Asthma is characterized by increased responsiveness of airways to various stimuli, variable airflow limitation, and reversible airway obstruction (Box 34-1). Given these features, asthma is a disease that is best characterized in a quantitative manner by tests of lung function. During acute episodes of asthma, marked decreases in flow rates together with hyperinflation of the lungs are seen in tests of lung mechanics. In addition, hypoxemia is a common finding in subjects with wheezing, whereas hypercapnia develops as a late consequence of severe airflow obstruction. Clinical signs and symptoms of obstruction resolve long before tests of lung function normalize, which may not occur for some time. In a subgroup of asthmatic patients, lung function will never completely normalize. In the chronic phase of the disease, serial tests of lung function help define a child's personal best lung function values, help support the diagnosis of asthma, give clues to alternate diagnoses and complicating problems, and help identify subjects with increased risk of future asthma attacks. Serial tests of lung function also help define the effects of various approaches to therapy. A fundamental knowledge of the pathophysiology of acute and chronic asthma is necessary to fully interpret functional studies and to provide effective

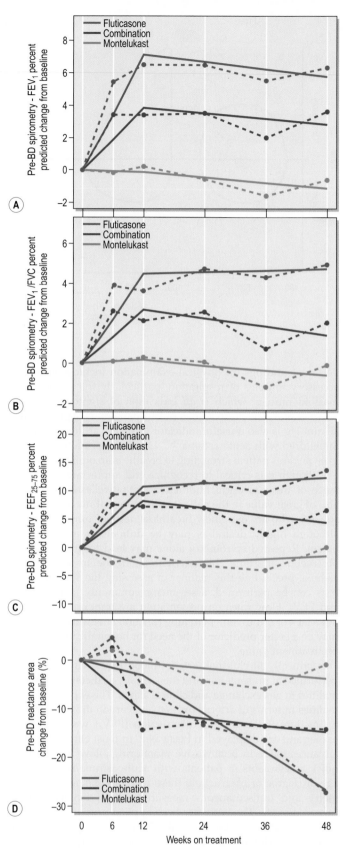

Figure 34-4 Changes in FEV$_1$ **(A)**, FEV$_1$/FVC **(B)**, FEF$_{25-75}$ **(C)**, and XA **(D)** over time are shown for three treatment groups as both mean data at each measurement point (dashed lines) and as a regression model with a change point at 12 weeks of therapy (solid lines). During the first 12 weeks of therapy, the slopes of FEV$_1$, FEV$_1$/FVC, and FEF$_{25-75}$ were significant in a positive direction for combination and fluticasone therapy. However, for these spirometric parameters, the pattern over the last period of therapy (12–48 weeks) was different, with all slopes close to zero (non-significant). Conversely, XA significantly improved in the fluticasone treatment group during the latter period, as reflected by the negative slope for change in XA. Pre-BD signifies measures were all performed before bronchodilator. (From Larsen GL, Morgan W, Heldt GP, et al. J Allergy Clin Immunol 2009;123:860–867.)

Functional Assessment of Asthma in Pediatric Patient

- Asthma is defined by physiologic abnormalities.
- Asthma pathology has physiologic correlates.
- Inflammatory stimuli may increase airway responsiveness.
- Decreases in airflow plus hyperinflation are seen in acute asthma.
- Normalization of lung function lags behind clinical recovery in acute asthma.
- Hypoxemia correlates with the level of airway obstruction in acute asthma.
- Carbon dioxide in arterial blood increases when airway obstruction is severe.
- Serial tests of lung function are valuable in following the course of asthma.

treatment for patients with this common yet potentially life-threatening condition.

Acknowledgments

This work was supported in part by National Institutes of Health grants HL-36577 and HL-67818.

References

1. Dunnill MS. The pathology of asthma, with special reference to changes in the bronchial mucosa. J Clin Pathol 1960;13:27–33.
2. Dunnill MS, Massarella GR, Anderson JA. A comparison of the quantitative anatomy of the bronchi in normal subjects, in status asthmaticus, in chronic bronchitis, and in emphysema. Thorax 1969;24:176–9.
3. Persson CGA. Centennial notions of asthma as an eosinophilic, desquamative, exudative, and steroid-sensitive disease. Lancet 1997;350:1021–4.
4. Richards W, Patrick JR. Death from asthma in children. Am J Dis Child 1965;110:4–23.
5. Cutz E, Levison H, Cooper DM. Ultrastructure of airways in children with asthma. Histopathology 1978;2:407–21.
6. Beasley R, Roche WR, Roberts JA, et al. Cellular events in the bronchi in mild asthma and after bronchial provocation. Am Rev Respir Dis 1989;139:806–17.
7. Vignola AM, Chanez P, Campbell AM, et al. Airway inflammation in mild intermittent and in persistent asthma. Am J Respir Crit Care Med 1998;157:403–9.
8. Djukanovic R, Roche WR, Wilson JW, et al. Mucosal inflammation in asthma. Am Rev Respir Dis 1990;142:434–57.
9. Ferguson AC, Wong FW. Bronchial hyper-responsiveness in asthmatic children. Correlation with macrophages and eosinophils in broncholavage fluid. Chest 1989;96:988–91.
10. Ferguson AC, Whitelaw M, Brown H. Correlation of bronchial eosinophil and mast cell activation with bronchial hyperresponsiveness in children with asthma. J Allergy Clin Immunol 1992;90:609–13.
11. Marguet C, Jouen-Boedes F, Dean TP, et al. Bronchoalveolar cell profiles in children with asthma, infantile wheeze, chronic cough, or cystic fibrosis. Am J Respir Crit Care Med 1999;159:1533–40.
12. Krawiec ME, Westcott JY, Chu HW, et al. Persistent wheezing in very young children is associated with lower respiratory inflammation. Am J Respir Crit Care Med 2001;163:1338–43.
13. Stein RT, Holberg CJ, Morgan WJ, et al. Peak flow variability, methacholine responsiveness and atopy as markers for detecting different wheezing phenotypes in childhood. Thorax 1997;52:936–7.
14. Wagers SS, Jaffe EF, Irvin CG. Development, structure, and physiology in normal and asthmatic lung. In: Adkinson NF Jr, Yuninger JW, Busse WW, et al, editors. Middleton's allergy: principles and practice. 6th ed. St Louis: Mosby; 2003.
15. Larsen GL, Brugman SM. Severe asthma in children. In: Barnes PJ, Grunstein MM, Leff A, editors. Asthma. Philadelphia: Lippincott-Raven; 1997.
16. Hargreave FE, Dolovich J, O'Byrne PM, et al. The origin of airway hyper-responsiveness. J Allergy Clin Immunol 1986;78:825–32.
17. Colasurdo GN, Larsen GL. Airway hyperresponsiveness. In: Busse WW, Holgate ST, editors. Asthma and rhinitis. 2nd ed. London: Blackwell Science; 2000.
18. Murray AB, Ferguson AC, Morrison B, et al. Airway responsiveness to histamine as a test for overall severity of asthma in children. J Allergy Clin Immunol 1981;68:119–24.
19. Avital A, Noviski N, Bar-Yishay E, et al. Nonspecific bronchial reactivity in asthmatic children depends on severity but not on age. Am Rev Respir Dis 1991;144:36–8.
20. Amaro-Galvez R, McLaughlin FJ, Levison H, et al. Grading severity and treatment requirements to control symptoms in asthmatic children and their relationship with airway hyperreactivity to methacholine. Ann Allergy 1987;59:298–302.
21. Larsen GL. Asthma in children. N Engl J Med 1992;326:1540–5.
22. Rakes GP, Arruda E, Ingram JM, et al. Rhinovirus and respiratory syncytial virus in wheezing children requiring emergency care. Am J Respir Crit Care Med 1999;159:785–90.
23. Hall WJ, Hall CB, Speers DM. Respiratory syncytial virus infection in adults. Clinical, virologic, and serial pulmonary function studies. Ann Intern Med 1978;88:203–5.
24. Lemanske RF Jr, Dick EC, Swenson CA, et al. Rhinovirus upper respiratory infection increases airway hyperreactivity and late asthmatic reactions. J Clin Invest 1989;83:1–10.
25. Bauer MA, Utell MJ, Morrow PE, et al. Inhalation of 0.3 ppm nitrogen dioxide potentiates exercise-induced bronchospasm in asthmatics. Am Rev Respir Dis 1986;134:1203–8.
26. Zwick H, Popp W, Wagner C, et al. Effects of ozone on the respiratory health, allergic sensitization, and cellular immune system in children. Am Rev Respir Dis 1991;144:1075–9.
27. Martinez FD, Antognoni G, Macri F, et al. Parental smoking enhances bronchial responsiveness in nine-year-old children. Am Rev Respir Dis 1988;138:518–23.
28. Fielder HMP, Lyons RA, Heaven M, et al. Effect of environmental tobacco smoke on peak flow variability. Arch Dis Child 1999;80:253–6.
29. Burr ML, Anderson HR, Austin JB, et al. Respiratory symptoms and home environment in children: a national survey. Thorax 1999;54:27–32.
30. Boulet LP, Cartier A, Thomson NC, et al. Asthma and increases in nonallergic bronchial responsiveness from seasonal pollen exposure. J Allergy Clin Immunol 1983;71:399–406.
31. Mussaffi H, Springer C, Godfrey S. Increased bronchial responsiveness to exercise and histamine after allergen challenge in children with asthma. J Allergy Clin Immunol 1986;77:48–52.
32. Wenzel SE, Larsen GL. Assessment of lung function: pulmonary function testing. In: Bierman CW, Pearlman DS, Shapiro GS, et al, editors. Allergy, asthma, and immunology from infancy to adulthood. 3rd ed. Philadelphia: WB Saunders; 1996.
33. Olive JT Jr, Hyatt RE. Maximal expiratory flow and total respiratory resistance during induced bronchoconstriction in asthmatic subjects. Am Rev Respir Dis 1972;106:366–76.
34. McFadden ER Jr, Kiser R, deGroot WJ. Acute bronchial asthma. Relations between clinical and physiologic manifestations. N Engl J Med 1973;288:221–5.
35. Expert Panel Report 3 (EPR-3). Guidelines for the diagnosis and management of asthma–summary report 2007. J Allergy Clin Immunol 2007;120:S94–138.
36. Bye MR, Kerstein D, Barsh E. The importance of spirometry in the assessment of childhood asthma. Am J Dis Child 1992;146:977–8.
37. Martin RJ. Nocturnal asthma. Clin Chest Med 1992;13:533–50.
38. Hetzel MR, Clark TJH, Branthwaite MA. Asthma: analysis of sudden deaths and ventilatory arrests in hospitals. Br Med J 1977;1:808–11.
39. Woolcock AJ, Read J. Lung volumes in exacerbations of asthma. Am J Med 1966;41:259–73.
40. Weng TR, Levison H. Pulmonary function in children with asthma at acute attack and symptom-free status. Am Rev Respir Dis 1969;99:719–28.
41. McFadden ER Jr, Lyons HA. Arterial-blood gas tension in asthma. N Engl J Med 1968;278:1027–32.
42. Weng TR, Langer HM, Featherby EA, et al. Arterial blood gas tensions and acid-base balance in symptomatic and asymptomatic asthma in childhood. Am Rev Respir Dis 1970;101:274–82.
43. Kikuchi Y, Okabe S, Tamura G, et al. Chemosensitivity and perception of dyspnea in patients with a history of near-fatal asthma. N Engl J Med 1994;330:1329–34.
44. Baker RR, Mishoe SC, Zaitourn FH, et al. Poor perception of airway obstruction in children with asthma. J Asthma 2000;37:613–24.
45. Downes JJ, Wood DW, Striker TW, et al. Arterial blood gas and acid-base disorders in infants and children with status asthmaticus. Pediatrics 1968;42:238–49.
46. Appel D, Rubenstein R, Schrager K, et al. Lactic acidosis in severe asthma. Am J Med 1983;75:580–4.

47. Eigen H, Bieler H, Grant D, et al. Spirometric pulmonary function in healthy preschool children. Am J Respir Crit Care Med 2001;163:619–23.

48. Jones MH, Castile RG, Davis SD, et al. Forced expiratory flows and volumes in infants: normative data and lung growth. Am J Respir Crit Care Med 2000;161:353–9.

49. Martinez FD, Morgan WJ, Holberg CJ, et al. Initial airway function is a risk factor for recurrent wheezing respiratory illnesses during the first three years of life. Am J Respir Crit Care Med 1991;143:312–6.

50. Tepper RS. Airway reactivity in infants: a positive response to methacholine and metaproterenol. J Appl Physiol 1987;62:1155–9.

51. Lesouef PN, Geelhoed GC, Turner DJ, et al. Response of normal infants to inhaled histamine. Am Rev Respir Dis 1989;139:62–6.

52. Geller DE, Morgan WJ, Cota KA, et al. Airway responsiveness to cold, dry air in normal infants. Pediatr Pulmonol 1988;4:90–7.

53. Goldstein AB, Castile RG, Davis SD, et al. Bronchodilator responsiveness in normal infants and young children. Am J Respir Crit Care Med 2001;164:447–54.

54. Hopp RJ, Bewtra A, Nair NM, et al. The effect of age on methacholine response. J Allergy Clin Immunol 1985;76:609–13.

55. Young S, LeSouef PN, Geelhoed GC, et al. The influence of a family history of asthma and parental smoking on airway responsiveness in early infancy. N Engl J Med 1991;324:1168–73.

56. Tepper RS, Rosenberg D, Eigen H. Airway responsiveness in infants following bronchiolitis. Pediatr Pulmonol 1992;13:6–10.

57. Montgomery GL, Tepper RS. Changes in airway reactivity with age in normal infants and young children. Am Rev Respir Dis 1990;142:1372–6.

58. Croner S, Kjellman N-IM. Natural history of bronchial asthma in childhood: a prospective study from birth up to 12–14 years of age. Allergy 1992;47:150–7.

59. Yunginger JW, Reed CE, O'Connell EJ, et al. A community-based study of the epidemiology of asthma: incidence rates, 1964–1983. Am Rev Respir Dis 1992;146:888–94.

60. Halonen M, Stern DA, Lohman C, et al. Two subphenotypes of childhood asthma that differ in maternal and paternal influences on asthma risk. Am J Respir Crit Care Med 1999;160:564–70.

61. Desager KN, Marchal F, van de Woestijne KP. Forced oscillation technique. In: Stocks J, Sly PD, Tepper RS, et al, editors. Infant respiratory function testing. New York: Wiley-Liss; 1996.

62. Larsen GL, Kang J-KB, Guilbert T, et al. Assessing respiratory function in young children: developmental considerations. J Allergy Clin Immunol 2005;115:657–66.

63. Duiverman EJ, Neijens HJ, Van der Snee-van Smaalen M, et al. Comparison of forced oscillometry and forced expirations for measuring dose-related responses to inhaled methacholine in asthmatic children. Bull Eur Physiopathol Respir 1986;22:433–6.

64. Klug B, Bisgaard H. Measurement of lung function in awake 2–4-year-old asthmatic children during methacholine challenge and acute asthma: a comparison of the impulse oscillation technique, the interrupter technique, and transcutaneous measurement of oxygen versus whole-body plethysmography. Pediatr Pulmonol 1996;21:290–300.

65. Hellinckx J, De Boeck K, Bande-Knops J, et al. Bronchodilator response in 3–6.5 years old healthy and stable asthmatic children. Eur Respir J 1998;12:438–43.

66. Guilbert TW, Morgan WJ, Zeiger RS, et al. Long-term inhaled corticosteroids in preschool children at high risk for asthma. N Eng J Med 2006;354:1985–97.

67. Kurland G, Michelson P. Bronchiolitis obliterans in children. Pediatr Pulmonol 2005;39:193–208.

68. Fan LL, Mullen ALW, Brugman SM, et al. Clinical spectrum of chronic interstitial lung disease in children. J Pediatr 1992;121:867–72.

69. Fan LL, Deterding RR, Langston C. Pediatric interstitial lung disease revisited. Pediatr Pulmonol 2004;38:369–78.

70. Christopher KL, Wood RP, Eckert C, et al. Vocal-cord dysfunction presenting as asthma. N Engl J Med 1983;308:566–70.

71. Davis RS, Brugman SM, Larsen GL. Use of videography in the diagnosis of vocal cord dysfunction: a case report with video clips. J Allergy Clin Immunol 2007;119:1329–31.

72. O'Connell MA, Sklarew PR, Goodman DL. Spectrum of presentation of paradoxical vocal cord motion in ambulatory patients. Ann Allergy Asthma Immunol 1995;74:341–4.

73. Gavin LA, Wamboldt M, Brugman S, et al. Psychological and family characteristics of adolescents with vocal cord dysfunction. J Asthma 1998;35:409–17.

74. Powell DM, Karanfilov BI, Beechler KB, et al. Paradoxical vocal cord dysfunction in juveniles. Arch Otolaryngol Head Neck Surg 2000;126:29–34.

75. Commey JOO, Levison H. Physical signs in childhood asthma. Pediatrics 1976;58:537–41.

76. Galant SP, Groncy CE, Shaw KC. The value of pulsus paradoxus in assessing the child with status asthmaticus. Pediatrics 1978;61:46–51.

77. Martell JAO, Lopez JGH, Harker JEG. Pulsus paradoxus in acute asthma in children. J Asthma 1992;29:349–352.

78. Schuh S, Johnson D, Stephens D, et al. Hospitalization patterns in severe acute asthma in children. Pediatr Pulmonol 1997;23:184–92.

79. Holmgren D, Sixt R. Transcutaneous and arterial blood gas monitoring during acute asthmatic symptoms in older children. Pediatr Pulmonol 1992;14:80–4.

80. Geelhoed GC, Landau LI, LeSouef PN. Predictive value of oxygen saturation in emergency evaluation of asthmatic children. Br Med J 1988;297:395–6.

81. Holmgren D, Sixt R. Effects of salbutamol inhalations on transcutaneous blood gases in children during the acute asthmatic attack: from acute deterioration to recovery. Acta Paediatr 1994;83:515–9.

82. Fuhlbrigge AL, Kitch BT, Paltiel AD, et al. FEV1 is associated with risk of asthma attacks in a pediatric population. J Allergy Clin Immunol 2001;107:61–7.

83. Bahceciler NN, Barlan IB, Nuhoglu Y, et al. Risk factors for the persistence of respiratory symptoms in childhood asthma. Ann Allergy Asthma Immunol 2001;86:449–55.

84. Larsen GL, Morgan W, Heldt GP, et al. Impulse oscillometry versus spirometry in a long-term study of controller therapy for pediatric asthma. J Allergy Clin Immunol 2009;123:860–7.

CHAPTER 35

Infections and Asthma

Theresa W. Guilbert • James E. Gern • Robert F. Lemanske, Jr

Respiratory infections can cause wheezing illnesses in children of all ages and also may influence the development and severity of asthma. Respiratory tract infections caused by viruses,[1-3] chlamydia[4-7] or mycoplasma[5,8-10] have been implicated in the pathogenesis of asthma. Of these respiratory pathogens, viruses have been demonstrated to be epidemiologically associated with asthma in several ways (Figure 35-1). First, certain viruses associated with infantile wheezing have been implicated as potentially being responsible for the inception of the asthmatic phenotype.[11,12] Second, in children with established asthma, viral upper respiratory tract infections (URIs) play a significant role in producing acute exacerbations that may result in healthcare utilization.[13-15] Furthermore, children who develop severe viral respiratory infections in the first 3 years of life are more likely to have asthma later in childhood.[3,11,16] Several host factors, including respiratory allergy[13,17] and virus-induced interferon responses[18-20] modify the risk of virus-induced wheezing. Treatment of virus-induced wheezing and exacerbations of asthma can be challenging and studies evaluating current treatment strategies are reviewed. For infections with other microbial agents, attention has focused on chlamydophila and mycoplasma,[5,7] as potential contributors to both exacerbations and the severity of chronic asthma. Finally, colonization of the upper airways in infancy with common bacterial pathogens has been associated with increased risk of subsequent asthma. We review these various associations as they pertain to both the pathogenesis and treatment of childhood asthma.

Epidemiology

Relationship of Virus-Induced Wheezing in Infancy to Childhood Asthma

One of the most common viral illnesses that leads to lower respiratory tract infection (LRI) and wheezing in infancy is respiratory syncytial virus (RSV). Using multiple virus detection methods, including polymerase chain reaction (PCR), Jartti and colleagues[21] investigated the etiology of wheezing illness in 293 hospitalized children. Of the 76 infants with virus detected, 54% had RSV, 42% had picornavirus (human rhinovirus [HRV] and enterovirus) and 1% had human metapneumovirus-1 (hMPV). In older children, respiratory picornaviruses dominated (65% of children aged 1 to 2 years and 82% of children aged ≥ 3 years).[21] From 1980 to 1996, the rates of hospitalization of infants with bronchiolitis increased substantially[22] and RSV was the etiology in about 70% of these episodes.

However, bronchiolitis is a severe form of RSV infection that occurs in a minority of children. By the age of 1 year, 50% to 65% of children will have been infected with this virus and by the age of 2 years, nearly 100%[23] Children aged 4 months and born close to the onset of the viral season are most prone to the development of lower respiratory tract symptoms,[24,25] and this is likely to be due to a developmental component (e.g. airway, lung parenchyma, and/or immunologic maturation).[23] Furthermore, infant birth 4 months before the winter virus peak predicts an increased likelihood of developing childhood asthma.[24] Additional risk factors for bronchiolitis include antiviral immune responses (both innate[26] and adaptive[27]), gender, lung size, and passive smoke exposure.[16]

Several large, long-term prospective studies of children have demonstrated that RSV bronchiolitis is a significant independent risk factor for recurrent wheezing and asthma, at least within the first decade of life.[12,28] A longitudinal, population-based cohort study has demonstrated that the association between RSV LRIs and both frequent (>3 episodes) and infrequent wheezing (<3 episodes) decreased markedly with age and becomes nonsignificant by the age of 13 years.[12] A decrease in the frequency of wheezing with increasing age after documented RSV infections has been observed by other investigators as well.[29,30] These data suggest that although RSV infections contribute substantially to the risk of recurrent wheezing and asthma in early childhood, other cofactors (e.g. genetic, environmental, developmental) also contribute to the initial expression of asthma or modification of the phenotype over time.

Although a bronchiolitis diagnosis during infancy is associated with an approximately 2-fold increased risk of early childhood asthma, this risk differs by season of bronchiolitis. Bronchiolitis occurring during HRV-predominant months (spring and fall) was associated with an estimated 25% increased risk of early childhood asthma compared with RSV-predominant (winter) months. However, the proportion of associated asthma after winter season bronchiolitis is greater than HRV-predominant months because of higher rates of bronchiolitis during the RSV season.[31] Another study by Kuesel and coworkers demonstrated that although RSV was associated with more severe LRI requiring hospitalization, HRV was associated with more than three times the number of both wheezing and nonwheezing LRI in infancy. These findings support the concept that HRV is also an important cause of bronchiolitis and appears to be most indicative of the risk for developing asthma.[11]

DOI: 10.1016/B978-1-4377-0271-2.00035-3

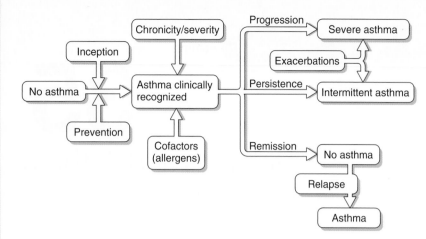

Figure 35-1 Infections and asthma. Infections can influence the pathophysiology of asthma in a number of ways. First, they may be involved in the inception of the asthmatic phenotype within the first decade of life. Second, once asthma is clinically recognized, viral infections may cause disease exacerbations in patients with both intermittent and persistent phenotypes. Third, if asthma goes into remission, it is possible that certain infections may contribute to disease relapse. Fourth, infections may contribute to disease chronicity and/or severity over time. Fifth, infections (based on their type, frequency, target organ involvement, and/or timing) may actually prevent the development of allergic sensitization and perhaps asthma as well. Finally, allergic sensitization and allergen exposures may act as important cofactors in the clinical expression of the asthmatic response to various infections.

Host factors such as atopy or decreased lung function in infancy may also potentiate the risk of recurrent wheeze and/or asthma. Premorbid measurements of lung function indicate that children with reduced levels of lung function in infancy appear to be at an increased risk of the development of chronic lower respiratory tract sequelae after viral infections[32] and an obstructive pattern of lung function into adulthood.[33] Whether reduced lung function alone is responsible for these developments is presently unknown. Children with early atopy (less than 2 years) were more likely to be diagnosed with current wheeze or asthma if they had an LRI with RSV or HRV in infancy.[3] Thus, viral infections may interact with atopy and reduced lung function in infancy to promote later asthma.

Viral Respiratory Infections and Acute Exacerbations of Asthma

The relationship between viral infections and and exacerbations of asthma has been clarified by the advent of sensitive diagnostic tests, based on the polymerase chain reaction (PCR), for viruses that are difficult to culture, such as HRV, hMPV, and bocaviruses. With the advent of these more sensitive diagnostic tools, information linking common cold infections with exacerbations of asthma has come from a number of sources. Prospective studies of subjects with asthma have demonstrated that up to 85% of exacerbations of wheezing or asthma in children are caused by viral infections.[15] Although many respiratory viruses can provoke acute asthma symptoms, HRVs are most often detected, especially during the spring and fall HRV seasons. In fact, the spring and fall peaks in hospitalizations because of asthma closely coincide with patterns of HRV isolation within the community.[14] HRV infections are frequently detected in children older than 2 years who present to emergency departments with acute wheezing[13] and in children hospitalized for acute asthma.[34] A newly discovered HRV species, HRV-C, is associated with asthma exacerbations in children during the fall and winter.[35-37] Influenza and RSV are somewhat more likely to trigger acute asthma symptoms in the winter but appear to account for a smaller fraction of total asthma flares. Other viruses that are less frequently associated with exacerbations of asthma include bocavirus, metapneumonvirus, and coronaviruses.[38] Together, these studies provide evidence of a strong relationship between viral infections, particularly those because of HRV, and acute exacerbations of asthma.

It is interesting that individuals with asthma do not necessarily have more colds, and neither the severity nor the duration of virus-induced *upper* respiratory symptoms is enhanced by respiratory allergies or asthma.[39,40] In contrast to findings in the upper airway, a prospective study of colds in couples consisting of one asthmatic and one normal individual demonstrated that colds cause greater duration and severity of *lower* respiratory symptoms in subjects with asthma.[40] These findings suggest that asthma is associated with fundamental differences in the lower airway, but not necessarily upper airway, manifestations of respiratory viral infections. In addition to provoking asthma, HRV infections can increase lower airway obstruction in individuals with other chronic airway diseases (e.g. chronic obstructive pulmonary disease and cystic fibrosis).[41,42] Thus, common cold viruses that produce relatively mild illnesses in most people can cause severe pulmonary problems in selected individuals.

Viral Respiratory Infections and the Hygiene Hypothesis

The 'hygiene hypothesis' postulates that some viral or bacterial infections might actually *protect* against the subsequent development of allergies and asthma. David Strachan first noted that the risk of the development of allergies and asthma is inversely related to the number of children in the family,[43] an observation that has been duplicated in a number of subsequent studies.[44-46] This finding has led to speculation that infectious diseases, which are more likely to be transmitted in large families or daycare centers,[47,48] could modulate the development of the immune system in a manner to reduce the chances of developing allergies. This hypothesis implies that the immune system is skewed toward a T helper cell type 2 (Th2)-like response pattern at birth. In support of this concept, there is experimental evidence to show that Th1-like interferon responses are depressed at birth[49] and are more likely to be depressed in children who develop recurrent wheezing.[20] According to this hypothesis, each viral infection would provide a stimulus for the development and/or activation of Th1-like immune responses. The result of this repetitive stimulation would be to change the polarization of the Th system away from a Th2 overexpression and thus reduce the risk for developing allergies (Figure 35-2).

However, there is no evidence that viral infections of the respiratory tract protect against either allergies or asthma, and in fact, as previously described, bronchiolitis and pneumonias in infancy indicate an increased risk of subsequent asthma. This has led to speculation that the site of infection might also be an important factor related to asthma risk, and it is possible the gastrointestinal infections are protective. Other epidemiologic and biologic factors that influence the risk of allergic sensitization and/or asthma include early exposure to pets, a farming

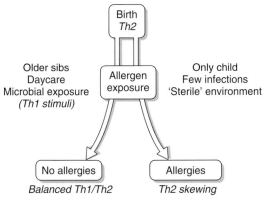

Figure 35-2 *The hygiene hypothesis.* According to this hypothesis, children are born with an immature immune system that is skewed toward T helper cell type 2 (*Th2*) responses. Exposure to infections or microbial products soon after birth provides Th1-like stimuli that help the immune system to develop balanced T cell responses. In the absence of these stimuli, the Th2 skewing persists, and with exposure to allergens in the environment, allergy and atopic disorders are likely to develop. (Modified from Gern JE, Busse WW. J Allergy Clin Immunol 2000; 106:201–212.)

lifestyle, alterations in bacterial flora of the gut, and increased use of antibiotics.[50] Furthermore, exposure to high levels of endotoxin in the home, such as occurs in farmhouses, is associated with reduced rates of allergy and an enhanced number of interferon-producing cells in peripheral blood.[51,52] Collectively, these studies suggest that exposure to microbes may have a greater effect than actual infections on immune development and the risk of atopy and asthma. Other epidemiologic and biologic factors that have been considered to influence the development of allergic sensitization and/or asthma are reviewed in detail in Chapters 2 and 6.

Can Chronic Infections Cause Asthma?

It has been proposed that chronic viral and bacterial infections or colonization with pathogenic bacteria could initiate chronic lower airway inflammation, impaired mucociliary clearance, increased mucus production and ultimately in asthma.[53,54] Organisms primarily implicated in this process include Adenovirus,[55] *Chlamydophila pneumoniae*,[4,5,7] *Mycoplasma pneumoniae*,[8–10] *S. pneumoniae*, *H. influenzae*, and *M. catarrhalis*.[54] Studies of chronic mycobacteria or chlamydophila infection and asthma in children have yielded conflicting results, probably in part due to the limitations of current diagnostics. Findings of diagnostic tests in the upper and lower airways are not always concurrent, and diagnosis of infection by serology leads to inaccuracies.

Historically, the first potential association between asthma and *C. pneumoniae* was reported in 1991 in 19 wheezing adult asthmatic patients, of whom 9 were found to have serologic evidence of current or recent infection with this organism.[6] In school-age children with wheezing, an unexpectedly high prevalence of low-grade *C. pneumoniae* infection in nasal aspirates has been reported.[56] The detection of *C. pneumoniae* infection by PCR and serology (secretory IgA) was similar during symptomatic and asymptomatic episodes (23% vs 28%, respectively). Children who reported multiple episodes also tended to remain PCR positive for *C. pneumoniae*, suggesting chronic infection. Further, *C. pneumoniae*-specific secretory IgA antibodies were more than 7 times greater in subjects who reported four or more exacerbations in the study compared with those who reported just one. In a study of 70 pediatric patients undergoing flexible fiberoptic

bronchoscopy, 40% PCR *C. pneumoniae*-positive samples were from patients with asthma. Culture of the blood samples revealed that a significantly higher proportion of asthma subjects (34.3%) were positive for Chlamydia compared to matched nonrespiratory control subjects (11%).[4] It is interesting to speculate that chronic chlamydophila infection promotes ongoing airway inflammation that increases susceptibility to other exacerbating stimuli such as viruses, allergens, or both.

Thus far, the most comprehensive evaluation of the role of both chlamydophila and mycoplasmal infections in chronic asthma was recently reported by Martin and colleagues.[53] This group of investigators evaluated 55 adult patients with chronic asthma (percent predicted forced expiratory volume in 1 second [FEV_1] = 69.3 [2.1%]) and 11 controls for infection with *Mycoplasma*, *C. pneumoniae*, and viruses. Bronchoalveolar lavage cell count and differential, as well as tissue morphometry, were also evaluated. Of the asthmatic patients, 56% had a positive PCR for *M. pneumoniae* (N = 25) or *C. pneumoniae* (N = 7), which was mainly found in lavage fluid or biopsy samples. Only 1 of 11 control subjects had a positive PCR for *Mycoplasma*. A distinguishing feature between patients with positive and negative PCR results was the significantly greater number of tissue mast cells in the group of patients who were positive on PCR. Cultures for both organisms were negative in all patients, and serologic confirmation correlated poorly with PCR results. In another study by Biscardi and colleagues, 119 children, aged 2 to 15 years, with a previous history of asthma and hospitalized for a severe asthma exacerbation were tested for acute infection due to *M. pneumoniae* or *C. pneumoniae* determined by positive results of serologic testing. Nasopharyngeal aspirate PCR was also performed. Acute *M. pneumoniae* infection by positive serology was found in 20% and *C. pneumoniae* infection was found in 3.4% of the patients during the current exacerbation. Of 51 patients experiencing their first asthma attack, acute *M. pneumoniae* infection was proven in 50% of the patients and *C. pneumoniae* in 8.3%. Of the children experiencing their first asthma attack and infected with *M. pneumoniae* or *C. pneumoniae*, 62% had asthma recurrences but only 27% without these infections had asthma recurrences.[9] Similar to the previous study, serologic confirmation correlated poorly with PCR results. Chronic chlamydophila infection may possibly promote ongoing airway inflammation that increases susceptibility to other exacerbating stimuli such as viruses, allergens, or both.

To further substantiate the contribution of *C. pneumoniae* to asthma, the results of pharmacologic intervention trials are noteworthy. In one study, roxithromycin was administered for 6 weeks to a group of adult asthmatic patients who had serologic evidence of concurrent infection with *C. pneumoniae* and a small but significant improvement was observed in both morning and evening peak expiratory flow rates; however, these improvements were not sustained several months after the discontinuation of therapy and no control group was included.[57] In a pediatric trial, 71 children aged 2 to 14 years with an acute episode of wheezing and 80 age-matched healthy children were studied. Sera for specific antibody levels and nasopharyngeal aspirates for the PCR detection of *M. pneumoniae* and *C. pneumoniae* were obtained on admission and after 4 to 6 weeks. All children with wheezing received a standard therapy with inhaled corticosteroids and bronchodilators for 5 to 7 days and 30.9% received a 10-day course of clarithromycin irrespective of serological and PCR results, on the judgement of the pediatrician in charge. During the 3-month follow-up period, among children with evidence of acute *M. pneumoniae* and/or *C. pneumoniae* infection, significantly more (69.2%) nonantibiotic-treated subjects showed recurrence of wheezing; conversely, none of the clarithromycin-treated patients showed a new episode of wheezing.[10] To date, the data are difficult to interpret because of the limited number of studies, difficulty in eradicating Chlamydia and Mycoplasma infection, and the fact that many of the macrolide antibiotics have antiinflammatory effects in addition to serving as antimicrobials.[58]

If *C. pneumoniae* infection does indeed contribute to asthma chronicity, disease severity, and instability, what mechanisms may contribute to these effects? In this regard, some investigators have proposed that the development of *C. pneumoniae*-specific immunoglobulin E (IgE) antibody causes the release of mediators that lead to bronchospasm, airway inflammation, and airway reactivity.[59] Unless the organism was eradicated with antibiotic therapy, antigenic stimulation leading to specific IgE production would persist, thereby explaining the protracted course of asthma in some patients that is unresponsive to the aggressive use of bronchodilators and steroids.[59] In addition, as indicated previously, a major *C. pneumoniae* antigen is heat shock protein 60 (cHSP60). This protein has been implicated in the induction of deleterious immune responses in human chlamydial infections and has been found to colocalize with infiltrating macrophages in atheromatous lesions. Recently, cHSP60 was found to be a potent inducer of macrophage inflammatory responses mediated through the innate immune receptor complex TLR4-MD2 (Toll-like receptor 4).[60] These latter findings suggest that chronic asymptomatic chlamydial infections may perpetuate ongoing airway inflammatory responses through both innate and adaptive immune responses.

As briefly introduced previously, *M. pneumoniae* also has been associated with both acute and chronic asthma. Various investigators have not been able to uniformly establish the potential for mycoplasmal infections to induce acute exacerbations of asthma. Although some have reported infection in up to 25% of children with wheezing,[61] others have not been able to substantiate these observations.[56] Indeed, when the same population of children was evaluated for the relative contributions of mycoplasmal (and chlamydial) infections to acute exacerbations, viral etiologies were by far the most frequently implicated.[12,56] It is possible that these data may be altered in the future as more sensitive and specific serologic diagnostic tests become available and/or culture techniques improve.

In contrast to the effects of pathogenic *Mycoplasma* species on acute asthma exacerbations, associations of this microbe with chronic asthma have been more securely established. Using PCR techniques on bronchial biopsy specimens, *Mycoplasma* species have been detected in 25 of 55 adult asthmatic subjects and only 1 of 11 controls.[24] Case reports of chronic asthma beginning with *M. pneumoniae* infection suggest that this infection is potentially a causative agent in some patients.[62] In this regard, possible causal mechanisms of *Mycoplasma*-induced airway inflammation have been investigated, including increased Th2 responses and inflammatory neuropeptides. Children with acute *M. pneumonia* have an elevated interleukin (IL)-4/interferon (IFN)-γ ratio compared with children with pneumococcal pneumonia or controls,[63] and mice experimentally infected with *M. pneumoniae* develop airway hyperresponsiveness (AHR), which is associated with decreased production of mRNA for IFN-γ.[64] In addition, asthmatic patients with *M. pneumoniae* infection detected by PCR have elevated levels of neurokinin 1, which responds to treatment with a macrolide antibiotic.[65]

One additional mechanism implicated in the pathogenesis of chronic asthmatic symptoms is latent adenovirus infection.[55] A latent infection occurs when a virus incorporates itself into the host cell DNA and continues to periodically express viral genes. Respiratory disease caused by adenoviruses can be followed by latent infection that persists for many years.[66] A Slovenic study demonstrated that 94% of children with steroid-resistant asthma had detectable adenovirus antigens compared with 0% of controls.[67] In adults, both with and without asthma, evidence of adenoviral infection has been reported to be as high as 50% of the individuals tested.[53]

A recent study by Bisgaard and coworkers found that neonates colonized in the hypopharyngeal region with *S. pneumoniae*, *H. influenzae*, or *M. catarrhalis*, or with a combination of these organisms, are at increased risk for recurrent wheeze early in life and the diagnosis of asthma at the age of 5 years.[54] Although these preliminary results are intriguing, additional studies are needed to establish causality and the specificity of these observations to asthma pathogenesis and to define immunoinflammatory mechanisms contributing to these associations in both adult and pediatric patients.

Sinus Infections and Asthma

The nature of the association between asthma and sinusitis in children (and adults) has been the subject of debate for many years. Much of the difficulty in defining this relationship results from the uncertainties in making the clinical diagnosis of sinusitis, because the signs and symptoms of sinusitis in children overlap with many common childhood respiratory disorders, including the common cold, allergic rhinitis, and asthma. As reviewed in Chapter 30, untreated sinus disease may contribute to unstable asthma control in some patients. Because bacterial infections are clearly involved in acute and chronic sinus disease, the mechanisms by which these microbes may promote AHR in the lower airway have been of great interest. These relationships are covered in depth elsewhere in this text and therefore are not further reviewed in this chapter.

Mechanisms of Virus-Induced Wheezing and Asthma

Several mechanisms have been proposed to explain how respiratory viruses cause wheezing illnesses and exacerbations of asthma (Box 35-1). First, viral infections damage airway epithelial cells and can cause airway edema and leakage of serum proteins into the airway. These effects, together with shedding of infected cells into the airway, can lead to obstruction and wheezing. In addition, virus-induced immune responses are necessary to clear

---

BOX 35-1 Key concepts

Proposed Mechanisms of Virus-Induced Asthma and Wheezing

- Virus-induced damage to airways.
- Airway edema and transudation of serum proteins.
- Respiratory viral infections may enhance underlying airway inflammation in asthma in at least two ways:
    Directly through infection of lower airway epithelial cells
    Indirectly after infection of the upper airway through the generation of systemic immune responses
- A characteristic feature of respiratory viral infections is their ability to enhance airway responsiveness in both normal and asthmatic individuals.
- Interactions between respiratory viral infections and allergic inflammation.

the viral infection, but could also contribute to airway dysfunction and symptoms by causing influx of inflammatory cells that adversely affect lower airway physiology. Respiratory viruses can enhance airway inflammation by directly infecting lower airway tissues, or possibly by infecting the upper airway and then inducing a systemic immune response that potentiates lower airway inflammation. Environmental factors may be important influences on the outcome of viral infections, and viral infections and other known triggers for asthma exert synergistic effects to cause acute exacerbations. Allergy is a strong risk factor for the development of asthma after virus-induced wheezing episodes in infancy, and is also closely associated with virus-induced exacerbations of asthma in older children and adults with asthma. For example, effects of colds on asthma may be amplified by exposure to allergens[17] and by exposure to greater levels of air pollutants.[68] Mechanisms underlying virus-induced wheezing episodes and asthma will be discussed in the following sections.

Viral Infections of the Lower Airway

Respiratory viruses such as RSV and influenza are well known to infect the lower airway, and both can cause bronchitis, bronchiolitis, and pneumonia. HRV has traditionally been considered to be an upper airway pathogen because of its association with common cold symptoms and the observation that HRV replicates best at 33–35°C, which approximates temperatures in the upper airway. In fact, lower airway temperatures have been directly mapped using a bronchoscope equipped with a small thermistor.[69] During quiet breathing at room temperature, airway temperatures are conducive to HRV replication down to fourth-generation bronchi and exceed 35°C only in the periphery of the lung. Moreover, HRV appears to replicate equally well in cultured epithelial cells derived from either upper or lower airway epithelium.[70] Finally, HRV has been detected in lower airway cells and secretions by several techniques after experimental inoculation.[71-73] Titers of infectious virus in lower sputum reach or exceed those found in nasal secretions in some individuals.[73] In addition to evidence from experimental infection models, HRV is frequently detected in infants and children with lower respiratory signs and symptoms, including children hospitalized for pneumonia.[74] Collectively, these findings suggest that respiratory viruses, including HRV, are likely to cause wheezing illnesses and exacerbations of asthma mainly by infecting lower airways and causing or amplifying lower airway inflammation.

Role of Virus-Induced Inflammation

Epithelial Cells

Respiratory viruses replicate primarily in upper and lower airway epithelial cells (Figure 35-3). Virus-induced injury to the epithelium can disrupt airway physiology through a number of different pathways (Box 35-2). For example, epithelial edema and sloughing together with mucus production can lead to airway obstruction and wheezing. The resultant epithelial damage can also increase the permeability of the mucosal layer,[75] which may facilitate contact of irritants and allergens with immune cells, leave neural elements exposed, and enhance viral replication in less differentiated basal epithelial cells.[76]

The processes associated with viral replication trigger both innate and adaptive immune responses within the epithelial cell. For viruses such as HRV, which infect relatively few cells in the airway, this may be the primary mechanism for airway symptoms and lower airway dysfunction.[77] Virus attachment to cell surface receptors can initiate some immune responses. For example, RSV infection activates signaling pathways in airway epithelial cells through the innate immune system through Toll-like receptor-4.[78] Apart from receptor activation, the development of oxidative stress during viral infections can activate epithelial cell responses.[79] Viral RNA binds to cell surface receptors (Toll-like receptor-3)[80] and intracellular proteins, such as the dsRNA-dependent protein kinase and retinoic acid-inducible gene I, to activate the innate antiviral immune response.[81] Through these pathways, viral replication stimulates the production of nitric oxide, activation of RNase L, and inhibition of protein synthesis within infected cells. In addition, innate antiviral responses induce chemokines that recruit inflammatory cells into the airway.[82] HRV-infected epithelial cells secrete RANTES and IFN-γ–inducible protein (IP)–10, which induce T cell chemotaxis.[83] Notably, IP-10 expression is augmented in asthma exacerbations caused by HRV and other viruses, and the level of IP-10 expression has been reported to differentiate between virus-induced and nonvirus-induced asthma exacerbations.[83]

Finally, viral respiratory infections can induce the synthesis of many of the factors that regulate airway and alveolar development and remodeling, including vascular endothelial growth factor (VEGF), nitric oxide (NO), and fibroblast growth factor (FGF).[84-87] How single or repeated bouts of virus-induced over-expression of these regulators of lung development and remodeling affects the ultimate lung structure and function are not known, but is of interest regarding the long-term effects on lung function and asthma.

Inflammatory Cells

Monocytes and macrophages can be activated by viruses to secrete proinflammatory cytokines such as IL-1, IL-8, IL-10, tumor necrosis factor (TNF)-α, and IFN-γ.[88-90] In animal models, respiratory viral infections lead to a prominent expansion of mature dendritic cells in the lung.[91] These lung dendritic cells have a strong facility to activate both naïve and memory T cells and to stimulate their proliferation. Increases in numbers of lung dendritic cells created from local precursors in the lung, survive past the resolution of disease in RSV infection.[92] Significantly, pulmonary dendritic cells express high levels of Toll-like receptors, and secrete large amounts of interferons in response to viral infection.

Acute respiratory viral infections are often accompanied by neutrophilia of upper and lower respiratory secretions, and products of neutrophil activation are likely to be involved in obstructing the airways and causing lower airway symptoms. Importantly, there is evidence that activated neutrophils, through the release of the potent secretagogue elastase, can up-regulate goblet cell secretion of mucus.[93] Additionally, changes in IL-8 levels in nasal secretions have been related to respiratory symptoms and virus-induced increases in AHR.[94,95]

P2X7 is a cation channel expressed by leukocytes and airway epithelial cells that is important to pathogen control and concomitant cellular inflammation. A recent study by Denlinger and coworkers demonstrated that attenuated P2X7 function is common in mild to moderate asthma.[96] This attenuated function is associated with reduced recruitment of neutrophils to the airway during HRV colds, and an increased risk of acute asthma symptoms, even after adjustment for inhaled corticosteroid treatment. Thus, attenuated P2X7 pore activity may be an important regulator of virus-induced neutrophilia, and potentially a novel biomarker for the loss of asthma control during HRV infections.

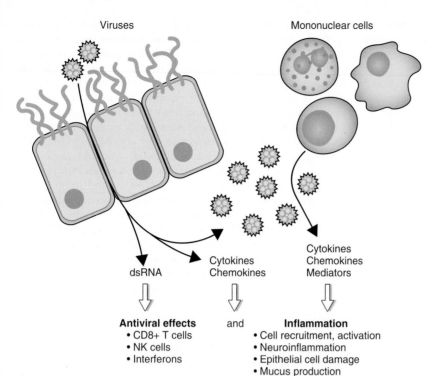

dsRNA

Cytokines
Chemokines

Cytokines
Chemokines
Mediators

Antiviral effects
- CD8+ T cells
- NK cells
- Interferons

and

Inflammation
- Cell recruitment, activation
- Neuroinflammation
- Epithelial cell damage
- Mucus production
- ↑ Vascular permeability

Figure 35-3 Virus-induced inflammation. Airway epithelial cells are the principal host cells for viral replication and, through the release of cytokines and chemokines, help to initiate the immune response to viral infection. In turn, these factors recruit mononuclear cells into the airway, and after the initial round of viral replication, these cells are activated by virus. Virus-induced cytokines, together with unique viral products such as double-stranded RNA (dsRNA), are potent inducers of antiviral responses. In addition, many of these factors promote airway inflammation and dysfunction through a number of mechanisms, as shown in the figure.

BOX 35-2 Key concepts

Components of the Immune Response to Viral Infections

- Airway epithelial cells serve as hosts for viral replication and help to initiate the innate immune response to infection.

- Innate and adaptive immune responses to viral infections promote viral clearance; however, both may augment ongoing local inflammatory responses as well.

- There is evidence that the effectiveness of the antiviral response depends on factors related to the host (developmental and genetic), virus (strain, virulence), and environment (allergens, pollutants, nutrition).

Lymphocytes are recruited into the upper and lower airways during the early stages of a viral respiratory infection, and it is presumed that these cells help to limit the extent of infection and to clear virus-infected epithelial cells. This is consistent with reports of severe viral LRIs in immunocompromised patients.[97] After virus inoculation, B cell responses to infection can be detected in the generation of mucosal IgA by day 3, followed by IgM, and finally IgG after 7 to 8 days.[98] Rapid induction of specific preformed neutralizing IgG to HRV serves to prevent or limit the degree of reinfection.

Relationship of Mononuclear Cell Responses to Outcome of Viral Infections

Several studies have tested the hypothesis that individual variations in cellular immune responses and patterns of cytokine production are related to the outcome of respiratory infections. In a study of children at high risk for the development of asthma based on parental history, reduced mitogen-induced production of IFN-γ from cord blood mononuclear cells ex vivo was associated with a significant increase in viral respiratory illnesses during infancy.[18] Moreover, reduced peripheral blood mononuclear cell (PBMC) production of IFN-γ, both during and months

after RSV, is a risk factor for subsequent asthma.[99] There is evidence in vitro that asthma is associated with impaired virus-induced secretion of interferons by airway and peripheral blood cells.[100-102] Together, these experimental findings suggest that the cellular immune response to respiratory viruses, and interferon responses in particular, can influence the clinical and virologic outcomes of infection.

Interactions between Viral Infections and Allergy

The impact that allergic sensitization may have on the asthmatic airway response to viral infection has generated much interest and research. Interactions between these two factors appear to be bidirectional and dynamic in that the atopic state can influence the lower airway response to viral infections,[16,103] viral infections can influence the development of allergen sensitization,[104,105] and interactions can occur when individuals are exposed simultaneously to both allergens and viruses.[11,106,107]

Atopy is a risk factor for the development of childhood asthma after virus-induced wheezing illnesses, and defining the mechanisms of this relationship has been of interest to many investigative groups.[108] It has also been suggested that atopy could be a significant predisposing factor for the development of acute bronchiolitis during RSV epidemics.[109] Although some have found that those children most likely to have persistent wheezing were born to atopic parents,[109-111] others have not found this.[112,113] Similarly, there is debate as to whether personal atopy is more prevalent *after* bronchiolitis.[12,104,113,114] Despite these uncertainties, it is clear that children who wheeze in early life and have atopic features such as allergic sensitization, atopic dermatitis, and either blood eosinophilia or allergen-specific IgE are at the highest risk for subsequent asthma. These observations have led to the development of predictive indices to estimate the risk of asthma after wheezing in infancy (Table 35-1).

There is convincing evidence to implicate respiratory allergy as a risk factor for wheezing with common cold infections later

Table 35-1 Active Predictive Indices

1. The child must have a history of four or more wheezing episodes with at least one physician diagnosis.
2. In addition, the child must have a history of four or more wheezing episodes with at least one confirmed by a physician.

mAPI: major criteria	Original API: major criteria
• Parental history of asthma	• Parental history of asthma
• Physician-diagnosed atopic dermatitis	• Physician-diagnosed atopic dermatitis
• **Allergic sensitization to ≥ 1 aeroallergen**	

mAPI: minor criteria	Original API: mcriteria
• **Allergic sensitization to milk, egg, or peanuts**	• **Physician-diagnosed allergic rhinitis**
• Wheezing unrelated to colds	• Wheezing unrelated to colds
• Blood eosinophils ≥ 4%	• Blood eosinophils ≥ 4%

Differences in indices are in bold

The original Asthma Predictive Index (API) was based on data from the Tucson Children's Respiratory Study and it had a positive predictive value for active asthma of 47.5% to 51.5% between the ages of 6 and 13 years.[163] Conversely, only 5% of children with a negative API result had active asthma between the ages of 6 and 13 years. The Prevention of Early Asthma in Kids trial[132] modified the published API to include allergic sensitization to aeroallergens and to foods and was used in place of MD-diagnosed allergic rhinitis as this can be difficult to diagnose in young children. It is expected that this modified index would have a similar positive predictive value as the original API for asthma. The modified index has since been adopted by the National Asthma Education and Prevention Program (NAEPP) 2007 Guidelines[136] to identify children at high risk of developing asthma and who may benefit from asthma controller therapy. From Guilbert et al.[162]

on in childhood. In studies conducted in an emergency department, risk factors for developing acute wheezing episodes were determined.[13] Individual risk factors for developing wheezing included detection of a respiratory virus, most commonly HRV, positive allergen-specific IgE (RAST), and presence of eosinophilic inflammation. Notably, viral infections and allergic inflammation synergistically enhanced the risk of wheezing. Furthermore, experimental inoculation with HRV is more likely to increase airway responsiveness in allergic individuals compared with nonallergic individuals.[115] Lastly, the risk of hospitalization among virus-infected individuals is increased in patients who are both sensitized and exposed to respiratory allergens.[17] These findings suggest that individuals with respiratory allergies or eosinophilic airway inflammation are at increased risk for wheezing with virus. This concept has been difficult to model using experimentally-induced colds, however, as allergen administration before inoculation did not enhance symptoms of the cold.[116,117]

Viral infections are postulated to interact with allergic inflammation leading to airway dysfunction through several mechanisms. For example, viral infections could damage the barrier function of the airway epithelium, leading to enhanced absorption of aeroallergens across the airway wall and enhanced inflammation.[118] Additionally, production of various cytokines (tumor necrosis factor [TNF]-α, IL-1β, IL-6), chemokines (CCL3, CCL5, CCL2, CXCL8), leukotrienes, and adhesion molecules (ICAM-1) may further up-regulate cellular recruitment, cell activation, and the ongoing inflammatory response.[119]

Effects of Viral Infections on Airway Hyperresponsiveness

Information derived from animal models, as well as clinical studies of natural or experimentally induced viral infections,

indicate that viruses can enhance airway hyperresponsiveness, which is one of the key features of asthma. Clinical studies of human volunteers inoculated with common cold viruses have generally shown that viral infections cause mild increases in airway responsiveness during the time of peak cold symptoms, and that these changes can last for several weeks.[120] A heightened sensitivity to inhaled irritants, as well as greater maximum bronchoconstriction in response to these stimuli have both been observed. The mechanism of virus-induced airway responsiveness is likely to be multifactorial, and contributing factors are likely to include impairment in the inactivation of tachykinins, virus effects on nitric oxide production, and virus-induced changes in neural control of the airways.[121]

Tachykinins, which are synthesized by sensory nerves, are potent bronchoconstrictors and vasodilators and, through these effects, have the potential to cause severe airway obstruction. Because airway epithelial cells help to regulate tachykinin levels through the production of the enzyme neutral endopeptidase, loss of this enzyme activity in epithelium that has been damaged by viral infection could lead to airway obstruction.[122] Nitric oxide can regulate both vascular and bronchial tone and can interfere with the replication of some viruses.[86] Nitric oxide synthesis is enhanced by viral infections.[123] but because of the many potential effects of nitric oxide on the lower airways, it is uncertain as to whether this is beneficial to lower airway function in asthma.

Viruses can also affect airway tone and responsiveness by enhancing vagally mediated reflex bronchoconstriction. A potential mechanism for this effect is virus interference in the function of the M2 muscarinic receptor.[124] The M2 receptors are part of an important negative feedback loop that limits the release of acetylcholine from vagal nerve endings. When the M2 receptor is damaged by viral infection or virus-induced interferon[125] bronchoconstriction is enhanced, leading to increased airway obstruction. Further delineation of this pathway may lead to novel treatments for virus-induced asthma symptoms that are refractory to standard therapy.

Treatment

Virus-Induced Wheezing in Infancy

Virus-induced coughing and wheezing lead to significant morbidity, and can be particularly difficult to treat. Potential therapies include the use of bronchodilators, antiinflammatory agents, and strategies based on an antiviral approach to either prevention or treatment of acute wheezing. Conventional therapy for virus-induced wheezing in young children commonly includes a step-wise addition of medications, typically starting with a bronchodilator. If lower respiratory tract symptoms become increasingly severe or respiratory distress develops, oral corticosteroids are often added. Recent clinical trials in the management of these wheezing episodes also have included the use of high-dose inhaled corticosteroids (ICS) (both prophylactically and as an acute intervention) and leukotriene receptor antagonists (Box 35-3). These strategies are reviewed in the following sections.

The Role of Bronchodilators and Corticosteroids for Acute Respiratory Syncytial Virus-Induced Bronchiolitis

The efficacy of various therapeutic interventions for the acute symptoms of wheezing, tachypnea, retractions, and hypoxemia

Treatment of Virus-Induced Asthma: Prevention and Intervention

- Inhaled corticosteroid (ICS) treatment after respiratory syncytial virus bronchiolitis does not significantly decrease the development of chronic lower airway symptomatology.
- Chronic treatment with ICS reduces the frequency and severity of intermittent virus-induced wheezing episodes in children with multi-trigger wheezing but does not completely prevent their occurrence. Conversely, in nonatopic children who wheeze only with viral infections, it has not been demonstrated that ICS given either prophylactically or as an acute intervention are effective in reducing the severity or frequency of virus-induced wheezing episodes.
- Treatment of virus-induced asthma exacerbations with oral corticosteroids significantly improves a number of outcome measures.
- The overall and comparative efficacy and the safety of the treatment of similar episodes with either high-dose ICS or leukotriene modifiers warrants further study.

that occur as a result of bronchiolitis has been controversial because of variations in study design, the inability to rapidly and conveniently measure pulmonary physiologic variables, the confounding of results by the inclusion of children with a history of multiple wheezing episodes (i.e. asthmatic phenotypes), and the choice of outcome measures that have been evaluated. In a Cochrane meta-analysis of this subject[126] bronchodilators were found to generate modest short-term improvements in clinical features of mild or moderately severe bronchiolitis; no differences in the rate or duration of hospitalization were noted. However, given the high costs and uncertain benefit of this therapy, the authors concluded that bronchodilators could not be recommended for routine management of first-time wheezers. Similarly, the recent American Academy of Pediatrics (AAP) bronchiolitis guidelines suggest that many children with bronchiolitis do not show a response to bronchodilators. However, a carefully monitored trial of β-adrenergic medication is an option and inhaled bronchodilators could be continued if there is a documented positive clinical response to the trial using an objective means of evaluation.[127]

The efficacy of therapy with either oral or parenteral corticosteroids was reviewed in a meta-analysis of studies that sought to evaluate this form of intervention.[128] A meta-analysis of 13 studies involving therapy with either oral or parenteral corticosteroids concluded that this approach demonstrated a pooled decrease in length of stay of 0.38 days. However, this decrease was not statistically significant. The review concluded: 'No benefits were found in either LOS [length of stay] or clinical score in infants and young children treated with systemic glucocorticoids as compared with placebo'. Two additional studies that evaluated inhaled corticosteroids in bronchiolitis[129,130] showed no benefit in the course of the acute disease. Thus, the AAP bronchiolitis guidelines recommend that corticosteroid medications should not be used routinely in the management of bronchiolitis as the safety of high-dose inhaled corticosteroids in infants is still not clear and an apparent benefit has not been demonstrated.[127] For the majority of cases, supportive treatment remains the standard of care for infants with bronchiolitis.

Effect of Corticosteroids for the Prophylactic Treatment of Recurrent Wheezing and Asthma after Bronchiolitis

Another controversial question is whether corticosteroid treatment can prevent respiratory sequelae after bronchiolitis. Several placebo-controlled trials that address the question of whether corticosteroid treatment can influence the degree of respiratory sequelae after bronchiolitis have been reviewed.[30,128] The majority (7 of 10) of these trials did not show any long-term effects (follow-up time, 6 months to 5 years) on postbronchiolitic wheezing, the development of various wheezing phenotypes (transient, persistent, or late onset), or a subsequent diagnosis of asthma. In the trials that did show some benefit, the positive effects observed were mainly over shorter time intervals after infection. One study[131] concluded that the greatest benefit was more likely to be seen in atopic children. This is similar to other studies of preschool children with recurrent, viral-induced wheezing which demonstrate that atopic children show response to inhaled corticosteroids (ICS).[132,133] Additionally, there is new data that infants who wheeze with HRV are less likely to develop recurrent wheezing if systemic corticosteroid therapy is initiated during the acute infection.[134] This finding, if confirmed, suggests a distinct pathogenesis and therapeutic approach for infants diagnosed with HRV wheezing illnesses.

Role of Oral Corticosteroids in Acute Exacerbations of Asthma in Young Children

Numerous studies have been undertaken to assess the role of corticosteroid therapy in acute episodes of asthma in children and adults. A recent meta-analysis of six trials involving 374 subjects assessed the benefit of systemic corticosteroids for the treatment of asthmatic patients discharged from an acute care setting after assessment and treatment of an acute asthmatic exacerbation.[135] A short course of corticosteroids following assessment for an asthma exacerbation significantly reduces the number of relapses to additional care, hospitalizations and use of short-acting β₂ agonist without an apparent increase in side-effects. Intramuscular and oral corticosteroids are both effective. As a reflection of such information, the most recent National Heart, Lung, and Blood Institute Guidelines for the Diagnosis and Management of Asthma[136] recommends the addition of corticosteroids for asthma exacerbations unresponsive to bronchodilators. These guidelines suggest that the introduction of oral prednisone or prednisolone, for a short course may reduce the duration of the exacerbation and prevent hospitalization. However, only a few pediatric studies have examined whether systemic corticosteroids reduce the severity of exacerbations in children who have bronchospasm exclusively with viral infections. Brunette and colleagues[137] explored the role of early intervention with oral corticosteroid therapy in 32 children under the age of 6 years (mean age, 38.4 months) with asthma typically provoked by viral URI. During the first year of this 2-year study, acute exacerbations were treated with oral bronchodilators initially, with the addition of prednisone for more severe attacks. In the second year, oral prednisone was administered at the first sign of a URI to a group of patients whose parents and caretakers were unblinded to the treatment intervention. The group receiving prednisone during the second year experienced fewer attacks, a 65% reduction in the number of wheezing days, a 61% decrease in emergency department visits, and a 90% decrease in hospitalizations. The administration of prednisone at the first sign of URI was not associated with greater overall prednisone use. Although this study suggests that early intervention with oral corticosteroids has the potential to significantly affect the morbidity associated with acute virus-induced asthma episodes, the unblinded study design makes these results less convincing.

Tal and colleagues[138] conducted an emergency department-based, double-blind, placebo-controlled trial of administration of a single dose of methylprednisolone intramuscularly and demonstrated a statistically significant decrease in hospitalization rate (20% in the methylprednisolone group vs 43% in the control group, $P < 0.05$); this effect was most pronounced in the group less than 24 months old (18% in the methylprednisolone group vs 50% in the control group, $P < 0.050$). Taken together, the results of these two studies suggest that early corticosteroid therapy, ideally started at home, should have an impact on the progression of asthma episodes and decrease the rate of hospitalization for asthma.

Conversely, a recent study comparing oral prednisolone to placebo in 687 hospitalized preschool children with virus-induced wheezing demonstrated no benefit in length of hospitalization, symptom scores, or albuterol use.[139] This study suggests that nonatopic preschool children (only 8% with physician-diagnosed 'hayfever') with severe wheezing episodes severe enough to warrant evaluations in a hospital setting may not respond to corticosteroids; however, the systemic corticosteroids were given during initial evaluation in the hospital setting when the exacerbation was already well underway. In addition, more than one third of these children had no prior history of wheezing.

Young children who experience frequent exacerbations of asthma may receive several short courses of systemic corticosteroids during each viral season and the potential toxicity of repeated courses of oral corticosteroids is a significant clinical concern. Individual courses of oral corticosteroids may be associated with behavioral side-effects. In addition, Dolan and colleagues[140] reported that 20% of children who received four or more short courses of oral corticosteroids in the past year had impaired responses to insulin-induced hypoglycemia. The potential toxicity of repeated courses of oral corticosteroids is a significant clinical concern and likely influences the behaviors of primary care physicians faced with young children who wheeze after having URI symptoms.

Role of Inhaled Corticosteroids in the Treatment of Acute Asthma Exacerbations

Due to the concern of side-effects from repeated doses of oral corticosteroids, the efficacy of ICS intervention for exacerbations has been evaluated in several studies. First, Wilson and Silverman[141] examined the use of beclomethasone dipropionate (750 µg 3 times daily for 5 days administered via metered-dose inhaler [MDI]) at the first sign of an asthma episode in children 1 to 5 years of age. Although failing to alter the need for additional therapy, ICS therapy was associated with improvement in asthma symptoms during the first week of the episode. Daugbjerg and colleagues[142] conducted a double-blind, placebo-controlled trial comparing the effects of inhaled bronchodilator alone or in combination with either high-dose ICS (budesonide nebulization 0.5 mg every 4 hours until discharge) or systemic corticosteroid (prednisolone) in children younger than 18 months who were admitted to a hospital with acute wheezing. Their results demonstrated earlier discharge from the hospital in both the inhalation and systemic corticosteroid-treated groups, as well as a significantly accelerated rate of clinical improvement in the budesonide-treated group compared with the oral cortico-

steroid- and noncorticosteroid-treated groups. Connett and Lenney[143] compared the efficacy of two doses of budesonide (800 or 1600 µg twice daily) via MDI and a spacer device initiated at the onset of upper respiratory tract symptoms in preschool-aged children with recurrent wheezing with URIs. Therapy was continued for up to 7 days or until patients were asymptomatic for 24 hours. Budesonide therapy was associated with decreased symptom scores during the first week of infection. A double-blind, placebo-controlled crossover study by Svedmyr and colleagues[144] involved the administration of budesonide (200 µg 4 times daily for 3 days, 3 times daily for 3 days, and then twice daily for 3 days) via MDI and spacer or placebo to children 3 to 10 years of age with a history of URI-associated deterioration of asthma. Although budesonide therapy had no significant impact on symptom scores, it was associated with significantly higher peak expiratory flow rates. In an emergency department-based study, Volovitz and colleagues[145] compared the effects of inhaled budesonide and oral prednisolone in children aged 6 to 16 years with acute asthma exacerbations. Patients received either budesonide 1600 µg by Turbuhaler or 2 mg/kg of oral prednisolone in the emergency department followed by a tapering dose of medication over the next 6 days. Both treatment groups had similar rates of improvement in the emergency department in terms of symptom scores and peak expiratory flow. However, over the next week, the budesonide-treated group had a more rapid improvement in asthma symptoms. Serum cortisol levels and response to corticotropin were significantly decreased in the prednisolone-treated group at the end of the week of therapy compared with the budesonide-treated group but returned to the normal range 2 weeks later. This study suggests that high-dose therapy with a potent ICS may be as effective as oral prednisolone and avoids hypothalamic-pituitary-adrenal axis suppression. Another study comparing the effects of high-dose ICSs and oral corticosteroids in children seen in an emergency department for severe, acute asthma (mean FEV_1, <40% predicted on presentation) found oral corticosteroids to be superior in terms of improvement in lung function and hospitalization rate.[146] However, these patients were clearly in the middle of severe exacerbations, and ICSs were not used early in the course of the illness. Another recent study of 129 nonatopic preschool children with moderate-to-severe virus-induced wheezing demonstrated a 50% reduction in use of rescue oral corticosteroids during wheezing episodes when high-dose fluticasone was used intermittently at the onset of illness compared to placebo.[147] This suggests a potential benefit of inhaled corticosteroid use in nonatopic children with recurrent wheeze; however, the authors recommended further studies to be done before this treatment strategy was adopted as a small, but statistically significant decrease in height growth was observed.

In summary, ICSs appear to improve asthma symptoms when administered for acute exacerbations of asthma. Although all of these studies provide useful information, they are limited by small numbers of patients and do not delineate features predictive of patients who would be expected to respond to a given therapy. In addition, the ideal drug, dosage, delivery system, and duration of therapy remain unclear. Improved delivery of a potent drug to the lower airways may be associated with a more favorable clinical response.

Role of Leukotrienes in Virus-Induced Wheezing

The cysteinyl leukotrienes have been identified as important mediators in the complex pathophysiology of asthma. Leukotrienes are detectable in the blood, urine, nasal secretions, sputum, and bronchoalveolar lavage fluid of patients with chronic asthma. In addition, leukotrienes are released during acute asthma episodes. Volovitz and colleagues[148] demonstrated elevated levels of leukotriene C_4 (LTC_4) in nasopharyngeal secretions from infants with acute bronchiolitis because of RSV compared with children with upper respiratory illnesses alone. In another study, van Schaik and colleagues[149] also examined leukotriene levels in nasopharyngeal samples from infants and young children with URIs without wheezing, bronchiolitis (first-time wheezers), or acute episodes of wheezing in children with prior wheezing episodes. These investigators found elevated levels of leukotrienes in nasopharyngeal samples from both first-time and recurrent viral wheezers compared with children with nonwheezing URIs. Finally, bronchoalveolar lavage samples obtained from young children (median age, 14.9 months) with recurrent wheezing contain increased numbers of epithelial and inflammatory cells, and also increased levels of cyclooxygenase and lipoxygenase pathway mediators.[150] Interestingly, the levels of these cells and mediators were unaffected by concurrent treatment with ICSs. Studies in vitro or in animal models also suggested that leukotrienes contribute to virus-induced wheezing and asthma. For example, RSV induces 5-lipoxygenase activity in bronchial epithelial cell lines,[151] and in a rat model, treatment with a leukotriene antagonist reduces RSV-induced airway edema in rats.[152]

The effect of a leukotriene receptor antagonist (LTRA) in modulating virus-induced wheezing has been evaluated in clinical studies. Initially, a pilot study demonstrated a 28-day treatment course of montelukast significantly reduced lower respiratory tract symptoms in infants who were hospitalized for RSV bronchiolitis.[153] However, a larger double-blind, placebo-controlled study of 979 children, aged 3 to 24 months, who had been hospitalized for a first or second episode of physician-diagnosed RSV bronchiolitis, were randomized to placebo or to montelukast at 4 or 8 mg/day for 4 weeks and 20 weeks. In this more definitive study, no significant differences were seen between montelukast and placebo groups in the percentage of symptom-free days over either treatment period. This study suggests that this class of compounds are not useful in the prevention of post-bronchiolitis respiratory symptoms. Many other mediators and cytokines have been found to be augmented during viral infection. Future studies will determine whether inhibition of specific components of virus-induced inflammation, such as proinflammatory cytokines (eg, IL-8) or mediators (leukotrienes, bradykinin), will be able to provide safe and effective relief from virus-induced wheezing and asthma.

The efficacy of LTRA in intermittent viral wheezing episodes in preschool children was studied in the Prevention of Viral Induced Asthma (PREVIA) trial.[154] PREVIA was a 1-year randomized double-blind placebo-controlled parallel group worldwide trial in 549 preschool children, aged 24 to 60 months, with intermittent asthma-like symptoms (15% with >2 days of symptoms/week and 16% >2 night awakening/month at baseline) that compared montelukast (4 mg daily) to matching placebo. Montelukast was better than placebo in reducing the rate of (−32%, p < 0.001) and time to first exacerbation/CSW episode (p = 0.024) and supplementary ICS courses (p = 0.027). However, because most exacerbations/CSW episodes were mild and did not require OCS, montelukast failed to reduce oral corticosteroid courses (p = 0.368). Post-hoc analyses did not demonstrate an effect of age or atopic status on response to therapy. In a more recent double-blind, placebo-controlled clinical trial, 220 children, aged 2 to 14 years with intermittent asthma, were randomized to receive a 12-month treatment with montelukast or placebo, initiated by parents at the onset of each upper respiratory tract infection or asthma symptoms for a minimum of 7 days. Emergency department visits were reduced by 45%, visits to all healthcare practitioners were reduced by 23%, and time of preschool/school and parental time off work was reduced by 33% for children who took montelukast for a median of 10 days.

Comparison of Role of ICS and Leukotrienes in Virus-Induced Wheezing

While both ICS and LTRA continuous treatment regimens have demonstrated efficacy in preschool children, comparisons between them have not been conducted with sufficient rigor in order to better clarify which treatment would be best suited for individual children based on various phenotypic or genotypic characteristics. In younger children (2 to 8 years of age) with mild asthma or recurrent wheezing, only one comparison trial of continuous treatment has been published.[155] In this study, the effects of ICS (once-daily budesonide inhalation suspension 0.5 mg) were compared to LTRA (once-daily oral montelukast 4 or 5 mg). No significant between-group differences were observed for the primary outcome (time to first additional asthma medication at 52 weeks); however, other secondary outcomes such as time to first additional asthma medication was longer and exacerbation rates were lower over a period of 52 weeks for budesonide versus montelukast. Time to first severe exacerbation (requiring oral corticosteroids) was similar in both groups. This study had some significant limitations, as ≈ 30% of children did not complete the study and one third of children had adherence rates less than 80%. In addition, a significant portion of children were ≥ 5 years of age and analyses were not stratified by age, making it difficult to extrapolate conclusions to the toddler wheezing age group. Finally, the study was not stratified by atopic status. A recent trial, Acute Intervention Management Strategies (AIMS), examined the effectiveness of episodic use of a high-dose inhaled corticosteroid, a leukotriene receptor antagonist, or placebo during respiratory tract illnesses in 238 preschool children with moderate-to-severe intermittent wheezing. Intermittent budesonide and montelukast modestly improved symptom scores during respiratory tract illnesses but did not improve episode-free days (EFDs) or decrease oral corticosteroid use. Children with positive asthma predictive indices or those who required oral corticosteroids for wheezing in the past year demonstrated the most benefit.[156]

Antiviral Strategies

Influenza vaccine is used as a prevention strategy to reduce virus-induced exacerbations of asthma in the winter. For RSV and HRV, which are more frequently associated with wheezing illnesses, vaccines are not available, and considering that there are well over 100 strains of HRV[35] standard vaccination techniques are not technically feasible for this virus. Although limited by high cost to treatment of high-risk groups, passive prophylaxis with neutralizing antibody to RSV can reduce the influence of more severe respiratory disease. It is encouraging that a small case-control study of premature infants treated with RSV immune globulin reported better lung function and less atopy and asthma in the treated group 7 to 10 years later.[157] In addition, in a European case-control study, infants treated with palivizumab had lower rates of recurrent wheezing compared with untreated controls.[158] Although interpretation of these studies is limited by the lack of randomization, the findings provide reason for optimism and additional preventive studies. Several antiviral agents are in development, and a number of anti-HRV compounds have been tested in clinical trials. These include molecules such as soluble ICAM and capsid-binding agents (e.g. pleconaril), which either hinder HRV binding to cellular receptors or inhibit uncoating of the virus to release RNA inside the cell[159-161] and inhibitors of HRV 3C protease. It is not clear whether these antiviral agents can prevent asthma exacerbations if given at the first sign of a cold.

Conclusions

Viral infections are important causes of wheezing illnesses in children of all ages, and progress is being made toward understanding the mechanisms by which viruses can cause acute wheezing, and perhaps even more importantly, how severe viral infections influence the pathophysiology of asthma in a number of ways (see Figure 35-1). Once these mechanisms are established, it may be possible to identify with greater certainty children who are at the greatest risk for wheezing with viral infections, or those children whose virus-induced wheezing is a preface to asthma. This would represent an important step forward in that preventive therapy could be focused to the groups with the greatest need. Of course, the other rationale for identifying pathogenic mechanisms of virus-induced wheeze is to identify targets for novel therapeutic strategies. Standard therapy for asthma is not satisfactory in that efficacy is low during respiratory infections, and in the case of systemic corticosteroids, side-effects can be significant. Given the close relationship between viral infections and wheezing illnesses in children, it would be attractive to apply antiviral strategies to the prevention and treatment of asthma, and both HRV and RSV are obvious targets. Unfortunately, attempts at developing an RSV vaccine have so far been unsuccessful, and vaccination to prevent HRV infection does not seem to be feasible because of the large number of serotypes. As an alternative, several types of antiviral agents are in development, and several compounds with activity against HRV have been tested in clinical trials.

The other potential therapeutic approach for respiratory viral infections would be to inhibit proinflammatory immune responses induced by the virus. This approach has proved to be effective because the systemic administration of glucocorticoids can reduce acute airway obstruction and the risk of hospitalization for virus-induced exacerbations of asthma. It remains to be demonstrated whether more focused inhibition of specific components of virus-induced inflammation, such as proinflammatory cytokines (e.g. IL-8) or mediators (leukotrienes, bradykinin), will be successful in reducing the severity of viral respiratory infections or exacerbations of asthma.

The evidence that asthma may be associated with a defective immune response to viruses and allergens also could lead to novel therapeutic strategies. Infancy seems to be a time during which the immune response is rapidly developing, and this process appears to be responsive to environmental stimuli, and perhaps dietary factors and lifestyle. It is intriguing that children exposed to rich microbial environments (exposure to pets, farm animals) are less likely to develop acute and chronic wheezing, suggesting that there are environmental factors that can positively modify immune development to strengthen antiviral responses in childhood. Future goals include the development of new treatments to enhance or supplement antiviral responses in infancy to treat acute wheezing episodes, and perhaps reduce the risk of subsequent asthma.

Acknowledgments

This work was supported by National Institutes of Health grants HL070831, AI070503, HL080072, RR025011.

Helpful Websites

The National Heart, Lung and Blood Institute website (www.nhlbi.nih.gov)

The American Academy of Allergy Asthma and Immunology website (www.aaaai.org)

The Childhood Asthma Research and Education Network website (www.asthma-carenet.org)

The Asthma Clinical Research Network website (www.acrn.org)

References

1. Gern JE. Viral respiratory infection and the link to asthma. Pediatr Infect Dis J 2008;27(10 Suppl):S97–103.
2. Gern JE, Bacharier LB, Lemanske RFJ. Infections and Asthma. In: Leung DYM, Sampson HA, Geha RS, Szefler SJ, editors. Pediatric allergy. St. Louis, Missouri: Mosby; 2003. p. 366–78.
3. Kusel MM, de Klerk NH, Kebadze T, et al. Early-life respiratory viral infections, atopic sensitization, and risk of subsequent development of persistent asthma. J Allergy Clin Immunol 2007;119:1105–10.
4. Webley WC, Salva PS, Andrzejewski C, et al. The bronchial lavage of pediatric patients with asthma contains infectious Chlamydia. Am J Respir Crit Care Med 2005;171:1083–8.
5. Sutherland ER, Brandorff JM, Martin RJ. Atypical bacterial pneumonia and asthma risk. J Asthma 2004;41:863–8.
6. Hahn DL, Dodge RW, Golubjatnikov R. Association of Chlamydia pneumoniae (strain TWAR) infection with wheezing, asthmatic bronchitis, and adult-onset asthma. JAMA 1991;266:225–30.
7. von HL. Role of persistent infection in the control and severity of asthma: focus on Chlamydia pneumoniae. Eur Respir J 2002;19:546–56.
8. Kraft M, Cassell GH, Henson JE, et al. Detection of Mycoplasma pneumoniae in the airways of adults with chronic asthma. Am J Respir Crit Care Med 1998;158:998–1001.
9. Biscardi S, Lorrot M, Marc E, et al. Mycoplasma pneumoniae and asthma in children. Clin Infect Dis 2004;38:1341–6.
10. Esposito S, Blasi F, Arosio C, et al. Importance of acute Mycoplasma pneumoniae and Chlamydia pneumoniae infections in children with wheezing. Eur Respir J 2000;16:1142–6.
11. Jackson DJ, Gangnon RE, Evans MD, et al. Wheezing rhinovirus illnesses in early life predict asthma development in high risk children. Am J Respir Crit Care Med 2008.
12. Stein RT, Sherrill D, Morgan WJ, et al. Respiratory syncytial virus in early life and risk of wheeze and allergy by age 13 years. Lancet 1999;354:541–5.
13. Rakes GP, Arruda E, Ingram JM, et al. Rhinovirus and respiratory syncytial virus in wheezing children requiring emergency care. IgE and eosinophil analyses. Am J Respir Crit Care Med 1999;159:785–90.
14. Johnston SL, Pattemore PK, Sanderson G, et al. The relationship between upper respiratory infections and hospital admissions for asthma: a time-trend analysis. Am J Respir Crit Care Med 1996;154(3 Pt 1):654–60.
15. Johnston SL, Pattemore PK, Sanderson G, et al. Community study of role of viral infections in exacerbations of asthma in 9–11 year old children. Br Med J 1995;310:1225–9.
16. Martinez FD, Wright AL, Taussig LM, et al. Asthma and wheezing in the first six years of life. The Group Health Medical Associates. N Engl J Med 1995;332:133–8.
17. Green RM, Custovic A, Sanderson G, et al. Synergism between allergens and viruses and risk of hospital admission with asthma: case-control study. Br Med J 2002;324:763.
18. Copenhaver CC, Gern JE, Li Z, et al. Cytokine response patterns, exposure to viruses, and respiratory infections in the first year of life. Am J Respir Crit Care Med 2004;170:175–80.
19. Ly NP, Rifas-Shiman SL, Litonjua AA, et al. Cord blood cytokines and acute lower respiratory illnesses in the first year of life. Pediatrics 2007;119:e171–8.
20. Gern JE, Brooks GD, Meyer P, et al. Bidirectional interactions between viral respiratory illnesses and cytokine responses in the first year of life. J Allergy Clin Immunol 2006;117:72–8.
21. Jartti T, Lehtinen P, Vuorinen T, et al. Respiratory picornaviruses and respiratory syncytial virus as causative agents of acute expiratory wheezing in children. Emerg Infect Dis 2004;10:1095–101.
22. Shay DK, Holman RC, Newman RD, et al. Bronchiolitis-associated hospitalizations among US children, 1980–1996. JAMA 1999;282:1440–6.
23. Openshaw PJ. Immunopathological mechanisms in respiratory syncytial virus disease. Springer Semin Immunopathol 1995;17:187–201.
24. Wu P, Dupont WD, Griffin MR, et al. Evidence of a causal role of winter virus infection during infancy in early childhood asthma. Am J Respir Crit Care Med 2008;178:1123–9.

25. Holberg CJ, Wright AL, Martinez FD, et al. Risk factors for respiratory syncytial virus-associated lower respiratory illnesses in the first year of life. Am J Epidemiol 1991;133:1135–51.

26. Smyth RL. Innate immunity in respiratory syncytial virus bronchiolitis. Exp Lung Res 2007;33:543–7.

27. Welliver RC Sr. The immune response to respiratory syncytial virus infection: friend or foe? Clin Rev Allergy Immunol 2008;34:163–73.

28. Sigurs N, Gustafsson PM, Bjarnason R, et al. Severe respiratory syncytial virus bronchiolitis in infancy and asthma and allergy at age 13. Am J Respir Crit Care Med 2005;171:137–41.

29. Kneyber MCJ, Steyerberg EW, de Groot R, et al. Long-term effects of respiratory syncytial virus (RSV) bronchiolitis in infants and young children: a quantitative review. Acta Paediatrica 2000;89:654–60.

30. Wennergren G, Kristjansson S. Relationship between respiratory syncytial virus bronchiolitis and future obstructive airway diseases. Eur Respir J 2001;18:1044–58.

31. Carroll KN, Wu P, Gebretsadik T, et al. The severity-dependent relationship of infant bronchiolitis on the risk and morbidity of early childhood asthma. J Allergy Clin Immunol 2009;123:1055–61.

32. Castro-Rodriguez JA, Holberg CJ, Wright AL, et al. Association of radiologically ascertained pneumonia before age 3 yr with asthma-like symptoms and pulmonary function during childhood: a prospective study. Am J Respir Crit Care Med 1999;159:1891–7.

33. Stern DA, Morgan WJ, Wright AL, et al. Poor airway function in early infancy and lung function by age 22 years: a non-selective longitudinal cohort study. Lancet 2007;370:758–64.

34. Heymann PW, Carper HT, Murphy DD, et al. Viral infections in relation to age, atopy, and season of admission among children hospitalized for wheezing. J Allergy Clin Immunol 2004;114:239–47.

35. Lee WM, Kiesner C, Pappas T, et al. A diverse group of previously unrecognized human rhinoviruses are common causes of respiratory illnesses in infants. PLoS ONE 2007;2:e966.

36. Lau SK, Yip CC, Tsoi HW, et al. Clinical features and complete genome characterization of a distinct human rhinovirus (HRV) genetic cluster, probably representing a previously undetected HRV species, HRV-C, associated with acute respiratory illness in children. J Clin Microbiol 2007;45:3655–64.

37. Miller EK, Edwards KM, Weinberg GA, et al. A novel group of rhinoviruses is associated with asthma hospitalizations. J Allergy Clin Immunol 2009;123:98–104 e1.

38. Calvo C, Garcia-Garcia ML, Pozo F, et al. Clinical characteristics of human bocavirus infections compared with other respiratory viruses in Spanish children. Pediatr Infect Dis J 2008;27:677–80.

39. Doyle WJ, Skoner DP, Fireman P, et al. Rhinovirus 39 infection in allergic and nonallergic subjects. J Allergy Clin Immunol 1992;89:968–78.

40. Corne JM, Marshall C, Smith S, et al. Frequency, severity, and duration of rhinovirus infections in asthmatic and non-asthmatic individuals: a longitudinal cohort study. Lancet 2002;359:831–4.

41. Smyth AR, Smyth RL, Tong CY, et al. Effect of respiratory virus infections including rhinovirus on clinical status in cystic fibrosis. Arch Dis Child 1995;73:117–20.

42. Seemungal TA, Harper-Owen R, Bhowmik A, et al. Detection of rhinovirus in induced sputum at exacerbation of chronic obstructive pulmonary disease. Eur Respir J 2000;16:677–83.

43. Strachan DP. Hay fever, hygiene, and household size. Br Med J 1989;299:1259–60.

44. Liu AH, Leung DY. Renaissance of the hygiene hypothesis. J Allergy Clin Immunol 2006;117:1063–6.

45. von Mutius E, Martinez FD, Fritzsch C, et al. Skin test reactivity and number of siblings. Br Med J 1994;308:692–5.

46. von Mutius E. The influence of birth order on the expression of atopy in families: a gene-environment interaction? Clin Exp Allergy 1998;28:1454–6.

47. Ball TM, Castro-Rodriguez JA, Griffith KA, et al. Siblings, day-care attendance, and the risk of asthma and wheezing during childhood. N Engl J Med 2000;343:538–43.

48. Oddy WH, de Klerk NH, Sly PD, et al. The effects of respiratory infections, atopy, and breastfeeding on childhood asthma. Eur Respir J 2002;19:899–905.

49. Prescott SL, Macaubas C, Smallacombe T, et al. Development of allergen-specific T cell memory in atopic and normal children. Lancet 1999;353:196–200.

50. Schaub B, Lauener R, von Mutius E. The many faces of the hygiene hypothesis. J Allergy Clin Immunol 2006;117:969–77; quiz 78.

51. Liu AH. Endotoxin exposure in allergy and asthma: reconciling a paradox. J Allergy Clin Immunol 2002;109:379–92.

52. Gereda JE, Leung DY, Thatayatikom A, et al. Relation between house-dust endotoxin exposure, type 1 T cell development, and allergen sensitisation in infants at high risk of asthma. Lancet 2000;355:1680–3.

53. Martin RJ, Kraft M, Chu HW, et al. A link between chronic asthma and chronic infection. J Allergy Clin Immunol 2001;107:595–601.

54. Bisgaard H, Hermansen MN, Buchvald F, et al. Childhood asthma after bacterial colonization of the airway in neonates. N Engl J Med 2007;357:1487–95.

55. Hogg JC. Role of latent viral infections in chronic obstructive pulmonary disease and asthma. Am J Respir Crit Care Med 2001;164(10 Pt 2):S71–5.

56. Cunningham AF, Johnston SL, Julious SA, et al. Chronic Chlamydia pneumoniae infection and asthma exacerbations in children. Eur Respir J 1998;11:345–9.

57. Black PN, Blasi F, Jenkins CR, et al. Trial of roxithromycin in subjects with asthma and serological evidence of infection with Chlamydia pneumoniae. Am J Respir Crit Care Med 2001;164:536–41.

58. Avila PC, Boushey HA. Macrolides, asthma, inflammation, and infection. Ann Allergy Asthma Immunol 2000;84:565–8.

59. Emre U, Sokolovskaya N, Roblin PM, et al. Detection of anti-Chlamydia pneumoniae IgE in children with reactive airway disease. J Infect Dis 1995;172:265–7.

60. Bulut Y, Faure E, Thomas L, et al. Chlamydial heat shock protein 60 activates macrophages and endothelial cells through Toll-like receptor 4 and MD2 in a MyD88-dependent pathway. J Immunol 2002;168:1435–40.

61. Henderson FW, Clyde WA Jr, Collier AM, et al. The etiologic and epidemiologic spectrum of bronchiolitis in pediatric practice. J Pediatr 1979;95:183–90.

62. Yano T, Ichikawa Y, Komatu S, et al. Association of Mycoplasma pneumoniae antigen with initial onset of bronchial asthma. Am J Respir Crit Care Med 1994;149:1348–53.

63. Koh YY, Park Y, Lee HJ, et al. Levels of interleukin-2, interferon-gamma, and interleukin-4 in bronchoalveolar lavage fluid from patients with Mycoplasma pneumonia: implication of tendency toward increased immunoglobulin E production. Pediatrics 2001;107:E39.

64. Martin RJ, Chu HW, Honour JM, et al. Airway inflammation and bronchial hyperresponsiveness after Mycoplasma pneumoniae infection in a murine model. Am J Respir Cell Mol Biol 2001;24:577–82.

65. Chu HW, Kraft M, Krause JE, et al. Substance P and its receptor neurokinin 1 expression in asthmatic airways. J Allergy Clin Immunol 2000;106:713–22.

66. Matsuse T, Hayashi S, Kuwano K, et al. Latent adenoviral infection in the pathogenesis of chronic airways obstruction. Am Rev Respir Dis 1992;146:177–84.

67. Macek V, Sorli J, Kopriva S, et al. Persistent adenoviral infection and chronic airway obstruction in children. Am J Respir Crit Care Med 1994;150:7–10.

68. Tarlo SM, Broder I, Corey P, et al. The role of symptomatic colds in asthma exacerbations: Influence of outdoor allergens and air pollutants. J Allergy Clin Immunol 2001;108:52–8.

69. McFadden ER Jr. Improper patient techniques with metered dose inhalers: clinical consequences and solutions to misuse. J Allergy Clin Immunol 1995;96:278–83.

70. Mosser AG, Brockman-Schneider R, Amineva S, et al. Similar frequency of rhinovirus-infectible cells in upper and lower airway epithelium. J Infect Dis 2002;185:734–43.

71. Gern JE, Galagan DM, Jarjour NN, et al. Detection of rhinovirus RNA in lower airway cells during experimentally induced infection. Am J Respir Crit Care Med 1997;155:1159–61.

72. Papadopoulos NG, Bates PJ, Bardin PG, et al. Rhinoviruses infect the lower airways. J Infect Dis 2000;181:1875–84.

73. Mosser AG, Vrtis R, Burchell L, et al. Quantitative and qualitative analysis of rhinovirus infection in bronchial tissues. Am J Respir Crit Care Med 2005;171:645–51.

74. Simons E, Schroth MK, Gern JE. Analysis of tracheal secretions for rhinovirus during natural colds. Pediatr Allergy Immunol 2005;16:276–8.

75. Ohrui T, Yamaya M, Sekizawa K, et al. Effects of rhinovirus infection on hydrogen peroxide-induced alterations of barrier function in the cultured human tracheal epithelium. Am J Respir Crit Care Med 1998;158:241–8.

76. Jakiela B, Brockman-Schneider R, Amineva S, et al. Basal cells of differentiated bronchial epithelium are more susceptible to rhinovirus infection. Am J Respir Cell Mol Biol 2008;38:517–23.

77. Hendley JO. The host response, not the virus, causes the symptoms of the common cold. Clin Infect Dis 1998;26:847–8.

78. Kurt-Jones EA, Popova L, Kwinn L, et al. Pattern recognition receptors TLR4 and CD14 mediate response to respiratory syncytial virus. Nat Immunol 2000;1:398–401.

79. Casola A, Burger N, Liu T, et al. Oxidant tone regulates RANTES gene expression in airway epithelial cells infected with respiratory syncytial virus: role in viral-induced interferon regulatory factor activation. J Biol Chem 2001;276:19715–22.

80. Alexopoulou L, Holt AC, Medzhitov R, et al. Recognition of double-stranded RNA and activation of NF-kappaB by Toll-like receptor 3. Nature 2001;413:732–8.

81. Edwards MR, Slater L, Johnston SL. Signalling pathways mediating type I interferon gene expression. Microbes Infect 2007;9:1245–51.

82. Gern JE, French DA, Grindle KA, et al. Double-stranded RNA induces the synthesis of specific chemokines by bronchial epithelial cells. Am J Respir Cell Mol Biol 2003;28:731–7.

83. Wark PA, Bucchieri F, Johnston SL, et al. IFN-gamma-induced protein 10 is a novel biomarker of rhinovirus-induced asthma exacerbations. J Allergy Clin Immunol 2007;120:586–93.

84. Lee CG, Yoon HJ, Zhu Z, et al. Respiratory syncytial virus stimulation of vascular endothelial cell growth Factor/Vascular permeability factor. Am J Respir Cell Mol Biol 2000;23:662–9.

85. Leigh R, Oyelusi W, Wiehler S, et al. Human rhinovirus infection enhances airway epithelial cell production of growth factors involved in airway remodeling. J Allergy Clin Immunol 2008;121:1238–45 e4.

86. Sanders SP. Asthma, viruses, and nitric oxide. Proc Soc Exp Biol Med 1999;220:123–32.

87. Dosanjh A, Rednam S, Martin M. Respiratory syncytial virus augments production of fibroblast growth factor basic in vitro: implications for a possible mechanism of prolonged wheezing after infection. Pediatr Allergy Immunol 2003;14:437–40.

88. Gern JE, Vrtis R, Kelly EA, et al. Rhinovirus produces nonspecific activation of lymphocytes through a monocyte-dependent mechanism. J Immunol 1996;157:1605–12.

89. Johnston SL, Papi A, Monick MM, et al. Rhinoviruses induce interleukin-8 mRNA and protein production in human monocytes. J Infect Dis 1997;175:323–9.

90. Panuska JR, Merolla R, Rebert NA, et al. Respiratory syncytial virus induces interleukin-10 by human alveolar macrophages. Suppression of early cytokine production and implications for incomplete immunity. J Clin Invest 1995;96:2445–53.

91. Brimnes MK, Bonifaz L, Steinman RM, et al. Influenza virus-induced dendritic cell maturation is associated with the induction of strong T cell immunity to a coadministered, normally nonimmunogenic protein. J Exp Med 2003;198:133–44.

92. Wang H, Peters N, Schwarze J. Plasmacytoid dendritic cells limit viral replication, pulmonary inflammation, and airway hyperresponsiveness in respiratory syncytial virus infection. J Immunol 2006;177:6263–70.

93. Cardell LO, Agusti C, Takeyama K, et al. LTB(4)-induced nasal gland serous cell secretion mediated by neutrophil elastase. Am J Respir Crit Care Med 1999;160:411–4.

94. Grunberg K, Timmers MC, Smits HH, et al. Effect of experimental rhinovirus 16 colds on airway hyperresponsiveness to histamine and interleukin-8 in nasal lavage in asthmatic subjects in vivo. Clin Exp Allergy 1997;27:36–45.

95. Gern JE, Martin MS, Anklam KA, et al. Relationships among specific viral pathogens, virus-induced interleukin-8, and respiratory symptoms in infancy. Pediatr Allergy Immunol 2002;13:386–93.

96. Denlinger LC, Shi L, Guadarrama A, et al. Attenuated P2X7 pore function as a risk factor for virus-induced loss of asthma control. Am J Respir Crit Care Med 2009;179:265–70.

97. Malcolm E, Arruda E, Hayden FG, et al. Clinical features of patients with acute respiratory illness and rhinovirus in their bronchoalveolar lavages. J Clin Virol 2001;21:9–16.

98. Message SD, Johnston SL. The immunology of virus infection in asthma. Eur Respir J 2001;18:1013–25.

99. Renzi PM, Turgeon JP, Marcotte JE, et al. Reduced interferon-gamma production in infants with bronchiolitis and asthma. Am J Respir Crit Care Med 1999;159(5 Pt 1):1417–22.

100. Papadopoulos NG, Stanciu LA, Papi A, et al. A defective type 1 response to rhinovirus in atopic asthma. Thorax 2002;57:328–32.

101. Contoli M, Message SD, Laza-Stanca V, et al. Role of deficient type III interferon-lambda production in asthma exacerbations. Nat Med 2006;12:1023–6.

102. Wark PA, Johnston SL, Bucchieri F, et al. Asthmatic bronchial epithelial cells have a deficient innate immune response to infection with rhinovirus. J Exp Med 2005;201:937–47.

103. Bardin PG, Fraenkel DJ, Sanderson G, et al. Amplified rhinovirus colds in atopic subjects. Clin Exp Allergy 1994;24:457–64.

104. Sigurs N, Bjarnason R, Sigurbergsson F, et al. Asthma and immunoglobulin E antibodies after respiratory syncytial virus bronchiolitis: a prospective cohort study with matched controls. Pediatrics 1995;95:500–5.

105. Frick OL. Effect of respiratory and other virus infections on IgE immunoregulation. J Allergy Clin Immunol 1986;78(5 Pt 2):1013–8.

106. Lemanske RF Jr, Dick EC, Swenson CA, et al. Rhinovirus upper respiratory infection increases airway hyperreactivity and late asthmatic reactions. J Clin Invest 1989;83:1–10.

107. Calhoun WJ, Dick EC, Schwartz LB, et al. A common cold virus, rhinovirus 16, potentiates airway inflammation after segmental antigen bronchoprovocation in allergic subjects. J Clin Invest 1994;94:2200–8.

108. Sly PD, Boner AL, Bjorksten B, et al. Early identification of atopy in the prediction of persistent asthma in children. Lancet 2008;372:1100–6.

109. Laing I, Reidel F, Yap PL, et al. Atopy predisposing to acute bronchiolitis during an epidemic of respiratory syncytial virus. Br Med J (Clin Res Ed) 1982;284:1070–2.

110. Rooney JC, Williams HE. The relationship between proved viral bronchiolitis and subsequent wheezing. J Pediatr 1971;79:744–7.

111. Zweiman B, Schoenwetter WF, Pappano JE Jr, et al. Patterns of allergic respiratory disease in children with a past history of bronchiolitis. J Allergy Clin Immunol 1971;48:283–9.

112. Pullan CR, Hey EN. Wheezing, asthma, and pulmonary dysfunction 10 years after infection with respiratory syncytial virus in infancy. Br Med J (Clin Res Ed) 1982;284:1665–9.

113. Murray M, Webb MS, O'Callaghan C, et al. Respiratory status and allergy after bronchiolitis. Arch Dis Child 1992;67:482–7.

114. Noma T, Mori A, Yoshizawa I. Induction of allergen-specific IL-2 responsiveness of lymphocytes after respiratory syncytial virus infection and prediction of onset of recurrent wheezing and bronchial asthma. J Allergy Clin Immunol 1996;98:816–26.

115. Gern JE, Calhoun W, Swenson C, et al. Rhinovirus infection preferentially increases lower airway responsiveness in allergic subjects. Am J Respir Crit Care Med 1997;155:1872–6.

116. Avila PC, Abisheganaden JA, Wong H, et al. Effects of allergic inflammation of the nasal mucosa on the severity of rhinovirus 16 cold. J Allergy Clin Immunol 2000;105:923–32.

117. de Kluijver J, Evertse CE, Sont JK, et al. Are rhinovirus-induced airway responses in asthma aggravated by chronic allergen exposure? Am J Respir Crit Care Med 2003;168:1174–80.

118. Sakamoto M, Ida S, Takishima T. Effect of influenza virus infection on allergic sensitization to aerosolized ovalbumin in mice. J Immunol 1984;132:2614–7.

119. Papadopoulos NG, Xepapadaki P, Mallia P, et al. Mechanisms of virus-induced asthma exacerbations: state-of-the-art: a GA2LEN and InterAirways document. Allergy 2007;62:457–70.

120. Cheung D, Dick EC, Timmers MC, et al. Rhinovirus inhalation causes long-lasting excessive airway narrowing in response to methacholine in asthmatic subjects in vivo. Am J Respir Crit Care Med 1995;152(5 Pt 1):1490–6.

121. Jacoby DB. Virus-induced asthma attacks. JAMA 2002;287:755–61.

122. Jacoby DB, Tamaoki J, Borson DB, et al. Influenza infection causes airway hyperresponsiveness by decreasing enkephalinase. J Appl Physiol 1988;64:2653–8.

123. Sanders SP, Siekierski ES, Richards SM, et al. Rhinovirus infection induces expression of type 2 nitric oxide synthase in human respiratory epithelial cells in vitro and in vivo. J Allergy Clin Immunol 2001;107:235–43.

124. Fryer AD, Jacoby DB. Parainfluenza virus infection damages inhibitory M2 muscarinic receptors on pulmonary parasympathetic nerves in the guinea-pig. Br J Pharmacol 1991;102:267–71.

125. Bowerfind WM, Fryer AD, Jacoby DB. Double-stranded RNA causes airway hyperreactivity and neuronal M2 muscarinic receptor dysfunction. J Appl Physiol 2002;92:1417–22.

126. Kellner JD, Ohlsson A, Gadomski AM, et al. Bronchodilators for bronchiolitis. Cochrane Database Syst Rev 2000(2):CD001266.

127. Diagnosis and management of bronchiolitis. Pediatrics 2006;118:1774–93.

128. Patel H, Platt R, Lozano JM, et al. Glucocorticoids for acute viral bronchiolitis in infants and young children. Cochrane Database Syst Rev 2004(3):CD004878.

129. de Blic J. [Use of corticoids in acute bronchiolitis in infants]. Arch Pediatr 2001;8(Suppl 1):49S–54S.

130. Chao LC, Lin YZ, Wu WF, et al. Efficacy of nebulized budesonide in hospitalized infants and children younger than 24 months with bronchiolitis. Acta Paediatr Taiwan 2003;44:332–5.

131. Reijonen T, Korppi M, Kuikka L, et al. Antiinflammatory therapy reduces wheezing after bronchiolitis. Arch Pediatr Adolesc Med 1996;150:512–7.

132. Guilbert TW, Morgan WJ, Zeiger RS, et al. Long-term inhaled corticosteroids in preschool children at high risk for asthma. N Engl J Med 2006;354:1985–97.

133. Teper AM, Kofman CD, Szulman GA, et al. Fluticasone improves pulmonary function in children under 2 years old with risk factors for asthma. Am J Respir Crit Care Med 2005;171:587–90.

134. Lehtinen P, Ruohola A, Vanto T, et al. Prednisolone reduces recurrent wheezing after a first wheezing episode associated with rhinovirus infection or eczema. J Allergy Clin Immunol 2007;119:570–5.

135. Rowe BH, Spooner CH, Ducharme FM, et al. Corticosteroids for preventing relapse following acute exacerbations of asthma. Cochrane Database Syst Rev 2007(3):CD000195.

136. Expert Panel Report 3 (EPR-3): Guidelines for the Diagnosis and Management of Asthma-Summary Report 2007. J Allergy Clin Immunol 2007;120(5 Suppl):S94–138.

137. Brunette MG, Lands L, Thibodeau LP. Childhood asthma: prevention of attacks with short-term corticosteroid treatment of upper respiratory tract infection. Pediatrics 1988;81:624–9.

138. Tal A, Levy N, Bearman JE. Methylprednisolone therapy for acute asthma in infants and toddlers: a controlled clinical trial. Pediatrics 1990;86:350–6.

139. Panickar J, Lakhanpaul M, Lambert PC, et al. Oral prednisolone for preschool children with acute virus-induced wheezing. N Engl J Med 2009;360:329–38.

140. Dolan LM, Kesarwala HH, Holroyde JC, et al. Short-term, high-dose, systemic steroids in children with asthma: the effect on the hypothalamic-pituitary-adrenal axis. J Allergy Clin Immunol 1987;80:81–7.

141. Wilson NM, Silverman M. Treatment of acute, episodic asthma in preschool children using intermittent high dose inhaled steroids at home. Arch Dis Child 1990;65:407–10.

142. Daugbjerg P, Brenoe E, Forchhammer H, et al. A comparison between nebulized terbutaline, nebulized corticosteroid and systemic corticosteroid for acute wheezing in children up to 18 months of age. Acta Paediatr 1993;82:547–51.

143. Connett G, Lenney W. Prevention of viral induced asthma attacks using inhaled budesonide. Arch Dis Child 1993;68:85–7.

144. Svedmyr J, Nyberg E, Asbrink-Nilsson E, et al. Intermittent treatment with inhaled steroids for deterioration of asthma due to upper respiratory tract infections. Acta Paediatr 1995;84:884–8.

145. Volovitz B, Bentur L, Finkelstein Y, et al. Effectiveness and safety of inhaled corticosteroids in controlling acute asthma attacks in children who were treated in the emergency department: a controlled comparative study with oral prednisolone. J Allergy Clin Immunol 1998;102(4 Pt 1):605–9.

146. Schuh S, Reisman J, Alshehri M, et al. A comparison of inhaled fluticasone and oral prednisone for children with severe acute asthma. N Engl J Med 2000;343:689–94.

147. Ducharme FM, Lemire C, Noya FJ, et al. Preemptive use of high-dose fluticasone for virus-induced wheezing in young children. N Engl J Med 2009;360:339–53.

148. Volovitz B, Welliver RC, De Castro G, et al. The release of leukotrienes in the respiratory tract during infection with respiratory syncytial virus: role in obstructive airway disease. Pediatr Res 1988;24:504–7.

149. van Schaik SM, Tristram DA, Nagpal IS, et al. Increased production of IFN-gamma and cysteinyl leukotrienes in virus-induced wheezing. J Allergy Clin Immunol 1999;103:630–6.

150. Krawiec ME, Westcott JY, Chu HW, et al. Persistent wheezing in very young children is associated with lower respiratory inflammation. Am J Respir Crit Care Med 2001;163:1338–43.

151. Behera AK, Kumar M, Matsuse H, et al. Respiratory syncytial virus induces the expression of 5-lipoxygenase and endothelin-1 in bronchial epithelial cells. Biochem Biophys Res Commun 1998;251:704–9.

152. Wedde-Beer K, Hu C, Rodriguez MM, et al. Leukotrienes mediate neurogenic inflammation in lungs of young rats infected with respiratory syncytial virus. Am J Physiol Lung Cell Mol Physiol 2002;282:L1143–50.

153. Bisgaard H. A randomized trial of montelukast in respiratory syncytial virus postbronchiolitis. Am J Respir Crit Care Med 2003;167:379–83.

154. Bisgaard H, Zielen S, Garcia-Garcia ML, et al. Montelukast reduces asthma exacerbations in 2- to 5-year-old children with intermittent asthma. Am J Respir Crit Care Med 2005;171:315–22.

155. Szefler SJ, Baker JW, Uryniak T, et al. Comparative study of budesonide inhalation suspension and montelukast in young children with mild persistent asthma. J Allergy Clin Immunol 2007;120:1043–50.

156. Bacharier LB, Phillips BR, Zeiger RS, et al. Episodic use of an inhaled corticosteroid or leukotriene receptor antagonist in preschool children with moderate-to-severe intermittent wheezing. J Allergy Clin Immunol 2008;122:1127–35 e8.

157. Wenzel SE, Gibbs RL, Lehr MV, et al. Respiratory outcomes in high-risk children 7 to 10 years after prophylaxis with respiratory syncytial virus immune globulin. Am J Med 2002;112:627–33.

158. Simoes EA, Groothuis JR, Carbonell-Estrany X, et al. Palivizumab prophylaxis, respiratory syncytial virus, and subsequent recurrent wheezing. J Pediatr 2007;151:34–42, e1.

159. Rotbart HA. Treatment of picornavirus infections. Antiviral Res 2002;53:83–98.

160. Turner RB, Dutko FJ, Goldstein NH, et al. Efficacy of oral WIN 54954 for prophylaxis of experimental rhinovirus infection. Antimicrob Agents Chemother 1993;37:297–300.

161. Turner RB, Wecker MT, Pohl G, et al. Efficacy of tremacamra, a soluble intercellular adhesion molecule 1, for experimental rhinovirus infection: a randomized clinical trial. JAMA 1999;281:1797–804.

162. Guilbert TW, Morgan WJ, Zeiger RS, et al. Atopic characteristics of children with recurrent wheezing at high risk for the development of childhood asthma. J Allergy Clin Immunol 2004;114:1282–7.

163. Castro-Rodriguez JA, Holberg CJ, Wright AL, et al. A clinical index to define risk of asthma in young children with recurrent wheezing. Am J Respir Crit Care Med 2000;162(4 Pt 1):1403–6.

Special Considerations for Infants and Young Children

Ronina A. Covar • Joseph D. Spahn

Recent advances in the etiology, mechanisms, and management of asthma have led to a better understanding of this disease and may in part be responsible for the stabilization of the steady increase in asthma morbidity and mortality noted since the 1980s.[1] Nonetheless, the burden of asthma in very young children is still enormous. Epidemiologic studies suggest that the cumulative prevalence of asthma is as high as 22% by the age of 4 years.[2,3] Some studies have hinted that pulmonary development in infancy can be adversely affected by asthma, resulting in a decrease in lung function of approximately 20% by adulthood.[4] Another important reason why asthma in infants and younger children deserves special consideration is the fact that rates of ambulatory, emergency department visits, and inpatient hospital discharges for children under the age of 4 years are greater than those of other age groups.[1] In addition, younger children with asthma are also more likely to be readmitted to the hospital for acute exacerbations.[5] Lastly, in a retrospective analysis of 49 asthmatic children whose mean age was 5.2 years (range 2 months to 16 years) admitted to a community-based pediatric intensive care unit over a 10-year period, as many as 75% were 6 years or younger.[6] The public health consequences of dealing with asthma in children include the number of missed work days parents/guardians incur in order to care for an acutely ill child.

Relevant clinical practice guidelines developed in recent years have addressed special challenges in the management of asthma in this age group.[7,8] Many issues are unique to this age group such as the presence of confounding factors or disease masqueraders, who and when to treat with controller therapy, what medications to use, how best to deliver the medications, and how to monitor the response to treatment (Box 36-1).

Confounding Factors

The first practical consideration in approaching the wheezing child is to assure that an alternative diagnosis is not present. In addition, infants and small children have a greater degree of bronchial hyperresponsiveness (BHR), which may predispose them to wheeze.[9]

The differential diagnosis of wheezing in infants and young children includes conditions such as foreign body aspiration, congenital airway anomalies, abnormalities of the great vessels, congenital heart disease, cystic fibrosis, recurrent aspiration, immunodeficiency, infections, ciliary dyskinesia, and mediastinal masses. Other clinical features, such as a neonatal onset of symptoms, associated failure to thrive, diarrhea or vomiting, and even focal lung or cardiovascular findings, suggest an alternative

diagnosis and require special investigations. Additional factors that should be taken into consideration include triggers for the respiratory symptoms and aggravating conditions such as nighttime occurrences, environmental exposure, physical exertion, feeding, positioning, and infections. Clearly, making the correct diagnosis is essential because the treatment for these conditions can vary substantially. For example, in children with significant gastroesophageal reflux, improvement in asthma symptoms with concomitant reduction in asthma medication use occurred after a prokinetic agent was instituted.[10] A practical approach that can be considered for a young child in whom asthma is strongly suspected is an empiric trial of asthma controller therapy while other evaluations are still being pursued (Figure 36-1).

Diagnostic and Monitoring Tools to Evaluate Asthma in Young Children

Preschool children present some diagnostic challenges inherent to their young age which means that a confirmation of a diagnosis can be difficult to make. Infants and young children are too young to reliably perform objective measures of disease activity. Furthermore, they are unable to provide their own history so clinicians have to depend on the parents/caregivers' reports. Werk and colleagues[11] sought to determine the factors that primary care pediatricians believe are important in establishing an initial diagnosis of asthma. Questionnaires on asthma diagnosis consisting of 20 factors obtained from the National Heart, Lung, and Blood Institute (NHLBI) National Asthma Education Prevention Program (NAEPP) Expert Panel Report 2 (EPR2) guidelines[12] and an expert local panel of subspecialists were sent to 862 active members of the Massachusetts American Academy of Pediatrics.[11] Over 80% of the respondents rated 5 factors as necessary or important in establishing the diagnosis of asthma: recurrent wheezing, symptomatic improvement following bronchodilator use, presence of recurrent cough, exclusion of other diagnoses, and suggestive peak expiratory flow rate findings. Of note, 27% of the respondents indicated that a child had to be older than 2 years; 18% indicated that fever must be absent during an exacerbation.

The diagnosis of asthma in young children is based largely on clinical judgment and an assessment of symptoms and physical findings. Because lung function measurements in infants and small children are difficult to perform, a trial of treatment is often a practical way to make a diagnosis of asthma in young children.

©2010 Elsevier Ltd, Inc, BV
DOI: 10.1016/B978-1-4377-0271-2.00036-5

Challenging Issues Pertinent to the Management of Recurrent Wheezing

- Focus on the care of infants and small children with suspected asthma deserves special considerations because of the potential to modulate the disease process early on and alleviate the increased morbidity associated with uncontrolled asthma in this age group.

- The clinical presentation of asthma in this age group is often similar to those of other conditions seen in early childhood.

- After confounders and masqueraders of asthma have been excluded in the evaluation of children with suspected asthma, recurrent wheezing in infants and young children still comprises a heterogeneous group of conditions with different risk factors and prognoses.

- The diagnosis of asthma in infants and small children is often based on clinical grounds and fraught with lack of clinically available tools that meet the criteria for the definition of asthma used in older children and adults, such as airway inflammation, bronchial hyperresponsiveness, and airflow limitation.

- The difficulties in the management of asthma include limited effective and convenient delivery devices, complete dependence on the care-givers to carry out the treatment regimen, and inadequate selection of medications completely devoid of adverse effects.

Monitoring Disease Activity and Response

Monitoring disease activity and response to therapy can also be difficult to objectively assess. Recently, a 5-item caregiver-administered instrument, the Test for Respiratory and Asthma Control in Kids (TRACK), was the first of its kind to have been validated as a tool to assess asthma control in young children with recurrent wheezing or respiratory symptoms consistent with asthma.[13] This questionnaire includes an assessment of both impairment and risk reflected in the NAEPP EPR3 asthma management guidelines.[7] The items include four impairment questions (three on symptom burden and activity limitations over a 4-week period and one question on rescue medication use over a 3-month period) and one risk question on oral corticosteroid use over a 12-month period. Each item has 5 descriptive ordinal responses which can be scored over a 5-point scale (0, 5, 10, 15, and 20; total score range 0–100). The screening ability of the entire scale showed areas under the receiver operating characteristic (ROC) curve of 0.88 and 0.82, respectively, in the development and validation samples; with a diagnostic accuracy of 81% and 78%, respectively. Based on the highest area under the ROC curve, a score of less than 80 provided the best cut-off point between sensitivity and specificity for uncontrolled asthma for this group.

At present, for adults and older children, easily performed lung function measures and noninvasive markers of airway inflammation can be used to make the diagnosis of asthma, monitor asthma control, or guide therapeutic decisions. The following section will highlight 'cutting-edge' techniques with the potential to measure lung function and airway inflammation in the young child.

Forced Oscillometry

Forced oscillometry is a pulmonary function technique that measures respiratory system resistance (Rrs) and reactance (Xrs) at several frequencies. It involves the application of sine waves through a loudspeaker to the airway opening via a mouthpiece, through which the subject breathes normally for short periods of time. Measurements are carried out during tidal breathing over a 30-second interval with at least 3 efforts recorded. Given its relative ease of use, it is a reproducible and suitable measure of lung function in younger children.[14] Marotta and colleagues performed pre- and post-bronchodilator spirometry and forced oscillometry in young children at risk for asthma and found no difference in baseline FEV_1 or resistance between children with asthma versus those without, the degree of bronchodilator response differentiated the two groups.[15] Some investigators believe that reactance at low frequencies is a reflection of peripheral airways function.[16]

Using three different lung function measures, Nielsen and Bisgaard evaluated the bronchodilator response of 92 children 2 to 5 years old, 55 of whom had asthma.[17] Children with asthma had diminished lung function compared to nonasthmatic children using any of the following measures: specific airway resistance (sRaw) utilizing whole body plethysmography or respiratory resistance utilizing either an interrupter technique (Rint) or impulse oscillation technique at 5 Hz (Rrs5). Both asthmatic and nonasthmatic children responded to terbutaline, although children with asthma reversed greater than the nonasthmatic children. The investigators found that sRaw utilizing body plethysmography best distinguished asthmatics from nonasthmatics based on bronchodilator response. They concluded that assessment of bronchodilator responsiveness using sRaw may help define asthma in young children.

Measurement of Bronchial Reactivity

As with measurements of airflow limitation, procedures to assess BHR in infants and young children have distinctive challenges. Measurement of BHR using cold air (4 minutes of isocapneic hyperventilation) or dry air (6 minutes of eucapneic hyperventilation) challenge with sRaw as an outcome may be useful, practical alternatives to auscultatory pharmacologic or exercise bronchoprovocation challenges which are more difficult to standardize in young children.[18] Using a dry air challenge, magnitude of response was associated with a wheeze phenotype. Persistent wheezers had a larger increase in sRaw following eucapneic hyperventilation challenge compared with never wheezers, but no significant differences between never wheezers, late-onset or transient wheezers were seen.[19]

Measures of Inflammation

Exhaled nitric oxide (eNO) levels are elevated in patients with asthma[20] and correlate positively with eosinophilic airway inflammation.[21] In addition, they rise during acute exacerbations[22] and fall following oral or inhaled corticosteroid therapy.[23,24]

Online[25] and offline[26] eNO measurements can be reliably obtained in very young children. Higher mean (±SEM) eNO concentrations (14.1 ± 1.8 ppb) were found in infants and young children (aged 7 to 33 months) presenting with an acute wheeze and a history of at least three prior wheezing episodes compared to first-time viral wheezers (aged 9 to 14 months) (8.3 ± 1.3 ppb, $P < 0.05$) and healthy matched controls (5.6 ± 0.5 ppb, $P < 0.001$). No differences in eNO measurements were seen between the two latter groups. In addition, eNO levels were reduced by 52% after steroid therapy to a level comparable to those of the healthy controls and first-time wheezers.[26]

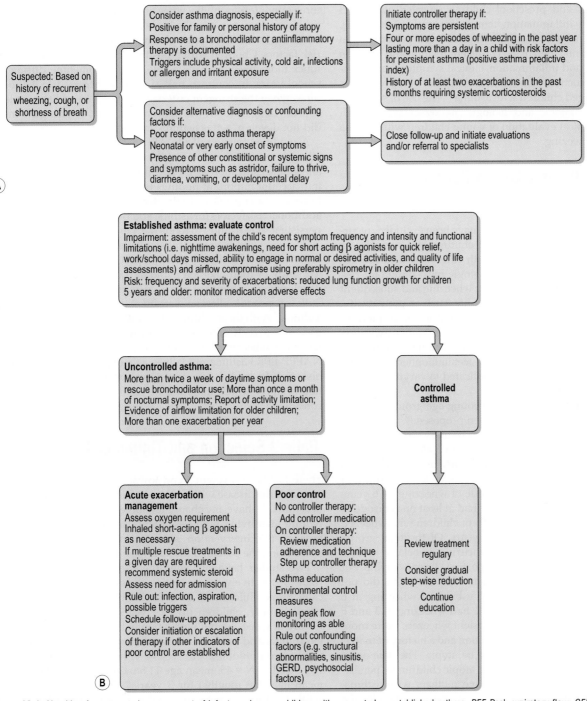

Figure 36-1 Algorithm for suggested management of infants and young children with suspected or established asthma. *PEF,* Peak expiratory flow; *GERD,* gastroesophageal reflux disease.

Unlike sophisticated measures of lung function and BHR, eNO can be easily and quickly measured. Its major disadvantage comes from the initial cost associated with buying the equipment.

In one of the few studies designed to specifically address the role of eosinophil cationic protein (ECP) in young children with recurrent wheezing, Carlsen and colleagues[27] found a strong correlation between serum ECP and response to albuterol (salbutamol) using the tidal flow volume loop technique in children 0 to 2 years of age. These investigators suggested that ECP may be measuring airway inflammation and may have some prognostic value in diagnosing asthma in infants and toddlers with recurrent wheezing. The major drawback for ECP is its lack of sensitivity and blood sample collection.

Although direct investigation of the airway using bronchoscopy and biopsy is the gold standard for establishing airway inflammation, it has limited clinical applicability, except when other pulmonary abnormalities are being considered. Understanding the underlying pathophysiology of the disease in children is critical in order to identify processes which can be impacted by interventions. Thickening of the bronchial epithelial reticular basement membrane (RBM) and eosinophilic airway inflammation are characteristic pathologic features of asthma found in children as young as 3 years old, but typically occurring between the ages of 6 to 16 years old.[28] It is unclear when airway thickening begins since routine biopsy studies are not performed in infants.[29] Studies on bronchoalveolar lavages obtained from wheezing infants and preschool children revealed an overall increase in airway inflammation, though it is rarely eosinophilic. In one study in which bronchial biopsies were performed on symptomatic infants, there is no consistent relationship between RBM thickening and inflammation, clinical symptoms and variable airflow obstruction;[30] similar to findings from biopsy studies in older school-aged children with asthma.[31] The use of sensitive, noninvasive physiologic and biologic markers is very much limited in the clinical evaluation of young children with asthma and recurrent wheezing.

Predicting Who Is Likely to Develop Persistent Asthma

After confounders and masqueraders have been excluded, recurrent wheezing in infants and young children still comprises a heterogeneous group of conditions with different risk factors and prognoses. Atopy appears to be the single most important risk factor in the development of persistent wheezing and subsequent asthma. Factors or exposures early in life, such as prematurity, fetal nutrition, duration of pregnancy, viral lower respiratory tract infections in the first years of life, cigarette smoke exposure, air pollution, postnatal nutrition, breast-feeding, family size, maternal age, socioeconomic status, acetaminophen exposure, and allergen exposure have been implicated to varying degrees. This is summarized in Chapter 2.

Several types of 'wheezers' in the young age group based on time of onset and persistence have been proposed.[19,32] The investigators from the Tucson Children's Respiratory Group enrolled over 1000 newborns served by a large health maintenance organization to evaluate factors involved in early-onset wheezing in relation to persistent wheezing at 6 years of life.[32] About half of the children had at least one episode of wheezing by 6 years of age. Nearly one third of the cohort had at least one episode of wheezing by 3 years of age. Only 40% of children who wheezed early had persistent wheezing at 6 years. Of the total group, 20% had at least one episode of wheezing associated with a respiratory tract infection during the first 3 years of life but had no wheezing at 6 years ('transient wheezers'), 14% did not wheeze during the first 3 years of life but had wheezing at 6 years ('late-onset wheezers'), and 15% had wheezing at 3 and 6 years ('persistent wheezer'). The 'transient wheezers' were more likely to have diminished airway function and a history of maternal smoking and were less likely to be atopic. The 'late-onset wheezers' had a similar percentage of atopic children to 'persistent wheezers' and were likely to have mothers with asthma. Hence, there seems to be a similar genetic predisposition for the asthma phenotype characterizing both 'persistent' and 'late-onset wheezers'. Essentially all of the current natural history studies have found that allergic disease or evidence of pro-allergic immune development are significant risk factors for persistent asthma.

An asthma predictive index (API) using a combination of clinical and easily obtainable laboratory data to help identify children aged ≤3 years with a history of wheezing at risk of developing persistent asthma was developed from the Tucson cohort.[33] Information on parental asthma diagnosis and prenatal maternal smoking status was obtained at enrollment, while the child's history of asthma and wheezing and physician-diagnosed allergic rhinitis or eczema, along with measurements of blood eosinophil count, were obtained at the follow-up visits. Two indices were used to classify the children. The stringent index required recurrent wheezing in the first 3 years plus one major (parental history of asthma or physician-diagnosed eczema) or two of three minor (eosinophilia, wheezing without colds, allergic rhinitis) risk factors, whereas the loose index required any episode of wheezing in the first 3 years plus one major or two of three minor risk factors. Children with a positive loose index were 2.6 to 5.5 times more likely to have active asthma sometime during the school years. In contrast, risk of asthma increased to 4.3 to 9.8 times when the stringent criteria were used. In addition, at least 90% of young children with a negative 'loose' or 'stringent' index did not develop 'active asthma' in the school-age years.

A modified version of the API (mAPI) incorporates inhalant allergen sensitization as an additional major risk factor, and food allergen sensitization as an additional minor risk factor to take into account important findings from other longitudinal natural history asthma studies.[34] In the Berlin Multicentre Allergy Study, additional risk factors for asthma and BHR at age 7 years included persistent sensitization to foods (i.e. hen's egg, cow's milk, wheat and/or soy) and perennial inhalant allergens (i.e. dust mite, cat), especially in early life.[35,36] In a prospective, randomized, controlled study of food allergen avoidance in infancy evaluating the development of atopy at age 7 years in a high-risk cohort, egg, milk or peanut allergen sensitization were risk factors for asthma.[37] With these additional considerations, a mAPI has been used in an early intervention study for young children with recurrent wheezing.[38] Henceforth, it has been adapted by the NAEPP EPR3 asthma guidelines as a requirement along with a history of four wheezing episodes per year lasting more than 24 hours, upon which initiation of controller therapy should be considered.[7]

Patient Selection and Timing of Treatment

There has been a recent trend toward intervening early in the course of the disease with the hope of altering the natural history of asthma. To have any chance for success, early intervention will require identifying high-risk infants and establishing effectiveness of the intervention strategy in young children while minimizing the potential for adverse effects.

Two studies have evaluated the effects of ketotifen and cetirizine, respectively, in preventing the onset of asthma in genetically prone children.[39,40] In a double-blind, placebo-controlled, parallel study, children up to 2 years of age without a prior history of wheezing but with a family history of asthma or allergic rhinitis and presence of elevated serum immunoglobulin E (IgE) were randomized to receive either ketotifen (0.5 to 1 mg twice daily) ($N = 45$, mean age 11.5 months) or placebo ($N = 40$, mean age 10.8 months) for 3 years.[39] Only 9% of children on active treatment compared to 35% of the placebo group developed frequent episodes of wheezing during the study period ($P = 0.003$). The other study, called the Early Treatment of the Atopic Child, was a randomized, double-blind, parallel group trial that compared cetirizine (0.25 mg/kg twice daily) and placebo.[40] The medications were administered for 18 months to infants between 1 and 2 years of age with atopic dermatitis and a family history of atopy. The primary outcome, which was the time to onset of asthma in the next 18 months after discontinuation of treatment, was not different between the two groups. Half of the children in both the cetirizine and placebo groups developed asthma (defined as three episodes of wheezing during the 36 months of follow-up) ($P = 0.7$). However, in the cetirizine group, infants with evidence of dust mite or grass pollen sensitivity were less likely to have asthma over the 18 months of treatment with a sustained effect for grass-sensitized infants over the 36 months of follow-up compared with those treated with placebo. Furthermore, in the placebo group there was an increased risk of developing asthma in those with baseline sensitivity to egg, house dust mite, grass pollen, or cat allergen. These two studies support the role of easily administered secondary preventive measures in delaying or even preventing the development of asthma in genetically predisposed children.

There have been recent studies that sought to determine if treatment with an inhaled corticosteroid (ICS) soon after the onset of early indicators of the disease would modify the course of asthma.[38,41-43] The study designs varied with respect to the eligibility criteria, age at entry, frequency of past wheezing episodes, and manner and duration of treatment (e.g. maintenance vs intermittent or as needed intervention).

The NHLBI Childhood Asthma Research and Education (CARE) network-sponsored 'Prevention of Early Asthma in Kids (PEAK)' study enrolled approximately 300 children aged 2 to 3 years with more than 3 episodes of wheezing and a positive mAPI to receive either fluticasone propionate 88 µg via pressurized metered dose inhaler (pMDI) or matching placebo twice daily for 2 years.[38] During the third year observation period of interest, no difference in either the proportion of children with active wheezing or measurement of lung function using forced oscillometry between the two treatment groups was found. However, during the first 2 years while on treatment, symptom control and asthma exacerbations were better for the active treatment group compared to the placebo group. A reduction in growth velocity during the first 8 months (6.6 ± 1.0 vs 7.3 ± 1.0 cm/year between 1 to 8 months, p = 0.005) and a smaller mean increase in height between 4 to 12 months (4.5 ± 1.1 vs 4.9 ± 1.1 cm, p = 0.001) were observed in the ICS group. However, during the second year of treatment, the growth velocity in the ICS group was greater than that in the placebo group (7.0 ± 0.8 vs 6.4 ± 0.9 cm/year, p = 0.001). Children in the ICS group had an average height percentile of 51.5 ± 29.2 compared to 56.4 ± 27.3 in the placebo group at the end of treatment (p < 0.001) and 54.4 ± 27.9 compared to 56.4 ± 26.9 at the end of observation (p = 0.03). The PEAK extension observational study will provide data on long-term effects on growth of ICS use.

Another study (Inhaled Fluticasone propionate in Wheezy INfants [IFWIN]) evaluated if ICS therapy for infants with a history wheezing could prevent active asthma and prevent loss of lung function in later childhood.[41] A total of 200 children (mean age at entry 1.2 years) from a birth study cohort with two documented episodes of wheeze or one prolonged episode of more than 1 month duration, and a parental history of atopy, were randomized to receive fluticasone propionate 100 µg or matching placebo twice daily. At the age of 5 years, no difference between the ICS and placebo groups in the proportion of children with current wheeze, physician-diagnosed asthma, and use of supplemental open-label ICS (fluticasone 100 µg twice daily) was found. Furthermore, the number of exacerbations, lung function (using sRaw through plethysmography with dynamic lung volumes and expiratory flow), and BHR (using eucapnic voluntary hyperventilation) were also not different between the groups. Children who were on ICS, particularly after 6 to 12 months, had transient reduction in growth velocity, and those who received both masked and open-label ICS had a slower rate of growth compared to either the 'masked treatment only' or 'open-label treatment only' groups.

While these two studies demonstrate that long-term treatment with ICS does not modify the course of asthma, they also raise the potential for systemic effects of this intervention which can limit its use for this purpose. Using ICS only for an acute illness and evaluating its long-term impact is attractive, not only because it is less imposing, but also because it may decrease the risk of growth retardation.

One study, the Prevention of Asthma in Childhood (PAC), sought to determine if early intervention using intermittent administration of an ICS, when initiated at the first episode of wheezing and during subsequent episodes, could alter the development of asthma.[42] Of 411 infants born to mothers with asthma enrolled at 1 month of age, approximately 300 children received at least one 14-day course of budesonide 400 µg/day or matching placebo administered via pMDI and holding chamber (mean age at the first course of study medication was 10.7 months). For every acute illness, children were to start treatment after 3 days of wheezing. Upon completion of this 3-year study, a similar percentage of symptom-free days between treatment groups (83% vs 82% for the budesonide and placebo groups, respectively) was found. In addition, 24% and 21% of children in the budesonide and placebo groups, respectively, had persistent wheezing. The mean duration of each acute wheezing episode was not reduced by budesonide therapy. Lung function using pre-and post-bronchodilator sRaw at age 3 years was comparable between the two treatment groups. Lastly, there was also no difference in height between the groups. Thus, intermittent ICS did not alter the natural history of asthma in infants at risk for asthma nor did it change the duration of the acute wheezing episodes.

The NHLBI CARE network recently completed the Acute Intervention Management Strategies (AIMS) study.[43] The study randomized 238 children aged 12 to 59 months who had at least two episodes of moderate-to-severe wheezing requiring either an urgent care visit and/or systemic steroid course in the context of a respiratory tract illness within the past year. Participants were randomized to receive one of the following for 7 days at the onset of symptoms: budesonide inhalation suspension (1.0 mg twice daily) or montelukast group (4 mg once daily) or conventional rescue bronchodilator therapy. The primary outcome was the proportion of episode-free days (i.e. days free from cough, wheeze, trouble breathing, asthma associated interference with daily activities or awakening from sleep, healthcare utilization due to wheezing, and use of asthma-related nonstudy medications) over the entire study period. Compared to conventional rescue bronchodilator therapy, neither budesonide nor montelukast initiated at early signs of illness increased the proportion of episode-free days over a 1-year period. In addition, no differential effect on oral corticosteroid rescue, asthma healthcare utilization, or quality of life was found. Nevertheless, both active study treatments demonstrated modest reductions in symptom severity score (such as wheezing, trouble breathing, or activity limitation) relative to conventional therapy, particularly among children with positive API or prior oral corticosteroid use.

These studies provide important information regarding ICS therapy in young children with recurrent wheezing episodes although the overall results regarding prevention of progression to persistent asthma are not convincing. ICS can be indicated to improve asthma control but should not be expected to prevent the development of asthma or persistent wheezing, even for high-risk subjects.

Management

Controller Therapy for Small Children with Persistent Asthma

The new versions of the NHLBI NAEPP EPR3[7] and the GINA[8] asthma guidelines acknowledge the special challenges unique to the management of asthma in preschool children; hence a

Table 36-1 Classifying Asthma Severity and Initiating Treatment in Children Aged 0 to 4 Years: Assessing Severity and Initiating Treatment for Patients Who Are Not Currently Taking Long-Term Control Medications

Components of Severity		Classification of Asthma Severity (0–4 yr)			
		Intermittent	**Persistent**		
			Mild	Moderate	Severe
Impairment	Symptoms	≤2 d/wk	>2 d/wk but not daily	Daily	Throughout the day
	Nighttime awakenings	0	1–2/mo	3–4/mo	>1/wk
	SABA use for symptoms (not EIB pretreatment)	≤2 d/wk	>2 d/wk but not daily	Daily	Several times per day
	Interference with normal activity	None	Minor limitation	Some limitation	Extremely limited
Risk	Exacerbations requiring systemic corticosteroids	0–1/yr	≥2 exacerbations in 6 mo requiring systemic corticosteroids, or ≥4 wheezing episodes/1yr lasting >1 d *and* risk factors for persistent asthma Consider severity and interval since last exacerbation Frequency and severity may fluctuate over time Exacerbations of any severity may occur in patients in any severity category		
Recommended step for initiating therapy		Step 1	Step 2	Step 3 and consider short course of oral systemic corticosteroids	
		In 2–6 weeks, depending on severity, evaluate level of asthma control that is achieved. If no clear benefit is observed within 4–6 weeks, consider adjusting therapy or alternative diagnoses			

Notes:
- The step-wise approach is meant to assist, not replace, the clinical decision-making required to meet individual patient needs.
- Level of severity is determined by both impairment and risk. Assess impairment domain by patient's/care-giver's recall of previous 2 to 4 weeks. Symptom assessment for longer periods should reflect a global assessment, such as inquiring whether a patient's asthma is better or worse since the last visit. Assign severity to the most severe category in which any feature occurs.
- At present, there are inadequate data to correspond frequencies of exacerbations with different levels of asthma severity. For treatment purposes, patients who had ≥2 exacerbations requiring oral systemic corticosteroids in the past 6 months, or ≥4 wheezing episodes in the past year, and who have risk factors for persistent asthma, may be considered the same as patients who have persistent asthma, even in the absence of impairment levels consistent with persistent asthma.

EIB, exercise-induced bronchospasm; SABA, short-acting β₂ agonist use

Adapted, with permission, from the National Asthma Education and Prevention Program: Expert Panel Report 3 (EPR 3). J Allergy Clin Immunol 2007; 120(Suppl):S94–138. Available at: http://www.nhlbi.nih.gov/guidelines/asthma/asthgdln.htm.

specific approach and treatment recommendations for preschool children with asthma are presented.[7,8] Both sets of guidelines now emphasize maintenance of asthma control as the goal for asthma management and use of ICS as the preferred therapy for persistent asthma. A comprehensive management is outlined in several components and/or sections and generally includes establishment of patient/doctor partnership and provision of education to enhance the patient's/family's knowledge and skills for self-management, identification and management of risk and precipitating factors and co-morbid conditions that may worsen asthma, adequate assessment and monitoring of disease activity, appropriate selection of medications to address the patient's needs, and management of asthma exacerbations.[7] The details of each of these elements are discussed in Chapter 33 of this book.

Key differences between the two clinical guidelines are apparent. The approach implemented by the NHLBI NAEPP EPR3 on starting controller therapy is based on the concept of asthma severity which is the intrinsic intensity of disease, and applicable for patients not receiving controller therapy. Please refer to Chapter 33. The guidelines have a separate set of criteria for various age groups and Table 36-1 summarizes the classification of asthma severity for children 0 to 4 years old. The classification of asthma severity is contingent upon the domains of impairment and risk and the level of severity is based on the most severe impairment or risk component. Impairment includes an assessment of the child's recent symptom frequency (daytime and nighttime), need for short-acting β₂ agonists for quick relief, and ability to engage in normal or desired activities. Risk refers to an

evaluation of the child's likelihood of developing asthma exacerbations. Of note, in the absence of frequent symptoms, 'persistent' asthma should be considered and therefore long-term controller therapy initiated for infants or children who have: 1) risk factors for asthma (i.e. using the mAPI: any of parental history of asthma, physician-diagnosed atopic dermatitis, or sensitization to aeroallergens OR two of the following: wheezing apart from colds, sensitization to foods, or peripheral eosinophilia) *AND* four or more episodes of wheezing over the past year that lasted longer than 1 day and affected sleep; 2) two or more exacerbations within 6 months requiring systemic corticosteroids.

On the other hand, in the GINA guidelines, upon establishing a diagnosis of asthma in young children which proposes the use of the original API, initiation of ICS is warranted for asthma that is 'not controlled' and the most important determinant of dosing is the clinician's judgment of the patient's response to therapy. Medication dose adjustment is appropriate based on levels of asthma control, although dose-response relationships are not well studied. Detailed recommendations using a step-wise approach for children 5 years and younger are not presented, unlike a step-wise approach utilized for older children, due to its acknowledgement of limited literature on treatment of asthma in the younger children.

The criteria for 'controlled', 'partly controlled', and 'uncontrolled' asthma according to the GINA guidelines are summarized in Table 36-2 and in contrast to the NAEPP EPR3, there is no separate distinction between different age groups. 'Controlled' asthma is characterized by daytime symptoms or rescue/reliever treatment less than 3 times a week and no nocturnal

Table 36-2 Assessing Asthma Control and Adjusting Therapy in Children Aged 0–4 Years

Components of Control		Classification of Asthma Control (0–4 yr)					
		Well controlled[a]	Controlled (all of the following)[b]	Not well controlled[a]	Partly controlled (any measure present in any week)[b]	Very poorly controlled[a]	Uncontrolled[b]
Impairment[a]	Daytime symptoms[ab]	≤2 d/wk	None (twice or less/week)	>2 d/wk	More than twice per week	Throughout the day	Three or more features of partly controlled asthma present in any week
	Nighttime awakenings[ab]	≤1/mo	None	>1/mo	Any	>1/wk	
	SABA use for symptoms (not EIB pretreatment)[ab]	≤2 d/wk	None (twice or less/week)	>2 d/wk	More than twice per week	Several times per day	
	Interference[a] or limitations[b] with normal activity	None	None	Some limitation	Any	Extremely limited	
Risk[a]	Exacerbations[ab] requiring oral systemic corticosteroids	0–1/yr	None	2–3/yr	One or more per year*	>3/yr	One in any week[†]
	Treatment-related adverse effects[a]	Medication side-effects can vary in intensity from none to very troublesome and worrisome. The level of intensity does not correlate to specific levels of control but should be considered in the overall assessment of risk					
Recommended action for treatment per NAEPP guidelines[a]		Maintain current treatment. Regular follow up every 1–6 months. Consider step down if well controlled for at least 3 months		Step up (1 step) and reevaluate in 2–6 weeks. If no clear benefit in 4–6 weeks, consider alternative diagnoses or adjusting therapy. For side-effects, consider alternative treatment options		Consider short course of oral systemic corticosteroids. Step up (1–2 steps), and Reevaluate in 2 weeks. If no clear benefit in 4–6 weeks, consider alternative diagnoses or adjusting therapy. For side-effects, consider alternative treatment options	

* Any exacerbation should prompt review of maintenance treatment to ensure that it is adequate.

[†] By definition, an exacerbation in any week makes that an uncontrolled asthma week.

Adapted from the [a]National Asthma Education and Prevention Program: Expert Panel Report 3 (EPR 3). Available at: http://www.nhlbi.nih.gov/guidelines/asthma/asthgdln.htm; and the [b]Global strategy for asthma management and prevention 2006. Available at: http://www.ginasthma.org.

Notes:
- The step-wise approach is meant to assist, not replace, the clinical decision-making required to meet individual patient needs.
- The level of control is based on the most severe impairment or risk category. Assess impairment domain by care-giver's recall of previous 2 to 4 weeks. Symptom assessment for longer periods should reflect a global assessment such as inquiring whether the patient's asthma is better or worse since the last visit.
- At present, there are inadequate data to correspond frequencies of exacerbations with different levels of asthma control. In general, more frequent and intense exacerbations (e.g. requiring urgent, unscheduled care, hospitalization, or ICU admission) indicate poorer disease control. For treatment purposes, patients who had ≥ 2 exacerbations requiring oral systemic corticosteroids in the past year may be considered the same as patients who have not-well-controlled asthma, even in the absence of impairment levels consistent with not-well-controlled asthma.

Before step-up therapy:
- Review adherence to medications, inhaler technique, and environmental control.
- If alternative treatment option was used in a step, discontinue it and use preferred treatment for that step.

symptoms/awakenings, limitations of activities, or exacerbations, and normal lung function (if reliable in 5-year-old children or older). 'Partly controlled' asthma has any of the following: daytime symptoms or rescue use more than twice a week, any nocturnal symptoms/awakenings or limitations of activities, an FEV$_1$ or peak flow rate less than 80% predicted or personal best (for older children), and one or more exacerbation per year. Lastly, 'uncontrolled' asthma is defined as presence of three or more features characteristic of 'partly controlled' asthma present in any week or exacerbation occurring once in any week.

In the NAEPP EPR3 guidelines for preschool children already on a controller medication, management is tailored based on the child's level of control. As with the classification of asthma severity, assessment of asthma control is based on both impairment and risk (Table 36-2). The three levels of asthma control are: 'well controlled', 'not well controlled', and 'very poorly controlled' asthma. Children whose asthma is not well controlled have daytime symptoms or need for rescue albuterol >2 days/week, nighttime symptoms more than once a month but not more than once a week, 'some limitation' with normal activity, had 2 to 3 exacerbations in the past year, and an FEV$_1$ of 60–80% of predicted (or FEV$_1$/FVC ratio 75–80%) for children 5 years of age or older. Children with very poorly controlled asthma have: symptoms 'throughout the day', nocturnal symptoms more than once

Table 36-3 Step-Wise Approach for Managing Asthma in Children Aged 0–4 Years

Intermittent asthma	Persistent asthma: daily medication* Consult with asthma specialist if step 3 or higher is required Consider consultation at step 2					
Step 1 *Preferred* SABA prn	**Step 2** *Preferred* Low-dose ICS *Alternative* Cromolyn or montelukast	**Step 3** *Preferred* Medium-dose ICS	**Step 4** *Preferred* Medium-dose ICS + either LABA or montelukast	**Step 5** *Preferred* High-dose ICS + either LABA or montelukast	**Step 6** *Preferred* High-dose ICS + either LABA or montelukast Oral systemic corticosteroids	**Step up if needed** (first check adherence, inhaler technique, and environmental control) **Assess Control** Step down if possible (and asthma is well controlled at least 3 mo)
Patient education and environmental control at each step						
Quick-relief medication for all patients: • SABA as needed for symptoms. Intensity of treatment depends on severity of symptoms • With viral respiratory infection: SABA q 4–6 hr up to 24 hr (longer with physician consult). Consider short course of systemic corticosteroids if exacerbation is severe or patient has history of previous severe exacerbations • Caution: frequent use of SABA may indicate the need to step up treatment						

*Alphabetical order is used when more than one treatment option is listed within either preferred or alternative therapy.

ICS, inhaled corticosteroid; *LABA*, inhaled long-acting β₂ agonist; *prn*, as needed; *SABA*, inhaled short-acting β₂ agonist
Adapted, with permission, from the National Asthma Education and Prevention Program: Expert Panel Report 3 (EPR 3). J Allergy Clin Immunol 2007; 120(Suppl):S94–138. Available at: http://www.nhlbi.nih.gov/guidelines/asthma/asthgdln.htm.

Notes:
• The step-wise approach is meant to assist, not replace, the clinical decision-making required to meet individual patient needs.
• If alternative treatment is used and the response is inadequate, discontinue it and use the preferred treatment before stepping up.
• If clear benefit is not observed within 4 to 6 weeks and patient/family medication technique and adherence are satisfactory, consider adjusting the therapy or alternative diagnosis.
• Studies on children aged 0 to 4 years are limited. Step 2 therapy is based on Evidence A. All other recommendations are based on expert opinion and extrapolation from studies in older children. The step-wise approach is meant to assist, not replace, the clinical decision-making required to meet individual patient needs.

weekly, need for rescue albuterol several times per day, 'extreme limitations' with normal activity, had ≥3 exacerbations in the past year, and for children aged at least 5 years, an FEV₁ of <60% of predicted or FEV₁/FVC ratio <75%. Using a validated questionnaire to monitor quality of life for older children is recommended and perhaps the TRACK questionnaire[13] discussed in an earlier section may now be applied for younger children.

Unlike the GINA guidelines, the NAEPP EPR3 provides an expanded step-wise treatment approach (Table 36-3) even for young children. The choice of initial therapy is based on assessment of asthma severity, and for patients who are already on controller therapy, modification of treatment is based on assessment of asthma control and responsiveness to therapy. A major objective of this approach is to identify and treat all 'persistent' and uncontrolled asthma with antiinflammatory controller medication. Management of intermittent asthma is short-acting inhaled β agonist *as needed* for symptoms and for pretreatment for those with exercise-induced bronchospasm (step 1). The type(s) and amount(s) of daily controller medications to be used are determined by the asthma severity and control rating. Even for young children, the preferred treatment for 'persistent asthma' is daily ICS therapy, with or without an additional medication. Alternative medications for step 2 include a leukotriene receptor antagonist (montelukast) or a nonsteroidal antiinflammatory agent (cromolyn). For young

children (≤4 years of age) with moderate and severe persistent asthma, medium dose ICS monotherapy is recommended and combination therapy of medium dose ICS plus either LABA or montelukast is to be initiated only as a step 4 treatment for uncontrolled asthma. Children with severe persistent asthma (treatment steps 5 and 6) should receive high-dose ICS and a long-acting β agonist or montelukast, and an oral corticosteroid, if required. A rescue course of systemic corticosteroids may be necessary at any step.

The 'step-up, step-down' approach initially introduced in the earlier versions of the NAEPP guidelines and slightly modified in the current iteration[7] is discussed in further detail in Chapter 33. The NAEPP guidelines emphasize initiating higher-level controller therapy at the outset to establish prompt control, with measures to 'step down' therapy once good asthma control is achieved. Initially, airflow limitation and the pathology of asthma may limit the delivery and efficacy of ICS such that stepping up to higher doses and/or combination therapy may be needed to gain asthma control. Asthma therapy can be stepped down after good asthma control has been achieved and ICS has had time to achieve optimal efficacy, by determining the least number or dose of daily controller medications that can maintain good control, thereby reducing the potential for medication adverse effects. If step-up therapy is being considered at any point, it is important to check delivery device technique and adherence, implement environmental control measures, and identify and treat co-morbid conditions.

Inhaled Corticosteroids

ICS are the preferred controller therapy for persistent asthma or asthma that is not controlled. Although there are 6 available ICS available, nebulized budesonide is the only US FDA-approved ICS for children less than 4 years of age. The initial studies with nebulized budesonide in young children with moderate to severe persistent asthma found nebulized budesonide to be superior to placebo in improving symptoms, decreasing exacerbations, reducing chronic oral prednisone use, or improving overall asthma control.[44,45]

Studies have also evaluated the efficacy and safety of nebulized budesonide in children with mild to moderate persistent asthma. The initial studies included older children and evaluated multiple budesonide dosages administered once or twice daily given over a 3-month period.[46-48] The efficacy of nebulized budesonide over placebo was consistently demonstrated with improvement in symptoms scores, reduction in rescue medication use, and improvement in morning peak expiratory flow rates in patients who could adequately perform the procedure. Improvement in symptom scores occurred as early as 2 weeks after starting budesonide.[48] Twice-daily dosing of 0.5 mg appeared to be somewhat more effective than 1 mg administered once daily. The investigators suggested that a dose of 0.25 mg/day may be sufficient for mild asthma, whereas subjects with moderate asthma should be treated with 0.5 to 1 mg/day and those with severe asthma dependent on oral steroids should be treated with 1 to 2 mg/day. No significant differences in basal cortisol levels or ACTH-stimulated cortisol levels were found between any of the active treatment groups and placebo.

Pharmacokinetics of Nebulized Budesonide in Small Children

Little is known regarding the amount of drug delivered, by any inhaled device and with any drug, to infants and young children with asthma. ICS have the potential for adverse effects, so it is important to deliver the smallest amount of drug required for response. Agertoft and colleagues evaluated the systemic availability and pharmacokinetics of nebulized budesonide in a group of preschool children (mean age 4.7 years) with chronic asthma.[49] Ten children underwent pharmacokinetic studies of both intravenously administered (125 μg) and inhaled budesonide (1 mg delivered by nebulization). The amount of nebulized budesonide delivered to the patient was calculated by subtracting the amount of drug remaining in the nebulizer, the amount emitted into the ambient air, and the amount found in the mouth after rinsing from the initial amount of budesonide in the nebulizer (the nominal dose). The mean dose to the subject was found to be 23% of the nominal dose (231 μg), while the systemic availability was only 6.1% of the nominal dose, or 61 μg. The clearance of budesonide was calculated to be 0.54 L/min with a $t_{1/2}$ of 2.3 hours, and V_{dss} of 55 L. The systemic availability in these small children was approximately half that seen in adults. In addition, the clearance of budesonide in these children was twice that of adults.

Efficacy of ICS Administered Via MDI with Holding Chamber and Mask

The GINA guidelines prefer the administration of ICS via a pressurized metered-dose inhaler (pMDI) with a spacer and facemask in small children with asthma. Bisgaard and colleagues

sought to determine whether fluticasone delivered via a pMDI with holding chamber and facemask was superior to placebo in improving asthma symptoms in young children with frequent asthma symptoms.[50] Children (N = 237; mean age = 28 months) were enrolled to receive fluticasone (100 μg/day or 200 μg/day) or placebo for 12 weeks. Fluticasone resulted in a dose-related improvement in asthma symptoms with fluticasone 200 μg/day more effective than placebo in 8 out of 10 diary card parameters (including wheezing, cough, and breathlessness), whereas fluticasone 100 μg/day resulted in significant improvements in 5 parameters. In addition, fewer children on fluticasone experienced asthma exacerbations and required a prednisolone burst. Fluticasone delivered via a holding chamber and mask has been shown to be effective for small children as a result of its high potency and its long retention time within the lung. Therefore, fluticasone can be utilized, and if a response is not seen, therapy should be discontinued. In those who respond, the dose should be titrated to the lowest effective dose.

What type of patient will respond favorably to ICS is an important question that has yet to be answered. A study by Roorda and colleagues using data from two large placebo-controlled studies evaluated the clinical features of preschool children likely to respond to fluticasone administered via a pMDI with holding chamber and facemask.[51] The investigators identified two clinical features that predicted a positive response to ICS therapy: frequent symptoms ($\geq$3 days/week) and a family history of asthma. The presence of eczema and the number of previous acute exacerbations were not associated with response to fluticasone. Eczema predisposes a child with recurrent wheezing to subsequent asthma,[33] but it does not appear to predict response to ICS therapy. It should be noted that a lack of response over a short course of treatment (12 weeks) does not necessarily mean that a response would not be seen over a much longer period of time (months to years).

The clinical efficacy and safety of intermittent ICS or systemic corticosteroid for young children with associated upper respiratory infection or viral-induced wheeze remain controversial. A recent study which evaluated 'as needed' high-dose fluticasone propionate (750 μg twice daily) given at the onset of an upper respiratory tract illness found lower rescue oral corticosteroid use in those on active treatment compared to placebo (8% vs 18%, respectively); although this was accompanied by a statistically significant difference in height and weight gain.[52] In another recent study, oral prednisolone was found not to be superior to placebo with respect to duration of hospitalization, clinician and parent symptom severity assessment, and hospital readmission for preschool children presenting to a hospital with viral-induced mild to moderate wheezing.[53]

ICS and Growth in Small Children

Few published studies have evaluated the effects of ICS on the linear growth of preschool children. Reid and colleagues in an open-label study, measured linear growth velocity in 40 children (mean age 1.4 years) before and during treatment with nebulized budesonide.[54] All of the children had 'troublesome' asthma despite treatment with an ICS administered with a pMDI with spacer and facemask or nebulized cromolyn before entry into the study. They were then administered 1 to 4 mg/day of nebulized budesonide depending on their level of asthma severity. The median intervals of time for linear growth determinations during the run-in period and nebulized budesonide treatments were 6 months and 1 year, respectively. The height standard deviation scores (SDSs) for the group during the run-in period were −0.21, at baseline −0.46, and after at least 6 months of nebulized budesonide −0.17. Note that an SDS of less than 0 denotes impaired growth velocity. Thus the subjects were growing at less than an impaired rate before nebulized budesonide therapy, and the institution of nebulized budesonide did not result in further growth suppression. In fact, there was a trend toward improved growth velocity while on nebulized budesonide.

Skoner and colleagues[55] evaluated the growth of children enrolled in 52-week open-label extension studies of the three efficacy studies of budesonide.[46-48] The dose of budesonide was either 0.5 mg once or twice daily with a taper to the lowest tolerated dose, and conventional asthma therapy consisted of any available therapy including ICS in two of the studies; in total, 670 children participated. The investigators found a modest impairment in growth in only one of the three extension studies. The extension study, where a decline in growth was noted, consisted primarily of young children with milder asthma who had not been on ICS before entry into the initial study. In contrast, the two extension studies that did not find growth impairment consisted of children with more severe disease and had allowed for ICS use as part of the conventional asthma therapy algorithm. The Skoner study suggests that modest growth suppression can occur in young children receiving nebulized budesonide who have not required ICS therapy in the past and that children with milder asthma may be at greater risk for growth suppression secondary to increased intrapulmonary deposition. Alternatively, the findings may be attributable to the fact that over twice as many children randomized to the conventional asthma therapy arm withdrew from the study because of poor asthma control.

The PEAK[38] and IFWIN[41] studies which used ICS via MDI with a holding chamber and mask mentioned in an earlier section have also provided important findings on the adverse effects of long-term ICS on growth in preschool children at risk for persistent asthma. It is still uncertain if there is a potential for catch-up or if the effects in very young children are cumulative. However, for young children with poor asthma control, the disease itself can negatively impact growth. The growth of 58 children (mean age 3.5 years for males, 4.4 years for females) with asthma was followed over a 5-year period.[56] Each child's asthma was classified as being in good, moderate, or poor control according to asthma symptoms during a 2-year observational period before the institution of ICS therapy. The group as a whole had diminished growth velocity to start the study, with a mean height velocity standard deviation (HVSD) score of −0.51. Children whose asthma was in good control had the least evidence for growth suppression before ICS therapy was instituted and continued to grow at the same rate as when on therapy (HVSD score −0.01 pre- vs −0.07 during treatment). In contrast, the subjects whose asthma was poorly controlled grew poorly before and after institution of ICS therapy (HVSD score −1.50 pretreatment vs −1.55 during treatment). Of interest, those with moderately controlled asthma demonstrated improved growth velocity while on ICS therapy, with their HVSD score increasing from −0.83 to −0.49. The investigators concluded that poor asthma control adversely impacts linear growth to a greater extent than ICS therapy.

Alternative and/or Adjunct Medications

The NHLBI NAEPP EPR3 guidelines[7] recommend cromolyn or montelukast as alternative therapy for younger children with mild persistent asthma and combination therapy using ICS plus either LABA or montelukast for younger children with moderate to severe persistent asthma (steps 4 and 5).

Cromolyn

Cromolyn (Intal) inhibits mediator release from mast cells. It inhibits both the early- and late-phase pulmonary components of the allergic response following inhalation of an allergen in sensitized subjects. A few studies have shown no added benefit with the use of cromolyn over placebo in young children with more severe disease.[57-59] Several efficacy studies that have found cromolyn to have beneficial effects were short-term trials and employed small numbers.[60-62] A meta-analysis of 22 control studies evaluating cromolyn in childhood asthma found it no better than placebo.[63] A multicenter, randomized, parallel-group, 52-week, open-label study in preschool children found nebulized cromolyn (20 mg four times daily) (N = 335) to be inferior to nebulized budesonide suspension (0.5 mg daily) (N = 168) using several outcome parameters.[64] Children who received inhaled budesonide suspension had a reduced rate of asthma exacerbations per year, longer time to first asthma exacerbation and first use of additional long-term controller therapy, nearly doubled improvements in nighttime and daytime symptom scores by the second week of treatment, and had lower use of rescue medications. Although there were no significant differences in the rates of hospitalization and emergency room visits between the two groups, significantly lower urgent-care or unscheduled physician visits and oral corticosteroid use were found in children who received the ICS. However, mean height increases from baseline in children randomized to inhaled budesonide and inhaled cromolyn were 6.69 and 7.55 cm, respectively. This difference of 0.86 cm is similar to the difference in height measurements seen in other studies with ICS therapy after 1 year of treatment in both younger and older children.[38,65,66]

Leukotriene Modifying Agents

Leukotrienes are potent proinflammatory mediators that induce bronchospasm, mucus secretion, and airway edema. In addition, they may be involved in eosinophil recruitment into the asthmatic airway.[67] Leukotriene modifiers (synthesis inhibitor or receptor antagonist) have beneficial effects in terms of reducing asthma symptoms and supplemental β agonist use while improving baseline pulmonary function.[68-70] The leukotriene receptor antagonists (LTRA) prevent the binding of LTD_4 to its receptor. This class has a pediatric indication and includes both montelukast (given once daily and has been approved for treatment of chronic asthma for children age 1 year and older) and zafirlukast (administered twice daily and is approved for children 7 years and older).

Safety and efficacy studies with the 4-mg chewable montelukast tablet in children aged 2 to 5 years with asthma have been published.[71-73] Almost 700 children, aged 2 to 5 years, were enrolled to receive montelukast or placebo for 12 weeks in a double-blind, multicenter, multinational study at 93 centers worldwide.[71] Montelukast was well tolerated and was not associated with any significant adverse effects. Montelukast was superior to placebo in reducing daytime symptoms including improvements in cough, wheeze, difficulty breathing, and activity level, and nighttime cough. In addition, montelukast therapy was associated with a reduction in rescue β agonist use and reduced need for prednisone for acute severe exacerbations.

Recent studies have been done to evaluate the long-term effects of an LTRA (continuous[72] and intermittent[73]), on the occurrence of exacerbations. In a 12-month, double-blind, parallel study which was designed to investigate the role of montelukast in the prevention of viral-induced asthma exacerbations in children aged 2 to 5 years with a history of intermittent asthma symptoms, subjects were randomized to receive daily oral montelukast 4 or 5 mg (by age) or placebo for 12 months.[72] During the trial, montelukast significantly reduced the rate of asthma exacerbations by 31.9% compared with placebo. Montelukast delayed the median time to first exacerbation by approximately 2 months and the rate ICS courses compared to placebo. In another study, 220 children aged 2 to 14 years were randomized to receive either intermittent montelukast or placebo at the onset of asthma or upper respiratory tract infection symptoms for a minimum of 7 days.[73] The montelukast group had 163 unscheduled healthcare resource utilizations for asthma compared with 228 in the placebo group (OR = 0.65, 95% CI:0.47–0.89). There was a nonsignificant reduction in specialist attendances and hospitalizations, duration of episode, and β agonist and prednisolone use. These studies suggest that intermittent or persistent therapy with montelukast for children with intermittent asthma symptoms is effective in reducing risk of exacerbations compared with placebo.

Long-Acting Inhaled β Agonists

Long-acting inhaled $β_2$ agonists (LABAs) are the alternative add-on therapy for children and adults with moderate and severe persistent asthma. They are not viewed as 'rescue' medications for acute episodes of bronchospasm, nor are they meant to replace inhaled antiinflammatory agents. Salmeterol has a prolonged onset of action with maximal bronchodilation approximately 1 hour following administration; formoterol has an onset of effect within minutes. Both medications have a prolonged duration of action of at least 12 hours. As such, they are especially well suited for patients with nocturnal asthma[74] and for individuals who require frequent use of short-acting β agonist inhalations during the day to prevent exercise-induced asthma.[75] There is an added advantage to the use of these alternative therapies for preschool children who may deserve an extended bronchodilatory coverage for exercise because they are constantly active. Salmeterol via the Diskus™ device is FDA-approved for children as young as 4 years of age (50 μg blister every 12 hours), whereas formoterol delivered via the Aerolizer™ is approved for use in children 6 years of age and older (12 μg capsule every 12 hours); both LABAs are also available as combination pMDI with an ICS (salmeterol and fluticasone [Advair HFA] and formoterol and budesonide [Symbicort HFA]). Although LABAs combined with ICS are recommended for young children in steps 4 to 6 of the NAEPP EPR3 guidelines (Table 36-3), they have limited application. The Diskus™ combination product is FDA-approved down to 4 years of age but its use requires adequate inspiratory effort to get an optimal delivery of the dry powder. While the pMDI can be used with a holding chamber, it is not currently approved for children younger than 12 years of age. The efficacy and safety of LABA or combination products in younger children with asthma are still uncertain due to lack of studies.

The US Food and Drug Administration (FDA) has requested the manufacturers of LABAs to update their product information warning sections regarding an increase in severe asthma episodes associated with these agents. This action is in response to data showing an increased number of asthma-related deaths in patients receiving LABA therapy in addition to their usual asthma care as compared with patients not receiving LABAs.

Treatment immediately prior to vigorous activity or exercise is usually effective. The combination of a SABA with either cromolyn or nedocromil is more effective than either drug alone. Montelukast may be effective for up to 24 hours. Salmeterol and formoterol may block exercise-induced bronchospasm for up to 12 hours. There is one study that has evaluated single-dose bronchoprotective effects of salmeterol given through a Babyhaler spacer device using a methacholine provocation challenge in infants less than 4 years old with recurrent episodes of wheezing.[76] Originally, 42 preschool children (age range 8 to 45 months) received one of the 25-, 50-, or 100-μg doses of salmeterol and a placebo dose 2 to 7 days apart in a double-blind, randomized fashion, but only 33 completed the study. The investigators found a dose-dependent bronchoprotective effect of salmeterol measured by treatment/placebo methacholine dose ratios. Significant improvements from placebo were found only for the 50- (2.5 fold) and 100- (4-fold) μg doses.

Issues Related to the Delivery of Medications to Infants and Small Children

There are unique challenges relating to the delivery of medications (both oral and inhaled) to infants and young children with asthma. Obviously, liquid preparations are tolerated by infants but chewable tablets/pills can already be consumed by toddlers. Montelukast is available as oral granules or chewable tablet and prednisone/prednisolone comes in either liquid formulations or orally disintegrating tablet preparations. With regard to inhaled medications, certain anatomic and physiologic characteristics of children younger than 6 years are worth considering. First, because infants display preferential nasal breathing and have small airways, low tidal volume, and high respiratory frequency, delivery of the drug to the lower airways is often inadequate.[77] Second, it is difficult if not impossible for young children to perform the maneuvers specified for optimal delivery of aerosol therapy such as slow inhalation through the mouth with a period of breath-holding for pMDIs or rapid and forceful inhalation required in the case of dry-powder inhalers (DPIs). Third, delivery devices appropriate for the young child are limited to those that require minimum cooperation from the child and must allow ease of administration for the caregivers. Although, at present, there are at least three inhaled aerosol delivery systems available for older children and adults, only two are used in this age group: the nebulizer and the pMDI with spacer/holding chamber and facemask. Because of the reliance on the subject's ability to generate a sufficient inspiratory flow and overcome the resistance required of DPIs, preschool-age children are unable to use them.

Within these two general types of delivery systems there are numerous products available that vary widely in performance. The pMDI with spacer or holding chamber is portable and inexpensive, takes less time to administer, and is likely to be better tolerated than delivery with a nebulizer. Dolovich and colleagues[78] published a comprehensive systematic review to determine if device selection affects clinical efficacy and safety. Randomized placebo-controlled trials that involved various devices for the delivery of β agonists, ICS and anticholinergic agents in different clinical settings (emergency department, in-patient, intensive care, and out-patient) and patient populations (pediatric and adult asthma, and COPD) were included. Reports in which the same drug delivered with different devices were analyzed. Their findings indicated that the drugs delivered via different formats are equally effective. Appropriate technique, cooperation, and convenience determine which delivery may be best.

Asthma clinical guidelines mention the use of inhaled short-acting β agonist either by pMDI or nebulizer treatment as an initial asthma exacerbation home intervention.[7,8] The Global Initiative for Asthma (GINA) guidelines[8] recommend the use of short-acting inhaled β agonist by pMDI (ideally with a spacer) for home management of mild, moderate, and severe exacerbations. The GINA guidelines also recommend nebulized treatments for severe exacerbations at home and for hospital-based management of acute asthma.

Data in young children clearly support the use of β agonists at higher doses administered via a pMDI with spacer for acute asthma.[79,80] In a study of 60 children between 1 and 5 years of age hospitalized for an asthma exacerbation, Parkin and colleagues found albuterol (400 to 600 μg, 4 to 6 puffs, based on weight) and ipratropium bromide (40 μg, 2 puffs), both delivered via pMDI with an Aerochamber and mask, to be as effective as nebulized albuterol (0.15 mg/kg) and ipratropium bromide (125 μg) administered over 15 minutes by facemask.[79] However, nearly one third of the subjects randomized to MDI eventually required a nebulized β agonist.

Two studies have evaluated lower respiratory tract deposition of radiolabeled albuterol administered to young children. Tal and colleagues showed that, on average, less than 2% of the nominal dose of the albuterol given by a pMDI with a spacer and mask to children less than 5 years old was deposited in the lower respiratory tract, with most of the drug remaining in the spacer.[81] Wildhaber and colleagues compared the lung deposition of radiolabeled albuterol from a nebulizer and a pMDI and spacer in 17 asthmatic children aged 2 to 9 years.[82] Both devices were delivering roughly 5% of the nominal dose to the lower airways. Because of the larger doses of albuterol administered via the nebulizer (2000 μg vs 400 μg) than the pMDI, a larger amount of drug was deposited in the airways using the nebulizer (108 μg vs 22 μg, respectively). In addition, both devices were approximately 50% less efficient in children less than 4 years old than the older children.

In general, β agonist administration by nebulization is still the delivery system of choice in the treatment of infants and young children with severe, acute asthma because it requires the simple technique of relaxed tidal breathing. In addition, oxygen can be used to power the nebulizer providing β agonist and supplemental oxygen simultaneously, and it does offer the capability to administer a controller agent and rescue β agonist at the same time.

With respect to controller therapy, the only available inhaled drugs that are FDA-approved for children under 4 years of age are drug solutions cromolyn and suspensions (budesonide) intended for nebulization. However, a pMDI with a spacer device, while not yet US FDA-approved for children younger than 4 years, is certainly more convenient and easier to administer.

There have been recent changes in drug formulation. The Montreal Protocol, adopted in 1987, mandated a complete elimination of the chlorofluorocarbon (CFC) propellant due to concerns about its damaging effect on the ozone layer. The US Food and Drug Administration had ruled that no CFC MDIs would be sold in the USA after 2008 so pMDIs now contain hydrofluoroalkane (HFA). However, the pMDI HFAs (even rescue short-acting β agonists) are approved for use only in children 4 years of age and older. There is no information available on the relationship between lung deposition from HFA pMDI and clinical efficacy in small children. In addition, no studies exist comparing inhaled medications administered via nebulizer and HFA pMDI with spacer and mask.

Additional factors which should be considered are the costs to the patient (including use of spacer attachments which are not reimbursable) and the use of multiple delivery devices which requires more time for the clinician staff to educate families on proper techniques. To address both issues, perhaps the same type of device can be used for all inhaled drugs for an individual patient. The decision should also incorporate which device the clinician is capable of teaching properly and what the patient/parent prefers. When a child presents with uncontrolled asthma, the assessment should first focus on technique and adherence.

Adherence

The issue of adherence in infants and small children is complicated because the child is entirely dependent on the care-giver to administer the medication. In an observational study of preschool children, Gibson and colleagues sought to evaluate adherence with inhaled prophylactic medications delivered through a large volume spacer using an electronic timer device. Adherence was only 50% with a range of 0% to 94%.[83] In addition, only 42% of the subjects received the prescribed medication on each study day, and reporting of symptoms in the diary cards did not correlate with good compliance with the prophylactic medication, nor was a correlation found between frequency of administration and adherence. In another study, parental reporting of symptom scores correlated with measured bronchodilator use in only 63% of preschool children.[84]

A few studies have attempted to determine why care-givers are unable to administer medications as prescribed. Lim and colleagues asked parents why they were reluctant to administer prophylactic medications (such as ICS) to their young children with asthma. Reasons cited included hesitancy to use medications for fear of dependence, side-effects, and overdosage.[85] Fortunately, patient education programs developed for parents of small children with asthma improve asthma morbidity and self-management outcome.[86,87]

Nonpharmacologic Intervention

Nonpharmacologic measures may be as important, not only for young children with established respiratory symptoms, allergies, and passive smoke exposure, but also in the primary and secondary prevention of asthma.[88-90] The first and probably the most important step toward controlling asthma in sensitized children is to avoid or reduce the patient's exposure to the offending allergen. The environmental interventions that seem to hold the most promise are those that target reducing exposure to indoor allergens and tobacco smoke. Specific environmental control measures are covered in Chapter 26.

Lastly, yearly influenza immunization is also strongly recommended for children 6 months of age and older with chronic pulmonary diseases, including asthma. Kramarz and colleagues evaluated the effectiveness of influenza vaccination in preventing influenza-related asthma exacerbations in children 1 to 6 years of age using a retrospective cohort study with the Vaccine Safety Datalink, which contains data on more than 1 million children enrolled in four large health maintenance organizations.[91] Of note, less than 10% of children with asthma were vaccinated against influenza in any of the years studied. Although the incidence rates of asthma exacerbation in those who were vaccinated were found to be higher in the vaccinated group than in those who were not vaccinated, the difference was thought to be largely confounded by asthma severity in the vaccinated group. Using a 'self-control' analysis to correct for this con-founder, the risks of asthma exacerbation during each of the influenza seasons were reduced by 22% to 41% with influenza vaccination.

Conclusions

There still exists a tremendous gap in our knowledge regarding the pathogenesis and management of asthma in older children and adults compared to the information available on this disease in infants and younger children. The findings of large population-based studies that included preschool children with recurrent wheezing demonstrate that they constitute a heterogeneous group. The diagnosis and management of infants and small children with asthma remain problematic, and numerous areas need to be explored. Currently, no clinically available objective measure of lung function, BHR, or airway inflammation exists that is applicable to this age group. The need to evaluate objectively the efficiency and safety of the various delivery devices and HFA formulation available for inhaled therapies to infants and young children persists. Again, this may be partly the result of the difficulty in evaluating lung deposition because it may require radiolabeled material or invasive techniques for pharmacokinetic analysis. Only a few medications have been approved for use in this population, and studies have demonstrated effects on asthma control using short-term parameters. Limited studies exist to investigate long-term effects specifically in reducing significant exacerbations and preventing the development of asthma in high-risk population, but still no data are available evaluating modulation of underlying inflammatory reaction and airway remodeling and prevention of deterioration in lung function over time, and induction of remission once disease is present. Yet, these are the ultimate goals which may motivate patients and families, if indeed interventions can really alter the natural history of their disease. These studies often require large sample size and monitoring over longer periods of time which require enormous resources, and use of practical, objective measures of disease activity which are still lacking.

Helpful Websites

The National Heart, Lung, and Blood Institute (http://www.nhlbi.nih.gov/guidelines/asthma/asthgdln.htm)

References

1. Akinbami LJ, Moorman JE, Garbe PL, et al. Status of childhood asthma in the United States, 1980-2007. Pediatrics 2009;123:S131-45.
2. Croner S, Kjellman N-I. Natural history of bronchial asthma in childhood. Allergy 1992;47:150-7.
3. Tariq SM, Matthews SM, Hakim EA, et al. The prevalence of and risk factors for atopy in early childhood: a whole population birth cohort study. J Allergy Clin Immunol 1998;101:587-93.
4. Martin AJ, Landau LI, Phelan PD. Lung function in young adults who had asthma in childhood. Am Rev Respir Dis 1980;122:609-16.
5. Mitchell EA, Bland JM, Thompson JMD. Risk factors for readmission to hospital for asthma in childhood. Thorax 1994;49:33-6.
6. Paret G, Kornecki A, Szeinberg A, et al. Severe acute asthma in a community hospital pediatric intensive care unit: a ten years' experience. Ann Allergy Asthma Immunol 1998;80:339-44.
7. National Asthma Education and Prevention Program. Expert Panel Report 3 (EPR 3): Guidelines for the Diagnosis and Management of Asthma – Summary Report 2007. J Allergy Clin Immunol 2007;120(Suppl):S94-138.
8. National Heart, Lung and Blood Institute/World Health Organization Workshop. Global strategy for asthma management and prevention. Bethesda, Md: National Institutes of Health; 2006. (www.ginasthma.org)
9. Young S, Le Souef PN, Geelhoed GC, et al. The influence of a family history of asthma and parental smoking on airway responsiveness in early infancy. N Engl J Med 1991;324:1168-73.
10. Ibero M, Ridao M, Artigas R, et al. Cisapride treatment changes the evolution of infant asthma with gastroesophageal reflux. Invest Allergol Clin Immunol 1998;8:176-9.
11. Werk LN, Steinbach S, Adams WG, et al. Beliefs about diagnosing asthma in young children. Pediatrics 2000;105:585-90.
12. Expert Panel Report II. Guidelines for the diagnosis and management of asthma. Bethesda, Md: National Heart, Lung, and Blood Institute/National Institutes of Health; 1997.
13. Murphy KR, Zeiger RS, Kosinski M, et al. Test for respiratory and asthma control in kids (TRACK): a caregiver-completed questionnaire for preschool-aged children. J Allergy Clin Immunology 2009;123:833-39.
14. Hellinckx J, Boeck K, Bande-Knops J, et al. Bronchodilator response in 3-6.5 years old healthy and stable asthmatic children, Eur Respir J 1998;12:438-43.
15. Marotta A, Klinnert MD, Price MR, et al. Impulse oscillometry provides an effective measure of lung dysfunction in 4-year-old children at risk for persistent asthma. J Allergy Clin Immunol 2003;112:317-22.
16. Delacourt C, Lorino H, Fuhrman C, et al. Comparison of the forced oscillation technique and the interrupter technique for assessing airway obstruction and its reversibility in children. Am J Respir Crit Care Med 2001;164:965-72.
17. Nielsen KG, Bisgaard H. Discriminitive capacity of bronchodilator response measured with three different lung function techniques in asthmatic and healthy children aged 2 to 5 years. Am J Respir Crit Care Med 2001;164:554-9.
18. Nielsen KG, Bisgaard H. Hyperventilation with cold versus dry air in 2- to 5-year-old children with asthma. Am J Respir Crit Care Med 2005;171:238-41.
19. Lowe LA, Simpson A, Woodcock A, et al. Wheeze phenotypes and lung function in preschool children. Am J Respir Crit Care Med 2005;171:231-7.
20. Artlich A, Busch T, Lewandowski K, et al. Childhood asthma: exhaled nitric oxide in relation to clinical symptoms. Eur Respir J 1999;13:1396-401.
21. Piacentini GL, Bodini A, Costella S, et al. Exhaled nitric oxide and sputum eosinophil markers of inflammation in asthmatic children. Eur Respir J 1999;13:1386-90.
22. Baraldi E, Azzolin NM, Zanconato S, et al. Corticosteroids decrease exhaled nitric oxide in children with acute asthma. J Pediatr 1997;131:381-5.
23. Carra S, Gagliardi L, Zanconato S, et al. Budesonide but not nedocromil sodium reduces exhaled nitric oxide levels in asthmatic children. Respir Med 2001;95:734-9.
24. Mattes J, Storm van's Gravesande K, Reining U, et al. NO in exhaled air is correlated with markers of eosinophilic airway inflammation in corticosteroid-dependent childhood asthma. Eur Respir J 1999;13:1391-5.
25. Buchvald F, Bisgaard H. FeNO measured at fixed exhalation flow rate during controlled tidal breathing in children from the age of 2 yr. Am J Respir Crit Care Med 2001;163:699-704.
26. Baraldi E, Dario C, Ongaro R, et al. Exhaled nitric oxide concentrations during treatment of wheezing exacerbation in infants and young children. Am J Respir Crit Care Med 1999;159:1284-8.
27. Carlsen KCL, Halvorsen R, Ahlstedt S, et al. Eosinophil cationic protein and tidal flow volume loops in children 0-2 years of age. Eur Respir J 1995;8:1148-54.
28. Saglani S, Payne D, Zhu J, et al. Early detection of airway wall remodeling and eosinophilic inflammation in preschool wheezers. Am J Respir Crit Care Med 2007;176:858-64.
29. Saglani S, Malmstrom K, Pelkonen A, et al. Airflow remodeling and inflammation in symptomatic infants with reversible airflow obstruction. Am J Respir Crit Care Med 2005;171:722-7.
30. Le Bourgeois M, Goncalves M, Le Clainche L, et al. Bronchoalveolar cells in children <3 years old with severe recurrent wheezing. Chest 2002;122:791-7.
31. Jenkins H, Cool C, Szefler S, et al. Histopathology of severe childhood asthma: a case series. Chest 2003;124:32-41.
32. Martinez FD, Wright AL, Taussig LM, et al. Asthma and wheezing in the first six years of life. N Engl J Med 1995;332:133-8.
33. Castro-Rodriguez JA, Holberg CJ, Wright AL, et al. A clinical index to define asthma in young children with recurrent wheezing. Am J Respir Crit Care Med 2000;162:1403-6.
34. Guilbert TW, Morgan WJ, Zeiger RS, et al. Atopic characteristics of children with recurrent wheezing at high risk for the development of childhood asthma. J Allergy Clin Immunol 2004;114:1282-7.
35. Kulig M, Bergmann R, Tacke U, et al. Long-lasting sensitization to food during the first two years precedes allergic airway disease. The

MAS Study Group, Germany. Pediatr Allergy Immunol 1998;9(2): 61–7.

36. Lau S, Illi S, Sommerfeld C, et al. Early exposure to house-dust mite and cat allergens and development of childhood asthma: a cohort study. Multicentre Allergy Study Group. Lancet 2000;356(9239):1392–7.

37. Zeiger RS, Heller S. The development and prediction of atopy in high-risk children: follow-up at age seven years in a prospective randomized study of combined maternal and infant food allergen avoidance. J Allergy Clin Immunol 1995;95:1179–90.

38. Guilbert T, Morgan W, Zeiger R, et al. Long-term inhaled corticosteroids in preschool children at risk for asthma. N Engl J Med 2006;354: 1985–97.

39. Bustos GJ, Bustos D, Bustos GJ, et al. Prevention of asthma with ketotifen in preasthmatic children: a three-year follow-up study. Clin Exp Allergy 1995;25:568–73.

40. Warner JO, Early Treatment of the Atopic Child Group. A double-blinded, randomized, placebo-controlled trial of cetirizine in preventing the onset of asthma in children with atopic dermatitis: 18 months' treatment and 18 months' posttreatment follow up. J Allergy Clin Immunol 2001;108:929–37.

41. Murray C, Woodcock A, Langley S, et al. For the IFWIN Study Team. Secondary prevention of asthma by the use of inhaled fluticasone propionate in wheezy infants (IFWIN). Lancet 2006;368:754–62.

42. Bisgaard H, Hermansen M, Loland L, et al. Intermittent inhaled corticosteroids in infants with episodic wheezing. N Engl J Med 2006;354: 1998–2005.

43. Bacharier LB, Phillips BR, Zeiger RS, et al. Childhood Asthma Research and Education Network of the National Heart, Lung, and Blood Institute. Episodic use of an inhaled corticosteroid or leukotriene receptor antagonist in preschool children with moderate-to-severe intermittent wheezing. J Allergy Clin Immunol 2008;122:1127–35.

44. DeBlic J, Delacourt C, LeBourgeois M, et al. Efficacy of nebulized budesonide in treatment of severe infantile asthma: a double blind study. J Allergy Clin Immunol 1996;98:14–20.

45. Ilangovan P, Pedersen S, Godfrey S, et al. Treatment of severe steroid-dependent preschool asthma with nebulized budesonide suspension. Arch Dis Child 1993;68:356–9.

46. Shapiro G, Mendelson L, Kraemer MJ, et al. Efficacy and safety of budesonide inhalation suspension (Pulmicort Respules) in young children with inhaled steroid-dependent, persistent asthma. J Allergy Clin Immunol 1998;102:789–96.

47. Kemp JP, Skoner DP, Szefler SJ, et al. Once-daily budesonide inhalation suspension for the treatment of persistent asthma in infants and young children. Ann Allergy Asthma Immunol 1999;83:231–9.

48. Baker JW, Mellon M, Wald J, et al. A multiple-dosing, placebo-controlled study of budesonide inhalation suspension given once or twice daily for treatment of persistent asthma in young children and infants. Pediatrics 1999;103:414–21.

49. Agertoft L, Andersen A, Weibull E, et al. Systemic availability and pharmacokinetics of nebulized budesonide in preschool children. Arch Dis Child 1999;80:241–7.

50. Bisgaard H, Gillies J, Groenewald M, et al. The effect of inhaled fluticasone propionate in the treatment of young asthmatic children: a dose comparison study. Am J Respir Crit Care Med 1999;160:126–31.

51. Roorda RJ, Mezei G, Bisgaard H, et al. Response of preschool children with asthma symptoms to fluticasone propionate. J Allergy Clin Immunol 2001;108:540–6.

52. Ducharme FM, Lemire C, Noya FJ, et al. Preemptive use of high-dose fluticasone for virus-induced wheezing in young children. N Engl J Med. 2009;360:339–53.

53. Panickar J, Lakhanpaul M, Lambert PC, et al. Oral prednisolone for preschool children with acute virus-induced wheezing. N Engl J Med 2009;360(4):329–38.

54. Reid A, Murphy C, Steen HJ, et al. Linear growth of very young asthmatic children treated with high-dose nebulized budesonide. Acta Paediatr 1996;85:421–4.

55. Skoner DP, Szefler SJ, Welch M, et al. Longitudinal growth in infants and young children treated with budesonide inhalation suspension for persistent asthma. J Allergy Clin Immunol 2000;105:259–68.

56. Ninan TK, Russell G. Asthma, inhaled corticosteroid treatment, and growth. Arch Dis Child 1992;67:703–5.

57. Tasche MJ, Van Der Wouden JC, Uijen JH, et al. Randomized placebo-controlled trial of inhaled sodium cromoglycate in 1–4 year old children with moderate asthma. Lancet 1997;350:1060–4.

58. Bertelsen A, Andersen JB, Busch P, et al. Nebulized sodium cromoglycate in the treatment of wheezy bronchitis. Allergy 1986;41: 266–70.

59. Furfaro S, Spier S, Drblik SP, et al. Efficacy of cromoglycate in persistently wheezing infants. Arch Dis Child 1994;71:331–4.

60. Hiller EJ, Milner AD, Lenney W. Nebulized sodium cromoglycate in young asthmatic children: double-blind trial. Arch Dis Child 1977;52: 875–6.

61. Glass J, Archer LNJ, Adams W, et al. Nebulized cromoglycate, theophylline, and placebo in preschool asthmatic children. Arch Dis Child 1981;56:648–51.

62. Cogswell JJ, Simpkiss MJ. Nebulized sodium cromoglycate in recurrently wheezy preschool children. Arch Dis Child 1985;60:736–8.

63. Tasche MJ, Uijen JH, Bernsen RM, et al. Inhaled disodium cromoglycate (DSCG) as maintenance therapy in children with asthma: a systematic review. Thorax 2000;55:913–20.

64. Leflein JG, Szefler SJ, Murphy KR, et al. Nebulized budesonide inhalation suspension compared with cromolyn sodium nebulizer solution for asthma in young children: results of a randomized outcomes trial. Pediatrics 2002;109:866–72.

65. Simons FE. A comparison of beclomethasone, salmeterol, and placebo in children with asthma. Canadian Beclamethasone Dipropionate-Salmeterol Xinafoate Study Group. N Engl J Med 1997;337:1659–65.

66. Verberne AA, Frost C, Roorda RJ, et al. One year treatment with salmeterol compared with beclomethasone in children with asthma. The Dutch Paediatric Asthma Study Group. Am J Respir Crit Care Med 1997;156:688–95.

67. Chung KF. Leukotriene receptor antagonists and biosynthesis inhibitors: potential breakthrough in asthma therapy. Eur Respir J 1995;8: 1203–13.

68. Israel E, Rubin P, Kemp JP, et al. The effect of inhibition of 5-lipoxygenase by zileuton in mild-to-moderate asthma. Ann Int Med 1993;119: 1059–66.

69. Liu MC, Dube LM, Lancaster J. Acute and chronic effects of a 5-lipoxy-genase inhibitor in asthma: a 6-month randomized multicenter trial. Zileuton Study Group. J Allergy Clin Immunol 1996;98: 859–71.

70. Spector SL, Smith LJ, Glass M. Effects of 6 weeks of therapy with oral doses of ICI 204, 219, a leukotriene D4 receptor antagonist, in subjects with bronchial asthma. ACCOLATE Asthma Trialists Group. Am J Respir Crit Care Med 1994;150:618–23.

71. Knorr B, Franchi LM, Bisgaard H, et al. Montelukast, a leukotriene receptor antagonist, for the treatment of persistent asthma in children aged 2 to 5 years. Pediatrics 2001;108:E48.

72. Bisgaard H, Zielen S, Garcia Garcia L, et al. Montelukast reduces asthma exacerbations in 2 to 5 year-old children with intermittent asthma. Am J Respir Crit Care Med 2005;171:315–22.

73. Robertson C, Price D, Henry R, et al. Short-course montelukast for intermittent asthma in children. Am J Respir Crit Care Med 2007;175: 323–9.

74. Fitzpatrick MF, Mackay T, Driver H, et al. Salmeterol in nocturnal asthma: a double-blind, placebo controlled trial of a long-acting inhaled beta 2 agonist. Br Med J 1990;301:1365–8.

75. Green CP, Price JF. Prevention of exercise-induced asthma by inhaled salmeterol xinafoate. Arch Dis Child 1992;67:1014–7.

76. Primhak RA, Smith CM, Yong SC, et al. The bronchoprotective effect of inhaled salmeterol in preschool children: a dose-ranging study. Eur Respir J 1999;13:78–81.

77. Newhouse MT. Pulmonary drug targeting with aerosols: principles and clinical applications in adults and children. Am J Asthma Allergy Pediatr 1993;7:23–35.

78. Dolovich MB, Ahrens RC, Hess DR, et al, American College of Chest Physicians; American College of Asthma, Allergy, and Immunology. Device selection and outcomes of aerosol therapy: evidence-based guidelines. Chest 2005;127:335–71.

79. Parkin PC, Saunders NR, Diamond SA, et al. Randomized trial spacer vs nebulizer for acute asthma. Arch Dis Child 1995;72:239–40.

80. Closa RM, Ceballos JM, Gomez-Papi A, et al. Efficacy of bronchodilators administered by nebulizers versus spacer devices in infants with acute wheezing. Pediatr Pulmonol 1998;26:344–8.

81. Tal A, Golan H, Grauer N, et al. Deposition pattern of radiolabeled salbutamol inhaled from a metered-dose inhaler by means of a spacer with mask in young children with airway obstruction. J Pediatr 1996;128:479–84.

82. Wildhaber JH, Dore ND, Wilson JM, et al. Inhalation therapy in asthma: nebulizer or pressurized metered-dose inhaler with holding chamber? In vivo comparison of lung deposition in children. J Pediatr 1999;135: 28–33.

83. Gibson NA, Ferguson AE, Aitchison TC, et al. Compliance with inhaled asthma medication in preschool children. Thorax 1995;50: 1274–9.

84. Ferguson AE, Gibson NA, Aitchison TC, et al. Measured bronchodilator use in preschool children with asthma. Br Med J 1995;310: 1161–4.

85. Lim SH, Goh DYT, Tan AYS, et al. Parents' perceptions towards their child's use of inhaled medications for asthma therapy. J Paediatr Child Health 1996;32:306–9.

86. Mesters I, Meertens R, Kok G, et al. Effectiveness of a multidisciplinary education protocol in children with asthma (0–4 years) in primary health care. J Asthma 1994;31:347–59.

87. Wilson SR, Latini D, Starr NJ, et al. Education of parents of infants and very young children with asthma: a developmental evaluation of the Wee Wheezers program. J Asthma 1996;33:239-54.

88. Gore C, Custovic A. Primary and secondary prevention of allergic airway disease. Paediatr Respir Rev 2003;4:213-24.

89. Arshad SH, Bateman B, Matthews SM. Primary prevention of asthma and atopy during childhood by allergen avoidance in infancy: a randomised controlled study. Thorax 2003;58:489-93.

90. Arshad SH, Bateman B, Sadeghnejad A, et al. Prevention of allergic disease during childhood by allergen avoidance: the Isle of Wight prevention study. J Allergy Clin Immunol 2007;119:307-13.

91. Kramarz P, Destefano F, Gargiullo PM, et al. Does influenza vaccination prevent asthma exacerbations in children? J Pediatr 2001;138:306-10.

CHAPTER
37

Inner City Asthma

Craig A. Jones • Loran T. Clement

During the past 30 years, inner city asthma has emerged as a story about the influence of modern society on health and disease. Although asthma prevalence and morbidity have increased in many countries worldwide, a disproportionate increase has occurred in westernized urban settings. Extensive multidiscipinary research efforts have been directed toward understanding the causes of this epidemic. In the USA, a desire to mitigate health-care-related financial pressures has certainly provided one important motivation. The annual direct cost of asthma care in the USA exceeds $10 billion, 50% of which is related to emergency department (ED)- or hospital-based care. Considerable effort has been focused on understanding and correcting a pattern of resource utilization that is expensive and episodic.

However, investigation of the urban asthma epidemic that has taken place goes beyond the motivations stemming from escalating health-care costs. To some degree, the study of inner city asthma offers a fundamental look at the way in which modern living and an urban environment influence the functions of the immune system. It is also a look at the way in which environmental, social, and economic factors can converge to influence health status and the course of a chronic disease. In addition, research studies of urban asthma have provided a novel view of the ways that modern societies prioritize, structure, and fund health-care delivery, as well as the way in which social and economic factors influence health-care utilization.

Prevalence, Morbidity, and Mortality of Asthma in Inner Cities

Asthma Prevalence

The International Study of Asthma and Allergies in Childhood Steering Committee has reported that the 12-month prevalence of symptoms of asthma among children 13 to 14 years of age in countries around the world varies from 1.6% to 36.8%, with the highest prevalence rates generally found in economically developed, 'westernized' societies.[1] In the USA, the principal source of national asthma prevalence data has been the National Health Interview Survey conducted by the National Center for Health Statistics. In 2006, the overall age-adjusted prevalence rate for current asthma in the USA was estimated to be 7.8%.[2] Among children, prevalence rates are considerably higher. Of US children, 13.5% have been diagnosed with asthma at some time in their lives, and the highest age-specific prevalence rate for any age group (10.9 %) is found for children 5 to 14 years of age.[2]

From 1980 through 1998, the overall age-adjusted asthma prevalence rate in the USA increased by 75%.[3] Although a plateau in asthma prevalence rates has been reported in recent years,[3,4] rates remain at historic highs. Furthermore, demographic analyses have consistently shown that the increased prevalence and morbidity of asthma have been disproportionate among various segments of the population.[2–7] The populations in the USA that have been most affected include the following:

- Children: Although increases in prevalence and morbidity across time have occurred in all age groups, the greatest proportionate rise has occurred in children.[3–7] From 1980 to 2005, asthma prevalence more than doubled in children between the ages of 0 and 17 years.[4] Increases in ED visits and hospitalizations due to asthma also occurred, and the number of children dying from asthma increased almost 3-fold from 1979 to 1996.
- Urban populations: The prevalence of asthma for people living in metropolitan areas in the USA (9.0–11.1%) is higher than that found for those living in nonurban areas (7.4%).[5]
- Ethnic minorities: Racial differences in asthma prevalence, morbidity, and mortality have consistently been found. The greatest increases in asthma prevalence have been seen among African Americans and people of Puerto Rican heritage. In 2005, the prevalence of asthma among children self-identified as black (12.8%) or Puerto Rican (19.2%) exceeded that reported for children self-identified as white (7.9%) or Asian (4.9%).[4]
- Low socioeconomic status (SES) populations: The prevalence of asthma is inversely correlated with family income; asthma prevalence varied from 9.8% among persons with family incomes of less than $15 000 to 5.9% in those with family incomes of greater than $75 000.[3,6]

Numerous efforts have been made to determine asthma prevalence rates for children living in various US cities.[8–13] The disparate, and often staggering, prevalence rates for current asthma or undiagnosed (probable) asthma reported for several US inner city populations are shown in Table 37-1. It is important to note that accurate measurements of asthma prevalence in inner city populations are problematic. Woolcock[14] has described five areas of difficulty: (1) the lack of a uniform definition of asthma, (2) the absence of a standardized questionnaire, (3) the nonspecific nature of bronchial provocation tests, (4) the variable nature of the disease at different ages, and (5) the seasonal nature of the illness. Because there also is no uniform definition of the term *inner city,* further variation in the environmental or demographic characteristics of different urban areas can be expected. As a

©2010 Elsevier Ltd, Inc, BV
DOI: 10.1016/B978-1-4377-0271-2.00037-7

Table 37-1 Asthma Prevalence Rates for Children Living in Selected US Inner Cities

Urban Area	Prevalence of Diagnosed Asthma	Prevalence of Undiagnosed (probable) Asthma	Reference
Bronx, New York	14.3%	4.2%	8
San Diego, California	14.7%	12.5%	9
Detroit, Michigan	17.4%	11.7%	10
St. Louis, Missouri	20.0%	24.0%	11
Chicago, Illinois	10.8%	30.1%	12

result, it remains difficult to ascertain, interpret, or compare asthma prevalence rates reported for different inner city populations. Nonetheless, although precise prevalence figures may be lacking, the evidence that asthma has disproportionately affected inner city children is compelling.

Asthma Morbidity

The increased prevalence of asthma has been accompanied by a significant rise in the number of ED visits and hospitalizations due to asthma. From 2001 to 2004, there were an estimated 1.8 million ED visits annually for asthma in the USA.[3,4] The ED visit rate for children was substantially higher than that for adults, and the rate for African Americans was more than three times higher than rates for non-Hispanic whites.[3–5,15] Factors associated with recurrent or increased use of the ED for asthma care included lower education, single-parent families, African American race, and residence in an urban setting.[15–17]

Comparable increases in the estimated number of asthma-related hospitalizations have been reported. Although recent data suggest that hospitalization rates have declined somewhat,[15] there were still 497 000 asthma hospitalizations in the USA in 2004. Rates have consistently been higher for children and African Americans than for other age or ethnic groups.[18] The most striking increases have occurred in inner city neighborhoods inhabited by ethnic minorities and/or persons of low SES.[4,15,18,19]

Asthma Mortality

From 1960 to 1978, the overall mortality rate for asthma in the USA declined by 7.8% per annum. Declines were observed for all age, gender, and ethnic groups.[2,20] In 1979, however, asthma mortality rates started to increase, and the overall age-adjusted mortality rate in 1998 was 55.6% higher than the rate reported in 1978.[21] Neither more frequent diagnosis nor aging of the population could account for this change.[20] Fortunately, it appears that this trend has abated for all age groups; from 2001 to 2003, the average number of children who died because of asthma each year declined to 200.[3,4]

Although increases in asthma mortality have been recorded for all major demographic groups, asthma-related deaths in the USA have occurred predominantly in large cities. Among urban dwellers, those who are at particularly high risk include persons of low SES and ethnic minorities.[4,22–24] Asthma mortality rates for

African Americans are particularly disturbing: age-adjusted mortality rates are more than three times greater for urban African Americans (particularly young African American males) than for whites.[23] Among children, the disparity appears to be even greater: African American children are more than four times as likely to die from asthma as white children.[4,25] In one US city, asthma mortality remained stable among non-Hispanic whites over a 23-year period but increased by 337% for African Americans.[24]

Causative or Contributory Factors

Urbanization

From the earliest analyses, it has been apparent that the pace and magnitude of the increases in asthma prevalence and morbidity (in the USA and elsewhere) have been greatest among urban populations.[26,27] The hypothesis that the 'urbanization' of a discrete population results in an increase in the prevalence and morbidity of asthma has stimulated considerable interest in identifying transcultural facets of urban life that may alter the prevalence and/or morbidity of this disease. Perhaps the most striking revelation from the hundreds of elegant, yet frequently inconclusive, analyses that have been conducted is the complexity of this issue.[13] Potential sources of variability and/or contradiction include the following:

- There are inconsistent definitions of asthma and variations in methodology.
- 'Inner cities' are not uniform, either in the USA or globally. The largest US cities differ considerably in climate, ethnic composition, air pollution, cultural practices, and a broad range of other attributes that have been implicated as possible risk factors.
- Most of the putative risk factors for inner city populations are prevalent in other settings. For example, the poverty rate in rural areas of the USA exceeds that found in metropolitan areas and closely approaches the rate found for inner city populations.[28] Rural children with asthma (from every ethnic group) face many of the same barriers that have been proposed to adversely affect the health of their urban counterparts; indeed, the prevalence and/or magnitude of these barriers is often greater for rural children, who are less likely to have health insurance, face greater geographic barriers to health-care, and are less likely to see an asthma specialist or be treated with long-term controllers.[29–31]

Some of the factors that have been most frequently found to be associated with the increased prevalence, morbidity, and mortality from asthma among inner city dwellers are discussed later. Although certain attributes, either individually or in combination, identify populations at risk, there continues to be uncertainty or even controversy concerning the role of these factors in the inner city asthma epidemic. Taken together, it appears likely that a variable array of different risk factors and barriers, which are probably unique to each child or family, combine to increase the risk of morbidity from this treatable disease.

Putative Factors in the Physical Environment

Since genetic change is highly unlikely in the short time span attending the inner city asthma explosion, exposures to environmental factors, including allergens and indoor and outdoor pollutants, have been postulated to have contributory roles.

Increased Allergen Exposure and Sensitization

Although little indication exists that the mechanisms involved in allergen sensitization are qualitatively different for those living in the inner city, a number of studies have suggested that sensitization and subsequent re-exposure to high levels of certain allergens commonly found in the inner city may play an important role in the inner city asthma epidemic. Two allergens (cockroach and dust mite) have been most extensively studied.

Cockroach Allergens

One allergen of particular interest is cockroach allergen.[32] High levels of this allergen have been demonstrated in many inner city homes in the USA, and cockroach allergy is common among poor inner city dwellers.[32-35] The risk of sensitization appears to be related to the concentration of allergen in bedrooms.[36] Although cockroach infestation, allergen exposure, and sensitization is certainly not unique to urban dwellings,[33,37] the number of homes with elevated allergen concentrations appears to be greater in at least some urban settings;[33-36] thus children living in the inner city may be more likely to be exposed and sensitized.

Important information about the possible role of inner city allergens has come from studies conducted by the National Cooperative Inner-City Asthma Study (NCICAS) group. Children with asthma symptoms who lived in urban neighborhoods where more than 30% of the households had incomes below the poverty level were enrolled. In a study investigating allergen sensitization and exposure, cockroach allergy was found to be a particularly significant factor in the morbidity of inner city asthma.[35] The asthma hospitalization rate for children who were cockroach sensitive and exposed to high levels of this allergen was more than 3-fold higher than seen for other children in this cohort. These children also had 78% more unscheduled visits to health-care facilities and significantly more days and nights with asthma symptoms. Both allergen sensitivity and exposure to high levels of cockroach allergen were required to produce increased asthma morbidity. Although comparable numbers of children were allergic to other common inner city allergens, such as dust mite and cat, no significant associations between any measure of asthma morbidity and high exposure to these allergens was noted. Comparable findings have been reported from the multi-center Inner-City Asthma Study.[33,34]

House Dust Mite Allergens

Exposure and sensitization to dust mite allergen are frequently high in inner city areas, where human crowding, high indoor humidity, and older carpeting or bedding provide ideal conditions for mite proliferation.[33,38] Exposure to high levels of dust mite allergen has been shown to be associated with asthma,[39] and in an analysis of 27 environmental agents that have been reported to play a role in the development of asthma, the Institute of Medicine concluded that exposure to dust mites was one of only two exposures (along with tobacco smoke) for which there was sufficient evidence to establish an etiologic role.[40] In both case-control and prospective cohort studies conducted in a variety of geographic settings, reducing dust mite allergen exposure has been found to mitigate asthma morbidity in sensitized subjects.[41-43] Although dust mite sensitization and exposure were not shown to affect asthma symptom frequency or the rate of hospitalization in other studies of inner city asthma,[33,35] it nonetheless seems likely that dust mite allergy plays a role in inner city asthma, particularly in locales that promote dust mite proliferation.[44]

Although the hypothesis that allergen sensitization and exposure are responsible for the increased morbidity of asthma in the inner city remains popular, some have questioned whether the epidemiologic evidence in support of this premise is suffi-

cient.[45,46,47] They argue that the data from population studies are equivocal and provide little consistent evidence that allergen exposure is associated with the asthma prevalence at the population level. They also note that there have been no longitudinal studies in which allergen exposure during infancy in a random population sample has been related to asthma risk after the age of 6 years. Indeed, two longitudinal studies that were conducted in populations chosen on the basis of a family history of asthma or allergy failed to show an association between allergen exposure and current asthma.[46,47] Others have suggested that factors unrelated to atopy are of primary importance because preschool wheezing disorders distinct from atopic asthma, such as virus-induced wheezing, have also increased in recent years.[48] Finally, there is little evidence that allergen concentrations, sensitization rates, or the magnitude of allergen exposure has increased during the 25 years in which the prevalence and morbidity of asthma in US cities increased so dramatically; indeed, cockroaches and dust mites have been shown to be present (and allergenic) in inner city environments for many decades.[49] Although changes in allergen sensitization and/or exposure per se are not solely responsible for the observed increases in asthma prevalence, it appears likely that these factors have contributed to the increases in inner city asthma morbidity.

Air Pollution

The possible role that air pollution may play in the inner city asthma epidemic has been the subject of a number of recent reviews.[50-53] The factors that have been studied most extensively have been (a) pollutant levels, (b) proximity to a source of pollution, and (c) particle size. Outdoor air pollutants that have been most widely studied include ozone, sulfur dioxide, nitrogen dioxide, volatile organic compound emissions, diesel exhaust particles, and particulate matter, a complex mixture of particles containing many components, including endotoxin. Laboratory and epidemiologic studies have linked high concentrations of these air pollutants with bronchial hyper-reactivity, pulmonary function decrements, and signs of increased asthma morbidity (e.g. increases in medication use, ED visits, and asthma-related hospitalizations). Indoor air pollution has received less attention, and environmental tobacco smoke (ETS; discussed later) is the only indoor air pollutant that has consistently been linked to disease activity.

Studies seeking to define the role of air pollutants in the increasing morbidity of inner city asthma have focused on two questions: (1) Does air pollution initiate (or induce) the appearance of asthma in an unaffected individual? (2) Are air pollutants responsible for the increased morbidity described for inner city inhabitants who already have the disease? It has been well documented that exposure to air pollutants in an urban environment can aggravate asthma symptoms (particularly in children with decreased lung capacity) and increase disease morbidity.[50-53] Whether exposure to air pollutants induces the appearance of asthma in an unaffected child remains uncertain. Although several studies have reported that children living in areas with high road density or vehicular traffic are more likely to develop asthma,[13,15,53] proof that air pollution was the causal factor has been problematic. Many investigators have concluded that, with the possible exception of tobacco smoke, it appears unlikely that either outdoor or indoor air pollution has contributed substantially to the initiation of asthma in healthy subjects or to the increases in asthma prevalence or morbidity that have been observed in recent decades in the inner cities.[50-53] Exposure to pollutant levels that evoke acute respiratory responses is uncommon in community air pollution. Furthermore, temporal correlations between the concentrations of most air pollutants and signs of increasing asthma morbidity have generally been poor. The striking increase in inner city asthma has occurred during a time when the concentrations of all major outdoor air pollutants have declined substantially, a trend apparent since the mid-1960s. Taken together, these data suggest that air pollution has not been a major factor in the increasing morbidity of asthma in inner city populations during the past 25 years.

Environmental Tobacco Smoke Exposure

Numerous studies have shown that children exposed to ETS have a considerably higher-than-average risk of developing asthma.[54] As noted previously, the Institute of Medicine has concluded that exposure to tobacco smoke was one of only two exposures (along with dust mite exposure) for which there was sufficient evidence to establish an etiologic role.[40] Exposure to ETS has also been shown to increase airway reactivity, the frequency of ED visits, and the risk of hospitalization for children with asthma.[55,56] Although the level of cigarette smoking has declined in the USA during the past two decades, smoking rates remain relatively high in certain subpopulations.[34,57] The role that ETS exposure may play in the increased prevalence and morbidity of asthma in the inner cities has not been precisely defined, but it is highly likely that exposure to ETS contributes to this problem.

Socioeconomic, Cultural, and Ethnic Factors

Low Socioeconomic Status

Almost all analyses of the risk factors associated with increased asthma morbidity in the USA have shown that inner city residents of low SES are disproportionately affected, in terms of both increased disease prevalence and increased rates of adverse clinical sequelae (ED use, hospitalization, and mortality). This relationship has been the subject of numerous reviews or commentaries.[13,15,26,58-60] The measures used to define low SES have varied somewhat; low family income has been the primary variable in almost all US studies, whereas occupational social class has been used more frequently in Great Britain.[60] Other parameters that have been used as indicators of low SES include low parental or personal education levels, health insurance status, or enrollment in Medicaid programs.

Although increased asthma morbidity has consistently been associated with low SES in most studies of urban populations in the USA, a review of 22 questionnaire-based studies of asthma in children from other countries revealed little consistency in the relationship between SES and asthma morbidity, although children with severe asthma generally had lower SES.[61] In addition, atopy, which continues to be the single most significant risk factor for the development of asthma, has frequently been found to be more prevalent among higher SES groups, and asthma severity and morbidity do not appear to be increased in individuals of lower SES (of any ethnicity) who live in rural environments of the USA. Thus it appears that the association of increased asthma morbidity with lower SES may be largely restricted to the inner cities of the USA.

Many of the problems faced by poor families are directly related to their economic privation. However, a number of other factors that have been linked to asthma (smoking, obesity, large family size, low birth weight, and minority ethnic background) are also more prevalent in populations of lower SES in the USA. In Box 37-1 some of the many environmental, socioeconomic, cultural, and psychosocial factors that have been reported to contribute to the morbidity of asthma in inner city children from families of lower SES are listed.

BOX 37-1

Factors Reported to Contribute to Asthma Morbidity in Children of Lower SES

Suboptimal Access to Medical Care
- No health insurance
- Limited access to primary care physicians
- Limited access to asthma specialists
- Lack of transportation to out-patient health-care facilities
- Poor access to asthma support groups
- Unable to afford medications

Inadequate Medical Care
- Improper or under-diagnosis
- Lack of recognition of asthma severity by physician
- Under-prescription of controller medications

Increased Frequency of other Contributory or Co-morbid Medical Conditions
- Obesity
- Low birth rate, preterm delivery
- More frequent upper respiratory infections

Inadequate Asthma Education
- Lack of understanding of the role of bronchial inflammation
- Lack of understanding of the importance of early intervention
- Overuse or inappropriate use of asthma medications
- Poor adherence to therapeutic regimens

Low Level of Education or Illiteracy

Psychosocial Dysfunction of Patient and Family
- Depression
- Mood and anxiety disorders
- Hopelessness and despair
- Stress from exposure to violence and crime
- Illicit drug use

Lack of Social Support
- Young maternal age
- Single-parent families
- Social isolation of care-givers
- Lack of childcare resources

Increased Exposure to Indoor or Outdoor Environmental Agents
- Dust mites
- Cockroaches
- Air pollutants
- Maternal cigarette smoking and/or exposure to tobacco smoke

Deprived Living Conditions
- Overcrowded living conditions
- Decrepit housing and physical decay

Asthma in Ethnic Minorities

During the latter half of the 20th century, the percentage of inner city residents belonging to ethnic minorities increased significantly in the USA. According to the 2000 US Census, the non-Hispanic white share of population in the largest 100 cities declined to 44%, the lowest level on record. Almost half of these cities no longer have majority white populations. Because these demographic changes correlated temporally with the increased asthma morbidity and mortality noted for inner city residents, numerous studies have been done to assess the basis for the disproportionate burdens borne by various ethnic minorities living in the inner cities.

The difficulties experienced by African Americans have been particularly well documented. As noted previously, the prevalence of asthma in African American children and adults is somewhat higher than that found for other ethnic populations.[4,13,15] In addition, disproportionately increased rates of ED use and hospital admissions for asthma have been repeatedly observed for inner city African American populations, and disturbing differences in asthma mortality rates (particularly for young African American males) have been well documented.[19,21-24,62,63] Whether these substantial differences are the result of independent ethnic factors or reflect the coexisting burdens resulting from lower SES or inner city environmental factors has been the subject of some debate. A number of epidemiologic studies have reported that the increased prevalence or morbidity of asthma is still significantly associated with race (African-American vs white) after adjusting for socioeconomic factors, environmental exposures, and other confounding factors.[23,63-65] In contrast, others have found that the increased risks in African-American children lost significance when other risk factors were included in multivariate linear regression models.[7,12,18] Although an unequivocal explanation for the increased problems faced by African Americans remains elusive, the disparate data from these studies clearly indicate that the disproportionately high measures of asthma morbidity in this population cannot be explained by biological factors, modest differences in prevalence, or the demographic shifts that have been reported.

Increased asthma prevalence and morbidity rates have also been reported for inner city Hispanic populations.[9,59,65-68] The Hispanic population (a grouping defined solely by cultural heritage) is racially and culturally diverse, and the prevalence and impact of asthma appear to vary among subgroups. In the USA, asthma prevalence, hospitalization, and mortality rates are highest for Hispanics of Puerto Rican ancestry.[4,13,66,67] Rates for Mexican Americans appear to be considerably lower, approaching those reported for non-Hispanic whites in some studies[67,68] but not others.[9] This variability may at least in part reflect the fact that asthma is often under-diagnosed in this population.[9,68] The basis for the increased morbidity of asthma in inner city Hispanics appears to be multi-factorial. Many of the factors that have been reported (low SES and lower educational attainment[60]) parallel those identified for other ethnic minorities. In addition, Hispanics are particularly likely to have poor access to medical care. In many areas of the USA, medical insurance coverage is considerably lower for Hispanic children than for African American or non-Hispanic white children.[9,69] Language barriers and/or culturally based beliefs about health and illness may be of greater significance than low SES or environmental exposures.[66,70]

When analyzing data from studies examining the disproportionate morbidity of asthma among ethnic minorities, it is important to note that epidemiologic studies cannot adequately quantify a variety of highly subjective factors that may nonetheless be extremely important. These include cultural factors, habits, traditions, or beliefs that may differ significantly among populations grouped by ethnicity. In addition, ethnicity may be a surrogate measure of discrimination that affects the nature or quality of health-care, even within systems where access is not a variable.[63,71] Finally, as discussed later, asthma-related medical care for ethnic minorities and the poor living in the inner cities of the USA may be inaccessible, inappropriate, or substandard in quality.

Inadequacies of the Health-Care Delivery System

Although many of the risk factors associated with inner city asthma extend beyond the traditional purview of US health-care systems, deficiencies in the availability or quality of the medical care received by inner city residents play a major and perhaps primary role in the increased morbidity of asthma experienced by this population. Although almost every attribute, process, and component of asthma care for inner city populations has been studied and described in detail, the current status of asthma care in the inner city can best be understood when it is first viewed in a broader context. The functions of urban health-care delivery systems and the manner in which they are used are influenced by a number of complex issues that converge to define life in the urban USA. These include the logistics of daily living for people of lower SES, interactions among people of diverse ethnic and cultural backgrounds, and the financial incentives that influence health-care providers and health service models.

From almost any perspective, the picture of asthma care that emerges from this mix of social, cultural, and economic influences is unsettling. In the USA it is largely a picture of African American and Hispanic children living in an environment that is defined and dominated by their lower socioeconomic standing. They often have only episodic contact with health-care professionals, and this typically occurs when they are acutely ill in a setting, such as an ED, that is neither structured nor inclined to provide disease-specific education, prescribe long-term anti-inflammatory medications, or engage in other preventative care practices. When inner city children do have contact with health-care providers in a more appropriate setting, their asthma severity may be underestimated, and they are often under-treated. Even if antiinflammatory medications are prescribed, adherence and outcomes are poor for those patients who do not have routine follow-up with a single, knowledgeable provider. Poor compliance is accentuated by the fact that many of these children are from single-parent households, and they are frequently responsible for their own daily care.

Appropriate, effective care for children with chronic diseases is typically a complex process that requires coordinated interactions among different components of the health-care delivery system. For inner city children with asthma, almost every link in this health-care delivery chain has been shown to be broken or deficient.

Inadequate Access to Health-Care
Lack of Health Insurance

A significant fraction (as high as 25%) of children in some urban areas do not have health insurance.[69,72] In comparison with children with insurance, uninsured children are more likely to lack a regular source of care, to rely on EDs for their care, and to go without care for chronic health conditions, including asthma.[72,73] The Institute of Medicine has cited lack of adequate health insurance as the single most important barrier to health-care services for children in the USA.[74]

Poor Access to Asthma Specialists

Patients receiving their asthma care from specialists have higher health-related quality of life measures and are considerably more likely to report using asthma controller therapy.[75-77] Access to care from asthma specialists is reduced for those who are poor (and, independently, for those who belong to an ethnic minority).[71]

Inappropriate Utilization of Health-care Resources

Numerous studies have shown that EDs are frequently the main source of health-care for inner city asthmatics.[78,79] In part, this can be directly attributed to the increased prevalence and/or severity of asthma among inner city residents. In addition, asthma patients without insurance or a primary care-giver may use the ED as a last resort, when asthma symptoms or exacerbations can no longer be ignored and emergency care is essential.

The need for repetitive emergency care has a number of untoward consequences. First, this may become habitual: the ED can become a familiar surrogate for a primary care provider. In one study, poor asthmatic subjects were four times more likely to attend an ED than other asthmatics with similar severity.[80] This pattern of inappropriate utilization, which is independent of health insurance status, may continue, even when more appropriate sources of out-patient care are available.[16,81,82] In addition, a wide variety of other socioeconomic barriers (e.g. transportation difficulties or problems in paying co-payments) have been shown to discourage the use of nonurgent health-care resources and to increase the number of ED visits for asthma care.[81] Certain 'cultural' attributes of the medical care delivery system also contribute to this phenomenon. Patterns of reimbursement by insurance companies or other payers, which often reimburse care provided in an ED more readily or fully than regular out-patient care, perpetuates this process. This 'crisis management' approach to care contributes to the higher admission rates for inner city asthmatics that are seen in urban EDs.[81,83] Reliance on an ED for asthma care has numerous other shortcomings. Children who receive care in an ED seldom receive significant education about long-term asthma control. They rarely receive written action plans, are unlikely to be started on controller medications, and provisions for follow-up care in regular facilities are sporadic and are associated with poor adherence.

What happens after a child leaves the ED, and why is the transition to regular out-patient preventive care so unusual? Detailed insight emerges from an NCICAS study examining follow-up care for inner city children who were seen in an ED for an acute exacerbation of asthma.[84] Only 29% of the patients were provided with a follow-up appointment at the time of the ED visit; 69% of these appointments were kept. An additional 39.9% were told to make an appointment. More than 78% of the caretakers tried to make an appointment, and 63% were able to do so: 95% of these appointments were kept. In contrast, for the 31% who were neither given an appointment nor told to make one, only 28% made a follow-up appointment. Caretaker-reported barriers to making an appointment included (1) their child was well, (2) lack of a suitable appointment time, (3) not knowing an appointment was needed, (4) busy telephone, (5) busy parent, and (6) cost. It is important to focus on the lessons learned from 'real world' studies such as this, because children will not have improved health status unless they become engaged in routine preventive health-care practices.

Inadequate Medical Care

Studies like NCICAS and ICAS demonstrate that it is essential to develop strategies that transition families from episodic care to routine out-patient care. However, at the present time, it is not clear that this would improve the health status of inner city children with asthma because it has been repeatedly documented that the quality of care delivered to poor inner city children who do gain access to primary medical care is typically suboptimal.[79,85-87] Frequently, the diagnosis of asthma is not made, even when children are experiencing daily respiratory symptoms.[10] Inner city children with asthma are rarely treated in accordance with nationally accepted standards of asthma care. Primary care physicians frequently report that they are unable to devote the time needed to provide disease-specific education, and written treatment plans outlining the steps that should be taken when an asthma exacerbation commences are seldom provided or explained.

The failure to prescribe antiinflammatory medications for children with persistent asthma is particularly common and consequential. It is widely accepted that the daily use of controller medications, such as inhaled corticosteroids, can reduce the number of asthma exacerbations and ED visits.[86-88] Numerous studies have shown that patients with persistent asthma (in all areas of the country, including the inner cities) are frequently not using the controller medications indicated for controlling disease activity. This may result because these medications are not prescribed, because prescriptions are not filled, or because patients fail to use the medications as directed. One of the more thorough descriptions of the use of controller medications by inner city children was reported as part of a school- and community-based intervention project.[86,87] Almost all participating children were from a low-income, single-parent family, and the care-giver was typically uneducated and unemployed. The majority (90%) of these families had insurance or Medicaid; thus, access to care and medication costs were not primary obstacles. Although the children in this study had frequent symptoms and substantial asthma-related morbidity, 20% had no medication or were using only over-the-counter remedies, and only 10% used any controller. The poor health status of these children resulted from the lack of a competent, familiar health-care provider and inadequate engagement of the parent or caretaker in maintenance therapy and competent decision-making; an ongoing relationship with a single physician was associated with increased use of antiinflammatory medications, and children were more likely to use these medications if the parent believed that the medications should be taken regularly.

In summary, the chronicle of inner city children with asthma is a story about barriers. It is a story about inadequate health-care delivery systems superimposed on the consequences of poverty, single-parent households, low literacy and caretaker awareness, and the difficulties of contemporary urban life in the USA. In this setting, children frequently lack access to medical care structured to meet the challenges posed by this chronic, but controllable, disease. Families often live in crowded conditions with high levels of exposure to environmental risk factors that are difficult to modify. Transportation difficulties, fears of losing a job, and other challenges of daily living frequently overshadow health-care as a routine priority.

Strategies for Inner City Asthma Interventions

One of the most notable aspects of the inner city asthma explosion in the USA relates to its timing. During the past three

- Increases in asthma prevalence, morbidity, and mortality rates during the concluding three decades of the 20th century have been disproportionately great in urban areas, particularly those of the USA.

- The pace and magnitude of these changes have been greatest for inner city dwellers of low socioeconomic status, members of ethnic minorities, and children.

- Deficiencies in the availability or the quality of preventive medical care received by inner city inhabitants have played a major role in the increased asthma morbidity experienced by this population.

- Sensitization and subsequent re-exposure to high levels of certain allergens commonly found in the inner city (e.g. cockroaches) may contribute to asthma morbidity.

- Although air pollution adversely affects asthma health status, levels of most pollutants have decreased in urban areas during the time period when inner city asthma prevalence and morbidity have increased, and associations between pollutant levels and asthma activity are inconsistent. Exposure to potential immune-modifying pollutants (e.g. diesel particulates, tobacco smoke) may be of etiologic significance.

- Taken together, current evidence suggests that the health status of inner city children with asthma in the USA is a chronicle of inadequate or inappropriate health-care superimposed on the social, educational, environmental, and cultural consequences of low socioeconomic status in an urban setting.

decades, air pollution has been reduced by more than 90%, the number of people who smoke has declined more than 30%, and advances in basic and medical sciences, intensive care practices, and drug development have provided knowledge and tools that would quite reasonably be expected to produce favorable results. Instead, almost every parameter of asthma morbidity in the inner cities of the USA has increased by more than 75%.

Efforts to understand and address this paradox have generally focused on the allocation of limited resources to produce a health-care delivery chain in which all of the essential links are intact – and capable of withstanding the strains produced in treating thousands of disadvantaged children with a chronic disease (Box 37-2). Strategies that have been tested include expanded access to specialty care, structured transitions from acute care sites to appropriate out-patient care, the use of asthma care coordinators and patient tracking, education programs for health-care providers, education programs for asthmatic children and their care-givers, school- and community-based outreach programs, and programs to reduce environmental risk factors.[86–100] Some of the general characteristics of selected interventions, with references, are summarized in Table 37.2.

Although these intervention models differ in rationale, goals, and approach, several general observations about inner city asthma interventions can be made. First, it appears that almost any intervention strategy results in improvements in some measure of the health status of inner city children with asthma; thus paying more attention to the problem is likely to produce benefits. Similarly, frequent contact and consistent follow-up are associated with superior outcomes; education or assistance provided by a single, familiar person is particularly meaningful. Efforts to educate patients and families about asthma are almost always useful (but seldom, if ever, sufficient to deal with all

aspects of this chronic disease). In contrast, it remains unclear whether allergen reduction strategies can improve clinical outcomes for inner city children; the challenge of eliminating allergens from a mobile and hardy pest like the cockroach from large urban areas appears to be particularly daunting.[97,98]

Many interventions have focused on utilizing people who are not professional health-care providers to help families in small study cohorts to overcome the consequences of their SES and urban living. Themes such as improving problem solving or communication skills, changing the family living environment and risk behaviors, or developing supportive social structures have been emphasized. Activities of this nature improve health status and enhance ongoing patient participation, which is extremely important.[94–96] Despite the merits of these goals, health-care delivery has been largely unaffected by this type of intervention, primarily because entities that pay for and deliver health-care have rarely adopted comparable strategies aimed at modifying social, cultural, and environmental factors.

Efforts to develop interventions that alter patterns of health-care utilization or physician practices have met with only modest success. Despite widespread efforts for almost two decades, it does not appear that asthma education programs directed solely at health-care providers have translated into significant changes in the health of inner city children or the quality of their asthma care. The limited time typically available to primary care physicians for individual patient interactions continues to be a significant barrier to improving the standard of asthma care provided in this setting.[99,100]

Although interventions structured to provide accessible, ongoing specialty care have consistently been shown to improve the health status of patients with asthma, the development of such programs has been thwarted by the assumption that direct specialty care interventions are likely to be too expensive to offer to large inner city populations. However, several recent studies have shown that specialty care can be provided to inner city children in a cost-effective fashion.[89–92] As an example, in Los Angeles, the California Chapter of the Asthma and Allergy Foundation of America, the Los Angeles County Department of Health Services, and the Los Angeles Unified School District entered into a partnership to develop a sustainable school-based health service model (the Breathmobile™ program) for inner city children with asthma. This program has evolved from a community outreach effort to an integrated disease-management model that has expanded both regionally and nationally (see Figure 37-1).[90] More than 7000 patients at eight national sites have been entered into this specialty-based program, ongoing patient participation has remained high, and significant reductions in measures of asthma morbidity and improvements in disease control have been achieved for inner city children receiving care in a 'real world' setting.[100]

Finally, it is important to note that most of these research efforts have evaluated intervention strategies that involve relatively small numbers of patients. The NCICAS Phase II study, which is the largest inner city intervention reported to date, included 515 patients, and the costs to scale and sustain this intervention were not reported. Although it is frequently anticipated that strategies shown to be effective in controlled trials will produce similar effects when incorporated into health-care delivery systems, most small interventions of demonstrated effectiveness have not translated into widespread, sustained changes in the health of inner city populations. This may reflect the fact that current health-care delivery models are primarily motivated by financial concerns and/or cost efficacy rather than by clinical efficacy. If intervention research is going to have an impact on inner city health-care delivery systems, it is important for these

Table 37-2 Intervention Strategies and Models

Strategic Goal	General Approach	Demonstrated Benefits	Reference
Enhanced access to specialty care	Provide ongoing access to asthma care specialists. Comprehensive care plans in accordance with national asthma care standards	1. Reduced acute care visits 2. Reduced hospitalizations 3. Increased preventative care 4. Possible cost reductions	89–92
Structured transition from acute care to out-patient care	Standardize and centralize acute asthma care. Arrange and monitor transition from acute care setting to out-patient settings that provide optimal preventive care	1. Reduced length of stay in ED and as in-patient 2. Reduced ED and in-patient re-admission rates	93
Patient and family education by specially trained social workers or peer counselors	Educate families, coordinate care activities, assist with allergen reduction efforts, and/or monitor self-management care practices	1. Fewer symptomatic days 2. Reduced hospitalizations 3. Possible reduction of acute care visits 4. Improved environmental control measures	94, 95
Community-based social networking and education	Establish informal social networks throughout a community to effect behavior changes, broaden patient education, and improve asthma management practices	1. Improved community awareness of asthma	96
Reduction of environmental risk factors	Conduct home visits for environmental evaluation and allergen reduction procedures	1. Reduced concentrations of some indoor allergens 2. Reduced acute care visits 3. Improved allergen avoidance practices	97, 98
Educate health-care providers	Distribute educational materials and conduct classes targeted to improve physician awareness and compliance with asthma care standards	1. Improved use of asthma controller therapy 2. Improved patient education and care practices	99, 100

efforts to be conducted on a scale and in a manner that evaluates both clinical and cost efficacy rather than simply responding to economic and business pressures.

Future Opportunites: Health-Care Reform

Viewed in its entirety, the complex social, financial, behavioral, environmental, health-care delivery, and biologic factors that contribute to increased asthma morbidity for urban children can appear overwhelming. For other complex public health issues (e.g. environmental exposures that have a broad health impact, such as air pollutants and tobacco smoke), detailed scientific work has frequently engendered public policy designed to reduce these risk factors. Unfortunately, a similar paradigm (e.g. using scientifically derived information to support sweeping societal changes) has not emerged for improving the health of inner city children with asthma. The burden borne by this unfortunate population remains unsettling.

In large part, the factors responsible for the high asthma-related morbidity for inner city children derive from fundamental health-care issues that affect the country as a whole. Indeed, increased morbidity and financial hardship associated with a potentially preventable (or controllable) chronic disease has become a common finding for a large portion of the US population. Accordingly, the need for effective, affordable health-care that addresses health disparities, minimizes disease-associated morbidity, and incorporates disease prevention is shared across American society.[101] Viewed in this context, improving the health of inner city children with asthma may be intimately linked to addressing the issues that affect the health and well-being of the entire American population.

Until recently, comprehensive health-care reform based on national health policy and the primacy of improving the health of the entire US population has regularly been thwarted by conflicting financial and political interests. However, a new sense of urgency and national consensus to address health-care delivery issues has emerged. In large part, the political will to reform health-care policies appears to be fueled by escalating health-care costs superimposed on the most severe economic downturn since the Great Depression. In this environment, the health-related interests of the country's poorest populations, including inner city children with asthma, may ironically be aligned with the financial priorities of some of the nation's largest businesses and political lobby groups that have previously opposed government-directed reforms.

As the nature and scope of health-care reform are debated, several core principles appear to have particular application and relevance for mitigating the problems that have been so clearly defined in research studies of inner city asthma:

- **Universal access to affordable health-care**. As previously noted, the lack of access to both primary and specialty health-care providers is clearly linked to poor asthma control, decreased use of long-term controllers, increased emergency and in-patient care, and worsening of other measures of asthma morbidity. Although providing health insurance and otherwise improving access to all pertinent health-care resources cannot alleviate all of the factors responsible for increased asthma morbidity, universal coverage to affordable health-care is nonetheless an essential component of any solution. Actions such as the recent renewal and expansion of State Children's Health Insurance Program (SCHIP), which provides new or ongoing coverage for 11 million children from lower socioeconomic backgrounds, are encouraging. Similarly, efforts by states, such as those implemented in Massachusetts, to achieve mandatory health coverage for all citizens, favorably affect urban residents with chronic diseases such as asthma.

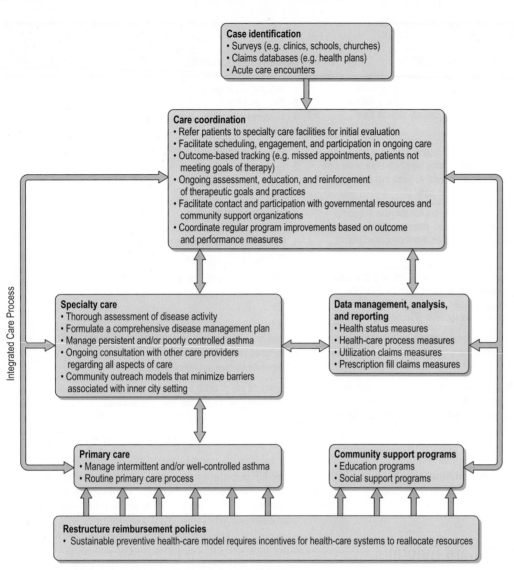

Integrated Care Process

Case identification
• Surveys (e.g. clinics, schools, churches)
• Claims databases (e.g. health plans)
• Acute care encounters

Care coordination
• Refer patients to specialty care facilities for initial evaluation
• Facilitate scheduling, engagement, and participation in ongoing care
• Outcome-based tracking (e.g. missed appointments, patients not
  meeting goals of therapy)
• Ongoing assessment, education, and reinforcement
  of therapeutic goals and practices
• Facilitate contact and participation with governmental resources and
  community support organizations
• Coordinate regular program improvements based on outcome
  and performance measures

Specialty care
• Thorough assessment of disease activity
• Formulate a comprehensive disease management plan
• Manage persistent and/or poorly controlled asthma
• Ongoing consultation with other care providers
  regarding all aspects of care
• Community outreach models that minimize barriers
  associated with inner city setting

**Data management, analysis,
and reporting**
• Health status measures
• Health-care process measures
• Utilization claims measures
• Prescription fill claims measures

Primary care
• Manage intermittent and/or well-controlled asthma
• Routine primary care process

Community support programs
• Education programs
• Social support programs

Restructure reimbursement policies
• Sustainable preventive health-care model requires incentives for health-care systems to reallocate resources

Figure 37-1 Algorithm for health service model for inner city asthma care.

• **Realignment of financial incentives and reimbursement rules.** The paucity of comprehensive asthma care programs in urban health-care systems is a logical consequence of current economic incentives. Under current private and Medicaid reimbursement rules, payments to health-care institutions are highest for ED and in-patient care. This provides an unmistakable incentive to allocate resources to high acuity service areas rather than toward developing comprehensive out-patient disease management programs, which are poorly reimbursed, if at all.

A contrasting approach that is presently gaining favor is to pay for medical care according to quality or outcomes. If the current emphasis on volume-based fee-for-service payments were reduced in favor of financial incentives for high quality, guideline-based care by primary care providers, treatment of chronic diseases such as asthma would undoubtedly improve. Importantly, it is essential that Medicare and Medicaid fully participate in payment reform if these efforts are to be effective and sustainable.

A wide variety of different schemes and models have been proposed or implemented. As an example, the Community Care Program in North Carolina features local health networks comprised of primary care providers, care coordinators, social services, hospitals, and local health departments that provide Medicaid patients with well-coordinated care.

Improved health and financial outcomes for lower socioeconomic populations have been demonstrated. For children with asthma, these networks have achieved a shift from episodic acute care to preventive care with improved control over health-care expenditures.

Creation of effective patient-centered medical homes. As shown in Box 37-3, effective care for asthma includes regular visits with qualified health-care professionals who provide consistent disease-specific education, implement appropriate therapeutic strategies, monitor compliance, and engage in preventive practices. Changes in reimbursement parameters would favor the emergence of primary care practices that operate with the staffing and health information technology needed to support effective guideline-based care and enhanced clinical tracking in accordance with standards established by the National Committee for Quality Assurance. This is particularly relevant for patients with asthma, many of whom receive care from primary care providers. In this setting, children are more likely to receive regular scheduled visits with a familiar provider, structured assessments of asthma control, implementation of self-management plans, and careful tracking of patient-oriented goals.

As efforts to define transformative national health policy are proceeding, it is likely that state-directed initiatives will facilitate the expansion and quality of health-care reforms. Thus, Vermont

BOX 37-3 Therapeutic principles

Standards of excellence in medical care should not be compromised.	Asthma care for disadvantaged children should be comprehensive and in full accordance with standards established by the National Asthma Education and Prevention Program (NAEPP).
Care should be provided by a physician with the appropriate knowledge, experience, and level of involvement.	The participation of a concerned asthma specialist is of demonstrated efficacy and offers the most effective and preferred approach.
The proper use of inhaled corticosteroids and other controller medications must be emphasized.	Considerable evidence indicates that any intervention that fails to achieve regular use of controller medications is unlikely to substantially alter asthma morbidity.
Care activities should be accessible, recurrent, and engaging.	Child and family members should have regular contact at a readily accessible site with a stable, familiar team of specially trained health-care providers and support personnel.
Adequate time for a meaningful patient-provider interaction is essential.	The time required for appropriate clinical assessment, effective patient education, and assistance with overcoming other barriers to care should be recognized and anticipated in advance.
Teaching is not the same as learning.	Patients and their families must achieve – and demonstrate – a thorough understanding of a written action plan and the purpose and correct use of every medication. This typically requires personal, one-on-one educational efforts that cannot be achieved with pamphlets or video presentations.
Outcomes and patient asthma-related behaviors should be monitored.	An integrated disease management program greatly facilitates patient identification, compliance with appointments and medication use, and targeted efforts to reduce inappropriate utilization of health-care resources or detrimental behaviors.

BOX 37-4 Key concepts

Intervention Strategies and Opportunities

- Effective inner city asthma interventions must incorporate key *therapeutic principles* that can be resourcefully applied within the context of the social, economic, and environmental realities of the contemporary urban setting.
- Intervention strategies designed to educate primary health-care providers or to alter existing patterns of health-care utilization have not produced significant improvements in the quality or regularity of preventative asthma care received by inner city children or translated into widespread changes in health-care delivery systems.
- The best opportunities to develop and establish models of care for inner city populations may lie within large health-care delivery systems and public hospitals that already have the necessary infrastructure and network resources.
- Current Medicaid reimbursement policies motivate resource allocation to emergency room and in-patient service areas. As the ultimate purchaser of health-care for poor inner city populations, Medicaid reimbursement should be restructured to provide economic incentives for establishing effective out-patient programs that emphasize preventative care.
- Health-care models structured to provide ongoing, comprehensive, specialty care are currently feasible and offer an effective approach to improve the health of inner city children with asthma.
- Future efforts toward primary prevention and disease modification may have the greatest impact on asthma health at a population level.

has implemented a broad range of reforms that address coverage as well as health-care delivery. Catamount Health highlights a private-public approach to expanding coverage through commercial insurers with state subsidies based on income. In addition, the Vermont Blueprint for Health includes an ambitious array of delivery system reforms that emphasize health maintenance, prevention, and control of chronic disease (including asthma). In pilot communities, commercial insurers and Medicaid have restructured payments to support quality care in patient-centered medical homes supported by multidisciplinary

Community Care Teams (CCTs). The CCT, which includes nurse coordinators, social workers, dieticians, behavioral health specialists, and public health prevention specialists, is a scalable entity that works closely with the medical homes to provide support for individual patients and to assist with panel management for the general population. Expanded application of health information technology allows coordinated care and population management across independent practices, clinics, and hospitals.

Comprehensive national reform has the potential to alleviate the disproportionate burden of asthma borne by inner city populations. To be effective, however, reform must align financial incentives with achieving clinical goals rather than promoting acute episodic care. Adopted reforms must support a comprehensive and well-coordinated approach that includes guideline-based preventive care in primary care settings, expanded access to specialty care for patients with poorly controlled disease, structured transitions from acute care sites to appropriate out-patient care, the use of care coordinators and social support services, health information technology that supports individual patient tracking as well as population management, effective education programs for health-care providers, effective education programs for asthmatic children and their care-givers, school- and community-based outreach programs, and programs to reduce environmental risk factors.[86–100] Although the challenges are substantial, bold and effective changes in national policy offer the best opportunity to mitigate the morbidity of asthma for inner city populations in the USA.

Helpful Websites

The Action Against Asthma website (http://www.aspe.hhs. gov/sp/asthma/index.htm)

The National Center for Health Statistics, Asthma website (http://www.cdc.gov/nchs/products/pubs/pubd/hestats/asthma/asthma.htm)

National Committee for Quality Assurance: Physician Practice Connections® – Patient-Centered Medical Home™ (http://www.ncqa.org/tabid/631/Default.aspx)

The American Recovery and Reinvestment Act 2009 (http://www.recovery.gov/)

Call to Action Health Reform 2009 (http://finance.senate.gov/healthreform2009/home.html)

Community Care of North Carolina (http://www.community-carenc.com/)

Massachusetts Commonwealth Connector (http://www.mahealthconnector.org/portal/site/connector/)

Vermont Blueprint for Health (http://healthvermont.gov/blueprint.aspx)

References

1. Beasley R, Keil U, von Mutius E, et al. Worldwide variation in prevalence of symptoms of asthma, allergic rhinoconjunctivitis, and atopic eczema: ISAAC. Lancet 1998;351:1225–32.

2. National Health Interview Survey (NHIS) Data. 2006 Asthma Data. National Center for Health Statistics, Center for Disease Control and Prevention. Available on the World Wide Web (accessed January 17, 2009): http://www.cdc.gov/asthma/nhis/06/data.htm.

3 Moorman JE, Rudd RA, Johnson CA, et al. National Surveillance for Asthma – United States, 1980–2004. MMWR 2007;56:1–53.

4. Akinbami LJ. The State of Childhood Asthma, United States, 1980–2005. Advance Data from Vital and Health Statistics; no. 381. Hyattsville, MD: National Center for Health Statistics, 2006.

5. Bloom B, Cohen RA. Summary Health Statistics for U.S. Children: National Health Interview Survey, 2006. Vital and Health Statistics; no. 234. National Center for Health Statistics, 2007.

6. Weitzman M, Gortmaker SL, Sobol AM, et al. Recent trends in the prevalence and severity of childhood asthma. JAMA 1992;268:2673–7.

7. Gergen PJ, Mullally DI, Evans III RE. National survey of prevalence of asthma among children in the United States, 1976 to 1980. Pediatrics 1988;81:1–7.

8. Crain EF, Weiss KB, Bijur PE, et al. An estimate of the prevalence of asthma and wheezing among inner-city children. Pediatrics 1994;94:356–62.

9. Christiansen SC, Martin SB, Schleicher NC, et al. Current prevalence of asthma-related symptoms in San Diego's predominantly Hispanic inner city children. J Asthma 1996;33:17–26.

10. Joseph CLM, Foxman B, Leickly FE, et al. Prevalence of possible undiagnosed asthma and associated morbidity among urban schoolchildren. J Pediatr 1996;129:735–42.

11. Nelson KA, Meadows L, Yan Y, et al. Asthma prevalence in low-income urban elementary school students in St. Louis, 1992 and 2004. J Pediatr 2009;154:111–1115.

12. Grant EN, Daugherty SR, Moy JN, et al. Prevalence and burden of illness for asthma and related symptoms among kindergartners in Chicago public schools. Ann Allergy Asthma Immunol 1999;83:113–20.

13. Federico MJ, Liu AH. Overcoming childhood asthma disparities of the inner-city poor. Pediatr Clin N Am 2003;50:655–75.

14. Woolcock AJ. Epidemiologic methods for measuring prevalence of asthma. Chest 1987;91:89S–92S.

15. Gold DR, Wright R. Population disparities in asthma. Annu Rev Public Health 2005;26:89–113.

16. Halfon N, Newacheck PW, Wood DL, et al. Routine emergency department use for sick care by children in the United States. Pediatrics 1996;98:28–34.

17. Rand CS, Butz AM, Kolodner K, et al. Emergency department visits by urban African American children with asthma. J Allergy Clin Immunol 2000;105:83–90.

18. Wissow LS, Gittelsohn AM, Szklo M, et al. Poverty, race and hospitalization for childhood asthma. Am J Public Health 1988;78:777–81.

19. Gergen PJ, Weiss KB. Changing patterns of asthma hospitalization among children: 1979–1987. JAMA 1990;264:1688–92.

20. Weiss KB, Wagener DK. Changing patterns of asthma mortality: identifying target populations at high risk. JAMA 1990;264:1683–7.

21. Murphy SL. Deaths: final data for 1998. National Vital Statistics Reports, National Center for Health Statistics, Center for Disease Control and Prevention, vol 48. July 24 2000.

22. Carr W, Zeitel L, Weiss K. Variations in asthma hospitalizations and deaths in New York City. Am J Public Health 1992;82:59–65.

23. Lang DM, Polansky M. Patterns of asthma mortality in Philadelphia from 1969 to 1991. N Engl J Med 1994;331:1542–6.

24. Targonski PV, Persky VW, Orris P, et al. Trends in asthma mortality among African Americans and whites in Chicago, 1968 through 1991. Am J Public Health 1994;84:1830–3.

25. Underlying cause of death dataset, 1996. National Center for Health Statistics. Action Against Asthma: A Strategic Plan for the Department of Health and Human Services, May 2000. Available on the World Wide Web (accessed January 30, 2009): http://aspe.hhs.gov/sp/asthma/index.htm.

26. Sly RM. Asthma in the inner city. Immunol Allergy Clin North Am 1991;11:103–51.

27. Galea S, Vlahov D. Urban health: evidence, challenges, and directions. Annu Rev Public Health 2005;26:341–65.

28. Dalaker J. U.S. Census Bureau, Current population reports, series P60–214, poverty in the United States: 2000. Washington, DC: U.S. Government Printing Office; 2001.

29. Schwartz DA. Etiology and pathogenesis of airway disease in children and adults from rural communities. Environ Health Perspectives 1999;107:393–401.

30. von Maffei J, Beckett WS, Belanger K, et al. Risk factors for asthma prevalence among urban and nonurban African American children. J Asthma 2001;38:555–64.

31. Yawn BP, Mainous III AG, Love MM, et al. Do rural and urban children have comparable asthma care utilization? J Rural Health 2001;17:32–9.

32. Arruda KL, Vailes LD, Ferriani VPL, et al. Cockroach allergens and asthma. J Allergy Clin Immunol 2001;10:419–28.

33. Gruchalla RS, Pongracic J, Plaut M, et al. Inner city asthma study: relationships among sensitivity, allergen exposure, and asthma morbidity. J Allergy Clin Immunol 2005;115:478–85.

34. Crain E, Walter M, O'Conner GT, et al. Home and allergic characteristics of children with asthma in seven US urban communities and design of an environmental intervention: the Inner-city Asthma Study. Environ Health Perspect 2002;110:939–45.

35. Rosenstreich DL, Eggleston PA, Kattan M, et al. The role of cockroach allergy and exposure to cockroach allergen in causing morbidity among inner-city children with asthma. N Engl J Med 1997;336:1356–63.

36. Sarpong SB, Hamilton RG, Eggleston PA, et al. Socioeconomic status and race as risk factors for cockroach allergen exposure and sensitization in children with asthma. J Allergy Clin Immunol 1996;97:1393–401.

37. Garcia DP, Corbert ML, Sublet JL, et al. Cockroach allergy in Kentucky: a comparison of inner city, suburban, and rural small town populations. Ann Allergy 1994;72:203–8.

38. Arlian LG, Bernstein D, Bernstein IL, et al. Prevalence of dust mites in the homes of people with asthma living in eight different geographic areas of the United States. J Allergy Clin Immunol 1992;90:292–300.

39. Sporik R, Holgate ST, Platts-Mills TAE, et al. Exposure to house-dust mite allergen (Der p I) and the development of asthma in childhood. N Engl J Med 1990;323:502–7.

40. Institute of Medicine. Clearing the air: asthma and indoor air exposures. National Academy of Sciences, January 19, 2000. Available on the World Wide Web (accessed February 3, 2009): http://books.nap.edu/catalog/9610.html.

41. Korsgaard J. Mite asthma and residency: a case-control study on the impact of exposure to house-dust mites in dwellings. Am Rev Respir Dis 1983;128:231–5.

42. Murray AB, Ferguson AC. Dust-free bedrooms in the treatment of asthmatic children with house dust or house dust mite allergy: a controlled trial. Pediatrics 1983;71:418–22.

43. Ehnert B, Lau-Schadendorf S, Weber A, et al. Reducing domestic exposure to house dust mite allergen reduces bronchial hyperreactivity in sensitive children with asthma. J Allergy Clin Immunol 1992;90:135–8.

44. Woodcock A, Custovic A. Allergen avoidance: does it work? Br Med Bull 2000;56:1071–86.

45. Platts-Mills TAE, Carter MC. Asthma and indoor exposure to allergens. N Engl J Med 1997;336:1382–4.

46. Pearce N, Pekkanen J, Beasley R. How much asthma is really attributable to atopy? Thorax 1999;54:268–72.

47. Pearce N, Douwes J, Beasley R. Is allergen exposure the major primary cause of asthma? Thorax 2000;55:424–31.

48. Kuehni CE, Davis A, Brooke AM, et al. Are all wheezing disorders in very young (preschool) children increasing in prevalence? Lancet 2001;357:1821–5.

49. Bernton HS, Brown H. Insect allergy – preliminary studies of the cockroach. J Allergy 1964;35:506–13.

50. Teague WG, Bayer CW. Outdoor air pollution: asthma and other concerns. Pediatr Clin North Am 2001;48:1167–83.

51. Koenig JQ. Air pollution and asthma. J Allergy Clin Immunol 1999;104:717–22.

52. Peden DB. Air pollution in asthma: effect of pollutants on airway inflammation. Ann Allergy Asthma Immunol 2001;87:12-7.
53. Holguin F. Traffic, outdoor air pollution, and asthma. Immunol Allergy Clin N Am 2008;28:577-88.
54. Strachan DP, Cook DG. Health effects of passive smoking. 6. Parental smoking and childhood asthma: longitudinal and case-control studies. Thorax 1998;53:204-12.
55. Chilmonczyk BA, Salmun LM, Megathlin KN, et al. Association between exposure to environmental tobacco smoke and exacerbations of asthma in children. N Engl J Med 1993;328:1665-9.
56. Evans D, Levison MJ, Feldman CH, et al. The impact of passive smoking on emergency room visits of urban children with asthma. Am Rev Respir Dis 1987;135:567-72.
57. Brownson RC, Jackson-Thompson J, Wilkerson JC, et al. Demographic and socioeconomic differences in beliefs about the health effects of smoking. Am J Public Health 1992;82:99-103.
58. Weiss KB, Gergen PJ, Crain EF. Inner city asthma: the epidemiology of an emerging US public health concern. Chest 1992;101:362S-7S.
59. Coultas DB, Gong Jr H, Grad R, et al. Respiratory diseases in minorities of the United States. Am J Respir Crit Care Med 1994;149:S93-S131.
60. Rona RJ. Asthma and poverty. Thorax 2000;55:239-44.
61. Mielck A, Reitmeir P, Wjst M. Severity of childhood asthma by socioeconomic status. Int J Epidemiol 1996;25:388-93.
62. Malveaux FJ, Houlihan D, Diamond EL. Characteristics of asthma mortality and morbidity in African-Americans. J Asthma 1993;30:431-7.
63. Lozano P, Connell FA, Koepsell TD. Use of health services by African-American children with asthma on Medicaid. JAMA 1995;274:469-73.
64. Nelson DA, Johnson CC, Divine GW, et al. Ethnic differences in the prevalence of asthma in middle class children. Ann Allergy Asthma Immunol 1997;78:21-6.
65. Ray NF, Thamer M, Fadillioglu B, et al. Race, income, urbanicity, and asthma hospitalization in California: a small area analysis. Chest 1998;113:1277-84.
66. Poma PA. The Hispanic health challenge. J Natl Med Assoc 1988;80:1275-7.
67. Carter-Pokras OD, Gergen JP. Reported asthma among Puerto Rican, Mexican American, and Cuban children, 1982 through 1984. Am J Public Health 1993;83:580-2.
68. New asthma estimates: tracking prevalence, health care, and mortality. National Center for Health Statistics, Asthma, October 2001. Available on the World Wide Web (accessed January 29, 2009): http://www.cdc.gov/nchs/products/pubs/pubd/hestats/asthma/asthma.htm.
69. Recent trends in health insurance coverage among Los Angeles County children. Los Angeles County Department of Health Services. LA Health 2000;3(1):October.
70. Bearison DL, Minian MA, Granowetter L. Medical management of asthma and folk medicine in a Hispanic community. J Pediatr Psychol 2002;27:385-92.
71. Zoratti EM, Havstad S, Rodriguez J, et al. Health service use by African Americans and Caucasians with asthma in a managed care setting. Am Rev Respir Crit Care Med 1998;158:371-7.
72. Newacheck PW, Stoddard JJ, Hughes DC, et al. Health insurance and access to primary care for children. N Engl J Med 1998;338:513-9.
73. Andrulis DP. Access to care is the centerpiece in the elimination of socioeconomic disparities in health. Ann Intern Med 1998;129:412-6.
74. Institute of Medicine. America's children: health insurance and access to care. Washington, DC: National Academy Press; 1998.
75. Vollmer WM, O'Hollaren M, Ettinger KM, et al. Specialty differences in the management of asthma: a cross-sectional assessment of allergists' patients and generalists' patients in a large HMO. Arch Intern Med 1997;157:1201-8.
76. Jatulis DE, Meng YY, Elashoff RM, et al. Preventive pharmacologic therapy among asthmatics: five years after publication of guidelines. Ann Allergy Asthma Immunol 1998;81:82-8.
77. Vilar ME, Reddy BM, Silverman BA, et al. Superior clinical outcomes of inner city asthma patients treated in an allergy clinic. Ann Allergy Asthma Immunol 2000;84:299-303.
78. Dales RE, Schweitzer I, Kerr P, et al. Risk factors for recurrent emergency department visits for asthma. Thorax 1995;50:520-4.
79. Crain EF, Kercsmar C, Weiss KB, et al. Reported difficulties in access to quality care for children with asthma in the inner city. Arch Pediatr Adolesc Med 1998;152:333-9.
80. Halfon N, Newacheck PW. Childhood asthma and poverty: differential impacts and utilization of health services. Pediatrics 1993;91:56-61.
81. Hanania NA, David-Wang A, Kesten S, et al. Factors associated with emergency department dependence of patients with asthma. Chest 1997;111:290-5.
82. Joseph CLM, Havstad SL, Ownby DR, et al. Racial differences in emergency department use persist despite allergist visits and prescriptions filled for antiinflammatory medications. J Allergy Clin Immunol 1998;101:484-90.
83. Stern RS, Weissman JS, Epstein AM. The emergency department as a pathway to admission for poor and high-cost patients. JAMA 1991;266:2238-43.
84. Leickly EF, Wade SL, Crain E, et al. Self reported adherence, management behavior, and barriers to care after an emergency department visit by inner city children with asthma. Pediatrics 1998;101:8.
85. Finkelstein JA, Brown RW, Schneider LC, et al. Quality of care for preschool children with asthma: the role of social factors and practice setting. Pediatrics 1995;95:389-94.
86. Busse WW, Mitchell H. Addressing issues of asthma in inner-city children. J Allergy Clin Immunol 2007;119:43-9.
87. Eggleston PA, Malveaux FJ, Butz AM, et al. Medications used by children with asthma living in the inner city. Pediatrics 1998;101:349-54.
88. Adams RJ, Fuhlbrigge A, Finkelstein JA, et al. Impact of inhaled antiinflammatory therapy on hospitalizations and emergency department visits for children with asthma. Pediatrics 2001;107:706-11.
89. Kelly CS, Morrow AL, Shults J, et al. Outcomes evaluation of a comprehensive intervention program for asthmatic children enrolled in Medicaid. Pediatrics 2000;105:1029-35.
90. Jones CA, Clement LT, Hanley-Lopez J, et al. The Breathmobile™ Program: Structure, implementation, and evolution of a large-scale, urban, pediatric asthma disease management program. Disease Management 2005;8:205-22.
91. Sperber K, Ibrahim H, Hoffman B, et al. Effectiveness of a specialized asthma clinic in reducing asthma morbidity in an inner city minority population. J Asthma 1995;32:335-43.
92. Battleman DS, Callahan MA, Silber S, et al. Dedicated asthma center improves the quality of care and resource utilization for pediatric asthma: a multicenter study. Acad Emerg Med 2001;8:709-15.
93. Evans III R, LeBailly S, Gordon KK, et al. Restructuring asthma care in a hospital setting to improve outcomes. Chest 1999;116:210S-6S.
94. Evans III R, Gergen PJ, Mitchell H, et al. A randomized clinical trial to reduce asthma morbidity among inner-city children: results of the National Cooperative Inner-City asthma study. J Pediatr 1999;135:332-8.
95. Persky V, Coover L, Hernandez E, et al. Chicago community-based asthma intervention trial: feasibility of delivering peer education in an inner-city population. Chest 1999;116:216S-23S.
96. Fisher EB, Strunk RC, Sussman LK, et al. Community organization to reduce acute care for asthma among African American children in low-income neighborhoods: the Neighborhood Asthma Coalition. Pediatrics 2004;114:116-23.
97. Carter MC, Perzanowski MS, Raymond A, et al. Home intervention in the treatment of asthma among inner-city children. J Allergy Clin Immunol 2001;108:732-7.
98. Wood RA, Eggleston PA, Rand C, et al. Cockroach allergen abatement with extermination and sodium hypochlorite cleaning in inner-city homes. Ann Allergy Asthma Immunol 2001;87:60-4.
99. Clark NM, Gong M, Schork MA, et al. Long-term effects of asthma education for physicians on patient satisfaction and use of health services. Eur Respir J 2000;16:15-21.
100. Jones CA, Clement LT, Morphew T, et al. Achieving and maintaining asthma control in an urban pediatric disease management program: The Breathmobile Program. J Allergy Clin Immunol 2007;119(6):1445-53.
101. Health Affairs 28, no. 1(2009):w1-w16 (published online 13 November 2008: 10.1377/hlthaff.28.1.w1).

38

Asthma in Older Children

Leonard B. Bacharier • Robert C. Strunk

Asthma is the most common chronic disorder of childhood, affecting approximately 9.1% of children 5 to 14 years of age,[1] with almost 6% of children in this age group reporting an episode of asthma or an asthma attack in the preceding 12 months.[1] However, estimates of wheezing in this age group approach 20% or greater in some areas of the USA and in many industrialized countries, further magnifying the impact of wheezing disease on children.

Epidemiology and Etiology

Prevalence of Childhood Asthma

In the USA, from 1980 to 2004, asthma prevalence in the general population increased from 3.1% to 7.1%, with increases from 4.4% in 1980 to 8.2% in 1995 and then 9.1% in 2004 in children 5 to 14 years of age.[1] Although the rise in asthma prevalence may reflect coding and classification issues, the influence of other factors, such as environmental exposures to allergens, infectious agents, endotoxin, vitamin D insufficiency, and tobacco smoke, must also be considered. Place of residence appears to influence asthma prevalence.[2] Furthermore, there appears to be an effect of gender on asthma prevalence, as the male-to-female ratio for asthma is 1.8:1 among children 2 years of age and under, but by puberty, asthma becomes more prevalent amongst females (M:F ratio of 0.8:1). The change in gender ratio is due to new cases of asthma developing in females during adolescence, not a decrease in males with asthma.[3]

Factors Influencing the Etiology of Asthma

A general pattern of factors influencing development of asthma seems to be emerging, including family history/genetics, smoking, diet, obesity, and inactivity, all of which seem to influence the development of asthma and disease outcomes (Table 38-1).

Socioeconomic Status

Many clinical or area studies have reported substantially higher rates of asthma prevalence, hospitalization, and mortality among racial and ethnic minorities. However, asthma is also most common among low socioeconomic groups, regardless of race. While black children have higher rates of asthma than white children, most studies have found that black race is not a signifi-

cant correlate of asthma after controlling for location of residence and socioeconomic status (SES). The basis for the effects of poverty and urban residence on asthma prevalence is not known. One potential factor is exposure and sensitization to allergens common in urban environments. Black children in inner city Atlanta are exposed to high levels of dust mite and cockroach allergen, and a high proportion of the children with asthma were sensitized to these allergens.[4] Litonjua and colleagues also concluded that a large proportion of racial/ethnic differences in asthma prevalence can be explained by factors related to income, area of residence, and level of education.[5]

Income is a determinant of access to healthcare, and frequently, the quantity and quality of healthcare available. Persons who have low income, regardless of race or ethnicity, are more likely to be uninsured, to encounter delays or be denied care, to rely on hospital clinics in emergency departments for health services, and to receive substandard care. The usual socioeconomic indicators, education and personal or household income, serve only as surrogates for more complicated correlates of individuals within populations and multiple factors that can impact both on prevalence of asthma and adverse outcomes from the disease.

Genetics

The genetic basis of asthma heritability has been extensively studied and the studies are yielding some understanding[6] (See Chapter 3). There is, as yet, no set genetic pattern that predicts presence of asthma or defines it severity.

Allergy

Studies by Williams and McNicol[7] of school children in Melbourne, Australia, have indicated both the increased incidence of asthma and asthma severity with increases in number of positive skin tests and total serum immunoglobulin E (IgE). The relationship between allergy and asthma has more recently been highlighted by the importance of aeroallergen sensitivity in the progression of frequent intermittent wheezing to persistent asthma in young children.[8] Several large epidemiologic studies have clearly indicated the importance of aeroallergen sensitization in asthma development among populations at risk. Sensitization to dust mite and mold was a predictor of asthma in rural Chinese individuals selected on the basis of having at least two siblings with physician-diagnosed asthma.[9] In a similar study, total serum IgE levels and positive skin tests to aeroallergens were correlated with current wheezing.[10] This association was present in children from nonatopic, asymptomatic probans, as well as in the expected atopic asthmatic probans, suggesting that

©2010 Elsevier Ltd, Inc, BV
DOI: 10.1016/B978-1-4377-0271-2.00038-9

Table 38-1	Factors that Influence Disease Development and Severity	
Factor	Disease Development	Disease Severity
Atopy	++++	++++
Allergen exposure	++	++++
Rhinitis	++	++
Sinusitis	?	+++
Infection (viral)	+	++++
Gastroesophageal reflux	−	++
Environmental factors		
Intrauterine tobacco smoke	++	?
Passive tobacco smoke	+	++
Air pollution	−	++
Psychological factors (including stress)	+	++++
Socioeconomic status	++	++++
Adherence	−	++++
Obesity	Adolescent females	++
Diet	?	?
Exercise	?	++*
Drugs (including ASA/NSAID)	−	++†

*While exercise is a common precipitant of asthma symptoms, improved physical conditioning can reduce asthma severity.
†Consider in the context of asthma, nasal polyposis, and severe sinus disease.

much of the increase in asthma prevalence is associated with specific IgE sensitization and is occurring in persons previously considered to be at low risk for developing asthma or atopy.

Demographic and Environmental Factors

Studies from Germany comparing the populations of East and West Germany have shown the prevalence of hay fever and asthma as significantly higher in West German children, suggesting that environmental factors explain the difference in prevalence in these ethnically similar populations.[11] Early exposure to infections (as with being in a daycare environment early in life) or exposure to endotoxin (as with growing up on a farm with close exposure to the farm animals) are associated with a decreased prevalence of asthma. In contrast, growing up in an urban environment or generally with an increased standard of living are associated with an increased prevalence of asthma[12] Such correlates are also present for atopic diseases other than asthma. In fact, Strachan, who noted that prevalence of hay fever was inversely related to family size, was the first to recognize the importance of early exposures on atopic disease.[13] In the USA, asthma is more prevalent in African-Americans and Puerto Ricans. These findings are not explained by the observations on the role of social class in European studies. Given the ethnic differences between African-Americans and whites, these studies may represent gene-by-environment interaction producing varied phenotypic outcomes.

Gene-Environment Interaction

Genetic factors cannot explain the rise in asthma prevalence, morbidity, or mortality.[14] However, a small change in the preva-

lence of relevant environmental exposures could explain a significant rise in disease prevalence among genetically susceptible individuals. Gene-environment interaction, defined as the co-participation of genetic and environmental factors, is particularly relevant to the etiology of asthma morbidity, especially in individuals who experience a disproportionate burden of environmental exposures.[15] Relevant exposures include smoking, stress, nutritional factors, infections, allergens, and occupational exposures. In addition, racial/ethnic variability in the distribution of genetic polymorphisms can potentially modify the response to pharmacotherapeutic agents, such as the β_2-adrenergic receptor.[16] A genetic polymorphism in the β_2-adrenergic receptor gene has been associated with asthma severity,[17] as well as with the susceptibility to develop asthma among individuals who smoked.[18]

Stress

Negative family characteristics such as family conflict and family dysfunction discriminated children who died of asthma from children with equally severe asthma who did not die.[19] Parenting difficulties have been associated with a higher risk for the development of asthma early in life.[20] In addition, children with the highest risk of developing early-onset asthma were those in families with both parenting problems and high stress. Evidence for a stress and asthma link has been demonstrated through temporal studies, as experiencing an acute negative life event increased children's risk for an asthma attack 4 to 6 weeks after the occurrence of the event.[21] Moreover, the combination of chronic and acute stress plays a role in the temporal association. Experiencing an acute life event among children who had ongoing chronic stress in their lives shortened the time frame in which children were at risk for an asthma attack to within 2 weeks of the acute event. The experience of daily life stressors is associated with same-day lower peak expiratory flow rate and greater self-report of asthma symptoms. Further, high levels of stress have been associated with detrimental biologic profiles, such as greater inflammatory responses after antigen challenge or in vitro stimulation of immune cells among children with or at risk for asthma.[22,23]

Children with asthma have been found to have higher rates of clinically significant family stress compared with healthy children.[24] Children whose families are more cohesive are more likely to have controlled, rather than uncontrolled, asthma.[25] Additionally, parenting difficulties early in a child's life, particularly during times of high stress, have been found to predict the onset of asthma in childhood.[20] Thus, strain in the family, both in terms of conflicts among family members and impact of illness on family relationships, could be associated with both increased asthma prevalence and poor asthma outcomes.

One psychological pathway that has been suggested to explain associations of SES with asthma is the differential experiences with stress that low and high SES children face. In healthy children, low SES has been associated with more frequent exposure to stressful life events, and children who live in low SES neighborhoods are more likely to report witnessing incidences of violence. Low SES also has been associated with more negative stress appraisals.[26]

Obesity

Obesity is linked with the development and severity of asthma in both children and adults, and weight reduction improves asthma severity and symptoms.[27,28] Similar to the results in industrialized countries, Celedon and colleagues found an association between overweight and presence of asthma or airway hyperresponsiveness among adults in China with either physician-diagnosed asthma or airway responsiveness to methacholine.[29] They also found an association between underweight (BMI 16 kg/m^2 or less) and asthma, which could be the result of an effect of asthma symptoms on nutrition or an effect of previous weight loss and development of asthma.

The relationship between obesity and asthma observed in adults has also been observed in adolescent females, but not males. Girls who were overweight or obese at age 11 years were more likely to have current wheezing at ages 11 and 15 years, but not at the ages of 6 to 8 years. The relationship between obesity and asthma is strongest among females beginning puberty before age 11 years. Females who became overweight or obese between 6 and 11 years are seven times more likely to develop new asthma symptoms at ages 11 and 13 years.[30] The mechanism of increased asthma with obesity is not clear. The strong gender differences observed[30,31] suggest that overweight status itself does not produce the asthma, as an effect directly attributable to weight should be seen in both boys and girls. Longitudinal studies[30] suggest that there is a more fundamental relationship as most of the asthma in obese adolescent girls was new onset asthma. In a study of young adults with asthma,[32] a lower level of physical activity did not explain the association between the incidence of asthma and gain in weight.

Infection

Viral respiratory infections are present in up to 85% of children with exacerbated asthma.[33] In addition to simply worsening asthma, there may be a more fundamental relationship between infection and presence of asthma. Such a relationship has been suggested by the finding of a higher than expected incidence of bronchial hyperresponsiveness in children who had whooping cough, croup, or bronchiolitis in their early years of life.[34]

The role of infections with *Mycoplasma pneumoniae* or *Chlamydia pneumoniae* in the underlying pathogenesis of asthma has been suggested (see Chapter 35). A conclusive association between development of *C. pneumoniae* or *M. pneumoniae* infection and onset of asthma, or even an association between the presence of the organism and more severe disease, remains to be established in large prospective studies.

Diet

Two independent birth cohorts have found that higher maternal intakes during pregnancy of vitamin D from both foods and supplements were associated with an almost 60% reduction of asthma and recurrent wheezing in children aged 3 to 5 years.[35,36] Some studies identified a relationship between a high dietary intake of vitamin C, A, and E with higher levels of lung function. A longitudinal analysis of decline in FEV-1 over a 9-year period in adults found the decline lower amongst those with a higher average vitamin C intake, but no relationship to magnesium or vitamins A or E.[37] The relationship between diet and atopy is not clearly understood, although there is some evidence for a relationship between concentrations of vitamin E and both allergen skin sensitization and IgE concentrations.[38]

Natural History of Asthma

Progression of Disease into Adulthood

More severe asthma can persist from childhood into adulthood without remission. Another important tendency in the natural history is for symptoms to remit in adolescence only to return again in adulthood. In general, the amount of wheezing in early adolescence seems to be a guide for severity in early adult years, with 73% of those with few symptoms at age 14 years continuing to have little or no asthma at age 28 years.[39] Similarly 68% of those with frequent wheezing at 14 years still suffered from recurrent asthma at age 28 years. Most subjects with frequent wheezing at 21 years continued to have comparable asthma at 28 years. In addition to the importance of symptoms in childhood, childhood degree of bronchial responsiveness in combination with a low FEV-1 were also related to the outcome of asthma in adulthood.[40] While many children become asymptomatic in adolescence, pulmonary function deficits associated with asthma and wheeze increase throughout childhood,[41] and a significant proportion of children free of symptoms and with normal FEV-1, and even FEV-1/FVC ratios, continue to have increases in bronchial reactivity.[42] This bronchial hyperresponsiveness is an independent risk factor for development of a low FEV-1 and associated symptoms in early adulthood.[43] What is perhaps most concerning about the persistence of childhood disease into adulthood is the development of chronic airflow obstruction, with loss of bronchodilator responsiveness[44] and a decline in FEV-1 over time greater than adults with asthma than asymptomatic peers.[45] These findings suggest that asthma, even uncomplicated by cigarette smoking, may be a precursor of a COPD-like syndrome in adults.

Duration of Disease is Associated with Degree of Abnormality in Pulmonary Function

Analysis of baseline data from the Childhood Asthma Management Program (CAMP) cohort demonstrated that longer duration of asthma was associated with lower levels of lung function in children with mild to moderate asthma aged 5 to 12 years. This association was independent of levels of atopy, presence of household allergens, and prior use of antiinflammatory medications. Duration of asthma was associated with lower levels of both pre- and postbronchodilator values for FEV-1 and FEV-1/FVC ratio.[46] While the values for FEV-1 both pre- and postbronchodilator were well within the normal range for children (93.9% predicted and 102.8% predicted, respectively), more than 50% of children with asthma had low FEV-1/FVC ratios, suggesting that airway obstruction was present and worsening even with duration of relatively mild-moderate asthma. The degree of bronchial hyperresponsiveness in these children was also related to duration of disease.[47] Since level of pulmonary function and degree of bronchial hyperresponsiveness are independent predictors of abnormal levels of lung function in adults who had childhood asthma, it is apparent that longer duration of disease in childhood is producing abnormalities of lung function predisposing adults to disease.

Morbidity and Mortality

In 2004, there were 2.4 million children aged 5 to 14 years, or 5.9% of this population group, with a self-reported asthma attack, with no decrease in prevalence since 1997[1] in spite of the much-improved therapies available. In this interval, the number of physician office visits for asthma doubled, from 1.7 to 3.3 million.[1]

Emergency department visits among children 5 to 14 years of age have increased approximately 15% from 1992 to 2004.[1] Rates among blacks are almost 3-fold higher than rates for whites. Asthma is the leading admitting diagnosis to children's hospitals,[1] and blacks have greater than 3-fold more hospitalizations than whites. Rates of hospitalizations in children aged 5 to 14 years have remained stable from 1980 to 2004, and are more than 3-fold lower than for younger children. A significant proportion of hospitalizations are repeat hospitalizations, with rehospitalization accounting for 20–25% of hospitalizations in a signal year and up to 43% of hospitalizations in one urban children's hospital within a 5- to 10-year period.[48] A lifetime history of hospitalizations was associated with family impacts (greater family strain and family conflict, greater financial strain), as well as caretaker characteristics of greater personal strain, beliefs about not being able to manage one's child's asthma.[49] Individual characteristics of the caretaker (lower sense of mastery, being less emotionally bothered by asthma) predicted greater likelihood of future asthma hospitalizations.[49]

The rate of deaths due to asthma in children aged 5 to 14 years increased more than 2-fold from 1980 (1.8 per million) to 1995 (3.4 per million) before stabilizing through 2002 (2.4 per million) and then decreasing in 2003 and 2004 to 2.6 per million.[1] Blacks have many more deaths than whites (2.9-fold in 2004). While death rate in children is relatively small compared to other age groups, physicians find that many, if not most, of these deaths are preventable with the major reason for death being late arrival associated with poor use of oral corticosteroids. Late arrival is often associated with psychological problems in the family or child, but can be associated with shortcomings in availability of medical care.

While there have been significant efforts toward understanding reasons that fatal and near-fatal asthma episodes occur, the identification of patients at risk for dying remains an art with no single set of criteria able to identify all patients who die. Prior history of severe events, especially respiratory failure requiring intubation, is an obvious risk factor. However, while as many as 25% of patients with a history of respiratory failure die in a 3- to 5-year follow-up, most patients who die have not had respiratory failure.[50] Most studies indicate that a high proportion of patients who have died have had severe asthma, but the number of patients with severe disease is large and only 1–3% will die over an extended follow-up period. The importance of psychological factors in poor outcomes from asthma[19] indicates that patient and family factors resulting in psychological dysfunction need to be identified as well.

There are certain time intervals when risk is increased. For example, patients may need extra care and communication in periods following hospitalization, as bronchial hyperresponsiveness persists after hospitalization much longer than abnormalities in spirometry, and oral steroids are being weaned, further increasing risk. Hospitalizations that occur in spite of optimally prescribed therapy are of special concern.

Differential Diagnosis of Asthma

The differential diagnosis of cough and wheeze is extensively reviewed in Chapter 35.

Evaluation

Figure 38-1 presents an algorithm for evaluation of a school-age or adolescent child who presents with chest symptoms of cough, wheeze, shortness of breath, chest tightness, or chest pain.

History

Historical elements should include specific symptoms, their frequency and severity, triggering factors, and response to therapy.

Age of onset of symptoms is important, as 80% of patients with asthma experience symptoms within the first 5 years of life. Thus, the adolescent presenting with recent onset of symptoms without a prior history warrants further evaluation of alternative diagnoses. Since asthma is a disorder characterized by repeated episodes of at least partially reversible airflow obstruction, failure of symptoms to improve with treatment including bronchodilators and corticosteroids should prompt evaluation for other processes, either a nonasthma diagnosis or a comorbid condition complicating underlying asthma.

A short series of questions focusing on recent symptom frequency is extremely informative in assessing the child with asthma. The Asthma Control Test (ACT) serves this purpose,[51,52] and when completed at each follow-up asthma visit, can serve as a rapid appraisal of asthma control over time.

Additional history should focus on identification of other comorbid conditions that may worsen asthma severity, including allergen exposure, rhinitis, sinusitis, and gastroesophageal reflux. Furthermore, an assessment of underlying psychosocial factors and adherence to medical regimen may provide valuable clues as to barriers in delivery and receipt of asthma care.

Physical Examination

Findings may include an increased anterior-posterior chest diameter in severe disease and expiratory wheezes and prolongation of the expiratory phase during exacerbation. Presence of nasal polyposis should prompt an evaluation for cystic fibrosis, regardless of the age of the child, as cystic fibrosis remains the leading cause of polyps in childhood. The primary focus of the exam should include careful evaluation to assure absence of findings suggestive of other diseases, such as the presence of crackles, digital clubbing, and hypoxemia, as well as to uncover factors that worsen disease, including nasal and sinus disease.

Laboratory Evaluation

Peripheral blood eosinophilia and/or elevated serum IgE levels are often found in children with asthma and can be helpful in evaluation of severe disease. Laboratory evaluation is helpful in excluding entities that comprise the differential diagnosis of asthma. Serum immunoglobulin levels (IgG, IgM, and IgA) may be helpful in evaluating for defects in humoral immunity predisposing to recurrent lower respiratory tract illness. Sweat chloride analysis is required to exclude cystic fibrosis. Children with bronchiectasis along with chronic otitis media and sinusitis may warrant an evaluation of ciliary structure and function. A purified protein derivative (PPD) skin test is helpful in excluding mycobacterial infection.

Allergy Skin Testing

Evaluation for allergen-specific IgE should be part of the evaluation of all children with persistent asthma, as proper identification of allergic sensitivities and instruction in environmental control measures may provide significant clinical benefit.

Radiology

All children with recurrent episodes of cough and/or wheeze should have a chest radiograph (anteroposterior and lateral views) performed to aid in exclusion of other diagnostic entities. Radiographic findings that may be seen with asthma include

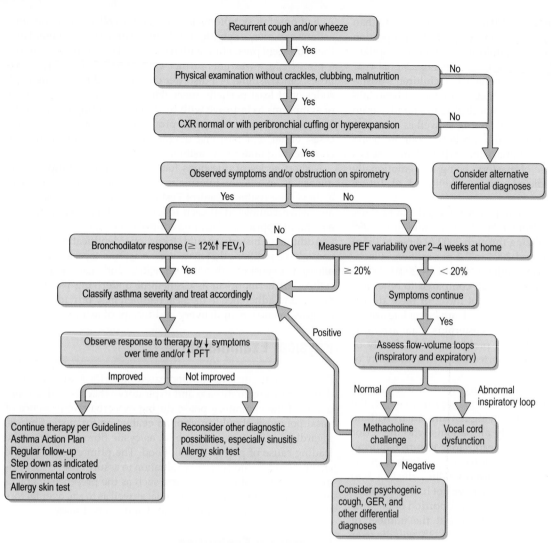

Figure 38-1 Algorithm for establishing diagnosis in children with recurrent cough and wheeze. *CXR*, chest X-ray; *FEV₁*, forced expiratory volume in 1 second; *PEF*, peak expiratory flow; *PFT*, pulmonary function test; *GER*, gastroesophageal reflux.

hyperexpansion, increased anteroposterior (AP) diameter, peribronchial cuffing, and areas of atelectasis (any lobe or subsegment can be involved). Findings of chronic changes, including bronchiectasis, should lead to further evaluation of alternate diagnoses.

Pulmonary Function Tests

With the help of well-trained and experienced pulmonary function technicians, children as young as 4 to 5 years of age should be capable of performing spirometry. Spirometry measures forced vital capacity (FVC), forced expiratory volume in 1 second (FEV_1), the ratio of FEV_1/FVC, as well as other measures of airflow including the forced expiratory flow between 25% and 75% of FVC (FEF_{25-75}). The FEV_1 is the most commonly used and reproducible measure of pulmonary function, whereas the FEF_{25-75} demonstrates much more intrapatient variability. Standards are widely available for most spirometric measures and allow for correction based upon patient age, gender, race, and height. The FEV_1/FVC ratio is an indicator of airflow obstruction and may be more sensitive in identifying airflow abnormalities in asthma than the FEV_1, as most children with asthma have FEV_1 within the normal range, even in the presence of severe disease (see the section on classification of asthma severity).

Asthma is characterized by airflow obstruction that is at least partially reversible by bronchodilator. Thus, spirometry is often performed before and 20 minutes following administration of a bronchodilator such as albuterol. An increase in the FEV_1 of at least 12% is considered to represent a significant change and exceeds that which is seen in nonasthmatic individuals.

Particular attention should be given to the inspiratory and expiratory flow-volume loops, as they are extremely helpful in excluding other patterns of airway obstruction.[53,54] For example, fixed airway obstruction (abnormalities on both the expiratory and inspiratory loops) can be seen with a mediastinal mass compressing a large airway or variable extrathoracic airway obstructive process (abnormalities just on the inspiratory loop) is seen with vocal cord dysfunction (VCD). Asthma produces variable intrathoracic obstruction (abnormalities on just the expiratory loop). Patients with VCD without asthma do not demonstrate intrathoracic airway obstruction, but may show blunting or truncation of the inspiratory loop consistent with variable extrathoracic obstruction. Variability between spirometric trials is not uncommon in patients with VCD, often consisting of normal and abnormal inspiratory loops during a single session.

In addition to spirometry, other tests of pulmonary function may aid in the evaluation of the child with asthma that is difficult to diagnose or control. Patients with asthma generally demonstrate normal total lung capacity (TLC) on lung volume testing by plethysmography, but may demonstrate evidence of air trapping as evidenced by elevated residual volumes (RV) and RV/TLC ratio. Measurement of diffusing capacity of carbon monoxide (DL_{CO}) is normal in patients with asthma, and abnormalities in DL_{CO} should prompt evaluation for interstitial lung diseases.

Challenge Testing

Some children present with atypical features of asthma and may pose greater challenges in confirming an asthma diagnosis. Thus, use of bronchial challenges with agents that provoke bronchoconstriction may be helpful in the diagnosis and management of the child with atypical symptoms, poor response to asthma medications, or lack of a response to bronchodilator during spirometry. Agents used for bronchoprovocation challenges include methacholine, histamine, adenosine, allergen, cold air, and exercise. Methacholine challenge has been widely used in epidemiologic and clinical trials of childhood asthma and has demonstrated an excellent safety record. Challenge studies should be performed in laboratories familiar with such procedures.

Bronchoscopy

In children with particularly severe disease or with poor response to conventional therapy, direct visualization of the airways along with bronchoalveolar lavage (BAL) may provide important clinical information. Such examinations may reveal the presence of previously undiagnosed foreign body aspiration or other intrinsic airway mass, infection, extrinsic airway compression, evidence of chronic aspiration, as well as indicators of airway inflammation (such as eosinophilia or neutrophilia).

Evaluation and Management of Factors that Increase the Severity of Disease

Overview

The most common precipitating factors are respiratory infections and weather changes. Drawing attention to these factors can help patients start increased treatment early in an exacerbation, as they will be looking for increasing symptoms that occur as an infection starts or as weather is changing rapidly. Exercise is also commonly identified as an exacerbating factor. Interestingly, although it is known that exposure to allergens and irritants can worsen asthma (see below), such exposures are much less commonly recognized as important.

Exposure to Inhalant Allergens

Exposure and allergic sensitization to cockroach was associated with a significantly greater risk of asthma hospitalization and greater healthcare utilization among 476 children aged 4 to 9 years who participated in the National Cooperative Inner-City Asthma Study.[55] Allergic sensitization to the mold Alternaria has been identified as a significant allergen in terms of increasing airway hyperresponsiveness[56] and was associated with a nearly 200-fold increased risk of respiratory arrest due to asthma,[57] emphasizing the importance of determining underlying allergic sensitivities in patients with asthma and providing patients with accurate and practical advice on allergen avoidance techniques.

The Childhood Asthma Management Program, comprised of 1041 children aged 5 to 12 years with mild-moderate asthma, found that allergic sensitization to tree pollen, weed pollen, Alternaria, cat dander, dog dander, or indoor molds was associated with greater airway hyperresponsiveness to methacholine.[58] A cross-sectional analysis of a birth cohort of 562 children studied at 11 years of age found that bronchial hyperresponsiveness significantly correlated with higher levels of total serum IgE.[59] Burrows and coworkers[60] found a close relationship between total serum IgE and both the severity and persistence of bronchial responsiveness in a longitudinal study of adolescents and adults. In CAMP, while sensitivity to tree, weed, Alternaria, cat, dog, and indoor mold allergens was associated with significantly increased sensitivity to methacholine, step-wise regression analysis indicated that only sensitivity to dog and cat dander and the outdoor fungus Alternaria had independent significant relationships. Together, these findings further the importance of control of these allergens in asthma symptoms.

A number of studies have followed children with asthma through childhood and adolescence into adulthood. Conclusions from the Melbourne, Australia study indicate that severity of asthma in adulthood is related to the presence of increased levels of atopy in childhood, with the presence of an atopic condition in childhood shifting the risk of asthma in later life toward more severe outcomes.

There is a clear association between sensitization to pets and current wheezing and bronchial hyperresponsiveness.[61] Dharmage and coworkers found that a high level of cat allergen in floor dust was associated both with an increased risk of being sensitized to cats and the presence of current asthma.[61] In the CAMP population, children sensitized to dog and exposed to high levels of dog allergen and sensitized to cat and exposed to high levels of cat allergen had a clearly increased risk of nocturnal awakenings.[62]

Two cohort studies provide evidence of a lower risk of asthma among children exposed to pets in early life compared with unexposed children.[63] Other studies find that individuals living with a pet have significantly less asthma or less severe bronchial hyperresponsiveness.[64] Studies showing protection from pet ownership are confounded by the likelihood that subjects with less severe asthma can keep the pets, whereas subjects with more severe disease are unable to hold pets.

Rhinitis

Rhinitis is common in children with asthma, with estimates of up to 80% of patients with asthma reporting upper airway symptoms. Whereas most rhinitis that worsens asthma is allergic, perennial rhinitis in nonatopic subjects can be a risk factor for more severe asthma.[65] Topical nasal steroid therapy for allergic rhinitis has also been shown to attenuate the increase in BHR during the grass pollen season[66] as well as decrease the risk of emergency department visits[67] or hospitalizations for asthma.[68] Thus treatment plans for patients with asthma and allergic rhinitis should consist of optimal management of concomitant allergic rhinitis (see Chapter 28).

Sinusitis

Sinusitis is often discovered in the search for factors responsible for an overall worsening of asthma unexplained by changes of environment or other obvious historical features. Although many of these patients present with symptoms of upper airway disease along with asthma, some have sinusitis as a significant contributor to difficult-to-control asthma with a paucity of symptoms suggestive of sinusitis.

Radiographic examination of the paranasal sinuses in children hospitalized for acute asthma exacerbations is positive in 30–60% of children, partly depending upon the diagnostic technique used (Water's view radiograph or computed tomography of the sinuses). The effect of antibiotic treatment of bacterial sinusitis on asthma control has been examined in several clinical studies, reducing asthma medication use, decreasing asthma symptoms, and improving bronchial hyperresponsiveness.[69,70] (See Chapter 35). Duration of antibiotic treatment should be individualized, but should continue until the patient is symptom-free for at least 7 days.

Gastroesophageal Reflux

Gastroesophageal reflux (GER) is common among patients with asthma, particularly adults, in whom the estimated prevalence of GER in asthma patients approaches 80%.[71] Studies of prevalence of GER in patients with asthma for the pediatric age group are limited, but include a 64% incidence of a positive pH probe study in a group of 25 children with asthma,[72] suggesting that GER may also be common among children with asthma.

In our experience, most young children and even adolescents with GER do not report symptoms classically associated with GER in adults, including heartburn, chest pain, dysphagia, or hoarseness. In fact, children rarely complain of symptoms even in the presence of significant GER demonstrated by pH probe studies. Thus, a high level of suspicion of underlying GER is necessary in the evaluation of the child with severe asthma, especially uncontrolled asthma associated with nocturnal symptoms. (See Chapter 41 on Severe Asthma for a more thorough discussion on diagnosis and management of GER.)

Environmental Exposures (Including Tobacco Smoke)

Passive exposure to tobacco smoke is a clear exacerbating factor in asthma, with increases in asthma prevalence and asthma severity among children exposed to parental smoking.[73] Maternal smoking is associated with small but statistically significant, and probably clinically important, deficits in pulmonary function among schoolchildren. Since most smokers begin smoking during the adolescent years, active personal tobacco smoke exposure must be considered in all adolescents with asthma, especially when the clinical course becomes more severe. Cigarette smoking has been reported to be associated with mild airway obstruction and slowed growth of lung function in adolescents without asthma.[74] Furthermore, asthma has been linked to an accelerated rate of decline in FEV_1 over time, and this rate is even greater among asthmatic individuals who smoke.[45]

Many patients report that their asthma is triggered by 'weather changes'. Weather changes may be accompanied by changes in airborne allergen exposures. However, multiple studies have failed to find a definitive link between airborne outdoor allergen levels (except for an occasional mold) and worsening asthma symptoms. Thus, the true link between weather changes and asthma attacks remains unknown. In addition to allergen exposure, epidemiological studies suggest an association between levels of air pollutants, including ozone, nitrogen oxides, carbon monoxide, and sulfur dioxide, and symptoms or exacerbations of asthma.

Vocal Cord Dysfunction

Vocal cord dysfunction (VCD), a functional respiratory tract disorder resulting from paradoxical adduction of the vocal cords, complicates the diagnosis and management of common respiratory tract problems, including asthma.[75] The recognition of VCD in a patient with atypical or difficult-to-control asthma is critical in minimizing symptoms and potential side-effects associated with treatment of severe asthma. The symptoms of VCD are not unique to the disorder and include cough, wheeze, stridor, dyspnea, hoarseness, and choking. Some patients report difficulty swallowing or tightness in the chest or throat. Patients with VCD often report difficulty 'getting air in' due to paradoxical adduction of the vocal cords during inspiration, in contrast to difficulty with exhalation as reported by asthmatics. However, patients with significant exacerbation of asthma do have diffuse airway narrowing and can have significant inspiratory limitation, which can dominate their perception of breathing difficulties. Cough is a common feature of VCD and must be differentiated from cough due to asthma or from postnasal drainage due to rhinosinusitis. Patients with VCD frequently complain of tightness in the throat and/or chest and may speak in a hoarse voice. Nocturnal symptoms are uncommon in uncomplicated VCD, but may occur in patients with both VCD and asthma. Exercise is a frequent precipitant of both VCD and asthma.

Upon presentation in an emergency department, increased work of breathing and decreased aeration caused by VCD can be difficult to distinguish from asthma. A recent report provides evidence that a normal level of oxygen saturation can be a clue that the cause of the distress is VCD rather than asthma.[76]

Spirometry and inhaled provocation challenges assist in the differentiation between VCD and asthma. Asthma typically produces abnormalities in the expiratory phase of the flow-volume loop, whereas VCD results in inspiratory loop abnormalities, such as blunting or truncation of the inspiratory loop due to variable extrathoracic airflow obstruction. Provocation challenges, either pharmacologic (methacholine or histamine) or exercise, are helpful in determining the presence or absence of airways hyperresponsiveness, a feature characteristic of asthma. Exercise challenges frequently reproduce the clinical symptoms and spirometric abnormalities consistent with VCD. If this approach fails to establish the diagnosis or if the patient does not respond to appropriate therapy, direct visualization of paradoxical vocal cord movement during symptomatic periods may be helpful in confirming the diagnosis of VCD. Characteristic findings include adduction of the true vocal cords during inspiration with a diamond-shaped opening at the posterior aspect of the glottis. Once the diagnosis of VCD has been established, attention should be focused toward reassurance and maneuvers directed at laryngeal relaxation (from speech therapy) and discovering underlying stress that is often involved in producing the problem (from psychology). In our experience, combining speech therapy and psychological evaluation is necessary for successful therapy for VCD. Maintenance therapy for VCD includes minimization of medication use for comorbid conditions frequently confused with VCD (i.e. asthma).

Psychologic Factors

Psychologic factors may be as, or even more important than medical factors in determining outcomes of asthma, particularly in children with more severe asthma. In a group of children with severe asthma, 50% had levels of fitness in the significant abnormal range.[77] Psychologic functioning as determined by structured interviews significantly correlated with cardiopulmonary function, but medical characteristics did not.[77] Similar to the findings in studies of fitness levels, school performance[78] and gross and fine motor coordination,[79] while generally in a normal range (in contrast to the findings of fitness), overall correlated with psychologic functioning but not medical characteristics of the asthma. Depression symptoms, cigarette smoking, and cocaine use occurred more frequently in adolescents reporting current asthma than in adolescents without asthma.[80] These results indicate a need to screen adolescents with asthma for depression.

At the level of characteristics of the individual caretaker, the beliefs that parents hold about their ability to manage their child's asthma, and the quality of life that they maintain while caring for a child with asthma, may be associated with asthma hospitalizations.[81] A health education intervention study conducted to improve asthma management skills and to build family self-confidence in the ability to manage asthma found that families that participated in the intervention reported better attack management strategies and preventive strategies compared to a control group.[82] Adults with asthma who have greater confidence or trust in the care they receive from their doctor report having better controlled asthma and are more likely to have mild, as opposed to severe, asthma.[83] Thus, parents who believe strongly that they cannot adequately care for their child's asthma may be more likely to bring their child to the hospital repeatedly for acute episodes.

Poor Adherence to Medical Regimen

Most patients receive suboptimal benefit from any given prescribed asthma regimen. This is often reflected as inadequate asthma control, and often leads to prescription of higher doses or additional controller medications based upon the assumption that the medication prescribed accurately reflects the medication the patient actually takes. However, since most patients miss substantial amounts of medications, even when participating in research studies examining medication adherence,[84] practitioners must focus on patient education regarding the importance of asthma medication use as directed and provision of a written plan of action which is practical for the patient. Complex regimens consisting of several medications given frequently during the day are less likely to be followed when compared to simple regimens with less frequent dosing requirements. When discussing asthma-related information and setting appropriate and achievable short- and long-term goals, excellence in communication between healthcare providers and patients is essential in establishing the foundation for asthma care and adherence to the recommended treatment approach.

The developmental level of the child complicates adherence in the pediatric population. Children's understanding of their asthma and the steps necessary to control the disease evolve over time. Thus, the action plan for each child must be individualized based upon the child's developmental stage. While children begin to acquire basic asthma skills decision-making abilities by the ages of 8 years, they remain unable to manage their asthma independently until about 16 years of age.

Obesity

Weight reduction in obese patients with asthma has been associated with improvement of lung function and other indicators of lung status[85] Similar to the importance of monitoring height in children with asthma, both as an indicator of general wellness

and effects of medications used to treat asthma, comprehensive care in children with asthma includes monitoring weight acquisition and encouraging weight reduction.

Exercise

Exercise-induced asthma (EIA) may lead to decreased participation in physical activities due to either exertional limitation or fear of symptom development. This may explain the finding that children with asthma are less physically fit than their nonasthmatic peers.[86] Despite these facts, asthma should not be perceived as a limitation on physical fitness, as evidenced by the prevalence of asthma among Olympic athletes approximating twice that of the general population.[87] Increased aerobic fitness decreases EIA, as better conditioned individuals require less increases in heart rate and ventilation for a given task.[86] Thus, although EIA may still occur, more physical work can be done before it begins (see Chapter 40).

Classification of Asthma Severity and Control

Asthma severity is currently classified as either intermittent or persistent disease (Table 38-2). While the distinction between intermittent and persistent disease, and even between the various levels of persistent disease, is arbitrary, it serves as a framework for severity classification and ultimately, treatment recommendations. Asthma severity is most easily assessed in a patient not receiving long-term control therapy and reflects the intrinsic intensity of the disease process. The assessment of asthma severity requires determination of morbidity in the domains of impairment and risk, where impairment reflects the frequency and intensity of symptoms and functional limitation experienced, and risk reflects the likelihood of asthma exacerbations. Four major features of asthma – daytime symptom frequency, nocturnal symptom frequency, interference with exercise, and pulmonary function – define levels of severity in the impairment domain, and exacerbations requiring systemic corticosteroids define severity in the risk domain. Nocturnal symptoms are a particularly important marker of more severe disease.[88]

Although most previous national and international guidelines provide lung function measures that are suggested as those which correspond to each level of asthma severity, these parameters do not appear to be entirely appropriate for the classification of childhood asthma, since most children with persistent asthma, even severe asthma, have FEV_1 measures within the normal range (≥80% predicted).[89] Current guidelines have improved on this by including the FEV_1/FVC ratio as an additional lung function parameter to help assess asthma severity.[88] Thus, clinicians and researchers should focus upon a combination of symptom frequency and medication use in assigning a level of asthma severity rather than relying solely on isolated measures of lung function (either FEV_1 or peak expiratory flow) as the primary determinants of asthma severity.

Once asthma therapy has been initiated, the ongoing assessment of asthma control becomes central to disease management. Asthma control is defined as the degree to which the manifestations of asthma are minimized by therapeutic intervention and the goals of therapy are met. Three levels of control (well controlled, not well controlled, and very poorly controlled) provide for gradations of control (Table 38-3) and emphasize the need to re-evaluate patients at every visit and adjust strategy if asthma is not well controlled or is very poorly controlled. The concepts of impairment and risk are central in determination of the level of

Table 38-2 Classification of Asthma Severity

		Intermittent		Persistent — Mild		Persistent — Moderate		Persistent — Severe	
		Age 5–11	Age ≥ 12	Age 5–11	Age ≥ 12	Age 5–11	Age ≥12	Age 5–11	Age ≥ 12
Impairment	Symptoms	≤2 days/week	≤2 days/week	>2 days/week but not daily	>2 days/week but not daily	Daily	Daily	Throughout the day	Throughout the day
	Nighttime awakenings	0	0	1–2/month	1–2/month	3–4/month	3–4/month	>1/week	>1/week
	Short-acting β_2 agonist use for symptom control	≤2 days/week	≤2 days/week	>2 days/week but not daily	>2 days/week but not daily	Daily	Daily	Several times per day	Several times per day
	Interference with normal activity	None	None	Minor limitation	Minor limitation	Some limitation	Some limitation	Extremely limited	Extremely limited
	Lung function	Normal FEV_1 between exacerbations; FEV_1 > 80% predicted; FEV_1/FVC > 85%	Normal FEV_1 between exacerbations; FEV_1 > 80% predicted; FEV_1/FVC normal	FEV_1 ≥ 80% predicted; FEV_1/FVC > 80%	FEV_1 < 80% predicted; FEV_1/FVC normal	FEV_1 60–80% predicted; FEV_1/FVC = 75–80%	FEV_1 > 60 but < 80% predicted; FEV_1/FVC reduced 5%	FEV_1 < 60% predicted; FEV_1/FVC < 75%	FEV_1 < 60% predicted; FEV_1/FVC reduced > 5%
Risk	Exacerbations (consider frequency and severity)	0–2/year		>2 exacerbations in 1 year					

Relative annual risk may be related to FEV_1.
Frequency and severity may fluctuate over time.
Exacerbations of any severity may occur in patients in any severity category

From National Asthma Education and Prevention Program. Expert Panel Report III: Guidelines for the diagnosis and management of asthma. Bethesda, MD: US Department of Health and Human Services; 2007.

Table 38-3 Classification of Asthma Control, ≥ 12 Years of Age

Components of Control		Classification of Asthma Control (Youths ≥ 12 Years of Age and Adults)		
		Well controlled	Not well controlled	Very poorly controlled
Impairment	Symptoms	≤2 days/week	>2 days/wk	Throughout the day
	Nighttime awakenings	≤2/month	1–3/week	≥4/week
	Interference with normal activity	None	Some limitation	Extremely limited
	Short-acting β₂ agonist use for symptom control	≤2 days/week	>2 days/week	Several times per day
	FEV₁ or peak flow	>80% predicted/personal best	60–80% predicted/personal best	<60% predicted/personal best
	Validated questionnaires			
	ATAQ	0	1–2	3–4
	ACQ	≤0.75	≥1.5	N/A
	ACT	≥20	16–19	≤15
Risk	Exacerbations (consider frequency and severity)	0–1/year	2–3/year	>3/year
	Progressive loss of lung function	Evaluation requires long-term follow-up		
	Treatment-related adverse effects	Medication side-effects can vary in intensity form none to very troublesome and worrisome. The level of intensity does not correlate to specific levels of control but should be considered in the overall assessment of risk.		

From National Asthma Education and Prevention Program. Expert Panel Report III: Guidelines for the diagnosis and management of asthma. Bethesda, MD: US Department of Health and Human Services; 2007.

BOX 38-1

The Goals of Asthma Treatment

Reducing Impairment

- Prevent chronic and troublesome symptoms (e.g. coughing or breathlessness in the daytime, in the night, or after exertion)
- Require infrequent use (≤2 days a week) of short-acting β2 agonist for quick relief of symptoms (not including prevention of exercise-induced bronchospasm)
- Maintain (near) normal pulmonary function
- Maintain normal activity levels (inducing exercise and other physical activity and attendance at work or school)
- Meet patients' and families' expectations of and satisfaction with care

Reducing Risk

- Prevent recurrent exacerbations of asthma and minimize the need for emergency department visits or hospitalizations
- Prevent loss of lung function; for children, prevent reduced lung growth
- Minimal or no adverse effects of therapy

Adapted from National Asthma Education and Prevention Program. Expert Panel Report III: Guidelines for the diagnosis and management of asthma. Bethesda, MD: US Department of Health and Human Services; 2007.

---

control. Similar to the assessment of asthma severity, the impairment domain for control includes daytime symptom frequency, nocturnal symptom frequency, interference with exercise, and pulmonary function while the risk domain includes exacerbations requiring systemic corticosteroids, progressive loss of lung function or reduced lung growth, or risk of adverse effects of medications. The incorporation of the use of standardized and validated tools to assess asthma control, such as the Asthma Control Test[51,52] and Asthma Control Questionnaire,[90] provide tools to identify and monitor patients whose level of asthma control falls below the goals of therapy, prompting consideration for adjustment of therapy.

To maximize the outcome of asthma therapy, goals must be high and be clearly communicated to the child and family. Achievable goals for nearly all children with asthma are outlined in Box 38-1. Routine re-assessment of patient attainment of these goals is a critical component of ongoing asthma care.

Perception of Bronchoconstriction

Presence of symptoms is an important determinant of severity determinations. Interpretation of symptom histories must be undertaken in the context of over-reporting in anxious individuals, under-reporting in children who do not want to be bothered by limitations that may be imposed if symptoms were fully reported, and under-reporting for children who do not perceive their level of bronchoconstriction, either acutely or chronically. The last of these possibilities is most worrisome because those asthma patients who have difficulty perceiving significant airway obstruction appear to be at risk for severe outcomes, such as hospitalization or even death. Review of studies in the literature on this subject do not provide clear guidelines on what patients to consider as possibly having inability to perceive bronchoconstriction, indicating that lung function should be measured at times of regular office visits and the relationship between level of lung function and current symptoms discussed. Finding of a discrepancy between the level of lung function and current symptoms can be an important part of the education and planning for future exacerbations as part of the visit; a child with no symptoms but with low lung function needs to be aware that any symptoms might mean severe problems are present. Such a child is one who might benefit from regular use of a peak flow meter, not stopping measurements when well as most children tend to do.

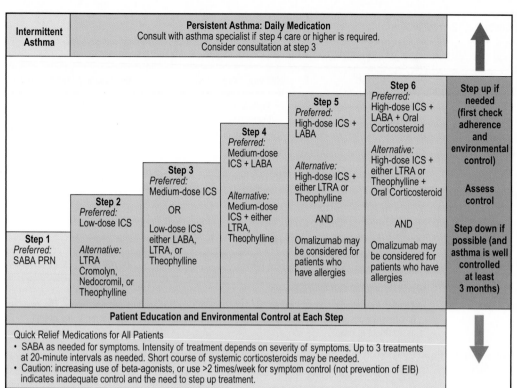

Figure 38-2 Step-wise approach for managing children 5 to 11 years of age with asthma. (From National Asthma Education and Prevention Program. Expert Panel Report III: Guidelines for the diagnosis and management of asthma. Bethesda, MD: US Department of Health and Human Services; 2007.)

Treatment of Childhood Asthma

Achieving optimal control of asthma requires a comprehensive approach that addresses the underlying pathophysiologic disturbances. Thus, in addition to the pharmacologic approach to asthma, one must minimize exposure to asthma triggers, including environmental allergens (see Chapter 26) and nonspecific airway irritants (such as tobacco smoke), and treat concomitant medical conditions which influence asthma severity (such as gastroesophageal reflux and rhinosinusitis). Equally important is providing asthma education, and support for the child and family for the process of chronic disease management.

Severity-Based Asthma Management

Once asthma has been diagnosed and a level of severity based upon the algorithm assigned, attention should be shifted toward the development of a comprehensive treatment plan. A central element to any treatment regimen is a written action plan, which provides the child and family with a clearly defined approach towards asthma management, including medications for routine daily use and a rescue plan for exacerbations, including medication modifications and signs of asthma symptom progression which should prompt contact with the healthcare provider or seeking of emergency care.

Pharmacologic Management

Currently, asthma medications are divided into two major categories – those that provide rapid relief of asthma symptoms (quick relievers) and those that serve to decrease airway inflammation and improve asthma on an ongoing basis (long-term controllers). The choice of medications for a given patient depends upon the level of asthma severity and control (Figure 38-2).

Intermittent asthma is managed with as-needed use of short-acting β_2 agonists by inhalation. However, all patients with persistent asthma should receive one, or potentially a combination of, controller medication(s) that possess antiinflammatory properties.

Controller Medications

The inflammatory nature of persistent asthma supports the use of medications aimed at decreasing, and ideally eliminating, airway inflammation. Thus, agents with antiinflammatory properties are essential in the treatment plan of all children with persistent asthma.

Inhaled Corticosteroids

Inhaled corticosteroids (ICS) are the most effective long-term controller medication for asthma in childhood. ICS therapy leads to significant improvement in asthma control as reflected by reductions in asthma symptom frequency and severity, exacerbation rates, hospitalizations, asthma death, quality of life and airway hyperresponsiveness. Short-term studies of ICS therapy have reported improvements in measures of lung function and reduction in inflammatory cells and other markers of inflammation within the airways.

The Childhood Asthma Management Program (CAMP), the largest and longest prospective clinical trial of ICS therapy in children, examined the effect of three treatment strategies in 1041 children with mild-to-moderate asthma.[91] Children received either (1) an inhaled corticosteroid (budesonide 200 µg bid), or (2) a nonsteroidal agent with antiinflammatory properties (nedocromil sodium 4 mg bid), or (3) a matching placebo for an average of 4.3 years of continuous therapy. All children received albuterol as needed for symptoms, and oral steroids for exacerbations. The primary outcome of the study was the FEV$_1$ after bronchodilator following a mean of 4.3 years of therapy. Children treated with ICS demonstrated an initial rise in FEV$_1$ over the first 6 to 12 months of the trial, but upon completion of the trial the ICS group and the placebo group did not differ in terms of FEV$_1$. Children who received ICS therapy experienced numerous clinical benefits not experienced by children who received placebo, including significant improvement in airway hyperresponsiveness, fewer asthma symptoms, less albuterol use, more days without an asthma episode, a longer time until need for oral corticosteroids for an asthma exacerbation, fewer courses of oral corticosteroids, fewer urgent care visits and hospitalizations, and less need for supplemental ICS therapy due to poor asthma control. The clinically meaningful improvements in control of asthma achieved during continuous treatment with inhaled corticosteroids do not persist after continuous treatment is discontinued.[92]

Evidence supporting ICS as the preferred maintenance therapy over montelukast in school-age children with mild persistent asthma (step 2) has come from several sources. A multi-center, randomized, double-blind trial demonstrated that clinical outcomes, pulmonary responses and inflammatory biomarkers improved more with fluticasone 100 µg twice daily compared to daily montelukast in children aged 6 to 17 years with mild-to-moderate persistent asthma.[93] The Pediatric Asthma Controller Trial (PACT), a year-long, randomized, double-blind trial in children aged 6 to 14 years with mild-to-moderate persistent asthma also demonstrated the superiority of the ICS fluticasone over montelukast therapy for asthma control days, exacerbations, quality of life, and pulmonary function.[94]

Guidelines for asthma management suggest that increasing levels of asthma severity or poor asthma control require increasing doses of ICS to achieve disease control. Several studies support a dose-response relationship for ICS. However, this relationship is nonlinear and is complicated by the dose–side-effect relationship. Low doses of ICS (as low as 200 µg/day of budesonide[95] or 50 µg bid of fluticasone propionate[96]) have been demonstrated to be effective in controlling asthma in children with persistent asthma. Furthermore, each child is likely to demonstrate his/her individual ICS dose-response relationship, as demonstrated in adults.[97] In addition, the rates of improvement of individual measures of asthma control vary, with symptom control and peak flow measures generally responding to low-dose ICS therapy within 2 to 4 weeks,[95] while treatment with higher doses for longer periods of time are necessary to maximize effect on airway hyperresponsiveness.[91] Thus, ICS dosing must be tailored to the individual patient's needs and response to therapy.

In general, ICS therapy is well-tolerated by the majority of patients. However, potential side-effects of ICS therapy include the effects of ICS upon skeletal growth and bone density, alteration of the hypothalamic-pituitary-adrenal (HPA) axis, local side-effects including oral candidiasis and hoarseness.

The effect of ICS therapy on growth during childhood has been extensively studied. However, many of the conclusions from these investigations are difficult to fully appreciate, as many studies are of short to intermediate durations (generally ranging from 8–12 weeks to 1 year). ICS therapy has been shown to result in short-term reductions in rates of linear growth in children, an effect which is most evident in prepubertal children. These effects are dose- and drug-dependent, with no significant effect on growth when low doses (100–200 µg/day of fluticasone propionate) are used for up to 1 year.[94,98] CAMP demonstrated that children receiving ICS therapy for 4 to 6 years grew 1.1 cm less than those receiving placebo. The growth effect was in the first year of treatment without additional effect as treatment continued. When adult height was predicted using standardized measures based upon current height, current age, bone age, and age at first menses (for females), the ICS-treated children and the placebo-treated children had similar projected final heights.[91] However, the effect of ICS therapy on growth persisted 5 years after regular ICS therapy was discontinued, with evidence that the effect is more pronounced in girls than boys.[92] Similar findings have been reported in other populations.[99-101] These results suggest that the effect of low-moderate dose ICS therapy on linear growth is transient and does not predict final adult height.

Numerous studies have examined the effect of ICS therapy on HPA axis function with conflicting results. While the available evidence suggests that low-moderate dose ICS therapy is generally not associated with alterations in HPA function,[102,103] the long-term effects of high dose ICS therapy in growing children remain unclear. The interaction between ICS use and bone mineral density (BMD) was studied thoroughly in CAMP; ICS therapy has the potential for reducing bone mineral accretion in male children progressing through puberty, although the ability of ICS to reduce the need for oral corticosteroid therapy (and the attendant reduction in BMD) largely outweighs this small risk.[104] The effect of high dose ICS therapy on BMD in growing children remains uncertain.

There has been some concern that ICS may cause the course of chicken pox to worsen, based upon case reports of death from chicken pox in individuals on high doses of *oral* steroids. There has been no case of death with ICS alone, but clinicians caring for children with persistent asthma should assure varicella immunity, either through prior natural infection or through vaccination, and be prepared to minimize ICS use, and add antiviral agents, should chicken pox occur in individuals on ICS.

Leukotriene Modifiers

The cysteinyl leukotrienes (LTC4/LTD4/LTE4) are mediators produced by eosinophils and mast cells and trigger many processes central to asthma – mucus secretion, bronchoconstriction, and increased vascular permeability. The clinical effects of agents which modulate leukotriene activity confirm the role of these mediators in the pathophysiology of asthma. Clinical trials have demonstrated the positive effects of LT antagonism on pulmonary function and clinical outcomes in children with asthma.[105]

Montelukast, a selective leukotriene receptor 1 antagonist, improved pulmonary function, reduced rescue albuterol use, improved quality of life, and decreased peripheral blood eosinophil counts over an 8-week period in children 6 to 14 years of age with moderate asthma compared with placebo.[105] Montelukast has also been shown to inhibit exercise-induced bronchoconstriction in children with mild-moderate asthma.[106] In addition to having positive effects as monotherapy, Leukotriene modifiers (LTMs) appear to have additive properties when given with ICS.[107,108]

The inflammatory nature of asthma currently demands that controller medications possess antiinflammatory properties. While the data regarding the antiinflammatory attributes of LTMs is limited compared to ICS, several studies strongly suggest that these agents decrease markers of allergic airway inflammation, including peripheral blood[105] and sputum eosinophils,[109] nitric oxide in exhaled air,[110,111] bronchial hyperreactivity,[112] and cellular infiltrates in bronchoalveolar lavage fluid following segmental allergen challenge.[113]

While the long-term effects of antileukotriene therapy are unknown, these agents possess desirable clinical and biological properties and deserve consideration in children with all levels of persistent asthma. These agents have excellent safety records in children and the oral delivery system makes these agents easy to administer to children. Recent trials have demonstrated that school-age children with mild-moderate persistent asthma receiving ICS therapy experience greater improvements in pulmonary function, albuterol use, and symptom control than patients receiving LTRA therapy.[94,114] Based upon these data, current Guidelines support the use of LTRA as an alternative to ICS as monotherapy in mild persistent asthma as well as adjunctive therapy in moderate-severe asthma.[88]

Long-Acting β agonists

Two long-acting β$_2$-adrenergic agonists (LABAs), salmeterol and formoterol, have been demonstrated to be safe and effective agents in children, both in terms of bronchodilation and prevention of exercise-induced bronchospasm. Their onsets of action differ, with formoterol having an onset similar to albuterol (3 minutes), while salmeterol has a slower onset of action (10–20 minutes). Following a single-dose administration, both agents demonstrate durations of action up to 12 hours. Following regular twice-daily administration, bronchodilation remains effective; however, a level of tolerance (or tachyphylaxis) develops, manifested as a loss of bronchoprotective properties to stimuli, such as exercise, methacholine, and allergen, although the clinical relevance of these findings is unclear.

The complementary actions of ICS and LABAs suggest that these agents should be effective when used in combination. Extensive data in adults confirm the superiority of the addition of a LABA to patients uncontrolled on ICS compared to increasing the dose of ICS alone.[115] However, such data are lacking in the pediatric population. The PACT trial also included a combination therapy arm consisting of fluticasone (100 μg once daily) plus the LABA salmeterol (50 μg twice daily).[94] This combination

of once-daily ICS therapy plus twice-daily LABA was associated with comparable asthma control to the twice-daily fluticasone approach in terms of the proportion of asthma control days and Asthma Control Questionnaire scores, but was inferior to fluticasone alone in terms of changes in lung function, airway hyperresponsiveness, and exhaled nitric oxide levels. Among children with asthma inadequately controlled by ICS alone, the addition of LABA led to improved lung function and symptom control compared to placebo.[116] In contrast, one study found no advantage with the addition of salmeterol to low-dose ICS therapy compared with a doubling of ICS dose in children with mild-moderate asthma.[117] Studies in adults also suggest that LABAs may facilitate ICS reduction in patients whose asthma is controlled on a moderate-to-high dose of ICS.[89,118] However, there is no evidence to date that the addition of a LABA to ICS therapy reduces significant asthma exacerbations in children.[119] The addition of LABA therapy may increase the risk of rare life-threatening or fatal asthma exacerbations, and thus should be carefully considered in children with asthma inadequately controlled with ICS therapy alone.[88] More clinical trials are necessary to fully determine the role of LABAs in the management of persistent asthma in childhood. However, the compelling evidence of the efficacy of ICS plus LABA therapy in older children and adults has led to the recommendation for the use of a combination of ICS and LABAs as preferred therapy in children 5 years of age and older whose asthma severity and/or control indicate the need for step 4 care (See Figure 38-3).[88]

Cromolyn and Nedocromil

Cromolyn sodium and nedocromil sodium are inhaled agents that are alternatives to ICS in the management of mild persistent asthma in children. Both drugs have been shown to possess antiinflammatory properties through nonsteroidal mechanisms, although the exact mechanisms for their actions remain unclear.

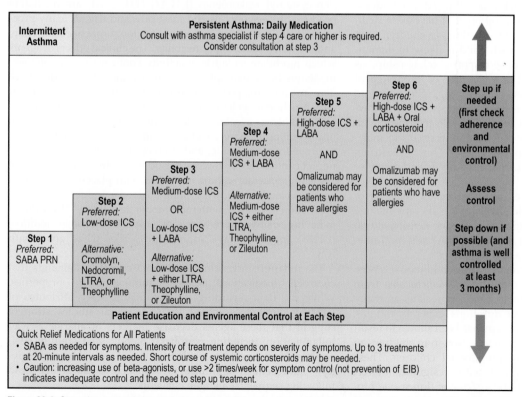

Figure 38-3 Step-wise approach for managing children ≥12 years of age with asthma. (From National Asthma Education and Prevention Program. Expert Panel Report III: Guidelines for the diagnosis and management of asthma. Bethesda, MD: US Department of Health and Human Services; 2007.)

Both agents are effective in the short-term prevention of exercise-induced bronchospasm. Several clinical trials have suggested beneficial effects with regular administration of cromolyn, although a meta-analysis suggests that there is insufficient evidence to support the use of cromolyn as maintenance therapy for asthma.[120] Nedocromil (8 mg/day) therapy for approximately 4 years in children with mild-moderate asthma resulted in a reduction in oral corticosteroid use and urgent care visits for asthma compared to placebo/albuterol for symptoms only, but did not affect lung function or rescue albuterol use compared with placebo.[91] These agents are generally well tolerated, with cough, sore throat and bronchoconstriction being the most common side-effects to cromolyn. Nedocromil is more commonly associated with bad taste, headache, and nausea than cromolyn.

Theophylline

Theophylline acts as an inhibitor of phosphodiesterase, although at therapeutic serum levels phosphodiesterase inhibition is weak yet bronchodilation occurs. Theophylline also inhibits the effects of adenosine, a molecule known to induce airway narrowing.

Theophylline is more effective than placebo in controlling asthma symptoms and pulmonary function, and is particularly effective in preventing nocturnal asthma symptoms. Current guidelines suggest theophylline as an alternative to ICS in children with mild persistent asthma and as an add-on therapy with a low-dose ICS in children with moderate-severe asthma.[88] Patients may experience deterioration of asthma control following withdrawal of theophylline from their regimen.[121,122]

Theophylline has the potential for significant toxicity occurring with increasing serum concentrations. The benefits of theophylline may be recognized at lower serum levels than previously recommended (a target range of 5–15 µg/mL).[88] Serum drug level monitoring is needed with doses above 12 mg/kg or if side-effects occur. Theophylline metabolism is age dependent, with younger children having greater rates of metabolism than older children and adolescents. Drug interactions may lead to decreased theophylline metabolism, and thus increased serum levels (such as macrolide antibiotics [erythromycin, clairithromycin], cimetidine, ciprofloxacin) or increased theophylline metabolism, and thus lower serum levels (such as carbamazepine, phenobarbital, phenytoin, and rifampin). Febrile illnesses may result in decreased theophylline clearance, whereas tobacco and marijuana smoking result in accelerated clearance. Side-effects of theophylline are often dose dependent and include anorexia, nausea, emesis, and headache. The effects of theophylline on psychomotor functioning and school performance have been examined and have generally shown no significant negative effect of theophylline on learning or behavior.[123]

Allergen Immunotherapy

Specific immunotherapy (SIT) is the repetitive parenteral injection of allergen extracts to reduce the manifestations of allergy caused by natural exposure to those allergens.

Although there is agreement that SIT offers clinical benefits to patients with allergic rhinitis, the role of SIT in asthma management remains controversial.[124,125] Clinical trials of SIT for asthma pose methodologic challenges, including the need for lengthy study durations, the difficulty of maintaining blinding, and the need for a multidimensional assessment of outcome. Nevertheless, a recent Cochrane Database review of randomized controlled trials of SIT in asthma[126] showed that SIT led to a significant reduction in asthma symptoms and medication requirement as well as improvement in specific and nonspecific bronchial responsiveness. Pulmonary function, however, was not consistently improved. Despite this evidence of efficacy, the benefit of SIT relative to other asthma therapies remains controversial, especially among multiply-sensitized asthmatics without prominent allergic rhinitis.[127]

SIT of monosensitized children may prevent the development of both additional sensitivities and asthma.[124] Specific immunotherapy to pollens in children aged 6 to 14 years with allergic rhinoconjunctivits without asthma led to fewer asthma symptoms after 3 years of therapy, suggesting that SIT can reduce the development of asthma in children with seasonal allergic rhinoconjuctivitis.[128]

Omalizumab

A humanized monoclonal antibody directed against IgE (anti-IgE or omalizumab) rapidly and significantly reduces circulating levels of IgE. Repeated subcutaneous administration of omalizumab has been demonstrated to be safe[129] and effective in permitting reduction of ICS dosing while preventing asthma exacerbations in placebo-controlled trials in both adults[130] and children[131] with moderate-severe persistent allergic asthma receiving ICS, as well as improving asthma-related quality of life.[132] Omalizumab is currently approved as an adjunctive therapy for children 12 years of age and older with moderate-severe persistent allergic asthma whose symptoms are inadequately controlled with ICS therapy, and the NAEPP Guidelines support its use when step 5 or 6 care is indicated.[88]

Quick Reliever Medications
β₂-Adrenergic Agonists

Rapid acting inhaled β_2-adrenergic receptor agonists are the most effective bronchodilator agents currently available and serve as the preferred treatment for acute symptoms and exacerbations of asthma as well as the prevention of exercise-induced asthma. These agents stimulate the β_2-adrenergic receptors located on bronchial smooth muscle and trigger a signaling cascade culminating in the generation of intracellular cyclic adenosine monophosphate (cAMP). In addition to relaxation of airway smooth muscle, β_2 agonists stimulate mucocilliary transport, modulate the release of mast cell mediators, and decrease edema formation.

β_2 agonists are available for inhalation (by metered dose inhalers and nebulizers), oral administration (syrup and sustained release tablets), and parenteral (subcutaneous and intravenous) administration. Inhalation is the preferred route of delivery, as it maximizes efficacy and minimizes side-effects. Several different β_2 agonists are currently available, and have comparable efficacy and safety properties. The single isomer preparation of albuterol, levalbuterol, has the theoretical advantage of possessing bronchodilatory properties (R-isomer of albuterol) without the presence of the nonbronchodilatory isomer (S-albuterol). Clinical trials with this agent demonstrate minimal, clinically relevant differences in bronchodilation or side-effects related to β-adrenergic receptor stimulation, such as tachycardia, tremor, and decreases in serum potassium levels compared to racemic albuterol.[133]

Anticholinergic Agents

Potential mechanisms by which cholinergic pathways contribute to asthma pathophysiology include bonchoconstriction through increased vagal tone, increased reflex bronchoconstriction due to stimulation of airway sensory receptors, and increased acetylcholine release induced by inflammatory mediators.[134] Patients with asthma experience lesser degrees of bronchodilation with

Follow this plan for After Hours patients only. Nurse may decide not to follow this home management plan if:
• Parent does not seem comfortable with or capable of following plan
• Nurse is not comfortable with this plan, based on situation and judgment
• Nurse's time does not allow for callbacks
In all cases, tell parent to call 9-1-1 if signs of respiratory distress occur during the episode
NOTE: If action plan has already been attempted without success, go to "RED ZONE - poor response" or "YELLOW ZONE - incomplete response" as symptoms indicate.

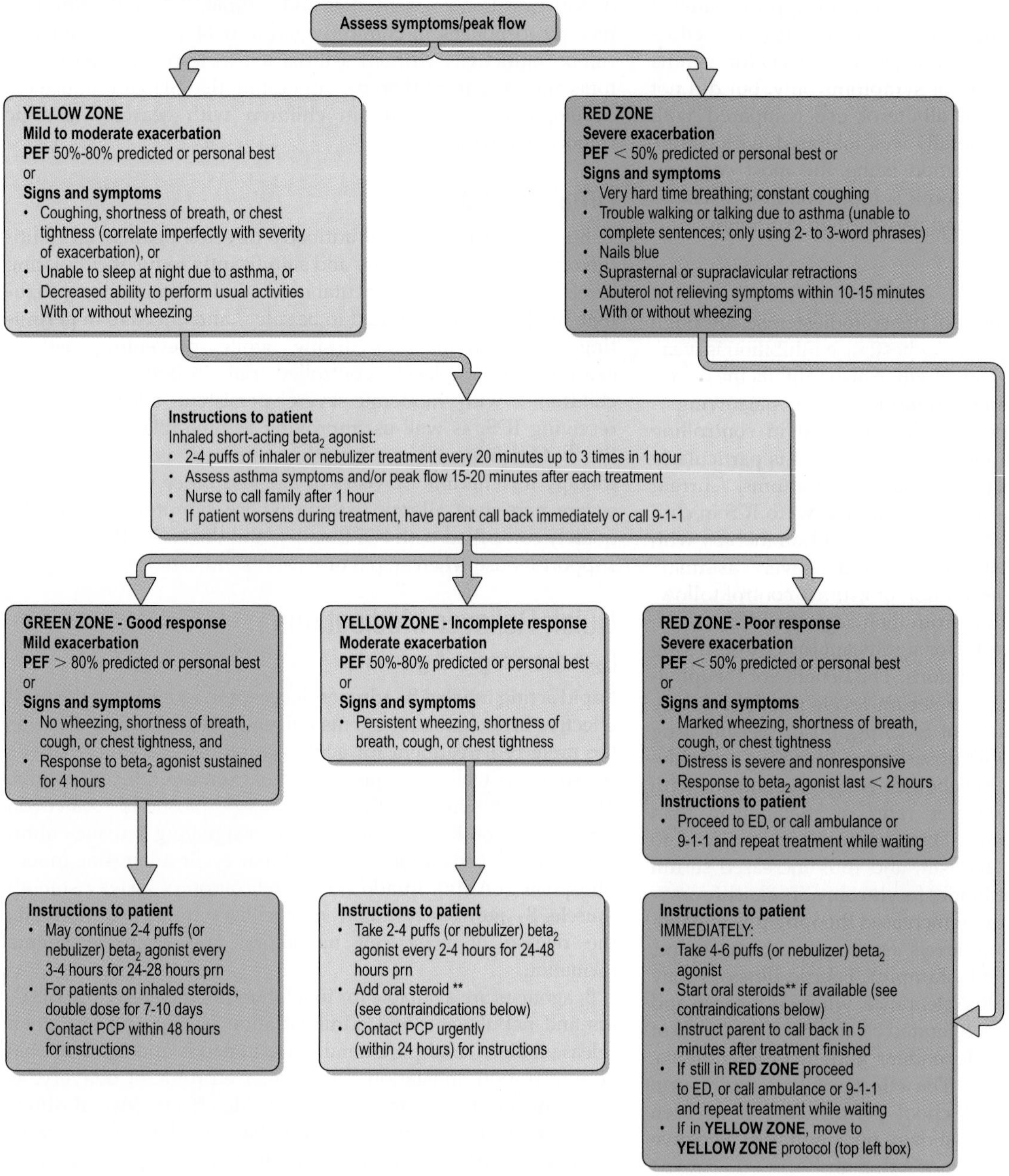

Assess symptoms/peak flow

YELLOW ZONE
Mild to moderate exacerbation
PEF 50%-80% predicted or personal best
or
Signs and symptoms
• Coughing, shortness of breath, or chest tightness (correlate imperfectly with severity of exacerbation), or
• Unable to sleep at night due to asthma, or
• Decreased ability to perform usual activities
• With or without wheezing

RED ZONE
Severe exacerbation
PEF < 50% predicted or personal best or
Signs and symptoms
• Very hard time breathing; constant coughing
• Trouble walking or talking due to asthma (unable to complete sentences; only using 2- to 3-word phrases)
• Nails blue
• Suprasternal or supraclavicular retractions
• Abuterol not relieving symptoms within 10-15 minutes
• With or without wheezing

Instructions to patient
Inhaled short-acting beta₂ agonist:
• 2-4 puffs of inhaler or nebulizer treatment every 20 minutes up to 3 times in 1 hour
• Assess asthma symptoms and/or peak flow 15-20 minutes after each treatment
• Nurse to call family after 1 hour
• If patient worsens during treatment, have parent call back immediately or call 9-1-1

GREEN ZONE - Good response
Mild exacerbation
PEF > 80% predicted or personal best
or
Signs and symptoms
• No wheezing, shortness of breath, cough, or chest tightness, and
• Response to beta₂ agonist sustained for 4 hours

YELLOW ZONE - Incomplete response
Moderate exacerbation
PEF 50%-80% predicted or personal best
or
Signs and symptoms
• Persistent wheezing, shortness of breath, cough, or chest tightness

RED ZONE - Poor response
Severe exacerbation
PEF < 50% predicted or personal best
or
Signs and symptoms
• Marked wheezing, shortness of breath, cough, or chest tightness
• Distress is severe and nonresponsive
• Response to beta₂ agonist last < 2 hours
Instructions to patient
• Proceed to ED, or call ambulance or 9-1-1 and repeat treatment while waiting

Instructions to patient
• May continue 2-4 puffs (or nebulizer) beta₂ agonist every 3-4 hours for 24-28 hours prn
• For patients on inhaled steroids, double dose for 7-10 days
• Contact PCP within 48 hours for instructions

Instructions to patient
• Take 2-4 puffs (or nebulizer) beta₂ agonist every 2-4 hours for 24-48 hours prn
• Add oral steroid ** (see contraindications below)
• Contact PCP urgently (within 24 hours) for instructions

Instructions to patient
IMMEDIATELY:
• Take 4-6 puffs (or nebulizer) beta₂ agonist
• Start oral steroids** if available (see contraindications below)
• Instruct parent to call back in 5 minutes after treatment finished
• If still in **RED ZONE** proceed to ED, or call ambulance or 9-1-1 and repeat treatment while waiting
• If in **YELLOW ZONE**, move to **YELLOW ZONE** protocol (top left box)

* Documentation faxed or given to PCP within 24 hours; phone or verbal contact sooner as indicated.
** Ask patient if preexisting conditions exist that may be contraindications to oral steroids (including type 1 diabetes, active chicken pox, chicken pox exposure or varicella vaccine within 21 days, MMR within 14 days). If so, nurse to contact PCP before initiating steroids. Oral steroid dosages: Child: 2 mg/kg/day, maximum 60 mg/day, for 5 days.

Date: _____

Signature _____

Figure 38-4 Algorithm for treatment of acute asthma symptoms. *PEF*, peak expiratory flow; *ED*, emergency department; *PCP*, primary care physician. (Courtesy of BJC Health System/Washington University School of Medicine, Community Asthma Program, January 2000.)

anticholinergic agents (such as atropine and ipratropium bromide) than with β₂ agonists. There is presently no indication for anticholinergic agents as a component for long-term asthma control. Evidence supports the use of ipratropium bromide in conjunction with inhaled β₂ agonists in the emergency depart-ment during acute exacerbations of asthma in children.[135,136] This effect is most evident in patients with very severe exacerbations. Addition of ipratropium has been shown to decrease rates of hospitalization[135] and duration of time in the emergency department.[136]

Systemic Corticosteroids

Systemic steroids are valuable in gaining control of asthma symptoms in patients under poor control. Although the onset of action of systemic corticosteroids is less rapid than inhaled bronchodilators, there is evidence that corticosteroids have a more rapid onset of action than that suggested by their primary mechanisms of action, namely inhibiting the function of inflammatory cells and the secretion of cytokines, chemokines and other proinflammatory mediators. Corticosteroids rapidly upregulate β_2-adrenoreceptor number and improve receptor function, likely leading to clinical improvement within 4 hours of administration.

Systemic corticosteroids hasten the resolution of acute exacerbations of asthma. Corticosteroid administration in the emergency department decreases admission rates for asthma[137] and shortens the length of stay in hospital. Dosing recommendations for acute asthma range from 1 to 2 mg/kg of body weight per day of prednisone. There is no significant difference in the efficacy of oral or parenteral corticosteroids in acute asthma,[138] unless the child is unable to tolerate oral medications due to vomiting. Given the well-described side-effect profile of repeated or continuous use of systemic corticosteroids, dosing should always be minimized. Rare patients with severe asthma may require regular steroid therapy to gain or maintain disease control. In these situations, alternate day dosing is associated with fewer adverse effects, but a very small percentage of patients with severe disease may still require daily steroid administration. Side-effects associated with chronic steroid use in severe asthma include hypertension, cushingoid features, decreased AM serum cortisol levels, osteopenia, growth suppression, obesity, hypercholesterolemia and cataracts.[139] There is no evidence for clinically significant HPA axis suppression following short 'bursts' of systemic steroids for acute exacerbations of asthma, and tapering is not required with courses of 10 to 14 days or less in duration. Furthermore, there is no evidence for increased susceptibility to common acute infections.[140]

Management of Acute Asthma Episodes

Asthma exacerbations occur frequently and may occur even in the context of regular use of long-term controller therapy. Most exacerbations, especially those that are mild in nature, can generally be managed without difficulty at home. However, success in out-patient care of acute asthma demands excellent preparation, including a written set of instructions to help guide patients and their families. The Asthma Action Plan is the central component for home asthma management. Patients must be instructed as to the early and accurate recognition of changes in asthma status, as early intervention is likely to lessen the severity and rate of progression of the episode. An algorithm which serves as the basis for the action plan and allows for telephone triage and recommendations is shown in Figure 38-4.

At the onset of asthma symptoms, including cough, chest tightness, wheeze, shortness of breath, or with a decline in peak expiratory flow (PEF) below 80% of personal best, initial therapy should include administration of a rapid-acting bronchodilator such as albuterol, either via metered dose inhaler (with a spacer device) or nebulizer. This treatment may be repeated up to three times in the first hour, with PEF measured before and after each albuterol administration. Patients who demonstrate rapid improvement following this intervention should be closely followed over the ensuing hours and days for signs of recurrence of symptoms, with particular attention to nocturnal awakenings. Given the potential for progression of symptoms, addition (or

---

increasing the dose) of an inhaled corticosteroid is often recommended. Increased use is continued until baseline status is achieved, and then for an additional 7 to 10 days because of the time needed for resolution of the increased inflammation produced during the exacerbation. Failure of this rescue approach to markedly reduce symptoms and improve PEF to >80% personal best should lead to institution of systemic corticosteroids. Several protocols for administration of oral corticosteroids are used commonly. One such approach is to give prednisone, 2 mg/kg/day (up to 60 mg), for 5 days. The approach used in the CAMP trial, 2 mg/kg/day (up to 60 mg) for 2 days followed by 1 mg/kg/day (up to 30 mg) for 2 days,[141] decreases overall steroid exposure and was very effective in resolving exacerbations in patients with mild to moderate asthma. This should be accompanied by frequent reassessment of clinical status and PEF as well as albuterol every 4 to 6 hours, more frequently if needed. Patients who do not improve with this approach are experiencing moderate-severe exacerbation and may need further evaluation and intervention, generally in the physician's office or in the emergency department. Signs of worsening respiratory distress should prompt emergent evaluation and therapy.

Conclusions

Asthma can significantly impact on the quality of life of both children and their families. Careful attention to details of determination of severity and applying an appropriate therapeutic regimen can bring about control of asthma symptoms in almost all children (see Box 38-2). In determining severity and applying the appropriate regimen, it is essential to establish good communication about the goals of therapy and understand the family dynamics to assure that the family can adhere to the therapeutic regimen prescribed. Ongoing evaluation based on communication of current symptoms, with regular assessment of the family's ability to adhere to therapeutic recommendations and the appropriateness of recommendations is necessary for long-term control of the disease and minimizing side-effects of medications. Review of actions to take during exacerbation, using the Asthma Action Plan as the central mechanism of communication, is part of regular visits for asthma.

References

1. Moorman JE, Rudd RA, Johnson CA, et al. National surveillance for asthma–United States, 1980–2004. MMWR Surveill Summ 2007;56:1–54.
2. von Mutius E. Allergies, infections and the hygiene hypothesis: the epidemiological evidence. Immunobiology 2007;212:433–9.
3. Mandhane PJ, Greene JM, Cowan JO, et al. Sex differences in factors associated with childhood- and adolescent-onset wheeze. Am J Respir Crit Care Med 2005;172:45–54.
4. Call RS, Smith TF, Morris E, et al. Risk factors for asthma in inner city children. J Pediatr 1992;121:862–6.
5. Litonjua AA, Carey VJ, Weiss ST, et al. Race, socioeconomic factors, and area of residence are associated with asthma prevalence. Pediatr Pulmonol 1999;28:394–401.
6. Vercelli D. Discovering susceptibility genes for asthma and allergy. Nat Rev Immunol 2008;8:169–82.
7. Williams H, McNicol KN. Prevalence, natural history, and relationship of wheezy bronchitis and asthma in children: an epidemiological study. Br Med J 1969;4:321–5.
8. Castro-Rodriguez JA, Holberg CJ, Wright AL, et al. A clinical index to define risk of asthma in young children with recurrent wheezing. Am J Respir Crit Care Med 2000;162(4 Pt 1):1403–6.
9. Celedon J, Palmer L, Weiss S, et al. Asthma, rhinitis, and skin test reactivity to aeroallergens in families of asthmatic subjects in Anqing, China. Am J Respir Crit Care Med 2001;163:1108–12.
10. Christie GL, Helms PJ, Godden DJ, et al. Asthma, wheezy bronchitis, and atopy across two generations. Am J Respir Crit Care Med 1999;159:125–9.
11. von Mutius E, Weiland SK, Fritzsch C, et al. Increasing prevalence of hay fever and atopy among children in Leipzig, East Germany. Lancet 1998;351:862–6.
12. von Mutius E, Martinez FD. Epidemiology of childhood asthma. In: Murphy S, Kelly H, editors. Pediatric asthma. New York: Marcel Dekker, Inc; 1999:363–431.
13. Strachan DP. Hay fever, hygiene, and household size. Br Med J 1989;299:1259–60.
14. Weiss ST. Gene by environment interaction and asthma. Clin Exp Allergy 1999;29(Suppl 2):96–9.
15. Sexton K, Gong Jr H, Bailar JC 3rd, et al. Air pollution health risks: do class and race matter? Toxicol Ind Health 1993;9:843–78.
16. Liggett SB. The pharmacogenetics of beta2-adrenergic receptors: relevance to asthma. J Allergy Clin Immunol 2000;105(2 Pt 2):S487–92.
17. Reihsaus E, Innis M, MacIntyre N, et al. Mutations in the gene encoding for the beta 2-adrenergic receptor in normal and asthmatic subjects. Am J Respir Cell Mol Biol 1993;8:334–9.
18. Wang Z, Chen C, Niu T, et al. Association of asthma with beta(2)-adrenergic receptor gene polymorphism and cigarette smoking. Am J Respir Crit Care Med 2001;163:1404–9.
19. Strunk R, Mrazek D, Fuhrmann G, et al. Physiologic and psychological characteristics associated with deaths due to asthma in childhood: a case-controlled study. JAMA 1985;254:1193–8.
20. Klinnert MD, Nelson HS, Price MR, et al. Onset and persistence of childhood asthma: predictors from infancy. Pediatrics 2001;108:E69.
21. Sandberg S, Paton JY, Ahola S, et al. The role of acute and chronic stress in asthma attacks in children. Lancet 2000;356:982–7.
22. Chen E, Hanson MD, Paterson LQ, et al. Socioeconomic status and inflammatory processes in childhood asthma: the role of psychological stress. J Allergy Clin Immunol 2006;117:1014–20.
23. Wright RJ, Finn P, Contreras JP, et al. Chronic caregiver stress and IgE expression, allergen-induced proliferation, and cytokine profiles in a birth cohort predisposed to atopy. J Allergy Clin Immunol 2004;113:1051–7.
24. Bussing R, Burket RC, Kelleher ET. Prevalence of anxiety disorders in a clinic-based sample of pediatric asthma patients. Psychosomatics 1996;37:108–15.
25. Meijer AM, Griffioen RW, van Nierop JC, et al. Intractable or uncontrolled asthma: psychosocial factors. J Asthma 1995;32:265–74.
26. Chen E, Matthews KA. Cognitive appraisal biases: an approach to understanding the relation between socioeconomic status and cardiovascular reactivity in children. Ann Behav Med 2001;23:101–11.
27. Beuther DA, Sutherland ER. Overweight, obesity, and incident asthma: a meta-analysis of prospective epidemiologic studies. Am J Respir Crit Care Med 2007;175:661–6.
28. Sin DD, Sutherland ER. Obesity and the lung: 4. Obesity and asthma. Thorax 2008;63:1018–23.
29. Celedon JC, Palmer LJ, Litonjua AA, et al. Body mass index and asthma in adults in families of subjects with asthma in Anqing, China. Am J Respir Crit Care Med 2001;164(10 Pt 1):1835–40.
30. Castro-Rodriguez JA, Holberg CJ, Morgan WJ, et al. Increased incidence of asthmalike symptoms in girls who become overweight or obese during the school years. Am J Respir Crit Care Med 2001;163:1344–9.
31. Shaheen SO, Sterne JAC, Montgomery SM, et al. Birth weight, body mass index and asthma in young adults. Thorax 1999;54:396–402.
32. Tobin MJ. Asthma, airway biology, and nasal disorders in AJRCCM 2001. Am J Respir Crit Care Med 2002;165:598–618.
33. Johnston SL, Pattemore PK, Sanderson G, et al. Community study of role of viral infections in exacerbations of asthma in 9–11 year old children [see comments]. Br Med J 1995;310:1225–9.
34. Mok JY, Simpson H. Symptoms, atopy, and bronchial reactivity after lower respiratory infection in infancy. Arch Dis Child 1984;59:299–305.
35. Camargo Jr CA, Rifas-Shiman SL, Litonjua AA, et al. Maternal intake of vitamin D during pregnancy and risk of recurrent wheeze in children at 3 y of age. Am J Clin Nutr 2007;85:788–95.
36. Devereux G, Litonjua AA, Turner SW, et al. Maternal vitamin D intake during pregnancy and early childhood wheezing. Am J Clin Nutr 2007;85:853–9.
37. McKeever TM, Scrivener S, Broadfield E, et al. Prospective study of diet and decline in lung function in a general population. Am J Respir Crit Care Med 2002;165:1299–303.
38. Fogarty A, Lewis S, Weiss S, et al. Dietary vitamin E, IgE concentrations, and atopy. Lancet 2000;356:1573–4.
39. Kelly W, Hudson I, Phelan P, et al. Childhood asthma in adult life: a further study at 28 years of age. Br Med J 1987;294:1059–62.
40. Roorda RJ, Gerritsen J, Van Aalderen WM, et al. Risk factors for the persistence of respiratory symptoms in childhood asthma. Am Rev Respir Dis 1993;148(6 Pt 1):1490–5.
41. Gold D, Wypij D, Wang X, et al. Gender- and race-specific effects of asthma and wheeze on level and growth of lung function in children in sex U.S. cities. Am J Respir Crit Care Med 1994;149:1198–208.
42. Blackhall MI. Ventilatory function in subjects with childhood asthma who have become symptom free. Arch Dis Child 1970;45:363–6.
43. Grol MH, Gerritsen J, Vonk JM, et al. Risk factors for growth and decline of lung function in asthmatic individuals up to age 42 years: a 30-year follow-up study. Am J Respir Crit Care Med 1999;160:1830–7.
44. Oswald H, Phelan PD, Lanigan A, et al. Childhood asthma and lung function in mid-adult life. Pediatr Pulmonol 1997;23:14–20.
45. Lange P, Parner J, Vestbo J, et al. A 15-year follow-up study of ventilatory function in adults with asthma. N Engl J Med 1998;339:1194–200.
46. Zeiger R, Dawson C, Weiss S, CAMP Research Group. Relationships between duration of asthma and asthma severity among children in the Childhood Asthma Management Program (CAMP). J Allergy Clin Immunol 1999;103(3 Pt 1):376–87.
47. Weiss ST, Van Natta ML, Zeiger RS. Relationship between increased airway responsiveness and asthma severity in the childhood asthma management program. Am J Respir Crit Care Med 2000;162:50–6.
48. Bloomberg G, Goodman G, Fisher E, et al. The profile of single admissions and readmissions for childhood asthma over a five year period at St. Louis Children's Hospital. J Allergy Clin Immunol 1997;99:S69.
49. Chen E, Bloomberg G, Fisher E, et al. Predictors to repeat hospitalizations in children with asthma: the role of psychosocial and socio-environmental factors. Health Psychology 2002; In press.
50. Strunk RC, Nicklas R, Milgrom H, et al. Risk factors for fatal asthma. In: Sheffer A, editor. Fatal asthma. New York: Marcel Dekker, Inc; 1998:31–44.
51. Liu AH, Zeiger R, Sorkness C, et al. Development and cross-sectional validation of the Childhood Asthma Control Test. J Allergy Clin Immunol 2007;119:817–25.

52. Nathan RA, Sorkness CA, Kosinski M, et al. Development of the asthma control test: a survey for assessing asthma control. J Allergy Clin Immunol 2004;113:59–65.

53. Miller RD, Hyatt RE. Evaluation of obstructing lesions of the trachea and larynx by flow-volume loops. Am Rev Respir Dis 1973;108:475–81.

54. Crapo RO. Pulmonary-function testing. N Engl J Med 1994;331:25–30.

55. Rosenstreich DL, Eggleston P, Kattan M, et al. The role of cockroach allergy and exposure to cockroach allergen in causing morbidity among inner-city children with asthma. N Engl J Med 1997;336:1356–63.

56. Downs SH, Mitakakis TZ, Marks GB, et al. Clinical importance of Alternaria exposure in children. Am J Respir Crit Care Med 2001;164:455–9.

57. O'Hollaren M, Yuninger J, Offord K, et al. Exposure to an aeroallergen as a possible precipitating factor in respiratory arrest in young patients with asthma. New Engl J Med 1991;324:359–63.

58. Nelson HS, Szefler SJ, Jacobs J, et al. The relationships among environmental allergen sensitization, allergen exposure, pulmonary function, and bronchial hyperresponsiveness in the Childhood Asthma Management Program. J Allergy Clin Immunol 1999;104(4 Pt 1):775–85.

59. Sears M, Burrows B, Flannery E, et al. Relation between airway responsiveness and serum IgE in children with asthma and in apparently normal children. N Engl J Med 1991;325:1067–71.

60. Burrows B, Sears M, Flannery E, et al. Relation of the course of bronchial responsiveness from age 9 to age 15 to allergy. Am J Respir Crit Care Med 1995;152:1302–8.

61. Dharmage S, Bailey M, Raven J, et al. Current indoor allergen levels of fungi and cats, but not house dust mites, influence allergy and asthma in adults with high dust mite exposure. Am J Respir Crit Care Med 2001;164:65–71.

62. Strunk RC, Sternberg A, Bacharier LB, et al. Nocturnal awakening due to asthma in children with mild to moderate asthma in the Childhood Asthma Management Program. J Allergy Clin Immunol 2002;110:395–403.

63. Nafstad P, Magnus P, Gaarder PI, et al. Exposure to pets and atopy-related diseases in the first 4 years of life. Allergy 2001;56:307–12.

64. Dekker C, Dales R, Bartlett S, et al. Childhood asthma and the indoor environment. Chest 1991;100:922–6.

65. Leynaert B, Bousquet J, Neukirch C, et al. Perennial rhinitis: an independent risk factor for asthma in nonatopic subjects: results from the European Community Respiratory Health Survey. J Allergy Clin Immunol 1999;104(2 Pt 1):301–4.

66. Foresi A, Pelucchi A, Gherson G, et al. Once daily intranasal fluticasone propionate (200 micrograms) reduces nasal symptoms and inflammation but also attenuates the increase in bronchial responsiveness during the pollen season in allergic rhinitis. J Allergy Clin Immunol 1996;98:274–82.

67. Adams RJ, Fuhlbrigge AL, Finkelstein JA, et al. Intranasal steroids and the risk of emergency department visits for asthma. J Allergy Clin Immunol 2002;109:636–42.

68. Crystal-Peters J, Neslusan C, Crown WH, et al. Treating allergic rhinitis in patients with comorbid asthma: the risk of asthma-related hospitalizations and emergency department visits. J Allergy Clin Immunol 2002;109:57–62.

69. Rachelefsky GS, Katz RM, Siegel SC. Chronic sinus disease with associated reactive airway disease in children. Pediatrics 1984;73:526–9.

70. Oliveira CA, Sole D, Naspitz CK, et al. Improvement of bronchial hyperresponsiveness in asthmatic children treated for concomitant sinusitis. Ann Allergy Asthma Immunol 1997;79:70–4.

71. Harding SM. Gastroesophageal reflux and asthma: insight into the association. J Allergy Clin Immunol 1999;104(2 Pt 1):251–9.

72. Martin ME, Grunstein MM, Larsen GL. The relationship of gastroesophageal reflux to nocturnal wheezing in children with asthma. Ann Allergy 1982;49:318–22.

73. Cook DG, Strachan DP. Health effects of passive smoking: summary of effects of parental smoking on the respiratory health of children and implications for research. Thorax 1999;54:357–66.

74. Gold DR, Wang X, Wypij D, et al. Effects of cigarette smoking on lung function in adolescent boys and girls. N Engl J Med 1996;335:931–7.

75. Bacharier LB, Strunk RC. Vocal cord dysfunction: a practical approach. J Respir Dis Pediatrician 2001;3:42–8.

76. Nolan PK, Chrysler M, Phillips G, et al. Pulse oximetry coupled with spirometry in the emergency department helps differentiate an asthma exacerbation from possible vocal cord dysfunction. Pediatr Pulmonol 2007;42:605–9.

77. Strunk RC, Mrazek DA, Fukuhara JT, et al. Cardiovascular fitness in children with asthma correlates with psychologic functioning of the child. Pediatrics 1989;84:460–4.

78. Gutstadt LB, Gillette JW, Mrazek DA, et al. Determinants of school performance in children with chronic asthma. Am J Dis Child 1989;143:471–5.

79. Bender BG, Belleau L, Fukuhara JT, et al. Psychomotor adaptation in children with severe chronic asthma. Pediatrics 1987;79:723–7.

80. Bender BG. Depression symptoms and substance abuse in adolescents with asthma. Ann Allergy Asthma Immunol 2007;99:319–24.

81. Grus CL, Lopez-Hernandez C, Delamater A, et al. Parental self-efficacy and morbidity in pediatric asthma. J Asthma 2001;38:99–106.

82. Clark N, Feldman C, Evans D. The impact of health education on frequency and cost of health care use by low income children with asthma. J Allergy Clin Immunol 1986;78:108–14.

83. Janson S, Reed ML. Patients' perceptions of asthma control and impact on attitudes and self-management. J Asthma 2000;37:625–40.

84. Bender BG, Rankin A, Tran ZV, et al. Brief-interval telephone surveys of medication adherence and asthma symptoms in the Childhood Asthma Management Program Continuation Study. Ann Allergy Asthma Immunol 2008;101:382–6.

85. Hakala K, Stenius-Aarniala B, Sovijarvi A. Effects of weight loss on peak flow variability, airways obstruction, and lung volumes in obese patients with asthma. Chest 2000;118:1315–21.

86. Strunk RC, Mascia A, Lipkowitz M, et al. Rehabilitation of a patient with asthma in the outpatient setting. J Allergy Clin Immunol 1991;87:601–11.

87. Weiler J, Layton T, Hunt M. Asthma in United States Olympic athletes who participated in the 1996 Summer Games. J Allergy Clin Immunol 1998;102:722–6.

88. National Asthma Education and Prevention Program. Expert Panel Report III: Guidelines for the diagnosis and management of asthma. Bethesda, MD: US Department of Health and Human Services; 2007.

89. Bacharier L, Mauger D, Lemanske RJ, et al. Classifying asthma severity in children: is measuring lung function helpful? J Allergy Clin Immunol 2002;109:S266.

90. Juniper EF, O'Byrne PM, Guyatt GH, et al. Development and validation of a questionnaire to measure asthma control. Eur Respir J 1999;14:902–7.

91. Childhood Asthma Management Program Research Group. Long-term effects of budesonide or nedocromil in children with asthma. N Engl J Med 2000;343:1054–63.

92. Strunk RC, Sternberg AL, Szefler SJ, et al. Long-term budesonide or nedocromil treatment, once discontinued, does not alter the course of mild to moderate asthma in children and adolescents. J Pediatr 2009;154:682–7.

93. Zeiger RS, Szefler SJ, Phillips BR, et al. Response profiles to fluticasone and montelukast in mild-to-moderate persistent childhood asthma. J Allergy Clin Immunol 2006;117:45–52.

94. Sorkness CA, Lemanske Jr RF, Mauger DT, et al. Long-term comparison of 3 controller regimens for mild-moderate persistent childhood asthma: The Pediatric Asthma Controller Trial. J Allergy Clin Immunol 2007;119:64–72.

95. Shapiro G, Bronsky EA, LaForce CF, et al. Dose-related efficacy of budesonide administered via a dry powder inhaler in the treatment of children with moderate to severe persistent asthma. J Pediatr 1998;132:976–82.

96. Peden DB, Berger WE, Noonan MJ, et al. Inhaled fluticasone propionate delivered by means of two different multidose powder inhalers is effective and safe in a large pediatric population with persistent asthma. J Allergy Clin Immunol 1998;102:32–8.

97. Szefler SJ, Martin RJ, King TS, et al. Significant variability in response to inhaled corticosteroids for persistent asthma. J Allergy Clin Immunol 2002;109:410–8.

98. Allen DB, Bronsky EA, LaForce CF, et al. Growth in asthmatic children treated with fluticasone propionate. Fluticasone Propionate Asthma Study Group. J Pediatr 1998;132(3 Pt 1):472–7.

99. Agertoft L, Pedersen S. Effect of long-term treatment with inhaled budesonide on adult height in children with asthma. N Engl J Med 2000;343:1064–9.

100. Silverstein MD, Yuninger JW, Reed CE, et al. Attained adult height after childhood asthma: effect of glucocorticoid therapy. J Allergy Clin Immunol 1997;99:466–74.

101. Van Bever HP, Desager KN, Lijssens N, et al. Does treatment of asthmatic children with inhaled corticosteroids affect their adult height? Pediatr Pulmonol 1999;27:369–75.

102. Chrousos GP, Harris AG. Hypothalamic-pituitary-adrenal axis suppression and inhaled corticosteroid therapy. 2. Review of the literature. Neuroimmunomodulation 1998;5:288–308.

103. Bacharier LB, Raissy HH, Wilson L, et al. Long-term effect of budesonide on hypothalamic-pituitary-adrenal axis function in children with mild to moderate asthma. Pediatrics 2004;113:1693–9.

104. Kelly HW, Van Natta ML, Covar RA, et al. Effect of long-term corticosteroid use on bone mineral density in children: a prospective longitudinal assessment in the childhood Asthma Management Program (CAMP) study. Pediatrics 2008;122:e53–61.

105. Knorr B, Matz J, Bernstein JA, et al. Montelukast for chronic asthma in 6- to 14-year-old children: a randomized, double-blind trial. Pediatric Montelukast Study Group. JAMA 1998;279:1181–6.

106. Kemp JP, Dockhorn RJ, Shapiro GG, et al. Montelukast once daily inhibits exercise-induced bronchoconstriction in 6- to 14-year-old children with asthma. J Pediatr 1998;133:424–8.

107. Simons FE, Villa JR, Lee BW, et al. Montelukast added to budesonide in children with persistent asthma: a randomized, double-blind, crossover study. J Pediatr 2001;138:694–8.

108. Phipatanakul W, Greene C, Downes SJ, et al. Montelukast improves asthma control in asthmatic children maintained on inhaled corticosteroids. Ann Allergy Asthma Immunol 2003;91:49–54.

109. Pizzichini E, Leff JA, Reiss TF, et al. Montelukast reduces airway eosinophilic inflammation in asthma: a randomized, controlled trial. Eur Respir J 1999;14:12–8.

110. Bisgaard H, Loland L, Oj JA. NO in exhaled air of asthmatic children is reduced by the leukotriene receptor antagonist montelukast. Am J Respir Crit Care Med 1999;160:1227–31.

111. Bratton DL, Lanz MJ, Miyazawa N, et al. Exhaled nitric oxide before and after montelukast sodium therapy in school-age children with chronic asthma: a preliminary study. Pediatr Pulmonol 1999;28:402–7.

112. Hakim F, Vilozni D, Adler A, et al. The effect of montelukast on bronchial hyperreactivity in preschool children. Chest 2007;131:180–6.

113. Calhoun WJ, Lavins BJ, Minkwitz MC, et al. Effect of zafirlukast (Accolate) on cellular mediators of inflammation: bronchoalveolar lavage fluid findings after segmental antigen challenge. Am J Respir Crit Care Med 1998;157(5 Pt 1):1381–9.

114. Ostrom NK, Decotiis BA, Lincourt WR, et al. Comparative efficacy and safety of low-dose fluticasone propionate and montelukast in children with persistent asthma. J Pediatr 2005;147:213–20.

115. Shrewsbury S, Pyke S, Britton M. Meta-analysis of increased dose of inhaled steroid or addition of salmeterol in symptomatic asthma (MIASMA). Br Med J 2000;320:1368–73.

116. Zimmerman B, D'Urzo A, Berube D. Efficacy and safety of formoterol Turbuhaler when added to inhaled corticosteroid treatment in children with asthma. Pediatr Pulmonol 2004;37:122–7.

117. Verberne AA, Frost C, Duiverman EJ, et al. Addition of salmeterol versus doubling the dose of beclomethasone in children with asthma. The Dutch Asthma Study Group. Am J Respir Crit Care Med 1998;158:213–9.

118. Fowler SJ, Currie GP, Lipworth BJ. Step-down therapy with low-dose fluticasone-salmeterol combination or medium-dose hydrofluoroalkane 134a-beclomethasone alone. J Allergy Clin Immunol 2002;109:929–35.

119. Bisgaard H. Effect of long-acting beta2 agonists on exacerbation rates of asthma in children. Pediatr Pulmonol 2003;36:391–8.

120. Tasche MJ, Uijen JH, Bernsen RM, et al. Inhaled disodium cromoglycate (DSCG) as maintenance therapy in children with asthma: a systematic review. Thorax 2000;55:913–20.

121. Brenner M, Berkowitz R, Marshall N, et al. Need for theophylline in severe steroid-requiring asthmatics. Clin Allergy 1988;18:143–50.

122. Baba K, Sakakibara A, Yagi T, et al. Effects of theophylline withdrawal in well-controlled asthmatics treated with inhaled corticosteroid. J Asthma 2001;38:615–24.

123. Bender BG, Ikle DN, DuHamel T, et al. Neuropsychological and behavioral changes in asthmatic children treated with beclomethasone dipropionate versus theophylline. Pediatrics 1998;101(3 Pt 1):355–60.

124. Bousquet J. Pro: Immunotherapy is clinically indicated in the management of allergic asthma. Am J Respir Crit Care Med 2001;164:2139–40; discussion 41–2.

125. Adkinson Jr NF. Con: Immunotherapy is not clinically indicated in the management of allergic asthma. Am J Respir Crit Care Med 2001;164:2140–1; discussion 1–2.

126. Abramson MJ, Puy RM, Weiner JM. Allergen immunotherapy for asthma. Cochrane Database Syst Rev 2000(2):CD001186.

127. Adkinson Jr NF, Eggleston PA, Eney D, et al. A controlled trial of immunotherapy for asthma in allergic children. N Engl J Med 1997;336:324–31.

128. Moller C, Dreborg S, Ferdousi HA, et al. Pollen immunotherapy reduces the development of asthma in children with seasonal rhinoconjunctivitis (the PAT-study). J Allergy Clin Immunol 2002;109:251–6.

129. Berger W, Gupta N, McAlary M, et al. Evaluation of long-term safety of the anti-IgE antibody, omalizumab, in children with allergic asthma. Ann Allergy Asthma Immunol 2003;91:182–8.

130. Busse W, Corren J, Lanier BQ, et al. Omalizumab, anti-IgE recombinant humanized monoclonal antibody, for the treatment of severe allergic asthma. J Allergy Clin Immunol 2001;108:184–90.

131. Milgrom H, Berger W, Nayak A, et al. Treatment of childhood asthma with anti-immunoglobulin E antibody (omalizumab). Pediatrics 2001;108:E36.

132. Lemanske Jr RF, Nayak A, McAlary M, et al. Omalizumab improves asthma-related quality of life in children with allergic asthma. Pediatrics 2002;110:e55.

133. Gawchik SM, Saccar CL, Noonan M, et al. The safety and efficacy of nebulized levalbuterol compared with racemic albuterol and placebo in the treatment of asthma in pediatric patients. J Allergy Clin Immunol 1999;103:615–21.

134. Martinati LC, Boner AL. Anticholinergic antimuscarinic agents in the treatment of airways bronchoconstriction in children. Allergy 1996;51:2–7.

135. Qureshi F, Pestian J, Davis P, et al. Effect of nebulized ipratropium on the hospitalization rates of children with asthma. N Engl J Med 1998;339:1030–5.

136. Zorc JJ, Pusic MV, Ogborn CJ, et al. Ipratropium bromide added to asthma treatment in the pediatric emergency department. Pediatrics 1999;103(4 Pt 1):748–52.

137. Scarfone RJ, Fuchs SM, Nager AL, et al. Controlled trial of oral prednisone in the emergency department treatment of children with acute asthma. Pediatrics 1993;92:513–8.

138. Becker JM, Arora A, Scarfone RJ, et al. Oral versus intravenous corticosteroids in children hospitalized with asthma. J Allergy Clin Immunol 1999;103:586–90.

139. Covar RA, Leung DY, McCormick D, et al. Risk factors associated with glucocorticoid-induced adverse effects in children with severe asthma. J Allergy Clin Immunol 2000;106:651–9.

140. Grant CC, Duggan AK, Santosham M, et al. Oral prednisone as a risk factor for infections in children with asthma. Arch Pediatr Adolesc Med 1996;150:58–63.

141. Childhood Asthma Management Program Research Group. The Childhood Asthma Management Program (CAMP): design, rationale, and methods. Childhood Asthma Management Program Research Group. Control Clin Trials 1999;20:91–120.

Asthma Education Programs for Children

Sandra R. Wilson • Harold J. Farber

Controlling persistent asthma in children requires multiple changes in lifestyle and behavior including: (1) reducing asthma triggers, (2) monitoring lung function, (3) following an asthma management plan, (4) taking asthma control medication daily, (5) recognizing an asthma flare promptly and escalating therapy appropriately, (6) effectively using the healthcare system and other resources, (7) ensuring effective communication among the child's adult care-givers, and (8) promoting positive adjustment of the child and other family members to the child's condition and resultant needs while not neglecting their own needs.[1] Effective education targets critical asthma management behaviors. Without effective education, parents and children frequently do not do what is necessary and may do things that are counterproductive, and as a result, the child's asthma is not well controlled.

Patient education is an essential component of asthma management. Consensus guidelines emphasize that patient education and a sound partnership between clinician, patient, and parent are essential, both for optimal disease outcome and for preventing asthma crises.[2] Failure to effectively educate patients and families can thwart the other components of medical management. Current asthma care guidelines state that asthma education should occur at all points of asthma care, from diagnosis through subsequent clinical contacts.[2]

Asthma education may occur in many settings. Education of the individual patient or family within the healthcare delivery setting can facilitate targeted behavior change. Small group education programs can be delivered in the context of the healthcare system, schools, and/or in the community. Mass media or community events can be used to deliver broad educational outreach to the larger public. Such outreach can help to set expectations and modify normative health beliefs.

Finally, education and motivation of behavior change on the part of public policy makers are also needed. Many actions to improve asthma control, such as reducing air pollution, eliminating involuntary tobacco smoke exposure, improving access to and quality of healthcare, and improving substandard housing, require changes in public policy.

Key Issues and Tools for Providing Asthma Education to Patients and Their Care-Givers

The criterion for determining whether education is effective is whether the patient actually understands the treatment plan and its rationale, has the necessary skills and is motivated to implement the treatment plan, and successfully puts this plan into action (Box 39-1). Simply providing information or demonstrating a task is insufficient; uptake of that information should be assessed. Can the patient and/or care-giver verbalize a correct understanding? Can s/he perform a correct return demonstration of the task? Documentation of effective education should provide evidence, not only that the education was delivered, but also that it was received and understood. Asthma control should be regularly assessed, as should patient understanding of what asthma control means. Moreover, where possible, medication refill rates should be objectively checked, and a determination made of whether adverse environmental exposures (e.g. to secondhand tobacco smoke) exist. Frequently, there are barriers for the patient and/or family in implementing the treatment plan. If so, further inquiry, skill development, resources, and/or modification of the treatment plan may be required.

Misunderstanding the role of long-term control medications (as being intended for treatment of asthma symptoms after they begin) is associated with nonadherence to daily use of these medications.[3] Low parental expectation of asthma outcomes is associated with suboptimal asthma control. Lack of daily routines for taking medication, concerns about medication side-effects, and a perception of one's child's asthma control that is discordant with 'control' as defined in asthma care guidelines, are all associated with nonadherence to regular use of long-term control medicine and with under-treatment.[4] Actions to reduce exposure to asthma triggers in the home or other places the child regularly spends time can be challenging. Confronting powerful addictions (such as tobacco), removing a household pet, undertaking significant expense, committing significant time, and/or changing routines may be required.

The US National Asthma Education and Prevention Program Expert Panel Report 3 (NAEPP EPR-3) recommends that five key educational messages be incorporated into every step of asthma care (Box 39-2). These include: (1) basic facts about asthma, (2) the role of medication(s) prescribed, (3) skills in using medications and devices, (4) controlling asthma triggers, and (5) when and how to take rescue actions.[2] However, the content of education is not the only issue in providing effective asthma education. Other issues must also be addressed, including:

- The setting(s) in which education will occur
- The overall nature of the patient-clinician communication
- Relevant characteristics of the target population, especially:
  - literacy level
  - language/cultural background
  - complex medical and/or social circumstances
- Educator selection, training and qualifications

©2010 Elsevier Ltd, Inc, BV
DOI: 10.1016/B978-1-4377-0271-2.00039-0

Box 39-1

Clinical Pearls

- Asthma education is a critical part of asthma care.
- Effective patient education does more than provide knowledge – it facilitates the specific behavioral, broader lifestyle, and environmental changes necessary to control asthma.
- Effective care of chronic asthma involves partnership among patient, family, and physician. Effective asthma education is the foundation of this partnership.
- A written asthma action plan should be provided to every asthma patient. It should include instruction for daily actions to maintain asthma control as well as how to recognize and manage deterioration in asthma control.

Box 39-2

Key Messages for Asthma Education

- Basic facts about asthma
  - What defines well-controlled asthma and the patient's current level of control
  - The contrast between airways of a person who has, and a person who does not have, asthma
  - What happens to the airways in an asthma flare-up
- Role of prescribed medication(s)
  - The difference between long-term control and quick-relief medications
- Patient skills
  - Taking medications correctly
    - Inhaler technique
    - Use of devices (spacer, valved holding chamber, nebulizer)
  - Self-monitoring
    - Assess level of asthma control
    - Recognize early signs and symptoms of worsening asthma
- Identifying and avoiding environmental exposures that worsen the patient's asthma
  - Allergens
  - Irritants
  - Tobacco smoke
  - Viral respiratory infections
- Using written asthma action plan to know when and how to do the following
  - Take daily actions to control asthma
  - Adjust medication in response to signs of worsening asthma
  - Seek medical care as appropriate

From National Heart, Lung and Blood Institute, National Asthma Education and Prevention Program: Expert Panel Report 3: guidelines for the diagnosis and management of asthma, Bethesda, MD, 2007, National Institutes of Health, National Heart, Lung and Blood Institute, Pub No. 08-4051. Also available: http://www.nhlbi.nih.gov/guidelines/asthma/asthgdln.pdf (accessed 6 Feb 2009).

- The specific content and tools to be used in the educational process
- How well asthma is managed in the setting/healthcare system in which the patients are receiving care
- Public policy that may facilitate or impede attempts to reduce the burden of asthma.

Box 39-3

Clark and Gong's Physician-Patient Communication Techniques to Facilitate Behavior Change

1. Attend to the patient:
   - Make eye contact
   - Sit rather than stand when conversing with the patient
   - Move closer to the patient, and lean slightly forward to attend to the discussion.
2. Elicit the patient's underlying concerns about the condition.
3. Construct reassuring messages that alleviate fears.
4. Address any immediate concerns expressed.
5. Engage in interactive conversation through use of open-ended questions, simple language, and analogies to teach important concepts.
6. Tailor the treatment regimen by eliciting and addressing potential problems in the timing, dose, or side-effects of the drugs recommended.
7. Use appropriate nonverbal encouragement and verbal praise when the patient reports using correct disease management strategies.
8. Elicit the patient's immediate objective related to controlling the disease and reach agreement with the family on a short-term goal.
9. Review the long-term plan for the patient's treatment:
   - The patient/parent should know what to expect over time
   - The patient/parent should know the situations under which the physician will modify treatment
   - The patient/parent should know the criteria for judging the success of the treatment plan.
10. Help the patient/parent plan in advance for decision-making about the chronic condition.

Adapted from Clark NM, Gong M. BMJ 2000;320:572–575.

Effective Patient-Provider Communication in the Clinical Setting

Education of the patient in the course of clinical care, beginning at the time of diagnosis and continuing at all subsequent clinical contacts, is the standard of care for asthma and is an essential part of good patient-provider communication. Clark and Gong cited 10 general techniques for effective physician-patient communication (Box 39-3).[5] These include engaging the patient/parent in interactive conversation through use of open-ended questions, simple language, and analogies to teach important concepts, tailoring the treatment regimen to the patient's/family's schedule, and discussing how side-effects will be managed. Teaching physicians to use these strategies was associated with better patient outcomes and greater patient satisfaction with care, an effect that was sustained over a 2-year follow-up.[6] Physicians who used these strategies spent no more time with patients than clinicians who did not receive the training.

Shared Treatment Decision-Making

Many experts believe in the importance of jointly developing treatment goals to promote patient adherence.[7,8] Tailoring the treatment regimen to the patient's and parent's goals and preferences is recommended by asthma management guidelines and is consistent with principles of effective patient-clinician com-

Box 39-4 Therapeutic principles

Patient Education

- Solicit and address patient/parent concerns, goals and treatment preferences.
- Present treatment options, discuss their benefits/deficiencies relative to patient/parent goals and preferences, and share treatment decisions with patient/parent.
- Keep messages simple and focused.
- Use simple written and pictorial materials to reinforce verbal messages:
  - Ensure literacy level is appropriate
  - Provide a written action plan, medication administration instructions, and environmental control instructions.
- Introduce, demonstrate, and obtain return demonstration for needed skills.
- Identify readiness to change, barriers to change, and opportunities to overcome barriers.
- Repeat and reinforce at every opportunity.

munication (Box 39-4). However, the underlying assumption of such recommendations, when carefully examined, is that the decision itself is being made by the clinician. Joint or shared development of the regimen goes further than simply observing the principles of good patient-provider communication or tailoring the physician-chosen regimen to the patient's lifestyle. Tailoring typically focuses on maximizing the convenience of the regimen and does not involve the patient or parent in choosing among the full range of available treatment options or in determining how well different options accommodate their preferences regarding asthma control, side-effects, taste, and cost as well as convenience.

Shared treatment decision–making, on the other hand, implies that (1) both the clinician and patient/parent are involved in the decision-making process, (2) both share information with each other, (3) both take steps to participate in the decision process by expressing treatment preferences, and (4) a decision is made that both patient/parent and physician agree to implement. A shared approach to treatment decision-making is distinguished from a decision-making model in which the clinician makes the basic decisions, and also from a decision-making model in which the physician provides information about the treatment options but the patient/parent makes the decision without discussion of the physician's recommendations.[9]

For adults with poorly controlled asthma, it has been demonstrated in a randomized controlled trial that involving the patient in a process of shared decision-making about the choice of an asthma treatment regimen is associated with substantially greater adherence to that regimen and with significantly better asthma outcomes compared with both patients who received identical care management, except that treatment was selected by the clinician, and with those who received their usual medical care (no specific educational or decision intervention).[10] In the shared treatment decision process, the clinician described the *medical* goals of treatment, but also elicited the *patient's* treatment goals and relative priorities regarding the medication regimen on four dimensions: (1) achieving asthma control, (2) avoiding medication side-effects, (3) regimen convenience, and (4) medication cost. In deliberation with the patient, the pros and cons of various options were evaluated in light of both participants' goals and preferences. Involvement of the patient in the treatment choice

did not result in suboptimal treatment choices. Clinical benefits included significantly lower use of rescue medication, better lung function and asthma-related quality of life, and lower healthcare utilization.

The benefits of involving parents in choosing asthma treatment for their child have not been specifically demonstrated in a comparably rigorous trial. However, this hypothesis is very plausible. The process of participating in treatment choice appears to generate 'buy-in' and commitment to implementing the treatment on the part of the adult patient, and by inference, would be expected to do so in parents of children with asthma.

Nonadherence also can be approached as a differential diagnosis within the context of a stage of change model.[11,12] If a patient or care-giver is not ready to make a change, motivational interviewing strategies may be helpful in encouraging the patient to identify his or her goals for treatment and can lead to discussion of barriers and potential benefits of change and the risks or problems associated with the status quo.[13] When the barriers are understood, alternative strategies may become apparent. For example, if the barrier is the adverse taste of the medication, the medication can be changed to one with a less unpleasant taste. Patients/parents may be ready to implement the desired changes; however, making the transition – from 'should do it' to 'is doing it' – may be difficult. If so, discussion can focus on implementation strategies such as establishing routines, positive reinforcement schedules, storing the medication in an easy to access location (such as near the toothbrush if brushing teeth is routine), ensuring an adequate supply of medicine, knowing how to tell when the inhaler is empty, etc. A survey of parents of children with asthma found that tailoring medical regimens to the family's daily routine, were associated with fewer emergency department (ED) visits.[4]

Nonadherence to a regimen chosen by the physician, and consequent poor asthma control, also are reasons to consider a shared decision approach and to reconsider the treatment regimen and the process by which it is selected. Continuation of the status quo (e.g., no or inconsistent medication use, poor control) is, in reality, always an option for the patient/parent and needs to be acknowledged and explicitly considered. If the pros and cons of the status quo relative to the patient's preferences and goals are discussed and compared with other treatment options, the evidence cited above indicates that patients typically choose, and subsequently use, a controller. Presentation of the full range of controller options (types of controllers, dose, delivery system, schedule, combination or not with a long-term β agonist, etc.) and discussion of their relative abilities to meet the patient's/parent's goals and preferences helps individuals find an acceptable regimen and commit to implementing it.

Health Literacy

Written materials are essential tools for asthma education and self-management, but too often are not written at a level patients comprehend. The National Assessment of Adult Literacy (2003) found that 43% of adults had basic or below basic literacy skills. Only 13% of the US adult population could be considered proficient readers (i.e. able to perform complex and challenging literacy activities).[14] Studies of adults bringing a child for medical care in a variety of settings have found their mean literacy skills to be at the seventh to eighth grade level.[15–17] Much of the patient education material located on the worldwide web, as well as materials produced by professional health organizations, require literacy skills greater than those possessed by the majority of adults.[18–20]

For parents with below-basic literacy, those who do not speak and/or read the language(s) in which written materials are available, and for young children in general, alternatives to printed text may be necessary.[21] Low and no-literacy materials are available as videotape and pictorial materials in the *Wee Wheezers* program[22] and as internet-based flash videos.[23,24] The need continues for high-quality asthma education materials that are readily understood by people with low or marginal literacy.

Visual Aids

Even for those with adequate or high literacy, pictorial material and well-chosen three-dimensional models can enhance and facilitate understanding and retention. For example, Figure 39-1 shows a simple visual aid, derived from a version used in a clinical trial with adults,[10] that clinicians can use with parents and children to help them understand how well or poorly the child's asthma is currently controlled. The green, yellow, and red sections correspond to the NAEPP EPR-3's asthma control levels of well controlled, not well controlled, and very poorly controlled.[2] On the first (blank) dial (Figure 39-1A), clinicians can ask parents or children (if old enough) to draw an arrow to indicate how well they feel the child's asthma is controlled. The clinician can then explain the second version of the dial that lists the medical criteria adopted by the EPR-3 for classifying control. The criteria shown in Figure 39-1B apply to children 5 to 11 years of age and define the specific frequency of symptoms and use of rescue medications, extent of activity limitation, and lung function values (where measured) that are considered indicative of different levels of control. Such a dial can be easily adapted for children aged 0 to 4 years by inserting the relevant EPR-3 criteria for that age group, or for children 12 years of age or older by inserting the criteria for adults). Since a child could be classified differently on different dimensions (e.g. lung function versus symptom frequency), the overall level of control is considered to be the lowest level implied by the child's status on any of the criterion dimensions. Because the EPR-3 criteria are written for a medical audience, they may need to be tailored for a low literacy population, and it is expected that the clinician would explain the criteria and any terminology the parent/child may not understand.

The arrows on the two dials in Figure 39-1 illustrate a not uncommon scenario in which the parent feels the child's asthma is well controlled whereas, from a medical standpoint, the fact that the child is using rescue medication daily and awakening frequently at night indicates that it is very poorly controlled. Drawing of an arrow on the second dial to indicate the patient's current level of asthma control using information supplied by the parent plus objective assessment where possible, can help clarify the concept of control as used by physicians, highlight any discrepancy between the medical evaluation of control and the parent/child's perception, and clarify the clinical goal of controlling asthma.

Small Group Asthma Education Programs

Education delivered to patients or parents in small groups led by a trained facilitator has been associated, in controlled trials, with improved asthma outcomes (Box 39-5).[25,26] The small-group format permits use of more powerful behavioral change methods, which are not as easily used either in a one-on-one encounter or in written materials alone, such as role playing and modeling, social comparison, and social support. Methods based on behav-

ioral science theory underlie the most effective programs, and such programs teach patients how to observe, judge, and react appropriately to changes in asthma status.[27]

Small group asthma education programs have been delivered in clinical settings as well as in schools, other community settings, and at asthma camps. When designing and implementing such programs, it is important to account for the needs and concerns of the target audience, focus on the key educational messages (Box 39-2), and utilize proven methods and group processes to achieve behavior change. Education of parents and/or children in groups offers the possibility of beneficial interaction among participants, and is not simply a more efficient means of didactic instruction. Programs should attend to the goals of treatment, what happens in the airways in a person with asthma, how to recognize and reduce asthma triggers, and the differing roles of controller and reliever medication. Specific skills also should be taught, including the use of inhaled medications and patient-relevant devices, recognizing early and late signs of deteriorating asthma control, and use of a written asthma action plan. Ideally, the asthma plan will be the result of shared clinician and patient decisions about the treatment regimen, will be consistent with current guidelines, and the demands of the regimen will fit into the family's daily routine. Fears and concerns should be elicited and coping strategies should be discussed. Strategies for communication with physicians and others in the healthcare system, school and childcare personnel, as well as family and friends, can be useful, especially when the program is not directly linked to the patient's medical care. Programs need to be age- and culture-appropriate. Although there is clear value in using successful programs as intended and as validated, they need to be selected and/or modified to fit individual situations and community needs.

A meta-analysis of asthma education programs for children found that, although single session programs showed reductions in morbidity measures, multisession programs demonstrated the greatest improvement in self-efficacy and the greatest reduction in number of ED visits.[27] Furthermore, culture-specific asthma education programs appear to be more effective than generic programs.[28,29] This finding is consistent with other research findings indicating that policies promoting cultural competence in medical practice are associated with improved asthma care quality, including improved adherence to asthma controller medications and improved patient satisfaction.[30]

The *Open Airways for Schools* and *Wee Wheezers* programs are among the most widely disseminated small-group pediatric asthma education programs in the USA.[31-33] The American Lung Association's *Open Airways for Schools* targets children 8 to 12

How well controlled is your child's asthma?

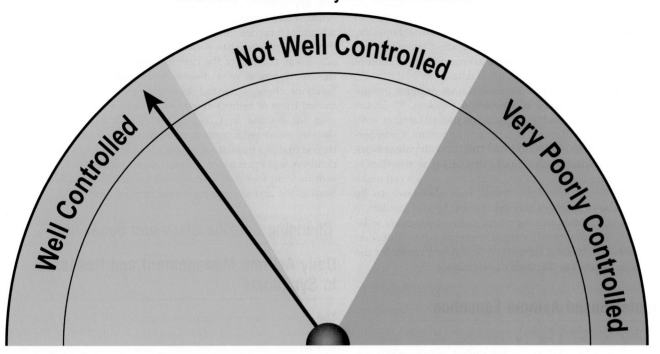

Dial for eliciting parent's/child's perception of child's asthma control, not showing medical criteria

A

How well controlled is your asthma?

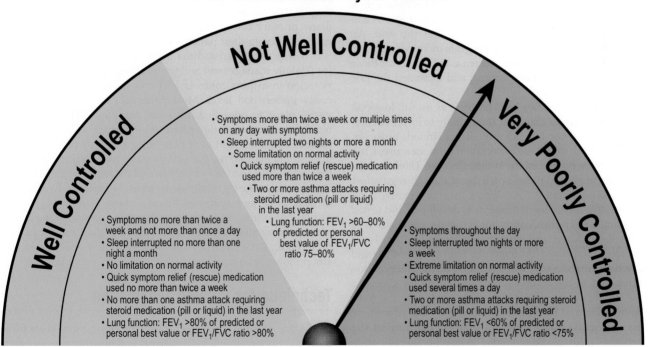

- Symptoms more than twice a week or multiple times on any day with symptoms
- Sleep interrupted two nights or more a month
- Some limitation on normal activity
- Quick symptom relief (rescue) medication used more than twice a week
- Two or more asthma attacks requiring steroid medication (pill or liquid) in the last year
- Lung function: FEV_1 >60–80% of predicted or personal best value of FEV_1/FVC ratio 75–80%

- Symptoms no more than twice a week and not more than once a day
- Sleep interrupted no more than one night a month
- No limitation on normal activity
- Quick symptom relief (rescue) medication used no more than twice a week
- No more than one asthma attack requiring steroid medication (pill or liquid) in the last year
- Lung function: FEV_1 >80% of predicted or personal best value or FEV_1/FVC ratio >80%

- Symptoms throughout the day
- Sleep interrupted two nights or more a week
- Extreme limitation on normal activity
- Quick symptom relief (rescue) medication used several times a day
- Two or more asthma attacks requiring steroid medication (pill or liquid) in the last year
- Lung function: FEV_1 <60% of predicted or personal best value or FEV_1/FVC ratio <75%

B

Criteria for classifying Asthma Control for children ages 5 to 11 years

Figure 39-1 Simple visual aids to: elicit parent/patient perceptions of asthma control (blank dial **[A]**); communicate the medical criteria for control and properly classify the child's asthma (criterion dial for 5- to 11-year-old children **[B]**).

years of age. The *Wee Wheezers* program, updated in 2003, and distributed by the Asthma and Allergy Foundation of American, targets children aged <7 years and their parents. Programs can rapidly become dated, particularly in terms of treatment options, and some popular, validated asthma education programs are more than 20 years old. It is important to ensure that the content of the program being used is kept up to date.

Implementation of asthma education classes presents unique challenges. Poor attendance is a common problem. Physician referral to the program and the expectation that all families with a child with asthma will attend is extremely important. Considerable flexibility is often needed to avoid conflict with parent work schedules and children's school and extracurricular activities in order to maximize accessibility and attendance, which can make staffing a challenge. Childcare needs may also have to be addressed.[34] Use of locations that are favored by and familiar to the parents and children may be useful. If the children are to be involved at some point or will simply be on-site while education of the parents is occurring, simple toys and refreshments for the children may encourage the family's attendance.

Computer-Based Asthma Education

The Baylor Asthma Care for Kids Educational Resource (BACKER) is an ED-based, computer guided, asthma education intervention implemented by asthma educators that includes both universal and tailored content.[35] The educator has the flexibility to navigate the content based on the individual child/family's needs and questions. BACKER utilizes educator prompts, tailored text, and video clips providing motivational messages and skills training. At the completion of the session, tailored education materials are generated (e.g. an asthma action plan and a report for the child's primary care provider). A follow-up telephone call occurs 1 to 2 weeks after the visit. An evaluation of BACKER found that the program increased parents' confidence in asthma management, decreased ED visits for those classified as having intermittent asthma, and increased the rate of asthma follow-up visits.[35]

Interactive computer games hold promise as useful, low-cost asthma education aids for children. Their ability to improve morbidity outcomes has not been clearly demonstrated; however, this may not be the appropriate expectation from their use. Children with asthma who played the *Watch, Discover, Think, and Act* computer game improved their knowledge about self-regulation, prevention, and treatment.[36] *The Asthma Files,* an interactive computer game with a secret-agent theme, was developed and tested in Nottingham, UK. The evaluation noted that the game was well accepted by the children, and their knowledge and asthma locus of control scores improved. At 6 months follow-up, oral steroid use and school absenteeism were reduced in the intervention group compared to the control group.[37] *Quest for the Code* is a widely distributed asthma video game developed by the Starbright Foundation and features the voices of several prominent celebrities. The game is currently available via the Internet site of the Starlight Children's Foundation.[38] A small-scale evaluation (n = 35) of this game in children aged 8 to 12 years with moderate-to-severe asthma noted improvements in child's self-efficacy scores.[39]

Asthma Care Management

For many patients, the severity of their asthma, complexity of their medical and psychosocial needs, or a combination of factors may necessitate not only supplementary asthma education, but also engagement of other resources to address broader issues. Asthma care managers are one such resource. They are generally advanced practice allied health personnel (nurses, respiratory therapists, pharmacists, social workers). In addition to providing education, the role of the care managers includes facilitation of the development of a disease management plan and of the behavior changes needed to implement it. Randomized controlled trials of asthma care management for children hospitalized for asthma in Glasgow, Scotland[40] and Boston, MA.[41] demonstrated reductions in re-admissions. A randomized controlled trial of a trained social worker intervention with inner city children with persistent asthma demonstrated a reduction in asthma symptom days and a trend toward reduced hospitalizations in the care management intervention group.[42]

Changing Specific Skills and Behaviours

Daily Asthma Management and Response to Symptoms

The daily asthma management regimen and how to recognize and handle worsening asthma are best documented in the form of a written Asthma Action Plan. Such plans are recommended by US and international asthma care guidelines[2,43] to convey key messages and provide a ready reference for patients when verbal instructions are forgotten or need to be shared with family members or care-givers. Having a written asthma action plan is associated with having fewer acute asthma events, fewer lost school days, lower symptom scores, decreased risk of hospitalization and ED visits, as well as with improved adherence to regular use of asthma control medication.[44-46] Unfortunately, many primary care providers have not adopted the practice of routinely giving their patients written plans.[47-49]

It is important that asthma action plans include instructions for (1) daily management and for recognizing and handling deterioration in asthma control,[2] and that (2) they be written at an easily understood level. Most patients/parents prefer simple, visual plans to ones that are more complex.[50] The most commonly used asthma action plans use the green/yellow/red zone format, with the green zone plan being the daily plan for avoiding asthma symptoms, the yellow zone plan indicating actions to take for mild asthma symptoms, and the red zone plan describing actions to take for moderate to severe symptoms. Evaluations of peak flow- and symptom-based asthma plans have yielded similar outcomes,[51] suggesting that in most situations the choice of monitoring method can be based on care-giver and/or patient preference. Patients who are poor symptom perceivers are among those who may benefit from peak flow monitoring.

Technique for Inhaled Medication

Ineffective or suboptimal technique for using inhaled medications is common among both patients and healthcare professionals, regardless of type of inhalation system (nebulizer, metered dose inhaler, or dry powder inhaler).[52,53] Poor technique can dramatically reduce medication delivery to the airways and is a common reason for poorly controlled asthma.[54]

Errors commonly observed with metered dose inhalers include blocking the mouthpiece with the tongue or teeth, lack of coordination of inhalation with actuation, lack of a deep inhalation and breath hold, failure to 'prime' the inhaler if needed, and continued use of the inhaler after the labeled number of doses has been exhausted. Some of the new hydroflouroalkane (HFA) metered dose inhalers also require regular cleaning of the canister sleeve (the mouthpiece unit, not the medication canister) to prevent clogging.

Errors with dry powder inhalers can include failure to load a dose of medication prior to inhalation, exhaling into the inhaler after the medication dose has been loaded, failure to exhale before actuation, failure to breath-hold after inhalation, incorrect positioning of the inhaler, and blocking the mouthpiece with the teeth or the tongue.[55]

Finally, common errors in using nebulizers include use of a 'blow by' technique (where the medication is blown in the general vicinity of the patient's face), inhaling through the nose while attempting to receive nebulized medication via a mouthpiece, and use of incompatible and/or malfunctioning equipment.

Although use of a valved holding chamber with mask or a nebulizer with mask can allow passive delivery of medication to infants and toddlers, crying impairs medication deposition.[56] When using a valved holding chamber with face mask, lack of a tight seal, resulting in even a small leak, will dramatically reduce medication delivery.[57]

When teaching inhaler use, it is important that the provider (1) be knowledgeable about the correct technique for the device, (2) explain and demonstrate correct technique for the patient/parent, and (3) obtain a return demonstration of correct technique from the patient and/or parent. Pre-post evaluation studies demonstrate improved inhaler technique after formal educational programs,[58,59] and even after brief educational interventions that used these methods.[60] Frequent repetition of evaluation and instruction is often needed to maintain correct technique over time.[61] Initial coaching that continues until performance is essentially error-free has been shown to result in good technique that persists well over time, even in older adults.[27,62]

Environmental Control Practices

Elimination of Secondhand Tobacco Smoke Exposure

Secondhand or involuntary tobacco smoke exposure is an important trigger of childhood asthma. Tobacco smoke exposure decreases the effectiveness of inhaled corticosteroid medication.[63,64] Tobacco smoking is common among young adults (24% of US adults aged 25 to 34 years are smokers), especially in lower education and income groups;[65] consequently, exposure of children with asthma is common.[66,67] Children can be exposed to smoke from many sources; however, primary care-giver smoking and childcare provider smoking are the major contributors to a child's total tobacco smoke exposure.[68] Although smoking bans in the home and car are associated with lower exposure,[69–71] they may not eliminate a child's exposure to secondhand tobacco smoke. Smoking cessation by the parents and care-givers, as well as avoiding places where others are smoking, are the most effective ways to eliminate a child's tobacco smoke exposure.

Perhaps the most important action that a pediatric healthcare provider can undertake to improve a child's asthma control is to ensure that his or her tobacco-dependent care-givers receive effective treatment for their tobacco dependence. Fortunately, effective treatments are available, although commonly underused.[72] By offering or referring for effective treatment, the provider can address the parent's tobacco dependence, thereby benefiting the health of both parent and child. Most parents who are willing to consider use of medication to treat their tobacco dependence would accept that recommendation and/or prescription from their child's doctor.[73] In fact, many younger adults do not have their own primary provider and may lack health insurance for themselves.[74] Consequently, their child's doctor may be their only path to treatment of their tobacco dependence.

Cotinine feedback plus behavioral counseling can be effective in reducing smoke exposure for children with high-risk asthma.[75] The tools provided in the *Clinical Effort Against Secondhand Smoke Exposure* program help pediatric healthcare clinicians address family tobacco use. The core aspects of the program are to Ask (about smoking status of family members and household smoking rules), Assist (in quitting smoking and establishing a smoke-free home and car), and Refer (to a tobacco dependence treatment program or quit line such as 1 800 QUIT NOW).[76,77] Use of any of the tobacco dependence treatment medications (nicotine replacement, bupropion, varenicline) is effective for increasing quit rates.[78] Combination therapy with two or more forms of tobacco dependence treatment improves effectiveness, and combining medication with a behaviorally focused program is more effective than either alone.[79] Use of individually titrated combination therapy was useful in the 'Tobacco-Free with FDNY' program.[80]

Control of Other Asthma Triggers

Most comprehensive, rigorously evaluated small-group asthma education programs have included education about identification and reduction of asthma triggers in the environment. Few have specifically evaluated the effectiveness of this educational component, and those that did so included home visits and assistance with environmental remediation. The ZAP Asthma program included a community health worker intervention to assess, assist, and reduce asthma triggers and included a one-time professional cleaning to reduce allergen levels.[81] Sustained reductions in dust mite allergen and transient reduction in cockroach allergen were achieved. The Inner-City Asthma Study evaluated the effectiveness of a multifaceted, home-based, environmental intervention for inner city children with goals of providing the child's caretaker with the knowledge, skills, motivation, equipment, and supplies necessary to perform comprehensive environmental remediation. The intervention reduced levels of dust mite and cockroach allergen, and consequently reduced days with asthma symptoms.[82]

Changing Asthma Care in Healthcare Systems

Healthcare systems can either facilitate or impair the behavioral changes that physicians and parents/patients need to make in order to control asthma, and can either support or undermine the effectiveness of patient education. Among the key determinants of healthcare system change are whether asthma care is focused on chronic care, whether financial incentives for patients and clinicians promote or discourage asthma follow-up, whether appropriate asthma education materials are readily available, and whether healthcare providers appropriately assess and treat the child's chronic asthma.

Clinical pathways are often used to coordinate care and reduce variation in practice when treating hospitalized patients with common diagnoses. Just as in diabetes, it is important to ensure that children and their families have the basic skills needed to manage their asthma prior to hospital discharge. In addition to standardizing acute care, an asthma clinical pathway should provide education, identify and offer strategies for reducing asthma-triggers, assess severity of chronic disease, initiate appropriate use of controller medication, provide a written asthma action plan, and ensure a smooth transition to out-patient care.[83] A controlled trial in hospitalized children with asthma, which provided them with an individual written asthma action plan, an educational session on the nature of asthma, the recognition of risk factors and how to avoid them, asthma medications and devices, found a decrease in re-hospitalization and urgent care for asthma in the intervention group.[84]

Changing Public Policy to Reduce the Burden of Asthma

To improve asthma outcomes requires behavior changes at the broader community level. Access to quality medical care, air quality, housing quality, and school operation are public policy issues. Air pollution exacerbates asthma.[85] Restriction of smoking in public places is essential to eliminate a child's involuntary tobacco smoke exposure.[86] School policies regarding access to asthma inhalers, maintaining indoor air quality, and motor vehicle idling, among others, can facilitate or impair asthma control.

Policy change can be advanced by advocacy organizations, community coalitions, voluntary health organizations, and government organizations. Researchers and disease specialists can collaborate with and provide education to members of advocacy organizations, voluntary health organizations, and policy makers to encourage policy changes needed to reduce the burden of asthma. They can help to ensure that policy changes promoted are evidence-based and relevant.[87]

Synthesis of relevant research into evidence-based policy proposals can facilitate implementation.[88] The US Environmental Protection Administration has developed the Indoor Air Quality Tools for Schools program to help schools maintain a healthy environment in school buildings.[89] Evidence-based expert consensus recommendations for an actionable public policy agenda for asthma have been developed by the American Lung Association with funding support from the US Centers for Disease Control and Prevention.[90]

Conclusions

Achieving asthma control requires behavioral and lifestyle changes on the part of patients and their families. An effective asthma education and management program not only provides information but focuses on the desired changes and uses evidence-based behavioral change strategies. Parental and patient involvement in determining the treatment regimen is also important to successful implementation of treatment at home. Asthma education must target patients in the variety of settings, including the clinic, emergency department, hospital, school, and community. Carefully developed and evaluated asthma education programs and materials exist that can be adopted or adapted for use.

References

1. Wilson SR, Mitchell JH, Rolnick S, et al. Effective and ineffective management behaviors of parents of infants and young children with asthma. J Pediatr Psychol 1993;18:63–81.

2. National Heart, Lung and Blood Institute, National Asthma Education and Prevention Program. Expert Panel Report 3: guidelines for the diagnosis and management of asthma. Bethesda, MD: National Institutes of Health, National Heart, Lung and Blood Institute, Pub No. 08-4051; 2007.

3. Farber HJ, Capra AM, Lozano P, et al. Misunderstanding of asthma medications: effects on adherence. J Asthma 2008;40:17–25.

4. Smith LA, Bokhour B, Hohman KH, et al. Modifiable risk factors for suboptimal control and controller medication underuse among children with asthma. Pediatrics 2008;122:760–9.

5. Clark NM, Gong M, Schork MA, et al. Impact of education for physicians on patient outcomes. Pediatrics 1998;101:831–6.

6. Clark NM, Cabana M, Kaciroti N, et al. Long-term outcomes of physician peer teaching. Clin Pediatr (Phila) 2008;47:883–90.

7. Hanson JE: Patient education in pediatric asthma. In: Murphy S, Kelly HW, editors. Pediatric asthma. Monticello, NY: Marcel Dekker; 1999.

8. Farber HJ, Boyette M. Control your child's asthma: a breakthrough program for the treatment nad management of childhood asthma. New York: Henry Holt; 2001.

9. Charles C, Gafni A, Whelan T. Shared decision-making in the medical encounter: what does it mean? (or it takes at least two to tango). Soc Sci Med 1997;44:681–92.

10. Wilson SR, Strub P, Buist AS, et al. Shared treatment decision-making improves adherence and outcomes in poorly controlled asthma. Amer J Resp and Crit Care Med 2010;181:566–77.

11. Farber HJ. High-quality asthma care: it's not just about drugs. The Permanente Journal 2005;9:32–6.

12. Norcross JC, Prochaska JO. Using the stages of change. Harv Ment Health Lett 2002;18:5–7.

13. Borrelli B, Riekert KA, Weinstein A, et al. Brief motivational interviewing as a clinical strategy to promote asthma medication adherence. J Allergy Clin Immunol 2007;120:1023–30.

14. Kutner M, Greenberg E, Jin Y, et al. Literacy in everyday life: results from the 2003 National Assessment of Adult Literacy. U.S. Department of Education, Washington, DC: National Center for Education Statistics; 2007. NCES 2007-480.

15. Davis TC, Mayeaux EJ, Fredrickson D, et al. Reading ability of parents compared with reading level of pediatric patient education materials. Pediatrics 1994;93:460–8.

16. Farber HJ, Johnson C, Beckerman RC. Young inner-city children visiting the emergency room (ER) for asthma: risk factors and chronic care behaviors. J Asthma 1998;35:547–52.

17. Moon RY, Cheng TL, Patel KM, et al. Parental literacy level and understanding of medical information, Pediatrics 1998;102:e25.

18. D'Alessandro DM, Kingsley P, Johnson-West J. The readability of pediatric patient education materials on the World Wide Web. Arch Pediatr Adolesc Med 2001;155:807–12.

19. Wallace LS, Lennon ES. American Academy of Family Physicians patient education materials: can patients read them? Fam Med 2004;36:571–4.

20. Freda MC. The readability of American Academy of Pediatrics patient education brochures. J Pediatr Health Care 2005;19:151–6.

21. Davis TC, Michielutte R, Askov EN, et al. Practical assessment of adult literacy in health care. Health Educ Behav 1998;25:613–24.

22. Asthma and Allergy Foundation of America. Wee Wheezers. (accessed January 29, 2009): http://www.aafa.org/display.cfm?id=4&sub=79&cont=434.

23. Calgary Health Region, Community Pediatric Asthma Service. iCAN Control Asthma Now. (accessed January 24, 2009): http://www.calgaryhealthregion.ca/ican/.

24. Venkayya R, Daher C, Tolpa T. What's Asthma All About? Neomedicus Inc., 2001. (accessed January 24, 2009): http://www.whatsasthma.org.

25. Guevara JP, Wolf FM, Grum CM, et al. Effects of educational interventions for self management of asthma in children and adolescents: systematic review and meta-analysis. Br Med J 2003;326:1308–9.

26. Wilson SR, Scamagas P, German DF, et al. A controlled trial of two forms of self-management education for adults with asthma. Am J Med 1993;94:564–76.

27. Clark NM, Valerio MA. The role of behavioural theories in educational interventions for paediatric asthma. Paediatr Respir Rev 2003;4:325–33.

28. Canino G, Vila D, Normand SL, et al. Reducing asthma health disparities in poor Puerto Rican children: the effectiveness of a culturally tailored family intervention. J Allergy Clin Immunol 2008;121:665–70.

29. Bailey EJ, Cates CJ, Kruske SG, et al. Culture-specific programs for children and adults from minority groups who have asthma. Cochrane Database of Syst Rev 1:CD006580, 2009.

30. Lieu TA, Finkelstein JA, Lozano P, et al. Cultural competence policies and other predictors of asthma care quality for Medicaid-insured children. Pediatrics 2004;114:e102–e110.

31. Evans D, Clark NM, Feldman CH, et al. A school health education program for children with asthma aged 8–11 years. Health Educ Q 1987;14:267–79.

32. Bruzzese JM, Markman LB, Appel D, et al. An evaluation of Open Airways for Schools: using college students as instructors. J Asthma 2001;38:337–42.

33. Wilson SR, Latini D, Starr NJ, et al. Education of parents of infants and very young children with asthma: a developmental evaluation of the Wee Wheezers program. J Asthma 1996;33:239–54.

34. Wilson SR, Knowles SB. Education and Support for Larger Groups. In: Castro M, Kraft M, editors. Clinical asthma. Philadelphia, PA: Elsevier Mosby; 2008.

35. Sockrider MM, Abramson S, Brooks E, et al. Delivering tailored asthma family education in a pediatric emergency department setting: a pilot study. Pediatrics 2006;117:S135–144.

36. Bartholomew LK, Gold RS, Parcel GS, et al. Watch, Discover, Think, and Act: evaluation of computer-assisted instruction to improve asthma self-management in inner-city children. Patient Educ Couns 2000;39: 269–80.

37. McPherson AC, Glazebrook C, Forster D, et al. A randomized, controlled trial of an interactive educational computer package for children with asthma. Pediatrics 2006;117:1046–54.

38. Starlight Children's Foundation: Quest for the code. (accessed January 24, 2009): http://asthma.starlightprograms.org/.

39. Delamater A, McCullough J, Castro M, et al. CD-ROM Intervention for Children with Asthma (abstract). Ann Behav Med 2006;31:S072.

40. Madge P, McColl J, Paton J. Impact of nurse-led home management training programme in children admitted to hospital with acute asthma: a randomized controlled study. Thorax 1997;52:223–8.

41. Greineder DK, Loane KC, Parks P. A randomized controlled trial of a pediatric asthma outreach program. J Allergy Clinical Immunol 1999;103: 436–40.

42. Evans R, Gergen PJ, Mitchell H, et al. A randomized clinical trial to reduce asthma morbidity among inner-city children: results of the National Cooperative Inner-City Asthma Study. J Pediatr 1999;135: 332–8.

43. Global Initiative for Asthma. Global Strategy for Asthma Management and Prevention, [Revised 2008]. 2008, National Institutes of Health, National Heart, Lung and Blood Institute. (accessed January 24, 2009): http://www.ginasthma.com.

44. Lieu TA, Quesenberry CP, Capra AM, et al. Outpatient management practices associated with reduced risk of pediatric asthma hospitalization and emergency department visits. Pediatrics 1997;100:334–41.

45. Finkelstein JA, Lozano P, Farber HJ, et al. Under-use of controller medications among Medicaid-insured children with asthma. Arch Pediatr Adolesc Med 2002;156:562–7.

46. Agrawal SK, Singh M, Mathew JL, et al. Efficacy of an individualized written home-management plan in the control of moderate persistent asthma: a randomized, controlled trial. Acta Paediatr 2005;94:1742–6.

47. Reeves MJ, Bohm SR, Korzeniewski SJ, et al. Children in western Michigan: how well does care adhere to guidelines? Pediatrics 2006;117: S118–26.

48. Sulaiman ND, Barton CA, Abramson MJ, et al. Factors associated with ownership and use of written asthma action plans in North-West Melbourne. Prim Care Respir J 2004;13:211–7.

49. Cabana MD, Chaffin DC, Jarlsberg LG, et al. Selective provision of asthma self-management tools to families. Pediatrics 2008;121: e900–e905.

50. Farber HJ, Smith-Wong K, Nichols L, et al. Patients prefer simple, visual asthma self management plan forms. The Permanente Journal 2001;5: 35–7.

51. Wensley D, Silverman M. Peak flow monitoring for guided self management in childhood asthma: a randomized controlled trial. Am J Respir Crit Care Med 2004;170:606–12.

52. Cochrane MG, Bala MV, Downs KE, et al. Inhaled corticosteroids for asthma therapy: patient compliance, devices, and inhalation technique. Chest 2000;117:542–50.

53. Scarfone RJ, Capraro GA, Zorc JJ, et al. Demonstrated use of metered-dose inhalers and peak flow meters by children and adolescents with acute asthma exacerbations. Arch Pediatr Adolesc Med 2002;156: 378–83.

54. Haughney J, Price D, Kaplan A, et al. Achieving asthma control in practice: understanding the reasons for poor control. Respir Med 2008;102:1681–93.

55. Lavorini F, Magnan A, Dubus JC, et al. Effect of incorrect use of dry powder inhalers on management of patients with asthma and COPD. Respir Med 2008;102:593–604.

56. Janssens HM, Tiddens HA. Aerosol therapy: the special needs of young children. Paediatr Respir Rev 2006;7:S83–5.

57. Janssens HM, Tiddens HA. Facemasks and aerosol delivery by metered dose inhaler-valved holding chamber in young children: a tight seal makes the difference. J Aerosol Med 2007;20:S59–63.

58. Prabhakaran L, Lim G, Abisheganaden J, et al. Impact of an asthma education programme on patients' knowledge, inhaler technique and compliance to treatment. Singapore Med J 2006;473:225–31.

59. Patterson EE, Brennan MP, Linskey KM, et al. A cluster randomised intervention trial of asthma clubs to improve quality of life in primary school children: the School Care and Asthma Management Project (SCAMP). Arch Dis Child 2005;90:786–91.

60. Basheti IA, Reddel HK, Armour CL, et al. Improved asthma outcomes with a simple inhaler technique intervention by community pharmacists (letter). J Allergy Clin Immunol 2007;119:1537–8.

61. Crompton GK, Barnes PJ, Broeders M, et al. The need to improve inhalation technique in Europe: a report from the Aerosol Drug Management Improvement Team. Respir Med 2006;100:1479–94.

62. Buist AS, Vollmer WM, Wilson SR, et al. A randomized clinical trial of peak flow monitoring versus symptom monitoring in older adults with asthma. Amer J Resp Crit Care Med 2006;174:1077–87.

63. Lazarus SC, Chinchilli VM, Rollings NJ, et al. Smoking affects response to inhaled corticosteroids or leukotriene receptor antagonists in asthma. Am J Respir Crit Care Med 2007;175:783–90.

64. Tomlinson JE, McMahon AD, Chaudhuri R, et al. Efficacy of low and high dose inhaled corticosteroid in smokers versus non-smokers with mild asthma. Thorax 2005;60:282–7.

65. Centers for Disease Control and Prevention. Behavioral Risk Factor Surveillance System (BRFSS) Prevalence and Trends Data Nationwide (States and DC) – 2007 Tobacco Use. (accessed February 1, 2009): http://apps.nccd.cdc.gov/brfss/age.asp?cat=TU&yr=2007&qkey=4394 &state=UB.

66. Pirkle JL, Flegal KM, Bernert JT, et al. Exposure of the US population to environmental tobacco smoke: the Third National Health and Nutrition Examination Survey, 1988 to 1991. JAMA 1996;275:1233–40.

67. Farber HJ, Wattigney W, Berenson G. Trends in asthma prevalence: the Bogalusa Heart Study. Ann Allergy Asthma Immunol 1997;78:265–9.

68. Farber HJ, Knowles SB, Brown NL, et al. Secondhand tobacco smoke in children with asthma: sources of and parental perceptions about exposure in children and parental readiness to change. Chest 2008;133: 1367–74.

69. Winkelstein ML, Tarzian A, Wood RA. Parental smoking behavior and passive smoke exposure in children with asthma. Ann Allergy Asthma Immunol 1997;78:419–23.

70. Halterman JS, Borrelli B, Tremblay P, et al. Screening for environmental tobacco smoke exposure among inner-city children with asthma. Pediatrics 2008;122:1277–83.

71. Wakefield M, Banham D, Martin J, et al. Restrictions on smoking at home and urinary cotinine levels among children with asthma. Am J Prev Med 2000;19:188–92.

72. Fiore MC, Jaen CR, Baker TB, et al. Treating tobacco use and dependence: 2008 Update. Clinical Practice Guideline No.18. Rockville, MD: US Department of Health and Human Services, Public Health Service, Agency for Healthcare Research and Quality; 2008.

73. Winickoff JP, Tanski SE, McMillen RC, et al. Child health care clinicians' use of medications to help parents quit smoking: a national parent survey. Pediatrics 2005;115:1013–7.

74. Hanson KL. Patterns of insurance coverage within families with children. Health Aff (Millwood) 2001;20:240–6.

75. Wilson SR, Farber HJ, Knowles S, et al. Results from the Lowering Environmental Tobacco Smoke (LETS) trial. Proc Am Thor Soc 2008;Abstract Issue;177:A53.

76. Massachusetts General Hospital, The Center for Child and Adolescent Health Policy: Clinical Effort Against Secondhand Smoke Exposure (CEASE). Boston, MA. (accessed February 1, 2009): http://www2. massgeneral.org/ceasetobacco/index.htm.

77. Winickoff JP, Park ER, Hipple BJ, et al. Clinical effort against secondhand smoke exposure: development of framework and intervention. Pediatrics 2008;122:e363–e375.

78. Eisenberg MJ, Filion KB, Yavin D, et al. Pharmacotherapies for smoking cessation: a meta-analysis of randomized controlled trials. CMAJ 2008;179:135–44.

79. Shah SD, Wilken LA, Winkler SR, et al. Systematic review and meta-analysis of combination therapy for smoking cessation. J Am Pharm Assoc 2008;48:659–65.

80. Bars MP, Banauch GI, Appel D, et al. 'Tobacco free with FDNY': the New York City Fire Department World Trade Center tobacco cessation study. Chest 2006;129:979–87.

81. Williams SG, Brown CM, Falter KH, et al. Does a multifaceted environmental intervention alter the impact of asthma on inner-city children? J Natl Med Assoc 2006;98:249–60.

82. Morgan WJ, Crain EF, Gruchalla RS, et al. Results of a home-based environmental intervention among urban children with asthma. N Engl J Med 2004;351:1068–80.

83. Glauber JH, Farber HJ, Homer CJ. Asthma clinical pathways: toward what end? (Commentary). Pediatrics 2001;107:590–2.

84. Wesseldine LJ, McCarthy P, Silverman M. Structured discharge procedure for children admitted to hospital with acute asthma: a randomised controlled trial of nursing practice. Arch Dis Child 1999;80: 110–4.

85. Friedman MS, Powell KE, Hutwagner L, et al. Impact of changes in transportation and commuting behaviors during the 1996 Summer Olympic Games in Atlanta on air quality and childhood asthma. JAMA 2001;285:897–905.

86. US Department of Health and Human Services: The health consequences of involuntary exposure to tobacco smoke: a report of the Surgeon General. Atlanta, GA: US Department of Health and Human Services, Centers for Disease Control and Prevention, Coordinating Center for Health Promotion, National Center for Chronic Disease Prevention and Health Promotion, Office on Smoking and Health; 2006.

87. Lavis JN, Robertson D, Woodside JM. How can research organizations more effectively transfer research knowledge to decision makers? Milbank Q 2003;81:221–48.

88. Lavis JN. Research, public policymaking, and knowledge-translation processes: Canadian efforts to build bridges. J Contin Educ Health Prof 2006;26:37–45.

89. US Environmental Protection Agency. Indoor air quality (IAQ) tools for schools program. (accessed February 8, 2009): http://www.epa.gov/iaq/schools.

90. American Lung Association. A national asthma public policy agenda. © 2009, American Lung Association.

Asthma and the Athlete

David A. Stempel

Asthma and the Athlete is an inclusive title that moves beyond the terms of exercise-induced bronchospasm, exercise-induced asthma (EIA), and activity-induced asthma. The focus of this chapter is the limitations on recreational and competitive exercise caused by childhood asthma. Children should have the potential to be a recreational or competitive athlete, unencumbered by the restrictions of illness. The goal applies even to the child banished to 'right field'. The impact of asthma on normal daily activity of all children, whether for an elite athlete or the majority of children at all other levels of skill, is the topic of this chapter.

The 2007 reports of both the National Asthma Education and Prevention Program (NAEPP) and the Global Initiative for Asthma (GINA) state that asthma symptoms associated with exercise are often manifestations of inadequately controlled asthma.[1,2] Patients who present with exercise as the only precipitant of asthma symptoms should be monitored regularly for evidence of persistent asthma. EIA is 'one expression of airway hyperresponsiveness, not a special form of asthma. EIA often indicates that the patient's asthma is not adequately controlled; therefore appropriate antiinflammatory therapy generally results in the reduction of exercise-related symptoms'.[3] Exercise is occasionally the only apparent trigger of asthma. One goal of asthma management is to 'enable most patients to participate in any activity they choose without experiencing symptoms'.[3] GINA recommends that physical activity be part of the therapeutic approach to EIA in addition to pharmacotherapy.

There is a continuum from the laboratory concept of exercise-induced bronchospasm to the clinical reality of the effect of asthma on daily physical activity. EIA may be formally defined as a 'transient narrowing of the airways that follows vigorous exercise'.[4] Exercise-induced asthma is the common term used to describe this form of asthma, but activity-induced asthma (AIA) is a more descriptive definition for children who wheeze with any type of exertion. Exercise is too limiting a term for the pediatric population because it focuses attention on formal exertion and not the frequent limitations imposed by asthma on a child's daily activities, which include multiple bursts of physical exertion from informal playground activities to competition in athletic events. Therapy for children needs to reflect the frequency of physical activity and on-demand need for bronchoprotection. Symptoms of asthma associated with activity occur in children with varying levels of exercise, only some of which is vigorous exercise. EIA is the term that will be used in this chapter because it is the present standard term in the literature and for the purposes of this chapter will include the large number of children who have persistent asthma and have exercise as a trigger and the smaller group of children who wheeze only with vigorous exertion.

EIA is defined from a physiologic perspective as intermittent airflow obstruction measured by a defined decline (usually 10–20%) in forced expiratory volume in 1 second (FEV_1) or peak expiratory flow rate (PEF). Exercise is a common, if not nearly universal, trigger of chronic asthma for children and adolescents. Persistent asthma, even in the absence of symptoms, or even during periods of remission, is frequently associated with inflammation.[5] Although most triggers of asthma induce increases in airway inflammation, the role of inflammation in acute EIA is less well defined. Because EIA occurs in children with persistent asthma, inflammation is frequently found in the child with incompletely controlled disease. Activity by itself is rarely the only trigger of asthma, and isolated EIA may suggest the need to search for an alternative diagnosis. Elite athletes without persistent asthma represent a small and unique phenotype of children with EIA. Whether exercise exists as a single trigger of asthma for the majority of children is not clear. The literature discusses the treatment of EIA in the absence of persistent asthma but does not describe whether these patients lack the inflammatory changes noted with the chronic forms of the disease (Box 40-1).

Markers of inflammation are noted during acute EIA and correlate with decline in lung function. A study in children with a mean age of 9.2 to 9.5 years demonstrated a significant correlation between the maximal fall in FEV_1 and the total blood eosinophil count.[6] Similar findings were noted in a study using exhaled nitric oxide (eNO) as a surrogate marker of inflammation. Increases in eNO correlated with the fall in FEV_1 following exercise challenge.[7]

The symptoms of EIA include any of the following associated with increased activity: shortness of breath, cough, wheeze, chest tightness, or difficulty breathing. Less frequently reported as symptoms of EIA are the lack of endurance and/or impairment in quality of life (Box 40-2). Similar to other forms of asthma, EIA is frequently under-recognized by the patient and parent, under-diagnosed by the healthcare professional, and therefore under-treated. For many children and adolescents, the only complaints may be the perception that they are out of shape or lack the interest to participate in exertional activities. Bronchial hyperresponsiveness (BHR) correlates with decreasing activity level in children with asthma.[8] It is unclear whether increasing disease severity further restricts a child's activity level or whether a more sedentary lifestyle has a further negative impact on BHR. Poor perception of the symptoms of EIA is common. Different activities will produce different degrees of airway narrowing. Godfrey

BOX 40-1 Key concepts

BOX 40-1 Key concepts

Exercise-induced asthma

- Exercise-induced asthma (EIA) occurs in most children and adolescents with persistent asthma.
- From 10–14% of children have EIA.
- The treatment of EIA begins with the treatment of persistent asthma.

BOX 40-2

Subjective and Objective Findings in Exercise-induced Asthma

Subjective Findings with Exertion

Wheezing

Cough

Shortness of breath

Perception of poor physical conditioning

Lack of interest in physical activities

Objective Findings with Exertion

Fall in lung function of 10–15%

Protection against a 15% fall in forced expiratory volume in 1 second

Protection with bronchodilators

BOX 40-3

Variables in Exercise-induced Asthma

Type of exercise

Duration of exercise

Ambient temperature

Ambient humidity

Associated triggers

Controller asthma medications

Bronchoprotective treatments

BOX 40-4

Assessment for Exercise-induced Asthma

History

Baseline spirometry

Exercise challenge

and colleagues[9] established a rank order exercise leading to EIA from the largest to the smallest effect on reduction in PEFR: free-range running, treadmill, bicycle ergometer, swimming, and walking. Ambient temperature and humidity also are discussed in this chapter, as are additional variables on the effect of the degree of fall in FEV_1 associated with EIA.

This chapter is divided into three sections: the definition, epidemiology, and differential of EIA; studies of the mechanism of disease; and the treatment of EIA.

Definition and Prevalence Definition and Prevalence

All children with persistent asthma should have their activity level assessed at the time of initial presentation and at follow-up visits. Up to 90% of children with persistent asthma have symptoms of EIA. In addition, all children with isolated EIA should be assessed for symptoms of persistent asthma. The reporting of EIA may vary depending on the type of exertion, the effort of the child, the duration of the activity, time of year and the ambient climate at the time of the activity. These and other variables are important when one compares the reported incidence of EIA[10] (Box 40-3). For children with asthma, exercise with concurrent allergen exposure or viral infection may further increase airway narrowing during activity.

EIA is found in virtually all children with a diagnosis of asthma.[11] Godfrey,[11] in his classic review article, describes the prevalence rate with testing and retesting. A fall of 10% to 15% in FEV1 and a 15% fall in PEFR are usually used as the standards for the diagnosis of EIA. False-positive test results in normal subjects without atopic backgrounds are uncommon. In children, a history of previous wheeze, a family history of asthma, and a diagnosis of allergic rhinitis all appear to be risk factors for greater bronchial reactivity with or without clinical EIA. The

therapeutic implication of children with allergic rhinitis who manifest a 15% fall in FEV_1 in the absence of any clinical symptoms or physical limitations raises the following important but unanswered questions. Would these children benefit from therapy? Are these children more likely to have later adult-onset asthma?

The appropriate diagnosis of EIA starts with the proper identification of children with chronic asthma (Box 40-4). A detailed history, including prior response to inhaled short-acting β agonists and measurement of lung function in children over 5 years of age, is helpful. Baseline FEV_1 in children with persistent asthma may be normal even in the presence of active disease.[12] Children with asthma, if appropriately questioned, will usually respond that they have physical activity limitations imposed by exercise. What is more important and more difficult to do is to assess the undiagnosed asthmatic population for the presence of EIA.

The formal diagnosis of EIA is usually made after a 10% to 15% fall in FEV_1. The lower value is selected for laboratory studies and the higher value for field testing.[4] The average decline in FEV_1 after exertion for normal individuals is 5% or less. In healthy school children, 92% have less than a 10% fall in PEFR and 98% have less than a 15% fall in PEFR.[11] Response to treatment is frequently defined as protection against a fall of greater than 10% to 15% after exercise challenge. The literature does not stipulate what the baseline fall in FEV_1 needs to be in studies designed to demonstrate efficacy other than children must demonstrate less than a 10% to 15% fall with exertion for purposes of prevention of EIA. It is difficult to compare different studies of children with EIA because of the variability of baseline parameters. Furthermore, when studying the addition of a second controller medication, there are no established effect size criteria for determining additional benefit.

Godfrey[11] described the classic response of lung function to an exercise challenge. During the initial minutes of the exercise challenge, there is a small increase in PEF, followed by a more significant fall in PEF and a gradual return to normal lung function with rest over a 1-hour period (Figure 40-1). This pattern is not applicable to a large number of children who start with their FEV_1 reduced below their personal best. These data are not well documented in the literature and further complicated by the fact

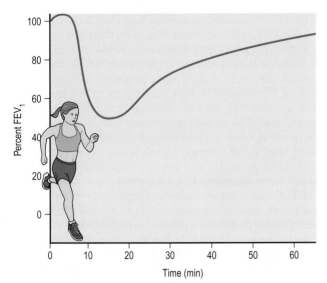

FIGURE 40-1 Change in forced expiratory volume in 1 second *(FEV₁)* after a 6-minute exercise challenge in a child with persistent asthma.

that children commonly have baseline lung function values that are greater than 100% of predicted.

The timing of the exercise challenge tests may alter the sensitivity of these tests in children. In a retrospective analysis of children being evaluated for EIA, those tested during the summer months had 50% fewer positive tests than those children tested during other seasons when symptoms of persistent asthma are more commonly reported in association with common viral illnesses. The children tested in this report all had normal baseline spirometry and none were on asthma controller medications. This data suggests that the challenge tests have a lower sensitivity during periods of decreased asthma activity and the authors recommend that testing be performed during symptomatic periods.[13]

The prevalence of EIA varies in reports from 45% to 94%.[14] Godfrey's[11] review reported that up to 86% of children with persistent asthma demonstrated EIA on testing. These data suggest that exercise is the most universal trigger of persistent asthma for children and adolescents. McFadden[15] reported in a survey of more than 400 consecutive patients with asthma that 94% indicated that they had airflow limitation associated with exercise. Children who no longer demonstrate active symptoms of asthma appear to retain some of their airway lability associated with exercise.[14] This may be related to the persistent finding of inflammation and increased submucosal collagen deposition found in this group of former childhood asthmatics.[3]

EIA is reported in 2.8% to 17% of elite world-class athletes. Weiler and colleagues[16] conducted a questionnaire of athletes competing for the USA in the 1996 summer Olympics. Of the athletes responding to the survey, 15.3% answered 'yes' to whether they had been told in the past that they had asthma or EIA.[16] When both history of asthma and previous use of asthma medications were combined, the rate increased to 16.7%. These results indicate a 50% increase in symptom report from the 1984 games, although the criteria differed somewhat in the earlier survey. The prevalence of EIA is greater with exercise at extremely high activity levels and in cold environments.[17] In this study, 10.4% of the athletes had the need for asthma medications at the time of the 1996 Olympic games. More females (19.9%) than males (14.3%) had a positive history of asthma or need for asthma medications. These results are higher than the approximately 10% lifetime prevalence of asthma for the US population recently reported.[18]

Hammerman and colleagues[19] reported on an assessment of high school athletes for asthma. They investigated 801 student athletes with a questionnaire, measurement of PEFR, and a free run challenge (a 15% drop in PEFR after an 8-minute run). Of the athletes responding to the questionnaire, 5.7% stated that they had asthma or EIA. All of these students had a positive exercise challenge. Of the known asthmatics, 85% had a positive exercise challenge despite using their prescribed medications. An additional 6.1% of these athletes had a positive exercise challenge and were identified as having undiagnosed asthma. Of these students who did not consider themselves as having asthma, 55% were identified by the questionnaire as having EIA. The prevalence of EIA was 16% of females and 9% of males. These findings again suggest that the prevalence of asthma may be greater than reported when more complete evaluations are performed and include the assessment of the effect of exercise on asthma.

Rupp and colleagues[20] demonstrated that baseline spirometry and questionnaire had significant false positive and false negative rates when used as a screening tool for EIA in a group of 166 high school athletes. Exercise challenge was used as the definitive test. Forty-eight students were considered at risk for EIA by history and screening spirometry. Twenty-two (13%) of these adolescents had positive exercise challenges. Of these students, 14, or 64%, were not identified by the screening survey or spirometry, suggesting the potential need to test all athletes. There are several explanations for the high rate of inaccuracy of screening. First, high school athletes are more likely to have higher than normal baseline lung function. There is also the possibility that there is a denial factor in the response to the questionnaire leading to the false-negative results.

A British Columbia study used a 'free running asthma screening test' and a questionnaire to assess EIA. This study screened 830 teenage volunteers.[21] In contrast to the previous study, the participants were not restricted to just the high school athletes. Exercise testing demonstrated that 13.2% of subjects had a 15% fall in PEFR after 6 minutes of activity that doubled their resting heart rate. The questionnaire alone failed to identify 34% of the students with EIA-positive tests even though they participated in a 15-minute workshop on asthma before filling out the survey. These two studies demonstrate the lack of specificity of questionnaires and support the need for formal exercise testing to reduce the false negative results of the surveys.

A large study was undertaken in Barcelona to look at the prevalence of asthma by history and to correlate bronchial responsiveness to exercise in 3000 school-age children aged 13 to 14 years. As in the previous studies, approximately 11% of children were noted to have positive exercise tests. In contrast, only 4% were noted to have 'current asthma' as defined by positive responses to the International Study of Asthma and Allergies in Childhood questionnaire and a history of bronchial responsiveness.[22] Present wheezing and treatment for respiratory symptoms in the past 12 months were the most predictive for positive exercise challenges. This discordance between positive challenge and the presence of active asthma symptoms by history confirms the need for more formal testing of EIA and affirms that underreporting or under-diagnosing of EIA, either alone or in the presence of persistent asthma, is common.

Differential Diagnosis

For the child who volunteers the history of EIA (wheeze, cough, dyspnea with activity), it is important to document the type of exercise, the duration of the activity, and the limitations placed by the associated respiratory difficulty. Response to various treatments is also important. More difficult to diagnose is the child with a sedentary lifestyle or the child with a preference for sedentary activities. Is this preference a response to the inability to breathe comfortably with exertion? For the child with asthma who avoids activity the frequent responsw to questions regarding activity level is that he or she is not in 'shape'. In addition, there are a group of children with EIA who have a significant fall in FEV_1 without symptoms. On the other side of the issue is the highly skilled nonasthmatic athlete who experiences rapid breathing with exertion that may be the normal physiologic response to activity and whose child, family, or physician is concerned that the diagnosis may be asthma.

The previous studies of the prevalence of EIA in high school students indicate that approximately 11% to 13% of adolescents with symptoms of cough and dyspnea associated with exercise have EIA. Empiric therapy may start with a trial of a short-acting inhaled β agonist. If this trial is successful, one has presumptive confirmation of the diagnosis of EIA. When the treatment fails, one needs to consider other diagnoses. Exercise-induced hyperventilation is included in the differential. Hammo and Weinberger[23] report a study of 32 children with uncertain diagnosis of EIA who had an exercise challenge consisting of treadmill running and monitoring of O_2 saturation and end-tidal CO_2. Four of the children had a classic asthma response to the challenge, and 17 had no significant change in any of the three study parameters. Of interest were the 11 children who complained of chest tightness without a significant fall in the FEV_1 or change in the O_2 saturation. These children had the largest fall: 23.2% in end-tidal CO_2. As a group they appeared to be highly competitive athletically and usually complained of dyspnea during times of peak performance.

Vocal cord dysfunction (VCD) should be considered in the differential of children with atypical EIA. EIA and VCD often occur concurrently. Patients with VCD may appear to be refractory to normal treatment for EIA. VCD differs from EIA in that the symptoms appear and resolve abruptly. VCD is associated with inspiratory wheeze and is more likely to occur during the day. In a report by Landwehr and colleagues,[24] the majority of the children studied had concurrent psychological difficulties. Abnormal movement of the arytenoid region during exercise has also been identified as a cause of exertional dyspnea associated with exercise. In this case it was associated with bronchial hyperreactivity and was responsive to speech therapy.[25] Additionally, the differential diagnosis needs to include fixed central airway obstruction and muscle disorders. EIA is distinguished from these illnesses by its more classic concave pattern of obstructive airways disease noted during the expiratory flow-volume curve. Finally, cardiac disease and other restrictive and obstructive respiratory disorders need to be considered in the differential of exertional dyspnea (Box 40-5).

Is there a gold standard for diagnosing EIA? The child with a positive history of EIA that is confirmed by an exercise challenge with a fall of 15% is an easy diagnosis. Less clear is the child with a 15% fall in FEV_1 without symptoms – does this child have EIA? What if this change in lung function is noted in a child with seasonal allergic rhinitis without symptoms of EIA? Is this underappreciated disease in a child with persistent asthma, or just evidence of increased BHR that deserves no active treatment? There is no definitive answer, although one might propose a therapeutic trial with either pretreatment with a short-acting β agonist or use of inhaled corticosteroids as controller therapy, as discussed later in this chapter. Methacholine hyperreactivity is present in most patients with a positive exercise test, but BHR is also found in the absence of EIA. Of interest is the fact that treatment of EIA may produce protection against the symptoms of exercise before there is improvement in exercise challenge, and this occurs before protection against nonspecific BHR.[26] Although there is a strong association between these two challenges, nonspecific bronchial hyperreactivity may lead to a high rate of false-positive values if it is used as a surrogate marker of EIA.

Mechanism of Disease

There are presently two main theories to explain the pathophysiology of EIA. The 'thermal hypothesis'[15] states that the transfer of heat from the airway mucosa to the airways and back to the mucosa during hyperpnea is the primary feature of the disease. In this theory, hyperventilation and exercise that ensures control of ambient temperature and humidity demonstrate the same degree of airway obstruction. The 'osmotic theory'[27] stresses that the exercising person has evaporation from the airway surface that leads to an osmotic gradient resulting in cell volume loss. This process then leads to bronchial smooth muscle contraction. Whether heat loss or water loss is the primary etiology of EIA, it is clear that breathing cold, dry air produces airway narrowing in the asthmatic patient.

The importance of inflammatory mediators in the pathophysiology of EIA has been controversial. Hallstrand and colleagues[28] exercise-challenged a group of 13 mild atopic asthmatics. Venous blood samples after exercise showed an increase in T helper cell type 2 lymphocyte activation with increased numbers of $CD23^+$ B cells and $CD25^+$ T cells. This study proposes an inflammatory mechanism for EIA. The variable attenuation of EIA by both a leukotriene receptor antagonist (LTRA) and histamine suggests a partial, varying, or incomplete involvement of these mediators in the pathophysiology of EIA. Prostaglandins have also been demonstrated to have a significant role in EIA.[29] In the osmotic hypothesis, it is suggested that the osmotic gradient caused by the water loss induces cells to release mediators that are implicated in the inflammatory process.

EIA occurs most commonly in the presence of persistent asthma. Airway inflammation is a universal characteristic of persistent asthma, whether the disease is active or asymptomatic. In addition, individuals demonstrating increased bronchial hyperreactivity to exercise and challenge (methacholine or histamine) have evidence of active airway inflammation. Patients with EIA have significantly higher levels of eosinophils and eosinophilic cationic protein in their sputum than asthmatics without EIA and with normal subjects. Furthermore, the severity of the EIA correlates with the percent of sputum eosinophils.[30]

Treatment

The vast majority of pediatric patients with EIA have underlying persistent asthma, with exercise as one of many triggers of their

---

BOX 40-5

Differential for Exercise-induced Asthma

Exercise-induced hyperventilation

Vocal cord dysfunction

Central airway obstruction

Cardiac disease

Other restrictive or obstructive pulmonary disease

Muscle disorders

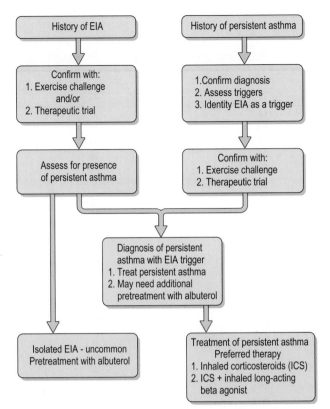

FIGURE 40-2 Clinical algorithm for exercise-induced asthma (EIA).

BOX 40-6

Treatment Options for Exercise-induced Asthma

Aerobic conditioning

Warm-up exercise

Treatment of persistent asthma

Pretreatment with or without persistent medications

EIA can be attenuated with physical conditioning alone or in the presence of active pharmacologic therapy. Aerobic conditioning has been demonstrated to improve aerobic fitness, reduce dyspnea associated with exertion, and improve the ventilatory capacity in patients with EIA.[31] Patients with EIA appear to have less difficulty if they perform warm-up exercise before exertion. Endogenous production of prostaglandin-2 may relax airway smooth muscle during this initial phase of activity[18] (Box 40-6).

The first step in the pharmacologic treatment of EIA is to gain control of the underlying airway inflammation in the child with persistent asthma. As mentioned in the beginning of this chapter, EIA occurs most often in children with persistent asthma for whom controller therapy is appropriate. Table 40-1 lists the studies in children of controller therapy and their impact on EIA. National and international guidelines state that inhaled corticosteroids are the most effective controller treatment for persistent asthma. This class of medication is associated with decreases in airway inflammation and improvement in BHR. Studies performed several decades ago looked at whether inhaled corticosteroids used prior to exercise could have a bronchoprotective effect. These trials were uniformly negative.

In contrast, studies of inhaled corticosteroids as a controller for persistent asthma demonstrate a consistent beneficial effect. A Cochrane review in 2007 based predominantly on pediatric studies reported that routine use of inhaled corticosteroids was associated with the prevention of EIA.[32] One of the early studies addressing the use of inhaled corticosteroids for EIA in persistent asthma was performed by Henriksen and Dahl.[33] They studied the effect of inhaled budesonide 200 µg twice daily and terbutaline alone and in combination in a group of children. The inhaled corticosteroid treated children had a significant, pre-exercise improvement in FEV_1 (19%) after 1 week of therapy. Terbutaline, budesonide, and the combination of the two therapies reduced the fall in FEV_1 by 30%, 51%, and 84%. The combination was thought to be additive and not synergistic. In addition, the authors found that the protection afforded by inhaled corticosteroids was related to its effect on BHR and not simply the improvement in lung function.

Another study investigated the dose-response protective effect of 100, 200, and 400 µg/day of budesonide. Children with moderate to severe asthma who were naïve to inhaled corticosteroids were studied and received increasing doses of budesonide every 4 weeks. There was a dose-dependent increase in FEV_1 between the three doses of budesonide, but the diary recordings of day and night PEF, day symptoms, and night symptoms improved after the use of budesonide for 4 weeks but did not differ among the three doses. In contrast, there was a dose-dependent protection against EIA. The maximum protection against the fall in FEV_1 after exercise for 100, 200, and 400 µg/day of budesonide was 54%, 64%, and 82%, respectively.[34] Greater improvement in FEV_1 was associated with greater bronchoprotection.

Jonasson and colleagues[35] studied a group of children with mild asthma and EIA. Their baseline FEV_1 was 100% of predicted. The children were placed on one of three doses of budeso-

disease. One can make the argument that EIA does not occur in the absence of persistent asthma. The initial preferred treatment in the NAEPP and GINA guidelines for children and adolescents with persistent asthma is the use of inhaled corticosteroids. The recognition of the importance of inflammation in the pathophysiology of asthma has led to the early introduction of inhaled corticosteroids as the most effective controller therapy for persistent asthma and therefore needs to be considered as the primary treatment for EIA in the presence of persistent asthma. The list of potential controller medications that may be beneficial in treating the underlying asthma includes inhaled corticosteroids, cromolyn, LTRAs, nedocromil, salmeterol, and theophylline. Three bronchoprotective therapies (medications to be used 15–120 minutes prior to exercise) include short-acting β agonist, cromolyn and LTRAs. Unfortunately, there are few comparative trials of these different controller or bronchoprotective agents (Figure 40-2).

In an attempt to compare the evidence from the literature in a uniform fashion comparing data from different trials, the baseline maximum fall in FEV_1 and the percent protection reported are the variables presented in this review. Area under the curve FEV_1 is reported in some studies, but because the common variable is percent maximal fall or percent protection of FEV_1, these will be the standards presented. These comparisons recognize the limitations imposed by the various challenges, the testing environment, and baseline characteristics of the study subjects. Some investigators have used protection against a 15% fall in FEV_1 as the standard for efficacy of a therapeutic agent. Other authors have reported the percent change. The heterogeneity of the baseline fall in lung function limits these comparisons. The baseline severity differs with baseline falls in FEV_1 of 15% to 20% in some studies and others have greater than 30%. Another variable reported in some recent studies has been the time to recovery from EIA.

Table 40-1 Pediatric Trials for the Treatment of Exercise-induced Asthma

Reference	Treatment	N	Maximum fall in FEV$_1$ (%)		Protection (%)	
Kemp et al[37] (CO)	Placebo	25	26			
	Montelukast	25	18		31	
Pearlman et al[39] (CO)	Placebo	39	16.7			
	Zafirlukast 5 mg	20	8.9		47	
	Zafirlukast 10 mg	19	11.1		34	
	Zafirlukast 20 mg	20	8.5		49	
	Zafirlukast 40 mg	19	10.2		6.5	
Hofstra et al[26] (PG)	Placebo	12	27.1			
	Fluticasone 100 µg	11	9.9		63	
	Fluticasone 250 µg	14	7.6		72	
Jónasson et al[35] (PG)	Placebo	14	16		21	
	Budesonide 100 µg	14	7		73	
	Budesonide 200 µg	14	7.5		70	
	Budesonide 100 µg twice daily	15	7		56	
Pederson and Hansen[34] (CO)	Budesonide 100 µg	19	25.7		54	
	Budesonide 200 µg	19	20.1		64	
	Budesonide 400 µg	19	9.9		83	
Vidal et al[45] (CO)	Baseline	20	24			
	Budesonide 400 µg twice daily	20	6		75	
	Montelukast 10 mg	20	12		50	
Pedersen[34] (CO)	Placebo	25	27.9			
	HFA Beclomethamone 50 µg, once daily	25	20.8		25	
	HFA Beclomethamone 100 µg, once daily	25	20.9		25	
Simons et al[45] Background twice daily BDP and once daily salmeterol (CO)			Day 1	Day 28	Day 1	Day28
	Placebo (1 hour)	13	24	16		
	Salmeterol (1 hour)	13	−7	4	130	75
	Placebo (9 hours)	13	18	15		
	Salmeterol (9 hours)	13	6	10	67	33

FEV$_1$, Forced expiratory volume in 1 second; CO, crossover study; PG, parallel group.

nide 100 or 200 µg once daily, 100 µg twice daily, or placebo. Budesonide improved both daily symptoms and protected against EIA. The protection with the three doses was similar and ranged from 58% to 74%.

Hofstra and colleagues[26] addressed the issue of whether the effect of inhaled corticosteroids on EIA was dose dependent or varied by the duration of the treatment. In this study, children were treated with either fluticasone propionate (FP) at doses of 100 or 250 µg twice daily or placebo for 6 months. The fall in FEV$_1$ after exercise was reduced by 71% to 79% and did not differ significantly with the dose or from week 3 to week 24. In contrast, the PD$_{20}$ methacholine increased significantly over time during the 6 months ($P = 0.04$) of the trial. The higher doses of fluticasone propionate correlated with greater protection ($P = 0.06$). The implication of this greater protection against methacholine noted with the higher dose of inhaled corticosteroid in the absence of greater clinical effect on bronchoprotection is difficult to explain. Sont and colleagues[36] also demonstrated a dose-response effect to inhaled corticosteroids when the dose was varied to reflect BHR. In that report there was greater protection against mild asthma exacerbations as BHR improved. Interestingly, in the study by Hofstra and colleagues,[26] there is no greater improvement in exercise challenge to correlate with the greater improvement in BHR.

Two pediatric studies looked at the effect of maintenance LTRA on EIA. The first study by Kemp and colleagues[37] evaluated 27 children with EIA treated with montelukast 5 mg for 2 days in a crossover fashion. The challenges were then performed

at 20 to 24 hours post dose. The percent maximum fall in FEV$_1$ was 26% for placebo and 18% for montelukast. There was a 31% inhibition of EIA with the active medication. The recovery time after the fall in lung function post-EIA was also reduced 38% for the montelukast-treated patients. These results are comparable to a 12-week study in adults by Leff and colleagues.[38] At the 12-week challenge, patients had a 31.6% inhibition of EIA and a recovery time that was reduced by 27%.

In another study, Pearlman and colleagues[39] assessed the effects of zafirlukast. The study subjects were controller naïve. There were two groups of patients, with each completing a three-way crossover. Group 1 was treated with 5 mg and 20 mg of zafirlukast and placebo. Group 2 was given 10 and 40 mg of zafirlukast, and there was a placebo arm. Study medications were given 4 hours before exercise challenge. Baseline FEV$_1$ was 88% to 91% of predicted. Maximum fall in FEV$_1$ with placebo was 16.3% to 17.1%, and with 5, 10, 20, and 40 mg of zafirlukast was 8.9%, 11.1%, 8.7%, and 10.2%, respectively.[39] The protection afforded by zafirlukast did not appear to be dose related. Overall, there was a 42% protective effect with zafirlukast.

Two studies from the adult literature have compared 8-week treatment of EIA with either montelukast or salmeterol as controller therapy. In an article by Edelman and colleagues,[40] patients were not allowed to use inhaled corticosteroids, and in the study by Villaran and colleagues,[41] only 6% and 14% of patients were on inhaled corticosteroids in addition to salmeterol and montelukast, respectively. (The present recommendation is to use long-acting bronchodilators only in combination with inhaled corticosteroids when they are administered on a daily basis.) These studies performed exercise challenge only at the approximate end of the dosing period, 9 and 21 hours for salmeterol and montelukast, respectively. In both studies, the percent protection was greater for montelukast. In the Edelman and colleagues study,[40] montelukast did not prevent a mean 15% fall in FEV_1 with exercise. Nelson and colleagues[42] noted that the bronchoprotective effect in EIA for salmeterol decreases between 9 and 12 hours post treatment. GINA and NAEPP guidelines do not recommend the use of long-acting β agonists (salmeterol and formoterol) as monotherapy for persistent asthma.

In a crossover study of 20 asthmatics with a median age of 17 years, patients were treated with either budesonide 400 µg twice daily or montelukast 10 mg daily. The baseline FEV_1 was 100% to 101% predicted in both groups with no change in baseline from either therapy prior to the exercise challenge. Both medications provided protection against EIA. Budesonide was effective in 80% of the patients, with a mean bronchoprotection of 75% compared to 50% for montelukast.[43] Although budesonide was more effective in a greater number of patients, both treatments had significant heterogeneity in their bronchoprotection, from 0% to 100%.

The role of dual controller therapy in protecting against pediatric EIA is addressed in the literature but there are no definitive conclusions and no licensed indication. Although adult studies have demonstrated greater improvement in lung function and symptom control with the addition of a long-acting bronchodilator to an inhaled corticosteroid than with an LTRA, these studies have not been replicated in children and adolescents.[42,44]

A study of children with persistent asthma treated with chronic inhaled corticosteroids[45] demonstrated a statistically significant bronchoprotective effect after 4 weeks of treatment with once daily salmeterol at 1 but not at 9 hours. In this study of 14 children on inhaled beclomethasone, 100 to 200 µg twice daily, with baseline FEV_1 of 98% to 106% predicted, the fall in FEV_1 at 9 hours was 9% with salmeterol and 15% with placebo. The patients on inhaled corticosteroids alone demonstrated a degree of protection against EIA, and the limited additional effect of salmeterol may be due to the small fall in lung function with exercise challenge in the placebo-treated patients. The difference between salmeterol and placebo was not statistically different with the addition of salmeterol to beclomethasone preventing a 15% fall in FEV_1. Two children on placebo exited the study because of worsening asthma.

A study investigated patients with persistent asthma and EIA with incomplete control of their EIA on FP 250 µg twice daily or the equivalent. These patients still had a greater than 20% decline in FEV_1 with exercise despite using inhaled corticosteroids. Patients were randomized for 4 weeks to chronic treatment with either FP 250 µg or FP 250 µg and salmeterol 50 µg combination (FSC) twice daily. They were exercise challenged on day 1 and at week 4 and at 1 and 8.5 hours post dosing. The study revealed that, at all time points, the combination FSC produced greater protection and no loss of bronchoprotection over the 4-week trial ($P < 0.016$).[46] At the 8.5 hour challenge on week 4, the FP monotherapy patients had an approximately 20% and the FSC patients had a 12% decline in FEV_1 with exercise challenge. These data are consistent with the data from the Simons and colleagues study,[45] but with the larger sample of nearly 100 patients in each cohort, a clinical and statistically different 40% greater protection is shown.

The use of antihistamines has been proposed as a potential treatment for EIA, although they have limited use in the treatment of persistent asthma. Badier and colleagues[47] investigated the effect of terfenadine 120 mg twice daily (at twice the recommended dose) and demonstrated an attenuation of hyperventilation-induced bronchospasm. Baki and Orhan[48] treated 11 children with 10 mg of loratadine and demonstrated a 42% reduction in EIA with the medication at 5 minutes post challenge. The authors caution that loratadine failed to prevent a 15% fall in FEV_1, the accepted standard that defines protection against EIA. Dahlen and colleagues[49] presented data on the use of zafirlukast 80 mg twice daily (4 times the recommended dosage), loratadine 10 mg twice daily (twice the recommended dosage), the combination of the two medications, and placebo in a four-way crossover trial. Subjects used these medications for 7 days before the exercise challenge. The mean FEV_1 at baseline was 90% predicted with a mean fall of 25.7% post exercise. Patients on placebo had a mean fall in FEV_1 with exercise of 21.6%; loratadine, 22.8%; zafirlukast, 13.9%; and the combination of the two active therapies, 10.3%. In this trial, there was no benefit from loratadine in preventing EIA either alone or in addition to zafirlukast. In general, the data with antihistamines remain inconclusive and do not support their role in the treatment of EIA.

The use of medications immediately prior to exertion has been the classic strategy for the treatment of EIA. Pretreatment can be used in the presence of controller therapy as demonstrated in the trial by Henriksen and Dahl or as an isolated treatment for children with exercise as the single trigger of asthma. For pretreatment of EIA, inhaled short acting β agonists are the standard of care. Two inhalations of a short-acting inhaled $β_2$ agonist 15 minutes prior to exercise provide many children with significant improvement in EIA for 1 to 2 hours.

Montelukast has been demonstrated to be effective when used 2 hours prior to exercise for preventing EIA. The studies have been conducted in adults and therefore the indication is for patients 15 years of age and older.[50,51] There are no comparative trials of albuterol and montelukast pretreatment for EIA that study these medications in their approved dosing. There is one crossover double-blind, double-dummy trial comparing albuterol prior to exercise and 3 to 7 days of montelukast pretreatment. The results indicated that albuterol was more effective in the prevention of EIA than montelukast.[52] This study did not compare the two medications as single doses prior to activity.

Long-acting bronchodilators such as salmeterol and formoterol may provide 8 to 10 hours of protection if used prior to activity to protect against EIA. Since the large majority of children with EIA have persistent asthma, this class of medications should be considered only in combination with inhaled corticosteroids as part of a daily controller medication program for patients not controlled on an inhaled corticosteroid alone. Cromolyn and nedocromil have been used as bronchoprotective therapies but with less demonstrated efficacy than albuterol. The literature on oral bronchodilators and inhaled anticholinergics for EIA is limited.[15]

Nonpharmacologic therapies have been suggested for EIA. The effect of physical training on blunting EIA has shown variable results. Warm-up exercise can attenuate EIA in some cases, but the effect has only a 30- to 40-minute duration of action. Additionally, there have been attempts to design devices that warm and humidify the air to alveolar conditions. These have shown some benefit but are generally not acceptable to the athletes.

Conclusions

There are multiple medical, physical and social reasons to have people exercise regularly. Healthy lifestyles include the need for regular exercise. Starting this pattern in childhood is important.

BOX 40-7 Therapeutic principles

Appropriate diagnosis

   Recognize exercise-induced asthma (EIA) as a component of most persistent asthma

   Assess for persistent asthma if history of isolated EIA

   Rule out other causes of exertional dyspnea

Ensure normal or near-normal physical activity level

Treat persistent asthma with 'step-wise approach'[49]

   Inhaled corticosteroids (low dose)

   ICS (low dose) plus inhaled, long-acting β_2 agonists

Pretreatment if needed with inhaled short-acting β_2 agonists

---

EIA is common and may effect between 10% to 14% of children. It is a nearly universal trigger of persistent childhood asthma. The history for EIA can be complicated by the lack of perception of significant airway obstruction during exercise by many children. Further, EIA may vary by intensity depending of the type of exercise and presence of other concurrent triggers of asthma. One must carefully identify those children with EIA from the group of children who report low level of activity because of lack of interest or because they are 'out of shape'. Baseline spirometry of children with persistent asthma is frequently normal. Formal exercise challenge, however, is important to identify those children with EIA who under-recognize their disease. Exercise testing should be considered when the diagnosis is unclear or if there appears to be a lack of bronchoprotection with inhaled albuterol.

The goal of treatment for EIA should be to improve exercise capacity or achieve normal activity level for all children and adolescents. Identification of the limits imposed by EIA and establishment of goals of therapy with the child and family should be the initial action. Inactivity in the presence of this diagnosis should not be accepted. Since EIA is most commonly a component of persistent asthma, therapy should start with control of the underlying persistent asthma (Box 40-7). Inhaled corticosteroids are the most effective initial treatment of both EIA and persistent asthma in children and adolescents as recommended in the NAEPP and GINA guidelines.[1,2] EIA is a common trigger of a prevalent disease that warrants proper diagnosis and treatment to assure the quality of life that all children and adolescents deserve.

References

1. National Institutes of Health. National Heart, Lung, and Blood Institute. National Education and Prevention Program. Expert Panel Report 3. Guidelines for the diagnosis and management of asthma. Summary report 2007. NIH Publication Number 08-5846. October 2007.
2. Global Initiative for Asthma. Global strategy for asthma management and prevention. Updated 2007. Available at http://www.ginasthma.org. Accessed January 16, 2008.
3. Global Initiative for Asthma. Global strategy for asthma management, Washington, DC, February 2002, U.S. Department of Health and Human Services. NIH Pub No. 02-3659.
4. Anderson SD, Holzer K. Exercise-induced asthma: is it the right diagnosis in the elite athlete? J Allergy Clin Immunol 2000;106:419–28.
5. Van Den Toorn LM, Overbeck SE, De Jongste JC, et al. Airway inflammation is present during clinical remission of atopic asthma. Am J Respir Crit Care Med 2001;164:2107–13.
6. Lee SY, Kim HB, Kim JH, et al. Eosinophils play a major role in the severity of exercise-induced bronchoconstricytion in children with asthma. Pediatr Pulmonol 2006;41:1161–6.
7. Nishio K, Odajima H, Motomura C, et al. Exhaled nitric oxide and exercise-induced bronchospasm assessed by FEV1 or FEF 25–75 in childhood asthma. J Asthma 2007;44:475–8.
8. Nystad W, Stigum H, Carlsen KH. Increase level of bronchial responsiveness in inactive children with asthma. Respir Med 2001;95:806–10.
9. Godfrey S, Silverman M, Anderson SD. Problems of interpreting exercise-induced asthma. J Allergy Clin Immunol 1973;52:199–209.
10. McFadden ER, Gilbert IA. Exercise-induced asthma. N Engl J Med 1994;330:1362–7.
11. Godfrey S. Exercise-induced asthma-clinical, physiological, and therapeutic implications. J Allergy Clin Immunol 1975;56:1–17.
12. Childhood Asthma Management Program Research Group. Long-term effects of budesonide or nedocromil in children with asthma. N Engl J Med 2000;343:1054–63.
13. Goldberg S, Schwartz S, Izbicki G. Sensitivity of exercise testing for asthma in adolescents is halved in the summer. Chest 2005;128:2408–11.
14. Spector SL, Nicklas RA, eds. Exercise-induced asthma in practice parameters for the diagnosis and treatment of asthma. J Allergy Clin Immunol 1995;96:831–5.
15. McFadden ER. Exercise-induced airway narrowing. In: Middleton E, Reed CE, Ellis EF, et al, editors. Allergy: principles and practice. 5th ed. St Louis: Mosby; 1998.
16. Weiler JM, Layton T, Hunt M. Asthma in the United States Olympic athletes who participated in the 1996 Summer games. J Allergy Clin Immunol 1998;102:722–6.
17. Becker A. Controversies and challenges of exercise-induced bronchoconstriction and their implications for children. Pediatr Pulmonol 2001;21S:S38–45.
18. Mannino DM, Homa DM, Akinbami LJ, et al. Surveillance for asthma-United States, 1980–1999. MMWR 2002;5:1–14.
19. Hammerman SI, Becker JM, Rogers J, et al. Asthma screening for high school athletes: identifying the undiagnosed and poorly controlled. Ann Allergy Asthma Immunol 2002;88:380–4.
20. Rupp NT, Brudno S, Guill MF. The value of screening for risk of exercise-induced asthma in high school athletes. Ann Allergy 1993;70:339–42.
21. Vacek L. Incidence of exercise-induced asthma in high school population in British Columbia. Allergy Asthma Proc 1997;18:89–91.
22. Busquets RM, Anto JM, Sunyer J, et al. Prevalence of asthma-related symptoms and bronchial responsiveness to exercise in children aged 13–14 yrs in Barcelona, Spain. Eur Respir J 1996;9:2094–8.
23. Hammo AH, Weinberger MW. Exercise-induced hyperventilation: a pseudoasthma syndrome. Ann Allergy Asthma Immunol 1999;82:574–8.
24. Landwehr LP, Wood II RP, Blager FB, et al. Vocal cord dysfunction mimicking exercise-induced bronchospasm in adolescents. Pediatrics 1996;98:971–4.
25. Bittleman DB, Smith RJH, Weiler JM. Abnormal movement of the arytenoid region during exercise presenting as exercise-induced asthma in an adolescent athlete. Chest 1994;106:615–6.
26. Hofstra WB, Neijens HJ, Duiverman EJ, et al. Dose-responses over time to inhaled fluticasone propionate treatment of exercise- and methacholine-induced bronchoconstriction in children. Pediatr Pulmonol 2000;29:415–23.
27. Anderson SA, Daviskas E. The mechanism of exercise-induced asthma is. ... J Allergy Clin Immunol 2000;106:453–9.
28. Hallstrand TS, Ault KA, Bates PW, et al. Peripheral blood manifestations of T(H)2 lymphocyte activation in stable atopic asthma and during exercise-induced bronchospasm. Ann Allergy Asthma Immunol 1998;80:424–32.
29. Anderson SA, Brannan JD. Exercise-induced asthma: is there still a case for histamine. J Allergy Clin Immunol 2002;109:771–3.
30. Yoshikawa T, Shoji S, Fujii T, et al. Severity of exercise-induced bronchoconstriction is related to airway eosinophilic inflammation in patients with asthma. Eur Respir J 1998;12:879–84.
31. Hallstrand TS, Bates PW, Schoene RB. Aerobic conditioning in mild asthma decreases the hyperpnea of exercise and impoves exercise and ventilatory capacity. Chest 2000;118:1460–9.
32. Koh MS, Tee A, Lasserson TJ, et al. Inhaled corticosteroids compared to placebo for exercise induced bronchoconstriction (Review). The Cochrane Collaboration. Accessed @ http://www.thecochranelibrary.com on March 27, 2009.
33. Henriksen JM, Dahl R. Effects of inhaled budesonide alone and in combination with low-dose terbutaline in children with asthma. Am Rev Respir Dis 1983;128:993–7.
34. Pederson S, Hansen OR. Budesonide treatment of moderate and severe asthma in children: a dose response effect. J Allergy Clin Immunol 1995;95:29–33.
35. Jonasson G, Carlsen K-H, Hultquist C. Low-dose budesonide improves exercise-induced bronchospasm in schoolchildren. Pediatr Allergy Immunol 2000;11:120–5.
36. Sont JK, Willems LNA, Bel EH, et al. Clinical control and histopathological outcome of asthma when using airway hyperresponsiveness as an additional guide to long-term treatment. Am J Respir Crit Care Med 1999;159:1043–51.

37. Kemp JP, Dockhorn RJ, Shapiro GG, et al. Montelukast once daily inhibits exercise-induced bronchoconstriction in 6- to 14-year-old children with asthma. J Pediatr 1998;133:424–8.

38. Leff JA, Busse WW, Pearlman D, et al. Montelukast, a leukotriene-receptor antagonist, for the treatment of mild asthma and exercise-induced asthma. N Engl J Med 1998;339:147–52.

39. Pearlman DS, Ostrom NK, Bronsky EA, et al. The leukotriene D_4-receptor antagonist zafirlukast attenuates exercise-induced bronchoconstriction in children. J Pediatr 1999;134:273–9.

40. Edelman JM, Turpin JA, Bronsky EA, et al. Oral montelukast compared with inhaled salmeterol to prevent exercise-induced bronchoconstriction. Ann Intern Med 2000;132:97–104.

41. Villaren C, O'Neill SJ, Helbling A, et al. Montelukast versus salmeterol in patient with asthma and exercise-induced bronchoconstriction. J Allergy Clin Immunol 1999;104:547–53.

42. Nelson HS, Busse WW, Kerwin E, et al. Fluticasone propionate/salmeterol combination provides more effective asthma control that low-dose inhaled corticosteroid plus montelukast. J Allergy Clin Immunol 2000; 106:1088–95.

43. Vidal C, Fernandez-Ovide E, Pineiro J, et al. Comparison of montelukast versus budesonide in the treatment of exercise-induced bronchoconstriction. Ann Allergy Asthma Immunol 2001;86:655–8.

44. Fish JE, Murray JJ, Boone EA, et al. Salmeterol powder provides significantly better benefit than montelukast in asthmatic patients receiving concomitant inhaled corticosteroid therapy. Chest 2001;120:423–30.

45. Simons FER, Gerstner TV, Cheang MS. Tolerance to the bronchoprotective effect of salmeterol in adolescents with exercise-induced asthma using concurrent inhaled glucocorticoid treatment. Pediatrics 1997;99: 655–9.

46. Dorinsky P, Kalberg C, Jones S, et al. Sustained protection against activity induced bronchospasm (AIB) during chronic treatment with the fluticasone propionate/salmeterol combination (FSC). Am J Respir Crit Care Med 2002;165:A568.

47. Badier M, Beaumont D, Orehek J. Attenuation of hyperventilation-induced bronchospasm by terfenadine: a new antihistamine. J Allergy Clin Immunol 1988;81:437–40.

48. Baki A, Orhan F. The effect of loratadine in exercise-induced asthma. Arch Dis Child 2002;86:38–9.

49. Dahlen B, Roquet A, Inman MD. Influence of zafirlukast and loratadine on exercise-induced bronchospasm. J Allergy Clin Immunol 2002;109: 789–93.

50. Pearlman DS, van Adelsberg J, Philip G, et al. Onset and duration of protection against exercise-induced bronchoconstriction by a single oral dose of montelukast. Ann Allergy Asthma Immunol 2006;97:98–104.

51. Philip G, Villarán C, Pearlman DS, et al. Protection against exercise-induced bronchoconstriction two hours after a single oral dose of montelukast. J Asthma 2007;44:213–7.

52. Raissy H, Harkins M, Kelly F, et al. Pretreatment with albuterol versus montelukast for exercise-induced bronchospasm in children. Pharmacotherapy 2008;28:287–94.

CHAPTER

41

New Insight into the Pathogenesis and Management of Refractory Childhood Asthma

Joseph D. Spahn

Introduction

Asthma is a chronic respiratory disease characterized by reversible airflow limitation and airway hyperresponsiveness to a variety of stimuli. Our understanding of the pathogenesis of asthma has evolved from that of a purely bronchospastic disease, to one in which airway inflammation plays a central role.[1,2] Glucocorticoids (GC) have broad antiinflammatory effects, and as such, have become first-line agents for both the acute and chronic manifestations of this disease.[3-5] Although the majority of patients with asthma have mild to moderate disease, approximately 5% to 10% have severe disease.[6] Severe or 'refractory' asthma, although uncommon, accounts for a significant proportion of the healthcare costs of asthma.[7,8] In addition, those with refractory asthma have the greatest morbidity in terms of impact on quality of life, emergency room (ER) visits, and hospitalizations. By definition, these asthmatics continue to have troublesome symptoms despite optimal conventional therapy including high-dose inhaled GC in combination with a long-acting β agonist (LABA), leukotriene modifying agents (LTMs), and oral GCs in some. At the extreme end of refractory asthma is a group of asthmatics that fail to adequately respond to oral GC therapy. These patients have been termed 'GC-insensitive' or 'GC resistant'. This chapter will address the complexity and heterogeneity of refractory asthma, highlighting the information available and areas of need with regard to the pathogenesis, evaluation, and management of refractory asthma.

Definition

Children with refractory asthma display evidence for ongoing disease activity despite optimal pharmacologic therapy. When attempting to define what constitutes refractory asthma, one must first distinguish between asthma severity and control. Although related, asthma control and asthma severity are often confused with each other. Severity is more reflective of the 'intrinsic' intensity of the disease and is less likely to vary over the long term, whereas control is reflective of disease activity based on levels of symptoms over a recent period of time. For example, one can have severe, but well-controlled asthma. In this situation, the child will often require high-dose inhaled GC therapy in combination with a LABA and/or LTM to maintain good asthma control. In contrast, a child with mild or moderate asthma may have frequent daytime symptoms and nocturnal awakening with asthma symptoms requiring frequently administered β agonists. In this case, the child has poorly controlled asthma. Once a controller agent is instituted, the patient's asthma control improves significantly. In an attempt to differentiate control from severity, the NAEPP EPR III has suggested that the need for, and daily dosage of inhaled GC required to maintain optimal asthma control, can be used to assess an individual's level of disease severity, while frequency of symptoms (day and night) can be used as a measure of control.[9]

The relationship between disease severity and level of asthma control was determined among a large cohort of asthmatics followed by primary care physicians.[10] Asthma control was ascertained by questionnaire with 42% reporting moderate or poor control based on frequency of symptoms. During the 1-year study period, 14.8% of the cohort reported ≥1 ER visit or hospitalization with a significant correlation noted between level of asthma control and ER visit and/or hospitalization (p < 0.001). The odds ratio (OR) for ER visit/hospitalization for an individual with good control was 0.5 vs 2.2 in patients with poor asthma control. Of importance, this association was independent of inhaled GC usage and dose (the surrogate marker of disease severity), before entry into the study. Poorly controlled asthmatics were six times more likely to report a hospital contact than patients with good control and three times more likely than patients with moderate control.

An NHLBI-sponsored workshop on severe asthma addressed the difficulties in making the diagnosis of refractory asthma.[6] The panel concluded that a refractory asthmatic should have at least three of the following criteria: (1) history of referral to an asthma specialist, (2) receiving maximal usual asthma therapy, including high-dose inhaled and oftentimes, oral GC therapy, (3) lung function abnormalities with FEV_1 values being consistently less than 70% of predicted, (4) persistent symptoms and decreased quality of life, or, (5) a history of previous respiratory failure/intubation, or near-fatal episode.

An FEV_1 of less than 70% of predicted may be 'setting the bar too low' to define refractory asthma in childhood, as many of these children may have values greater than 70% of predicted. In a retrospective cohort analysis of 3452 asthmatic children, Fulbrigge and colleagues determined that the FEV_1 was greater than 100% of predicted in 43% of the subjects studied while 5.5% of the values ranged from 60 and 80% and only 0.7% of the FEV_1

©2010 Elsevier Ltd, Inc, BV
DOI: 10.1016/B978-1-4377-0271-2.00041-9

values were <60% of predicted.[11] Similarly, in a cross-sectional evaluation of 2728 children with stable asthma referred to National Jewish Health from 1999 to 2002, the mean FEV_1 was 92.7% predicted with 19% of values 60% to 80% and only 3.1% were ≤60% of predicted.[12] Additionally, Bacharier and colleagues[13] reported FEV_1 values of greater than 100% predicted in 49% of 219 asthmatic children evaluated at two academic asthma clinics; with mean FEV_1 values of 97%, 101%, and 94% of predicted in those with mild, moderate and severe persistent asthma respectively. As a result of these studies, the NHLBI Guidelines[9] allows the use of the FEV_1/FVC ratio in assessing both severity and control in patients with asthma, as it is a more sensitive measure of airflow limitation, especially in children.

Clinical Characteristics of Refractory Asthma in Childhood

We have begun to understand the prevalence, pathophysiology and natural history of refractory asthma in childhood. Bratton and colleagues prospectively studied children with severe asthma referred for treatment in a multidisciplinary day program. They found a male predominance (56% male) with 17% minority, and 25% of lower socioeconomic status.[8] Age of onset of asthma was a median of 2 years. Over 80% were classified as atopic by skin testing and 65% had a cat or dog in the home. Comorbidity was frequent with rhinosinusitis (90%), gastroesophageal reflux disease (57%) and atopic dermatitis (21%) the most common concurrent conditions. The median lifetime hospital admissions numbered 6.5 per patient. In addition, a significant percentage had experienced cyanotic episodes (64%), loss of consciousness (30%) or intubation for respiratory arrest (25%). Sixty-six percent of patients were taking oral GCs on admission with a median dose of 10 µg/day for adolescents and 6.3 mg/day for school-age children. Steroid side-effects were reported in 79%, with nearly 50% obese, a comorbid condition receiving increasing attention in the literature.[14,15] Despite significant asthma morbidity, the median FEV_1 was 80% predicted, a value considered within normal limits.

A retrospective review of 164 consecutive pediatric admissions to National Jewish Health for refractory asthma was undertaken to examine response to optimized therapy.[16] The cohort studied had a median age of 14 years with a median duration of asthma of 11.9 years. Over 50% required chronic oral GC therapy (median 15 mg/d), and all were on high-dose inhaled GC (median 1500 µg/d) therapy on admission. The cohort studied had a median FEV_1 77% of predicted, and 73% were atopic.

Fifty percent of the study cohort required a prednisone 'burst' secondary to poor asthma control during their evaluation. Of those who received a prednisone burst, nearly one quarter (24%), failed to display an appropriate improvement in their baseline lung function (<15% increase in AM FEV_1) and were considered GC-insensitive. Risk factors associated with GC insensitivity included: chronically administered prednisone at an earlier age, higher maintenance prednisone requirement, and African American ethnicity. Furthermore, two distinct spirometric patterns were noted among the children with GC-insensitive asthma. Those with a 'chaotic' pattern displayed wide swings in lung function with no associated improvement in baseline lung function during the prednisone burst, while the 'nonchaotic' subjects had no improvement in baseline lung function and displayed little diurnal variability. Children with GC insensitive asthma are at the extreme end of refractory asthma as evidenced by their need for prednisone at a much earlier age and their higher maintenance prednisone requirement.

Pathogenesis of Refractory Asthma

Until recently, the majority of studies evaluating the pathogenesis of asthma utilized adults with mild to moderate asthma, many receiving only short-acting β agonists (SABA). These studies, utilizing flexible bronchoscopy with bronchoalveolar lavage (BAL) and/or endobronchial biopsy, uniformly demonstrated airway epithelial desquamation and inflammatory cell infiltration consisting of eosinophils, mast cells, and activated T lymphocytes. In addition, varying degrees of airway remodeling characterized by reticular basement membrane thickening, goblet cell hyperplasia, smooth muscle hypertrophy and hyperplasia, and angiogenesis was found. Over the past 5 years, studies evaluating refractory asthmatics have provided us with an enhanced understanding of the heterogeneity of airway inflammation and remodeling in patients receiving treatment.

Vrugt and colleagues were among the first to evaluate the pathophysiology of refractory asthma by performing bronchoscopy with biopsy in 15 adults with steroid-dependent asthma compared to 10 mild asthmatics, and 10 nonasthmatic controls.[17] The investigators found subjects with refractory asthma to have fewer airway eosinophils with greater numbers of activated T cells compared to those with mild asthma. Associated with the increase in activated T cells were greater numbers of cells expressing IL-5, an important cytokine for eosinophil recruitment and activation. No differences were found in the number of neutrophils among the groups studied, nor were differences noted in total number of CD3 and CD4 positive cells.

Wenzel and colleagues[18] obtained endobronchial biopsies on 34 refractory asthmatics requiring chronic oral GC therapy, 11 moderate, and 10 mild asthmatics, plus 11 nonasthmatic controls. Subjects with refractory asthma could be separated into those with and without airway eosinophilia. Those with airway eosinophilia had elevated T lymphocytes, mast cells, and macrophages, and a greater degree of sub-basement membrane thickening compared to those without eosinophilia. Refractory asthmatics with airway eosinophilia were also more likely to have required intubation secondary to respiratory failure, while subjects without eosinophilia had a lower baseline FEV_1. Lastly, the investigators found airway neutrophilia in all of the subjects with refractory asthma independent of their eosinophil status.

Benayoun and colleagues[19] obtained endobronchial biopsies on 15 subjects with refractory asthma, 15 with mild to moderate asthma, 10 with intermittent asthma, and 10 nonasthmatic controls. Surprisingly, neither the extent of airway inflammatory cells nor degree of airway epithelial damage differentiated subjects with refractory asthma from those with mild and moderate asthma. Rather, refractory asthmatics were more likely to have structural changes characterized by increased numbers of airway fibroblasts, deposition of type III collagen, larger mucous glands, greater airway smooth muscle (ASM) area and ASM size, and increased myosin light-chain kinase expression.

These studies demonstrate the pathologic heterogeneity of refractory asthma. Vrugt and colleagues[17] found persistent T cell activation, without associated eosinophilia and neutrophilia; Wenzel and colleagues[18] found elevated neutrophils with or without eosinophilia, while Benayoun and colleagues[19] found exaggerated structural changes to the airways of patients with refractory asthma. These studies offer intriguing insight into the pathology of severe asthma, and may eventually lead to 'targeted therapy' based on asthma phenotype.

Recent bronchoscopic studies in children with refractory asthma shed light on this phenotype of childhood asthma. Payne and colleagues[20] studied the relationship between exhaled nitric oxide (eNO) and airway eosinophilia in 31 children with refractory asthma following a 2-week prednisolone course. They found no active airway inflammation in the majority of children following a 2-week prednisolone course. In the minority with persistent airway eosinophilia, the investigators found significant correlations between eNO and tissue eosinophils ($r = 0.54$; $p = 0.03$).

Jenkins and colleagues[21] reported on a series of 6 children with refractory asthma, ranging in age from 6 to 17 years, who underwent bronchoscopy with endobronchial biopsy. In every case, the bronchial biopsies confirmed asthma, with no other lung diseases diagnosed. In 5 of 6 cases, active airway inflammation was absent, with few if any, eosinophils, neutrophils or T lymphocytes noted. Despite absence of airway inflammation, all children had significant airway remodeling characterized by thickening of the basement membrane, smooth muscle hypertrophy and hyperplasia, and goblet cell hyperplasia.

In both studies, children with refractory asthma had significant remodeling of their airways. This would suggest that airway remodeling may occur independent of airway inflammation and that it is likely to occur early in the course of refractory asthma. In addition, significant remodeling may occur despite chronically administered inhaled and oral GC therapy. Lastly, persistent eosinophilia occurs in a minority of children with refractory asthma who remain symptomatic despite oral GC therapy.

Evaluation of the Child With Refractory Asthma

When evaluating any patient with difficult-to-control asthma, in addition to obtaining a thorough history including the patient's past history, current symptoms, and medication use, physical examination, spirometry, and complete pulmonary function studies, the following questions should be specifically addressed (Box 41-1 and Box 41-2).

Question 1: Does the Patient Have Asthma?

As there are many 'masqueraders' of asthma, the first step in evaluating a child with refractory asthma is to ensure that the child indeed has asthma (Box 41-3). A history of acute and reversible episodes of cough, wheezing, or shortness of breath with clearly defined triggers and precipitants support the diagnosis of

asthma, as does a history of bronchial hyperresponsiveness (BHR).[3] BHR is best manifest clinically by exercise- or cold air-induced bronchoconstriction.[22] In children with suspected refractory asthma, lung function studies should also be performed to include spirometry with flow volume loops. As noted above, some children with refractory asthma can have an FEV_1 value within the normal range during periods of stability. A more sensitive measure of airflow obstruction is the FEV_1/FVC ratio, which can now be used to assess asthma severity and control, based upon the NAEPP EPR III asthma guidelines.[9]

Asthma is not the only pulmonary disorder characterized by airflow obstruction and wheezing. The most common childhood conditions in which wheezing may be present include aspiration syndromes, tracheobronchialmalacia, foreign body aspiration, bronchiectasis secondary to ciliary dyskinesia, humoral immunodeficiency, bronchopulmonary dysplasia, cystic fibrosis, allergic bronchopulmonary mycoses, or alpha-1-antitrypsin deficiency, and vocal cord dysfunction in older children and adolescents.

Although the diagnostic evaluation necessary to rule out all of the above abnormalities is beyond the scope of the chapter, a thorough history, physical exam, chest X-ray, and measure of pulmonary function utilizing spirometry (including the flow-volume loop) will significantly limit the number of possibilities and thus the number of tests required to make the diagnosis.

Question 2: Are Other Conditions Contributing to Poor Asthma Control?

Since most children with refractory asthma are atopic, the question of ongoing allergen exposure is paramount for many patients. Special consideration is also given to gastroesophageal reflux and sinusitis because they are frequently encountered in this population and are thought to contribute to poor asthma control. Finally, vocal cord dysfunction (VCD) can also accompany asthma. Since VCD does not generally respond to medications for asthma, it can be misperceived as refractory asthma by both the patient and physician leading to inappropriate escalation of medical treatment.

Ongoing Allergen Exposure

Chronic allergen exposure significantly contributes to the persistence of airway inflammation in atopic asthmatics. Thus, strict allergen avoidance can result in decreased airway inflammation and improved asthma control, which in turn, can lessen the need for chronic glucocorticoid therapy[23,24] Where avoidance is impossible, immunotherapy can be considered; recognizing that immunotherapy in refractory childhood asthma is incompletely studied and may be associated with greater potential for severe systemic reactions than in milder disease.[25,26] In fact, immunotherapy is contraindicated in many children with refractory asthma because of their disease lability.[27] If attempted, immunotherapy must be conducted with pulmonary function monitoring in a setting where adverse reactions can be handled.

Gastroesophageal Reflux Disease

Recent studies show a prevalence of gastroesophageal reflux disease (GERD) in children with asthma, ranging from 47 to 75%,[8,28–31] which is similar to adults with asthma, and about 2–4 times the prevalence in the general population. Respiratory symptoms in asthmatic adults are often associated with reflux. Field and colleagues found that 41% of adult asthmatics noted reflux-associated respiratory symptoms, prompting 28% to use their inhalers.[32] Similarly, Harding noted that 79% of respiratory symptoms were temporally associated with esophageal acidification during 24-hour esophageal pH testing.[33] In our experience, asthmatic children will often deny heartburn, regurgitation, and dysphagia on initial questioning, but may report symptoms once attention is directed to GERD symptoms. Additionally, an increasing cognizance of extrapulmonary and atypical manifestations of GERD should raise suspicion of its presence.[34-38] Nonetheless, GERD can be silent in as many as 33% of adults with asthma,[33,39] and 44% of infants with daily wheezing.[30] As such, GERD must always be considered, even in the absence of symptoms, in the treatment of any patient with asthma, and particularly with severe asthma and escalating need for medications. Although there is a clear association of asthma and GERD, there is debate as to the importance of GERD in asthma control. Disparity in methods of diagnosis, measurement of outcomes and stratification by disease severity (both GERD and/or asthma) among studies may be at the heart of conflicting results. Several studies support the hypothesis that the degree of esophageal damage may be an important determinant in the possible relationship between GERD and asthma; nocturnal reflux is more damaging to the esophagus than upright reflux because of prolonged acid contact time. Several studies in children and adults suggest that severe nocturnal asthma is more likely to be associated with GERD than daytime asthma.[40,41] In a recent study by Cuttitta and colleagues of adult nocturnal asthmatics with moderate to severe GERD, reflux was significantly and temporally associated with enhanced lower airways resistance.[42]

Determining the significance of GERD in asthma is further complicated by the fact that physiologic alterations often seen in asthma, particularly severe asthma, can clearly promote GERD. These include an increase in transient lower esophageal sphincter (LES) relaxations, LES hypotonia and esophageal dysmotility which may be increased due to autonomic dysfunction in asthma.[43] Furthermore, the LES pressure augmented by the crural diaphragm normally prevents GERD, but this augmentation is prevented by hyperinflation and hiatal hernia, or LES pressure is overcome by increased negative intrathoracic pressures (e.g. in bronchospasm, cough, upper airway resistance syndrome and obstructive apnea), increased intraabdominal pressures (e.g. in obesity) and in steroid-induced myopathy.[8]

Vagally mediated reflexive alterations of respiratory function (respiratory rate, minute ventilation, resistance and the sensation of dyspnea) have been demonstrated during acid infusion into the esophagus. Esophageal acidification has also been associated with heightened nonspecific hyperresponsivity of the airways to bronchoconstrictors, thus 'priming' the airway to other triggers.[44] Finally, microaspiration of acid into the airways may also contribute to lower airway abnormalities. Jack and colleagues[45] simultaneously monitored proximal esophageal and tracheal pH (via a probe inserted percutaneously into the trachea) in a small number of patients with severe asthma. Of 37 documented episodes of prolonged (i.e. >5 min) proximal acid reflux, 5 of these were associated with tracheal acidification and significant deterioration in pulmonary function. Episodes that did not result in tracheal acidification had much less effect on pulmonary function.

Thus asthma, particularly severe asthma, can predispose to GERD just as GERD can contribute to asthma severity in a seemingly vicious cycle. Although several studies have shown improvement in asthma control following institution of treatment of GERD with proton pump inhibitors (PPIs),[46-49] a large study of adults with poorly controlled asthma found esomeprazole to be of little help in improving asthma control, even in subjects with documented GERD.[50] While diagnostic testing may not be required prior to empiric PPI treatment for symptomatic patients, both confirmation of the diagnosis where desired, and/or verification of acid suppression following a 3-month course of PPI therapy requires 24-hour esophageal pH probe monitoring. Other tests, such as barium swallow and endoscopy, while providing important data, are neither sensitive nor specific for the diagnosis of GERD.[31]

As noted above, response among asthmatics to PPI therapy is heterogeneous and lack of response may result from nonsuppression of acid production on conventional PPI dosing. For severe GERD or refractory asthma with GERD, b.i.d. dosing of a PPI for 3 months is recommended (e.g. lansoprazole 30 mg b.i.d in adolescents, and 0.7–1.0 mg/kg b.i.d. up to this dose in younger children using either the sachet or opened capsule delivered in a variety of vehicles, such as applesauce.[49] Longer-term maintenance PPI treatment (often given as half the dose above once a day) is required in many patients. Recommendations are to elevate the head of the bed by 6 inches, abstain from eating 2 hours before bedtime, and avoid spicy and fatty foods, and caffeinated and carbonated beverages. Some adult patients have been shown to require the addition of H_2 blockers for acid suppression at night,[51] and prokinetic agents (e.g. metoclopramide) are employed if regurgitation is prominent.

Both surgery and medical antireflux therapy can result in improvement in many patients with refractory asthma.[32,48] Predictors of response to either form of therapy are identified as presence of regurgitation, proximal esophageal acid acidification, esophagitis healing on medical therapy, noted association of reflux with respiratory symptoms and obesity.[52] At this time, we consider surgery for those patients with severe asthma in whom persistent, documented GERD improves with PPIs but requires very protracted therapy, for those with documented GERD unwilling or unable to comply with medical therapy, and for those in whom life-threatening disease warrants definite treatment.

Sinusitis

Radiographic evidence for sinus disease is also commonly seen in asthma. Data link the physiology of the upper and lower airways and support the hypothesis that the same pathology underlies both sinusitis and asthma.[53,54] Studies demonstrate that inflammation of the nose and sinuses is associated with lower airway hyperresponsiveness and that nasal allergen challenge can result in airway hyperresponsiveness.[55-57] Mechanisms for these effects include systemic signals emanating from upper airway inflammation, 'cross-talk' via shared naso-bronchial or pharyngeal-bronchial innervation, and/or seeding of the lower airway by injurious mediators of inflammation by postnasal drainage.

Importantly, treatment of the upper airway, generally with nasal corticosteroids, has in several studies, led to amelioration of lower airway hyperreactivity.[58-61] Significant improvement in asthma control can occur in patients whose sinus disease has been successfully managed.[62-64] A screening sinus CT scan provides greater resolution and thus greater sensitivity than conventional sinus radiographs.[65] If a suspected refractory asthmatic displays evidence for sinusitis, aggressive topical therapy to include nasal saline irrigation and intranasal GCs should be instituted along with a 3-week course of antibiotics. Our experience with sinus surgery in patients with severe asthma has been disappointing. Surgery often results in temporary improvement with gradual recurrence of symptoms. Certainly, surgery is indicated for defined obstructive anatomic abnormalities, however, sinus surgery for mucosal disease is much less likely to be helpful. In these cases we rely heavily on medical management consisting of nasal saline irrigations, topical nasal steroids, and intermittent antibiotics.

Vocal Cord Dysfunction

Since the first descriptions of vocal cord dysfunction (VCD), defined as inappropriate, or paradoxical, adduction of the vocal cords during inspiration, it has emerged as a frequent masquerader of asthma.[66-68] Approximately 10–20% of severe asthma patients referred to our tertiary referral center are diagnosed with vocal cord dysfunction rather than asthma (unpublished data). At the same time, there has been a growing appreciation that VCD can also occur with asthma.[69] VCD has been identified in 10% of children with severe asthma treated at National Jewish.[8] In either case, frequent or unremitting symptoms can be misinterpreted as refractory asthma leading to over-treatment.[70-75]

VCD is frequently triggered by many of the usual asthma triggers (e.g. irritants, exercise, postnasal drip, GERD, emotions), and as such, it is easily mistaken by patients and physicians as asthma.[76-80] Questioning the patient for symptoms prominent in the throat and on inspiration suggest this diagnosis,[70,81,82] however, many patients are unable to localize symptoms to the throat. A history of nocturnal abatement of symptoms, and lack of response to bronchodilators may guide the diagnosis. The findings of stridor or inspiratory wheeze that is loudest at the neck, but often radiating throughout the chest during an acute episode is also suggestive of the diagnosis. Since all routine monitoring of expiratory function in asthma requires maximal inspiration prior to a maximal expiratory effort, both PEFR and FEV_1 can be falsely decreased and thus misleading in subjects with VCD. Because the FVC may also be falsely diminished, the FEV_1/FVC ratio will often remain in the normal range and the expiratory flow volume loop will not have the 'classic' scooped appearance that is characteristic of distal airflow limitation noted with asthma. Inspection of the inspiratory flow volume loop is indispensable in the interpretation of forced expiratory maneuvers. Persistent truncation or irregularity of the flow volume loop on inspiration, and an $FIF_{50}/FEF_{50} \leq 1$ is highly suggestive of VCD, but may only be present during a symptomatic episode. The current gold standard remains direct visualization of vocal cord motion by flexible rhinolaryngoscopy during a symptomatic episode.[69,71,83] Provocative challenges with methacholine or exercise are often required to elicit VCD, though a negative challenge does not rule out VCD. Its demonstrated presence, with or without bronchospasm and expiratory wheezing, substantiates whether VCD is a masquerader of asthma or an attendant contributor to refractory symptoms.

A number of treatment modalities (e.g. speech therapy, hypnosis, heliox, topical anesthetics) have been used to abort acute episodes; to help patients learn to distinguish VCD from asthma, and for long-term control.[84,85] Psychosocial evaluation is recommended if symptoms persist.[76] Accurate assessment of lower airways symptoms, function and degree of reactivity (in natural circumstances or in the challenge laboratory setting) is often not possible until VCD is controlled.

Question 3: What is the Patient's Level of Asthma Severity and Control?

Once the diagnosis of asthma is established, and other disorders that can mimic or exacerbate asthma have been addressed, determine the level of asthma severity and control by inquiring about the frequency and severity of exacerbations, including history of previous ER visits, hospitalizations, and whether there have been life-threatening episodes, such as loss of consciousness, seizures, and need for intubation and mechanical ventilation secondary to respiratory failure or arrest. In addition, inquire as to the interventions required during exacerbations and chronically to maintain adequate control. Also, ask about the dose and duration of inhaled GC and, if applicable, the dose of systemic GC required to maintain adequate control of symptoms and lung function.

Questions designed to address asthma control include the frequency of daytime symptoms, nocturnal awakenings with asthma symptoms, impact on quality of life, variability in lung function, and the frequency with which the patient requires rescue therapy SABA therapy. Need for frequent SABA is a 'red-flag' and must be addressed, especially in light of reports that have implicated overuse of SABA therapy as contributing to asthma morbidity and mortality.[86-88]

Question 4: Is the Patient's Current Asthma Medication Regimen Sufficient for Asthma Control?

Optimal control of a child's asthma should allow normal or near normal daily activities, including participation in gym class and other athletic activities, normal sleep with no nocturnal awakening due to asthma, little need for rescue SABA therapy, and few severe exacerbations requiring oral rescue GCs, ER visits, or hospitalizations. An obvious reason for poor asthma control is suboptimal controller medication use. According to the NHLBI guidelines,[9] all patients with persistent asthma should be on a controller agent, with inhaled GCs considered first-line agents. With increasing asthma severity, and in subjects with poorly controlled asthma, the inhaled GC dose is increased, and combination therapy with LABAs, LTMs, or theophylline, is recommended. Several studies in adults with moderate to severe asthma have demonstrated the superiority of adding a LABA to an inhaled GC vs doubling the dose of inhaled GC. Combination LABA plus inhaled GC provides better symptom control and lung function and results in fewer asthma exacerbations.[89-92] As such, patients who are suboptimally controlled on an inhaled GC would be likely to benefit from the addition of a LABA to the inhaled GC. There has been recent controversy regarding the safety of LABA therapy[93] and there continues to be a paucity of studies evaluating combination LABA/inhaled GC therapy in children with asthma.

Even children with well-controlled asthma are at risk for developing an acute asthma exacerbation, and in this situation, a short course of oral GC therapy is recommended. Unfortunately, patients with refractory asthma often require chronically administered oral GC therapy to maintain adequate symptom control. In these 'steroid-dependent' asthmatics, the goal of therapy is directed at administering the lowest possible dose while maintaining sufficient control of asthma symptoms. Alternate-day dosing is preferable to daily dosing as the incidence of long-term steroid-associated adverse effects can be minimized with this strategy. Short courses of high-dose oral/parenteral therapy should be used as needed for severe exacerbations in the steroid-dependent asthmatic and tapered, based on clinical response and objective measures of pulmonary function.

Question 5: Is the Patient Inhaler Technique Adequate? And is Poor Adherence a Contributing Factor?

Technique with Inhaled Medications

In addition to investigating for poor compliance, one must evaluate inhaled medication technique. The development and proper use of potent, inhaled GCs has allowed a significant number of severe asthmatics to reduce or discontinue chronically administered oral steroids.[94,95] In order to maximize effectiveness while decreasing the potential for local and systemic effects, all inhaled GCs delivered via a pressurized metered dose inhaler (pMDI) should be administered with a spacer device. These devices not only obviate the need for coordination between actuating the device and inhaling the medication, they also enhance GC delivery to the peripheral airways.[96,97] In addition, the incidence of local side-effects such as oral candidiasis and dysphonia can be significantly reduced.[98] The newer dry powder inhalation devices (DPI) do not require a spacer device. Rinsing the mouth and spitting out orally deposited corticosteroid is recommended to prevent undesirable local and systemic absorption.

Medication Adherence

Not surprisingly, poor adherence with GC therapy can be a significant contributing factor for poor response, yet it is often difficult to substantiate.[99-101] Studies have documented poor adherence with inhaled GC therapy in both children and adults with asthma.[102,103] Rand and colleagues[99] evaluated adherence with a pMDI and found that although 75% of the study participants reported using their MDIs as directed, only 15% of the participants actually used the pMDI as instructed. In a study designed to evaluate peripheral markers of inflammation in 8 subjects with steroid-dependent asthma (mean prednisone dose 20 mg daily), we found that 6 had measurable AM cortisol levels at baseline and 4 subjects had levels well within the normal range.[104]

Apter and colleagues[105] sought to identify the risk factors associated with poor adherence in 50 adults with moderate to severe asthma on routinely administered inhaled GC therapy. Adherence was monitored electronically utilizing the Chronolog® device over a 6-week period. The subjects were told that the Chronolog® recorded the time and date of each actuation of their inhaled GC, but they were not told the specific purpose of the study. Mean adherence for the study was 63%, while 'good adherence' (defined as adherence of greater than 70%) occurred in approximately 50% of subjects. Risk factors associated with poor adherence were socioeconomic (<12 years of formal education, income of <$20,000/yr, minority status, and Spanish as a primary language) and poor patient-clinician communication. Adherence was not related to asthma severity, gender, health beliefs, or knowledge of inhaled GCs.

Even under the best of circumstances, adherence with inhaled GC therapy remains suboptimal. This is a major issue as poor adherence with inhaled GC therapy has been shown to be associated with increased asthma morbidity.[103] As clinicians, we must be cognizant of the educational level of our patients. The evaluation of any child with suspected refractory asthma must include assurance of appropriate medication adherence and proper technique with inhaled medications. A pre-dose AM plasma cortisol level can be useful in assessing compliance in patients with steroid-dependent asthma. If a patient has a normal AM cortisol level despite chronically administered oral steroid therapy, the most likely explanation is inadequate adherence. Other possibilities would include assay interference with exogenous glucocorticoids or primary cortisol resistance.[106,107] A sensitive and specific high pressure liquid chromatography (HPLC) system can be used to reliably measure cortisol levels with little risk of interference from oral or inhaled glucocorticoid therapy.[108]

Question 6: What Factors Contribute to Poor Response to Glucocorticoid Therapy?

If the above conditions are recognized and adequately treated, and the patient continues to display evidence for poorly con-

Cellular, Molecular, and Pharmacologic Abnormalities Associated with Poor Response to Glucocorticoid Therapy

Cellular Abnormalities

1. Diminished ability of GCs to inhibit phytohemagglutinin-induced lymphocyte proliferation
2. Increased numbers of circulating T cells bearing surface activation markers (HLA-DR, CD25) and elevated serum levels of sIL-2R
3. Increased mRNA expression of IL-2 and IL-4 from BAL lymphocytes
4. Failure of glucocorticoids to inhibit mRNA IL-4 expression from BAL lymphocytes
5. Blunted eosinopenic response following the administration of glucocorticoids

Molecular Abnormalities of the Glucocorticoid Receptor

1. Diminished ligand binding affinity
2. Diminished DNA binding affinity
3. Diminished glucocorticoid receptor number
4. Up-regulation of glucocorticoid receptor beta

Other Etiologies for Poor Response to GC

1. Poor adherence with glucocorticoid therapy
2. Pharmacokinetic abnormality (poor absorption ± rapid clearance)

---

trolled asthma despite high-dose inhaled ± oral GC therapy, further evaluation as described below should be undertaken (Box 41-4).

Does the Child Have GC-Insensitive Asthma?

GC-insensitive asthmatics comprise a subgroup of patients with refractory asthma who do not adequately respond to systemically administered GC. These children are characterized by either persistent respiratory symptoms, frequent nocturnal awakenings with asthma, chronic airflow limitation, and life-threatening acute asthma exacerbations. More importantly, these individuals will fail to respond to a short course of high-dose oral GC therapy. Specifically, a patient with GC-insensitive asthma will fail to display a 15% improvement in FEV_1 following a 7- to 14-day course of high dose (≥40 mg daily) oral GC therapy.

Once the diagnosis of GC-insensitive asthma has been established, and all other contributing factors adequately addressed, an attempt should be made to identify etiologies for this apparent resistance. In our experience, poor adherence to the prescribed medical regimen, especially inhaled and oral GC therapy is the most likely factor. If poor compliance has been ruled out, then further evaluation as described below can be helpful.

Does the Child Have a Pharmacokinetic Abnormality?

Abnormal GC pharmacokinetics can be a contributing factor in children with refractory asthma who display fewer than expected GC-associated adverse effects.[108] Rapid oral GC clearance may be related to poor absorption, rapid elimination, or failure to convert prednisone to prednisolone. In our experience, approximately 25% of patients with poorly controlled asthma will have an identifiable GC pharmacokinetic abnormality characterized by poor absorption and/or rapid clearance. Poor absorption is relatively

uncommon, occurring in less than 10% of subjects studied, and will require a more detailed study, such as multiple samples or a liquid prednisolone dose, to fully differentiate rapid clearance from poor absorption. In patients who display poor absorption of prednisone or methylprednisolone, one must assess the possibility of a drug interaction with adsorbents such as antacids. If a patient has impaired absorption, a liquid prednisolone formulation should be substituted in place of a tablet. Liquid preparations such as Orapred® have been shown to be more rapidly and more completely absorbed than tablet preparations.

Drug interactions, especially the older anticonvulsants such as phenobarbital, phenytoin, and carbamazepine[109] and the antituberculosis agent, rifampin[110] can result in rapid GC clearance. Lastly, a group of patients have been identified as having inherently rapid clearance.[108] If rapid clearance is associated with a drug interaction, one can attempt to discontinue the medication responsible for rapid clearance (if possible) or one can alter either the formulation (i.e. methylprednisolone in place of prednisone or vice versa), or increase the dose or frequency of GC administration. Of note, methylprednisolone is much more susceptible to enzyme induction by the above anticonvulsants than prednisolone, and should be avoided with these drugs.

Does the Child Have an Abnormality in Glucocorticoid Receptor (GCR) Binding Affinity, Number or Function?

Studies in patients with refractory asthma suggest that abnormalities in GCR number, GCR binding (ligand and/or DNA binding), or up-regulation of an alternatively spliced, inactive form of the GCR, termed GRβ, contribute to the poor response to GC therapy noted in some patients with GC-insensitive asthma. These defects appear to be functional, rather than genetic, in that chemical mutational analyses of the GCR from steroid-insensitive asthmatics failed to reveal mutations that would explain the phenomenon.[111]

Management of Refractory Childhood Asthma

Nonpharmacologic Interventions

Addressing the many issues and confounding factors that can contribute to poor asthma control is essential. Concurrent with this, successful management of any refractory asthmatic patient begins with frequent clinic visits and objective measures of pulmonary function performed daily at home and during clinic visits. Home monitoring of peak expiratory flow prior to and following inhaled bronchodilator therapy can be especially helpful in identifying worsening asthma control in subjects with poor symptom perception. Spirometry provides valuable information regarding the child's level of pulmonary function and can be helpful in ruling out disorders such as vocal cord dysfunction.[112,113] Yearly evaluation of lung function assessment utilizing body box plethysmography is also important as information regarding the degree of hyperinflation, air-trapping, and increased airway resistance can be monitored. Other measures of pulmonary function, such as pressure volume curves in children with suspected loss of lung elasticity, methacholine challenges, and exercise challenge studies with albuterol pretreatment can also provide useful information. We have observed that some children with refractory asthma have pressure volume curves that are shifted upward and to the left, suggestive of a loss of elastic recoil.[114,115] These children often present with histories of life-threatening events, but will have normal, or at times, supranormal FEV_1 values when stable. Whether this observed abnormality is an acquired and reversible finding, and whether loss of elastic lung recoil pressure contributes to life-threatening exacerbations of asthma, remains unknown.

A multidisciplinary approach to the management of the refractory asthmatic should be undertaken. Children with refractory asthma remain poorly controlled despite optimal use of conventional asthma medications. In addition, they often have steroid-induced adverse effects such as growth suppression, myopathy and osteoporosis as a consequence of chronic high-dose inhaled and often oral GC use. Thus, a comprehensive approach that incorporates all aspects of disease management is essential for these challenging patients. This approach helps address other conditions which may confound the diagnosis or aggravate the disease, ensure that the patient is receiving an adequate antiinflammatory and bronchodilator treatment regimen with demonstrated good technique and compliance, and lastly, addresses the issue of psychosocial stress associated with severe chronic illness and its effect on the patient and the patient's family. A close working relationship among the patient, family, physician, and psychologist is also of critical importance.

Pharmacologic Therapy

The therapeutic goals of refractory asthma are similar to those of other types of asthma. These goals include utilizing SABAs as needed to relieve airflow obstruction, protecting the airway from irritating stimuli and subsequent airway inflammation, and utilizing antiinflammatory medications to treat ongoing airway inflammation. Unfortunately, refractory asthmatics often continue to display evidence for poor asthma control despite utilizing the above measures. Thus, the management of the refractory asthmatic often requires chronically administered oral GC therapy and in some cases, alternative agents.

Systemic Glucocorticoid Therapy

Although the vast majority of asthmatics can achieve optimal control on inhaled GC therapy, refractory asthmatics often require both chronically administered oral glucocorticoid therapy and high-dose inhaled GC therapy, for adequate symptom control. Chronically administered oral GC therapy can be associated with debilitating adverse effects such as adrenal suppression, growth suppression, osteoporosis, cataracts, hypertension, diabetes mellitus, myopathy, obesity, and cushingoid features.[116] As such, an attempt should be made to establish the patient's minimal effective oral GC dose. This entails performing a gradual oral GC taper with close monitoring of the patient's symptoms and pulmonary function. The daily oral GC dose should be tapered by 5 mg per week until 20 mg on alternate days is reached or until breakthrough asthma symptoms or declining pulmonary function is observed. Since most patients will have some degree of adrenal suppression, the GC taper is then slowed down with weekly reductions of 2.5 mg every other week with periodic measurement of AM cortisol levels to assess adrenal recovery. If, during the GC taper, the patient develops increasing asthma symptoms and/or diminished pulmonary function, the threshold dose is established and no further tapering should occur. Of note, the threshold GC requirement is dynamic and likely to change over time, depending on time of year, changes in intrinsic disease severity, and increasing age. If a child's threshold dose is determined to be greater than 20 mg of prednisone (or its equivalent) on alternate days, consideration for alternative asthma medications is warranted as the adverse

effects profile of prednisone at ≥20 mg administered on alternate days becomes unacceptable. However, all alternative antiinflammatory therapies carry their own risk for adverse effects and/or significant financial burden, which precludes their use in all but the most refractory patients.

High-Dose Second-Generation Inhaled Glucocorticoid Therapy

High-dose, second-generation inhaled GC therapy can result in significant reductions in the dose of oral GC needed to control asthma in adults with steroid-dependent asthma. This is likely to be due to the fact that second-generation GCs display greater topical to systemic potencies compared to other inhaled GCs, with the end result a better therapeutic index. The superior therapeutic index is the result of increased antiinflammatory potency of these compounds on a microgram to microgram basis, and reduced oral bioavailability due to extensive first pass metabolism.[117] Studies with fluticasone propionate, budesonide and mometasone furoate have shown these medications to result in varying degrees of oral GC dose reduction and improved asthma control in adults with oral GC-dependent asthma.[118-120] The ability of these second-generation inhaled GCs to result in significant oral steroid-sparing effects appears to be unique to these compounds in that similar effects have not been noted with the other available inhaled GCs.[121] Though useful in reducing the need for oral GCs, high-dose inhaled GC therapy can also result in adverse effects. As such, high-dose inhaled GC therapy warrants ongoing assessment of benefit and monitoring for GC-associated adverse effects.

Leukotriene Modifying Agents

The leukotriene modifying agents (synthesis inhibitors and receptor antagonists) are a frequently used class of asthma controller medications. Studies in subjects with mild and moderate asthma show these medications to be less effective than inhaled GCs in nearly every parameter studied.[122] In patients with moderate to severe asthma, a recently published study found montelukast to result in a modest, yet statistically significant reduction in inhaled GC dosage required to optimize asthma control.[123] In severe asthmatics who remained symptomatic despite therapy with high-dose inhaled GC and LABA therapy, Robinson and colleagues[124] found montelukast to offer no added clinical benefit compared to placebo. Whether the addition of an LTM will offer benefit in children already on combination inhaled GC/LABA therapy remains to be determined.

Theophylline

Although theophylline is an effective asthma controller medication, it is rarely used in children due to its potential for severe toxicity.[125] Because theophylline has steroid-sparing effects in individuals with steroid-dependent asthma, it can be attempted in select patients with severe asthma.[126] Theophylline has a narrow therapeutic window; consequently, levels need to be routinely monitored, especially during viral illnesses associated with fever, or if medication known to delay theophylline clearance, such as macrolide antibiotics, cimetidine, antifungals, oral contraceptives, and ciprofloxacin, are being used concurrently.[127]

Alternative Asthma Therapies

Methotrexate

When given in low doses, methotrexate displays antiinflammatory effects. As a result, methotrexate has been used to treat many autoimmune diseases for decades. Methotrexate has been extensively studied in adults with refractory asthma. Unfortunately, because the published data have yielded contrasting results, it is difficult to determine its true effectiveness in asthma.[128,129] A meta-analysis of all controlled studies evaluating the effectiveness of methotrexate in steroid-dependent asthma found it to display modest steroid-sparing effects.[130] Methotrexate at the doses used to treat asthma is relatively safe, with a low frequency of adverse effects. Rare, but significant, adverse effects include serious infection, pulmonary fibrosis, and liver toxicity.

Cyclosporine A

Cyclosporine (CyA) is a potent immunosuppressive agent that, when used in low doses, is an effective therapy for many autoimmune diseases. In a 12-week crossover study, Alexander and colleagues[131] found CyA to be effective in adults with severe asthma, with improvements in lung function and reductions in the frequency of asthma exacerbations. In contrast, Nizankowska and colleagues[132] failed to find CyA to be effective in improving lung function or reducing the oral GC dose requirement in an equally severe cohort of asthma.

CyA has several potential serious adverse effects, including nephrotoxicity, hypertension, and immunosuppression. Although CyA appears to be ideally suited for the treatment of refractory asthma, the potential for severe and potentially irreversible nephrotoxicity has limited its use in children with refractory asthma. In fact, there are no published controlled studies evaluating the safety or effectiveness of CyA in children with refractory asthma. An inhaled form of CyA is unlikely to be developed for the treatment of asthma since inhaled delivery can cause bronchospasm.

Intravenous Immunoglobulin (IVIG)

A number of small, uncontrolled studies have found IVIG to be an effective agent in children with refractory asthma. Mazer and colleagues[133] were the first to report the effectiveness of monthly high-dose (2 g/kg) IVIG therapy in steroid-dependent children. IVIG therapy was associated with a 3-fold reduction in oral GC requirement, reduction in symptoms, and improvement in lung function. In addition, significant reductions in serum immunoglobulin E (IgE) levels and percutaneous reactivity to aeroallergens were also noted. Another uncontrolled study designed to investigate the mechanisms of GC dose reduction associated with IVIG found IVIG to act synergistically with dexamethasone (Dex) to suppress lymphocyte stimulation in vitro.[134] In this study, IVIG therapy was also associated with reductions in chronic oral GC requirement, number of oral GC bursts, and hospitalizations during the 6-month study, compared to the 6-month period prior to enrollment into the study.

Two small, placebo-controlled studies of IVIG have also been performed. Salmun and colleagues[135] evaluated the effectiveness of IVIG on prednisone reduction in 28 adolescents with steroid-dependent asthma and found IVIG to result in a greater reduction in prednisone than those who received placebo. In contrast, Kishiyama and colleagues[136] found high-dose IVIG to be no more effective than placebo in prednisone reduction, or any other variable studied in adults with severe asthma. These investigators also found an unacceptably high rate of adverse reactions; 19% of subjects who received high-dose IVIG (2 g/kg) developed aseptic meningitis.

In summary, there are conflicting reports regarding the efficacy and safety of IVIG therapy in severe asthma. Definitive studies, i.e. large, randomized, placebo-controlled trials have not been performed to determine its true efficacy. In our experience, children and adolescents are more likely to respond to IVIG, as

are patients with the greatest oral GC requirement. Thus, IVIG may be an effective therapy in a highly selected patient population. Although the safety profile of IVIG is acceptable, adverse effects can occur and include anaphylaxis, headache, aseptic meningitis, and the remote potential for blood-borne infection. Lastly, its use is often cost prohibitive.

Omalizumab (Anti-IgE)

Omalizumab is a humanized murine monoclonal antibody to IgE that inhibits its binding to the high affinity IgE receptor on mast cells and basophils. Omalizumab reduces approximately 95% of circulating free IgE and inhibits both the early- and late-phase asthmatic responses following an allergen challenge.[137] Milgrom and colleagues[138] studied 317 asthmatics with moderate to severe asthma, all of whom were on inhaled GC, with 10% also requiring chronic oral GC therapy. The subjects received omalizumab or placebo every 2 weeks for 20 weeks. The inhaled and oral GC doses were held stable during the first 12 weeks and then tapered as tolerated in the ensuing 8 weeks of the trial. Omalizumab was associated with improved symptom scores, fewer asthma exacerbations, and oral GC dose reduction compared to placebo. Omalizumab has also been shown to be both safe and effective in reducing the inhaled GC requirement of children ≥12 years of age with moderate to severe asthma.[139] Omalizumab is currently undergoing studies in children 6 to 11 years of age with severe asthma.

Tumor Necrosis-Alpha (TNFα) Inhibition

A small open-label study found etanercept (a soluble TNFα receptor) therapy to result in a significant reduction in asthma symptoms and BHR in adults with steroid-dependent asthma.[140] Etanercept was also evaluated in a small, double-blind, placebo-controlled, cross-over study in 10 adults with refractory asthma. Etanercept therapy resulted in improved symptom control and a reduction in BHR, while also improving baseline FEV$_1$.[141] Infliximab, a recombinant human-murine chimeric monoclonal antibody (mAb) was studied in a double-blind, placebo-controlled, parallel-group study of 38 adults with moderate persistent asthma who remained poorly controlled on inhaled GC therapy. While infliximab had no effect on AM PEF (the primary endpoint) or FEV$_1$, it was associated with a decrease in the number of exacerbations and the time to an exacerbation.[142] A recent, large, placebo-controlled study evaluating golimumab, a fully human mAb to TNFα, in severe persistent asthma found its adverse effects to outweigh any potential beneficial effects. This study was discontinued prematurely due to the increased risk of serious adverse effects, namely infection.[143]

Antiinterleukin-5 (IL-5) Antibodies

Monoclonal antibodies directed against IL-5 prevent allergen-induced airway eosinophilia and BHR in both murine and primate models of asthma. Earlier studies evaluating humanized anti-IL-5 mAb in adults with asthma had shown dramatic reductions in circulating and airway eosinophils, with no accompanying reduction in the late-phase asthmatic response, allergen-driven BHR, or improvement in baseline lung function.[144,145] A recent, placebo-controlled study evaluated the effectiveness of mepolizumab, a humanized anti-IL-5 mAb, in 362 asthmatics who continued to be symptomatic despite treatment with inhaled GCs.[146] While mepolizumab therapy resulted in significant reductions in circulating and sputum eosinophils, it had no effect on any clinical end-point studied including AM PEF, FEV$_1$, symptom scores, exacerbations, or quality of life.

Two recent studies evaluated the effect of mepolizumab on patients with severe asthma who had sputum eosinophilia (>3%)

despite chronic GC therapy (inhaled ± oral). The first study enrolled 61 subjects who received monthly infusions of mepolizumab or placebo for 12 months. Mepolizumab-treated subjects had fewer asthma exacerbations and had better quality of life measures than placebo-treated patients.[147] The second study enrolled 20 subjects with eosinophilia, despite chronic prednisone use, to monthly infusions, for 5 months, of mepolizumab or placebo. Mepolizumab therapy was associated with significantly fewer exacerbations and a greater reduction in prednisone requirement while maintaining lung function.[148] Of note, severe asthma with persistent eosinophilia, despite GC therapy, appears to comprise of a very small phenotype of refractory asthma as less than 3% of eligible subjects with severe asthma had persistent sputum eosinophilia after treatment with ≥4 weeks of prednisone with doses ranging from to 5 to 25 mg.

Miscellaneous Alternative Agents

Studies evaluating the effectiveness of oral gold (auranofin) in adults with steroid-dependent asthma have demonstrated modest GC-sparing effects.[149] Whether auranofin is an effective agent in children with refractory asthma has yet to be determined. Auranofin has an acceptable safety profile with the most common reported adverse effect being diarrhea. Nebulized lidocaine has been studied in both adults and children with steroid-dependent asthma.[150,151] These small open-label studies have shown nebulized lidocaine to display significant steroid-sparing effects. Because nebulized lidocaine can cause bronchospasm, a low dose should be administered under supervision when initiating this form of therapy. Lastly, placebo-controlled studies of nebulized lidocaine in the treatment of refractory asthma have yet to be performed.

Conclusions

Refractory asthmatics comprise a subpopulation of asthmatics who continue to have frequent symptoms and exacerbations despite optimal pharmacologic therapy. These patients require frequent systemic courses of GCs and many require chronically administered oral GC to control their disease. As a result, refractory asthmatics will experience substantial GC-associated adverse effects in addition to the morbidity associated with their disease. At the extreme end of refractory asthma are GC-insensitive asthmatics, who fail to adequately respond to aggressive courses of high-dose oral and inhaled GC therapy. Persistent immune activation and airway inflammation that is resistant to GC therapy appears to contribute to the immunologic abnormalities underlying some patients with refractory asthma. Although much insight into the pathogenesis of refractory asthma has been gained, several issues remain unresolved. First, ongoing airway inflammation is thought to contribute to refractory asthma but at present, we have yet to develop a noninvasive way to determine the extent of airway inflammation. Second, significant airway remodeling can occur in children as young as 6 years of age. Structural changes to the airway may also significantly contribute to ongoing respiratory symptoms, persistent BHR, and diminished lung function despite aggressive treatment with antiinflammatory agents. Indeed, GC-independent mechanisms may be involved in the pathogenesis of severe asthma. More information is needed on the pathology of refractory asthma to determine whether ultrastructural abnormalities are present that may be irreversible. In this regard, it is possible that aggressive courses of antiinflammatory or immunomodulator therapy can suppress acute inflammation, but airway remodeling may predispose the patient to residual symptoms, and the development of irreversible airway disease. What is clear is that more effort must be placed on understanding the etiology of refractory asthma in children in order to guide pharmacotherapy for this challenging group of patients. It is hoped that by better understanding the mechanisms involved in the pathogenesis of refractory asthma, specific treatment modalities will be developed for this group of severe asthmatics.

References

1. Robinson DS, Hamid Q, Ying S, et al. Predominant T_{H2}-like bronchoalveolar T lymphocyte population in atopic asthma. N Engl J Med 1992;326:298–304.
2. Bousquet J, Chanez P, Lacoste JY, et al. Eosinophilic inflammation in asthma. N Engl J Med 1990;323:1033–9.
3. Spahn JD, Covar R, Szefler SJ. Glucocorticoids: clinical pharmacology. In: Adkinson NK, Bochner BS, Busse WW, Holgate ST, Lemanske RF, Simons FER, editors. Middleton's allergy: principles and practice. 7th edition. Philadelphia, PA: Mosby/Elsevier Inc; 2009, p. 1575–89.
4. Global Strategy for asthma management and prevention (updated 2006): Global Initiative for Asthma (GINA). http://ginasthma.org. Accessed June 23, 2008.
5. Szefler SJ. Glucocorticoid therapy for asthma: clinical pharmacology. J Allergy Clin Immunol 1991;88:147–65.
6. Busse WW, Banks-Schlegel S, Wenzel SE. Pathophysiology of severe asthma. J Allergy Clin Immunol 2000;106:1033–42.
7. Antonicelli L, Bucca C, Neri M, et al. Asthma severity and medical resource utilisation. Eur Respir J 2004;723:729.
8. Bratton DL, Price M, Gavin L, et al. Impact of a multidisciplinary day program on disease and healthcare costs in children and adolescents with severe asthma: a two-year follow- up study. Pediatr Pulmonol 2001;31:177–89.
9. Expert panel report 3. Guidelines for the diagnosis and management of asthma. Bethesda, Maryland: National Institutes of Health, National Asthma Education and Prevention Program; 2007. NIH Publication No. 08–4051. http://www.nhlbi.gov/guidelines/asthma/asthgdln.pdf. Accessed June 23, 2009.
10. Van Ganse E, Boissel JP, Gormand F, et al. Level of control and hospital contacts in persistent asthma. J Asthma 2001;38:637–43.
11. Fuhlbrigge AL, Kitch BT, Paltiel D, et al. FEV1 is associated with risk of asthma attacks in a pediatric population. J Allergy Clin Immunol 2001;107:61–7.
12. Paull K, Covar R, Jain N, et al. Do the NHLBI lung function criteria apply to children? A cross-sectional evaluation of childhood asthma at National Jewish Medical Center 1999–2002. Pediatr Pulmonol 2005;39:311–317.
13. Bacharier LB, Mauger DT, Lemanske RF, et al. Classifying asthma severity in children: is measuring lung function helpful? J Allergy Clin Immunol 2002;109:S266.
14. Beckett WS, Jacobs DR Jr., Yu X, et al. Asthma is associated with weight gain in females but not males, independent of physical activity. Am J Respir Crit Care Med 2001;164:2045–50.
15. von Kries R, Hermann M, Grunert VP, et al. Is obesity a risk factor for childhood asthma? Allergy 2001;56:318–22.
16. Chan MT, Leung DY, Szefler SJ, et al. Difficult-to-control asthma: clinical characteristics of steroid-insensitive asthma. J Allergy Clin Immunol 1998;101:594–601.
17. Vrugt B, Wilson S, Underwood J, et al. Mucosal inflammation in severe glucocorticoid-dependent asthma. Eur Respir J 1999;13:1245–52.
18. Wenzel SE, Schwartz LB, Langmack EL, et al. Evidence that severe asthma can be divided pathologically into two inflammatory subtypes with distinct physiologic and clinical characteristics. Am J Respir Crit Care Med 1999;160:1001–8.
19. Benayoun L, Druilhe A, Aubier M, et al. Airway structural alterations selectively associated with severe asthma. Am J Respir Crit Care Med 2003;167:1360–8.
20. Payne DN, Adcock IM, Wilson NM, et al. Relationship between exhaled nitric oxide and mucosal eosinophilic inflammation in children with difficult asthma, after treatment with oral prednisolone. Am J Respir Crit Care Med 2001;164:1376–81.
21. Jenkins HA, Cool C, Szefler SJ, et al. The histopathology of severe childhood asthma: a case series. Chest 2003;124:32–41.
22. Standards for the diagnosis and care of patients with chronic obstructive pulmonary disease (COPD) and asthma. This official statement of the American Thoracic Society was adopted by the ATS Board of Directors, November 1986. Am Rev Respir Dis 1987;136:225–44.
23. Platts-Mills TA, Tovey ER, Mitchell EB, et al. Reduction of bronchial hyperreactivity during prolonged allergen avoidance. Lancet 1982;2:675–8.

24. Simon HU, Grotzer M, Nikolaizik WH, et al. High altitude climate therapy reduces peripheral blood T lymphocyte activation, eosinophilia, and bronchial obstruction in children with house-dust mite allergic asthma. Pediatr Pulmonol 1994;17:304–11.

25. Bousquet J, Michel FB. Specific immunotherapy in asthma: is it effective? J Allergy Clin Immunol 1994;94:1–11.

26. Creticos PS. The consideration of immunotherapy in the treatment of allergic asthma. J Allergy Clin Immunol 2000;105:S559–74.

27. Reid MJ, Lockey RF, Turkeltaub PC, et al. Survey of fatalities from skin testing and immunotherapy 1985–1989. J Allergy Clin Immunol 1993;92: 6–15.

28. Tucci F, Resti M, Fontana R, et al. Gastroesophageal reflux and bronchial asthma: prevalence and effect of cisapride therapy [see comments]. J Pediatr Gastroenterol Nutr 1993;17:265–70.

29. Shapiro GG, Christie DL. Gastroesophageal reflux in steroid-dependent asthmatic youths. Pediatrics 1979;63:207–12.

30. Sheikh S, Stephen T, Howell L, et al. Gastroesophageal reflux in infants with wheezing. Pediatr Pulmonol 1999;28:181–6.

31. Balson BM, Kravitz EK, McGeady SJ. Diagnosis and treatment of gastroesophageal reflux in children and adolescents with severe asthma. Ann Allergy Asthma Immunol 1998;81:159–64.

32. Field SK, Underwood M, Brant R, et al. Prevalence of gastroesophageal reflux symptoms in asthma. Chest 1996;109:316–22.

33. Harding SM, Guzzo MR, Richter JE. 24-h esophageal pH testing in asthmatics: respiratory symptom correlation with esophageal acid events. Chest 1999;115:654–9.

34. Theodoropoulos DS, Ledford DK, Lockey RF, et al. Prevalence of upper respiratory symptoms in patients with symptomatic gastroesophageal reflux disease. Am J Respir Crit Care Med 2001;164: 72–6.

35. Jailwala JA, Shaker R. Oral and pharyngeal complications of gastroesophageal reflux disease: globus, dental erosions, and chronic sinusitis. J Clin Gastroenterol 2000;30:S35–8.

36. Ulualp SO, Toohill RJ, Hoffmann R, et al. Possible relationship of gastroesophagopharyngeal acid reflux with pathogenesis of chronic sinusitis. Am J Rhinol 1999;13:197–202.

37. Halstead LA. Role of gastroesophageal reflux in pediatric upper airway disorders. Otolaryngol Head Neck Surg 1999;120:208–14.

38. Stein MR, Baker J. Prevalence of gastroesophageal reflux (GER) in rhinitis. Part II. J Allergy Clin Immunol 2000;105:S198.

39. Irwin RS, Curley FJ, French CL. Difficult-to-control asthma: contributing factors and outcome of a systematic management protocol. Chest 1993;103:1662–9.

40. Gustafsson PM, Kjellman NI, Tibbling L. Oesophageal function and symptoms in moderate and severe asthma. Acta Paediatr Scand 1986;75:729–36.

41. Martin ME, Grunstein MM, Larsen GL. The relationship of gastroesophageal reflux to nocturnal wheezing in children with asthma. Ann Allergy 1982;49:318–22.

42. Cuttitta G, Cibella F, Visconti A, et al. Spontaneous gastroesophageal reflux and airway patency during the night in adult asthmatics. Am J Respir Crit Care Med 2000;161:177–81.

43. Lodi U, Harding SM, Coghlan HC, et al. Autonomic regulation in asthmatics with gastroesophageal reflux [see comments]. Chest 1997;111: 65–70.

44. Hamamoto J, Kohrogi H, Kawano O, et al. Esophageal stimulation by hydrochloric acid causes neurogenic inflammation in the airways in guinea pigs. J Appl Physiol 1997;82:738–45.

45. Jack CIA, Calverley PMA, Donnelly RJ, et al. Simultaneous tracheal and oesophageal pH measurements in asthmatic patients with gastro-oesophageal reflux. Thorax 1995;50:201–4.

46. Field SK, Sutherland LR. Does medical antireflux therapy improve asthma in asthmatics with gastroesophageal reflux? A critical review of the literature. Chest 1998;114:275–83.

47. Levin TR, Sperling RM, McQuaid KR. Omeprazole improves peak expiratory flow rate and quality of life in asthmatics with gastroesophageal reflux [see comments]. Am J Gastroenterol 1998;93:1060–3.

48. Kiljander TO, Salomaa ER, Hietanen EK, et al. Gastroesophageal reflux in asthmatics: a double-blind, placebo-controlled crossover study with omeprazole. Chest 1999;116:1257–64.

49. Chun AH, Erdman K, Zhang Y, et al. Effect on bioavailability of admixing the contents of lansoprazole capsules with selected soft foods. Clin Ther 2000;22:231–6.

50. The American Lung Association Asthma Clinical Research Centers. The efficacy of esomeprazole for treatment of poorly controlled asthma. N Engl J Med 2009;360:1487–99.

51. Peghini PL, Katz PO, Bracy NA, et al. Nocturnal recovery of gastric acid secretion with twice-daily dosing of proton pump inhibitors [see comments]. Am J Gastroenterol 1998;93:763–7.

52. Kiljander T, Salomaa ER, Hietanen E, et al. Asthma and gastro-oesophageal reflux: can the response to anti-reflux therapy be predicted? Respir Med 2001;95:387–92.

53. Togias AG. Systemic immunologic and inflammatory aspects of allergic rhinitis, J Allergy Clin Immunol 2000;106:S247–250.

54. Christodoulopoulos P, Cameron L, Durham S, et al. Molecular pathology of allergic disease. II. Upper airway disease, J Allergy Clin Immunol 2000;105:211–23.

55. Leone C, Teodoro C, Pelucchi A, et al. Bronchial responsiveness and airway inflammation in patients with nonallergic rhinitis with eosinophilia syndrome. J Allergy Clin Immunol 1997;100:775–80.

56. Bucca C, Rolla G, Scappaticci E, et al. Extrathoracic and intrathoracic airway responsiveness in sinusitis. J Allergy Clin Immunol 1995;95: 52–9.

57. Corren J, Adinoff AD, Irvin CG. Changes in bronchial responsiveness following nasal provocation with allergen. J Allergy Clin Immunol 1992;89:611–8.

58. Watson WTA, Becker AB, Simons FE. Treatment of allergic rhinitis with intranasal corticosteroids in patients with mild asthma: effect on lower airway responsiveness. J Allergy Clin Immunol 1993;91:97–101.

59. Corren J, Adinoff AD, Buchmeier AD, et al. Nasal beclomethasone prevents the seasonal increase in bronchial responsiveness in patients with allergic rhinitis and asthma. J Allergy Clin Immunol 1992;90:250–6.

60. Aubier M, Levy J, Clerici C, et al. Different effects of nasal and bronchial glucocorticosteroid administration on bronchial hyperresponsiveness in patients with allergic rhinitis. Am Rev Res Dis 1992;146:122–6.

61. Welsh PW, Stricker WE, Chu C-P, et al. Efficacy of beclomethasone nasal solution, flunisolide, and cromolyn in relieving symptoms of ragweed allergy. Mayo Clin Proc 1987;62:125–34.

62. Rachelefsky GS, Katz RM, Siegel SC. Chronic sinus disease with associated reactive airway disease in children. Pediatrics 1984;73:526–9.

63. Rachelefsky CS, Goldberg M, Katz RM, et al. Sinus disease in children with respiratory allergy. J Allergy Clin Immunol 1978;61:310–4.

64. Foresi A, Pelucchi A, Gherson G, et al. Once daily intranasal fluticasone propionate (200 micrograms) reduces nasal symptoms and inflammation but also attenuates the increase in bronchial responsiveness during the pollen season in allergic rhinitis. J Allergy Clin Immunol 1996;98: 274–82.

65. McAlister WH, Lusk R, Muntz HR. Comparison of plain radiographs and coronal CT scans in infants and children with recurrent sinusitis. Am J Roentgenol 1989;153:1259–64.

66. Christopher KL, Wood RP 2nd, Eckert RC, et al. Vocal-cord dysfunction presenting as asthma. N Engl J Med 1983;308:1566–70.

67. Corren J, Newman KB. Vocal cord dysfunction mimicking bronchial asthma. Postgrad Med 1992;92:153–6.

68. Thomas PS, Geddes DM, Barnes PJ. Pseudo-steroid resistant asthma. Thorax 1999;54:352–6.

69. Brugman SM, Howell JH, Mahler JL, et al. The spectrum of pediatric vocal cord dysfunction. Am Rev Respir Dis 1994;149:A353.

70. Newman KB, Mason UG 3rd, Schmaling KB. Clinical features of vocal cord dysfunction, Am J Respir Crit Care Med 1995;152:1382–6.

71. Elshami AA, Tino G. Coexistent asthma and functional upper airway obstruction. Case reports and review of the literature. Chest 1996;110: 1358–61.

72. Wood RP, Milgrom H. Vocal cord dysfunction. J Allergy Clin Immunol 1996;98:481–5.

73. Meltzer EO, Orgel HA, Kemp JP, et al. Vocal cord dysfunction in a child with asthma. J Asthma 1991;28:141–5.

74. Wood RP 2nd, Jafek BW, Cherniack RM. Laryngeal dysfunction and pulmonary disorder. Otolaryngol Head Neck Surg 1986;94:374–8.

75. Barnes PJ, Woolcock AJ. Difficult asthma. Eur Respir J 1998;12:1209–18.

76. Gavin LA, Wamboldt M, Brugman S, et al. Psychological and family characteristics of adolescents with vocal cord dysfunction. J Asthma 1998;35:409–17.

77. Goldberg BJ, Kaplan MS. Non-asthmatic respiratory symptomatology. Curr Opin Pulm Med 2000;6:26–30.

78. Landwehr LP, Wood RP 2nd, Blager FB, et al. Vocal cord dysfunction mimicking exercise-induced bronchospasm in adolescents. Pediatrics 1996;98:971–4.

79. Perkner JJ, Fennelly KP, Balkissoon R, et al. Irritant-associated vocal cord dysfunction. J Occup Environ Med 1998;40:136–43.

80. Loughlin CJ, Koufman JA. Paroxysmal laryngospasm secondary to gastroesophageal reflux. Laryngoscope 1996;106:1502–5.

81. O'Connell MA, Sklarew PR, Goodman D. Spectrum of presentation of paradoxical vocal cord motion in ambulatory patients. Ann Allergy Asthma Immunol 1995;74:341–4.

82. Place R, Morrison A, Arce E. Vocal cord dysfunction. J Adolesc Health 2000;17:125–29.

83. Nastasi KJ, Howard DA, Raby RB, et al. Airway fluoroscopic diagnosis of vocal cord dysfunction syndrome. Ann Allergy Asthma Immunol 1997;78:586–8.

84. Anbar RD, Hehir DA. Hypnosis as a diagnostic modality for vocal cord dysfunction. Pediatrics 2000;106:E81.

85. Weir M. Vocal cord dysfunction mimics asthma and may respond to heliox. Clin Pediatr (Phila) 2002;41:37–41.

86. Martin RJ. Managing the patient with intractable asthma. Hosp Pract (Off Ed) 1996;31:61–64, 69–74, 79–80.

87. Sears MR, Taylor DR, Print CG, et al. Regular inhaled beta-agonist treatment in bronchial asthma. Lancet 1990;336:1391–6.

88. Spitzer WO, Suissa S, Ernst P, et al. The use of b-agonists and the risk of death and near death from asthma. N Eng J Med 1992;326:501–6.

89. Greening AP, Ind PW, Northfield M, et al. Added salmeterol versus higher-dose corticosteroid in asthma patients with symptoms on existing inhaled corticosteroid. Allen & Hanburys Limited UK Study Group. Lancet 1994;344:219–24.

90. Woolcock A, Lundback B, Ringdal N, et al. Comparison of addition of salmeterol to inhaled steroids with doubling of the dose of inhaled steroids. Am J Respir Crit Care Med 1996;153:1481–8.

91. Kavuru M, Melamed J, Gross G, et al. Salmeterol and fluticasone propionate combined in a new powder inhalation device for the treatment of asthma: a randomized, double-blind, placebo-controlled trial. J Allergy Clin Immunol 2000;105:1108–16.

92. O'Byrne PM, Barnes PJ, Rodriguez-Roisin R, et al. Low dose inhaled budesonide and formoterol in mild persistent asthma: the OPTIMA randomized trial. Am J Respir Crit Care Med 2001;164:1392–7.

93. Nelson HS, Weiss ST, Bleecker ER, et al. The salmeterol multicenter asthma research trial: a comparison of usual pharmacotherapy for asthma or usual pharmacotherapy plus salmeterol. Chest 2006;129:15–26.

94. Cameron SJ, Cooper EJ, Crompton GK, et al. Substitution of beclomethasone aerosol for oral prednisolone in the treatment of chronic asthma. Br Med J 1973;4:205–7.

95. Tarlo SM, Broder I, Davies GM, et al. Six-month double-blind, controlled trial of high dose, concentrated beclomethasone dipropionate in the treatment of severe chronic asthma. Chest 1988;93:998–1002.

96. Whelan AM, Hahn NW. Optimizing drug delivery from metered-dose inhalers. DICP 1991;25:638–45.

97. Newman SP. Therapeutic aerosols. In: Clarke SW, Pavia D, editors. Aerosols and the lung: clinical and experimental aspects. Butterworths; 1984, p. 197–224.

98. Toogood JH, Jennings B, Baskerville J, et al. Clinical use of spacer systems for corticosteroid inhalation therapy: a preliminary analysis. Eur J Respir Dis Suppl 1982;122:100–7.

99. Rand CS, Wise RA, Nides M, et al. Metered-dose inhaler adherence in a clinical trial. Am Rev Respir Dis 1992;146:1559–64.

100. Anderson RJ, Kirk LM. Methods of improving patient compliance in chronic disease states. Arch Intern Med 1982;142:1673–5.

101. Mellins RB, Evans D, Zimmerman B, et al. Patient compliance: are we wasting our time and don't know it? Am Rev Respir Dis 1992;146:1376–7.

102. Kelloway JS, Wyatt RA, Adlis SA. Comparison of patients' compliance with prescribed oral and inhaled asthma medications. Arch Intern Med 1994;154:1349–52.

103. Milgrom H, Bender B, Ackerson L, et al. Noncompliance and treatment failure in children with asthma. J Allergy Clin Immunol 1996;98:1051–7.

104. Spahn JD, Leung DYM, Surs W, et al. Reduced glucocorticoid binding affinity in asthma is related to ongoing allergic inflammation. Am J Respir Crit Care Med 1995;151:1709–14.

105. Apter AJ, Reisine ST, Affleck G, et al. Adherence with twice-daily dosing of inhaled steroids: socioeconomic and health-belief differences, Am J Respir Crit Care Med 1998;157:1810–7.

106. Chrousos GP, Vingerhoeds A, Brandon D, et al. Primary cortisol resistance in man: a glucocorticoid receptor-mediated disease. J Clin Invest 1982;69:1261–9.

107. Hurley DM, Accili D, Stratakis CA, et al. Point mutation causing a single amino acid substitution in the hormone binding domain of the glucocorticoid receptor in familial glucocorticoid resistance. J Clin Invest 1991;87:680–6.

108. Hill MR, Szefler SJ, Ball BD, et al. Monitoring glucocorticoid therapy: a pharmacokinetic approach. Clin Pharmacol Ther 1990;48:390–8.

109. Bartoszek M, Brenner AM, Szefler SJ. Prednisolone and methylprednisolone kinetics in children receiving anticonvulsant therapy. Clin Pharmacol Ther 1987;42:424–32.

110. Udwadia ZF, Sridhar G, Beveridge CJ, et al. Catastrophic deterioration in asthma induced by rifampicin in steroid- dependent asthma. Respir Med 1993;87:629.

111. Lane SJ, Arm JP, Staynov DZ, et al. Chemical mutational analysis of the human glucocorticoid receptor cDNA in glucocorticoid-resistant bronchial asthma. Am J Respir Cell Mol Biol 1994;11:42–8.

112. Spahn JD, Chipps BE. Medical progress: office-based objective measures in childhood asthma. J Pediatr 2006;148:11–15.

113. Martin RJ, Blager FB, Gay M, et al. Paradoxic vocal cord motion in presumed asthmatics. Semin Respir Med 1987;8:332–7.

114. Liu AH, Brugman SM, Schaeffer EB, et al. Reduced lung elasticity may characterize children with severe asthma. Am Rev Respir Dis 1990;141:A906.

115. Gelb AF, Licuanan J, Shinar CM, et al. Unsuspected loss of lung elastic recoil in chronic persistent asthma. Chest 2002;121:715–21.

116. Covar RA, Leung DY, McCormick D, et al. Risk factors associated with glucocorticoid-induced adverse effects in children with severe asthma. J Allergy Clin Immunol 2000;106:651–9.

117. Lipworth BJ. New perspectives on inhaled drug delivery and systemic bioactivity. Thorax 1995;50:105–10.

118. Noonan M, Chervinsky P, Busse WW, et al. Fluticasone propionate reduces oral prednisone use while it improves asthma control and quality of life. Am J Respir Crit Care Med 1995;152:1467–73.

119. Nelson HS, Bernstein IL, Fink J, et al. Oral glucocorticosteroid-sparing effect of budesonide administered by Turbuhaler: a double-blind, placebo-controlled study in adults with moderate-to-severe chronic asthma. Pulmicort Turbuhaler Study Group. Chest 1998;113:1264–71.

120. Fish JE, Karpel JP, Craig TJ, et al. Inhaled mometasone furoate reduces oral prednisone requirements while improving respiratory function and health-related quality of life in patients with severe persistent asthma. J Allergy Clin Immunol 2000;106:852–60.

121. Hummel S, Lehtonen L. Comparison of oral-steroid sparing by high-dose and low-dose inhaled steroid in maintenance treatment of severe asthma. Lancet 1992;340:1483–7.

122. Malmstrom K, Rodriguez-Gomez G, Guerra J, et al. Oral montelukast, inhaled beclomethasone, and placebo for chronic asthma: a randomized, controlled trial. Montelukast/Beclomethasone Study Group. Ann Intern Med 1999;130:487–95.

123. Lofdahl CG, Reiss TF, Leff JA, et al. Randomised, placebo controlled trial of effect of a leukotriene receptor antagonist, montelukast, on tapering inhaled corticosteroids in asthmatic patients. BMJ 1999;319:87–90.

124. Robinson DS, Campbell D, Barnes PJ. Addition of leukotriene antagonists to therapy in chronic persistent asthma: a randomised double-blind placebo-controlled trial. Lancet 2001;357:2007–11.

125. Weinberger M. The value of theophylline for asthma, Ann Allergy 1989;63:1–3.

126. Brenner M, Berkowitz R, Marshall N, et al. Need for theophylline in severe steroid-requiring asthmatics. Clin Allergy 1988;18: 143–50.

127. Hendeles L, Weinberger M, Szefler S, et al. Safety and efficacy of theophylline in children with asthma. J Pediatr 1992;120:177–83.

128. Mullarkey MF, Blumenstein BA, Andrade WP, et al. Methotrexate in the treatment of corticosteroid-dependent asthma: a double-blind crossover study. N Engl J Med 1988;318:603–7.

129. Erzurum SC, Leff JA, Cochran JE, et al: Lack of benefit of methotrexate in severe, steroid-dependent asthma: a double-blind, placebo-controlled study. Ann Intern Med 1991;114:353–60.

130. Aaron SD, Dales RE, Pham B. Management of steroid-dependent asthma with methotrexate: a meta-analysis of randomized clinical trials. Respir Med 1998;92:1059–65.

131. Alexander AG, Barnes NC, Kay AB. Trial of cyclosporin in corticosteroid-dependent chronic severe asthma. Lancet 1992;339:324–8.

132. Nizankowska E, Soja J, Pinis G, et al. Treatment of steroid-dependent bronchial asthma with cyclosporin. Eur Respir J 1995;8:1091–9.

133. Mazer BD, Gelfand EW. An open-label study of high-dose intravenous immunoglobulin in severe childhood asthma, J Allergy Clin Immunol 1991;87:976–83.

134. Spahn JD, Leung DY, Chan MT, et al. Mechanisms of glucocorticoid reduction in asthmatic subjects treated with intravenous immunoglobulin. J Allergy Clin Immunol 1999;103:421–6.

135. Salmun LM, Barlan I, Wolf HM, et al. Effect of intravenous immunoglobulin on steroid consumption in patients with severe asthma: a double-blind, placebo-controlled, randomized trial. J Allergy Clin Immunol 1999;103:810–5.

136. Kishiyama JL, Valacer D, Cunningham-Rundles C, et al. A multicenter, randomized, double-blind, placebo-controlled trial of high-dose intravenous immunoglobulin for oral corticosteroid-dependent asthma. Clin Immunol 1999;91:126–33.

137. Fahy JV, Fleming HE, Wong HH, et al. The effect of an anti-IgE monoclonal antibody on the early- and late-phase responses to allergen inhalation in asthmatic subjects. Am J Respir Crit Care Med 1997;155:1828–34.

138. Milgrom H, Fick RB, Reimann JD, et al. Treatment of allergic asthma with monoclonal anti-IgE antibody. rhuMAb-E25 Study Group. N Engl J Med 1999;341:1966–1973.

139. Milgrom H, Berger W, Nayak A, et al. Treatment of childhood asthma with anti-immunoglobulin E antibody (omalizumab). Pediatrics 2001;108:E36.

140. Howarth PH, Babu KS, Arshad HS, et al. Tumour necrosis factor (TNFa) as a novel therapeutic target in symptomatic corticosteroid dependent asthma. Thorax 2005;60:1012–8.

141. Berry MA, Hargadon B, Selley M, et al. Evidence of a role of tumor necrosis in refractory asthma. N Engl J Med 2006;354:697–708.

142. Erin EM, Leaker BR, Nicholson GC, et al. The effects of a monoclonal antibody directed against tumor necrosis factor-a in asthma. Am J Respir Crit Care Med 2006;174:753–62.

143. Wenzel SE, Barnes PJ, Bleecker ER, et al. A randomized, double-blind, placebo-controlled study of tumor necrosis-a blockade in severe persistent asthma. Am J Respir Crit Care Med 2009;179:549–58.

144. Leckie MJ, tenBrinke A, Khan J, et al. Effects of an interleukin-5 blocking monoclonal antibody on eosinophils, airway hyper-responsiveness, and the late asthmatic response. Lancet 2000;356:2144–2148.

145. Kips JC, O'Conner BJ, Langley SJ, et al. Effect of SCH55700, a humanized anti-human interluekin-5 antibody in severe persistent asthma: a pilot study. Am J Respir Crit Care Med 2003;167:1655–9.

146. Flood-Page P, Swenson C, Faiferman I, et al. A study to evaluate safety and efficacy of mepolizumab in patients with moderate persistent asthma. Am J Respir Crit Care Med 2007;176:1062–71.

147. Haldar P, Brightling CE, Hargadon B, et al. Mepolizumab and exacerbations of refractory eosinophilic asthma. N Engl J Med 2009;360:973–84.

148. Nair P, Pizzichini MMM, Kjarsgaard M, et al. Mepolizumab for prednisone dependent asthma with sputum eosinophilia. N Engl J Med 2009;360:985–993.

149. Bernstein IL, Bernstein DI, Dubb JW, et al. A placebo-controlled multicenter study of auranofin in the treatment of patients with corticosteroid-dependent asthma. Auranofin Multicenter Drug Trial. J Allergy Clin Immunol 1996;98: 317–24.

150. Decco ML, Neeno TA, Hunt LW, et al. Nebulized lidocaine in the treatment of severe asthma in children: a pilot study. Ann Allergy Asthma Immunol 1999;82:29–32.

151. Hunt LW, Swedlund HA, Gleich GJ. Effect of nebulized lidocaine on severe glucocorticoid-dependent asthma. Mayo Clin Proc 1996;71: 361–8.

CHAPTER

42

Communication Strategies to Improve Adherence with Asthma Medications

Bruce G. Bender

Nonadherence is a Major Threat to Treatment Success

Patient adherence with asthma self-management plans, as with all chronic medical conditions, is often poor. Adherence to daily asthma medication regimens averages about 50% or less for chronic conditions in general,[1] including patients with asthma.[2,3] *Adherence,* as defined in these studies, means that about half of the prescribed medication was taken, although it does not necessarily signify that it was taken in the appropriate manner. In addition, the report of 50% medication adherence reflects the average of groups of patients studied but does not translate into a uniform pattern of taking every other dose of medication. Individual adherence patterns include widely varying behaviors, with some patients taking close to all their medications at the appropriate time and others taking almost no medication.[3] Individual adherence fluctuates greatly over time, often with periods of time during which patients take no medication for varying periods, often for days or weeks at a time.[4] Further, asthma medication adherence may be on the decline. A 1993 review of 10 published studies found that adherence had averaged 48%.[5] Recently published studies have reported mean inhaled corticosteroid (ICS) adherence at 34% in adults[6] and 40% in children.[7] Decreasing ICS adherence is followed by worsening asthma symptoms in children.[8] Because most adherence research is conducted on patients who volunteer to participate in studies and know that their adherence is being monitored, these numbers may be inflated. One medication refill study, reflecting the behavior of 5500 adult and pediatric patients using a national pharmacy chain, found mean ICS adherence of 22.2% over 12 months.[9]

What Happens When Patients are Nonadherent?

Depending on the duration of action and the drug side-effects profile, periods of nonadherence may have several potential consequences, including waning drug action, hazardous rebound effects when administration stops abruptly, and overdose effects when administration of full-strength drugs suddenly resumes.[4] In studies of metered-dose inhaler (MDI) use among children with asthma, inhalers were not used on 48% of study days and abandonment of medication typically occurred for several consecutive days.[10] The consequences of such start-and-stop adher-

ence patterns are unknown. Time to onset of the effectiveness of ICSs in the treatment of mild-to-moderate asthma is about 3 weeks, with faster impact (3 days) reflected on morning peak expiratory flow values in patients with severe asthma.[11] It remains to be determined how varying patterns of adherence translate into asthma control and whether, for example, control in patients with relatively high adherence who fail to use their medication for 1 week or longer is poorer than in patients who use less total medication but with better regularity.[12]

While the assumption that under-use of asthma controller medication can result in less control over the disorder is accurate, conclusions about the amount of medication required by any individual child are difficult to establish largely because of individual variations in disease characteristics, medication requirements, and drug metabolism rates. The prevailing standard, as reflected by the NAEPP guidelines for the diagnosis and management of asthma, is that increased medication administration is the correct response to inadequate symptom control.[13] The potential benefit of medication escalation on the part of the physician is realized only if the patient responds by adhering to the new regimen. Although some studies have defined nonadherence as less than 75% of medication taken, it is impossible to establish a minimum level of adherence that is sufficient for all patients. Evidence exists that ICSs are highly effective in controlling asthma, that some benefit persists even at relatively low dosing frequency, and that a dose-response relationship exists between degree of adherence and degree of benefit. Suissa and colleagues,[14] for example, conducted a nested case-control study of patients with severe asthma and found that a decreasing number of ICS pharmacy refills was associated with increasing risk of death from asthma. As few as three ICS canisters per year reduced risk by one half, with increasing protection gained as refills increased up to a full adherence level of 12 canisters per year. Clearly, as adherence levels drop, asthma becomes less controlled. For example, in a 3-month study, children with a median ICS adherence of 14% had asthma exacerbations requiring urgent office visits and oral steroid bursts, whereas those with adherence levels of 68% remained medically stable.[15] Even children with relatively mild asthma demonstrated increased asthma symptoms as adherence declined.[8] Nonadherent adults with asthma had more airway obstruction than adherent patients.[16] In large studies of managed care populations, decreasing use of ICSs has been linked to increased risk of hospitalization.[17] Children who did not adhere to their asthma treatment regimen had poorer asthma control and required more urgent-care visits, steroid bursts, and hospitalizations.[15,18] Tragically,

DOI: 10.1016/B978-1-4377-0271-2.00042-0

nonadherence has been associated with asthma-related deaths in children, particularly where psychologic dysfunction was observed in the patient or the patient's family.[19]

What Can be Done to Change Patient Behavior?

Numerous strategies to improve patient adherence have been tested, many in carefully conducted randomized clinical trials. While most of these interventions have been able to change patient or parent behavior, changes are often small and difficult to sustain. Further, effective interventions are often costly and require large amounts of healthcare provider time or supplementary staff. A Cochrane Collection meta-analysis of 69 randomized trials of adherence interventions, covering a large range of ages and diseases, reported that four of ten produced an effect on both adherence and at least one clinical outcome. All involved complex interventions combining components such as information giving, reminders, self-monitoring, reinforcement, counseling, psychological therapy, crisis intervention, and telephone follow-up.[20] A meta-analysis of 70 controlled studies of interventions to improve adherence across various chronic pediatric conditions, including asthma, diabetes, cystic fibrosis, cancer, sickle cell disease, and gastrointestinal disorders, revealed moderate effect size in multicomponent behavioral interventions and small effect size from interventions limited to education and instruction.[21] Multicomponent behavioral programs again included a variety of interventions such as behavioral reinforcement, social support, computer and technology-based components, homework assignments, and family and individual psychological counseling.

A recent consensus report from a group of 20 internationally recognized experts on adherence emphasized the essential importance of identifying simple, brief interventions that could be delivered by healthcare providers during the course of routine office care.[22] The challenge, then, becomes one of identifying interventions that are not costly, do not require a large amount of healthcare provider time, and can be implemented during routine office visits. Do such interventions exist, and are they evidence-based? A considerable amount of evidence indicates that key communication strategies exist that can change parent and patient behavior and are evidence-based, time efficient, and teachable to busy healthcare providers.

Evidence Basis for Changing Health Behaviors: The Health Beliefs Model

Behavioral scientists have long adopted a translational research approach to understanding and changing health behaviors. Much like 'bench' research, the process begins with studies that document frequencies, predictors, and moderators of health behaviors. This information is used to build models, or theories, that explain health behaviors. Such models of behavior change are used, in turn, to translate theory to the 'bedside' by allowing behavioral scientists to develop and test interventions that change peoples' health behavior.

One of the earliest, longest-standing, and most utilized models has been the Health Beliefs Model.[23,24] The Heath Beliefs Model has evolved over time with the accumulation of evidence from many studies of health behavior, but its core thesis remains the same: the probability that a person will change their behavior will depend on their perception of risk and benefit (Figure 42-1). Parents who perceive a favorable benefit-to-risk ratio of ICS are more likely to administer the medication to their child.[25] A

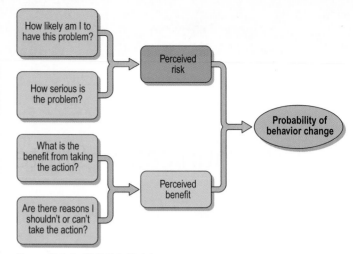

Figure 42-1 Health Beliefs Model.

patient with high blood pressure is more likely to take antihypertensive medication if they perceive that high blood pressure is dangerous, and if they believe that the medication will reduce that risk while not introducing other risks, such as side-effects. The probability of behavior change, in this case taking daily antihypertensive medication, is further influenced by self-efficacy and cues to action. Self-efficacy reflects the person's belief that they can change their behavior, particularly where the behavior change is difficult, such as losing weight or stopping smoking. Cues to action are essentially environmental influences, such as public service announcements that portray the dangers of high blood pressure, the availability of free blood pressure screening, or advice from a physician.

Health Beliefs Model (Figure 42-1) has evolved and spun off a number of related theories of health behavior change. These include *patient-centered care, motivational interviewing, readiness to change,* and *shared decision-making*. Each has produced evidence of the effectiveness of very specific communication strategies. These strategies are discussed below, along with evidence from each model that supports its use. The collective group of six strategies is presented here as an integrated program that can guide provider behavior during patient visits to increase treatment effectiveness and outcomes. Further, these strategies can enhance satisfaction from the encounter for both the family and the healthcare provider.

Six Communication Strategies for Changing Patient Behavior

1. Build a Relationship

Promoting strong adherence begins with the development of patient trust in the provider-patient relationship. Patients and parents are more likely to increase and accurately report their adherence levels, and to express satisfaction with their care, where healthcare providers demonstrate thorough information sharing, interpersonal sensitivity, and partnership-building.[26] *Patient-centered care* embraces the concept that trust is established where the provider demonstrates genuine interest in and concern about the patient and considers the family's cultural traditions, personal preferences and values, current situations, and lifestyle. Trust begins with communication, including listening and exploring concerns. The first moment of interaction when the provider and patient come together sets the tone for the communication that will follow. Consensus recommendations indicate that very basic elements of communication that establish this foundation include adopting a friendly tone, greeting the family with a smile, and being aware of tone, pace, eye contact, and other elements of nonverbal communication that establish genuine interest in the patient (Box 42-1).[27] Further, patients will be more adherent when physicians provide more information and are nonjudgmental, supportive, and understanding.[28] Patient-centered care has been shown to improve health outcomes for a number of disorders including diabetes,[29] hypertension,[30] obesity[31] and asthma.[32]

Demonstration of interest and concern includes asking questions that allow the patient or parent to tell the physician about their worries, symptoms, and hopes for the visit. In a survey study, 865 patients from three primary care practices completed a questionnaire inquiring about what the patient desired in a consultation with their physician. Factor analysis of the results identified three primary domains: (1) *communication*, which included listening, exploring concerns, and providing information with clear explanations; (2) *partnership*, which included discussion with the physician to achieve common ground and mutual agreement about the problem and treatment; and (3) *health promotion*, which included information and encouragement to maintain health and reduce risks of future illness.[33] A systematic review of relevant literature revealed that physician questioning is an important part of effective communication that can exert positive influence on the patient's emotional well-being, symptom resolution, and functional and physiologic improvement.[34] This approach has advantages for both the family and the provider. Taking the time to ask and answer patient questions is associated with greater physician job satisfaction and higher rates of adherence to medical treatment,[35] and lower rates of medical errors.[36]

The NAEPP Guidelines for the diagnosis and management of Asthma[13] provide examples of questions that can be asked in the initial visit and help set the stage for positive communication (Box 42-2).

2. Focus on Listening

Healthcare providers who want to be helpful to their patients by sharing important information about an illness, test results, and treatment plans, are often well-practiced at giving information, but may not always be as cognizant of the importance of listening. Time pressures add to the sense that the encounter must be brief and efficient, a tendency to ask questions that that can be answered 'yes' or 'no' to limit discussion, and a desire to move briskly toward completion of the visit. The result may be that the family's concerns are not heard. The family's unheard concerns often undermine adherence.

In the context of the Health Beliefs Model, the parent's decision about whether or not to follow a treatment plan is largely influenced by their perception of the risks associated with the disease, and the risks and benefits introduced by the treatment.[37] For patients or parents of patients with asthma, concerns often include fears about medication side-effects, a perception that the medication is not helping, concerns about long-term dependence on the medication, and the cost of the medication.[38] In a study of parents of 67 children with asthma, increased concerns about risks of taking asthma medications were associated with lower adherence; fewer concerns combined with a perception of benefit from the child's medication was associated with higher adherence.[25] When the patient or parent voices their concerns, the healthcare provider has an opportunity to discuss these concerns and perceptions, to provide more information, and to discuss treatment options. When the discussion leads to a shift in the family's perception of the relative benefits of the medication over its risks, increased adherence is likely to follow.[25,39]

Patients who do not perceive a positive benefit-to-risk advantage to their treatment are likely to be ambivalent and uncommitted to a daily treatment regimen. Evidence of this ambivalence is seen in the finding that over half of 5500 patients who filled an ICS prescription once did not return to refill within 12 months.[9] The technique of *motivational interviewing* is designed to increase patient and parent motivation by strategically helping to overcome ambivalence while avoiding confronting or lecturing the patient.[40] At the core of this technique are four important listening strategies: open-ended questions, affirmations, reflective listening, and summary statements:[41]

1. *Open-ended questions* allow the patient and parent to 'tell their story', and contrast with closed-ended questions, which force the family into a yes-no response (e.g. 'Tell me about how you are using the asthma medication' rather than 'Are you taking your medication?').

2. *Affirmations* are positive statements that help to build rapport and encourage behavior change (e.g. 'I can see that you are really trying to get your child's asthma under control').

3. *Reflective listening*, arguably the most challenging of these listening skills, involves stating back to the patient and parent what the healthcare provider believes they have heard from the family. Reflective listening helps to ensure that the provider understands the patient's perspective while emphasizing positive statements about change. The seven types of reflective listening, from simplest to most complex, are listed in Table 42-1.

Table 42-1 Types of Reflections Used in Motivational Interviewing

	Patient	HCP
1. Repeating Use to diffuse resistance	'I don't want to take my medication.'	'You don't want to take your medication.'
2. Rephrasing Slightly alter what the patient says to provide the patient with a different point of view	'I want to take my medication, but I have trouble fitting it into my day.'	'Taking your medication is important to you.'
3. Empathic reflection Provide understanding for the patient's situation	'You've probably never had to deal with anything like this.'	'It's hard to imagine how I could possibly understand.'
4. Reframing Help the patient think about his or her situation differently.	"I've tried to take my medication consistently, but I just can't seem to pull it off."	"You are persistent, even in the face of discouragement. Controlling your asthma is really important to you."
5. Feeling reflection Reflect the emotional undertones of the conversation	'I know that not taking medication is bad for my asthma.'	'You're worried about your asthma getting worse.'
6. Amplified reflection Reflect what the client has said in an exaggerated way. This encourages the client to argue less and can elicit the other side of the client's ambivalence	'My mom is totally exaggerating my symptoms. My asthma isn't that bad.'	'There's no reason to be concerned about your asthma.' (said without sarcasm)
7. Double-sided reflection Acknowledge both sides of the patient's ambivalence	'Taking medications just takes away my freedom. It's such a hassle.'	'On the one hand, you find that medication takes away your freedom. On the other hand, you said that your asthma symptoms limit your freedom by preventing you from doing things you enjoy. What do you make of this?'

Reprinted with permission, Borrelli B, Riekert K, Weinstein A, Rathier L. J Allergy Clin Immunol 2007;120:1023–1030.

4. *Summary statements* are longer summaries of what the provider has heard from the patient or parent, and serve the purpose of providing a recap of key points, highlighting the family's ambivalence, and gently moving the patient toward a positive change (e.g. 'You'd like to really get your child's asthma under better control, and you think this medication is helping, but you are not convinced that this medication is safe enough to take for a long period of time'). Both reflective listening and summary statements help to crystallize where a behavior change is needed, and help to transition the discussion toward action.

3. Collaborate on the Treatment Plan

Patient-centered care presumes that the provider is willing to put aside a paternalistic approach in which the patient is told what is wrong with them and what they need to do, and instead work toward a partnership in which the patient is heard, a discussion occurs, and the two parties agree, both on the goals of treatment as well as the treatment itself.[42] To accomplish this partnership, the provider must engage and listen to the patient and parent, showing sensitivity, interest, concern, and comprehension of the family's message. Differences in goals and expectations must be discussed and resolved before the treatment plan is finalized. The partnership approach is favored by many patients. For example, a survey of patients following a consultation showed increased satisfaction where physicians were 'interested in what I think the problem is', 'interested in what treatment I want', and would 'discuss and agree with me on treatment'.[33] The NAEPP guidelines emphasizes the importance of this relationship and provide recommendations toward establishing a partnership with the patient and family (Box 42-3).

BOX 42-3

Steps to Develop an Active Partnership with the Patient and Family

- Establish open communications.
- Identify and address patient and family concerns about asthma and asthma treatment.
- Identify patient/parent/child treatment preferences regarding treatment and barriers to its implementation.
- Develop treatment goals together with patient and family.
- Encourage active self-assessment and self-management of asthma.
- Encourage adherence by:
  - Choosing a treatment regimen that achieves outcomes and addresses preferences that are important to the patient/parent (Evidence B).
  - Reviewing the success of the treatment plan with the patient/parent at each visit and making adjustments as needed (Evidence B).
- Tailor the asthma self-management teaching approach to the needs of each patient.
- Maintain sensitivity to cultural beliefs and ethnocultural practices (Evidence C).

From NAEPP Guidelines for the diagnosis and management of asthma, Expert Panel Report 3, 2007.

Establishing a partnership between the provider and family necessarily reflects a shift of authority within which the physician takes into account the patient's concerns and preferences before making treatment recommendations. The degree to which the provider defers to the patient or parent will depend both on the physician and family. Many physicians are most comfortable maintaining control of the treatment plan, and may do so while still adopting a sensitive patient-centered focus. Other physicians may be comfortable taking the partnership a step further, allowing the patient more control over the choice of treatment plan. This approach is adopted in the *shared decision-making* model, a communication approach that attempts to increase concordance about treatment choices and goals by promoting greater involvement of the individual patient in deliberations about treatment options.[43] A recent NHLBI-funded study evaluated the effectiveness of shared decision-making in improving outcomes in adults aged 18 to 70 years with poorly controlled, mild to moderate persistent asthma. Healthcare providers were randomly assigned to one of three training conditions: (1) usual care (no training), (2) management by guidelines (training in following the evidence-based guidelines), and (3) shared decision-making (training in guidelines combined with shared decision-making). In the group of 170 patients of providers trained in shared decision-making, controller medication adherence improved from 40% at baseline to 70% following the intervention, significantly more than for the 331 patients in the other two conditions.[44] Not all patients may prefer a shared decision-making approach. In a study where patients evaluated videos of two different types of consultations with a physician, one shared decision and one in which the physician was more directive, the directed approach was often preferred by older patients while the shared decision approach was often preferred by younger patients and those with higher education levels.[45]

4. Assess Patient and Parent Readiness to Change

Motivating patients and parents to change health behaviors is a significant challenge. Providers may be frustrated by a perceived failure of patients to follow instructions and treatment plans, even when their health clearly hangs in the balance, and may consequently avoid discussing the patient's behavior. For example, only 32% of physicians make a regular practice of inquiring about their patients' smoking status.[46] However, providers can help motivate patients to stop smoking and make other behavior changes when they adopt more effective communication strategies and a less failure-oriented view of how people change their behavior. The *stages-of-change* model recognizes that patients and parents vary in their readiness to change, and that change typically occurs through a number of stages that include (1) precontemplation (the patient is unaware of the problem or not ready to deal with it), (2) contemplation (the patient acknowledges the problem and is seriously thinking about overcoming it), (3) action (the patient is ready to start overcoming the problem and has made a commitment to behavior change), and (4) maintenance (the patient is maintaining change and working to prevent relapse).[40,47] When discussing a health problem, patients and parents may identify their own readiness to take on a health behavior change, including adherence to their treatment plan. The family's confidence in making a behavior change is predictive of their likely level of adherence.[48] Therefore, a helpful exercise asks families to estimate their motivation and confidence, and consequently allows the provider to calibrate their approach.[41] Specifically, the physician can ask 'On a scale of 1 to 10, how motivated are you to use this medication every day' followed by 'On a scale of 1 to 10, how confident are you that you can do this?' The physician and family may then discuss what might help to increase the family's commitment and confidence. Within this partnership approach, the provider is less authoritative and allows the patient and parent to help determine how change will occur.[39]

Another communication approach which builds on the stages-of-change model is the '5 As', standing for Ask, Advise, Assess, Assist, and Arrange.[49] This brief intervention strategy allows the physician to regularly raise the question of a change in health behavior, listening for the patient's commitment and readiness to take on the change and providing assistance and referral as needed. Use of this approach is also time efficient, allowing the provider to address an 'A' in 1 to 3 minutes during an office visit. The 5 As are widely recommended for helping patients to stop smoking, but have also been adopted to help make changes in a variety of other health behaviors including changing diet[50] and exercise behaviors.[51]

5. Manage Time

With limitations in insurance reimbursement and a consequent need to see larger numbers of patients, physicians often experience significant pressure to limit the time they spend with each patient. Discussions about changing patient health behavior, therefore, are sometimes greeted with the concern that improved communication will mean large increases in time for each patient encounter. However, strategic time management and adoption of brief-but-effective communication strategies often results in meaningful changes in patient and parent motivation without increased encounter time. For example, a large randomized trial tested the effectiveness of educating primary care pediatricians in two interactive seminars that provided training in asthma-management guidelines and communication skills. Half of the 100 pediatricians received the training. Compared to the control pediatricians, patients of the trained group reported more discussion about personal concerns and goals for treatment during office visits, and experienced fewer symptom days and emergency department visits over the ensuing year. Assessments of time spent with the family revealed that those pediatricians who had received the training spent no more time than control physicians during the initial visit, acute asthma visits, or well-child visits.[52]

Effective time management begins with setting the agenda at the beginning of the visit. This includes asking the patient what they hope to accomplish ('What brings you here today?'; 'What are you hoping I might be able to do to help?'). The 'patient agenda' may differ from the 'physician agenda'.[42] Patients and parents may be reluctant to voice their agenda, feeling intimidated or worried about how their concerns will be heard by the physician.[42] However, when physicians proceed with their own presumed agenda and fail to elicit the family's agenda, outcomes are often less successful.[53] Asking families to voice their agenda does not carry with it a presumption that the provider can address all concerns in the allotted time. Simply listening to and acknowledging the patient's concerns often provides an emotional relief to the patient. The provider must establish priorities with the patient or parent for this visit ('What is at the top of your list?'), consider the time available, and make a plan that may include data collection and a follow-up visit.[54] It may be helpful for the provider to explicitly establish the boundaries for the visit and remind the patient of the time available.[55] ('We have about 15 minutes today, so let's decide together what is most important to accomplish. Then I'll order some tests and we'll have you schedule a follow-up visit. Would that be OK?'). Establishing interest in and concern for the patient does not mean giving unlimited time for the visit. Employing the techniques of reflective listening allows a means for the physician to summarize the information or concerns expressed by the patient or parent and move toward completion of the visit. An additional communication strategy that is helpful both to managing time and assuring that the patient or parent understands what the provider means to communicate is the 'teach back' method.[56] This method consists of asking the patient to repeat *in their own words* what has been decided and what they need to do when they leave the office, and allows the provider to check the understanding of all plans and instructions ('I want to see if I have done a good job of explaining all of this to you. Can you tell me what we decided today, and what you're going to do about your child's asthma this week?').

6. Follow-Up

Providers have limited opportunity to influence patient behavior once they leave the office. However, if strong communication in the office has set the stage for motivating health-promoting behavior, follow-up contact can reinforce this motivation. Follow-up interventions may include return visits to the clinic, telephone calls, and other media-based interventions.

NAEPP guidelines recommend follow-up visits at 2 to 6 weeks after the initiation of controller-medication therapy, and intervals of 1 to 6 month for asthma well-care visits. Because a large number of patients are almost immediately nonadherent following initial controller therapy prescription,[9] investment of efforts to increase adherence at the point of initiation of controller treatment may yield greatest return. Each follow-up visit provides an opportunity for discussion of the family's perceptions and concerns about treatment and, if necessary, re-negotiation of the treatment plan. NAEPP guidelines include recommendations for questions that can be asked at follow-up visits that invite increased communication, provider-patient collaboration, and treatment adherence (Box 42-4).

Other follow-up strategies to increase patient adherence include telephone calls and media-based interventions. Telephone follow-up between clinic appointments is one of the least costly means of maintaining contact with patients and parents, monitoring progress, and reinforcing medication adherence. Telephone follow-up can be made by any member of the clinic staff, can be brief, can query about medication filling and use, and can invite patient or parent questions following a clinic visit. Evidence indicates that such interventions are effective in changing behavior. For example, half of 500 older patients with chronic conditions were randomly assigned to an intervention group that received a telephone call from a pharmacist who inquired about the patient's medication use, medication-related problems, and adherence. Nonadherence in the telephone-intervention group was reduced by 44% relative to the control group.[57] Patients who received bi-monthly telephone calls were more adherent to anti-hypertensive treatment than a no-call control group. Combining telephone calls with letters about their medication improved adherence in adults with asthma.[58] A study of patients with various medical and psychiatric conditions revealed that patients attended more clinic visits with telephone prompting, patient reminder letters, and providing the patient with information about the reason for the appointment.[59] Other technology-based follow-up interventions have begun to appear in the literature and suggest the possibility of additional new, cost-efficient strategies to improve adherence. In a randomized study of a computerized speech recognition program designed to call patients with asthma to inquire about disease control and promote adherence, patients who received the calls were significantly more likely to use their ICS and to have a routine asthma follow-up visit.[60] A similar system has been developed to promote diabetes self-management.[61] Text messaging has been used to support adolescents with asthma[62] and diabetes.[63] Email interventions have been introduced to improve blood pressure treatment adherence,[64] and a variety of web-based interventions have been employed to improve smoking cessation outcomes[65] weight loss,[66] hypertension,[64] and COPD.[67]

Conclusions

A large proportion of patients with asthma take less than half of their prescribed controller medication, and surprisingly, many stop taking their controller medication altogether after an initial filling at their pharmacy. Decreasing use of inhaled corticosteroids has been linked to worsening asthma symptoms and increased risk of hospitalization and death. Many interventions to improve patient adherence have been tested in controlled clinical trials; while some interventions increase adherence, many are complex, costly, time consuming, and nearly impossible to adopt in independent primary care and allergy practices. Nonetheless, four decades of behavioral research and modeling have produced a number of communication strategies that may be used by healthcare providers to effectively change health behavior. From these, six key communication strategies with significant empirical support have been extracted and are presented here. These include: (1) build a relationship, (2) focus on listening, (3) assess patient and parent readiness to change, (4) collaborate on the treatment plan, (5) manage time, and (6) follow up. These communications strategies do not require a large amount of healthcare provider time, can be implemented during routine office visits, and can change patient behavior. Realistically, these strategies will not transform every nonadherent patient into an effective illness self-manager, but employment of these strategies will improve adherence in many families. Furthermore, they can be used to effect change in other health behaviors, such as smoking cessation or weight loss. Finally, beyond behavior change, enhanced communication has been

---

BOX 42-4

Monitoring Patient–Provider Communication and Patient Satisfaction

- 'What questions have you had about your child's asthma daily self-management plan and action plan?'
- 'What problems have you had following the daily self-management plan? The action plan?'
- 'How do you feel about making your own decisions about therapy?'
- 'Has anything prevented you from getting the treatment you need for your asthma from me or anyone else?'
- 'Have the costs of your child's asthma treatment interfered with your ability to get asthma care?'
- 'How satisfied are you with your asthma care?'
- 'How can we improve your asthma care?'

From NAEPP Guidelines for the diagnosis and management of asthma, Expert Panel Report 3, 2007.

repeatedly shown to improve satisfaction in the interaction for both the family and the provider.

References

1. Valenti W. Treatment adherence improves outcomes and manages costs. IDS Read 2001;11:77–80.
2. Baum D, Creer T. Medication compliance in children with asthma. J Asthma 1986;23:49–59.
3. Bender B, Milgrom H, Rand Cea. Psychological factors associated with medication nonadherence in asthmatic children. J Asthma 1998;35:347–53.
4. Urquhart J. Role of patient compliance in clinical pharmacokinetics. Clin Pharmacokinet 1994;27:202–15 clinical.
5. Creer T, Bender B. Psychological Disorders Research and Clinical Applications. Vol Research. Washington DC: American Psychological Association; 1993.
6. Le T, Bilderback A, Bender B, et al. Do asthma medication beliefs mediate the relationship between minority status and adherence to therapy? J Asthma 2008;45:33–7.
7. Walders N, Kopel S, Koinis-Mitchell D, et al. Patterns of quick-relief and long-term controller medication use in pediatric asthma. J Pediatr 2005;146:177–82.
8. Bender B, Rankin A, Tran S, et al. Brief interval telephone surveys of medication adherence and asthma symptoms in the Childhood Asthma Management Program Continuation Study. Ann Allergy Asthma Immunol 2008;101:382–6.
9. Bender B, Pedan A, Varasteh L. Adherence and persistence with fluticasoe propionate/salmeterol combination therapy. J Allergy Clin Immunol 2006;118:899–904.
10. Bender B, Wamboldt F, O'Connor S, et al. Measurement of children's asthma medication adherence by self-report, mother report, canister weight, and Doser CT. Ann Allergy Asthma Immunol 2000;85:416–21.
11. Szefler S, Boushey H, Pearlman D. Time to onset of effect of fluticasone propionate in patients with asthma. Allergy Clin Immunol 1999;103:780–8.
12. Bender B. Psychosocial factors mediating asthma treatment outcomes. London: Martin Dunitz Ltd; 2001.
13. National Heart Lung, and Blood Institute. Expert Panel report 3: guidelines for the diagnosis and management of asthma. Washington, DC: U.S. Department of Health and Human Services; 2007.
14. Suissa S, Ernest P, Benayoun S, et al. Low-dose inhaled corticosteriods and the prevention of death from asthma. N Engl J Med 2000;343:332–6.
15. Milgrom H, Bender B, Ackerson L, et al. Non-compliance and treatment failure in children with asthma. J Allergy Clin Immunol 1996;98:1051–7.
16. Horn C, Clar T, Cochrane G. Compliance with inhaled therapy and morbidity from asthma. Respir Med 1990;84:67–70.
17. Williams KL, Pladevall M, Xi H, et al. Relationship between adherence to inhaled corticosteriods and poor outcomes among adults with asthma. J Allergy Clin Immunol 2004;114:1288–93.
18. Bender B, Milgrom H, Rand C. Nonadherence in asthmatic patients: is there a solution to the problem? Ann Allergy Asthma Immunol 1997;79:177–86.
19. Strunk R. Identification of patients at risk and intervention. J Allergy Clin Immunol 1987;80:472–7.
20. Kahana S, Drotar D, Frazier T. Meta-analysis of psychological interventions to promote adherence to treatment in pediatric chronic health conditions. J Pediatr Psychol 2008;33:590–611.
21. Haynes R, Ackloo E, Sahota N, et al. Interventions for enhancing medication adherence. The Cochrane Collaboration 2008;2:1–19.
22. Van Dulmen S, Sluijs E, Van Dijk L, et al. International expert forum on patient adherence furthering patient adherence: a position paper of the international expert forum on patient adherence based on an internet forum discussion. BMC Health Serv Res 2008 Feb 27;(paper):8–47.
23. Rosenstock I. Why people use health services. Milbank Memorial Fund Quarterly 1966;44:94–124.
24. Becker M. The health belief model and personal health behavior. Health Education Monographs 1974;2:324–473.
25. Conn K, Halterman J, Fisher S, et al. Parental beliefs about medications and medication adherence among urban children with asthma. Ambul Pediatr 2005;5:306–10.
26. DiMatteo M. The role of effective communication with children and their families in fostering adherence to pediatric regimens. Patient Educ Couns 2004;55:339–44.
27. Makoul G. Essential elements of communication in medical encounters: the Kalamazoo Consensus Statement. Paper presented at: Bayer-Fetzer Conference on Physician-Patient Communication in Medical Education, 2001.
28. Hall J, Roter D, Katz N. Meta-analysis of correlates of provider behavior in medical encounters. Med Care 1988;26:657–75.
29. Kinmonth A, Woodcock A, Griffin S, et al. Randomized controlled trial of patient centered care of diabetes in general practice: impact on current well-being and future disease risk. The Diabetes Care From Diagnosis Research Team. Br Med J 1998;317:1202–8.
30. Boulware L, Daumit G, Frick K, et al. An evidence-based review of patient-centered behavioral interventions for hypertension. Am J Prev Med 2001;21:221–32.
31. Ockene I, Hebert J, Ockene J, et al. Effect of physician delivered nutrition counseling training and an office-support program on saturated fat intake, weight, and serum lipid measurements in a hyperlipidemic populations: Worcester Area of Trail for Counseling in Hyperlipidemia (WATCH). Arch Intern Med 1999;159:725–31.
32. Wilson S, Strub P, Buist A, et al. Does involving patients in treatment decisions improve asthma controller medication adherence? Paper presented at: 102nd International Conference of the American Thoracic Society. California: San Diego; 2006.
33. Little P, Everitt H, Williamson I, et al. Preferences of patients for patient centred approach to consultation in primary care: observational study. Br Med J 2001;322:468–72.
34. Stewart M. Effective physician-patient communicaiton and health outcomes: a review. Can Med Assoc 1995;152:1423–32.
35. DiMatteo R, Sherbourne C, Hays R, et al. Physicians' characteristics influence patients' adherence to medical treatment: results form the medical outcomes study. Health Psychol 1993;12:93–102.
36. Woolf S, Kuzel A, Dovey S, et al. A string of mistakes: the importance of cascade analysis in describing, counting, and preventing medical errors. Ann Fam Med 2004;2:317–26.
37. Rosenstock I. Historical Origins of the Health Belief Model. Health Education Monographs 1974;2(4).
38. Bender B, Bender S. Barriers to asthma treatment adherence: responses to interviews, focus groups, and questionnaires. Immunol Allergy Clin North Am 2005;25:107–30.
39. Horne R. Compliance, adherence, and concordance implications of asthma treatment. Chest 2006;130:65S–72S.
40. Miller W, Rollnick S. Motivational interviewing: preparing people to change addictive behavior. New York: Guilford; 1991:191–202.
41. Borrelli B, Riekert K, Weinstein A, et al. Brief motivational interviewing as a clinical strategy to promote asthma medication adherence. J Allergy Clin Immunol 2007;120:1023–30.
42. Irwin R, Richardson N. Patient-focused care: using the right tools. Chest 2006;130:73–82.
43. Bosworth H, Olsen M, Neary Aea. Take control of your blood pressure (TCYB) study: a multifactorial tailored behavioral and educational intervention for achieving blood pressure control. Patient Edu Couns 2008;70:338–47.
44. Wilson S. Does shared treatment decision-making improve asthma adherence and outcomes? Paper presented at: American Thoracic Society. San Diego, CA; 2006.
45. McKinstry B. Do patients wish to be involved in decision making in consultation? A cross sectional survey with video vignettes. Br Med J 2000;321:867–71.
46. Ferketich AK, Khan Y, Wewers ME. Are physicians asking about tobacco use and assisting with cessation? Results from the 2001–2004 national ambulatory medical care survey (NAMCS). Prev Med 2006;43:472–6.
47. Prochaska J, DiClemente C, Norcross J. In search of how people change. Am Psychol 1992;47:1102–4.
48. Guevara J, Wolf F, Grum C, et al. Effects of educational interventions for self management of asthma in children and adolescents. Br Med J 2003;326:1308–9.
49. Schroeder S. We can do better-improving the health of the American people. N Engl J Med 2007;357:1221–8.
50. Ockene J, Ockene I, Quirk Mea. Physician training for patient-centered nutrition counseling in a lipid intervention trial. Ann Behav Med intervention 1995;23:563–70.
51. Pinto B, Lynn H, Marcus B, et al. Physician-based activity counseling: Intervention effects on mediators of motivational readiness for physical activity. Ann Behave Med 2001;23:2–10.
52. Cabana M, Slish K, Evans D, et al. Impact of physician asthma care education on patient outcomes. Pediatrics 2006;117:2149–57.
53. Barry C, Bradley C, Britten N, et al. Patients' unvoiced agendas in general practice consultations: qualitative study. Br Med J 2000;520:1246–50.
54. Smith R. Patient-centered interviewing an evidence-based method. 2nd ed. Lippincott Williams & Wilkins; 2002:35–71.
55. Marvel M, Epstein R, Flowers K, et al. Soliciting the patient's agenda: have we improved? JAMA 1999;281:283–7.
56. Villaire M, Mayer G. Low health literacy: the impact on chronic illness management. Prof Case Manag 2007;12:213–6.
57. Clifford S, Barbara N, Horne R. Understanding different beliefs held by adherers, unintentional nonadherers, and intentional nonadherers:

application of the Necessity-Concerns Framework. J Psychosom Res 2008;64:41–6.

58. Inui T, Yourtee E, Williamson J. Improved outcomes in hypertension after physician tutorials. Ann Intern Med 1976;84:646–51.

59. Roter D, Hall J, Kern D. Improving physicians' interviewing skills and reducing patients' emotional distress: a randomized clinical trail. Arch Intern Med 1995;155:1877–84.

60. Vollmer W, Kirshner M, Peter SD, et al. Use and impact of an automated telephone outreach system for asthma in a managed care setting. Am J Manag Care 2006;12:725–33.

61. Goldman R, Sanchez-Hernandez M, Ross-Degnan D, et al. Developing an automated speech-recognition telephone diabetes intervention. In J Qual Health Care 2008;20:264–70.

62. Neville R, Greene A, McLeod J, et al. Mobile phone text messaging can help young people manage asthma. Br Med J 2002;325:600.

63. Franklin V, Waller A, Pagliari C, et al. A randomized controlled trail of Sweet Talk: a text-messaging system to support young people with diabetes. Diabet Med 2006;23:1332–8.

64. Green B, Ralston J, Fishman P, et al. Electronic communications and home blood pressure monitoring (e-BP) study design delivery, and evaluation. Contem Clin Trials 2008;29:376–95.

65. Stoddard J, Augustson E, Moser R. Effect of adding a virtual community (bulletin board) to smokefree.gov: randomized controlled trial. J Med Internet Res 2008;10:e53 virtual.

66. Brantley P, Appel L, Hollis J, et al. Design considerations and rationale of a multi-center trial to sustain weight loss: the Weight Loss Maintenance Trial. Clin Trials 2007;5:546–56.

67. Borycki E, Kushniruk A. Development of a virtual self-management tool for COPD patients: towards a user needs ontology. AMIA Annu Symp Proc 2007Oct 11;879.

New Directions in Asthma Management

Stanley J. Szefler

Recent statistics indicate that the concerted effort to halt the trend of increasing asthma mortality and morbidity has been successful because both of those areas have reached a plateau and show some indication of decline in recent years.[1] A strategy to establish a further decline in morbidity and mortality would be to recognize patients at risk for persistent asthma or asthma exacerbations and to intervene early. This review will highlight new information available on asthma pathogenesis and treatment that will help shape a new direction in managing childhood asthma.

At this time, asthma is characterized as a chronic inflammatory disease. Inhaled glucocorticoids, the most potent antiinflammatory asthma medications, have emerged as the cornerstone for the management of persistent asthma. Since the early 1980s substantial gains have been made in understanding the pathogenesis of asthma.[2] This effort has resulted in the introduction of new medications and delivery systems, as well as new initiatives to improve medication labeling for young children to facilitate early intervention. Consequently, new opportunities have emerged to improve the overall management of childhood asthma.

New directions include recognizing asthma in its early stages and taking steps to intervene earlier with environmental control and long-term control therapy. This movement will continue to lead to better methods to diagnose asthma and a critical analysis of the role of early intervention in altering the natural history of asthma. Although inhaled glucocorticoid therapy has played a major role in stabilizing the rise in asthma morbidity and mortality, there is still much to learn regarding its efficacy in preventing progression of asthma and thus altering the natural history of the disease.[3]

This review will begin by briefly summarizing the recommended principles of asthma management as a stepping stone to discussing methods that could strengthen the areas of weakness. To advance to a level where we can speak of a 'cure' for asthma, we must be able to take a proactive approach and recognize the disease early and intervene appropriately (Box 43-1).

Phase of Rapid Evolution

Principles of inhaled glucocorticoid therapy dosing emerged in the late 1970s along with clear evidence of efficacy in the management of asthma for both adults and children.[4] In the mid-1990s several important new classes of medications became available. Long-acting β_2-adrenergic agonists, salmeterol and formoterol, with a 12-hour duration of action, were introduced. To limit the adverse effects of short-acting β agonists, the stereoisomer of albuterol, levalbuterol, was developed. In addition, the class of leukotriene modifiers was added.

One of the oral leukotriene antagonists, montelukast, has emerged as a popular first-line long-term control therapy in children with asthma because of the availability of dosage guidelines and the demonstration of its safety in children as young as 1 year of age. In addition, renewed interest has developed for the combination of medications in one formulation, such as an inhaled steroid and a long-acting β-adrenergic agonist, based on evidence of additive effects, convenience for the patient, and the potential to further reduce the risk for significant exacerbations.[5] For severe asthma, omalizumab or antiimmunoglobulin E (anti-IgE) was approved for use in children 12 years and older. With the availability of numerous choices for medication selection, it is important to organize the approach to a treatment plan.

Current Management of Childhood Asthma

Current guidelines emphasize environmental control, objective monitoring, cooperative management, and a step-wise approach to pharmacotherapy as the core elements of asthma management. Asthma is now classified as *intermittent, mild persistent, moderate persistent,* and *severe persistent* based on symptoms, nighttime episodes, and pulmonary function. However, the most recent guidelines now focus on asthma control and have consisted of updated versions of the Global Initiative for Asthma and the National Heart, Lung, and Blood Institute (NHLBI) Guidelines for the Diagnosis and Management of Asthma.[6–8]

The updated National Asthma Education and Prevention Program (NAEPP) guidelines include an attempt to focus on the concept of asthma control and continue to address the needs of childhood asthma with evidence-based reviews.[8] The evidence for various steps in asthma management for children less than 5 years of age has been weak, primarily due to the relative paucity of studies in this age group as compared to older children and adults. To date, many assumptions continue to be based on adult studies and ultimately relegated to expert opinion. Studies are in progress to fill gaps in information as investigators and the pharmaceutical industry realize the need for improved dosing guidelines as well as new medications for this age group.

The updated version of the NAEPP guidelines still places inhaled glucocorticoids as the cornerstone of long-term control therapy in both children and adults.[8] The preferred additive therapy for inadequate control with a low dose of inhaled glucocorticoid is a long-acting β_2-adrenergic agonist although some would argue that the more appropriate step to take, especially

©2010 Elsevier Ltd, Inc, BV

DOI: 10.1016/B978-1-4377-0271-2.00043-2

in children, is to increase the dose of inhaled glucocorticoid monotherapy. Leukotriene antagonists are considered alternative first-line therapy and alternative supplementary long-term control therapy once inhaled glucocorticoids have been initiated. Two major areas that require ongoing research include the appropriate time to initiate long-term control therapy and the management of severe persistent asthma in children. Currently, several medications are now labeled for use in young children, specifically nebulized budesonide and montelukast for children as young as 1 year of age. There is a need for an easily administered, long-acting β_2-adrenergic agonist with specific labeling for use in children under 5 years of age.

Special Problems for Managing Asthma in Young Children

Current therapy is based on the belief that chronic inflammation is a major feature of asthma. Because persistent asthma can occur early in life, attention continues to move toward early recognition and early intervention. It was assumed that early treatment with inhaled glucocorticoid therapy could modify the disease process and the natural history of asthma, however, a recent prospective study indicated that inhaled glucocorticoids effectively control emerging asthma but do not alter the natural course of the disease.[9]

Although the approach to asthma control in young children is similar to that in older children and adults, there are limitations to the evaluation of asthma in young children. Assessment is primarily based on symptoms because pulmonary function cannot be measured reliably in young children. Environmental control measures can be applied if allergen sensitivity is defined and exposure confirmed. In addition, limiting exposure to viral respiratory infections could also reduce the frequency of significant acute exacerbations but this is difficult to achieve in daycare settings and schools. Pharmacotherapy can also be a challenge because the route of administration for inhaled medication administration must be adjusted to patient cooperation. First-line therapy may begin with low-dose inhaled glucocorticoid via nebulizer or a spacer/holding chamber and facemask.[8]

Current global guidelines and recent revisions to the US guidelines recommend an inhaled glucocorticoid by spacer/facemask or nebulized administration as first-line therapy in young children with persistent asthma. Comparative studies are needed to determine whether the inhaled glucocorticoid by metered-dose inhaler with spacer/facemask or nebulized administration is the preferred route of administration. In the USA, no inhaled glucocorticoid in the dry powder or metered-dose inhaler formulation is approved for use in children younger than 4 years of age. Because it is not feasible to administer a dry powder formulation to young children based on the necessary inspiratory flow rate, it will be important to evaluate the new hydrofluoroalkane preparations for use in young children.

For moderate persistent asthma, it is now recommended that a medium dose of inhaled glucocorticoid be administered or that a long-acting β-adrenergic agonist be added if low-dose inhaled glucocorticoid therapy is inadeqaute.[8] The latter recommendation is primarily based on conclusions derived from adult studies. A recently published study in the NIH/NHLBI Childhood Asthma Research and Education (CARE) Network addressed this specific question regarding comparative effectiveness of medium-dose inhaled glucocorticoid, or low-dose inhaled glucocorticoid combined with either long-acting β_2-adrenergic agonist (LABA) or leukotriene receptor antagonist (LTRA).[10] This study reported that nearly all children had a differential response to each of the three step-up treatments. LABA step-up therapy, when added to low-dose inhaled corticosteroid (ICS), was significantly more likely to provide the best response than either 2.5 times the dose of ICS or LTRA added to low-dose ICS. However, it was also observed that many children had a best response to ICS or LTRA step-up treatment options. This observation highlights the need to regularly monitor asthma therapy and perhaps consider another option within Step 3 treatment before advancing to Step 3 therapy. Unfortunately, there is no LABA approved for use in children younger than 5 years of age. It would be useful to evaluate the combination of budesonide and formoterol now currently available in metered-dose inhaler formulation for younger children or to develop a nebulized form of combination inhaled glucocorticoid and LABA for use in younger children.

Alternatively, an LTRA could be added to an inhaled glucocorticoid. For more severe asthma, high-dose inhaled glucocorticoids are recommended, and if needed, systemic glucocorticoid with adjustment to the lowest dose, either daily or on alternate days sufficient to stabilize symptoms, should be used. This step-care algorithm will continue to be refined as more information is obtained on the efficacy of the available approved medications for young children.

New Insights

Several studies provide important insight for the management of persistent asthma. These studies solidify the role of inhaled glucocorticoids as first-line therapy in the management of persistent asthma and also point to some limitations in the efficacy of inhaled glucocorticoids. These concepts should now be considered in the individualized management of asthma. It is also important that new treatment strategies address the limitations of inhaled glucocorticoids in altering the natural history of asthma and reversing pulmonary function in long-standing, poorly controlled asthma.

Outcomes Following Long-Term Inhaled Glucocorticoid Administration

The series of publications from the Childhood Asthma Management Program (CAMP) Research Group provide many new

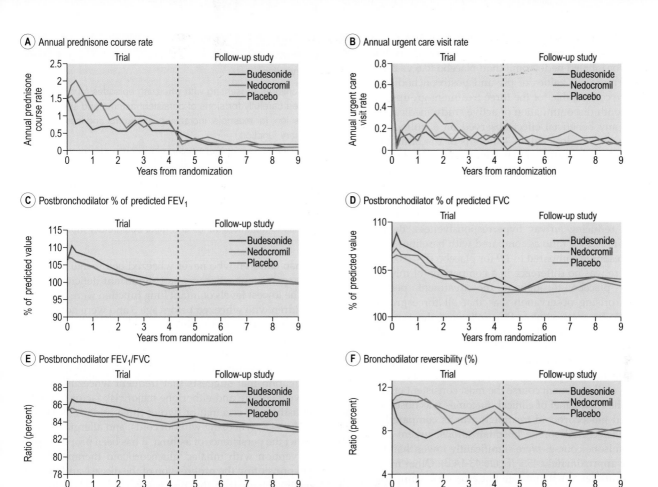

Figure 43-1 Mean values for measures of morbidity, lung function after the use of a bronchodilator, and bronchodilator reversibility during 9 years of follow-up after randomization to the budesonide, nedocromil, and placebo groups: **(A)** annual prednisone course rate; **(B)** annual urgent care visit rate; **(C)** postbronchodilator FEV_1 % of predicted; **(D)** postbronchodilator FVC % of predicted; **(E)** postbronchodilator FEV_1/FVC; **(F)** bronchodilator reversibility. All data to the left of the vertical line on each graph were obtained during the trial when participants were treated regularly with budesonide 200 µg *bid*, nedocromil 4 mg *bid*, or placebo. All data to the right of the vertical line on each graph were obtained during the post-trial follow-up period after regular treatment with study medications was discontinued. (From Strunk RC, Sternberg AL, Szefler SJ, et al. J Pediatr 2009;154:682–687.)

insights into the efficacy of long-term control therapy.[11–15] The major outcome reports, in particular, generate a number of questions to be considered in future studies.[14,15] This trial was initiated in 1991 in order to evaluate whether continuous long-term treatment with either an inhaled glucocorticoid (budesonide) or an inhaled nonsteroid (nedocromil) control medication could improve lung growth safely over a 4- to 6-year treatment period compared to treatment based on the frequency and severity of symptoms (albuterol as needed). In 1999, treatment was discontinued and participants continue to be followed in this study. The outcomes following the first 5 years of discontinued therapy were recently published (Figure 43-1).[15]

Postbronchodilator FEV_1% predicted was selected as the primary outcome and the parameter to assess lung growth because it is a measure of maximal lung capacity. This technique minimizes the effects of factors that influence airway constriction and has less variability over time than the prebronchodilator measurements applied in previous studies. The results of the CAMP trial showed that budesonide treatment improved postbronchodilator FEV_1% predicted from a mean 103.2% predicted to 106.8% predicted within 2 months, but this measurement gradually diminished to 103.8% predicted by the end of the treatment period (Figure 43-1D).[14,15] At the end of the treatment period and during follow-up after discontinuation of treatment, the postbronchodilator FEV_1% predicted in the budesonide group was not significantly different from that in the placebo group.

The nedocromil group was similar to the placebo group in this measure throughout the study period and follow-up.

The finding that neither budesonide nor nedocromil improved lung function, as measured by the percent predicted value for FEV_1 after the administration of a bronchodilator, was not expected. However, previous studies did not examine postbronchodilator FEV_1 measurements. In fact, there are few studies in childhood asthma that utilized postbronchodilator FEV_1 as an outcome measure. Because a decline in FEV_1% predicted has been interpreted as an indication of airway remodeling, the CAMP study results raised questions about whether airway remodeling is occurring in this population of mild to moderate persistent asthma and whether inhaled glucocorticoids have any effect on preventing this change in airway pathology. The CAMP results indicate that FEV_1% predicted did not decline in either the placebo group or the inhaled nedocromil group. Furthermore, the temporary increase in postbronchodilator FEV_1% predicted after initiating treatment was not sustained over the treatment period and was comparable to the placebo group at the end of the study. It was subsequently observed that a subset of the CAMP population, approximately 25%, were susceptible to a loss of pulmonary function (as defined by postbronchodilator % predicted) over time and likely due to airway remodeling despite ongoing inhaled glucocorticoid therapy.[16]

For inhaled nedocromil the only difference in pre- and postbronchodilator spirometry as compared with placebo was observed with prebronchodilator FEV$_1$ (liters). The end result indicated the difference at the end of treatment from the baseline value was less for inhaled nedocromil than placebo (0.6 vs 2.4, P = 0.02). Furthermore, all values of pre-and postbronchodilator spirometry were comparable for the three treatment groups following the 4-month discontinuation of active study medication, indicating that any beneficial effect observed on a pulmonary function parameter was lost within 4 months of discontinuing treatment. This is an important observation because it suggests that inhaled glucocorticoids do not have a sustaining effect on the natural history of asthma.

The most distinct effect observed on a measure of pulmonary function was the significant and consistent effect of inhaled budesonide on reducing airway hyperresponsiveness. By the end of treatment the PC$_{20}$ ratio as compared with baseline was 3 for inhaled budesonide compared to 1.9 for placebo (P < 0.001).[14] Once again, there was no difference in a comparison of inhaled nedocromil to placebo throughout the treatment period. However, a surprising observation was that all three groups were comparable for methacholine PC$_{20}$ following the 4-month washout phase and 5-year follow-up.[14,15] Therefore, this additional surrogate marker of airway remodeling is not permanently affected by inhaled glucocorticoid therapy as compared to the other two treatment options.

During the overall treatment course the most consistent effects on changes in the total panel of clinical outcomes was observed with the inhaled glucocorticoid treatment arm as compared to placebo. For inhaled budesonide hospitalizations, urgent care visits, and prednisone courses were significantly lower than the placebo arm by approximately 45% (Figure 43-1A,B). Other measures showing a difference with inhaled budesonide as compared with placebo included lower symptom score, higher number of episode-free days per month, and less albuterol inhalations per week. Treatment with inhaled nedocromil demonstrated effects only on reduction of urgent care visits and prednisone courses as compared to placebo.

The CAMP results challenged conclusions that have been derived in short-term studies, especially those related to pulmonary function and body development measures. The study alleviated growing concerns regarding the long-term effect of inhaled glucocorticoid therapy on body development by showing that the only detectable adverse effect was a transient reduction in growth velocity limited to 1 cm in the first year of treatment. This effect on growth has been persistent but did not progress.[14,15]

It is also clear that the medications used in CAMP did not completely eliminate the morbidity associated with asthma, and there is certainly room for improvement. The rich CAMP database continues to be evaluated as the ongoing CAMP Continuation Studies progress, now 18 years after the start of the study. This cohort study enables follow-up for an additional 14 years for those who were managed intensively for the 4- to 6-year treatment phase. The CAMP Continuation Studies are specifically designed to evaluate the long-term effects of long-term treatment on lung development and growth. The CAMP subjects are currently being followed into late adolescence and early adulthood in an attempt to define maximal lung and body growth parameters.

Early Recognition and Intervention

Reports from the Tucson Children's Respiratory Study show that children who wheezed during lower respiratory tract illnesses in the first 3 years of life and were still wheezing at age 6 ('persistent wheezers') had slightly but not significantly lower levels of lung

function than children who never wheezed before age 6. By age 6, however, persistent wheezers had significant deficits in lung function. The lowest levels of infant lung function were observed among children who wheezed before age 3 and were not current wheezers at age 6 ('transient wheezers').[17-19]

Information was derived on the risk factors for persistent asthma based on the natural history observed in this series of participants.[20] An Asthma Predictive Index was established from this investigation that suggests that frequent wheezing during the first 3 years of life and either one major risk factor (parental history of asthma or eczema) or two of three minor risk factors (eosinophilia >4%, wheezing without colds, and allergic rhinitis) could predict the persistence of asthma. It has been proposed that early intervention with inhaled glucocorticoid therapy can be effective in preventing the progression of the disease and the risk for irreversible changes in the airways that could contribute to the persistence of symptoms (Box 43-2).

In addition, long-term follow-up in the Tucson Children's Respiratory Study showed that patterns of wheezing prevalence and levels of lung function were established by age 6 years and did not appear to change significantly by age 16 years in children who started having asthma-like symptoms during the preschool years.[19] A recently published study by Guilbert and colleagues[9] from the NHLBI Childhood Asthma Research and Education (CARE) Network examined the effect of early intervention on altering the course of asthma. The Asthma Predictive Index was used in this study to identify infants at risk for developing asthma. Inhaled glucocorticoid or placebo was then initiated and continued for a 2-year treatment period. In the third year, study treatment was discontinued. Although inhaled glucocorticoid had a significant impact on improving asthma control during the treatment period as compared to placebo, this effect was rapidly lost after discontinuing inhaled glucocorticoid therapy. Therefore, it was concluded that inhaled glucocorticoids do not alter the natural course of asthma. It will be important to define therapeutic interventions that are effective in altering the natural history of asthma in order to advance treatment for this age group.

Variable Response to Inhaled Glucocorticoid Therapy

A study conducted by the NHLBI Asthma Clinical Research Network described the significant variability in response to inhaled glucocorticoids in adults with persistent asthma and reduced pulmonary function.[21] This study examined 30 adult subjects with persistent asthma with FEV$_1$ between 55% and 85% predicted and reported the effect of increasing doses of inhaled glucocorticoids. Multiple parameters of response were examined.

This study reported several key observations. First, near maximal FEV_1 and methacholine PC_{20} effects occurred with low-medium dose for both inhaled glucocorticoids used in this study, namely inhaled fluticasone propionate and inhaled beclomethasone dipropionate administered via metered-dose inhaler with a spacer device. High-dose inhaled glucocorticoid therapy did not significantly increase the efficacy measures that were evaluated, but increased the systemic effect measure of overnight plasma cortisol. Second, significant intersubject variability in response occurred with both inhaled glucocorticoids. The investigators cautioned that perhaps higher doses of inhaled glucocorticoids may be necessary to manage more severe patients or to achieve goals of therapy not evaluated in this study, such as prevention of significant asthma exacerbations.

Of interest, approximately one third of the subjects had a good response (>15%) as determined by improvement in FEV_1 over the baseline, whereas another third had a marginal response (5% to 15%) and the final third failed to respond (>5%). The same pattern was observed with methacholine PC_{20} improvement. The FEV_1 improvement did not correlate to the PC_{20} improvement in this group of subjects. However, certain biomarkers, such as exhaled nitric oxide (eNO) and sputum eosinophils, and asthma characteristics, such as duration of asthma and bronchodilator response, were associated with the two response parameters.[21] The NHLBI Asthma Clinical Research Network conducted an additional study to confirm the variability in response to inhaled glucocorticoids and to determine if any of the previously defined biomarkers could predict response to treatment. Of interest, the variability in response to inhaled glucocrticoids was confirmed, but only albuterol pulmonary function response and low FEV_1/FVC but not eNO was a predictor of pulmonary response to inhaled glucocorticoid.[22]

As previously indicated, the preferred long-term controller for the management of persistent asthma in all age groups including children is inhaled glucocorticoids. However, many parents and physicians are still concerned regarding potential adverse effects of inhaled glucocorticoids. Therefore, the NHLBI CARE Network conducted studies to examine the variability of response to ICS and LTRA in children. Using pulmonary function as an indicator of response, this study concluded that children with low pulmonary function or high levels of markers associated with allergic inflammation, including elevated eNO, should receive ICS therapy instead of a LTRA.[23]

A follow-up report using another marker of response, asthma control days (ACD), concluded that eNO as a predictor of response, might help to identify individual children not receiving controller medication who achieve a greater improvement in ACD with an ICS compared to a LTRA.[24]

The observations in children were confirmed by a subsequent prospective study in children with mild to moderate asthma to examine the effect of ICS, LTRA, and combination ICS and LABA on ACD, pulmonary function and exacerbations.[25] In a secondary analysis of the findings from this study, Knuffman and colleagues[26] reported that a parental history of asthma, increased eNO levels, low methacholine PC_{20} values, or a history of ICS use is associated with the best long-term outcomes with ICS therapy as compared with treatment with LTRA. These observations help pave the way for using biomarkers and asthma characteristics as predictors of response to long-term controller therapy.

Difficult-to-Control Asthma

Unfortunately, there has been only limited activity in the area of understanding and managing severe persistent asthma in chil-

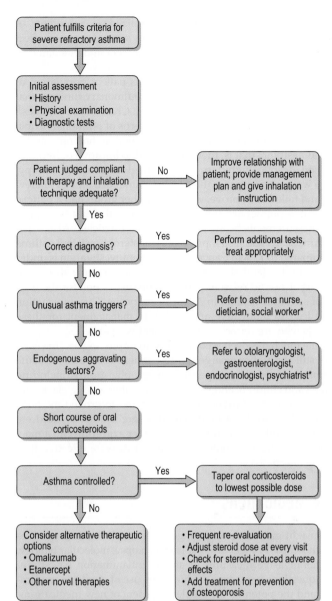

*If asthma remains uncontrolled, continue left column of algorithm

Figure 43-2 Algorithm for the approach to asthma management. (Modified from van Veen IH, Bel EH. The difficult-to-treat asthma patient. In: Castro M, Kraft M, eds. Clinical asthma. St. Louis: Mosby; 2008:323–331.)

dren. A review by van Veen and Bel[27] provides a summary of the current understanding of this concerning patient population. van Veen and Bel[27] developed an algorithmic approach to the evaluation and management of patients with difficult-to-control asthma (Figure 43-2). Once the features of diagnosis, behavior, and environmental control are addressed, the remaining issues center around appropriate medication use. Considerations must be given to the appropriate combination of bronchodilator and anti-inflammatory therapy along with decisions about dose, delivery device for inhaled medications, and timing of treatment before considering alternative therapeutic options.

Nevertheless, a report by Sont and colleagues[28] indicates that a treatment approach for the use of inhaled glucocorticoids that is guided by measures of airway hyperresponsiveness leads to better overall asthma control, as indicated by improved pulmonary function and reduced symptoms. The additional benefit could also be a reduction in airway collagen deposition. While induced sputum eosinophils[29] have proven useful as a guide to reduce asthma exacerbations when utilized as a monitor of inflammation, eNO has not shown the same degree of effect when added to guidelines-based management and evaluated in adolescents and young adults from the inner city.[30]

Another interesting observation in this patient population of severe asthma is the variable pattern of pulmonary function that can persist despite optimal management. Chan and colleagues[31] found that there were basically two patterns of pulmonary function in the population of patients classified as having steroid-resistant asthma, that is, those who failed to improve pulmonary function despite high-dose daily oral glucocorticoid therapy. There was one group of patients who maintained an FEV$_1$ below 70% and failed to improve, whereas another group had a pattern of variable pulmonary function throughout the day with periodic measurements below an FEV$_1$ of 70% predicted. Also, African-Americans had a 38% prevalence of steroid-resistant asthma as compared to 12% in Caucasians. Further investigation is under way to understand the underlying mechanisms for these two patterns of steroid resistance and the predisposition for the high rate of steroid resistance in African-Americans. This information could lead to innovative approaches to management for these patients who are refractory to treatment with steroids.

While much has been accomplished in improving asthma care, there still are higher emergency department visit rates for acute asthma observed among specific demographic groups, including women and children, and widening disparities among black subjects, that calls for further investigation and improved methods of care.[32] In a study of moderate to severe asthma in children, Strunk and colleagues[33] found that neither azithromycin, a macrolide antibiotic, or montelukast, an LTRA, were effective ICS-sparing alternatives.

New Medications

The insight gained through ongoing research that incorporates bronchoscopy, bronchoalveolar lavage, biopsy, molecular biology, and noninvasive measures of airway inflammation has stimulated questions regarding the judicious use of available medications and the potential for the development of new medications. Identification of predominant mediators associated with airway inflammation, especially those associated with allergic inflammation, such as interleukin (IL)-4, IL-5, IL-13 and interferon gamma, have resulted in the development of pharmaceutical agents to counteract the activity of these pathways of inflammation. To date, these approaches have provided only limited success but there are other strategies being considered.[34-38]

Although most of the early attempts at selective therapy have been disappointing, continuous assessment regarding the trial design is needed to link the treatment with the population most likely to see a benefit.

Pharmacogenetics

A new area of genetics has emerged, namely pharmacogenetics, that is designed to understand the relationship of genetics to medication response. It is becoming increasingly important to define risk factors for patients who are likely to develop persistent asthma, patients predisposed to severe life-threatening exacerbations, patients with severe persistent asthma requiring extensive therapy, and patients with steroid insensitive asthma. Advances in genetic associations could help define relevant asthma phenotypes associated with response to medications and pave the way for individualized treatment approaches based on

the identification of an asthma phenotype. The response to these medications could be related to genetic polymorphisms altering the site of action such as the drug receptor, or the availability of the drug at the site of action such as in relation to cytochrome P$_{450}$-dependent metabolic pathways.

Knowledge regarding genetics and the resultant complex disease of asthma continues to develop with information related to the effect of the environment on gene environment interactions, the contribution of TH$_2$ immunity gene variants to allergic inflammation, and the role of filaggrin mutations in atopic dermatitis.[39-41] To date, six genes have been identified by means of positional cloning as linking with asthma: *ADAM33, GRPA, PHF11, DPP1V, HLA-G,* and *CYF1P2*.[40] However, application of this information to clinical practice awaits confirmation through validation and replication studies.

In addition, genetic association of acidic mammalian chitinase, CHIA, with atopic asthma and serum total IgE levels in an Indian population;[42] increased susceptibility to asthma and poor asthma control in children and young adults with genetic variation at a locus controlling ORMDL3 expression;[43] increased serum tissue growth factor (TGF)β1 levels and airflow obstruction with C-509T polymorphism;[44] and functional relevant toll-like receptor (TLR)1 and TLR6 and a potential protective role in childhood asthma have been reported.[45] Also, Hunninghake and colleagues[46] observed that dust mite allergen levels modified the effect of IL10 SNPs on allergy and asthma exacerbations and Weidinger and colleagues[47] observed that filaggrin (FLG) mutations affect the development of eczema and confer significant risks of asthma in the context of eczema. Bouzigon and colleagues[48] reported an increased risk of asthma associated with 17q21 genetic variants related to early-onset asthma with increased risk through early-life exposure to environmental tobacco smoke.

Therefore the benefit of a medication could be tied to an active disease pathway influenced by a specific drug, for example, leukotriene synthesis and leukotriene antagonists as well as cytokine synthesis and an alteration of the glucocorticoid receptor. Failure to respond to treatment could be caused by excessive activity of this pathway or possibly alternative pathways involved in the disease. This area is in its infancy but holds promising opportunities for understanding the variability in response to treatment as well as insights into developing individualized treatment programs.

Conclusions

We now have answers to many questions regarding the effect of various long-term control treatment options available for managing childhood asthma through the studies conducted in the NIH asthma networks and other centers. It is possible that early indicators of asthma, such as increased symptoms or altered lung growth in children could prompt early intervention. With the right intervention it is feasible to control the disease in most children and thus, in a sense, a remission or relative 'cure' is achieved. Current interest regarding early pharmacologic intervention options centers around the comparative effects of ICS monotherapy and combination therapy with ICS and LABA or LTRA; however, none of these treatment options appear to be sufficient to control asthma progression (Box 43-3; see Box 43-2).

On the other extreme, patients with severe asthma have low and irreversible pulmonary function. Their disease often has its onset in early childhood. Does this information suggest that children who manifest low pulmonary function and persistent symptoms in the presence of antiinflammatory therapy are at increased risk for further disease progression? If so, it will be

BOX 43-3 Therapeutic principles

Persistent Asthma

- Establish follow-up after an initial wheezing episode.

- With each wheezing episode, assess risk criteria for persistent asthma.

- If the patient demonstrates frequent wheezing episodes and fits the high-risk profile, assess for allergen sensitivity and exposure.

- If environmental control is inadequate, begin intervention with low-dose inhaled glucocorticoids.

- Follow response by assessing both clinical control and pulmonary function.

- Increase dose of inhaled glucocorticoids or add long-acting β_2-adrenergic agonist if asthma control is inadequate or pulmonary function is compromised.

- Titrate therapy after control is established and pulmonary function maximized.

- If asthma control is established, consider stepping down therapy, but not prior to a known period of increased risk for an asthma exacerbation, such as the fall season.

important to recognize these patients and provide more effective interventions at critical stages of their disease progression. Furthermore, it would then be important to measure persistent inflammation and use this as another gauge to adjust therapy.

Once persistent asthma is established, it may be necessary to measure the response to treatment by evaluating the individual parameters of response, for example, symptoms, pulmonary function, and progression. Recent studies have clearly demonstrated that certain patients may respond to conventional treatment, such as inhaled glucocorticoids, in one category, for example, improvement in FEV_1, but not another, such as reduction in airways hyperresponsiveness.[21] Recognizing this deficiency in selective responses could prompt direction of treatment to improving individual response categories.

This review has concentrated on the current understanding of the therapeutic intervention and the possibilities it provides for improving asthma management and potentially inducing a remission or cure for the disease. However, none of this is possible without an integrated approach to patient care. There are serious deficiencies in the healthcare system that influence access to healthcare. The recent observation of an actual decline in asthma mortality and morbidity is encouraging but could be deceiving since it is not true for all racial/ethnic groups. Concerted efforts are now being directed toward understanding this phenomenon and recommendations have been made to integrate the various national resources available to improve outcomes of asthma care for children in the USA. Perhaps the application of electronic medical records and additional methods of surveying disease management will prompt improvements in medical care.

References

1. Moorman JE, Rudd RA, Johnson CA, et al. National surveillance for asthma—United States, 1980–2004. MMWR 2007;56:1–54.

2. Hamid QA, Minshall EM. Molecular pathology of allergic disease. I. Lower airway disease. J Allergy Clin Immunol 2000;105:20–36.

3. Suissa S, Ernst P. Inhaled corticosteroids: impact on asthma morbidity and mortality. J Allergy Clin Immunol 2001;107:937–44.

4. Spahn JD, Szefler SJ. Inhaled glucocorticoids from combination therapy for asthma and COPD. In: Martin RJ, Kraft M, editors. Lung biology in health and diseases series. New York: Marcel Dekker; 2000.

5. Matz J, Emmett A, Rickard K, et al. Addition of salmeterol to low-dose fluticasone versus higher-dose fluticasone: an analysis of asthma exacerbations. J Allergy Clin Immunol 2001;107:783–9.

6. Global Initiative for Asthma. Global strategy for asthma management and prevention. Available from www.ginasthma.com; 2008 [Accessed 05.09].

7. Expert Panel Report 3 (EPR-3). Guidelines for the Diagnosis and Management of Asthma – Summary Report 2007. J Allergy Clin Immunol 2007;120:S94–138.

8. National Institutes of Health. National Heart, Lung, and Blood Institute. National Asthma Education and Prevention Program. Expert Panel Report 3: Guidelines for the Diagnosis and Management of Asthma. August 2007. NIH Publication No. 07–4051, http://www.nhlbi.nih.gov/guidelines/asthma/index.htm.

9. Guilbert TW, Morgan WJ, Zeiger RS, et al. Two year inhaled corticosteroid treatment on subsequent asthma in high-risk toddlers. N Engl J Med 2006;354:1985–97.

10. Lemanske RF Jr, Mauger DT, Sorkness CA, et al. Step-up therapy for children with uncontrolled asthma while receiving inhaled corticosteroids. N Engl J Med 2010;362 (published online March 2, 2010 as article (10.1056/NEJMoal001278) at www.nejm.org.

11. Zeiger RS, Dawson C, Weiss S. Relationships between duration of asthma and asthma severity among children in the Childhood Asthma Management Program (CAMP). J Allergy Clin Immunol 1999;103:376–87.

12. Nelson HS, Szefler SJ, Jacobs J, et al. The relationships among environmental allergen sensitization, allergen exposure, pulmonary function, and bronchial hyperresponsiveness in the Childhood Asthma Management Program. J Allergy Clin Immunol 1999;104:775–85.

13. Bender BG, Annett RD, Ikle D, et al. Relationship between disease and psychological adaptation in children in the Childhood Asthma Management Program and their families: CAMP Research Group. Arch Pediatr Adolesc Med 2000;154:706–13.

14. The Childhood Asthma Management Program Research Group. Long-term effects of budesonide or nedocromil in children with asthma. N Engl J Med 2000;343:1054–63.

15. Strunk RC, Sternberg AL, Szefler SJ, et al. Long-term budesonide or nedocromil treatment, once discontinued, does not alter the course of mild to moderate asthma in children and adolescents. J Pediatr 2009;154:682–7.

16. Covar RA, Spahn JD, Murphy JR, et al. Progression of asthma measured by lung function in the Childhood Asthma Management Program. Am J Respir Crit Care Med 2004;170:235–41.

17. Martinez FD, Wright AL, Taussig LM, et al. Asthma and wheezing in the first six years of life. N Engl J Med 1995;332:133–8.

18. Martinez FD. Development of wheezing disorders and asthma in preschool children. Pediatrics 2002;109:362–7.

19. Morgan WJ, Stern DA, Sherrill DL, et al. Outcome of asthma and wheezing in the first 6 years of life. Am J Respir Crit Care Med 2005;172:121258.

20. Castro-Rodriguez JA, Holberg CJ, Wright AL, et al. A clinical index to define risk of asthma in young children with recurrent wheezing. Am J Respir Crit Care Med 2000;162:1403–6.

21. Szefler SJ, Martin RJ, King TS, et al. for the Asthma Clinical Research Network of the National Heart, Lung, and Blood Institute. Significant variability in response to inhaled corticosteroids for persistent asthma. J Allergy Clin Immunol 2002;109:410–8.

22. Martin RJ, Szefler SJ, King TS, et al. The Predicting Response to Inhaled Corticosteroid Efficacy (PRICE) trial. J Allergy Clin Immunol 2007;119:73–80.

23. Szefler SJ, Phillips BR, Martinez FD, et al. Characterization of within-subject responses to fluticasone and montelukast in childhood asthma. J Allergy Clin Immunol 2005;115:233–42.

24. Zeiger RS, Szefler SJ, Phillips BR, et al. Response profiles to fluticasone and montelukast in mild-to-moderate persistent childhood asthma. J Allergy Clin Immunol 2006;117:45–52.

25. Sorkness CA, Lemanske RF, Mauger DT, et al. Long-term comparison of 3 controller regimens for mild-moderate persistent childhood asthma: The Pediatric Asthma Controller Trial. J Allergy Clin Immunology 2007;119:64–72.

26. Knuffman JE, Sorkness CA, Lemanske RF, et al. Phenotypic predictors of long-term response to inhaled corticosteroid and leukotriene modifier therapies in pediatric asthma. J Allergy Clin Immunology 2009;123:411–6.

27. van Veen IH, Bel EH. The difficult-to-treat asthma patient. In: Castro M, Kraft M, editors. Clinical asthma. St. Louis: Mosby; 2008. p. 323–31.

28. Sont JK, Willems LNA, Bel EH, et al. and the AMPUL Study Group. Clinical control and histopathologic outcome of asthma when using airway hyperresponsiveness as an additional guide to long-term treatment. Am J Respir Crit Care Med 1999;159:1043–51.

29. Green RH, Brightling CE, McKenna S, et al. Asthma exacerbations and sputum eosinophil counts: a randomized controlled trial. Lancet 2002;360:1715–21.

30. Szefler SJ, Mitchell H, Sorkness CA, et al. Adding exhaled nitric oxide to guideline-based asthma treatment in inner-city adolescents and young adults: a randomized controlled trial. Lancet 2008;372:1065–72.

31. Chan MT, Leung DYM, Szefler SJ, et al. Difficult-to-control asthma: clinical characteristics of steroid-insensitive asthma. J Allergy Clin Immunol 1998;101:594–601.

32. Ginde AA, Espinola JA, Camargo CA. Improved overall trends but persistent racial disparities in emergency department visits for acute asthma, 1993–2005. J Allergy Clin Immunol 2008;122:313–8.

33. Strunk RC, Bacharier LB, Phillips BR, et al. Azithromycin or montelukast as inhaled corticosteroid-sparing agents in moderate to severe childhood asthma study. J Allergy Clin Immunology 2008;122:1138–44.

34. Adcock IM, Caramori G, Chung KF. New targets for drug development in asthma. Lancet 2008;372:1073–87.

35. Casale TB, Stokes JR. Immunomodulators for allergic respiratory disorders. J Allergy Clin Immunol 2008;121:288–96.

36. Cousins DJ, McDonald J, Lee TH. Therapeutic approaches for control of transcription factors in allergic disease. J Allergy Clin Immunol 2008;121:803–9.

37. Bhavsar P, Ahmad T, Adcock IM. The role of histone deacetylases in asthma and allergic diseases. J Allergy Clin Immunol 2008;121:580–4.

38. Chatila TA, Li N, Garcia-Lloret M, et al. T cell effector pathways in allergic diseases: transcriptional mechanisms and therapeutic targets. J Allergy Clin Immunol 2008;121:812–23.

39. Holloway JW, Yang IA, Holgate ST. Interpatient variability in rates of asthma progression: can genetics provide an answer? J Allergy Clin Immunol 2008;121:573–9.

40. Steinke JW, Rich SS, Borish L. Genetics of allergic disease. J Allergy Clin Immunol 2008;121:S384-7.

41. Vercelli D. Advances in asthma and allergy genetics in 2007. J Allergy Clin Immunol 2008;122:267–71.

42. Chatterjee R, Batra J, Das S, et al. Genetic association of acidic mammalian chitinase with atopic asthma and serum total IgE levels. J Allergy Clin Immunol 2008;122:202–8.

43. Tavendale R, Macgregor DF, Mukhopadhyay S, et al. A polymorphism controlling *ORMDL3* expression is associated with asthma that is poorly controlled by current medications. J Allergy Clin Immunol 2008;121:860–3.

44. Ueda T, Niimi A, Matsumoto H, et al. *TGFB1* promoter polymorphism C-509T and pathophysiology of asthma. J Allergy Clin Immunol 2008;121:659–64.

45. Kormann MSD, Depner M, Hartl D, et al. Toll-like receptor heterodimer variants protect from childhood asthma. J Allergy Clin Immunol 2008;122:86–92.

46. Hunninghake GM, Soto-Quirós ME, Lasky-Su J, et al. Dust mite exposure modifies the effect of functional *IL10* polymorphisms on allergy and asthma exacerbations. J Allergy Clin Immunol 2008;122:93–8.

47. Weidinger S, O'Sullivan M, Illig T, et al. Filaggrin mutations, atopic eczema, hay fever, and asthma in children. J Allergy Clin Immunol 2008;121:1203–9.

48. Bouzigon E, Corda E, Aschard H, et al. Effect of 17q21 variants and smoking exposure in early-onset asthma. N Engl J Med 2008;359:1985–94.

CHAPTER

44

Mucosal Immunology: An Overview

M. Cecilia Berin • Mirna Chehade

The gastrointestinal (GI) tract is the largest immunologic organ in the body. The small intestine itself has the largest surface area in the GI tract due to structural features including villi and microvilli. The purpose of this extensive surface is to facilitate nutrient absorption from ingested foods. From the stomach to the rectum, a single layer of columnar epithelial cells separates the external environment of the GI lumen from the body proper. The lumen contains a myriad of microorganisms and dietary proteins. The challenge from an immune perspective is to guard the extensive surface area of the GI tract from breaches by microorganisms, in particular, pathogenic microorganisms. In the small intestine, the main antigenic load is from ingested food. Along the proximal to distal axis the food antigen load decreases as it is digested and absorbed, but the microbial load increases. In the large intestine, there are 10^{10}–10^{12} organisms per gram of dry luminal contents.[1] The intestinal immune system must remain nonreactive or tolerant to antigens from food or commensal flora, yet retain the ability to mount a protective immune response to enteropathogens. This function is accomplished by the gastrointestinal associated lymphoid tissue (GALT) that has adapted to its unique environment.

Structure of the Gastrointestinal Associated Lymphoid Tissue (GALT)

The gastrointestinal tract has several types of organized lymphoid tissue comprising the GALT. Underlying the intestinal epithelial layer is a loose connective tissue stroma called the lamina propria (LP), containing a resident population of CD4 and CD8 T lymphocytes, plasma cells, macrophages, dendritic cells (DCs), and eosinophils. The LP of the small and large intestine is drained via lymphatics that empty into the mesenteric lymph nodes (MLNs). Migratory DCs capture antigens in the LP and deliver those antigens to the MLN. The MLN is a typical secondary lymph node with organized B cell follicles and paracortical T cell areas. Peyer's patches (PPs) are lymph nodes found within the mucosal wall and so have direct access to the intestinal lumen. PPs are large and visible by eye as bulges on the serosal surface of the intestine. In addition to PPs, the intestine contains smaller structures called isolated lymphoid follicles (ILF), each containing a single B cell follicle with an overlying follicular epithelium. Mouse intestine contains an abundance of these small organized structures.[2,3] An immature form of the ILF is the cryptopatch, comprised of clusters of lymphocyte precursors. Bacterial signals promote the enlargement of the ILFs through

the recruitment of B cells.[4,5] The MLN, PP, and ILF comprise the inductive sites in the gastrointestinal tract. In addition, T lymphocytes are normally found between epithelial cells (intraepithelial lymphocytes, or IELs). IELs are predominantly CD8$^+$ T cells in the small intestine, and have an oligoclonal repertoire. The immune cells of the LP and the IELs comprise the effector cells of the GALT, and are responsible for both the maintenance of tolerance to harmless antigens and immunity against pathogens. Figure 44-1 shows a schematic of the structure of the GALT.

Mechanisms of Antigen Sampling in the Intestinal Mucosa

Food protein antigens are digested by a combination of gastric acid, pancreatic proteases, and brush border peptidases, resulting in a mixture of amino acids and di- and tri-peptides, which are then absorbed by the intestinal epithelial cells. Dietary antigens that escape proteolysis in the lumen can be taken up by the intestine in various ways. Soluble antigens are taken up by enterocytes via fluid phase endocytosis by the microvillous membrane, transported in small vesicles and larger phagosomes, and then digested when lysosomes combine to form phagolysosomes. Intact molecules that remain after digestion are deposited in the extracellular space by exocytosis.[6] As a result, approximately 2% of intact proteins reach the intestinal lymph and portal circulation under physiologic conditions.[7]

Particulate antigens are poorly sampled by enterocytes, where the glycocalyx provides a barrier to even relatively small particles.[8] PPs are overlaid by specialized epithelial cells, referred to as membranous or microfold (M) cells.[9] M cells that overlay PPs have a reduced glycocalyx layer and shortened microvilli that allow for binding of particles that cannot adhere to enterocytes.[8] In addition, they have a sparse, flattened cytoplasm and enhanced endocytic activity, allowing rapid antigen delivery into the subepithelial dome region of the PP. The subepithelial dome is rich in DCs that process and present antigen to T lymphocytes or transfer antigen to B lymphocytes.

The intestinal mucosa is densely populated with a network of DCs that function to acquire antigen, migrate to T cell areas of lymph nodes, and present antigen to naïve T cells. They can acquire this antigen after it has been transcytosed across enterocytes or M cells as outlined above. In addition, DCs have been shown to extend dendrites between enterocytes into the intestinal lumen.[10,11] These dendrites are functional, as antigen sampling extensions can acquire luminal bacteria.[10,11]

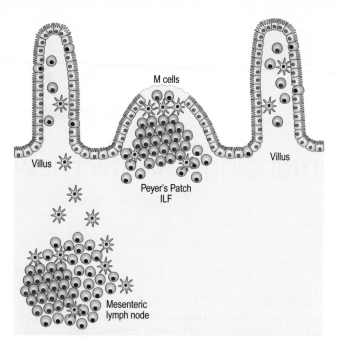

Figure 44-1 Structure of the GALT. Organized lymphoid structures in the gastrointestinal tract include the mesenteric lymph node (*MLN*) that drains the mucosa via the lymphatics. Peyer's patches and isolated lymphoid follicles (*ILF*) are present within the mucosal wall and are covered by specialized antigen sampling cells called M cells. Dendritic cells (orange) continuously migrate from the lamina propria into the MLN to present antigen. Organized lymphoid structures contain B cell follicles surrounded by T cell areas. Within the lamina propria are scattered T cells (green), B cells (red) and dendritic cells. A population of intraepithelial lymphocytes is also found through the gastrointestinal tract. A single layer of columnar epithelium separates the mucosal immune system from the luminal contents.

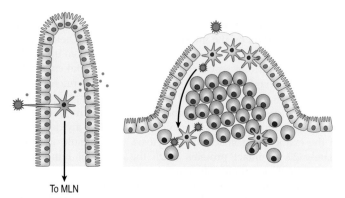

Figure 44-2 Antigen uptake in the intestine. In the normal mucosa (left), antigen can reach subepithelial dendritic cells (DCs) by two routes. DCs can send extensions between enterocytes to sample particulate antigens directly from the lumen. Alternatively, soluble antigens can be taken up by fluid phase endocytosis by enterocytes and be deposited in the lamina propria for uptake by macrophages or DCs. DCs migrate from the lamina propria to the mesenteric lymph node (*MLN*), where antigen can be presented to naïve T cells. In the Peyer's patch (right), M cells are specialized for uptake of particulate antigens, that are delivered to DCs in the subepithelial space. These DCs can then traffic to the interfollicular areas of the Peyer's patch for presentation to T cells (green) or interacting with B cells (red).

Antigen transport across the intestinal barrier has been shown to be altered by immunization or allergic sensitization, either enhancing[12,13] or inhibiting[14] uptake. As discussed in detail later, IgA, IgG, and IgE-facilitated antigen sampling have been documented in the intestinal mucosa. Figure 44-2 outlines these major pathways of antigen uptake.

Normal Immune Response to Sampled Antigens in the Intestine

Food contains a diverse mix of antigens that are capable of stimulating immune responses if administered by other routes. Administration of antigens by the oral route is one of the most effective means of inducing tolerance. The process of oral tolerance was first defined experimentally in laboratory rodents that displayed systemic unresponsiveness to immunization with antigens which they had previously been fed. Tolerance can be transferred to a naïve animal by transferring T lymphocytes,[15,16] demonstrating that this is an active immune-mediated process. Oral tolerance has also been demonstrated in humans by feeding a neoantigen[17,18] prior to immunization.

Different types of regulatory CD4$^+$ T cells have been shown to be important for oral tolerance induction to an antigen.[15,16] These cells may be divided into three subgroups: T-helper 3 (Th3) cells, T-regulatory cells 1 (Tr1) and CD4$^+$CD25$^+$ cells. Th3 cells were first described when low doses of myelin basic protein (MBP) were administered orally to animals and isolated MBP-specific CD4$^+$ T cell clones from the mesenteric lymph nodes of these animals. Adoptive transfer of these cells suppressed experimental allergic encephalomyelitis.[19] Th3 cells produce TGF-β with various amounts of IL-4 and IL-10. Inhibition of TGF-β with neutralizing antibodies can abrogate tolerance responses.[20,21] Tr1 cells secrete IL-10, which also drives generation of these cells. IL-10 was shown to suppress antigen-specific immune responses, and prevent colitis in a mouse model.[22] Although there is evidence that IL-10 is induced by antigen feeding,[23,24] there is no functional data yet demonstrating that IL-10 is required for oral tolerance responses. Natural T-regulatory cells are CD4$^+$CD25$^+$ T cells that arise from the thymus and are characterized by Foxp3 expression, naïve phenotype, low proliferative capacity and IL-2 production. There are data both for and against a role for naturally occurring T regulatory cells in oral tolerance.[20,25] Feeding mice induces a population of antigen-specific T-regulatory cells that express similar markers as natural T-regulatory cells (CD25$^+$, Foxp3$^+$, and CTLA-4) and mediate regulatory responses via TGF-β but not IL-10.[20]

Naïve T cells must be instructed to become regulatory in phenotype rather than effector Th1, Th2 or Th17 cells. There is growing evidence that the way in which food antigens are presented to the naïve T cells by antigen presenting cells, such as DCs and macrophages, is a critical factor promoting the development of regulatory T cells in the intestine.

The Role of Intestinal Dendritic Cells in Tolerance and Immunity

An abundant network of DCs surrounds the epithelium and fills the lamina propria. The role of DCs in both tolerance and immunity in the intestinal mucosa was first explored using the growth factor Flt3L to expand the DC population in mice. Flt3L treatment enhanced tolerance responses to an innocuous antigen when it was delivered orally.[26] In addition, when antigen was administered with adjuvant to elicit protective immunity, DC expansion also enhanced that response.[27] These studies show that, like elsewhere in the body, DCs are essential for the initiation of an active CD4$^+$ T cell response, whether regulatory, or effector Th1, Th2 or Th17 in nature.

DCs are not a homogenous population. Data suggest that there may be subset specialization, such that there may be tolerogenic

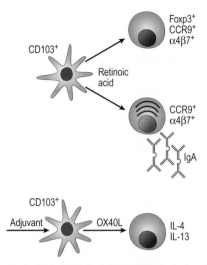

Figure 44-3 Function of CD103⁺ DCs in the intestine. A subset of DCs in the lamina propria expresses CD103. These are migratory DCs that acquire antigen and traffic to the MLN. In normal conditions, CD103⁺ DCs prime naïve T cells and B cells to generate a gut-homing phenotype expressing CCR9 and α4β7. CD103⁺ DCs promote the generation of regulatory T cells expressing Foxp3, and promote IgA secretion from B cells. In the presence of the strong mucosal adjuvant cholera toxin, CD103⁺ DCs up-regulate OX40L and induce Th2-skewing from responder T cells.

and immunogenic DC subsets.[28] DC subsets in the PP and MLN can be grouped based on surface expression of CD11b and CD8α.[29,30] CD11b⁺ DCs from the PP promote naïve T cells to produce IL-4 and IL-10 whereas CD8α⁺ and CD11b⁻CD8α⁻ DCs are better IL-12 (p70) producers.[31] These findings suggest that CD11b⁺ DCs may have greater potential to function as tolerogenic DCs through promotion of IL-10 producing T cells. Plasmacytoid DCs in the MLN also promote the development of regulatory T cells,[32] and recently, in vivo data has demonstrated a role for liver plasmacytoid DCs in the generation of oral tolerance.[33] Another potentially tolerogenic DC subset expresses the marker CD103, the αE integrin that together with β7 recognizes E-cadherin on epithelial cells. This subset promotes the development of Foxp3⁺ regulatory T cells via release of retinoic acid.[34] The majority of evidence suggests that CD103 is a marker of LP-derived DCs.[34,35] In vivo administration of the mucosal adjuvant cholera toxin can modify these CD103⁺ DCs into highly immunogenic DCs.[36] Therefore the tolerogenic versus immunogenic phenotype of the CD103⁺ DCs is regulated by the immune environment in the lamina propria of the gastrointestinal tract, rather than being a fixed characteristic of this subset. Figure 44-3 highlights the main features of this CD103⁺ DC subset.

Subsets in the intestine can also be differentiated by chemokine receptor expression. DCs expressing CX₃CR1 can be found in both LP and PP,[11] but DCs expressing CCR6 are found only in the PP.[37] The CCR6⁺, but not CX₃CR1⁺ DCs were found to be responsible for early T cell responses to *Salmonella* infection, again demonstrating functional specialization of DC subsets.[37]

Macrophages Have a Regulatory Phenotype in the Intestine

Macrophages are the most abundant phagocytic cells that are resident in the small and large intestinal LP. They form a band of cells directly beneath the surface epithelium distinct from the localization of DCs.[38] Like DCs, macrophages can take up antigen and present it to T lymphocytes; however, macrophages are not migratory, and do not reach lymph nodes for interaction with naïve T cells. Macrophages from the human intestine are adept at both phagocytosis and killing of microbes after uptake.[39,40] Therefore, they function as a secondary barrier after the epithelium in preventing the influx of microbes from the gut lumen into the body proper. Macrophages from the intestinal mucosa of mouse and human are nonresponsive to microbial stimuli compared to monocytes or macrophages from other sites.[40,41] This was shown to be due to TGF-β released from the intestinal stroma in humans[40] or autocrine effects of IL-10 in the mouse.[41] IL-10 is clearly important for immune homeostasis in the intestine as mice lacking IL-10 develop spontaneous colitis,[42] as do mice lacking the signaling machinery downstream of IL-10 specifically in the monocyte/macrophage/DC lineage.[43]

Toll-Like Receptor (TLR) Signaling in the Intestine

The intestinal mucosa, in particular, in the large intestine, is continually challenged with a heavy load of microbial products. Pathogen-associated molecular patterns (PAMPs) that are ligands for the TLRs are not restricted to pathogenic microbes, and are expressed by commensal bacteria. A critical question in mucosal immunology is how the intestinal immune system can differentiate pathogens from commensal organisms. For the most part, commensal organisms are restricted to the lumen of the gastrointestinal tract, and epithelial cells preferentially respond to TLR signaling at their basal surface.[44,45] Commensals are normally taken up by DCs in the PP or MLN in small numbers for the induction of IgA responses.[46] Macrophages and DCs isolated from the intestine have been shown to be globally unresponsive to stimulation through TLRs. One exception to this is TLR5. A subset of DCs in the mouse intestine expressing CD11c and CD11b have been shown to be highly responsive to flagellin, the ligand for TLR5.[47] When stimulated with flagellin, these DCs support the production of IgA from B cells and the development of effector Th17 CD4⁺ T cells.

Despite the lack of inflammatory responses, the commensal flora has significant impact on the development of the mucosal immune system. Germ-free mice have under-developed lymphoid tissue,[48] and reconstitution of germ-free mice with normal flora results in a significant modification of gene expression in the intestinal mucosa in the absence of any frank inflammation.[49] It was recently shown that constitutive signaling via the receptor TLR9 promotes the development of effector CD4⁺ T cells in the intestine and suppresses development of Foxp3⁺ CD4⁺ T regulatory cells.[50] Given that the commensal flora plays such an important role in shaping the mucosal immune system, it is also likely that signals from the flora will influence the development of tolerance versus allergic sensitization to food proteins.

Homing of Lymphocytes to the Intestine

Lymphocytes that differentiate in the inductive sites of the GALT into effector or regulatory T cells, or IgA-producing B cells home preferentially to the intestinal lamina propria to carry out their function. Targeted homing of lymphocytes is determined by expression of specific adhesion molecules and chemokine receptors.[51] Homing to the intestine is mediated by the adhesion molecule α4β7 binding to MAdCAM on high endothelial venules.[52] In addition, the chemokine receptor CCR9 promotes migration to the small intestine where constitutive expression of the ligand CCL25 is found.[53,54] Migration to the large intestine is promoted by the chemokine receptor CCR10 binding to its ligand CCL28.[55,56]

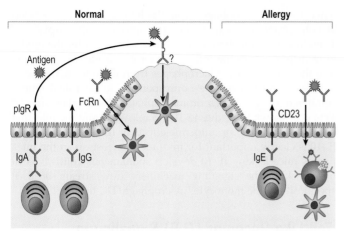

Figure 44-4 Immunoglobulin secretion and antibody-facilitated antigen uptake in the intestine. Epithelial cells express receptors for IgA (pIgR), IgG (FcRn), and IgE (CD23). All three receptors can facilitate the secretion of their respective immunoglobulins in a basal-to-apical direction. IgA can facilitate uptake of antigen by M cells through an as-yet-unidentified receptor. FcRn captures IgG-antigen complexes for delivery to dendritic cells (DCs) and promotes the amplification of antigen-specific immune responses. When allergen-specific IgE is produced and secreted (i.e. during food allergy), IgE-allergen complexes can be captured from the apical side by CD23 and transported to the basal side of the epithelium. IgE-allergen complexes can then degranulate effector cells or induce the migration of DCs through epithelial-derived chemokines.

Lymphocytes and IgA antibody secreting cells activated within the GALT preferentially home back to the LP,[57,58] where the cognate antigen is most likely to be re-encountered. The intestinal migratory phenotype is imprinted on lymphocytes by the CD103[+] population of DCs in the MLN.[59] The mechanism of this imprinting involves secretion of retinoic acid from the DC.[34] Epithelial cells and DCs express retinal dehydrogenase enzymes that can convert dietary vitamin A into retinoic acid, and dietary vitamin A has been proposed as an important factor in maintaining the localized tolerogenic milieu of the gastrointestinal tract.[34,60]

Humoral Immune Responses in the Intestine

The intestinal mucosa is a rich site of antibody production, particularly secretory IgA. Naïve B cells in the MLN and PP are activated by binding to their antigen, proliferate, and with T cell help, differentiate into antibody-secreting cells or memory B cells. GALT DCs promote the differentiation of B cells into IgA-secreting cells, as well as up-regulate CCR9 and α4β7 on B cells to promote gut homing.[57] CCR10 is also expressed on a subset of antibody-secreting cells and contributes to mucosal homing.[55,61] Immunoglobulins play an important role in neutralization of pathogens, and also function, together with epithelial-expressed receptors, as specific antigen sampling mechanisms in the intestinal mucosa. IgA is the most abundant immunoglobulin produced within the intestinal mucosa, but there is also evidence for a significant contribution of IgG to host defense against enteropathogens. In the context of food allergy, IgE and its receptor CD23 also come into play as an antigen sampling mechanism and inducer of inflammatory reactions in the intestine. Figure 44-4 shows a schematic of the function of these immunoglobulin receptors in the intestine.

IgA/pIgR

Eighty percent of IgA-secreting cells are found in the gastrointestinal mucosa, and daily production of IgA outpaces that of all other immunoglobulin isotypes combined.[62] IgA in plasma occurs primarily as monomers, but IgA in mucosal secretions is comprised of polymeric IgA (2–4 molecules) joined at the Fc region by a joining 'J' chain and secretory component (SC) that is a fragment of the polymeric Ig receptor (pIgR). There are two IgA subclasses, IgA1 and IgA2, that differ in their resistance to intestinal proteases (IgA2 being more resistant than IgA1). pIgR is expressed on the intestinal epithelium and transports polymeric IgA from the basolateral face into the intestinal lumen. Pentameric IgM is also transported into the lumen via the pIgR. Specificity for the polymeric form of the immunoglobulins is conferred by the J chain that connects the Ig subunits. Each molecule of pIgR can only perform one transport of Ig, as the extracellular portion is cleaved to form SC. In addition to secreting immunoglobulin polymers into the lumen, pIgR can also transport immune complexes formed in the LP. Thus IgA could secrete antigens that have already penetrated the epithelial barrier. Neutralization of viruses and LPS within the epithelium by IgA has also been demonstrated. Thus, a main function of IgA is to prevent or reverse entry of antigens into the intestinal mucosa.

Secretory IgA has been shown to selectively bind to M cells via the constant domains,[63] to a receptor that has not yet been identified but is distinct from the known IgA receptors pIgR and FcαRI. Antigens tagged to IgA are taken up by M cells and delivered to DCs in the PP[64] where they induce an immunoglobulin response. Thus IgA may selectively allow for controlled entry of antigens into the PP while preventing broad access to the remaining intestinal mucosa.

IgG/FcRn

Like IgA, IgG is also found in intestinal secretions in significant quantities. In rodents, the neonatal Fc receptor for IgG (FcRn) is expressed in the intestine prior to weaning and facilitates the transfer of passive immunity from the mother via colostrum. In humans, passive immunity is delivered via the placenta, but FcRn is expressed in the intestine and is maintained throughout adult life.[65] This suggests a function for FcRn beyond transfer of passive immunity. In vitro systems have shown that FcRn functions as a bi-directional transporter of IgG.[66] The development of transgenic mice expressing human FcRn into adulthood has uncovered a critical role for FcRn as an antigen sampling mechanism in vivo. IgG is secreted into the intestinal lumen via FcRn, where it binds to its antigens and can be recaptured by FcRn and transported into the intestinal LP.[67] Antigen is then delivered to subepithelial DCs that can generate a functional T cell response. This pathway was subsequently shown to promote clearance of the murine enteric pathogen *Citrobacter rodentium*.[68]

IgE/CD23

IgE is not generally thought of as a secretory immunoglobulin, but it can be detected in the intestinal secretions and stool of subjects with food allergy.[69,70] The low affinity IgE receptor CD23 is constitutively expressed by human intestinal epithelial cells.[71,72] Similar to studies with FcRn, CD23 has been shown to function as a bi-directional transporter of IgE in in vitro systems.[71] In addition, IgE-allergen complexes can be captured from the apical side of epithelial monolayers in a CD23-dependent manner, and these transported complexes degranulate allergic effector cells. Transported IgE-allergen complexes can also trigger chemokine release from the intestinal epithelium that supports the recruitment of DCs.[73] The in vivo relevance of this pathway has not yet been determined, but may be an important antigen sampling pathway in IgE-mediated immunity to helminth infection, or participate in pathological reactions to food allergens.

Conclusions

The mucosal immune system is tightly regulated to prevent inappropriate immune reactions to food antigens or the commensal flora, and is responsible for guarding a vast surface area against pathogenic entry. Antigens can gain access to the mucosal immune system by a number of different mechanisms including direct DC uptake and antibody-facilitated antigen uptake. The normal response to food antigens is an active tolerance response mediated by regulatory T cells, which are induced by IL-10, TGF-β and retinoic acid secreted by resident DCs and macrophages. These immune mechanisms are critical for the prevention of food- or flora-induced pathology.

References

1. Whitman WB, Coleman DC, Wiebe WJ. Prokaryotes: the unseen majority. Proc Natl Acad Sci U S A 1998;95:6578–83.
2. Williams IR. CCR6 and CCL20: partners in intestinal immunity and lymphorganogenesis. Ann N Y Acad Sci 2006;1072:52–61.
3. Forster R, Pabst O, Bernhardt G. Homeostatic chemokines in development, plasticity, and functional organization of the intestinal immune system. Semin Immunol 2008;20:171–80.
4. Lorenz RG, Chaplin DD, McDonald KG, et al. Isolated lymphoid follicle formation is inducible and dependent upon lymphotoxin-sufficient B lymphocytes, lymphotoxin beta receptor, and TNF receptor I function. J Immunol 2003;170:5475–82.
5. Bouskra D, Brezillon C, Berard M, et al. Lymphoid tissue genesis induced by commensals through NOD1 regulates intestinal homeostasis. Nature 2008;456:507–10.
6. Walker WA, Isselbacher KJ. Uptake and transport of macromolecules by the intestine. Possible role in clinical disorders. Gastroenterology 1974;67:531–50.
7. Warshaw AL, Walker WA, Isselbacher KJ. Protein uptake by the intestine: evidence for absorption of intact macromolecules. Gastroenterology 1974;66:987–92.
8. Frey A, Giannasca KT, Weltzin R, et al. Role of the glycocalyx in regulating access of microparticles to apical plasma membranes of intestinal epithelial cells: implications for microbial attachment and oral vaccine targeting. J Exp Med 1996;184:1045–59.
9. Wolf JL, Bye WA. The membranous epithelial (M) cell and the mucosal immune system. Annu Rev Med 1984;35:95–112.
10. Rescigno M, Urbano M, Valzasina B, et al. Dendritic cells express tight junction proteins and penetrate gut epithelial monolayers to sample bacteria. Nat Immunol 2001;2:361–7.
11. Niess JH, Brand S, Gu X, et al. CX3CR1-mediated dendritic cell access to the intestinal lumen and bacterial clearance. Science 2005;307:254–8.
12. Bockman D, Winborn W. Light and electron microscopy of intestinal ferritin absorption: observations in sensitized and non-sensitized hamster (Mesocricetus auratus). Anat Rec 1965;155:603–22.
13. Berin MC, Kiliaan AJ, Yang PC, et al. Rapid transepithelial antigen transport in rat jejunum: impact of sensitization and the hypersensitivity reaction. Gastroenterology 1997;113:856–64.
14. Walker WA, Isselbacher KJ, Bloch KJ. Intestinal uptake of macromolecules. II. Effect of parenteral immunization. J Immunol 1973;111:221–6.
15. Chen Y, Inobe J, Weiner HL. Induction of oral tolerance to myelin basic protein in CD8-depleted mice: both CD4+ and CD8+ cells mediate active suppression. J Immunol 1995;155:910–6.
16. Garside P, Steel M, Liew FY, et al. CD4+ but not CD8+ T cells are required for the induction of oral tolerance. Int Immunol 1995;7:501–4.
17. Kraus TA, Toy L, Chan L, et al. Failure to induce oral tolerance to a soluble protein in patients with inflammatory bowel disease. Gastroenterology 2004;126:1771–8.
18. Husby S, Mestecky J, Moldoveanu Z, et al. Oral tolerance in humans. T cell but not B cell tolerance after antigen feeding. J Immunol 1994;152:4663–70.
19. Chen Y, Kuchroo VK, Inobe J, et al. Regulatory T cell clones induced by oral tolerance: suppression of autoimmune encephalomyelitis. Science 1994;265:1237–40.
20. Mucida D, Kutchukhidze N, Erazo A, et al. Oral tolerance in the absence of naturally occurring Tregs. J Clin Invest 2005;115:1923–33.
21. Neurath MF, Fuss I, Kelsall BL, et al. Experimental granulomatous colitis in mice is abrogated by induction of TGF-beta-mediated oral tolerance. J Exp Med 1996;183:2605–16.
22. Groux H, O'Garra A, Bigler M, et al. A CD4+ T cell subset inhibits antigen-specific T cell responses and prevents colitis. Nature 1997;389:737–42.
23. Tsuji NM, Mizumachi K, Kurisaki J. Interleukin-10-secreting Peyer's patch cells are responsible for active suppression in low-dose oral tolerance. Immunology 2001;103:458–64.
24. Gonnella PA, Chen Y, Inobe J, et al. In situ immune response in gut-associated lymphoid tissue (GALT) following oral antigen in TCR-transgenic mice. J Immunol 1998;160:4708–18.
25. Dubois B, Chapat L, Goubier A, et al. Innate CD4+CD25+ regulatory T cells are required for oral tolerance and inhibition of CD8+ T cells mediating skin inflammation. Blood 2003;102:3295–301.
26. Viney JL, Mowat AM, O'Malley JM, et al. Expanding dendritic cells in vivo enhances the induction of oral tolerance. J Immunol 1998;160:5815–25.
27. Williamson E, Westrich GM, Viney JL. Modulating dendritic cells to optimize mucosal immunization protocols. J Immunol 1999;163:3668–75.
28. Kelsall B. Recent progress in understanding the phenotype and function of intestinal dendritic cells and macrophages. Mucosal Immunol 2008;1:460–9.
29. Iwasaki A, Kelsall BL. Localization of distinct Peyer's patch dendritic cell subsets and their recruitment by chemokines macrophage inflammatory protein (MIP)-3alpha, MIP-3beta, and secondary lymphoid organ chemokine. J Exp Med 2000;191:1381–94.
30. Kelsall BL, Strober W. Distinct populations of dendritic cells are present in the subepithelial dome and T cell regions of the murine Peyer's patch. J Exp Med 1996;183:237–47.
31. Iwasaki A, Kelsall BL. Unique functions of CD11b+, CD8 alpha+, and double-negative Peyer's patch dendritic cells. J Immunol 2001;166:4884–90.
32. Bilsborough J, George TC, Norment A, et al. Mucosal CD8alpha+ DC, with a plasmacytoid phenotype, induce differentiation and support function of T cells with regulatory properties. Immunology 2003;108:481–92.
33. Goubier A, Dubois B, Gheit H, et al. Plasmacytoid dendritic cells mediate oral tolerance. Immunity 2008;29:464–75.
34. Jaensson E, Uronen-Hansson H, Pabst O, et al. Small intestinal CD103+ dendritic cells display unique functional properties that are conserved between mice and humans. J Exp Med 2008;205:2139–49.
35. Worbs T, Bode U, Yan S, et al. Oral tolerance originates in the intestinal immune system and relies on antigen carriage by dendritic cells. J Exp Med 2006;203:519–27.
36. Blazquez AB, Berin MC. Gastrointestinal dendritic cells promote Th2 skewing via OX40L. J Immunol 2008;180:4441–50.
37. Salazar-Gonzalez RM, Niess JH, Zammit DJ, et al. CCR6-mediated dendritic cell activation of pathogen-specific T cells in Peyer's patches. Immunity 2006;24:623–32.
38. Pavli P, Maxwell L, Van de Pol E, et al. Distribution of human colonic dendritic cells and macrophages. Clin Exp Immunol 1996;104:124–32.
39. Smith PD, Janoff EN, Mosteller-Barnum M, et al. Isolation and purification of CD14-negative mucosal macrophages from normal human small intestine. J Immunol Methods 1997;202:1–11.
40. Smythies LE, Sellers M, Clements RH, et al. Human intestinal macrophages display profound inflammatory anergy despite avid phagocytic and bacteriocidal activity. J Clin Invest 2005;115:66–75.
41. Denning TL, Wang YC, Patel SR, et al. Lamina propria macrophages and dendritic cells differentially induce regulatory and interleukin 17-producing T cell responses. Nat Immunol 2007;8:1086–94.
42. Kuhn R, Lohler J, Rennick D, et al. Interleukin-10-deficient mice develop chronic enterocolitis. Cell 1993;75:263–74.
43. Takeda K, Clausen BE, Kaisho T, et al. Enhanced Th1 activity and development of chronic enterocolitis in mice devoid of Stat3 in macrophages and neutrophils. Immunity 1999;10:39–49.
44. Lee J, Mo JH, Katakura K, et al. Maintenance of colonic homeostasis by distinctive apical TLR9 signalling in intestinal epithelial cells. Nat Cell Biol 2006;8:1327–36.
45. Gewirtz AT, Navas TA, Lyons S, et al. Cutting edge: bacterial flagellin activates basolaterally expressed TLR5 to induce epithelial proinflammatory gene expression. J Immunol 2001;167:1882–5.
46. Macpherson AJ, Uhr T. Induction of protective IgA by intestinal dendritic cells carrying commensal bacteria. Science 2004;303:1662–5.
47. Uematsu S, Jang MH, Chevrier N, et al. Detection of pathogenic intestinal bacteria by Toll-like receptor 5 on intestinal CD11c+ lamina propria cells. Nat Immunol 2006;7:868–74.

48. Cebra JJ, Periwal SB, Lee G, et al. Development and maintenance of the gut-associated lymphoid tissue (GALT): the roles of enteric bacteria and viruses. Dev Immunol 1998;6:13–8.

49. Hooper LV, Wong MH, Thelin A, et al. Molecular analysis of commensal host-microbial relationships in the intestine. Science 2001;291:881–4.

50. Hall JA, Bouladoux N, Sun CM, et al. Commensal DNA limits regulatory T cell conversion and is a natural adjuvant of intestinal immune responses. Immunity 2008;29:637–49.

51. Kunkel EJ, Butcher EC. Chemokines and the tissue-specific migration of lymphocytes. Immunity 2002;16:1–4.

52. Williams MB, Butcher EC. Homing of naive and memory T lymphocyte subsets to Peyer's patches, lymph nodes, and spleen. J Immunol 1997;159:1746–52.

53. Stenstad H, Ericsson A, Johansson-Lindbom B, et al. Gut-associated lymphoid tissue-primed CD4+ T cells display CCR9-dependent and -independent homing to the small intestine. Blood 2006;107:3447–54.

54. Svensson M, Marsal J, Ericsson A, et al. CCL25 mediates the localization of recently activated CD8alphabeta(+) lymphocytes to the small-intestinal mucosa. J Clin Invest 2002;110:1113–21.

55. Kunkel EJ, Kim CH, Lazarus NH, et al. CCR10 expression is a common feature of circulating and mucosal epithelial tissue IgA Ab-secreting cells. J Clin Invest 2003;111:1001–10.

56. Pan J, Kunkel EJ, Gosslar U, et al. A novel chemokine ligand for CCR10 and CCR3 expressed by epithelial cells in mucosal tissues. J Immunol 2000;165:2943–9.

57. Mora JR, Iwata M, Eksteen B, et al. Generation of gut-homing IgA-secreting B cells by intestinal dendritic cells. Science 2006;314:1157–60.

58. Johansson-Lindbom B, Svensson M, Wurbel MA, et al. Selective generation of gut tropic T cells in gut-associated lymphoid tissue (GALT): requirement for GALT dendritic cells and adjuvant. J Exp Med 2003;198:963–9.

59. Johansson-Lindbom B, Svensson M, Pabst O, et al. Functional specialization of gut CD103+ dendritic cells in the regulation of tissue-selective T cell homing. J Exp Med 2005;202:1063–73.

60. Mucida D, Park Y, Cheroutre H. From the diet to the nucleus: vitamin A and TGF-beta join efforts at the mucosal interface of the intestine. Semin Immunol 2009;21:14–21.

61. Feng N, Jaimes MC, Lazarus NH, et al. Redundant role of chemokines CCL25/TECK and CCL28/MEC in IgA+ plasmablast recruitment to the intestinal lamina propria after rotavirus infection. J Immunol 2006;176:5749–59.

62. Mora JR, von Andrian UH. Differentiation and homing of IgA-secreting cells. Mucosal Immunol 2008;1:96–109.

63. Mantis NJ, Cheung MC, Chintalacharuvu KR, et al. Selective adherence of IgA to murine Peyer's patch M cells: evidence for a novel IgA receptor. J Immunol 2002;169:1844–51.

64. Corthesy B. Roundtrip ticket for secretory IgA: role in mucosal homeostasis? J Immunol 2007;178:27–32.

65. Israel EJ, Taylor S, Wu Z, et al. Expression of the neonatal Fc receptor, FcRn, on human intestinal epithelial cells. Immunology 1997;92:69–74.

66. Dickinson BL, Badizadegan K, Wu Z, et al. Bidirectional FcRn-dependent IgG transport in a polarized human intestinal epithelial cell line. J Clin Invest 1999;104:903–11.

67. Yoshida M, Claypool SM, Wagner JS, et al. Human neonatal Fc receptor mediates transport of IgG into luminal secretions for delivery of antigens to mucosal dendritic cells. Immunity 2004;20:769–83.

68. Yoshida M, Kobayashi K, Kuo TT, et al. Neonatal Fc receptor for IgG regulates mucosal immune responses to luminal bacteria. J Clin Invest 2006;116:2142–51.

69. Brown WR, Borthistle BK, Chen ST. Immunoglobulin E (IgE) and IgE-containing cells in human gastrointestinal fluids and tissues. Clin Exp Immunol 1975;20:227–37.

70. Belut D, Moneret-Vautrin DA, Nicolas JP, et al. IgE levels in intestinal juice. Dig Dis Sci 1980;25:323–32.

71. Li H, Nowak-Wegrzyn A, Charlop-Powers Z, et al. Transcytosis of IgE-antigen complexes by CD23a in human intestinal epithelial cells and its role in food allergy. Gastroenterology 2006;131:47–58.

72. Kaiserlian D, Lachaux A, Grosjean I, et al. Intestinal epithelial cells express the CD23/Fc epsilon RII molecule: enhanced expression in enteropathies. Immunology 1993;80:90–5.

73. Li H, Chehade M, Liu W, et al. Allergen-IgE complexes trigger CD23-dependent CCL20 release from human intestinal epithelial cells. Gastroenterology 2007;133:1905–15.

CHAPTER

45

Evaluation of Food Allergy

S. Allan Bock • Hugh A. Sampson

Introduction

The evaluation of food allergy has become increasingly scientific over the past three decades. In 1976, May published the first of his studies using the double-blind, placebo-controlled oral food challenge,[1] which has become the 'gold standard' for diagnosing all forms of adverse food reactions. This procedure has made the identification of food allergy/hypersensitivity particularly accurate compared to other diagnostic methods in the field of allergy.

The commonly accepted definitions of adverse reactions to food will be used throughout this chapter, although the recent European Academy of Allergy and Clinical Immunology (EAACI) task force nomenclature will be noted in parentheses here and in Table 45-1.[2,3] Adverse food reactions (food hypersensitivity) include any abnormal reactions resulting from the ingestion of a food. They may be the result of food intolerances, such as lactose intolerance (nonallergic food hypersensitivity) or a food hypersensitivity/allergy (food allergy). Food hypersensitivities/allergies may be due to immunoglobulin E (IgE) or non-IgE-mediated immune mechanisms. Toxic reactions (food poisoning) may mimic immunologic food reactions, but are due to either an inherent property of the food (e.g. pharmacologic quantities of a substance such as tyramine in aged cheese or an additive such as sulfite in wine) or contamination (e.g. scrombroid fish poisoning). Food aversions or psychological adverse reactions may imitate some allergic reactions and may occur in both truly allergic individuals and those who are not allergic.

Prevalence

The prevalence of food allergy depends to some extent on the population being examined and the methods of ascertainment. In surveys of the general public, 15% to 25% of individuals consider themselves to be 'allergic' to one or more foods.[4] When reviewing studies on prevalence, it is important to distinguish between (1) sensitization studies, (2) survey studies, (3) studies of particular foods, and (4) studies that incorporate some type of objective evaluation of clinical reactivity.[5-10] Food allergy is more frequent in young children and the prevalence of true immunologically mediated food allergy is about 6% of infants less than 3 years of age. As children approach school age the prevalence decreases, although recent natural history studies suggest that in some populations, the resolution of a food allergy may be more delayed.[11,12] Nevertheless, for most foods the probability of resolution is high, except for allergy to peanut, tree nuts and seafood.

In the USA, about 3–4% of the general population has food allergy, or about 12 million Americans.[13] With respect to food-induced anaphylaxis, surveys from Olmstead County, MN, suggest an increase from about 30/100 000 per year to 50/100 000 per year over the past decade.[14,15]

Differential Diagnosis (Box 45-1)

IgE-Mediated Reactions

Skin Symptoms

Urticaria is frequently attributed to 'allergy', but there are patterns of urticaria that are very suggestive of a food reaction. Prompt onset of urticaria following a meal and lasting minutes to hours is much more likely to be due to food allergy than symptoms that last for days. Chronic urticaria is rarely due to food allergy, but since exceptions always occur, the history should be reviewed carefully and in detail. Occasionally, children become allergic to a food ingested on a daily basis. Food additives have been reported to cause chronic urticaria in adults, but there are no systematically confirmed reports in children.[16]

Atopic dermatitis has been shown to be exacerbated by food allergies in numerous, carefully controlled studies using double-blind, placebo-controlled food challenges, beginning with Sampson's studies in the 1980s and continuing to the present.[17] (This subject is covered in more detail in Chapter 51.) Food allergic reactions have been shown to trigger atopic dermatitis in 30–40% of children with moderate to severe atopic dermatitis.[18] In some situations, the onset of symptoms is subtle and somewhat delayed, with irritability and then scratching being the first symptoms to appear, followed by erythema and/or urticaria preceding the more typical morbilliform eruption that may be most prominent the day after the offending food is consumed.

Gastrointestinal Symptoms (see also Chapters 48 and 49)

The immediate gastrointestinal (GI) symptoms include nausea, crampy abdominal pain, vomiting and diarrhea. Nausea and vomiting may occur almost immediately (while the food is being consumed) and should raise suspicion of a food allergic reaction, especially in an individual known to have food allergy. Rapid resolution of the GI symptoms and the prompt return of appetite help distinguish food allergic reactions from infections and toxic causes that typically result in more prolonged symptoms.

DOI: 10.1016/B978-1-4377-0271-2.00045-6

Table 45-1 Adverse Reaction to Food Terminology

US Terminology	EAACI Task Force/WAO
Adverse food reaction	Food hypersensitivity
Food intolerance (e.g. lactase deficiency)	Non-allergic food hypersensitivity
Food hypersensitive/allergies	Food allergy

BOX 45-1

Differential Diagnosis of Adverse Reactions to Foods

Immune

IgE-Mediated

Immediate (gastrointestinal, respiratory, cutaneous, ocular, cardiovascular, anaphylactic)

Immediate and late-phase (atopic dermatitis, allergic gastrointestinal disorders)

Oral allergy syndrome or pollen-food allergy syndrome

Non-IgE Immune-Mediated

Celiac disease, Dermatitis herpetiformis

Food protein-induced gastrointestinal illnesses

– Food protein-induced enterocolitis

– Eosinophilic esophagitis, gastroenteritis (allergic)

– Allergic colitis/proctocolitis

– Food protein-induced enteropathy (milk, soy, others)

Food-induced pulmonary hemosiderosis (Heiner's syndrome)

Toxic Reactions

Toxic reactions (food poisoning, e.g. scrombroid fish poisoning)

Non-toxic Reactions

Intolerances

– Carbohydrate malabsorption (e.g. lactase deficiency, sucrase-isomaltase deficiency)

Psychological Reactions (Strongly Held Beliefs)

Diarrhea may occur promptly and explosively or it may be delayed by several hours. Whether colic is due to food allergy remains controversial, but the literature contains some studies suggesting an allergic mechanism, although the reproducibility of these observations is questioned.[19–22] It is possible to help families determine the role of food in colic by recommending a brief elimination diet that is carefully monitored and nutritionally adequate. The subject of chronic constipation as a response to immediate hypersensitivity food allergy is equally controversial and less convincing. There are too few adequately controlled studies to establish an evidence base, but again it may be possible to clarify the situation with a brief elimination diet and challenge.[23,24]

The oral allergy syndrome (pollen-food allergy syndrome) is a common disorder in which oral symptoms of pruritus and mild edema in the mouth and throat occur promptly with the ingestion of certain raw fruits and vegetables. The reactions are due to IgE antibodies formed to certain aeroallergens, e.g. birch and ragweed pollens, which cross-react with certain food proteins, e.g. apples and bananas, respectively. In order to make the diagnosis, it is often necessary to use fresh foods to perform skin testing, as noted below.[25]

Respiratory Symptoms (see Chapter 50)

Respiratory symptoms, including those involving the upper respiratory tract (sneezing, rhinorrhea, nasal congestion/blockage), ocular symptoms (pruritus and tearing), and lower respiratory symptoms (stridor, hoarse voice, cough and wheezing) are often accompanied by GI and cutaneous symptoms. While asthma as the sole manifestation of an allergic reaction to food is uncommon, it should be thought of immediately in individuals with known food allergy and acute wheezing. There is evidence that food allergy predisposes individuals to more severe asthma attacks and even hospitalization.[26,27] It is important to note that recent case series strongly suggest that asthma, especially poorly controlled asthma, is a major risk factor for fatal food allergic reactions.[28–31]

Cardiovascular Symptoms

Food allergic reactions may manifest as isolated cardiovascular collapse and may result in death. In older adults, such reactions may not be immediately appreciated. This fact makes it especially crucial that individuals with known food allergy, even if previous reactions have not been severe, carry identifying information that can be quickly found so that prompt and potentially life-saving measures may be instituted without delay.

Anaphylaxis (see also Chapter 50)

While not yet universally accepted, there has been a recent attempt to create a definition and diagnostic criteria of anaphylaxis that will be universally accepted, put into practice and used to test research hypotheses: 'anaphylaxis is a serious allergic reaction that is rapid in onset and may cause death'.[32] The clinical criteria for diagnosing anaphylaxis are outlined in Box 45-2. Acceptance and use of these criteria should aid emergency responders in the rapid identification of anaphylaxis and prompt the institution of resuscitative measures.

Non-IgE Immune-Mediated

The majority of non-IgE-mediated immune reactions described involve the GI tract. Celiac disease is often classified as an autoimmune process, although it is actually initiated by a hypersensitivity response to gluten. It may be accompanied by the skin manifestations of dermatitis herpetiformis. The genetics are being unraveled (occurs only in individuals with HLA-DQ2 or DQ8 haplotypes) and improved serological methods are now available for confirming the diagnosis without necessarily undertaking a small bowel biopsy.[33] However, this disease requires a life-long change in dietary habits, i.e. a strict gluten-free diet, to avoid the increased risk of GI malignancies and lymphoma, so accurate diagnosis is essential. The eosinophilic GI disorders are discussed in detail in Chapter 49. Studies indicate that the prevalence of eosinophilic esophagitis, like other hypersensitivity disorders, is increasing.[34] Genomic studies are providing insight into the immunopathogenic mechanism underlying this disorder.[35,36] In a majority of pediatric patients, food allergy is a significant trigger, while in older patients this has been difficult to demonstrate.[37,38] A seasonal pattern in some patients has suggested a role for swallowed aeroallergens.[39]

Food protein-induced enterocolitis syndrome (FPIES), which presents with repetitive vomiting about 2 to 3 hours following allergen ingestion, appears to be becoming more common and is being attributed to an increasing list of foods.[40] Milk and soy were most often responsible in the past, but now grains, meats,

Clinical Criteria for Diagnosing Anaphylaxis

Anaphylaxis is highly likely when any one of the following 3 criteria are fulfilled:

1. Acute onset of an illness (minutes to several hours) with involvement of the skin, mucosal tissue, or both (e.g. generalized hives, pruritus or flushing, swollen lips-tongue-uvula)

   And at least one of the following:
   - Respiratory compromise (e.g. dyspnea, wheeze-bronchospasm, stridor, reduced PEF, hypoxemia)
   - Reduced BP or associated symptoms of end-organ dysfunction (e.g. hypotonia [collapse], syncope, incontinence)

2. Two or more of the following that occur rapidly after exposure to a likely allergen for that patient (minutes to several hours):
   - Involvement of the skin-mucosal tissue (e.g. generalized hives, itch-flush, swollen lips-tongue-uvula)
   - Respiratory compromise (e.g. dyspnea, wheeze-bronchospasm, stridor, reduced PEF, hypoxemia)
   - Reduced BP or associated symptoms (e.g. hypotonia [collapse], syncope, incontinence)
   - Persistent gastrointestinal symptoms (e.g. crampy abdominal pain, vomiting)

3. Reduced BP after exposure to known allergen for that patient (minutes to several hours):
   - Infants and children: low systolic BP (age specific) or greater than 30% decrease in systolic BP*
   - Adults: systolic BP of less than 90 mm Hg or greater than 30% decrease from that person's baseline

*Low systolic BP for children is less than 70 mmHg from one month to one year, less than (70 mmHg + [2 times age]) from 1–10 years and less than 90 mmHg from 11–17 years.
PEF: peak expiratory flow; *BP*: blood pressure
From: Sampson HA et al. Second symposium on the definition and management of anaphylaxis: summary report. Second National Institute of Allergy and Infectious Disease/Food Allergy and Anaphylaxis Network symposium. J Allergy Clin Immunol 2006;117(2):391–397.

fruits and vegetables are increasingly the cause of these reactions.[41]

Toxic Reactions

The prototypic toxic adverse reaction to food is food poisoning. Bacterial contamination commonly provokes nausea, abdominal cramping and diarrhea, whereas scrombroid fish poisoning is less common and closely mimics an allergic reaction to food. In addition to the GI symptoms that occur, individuals may present with flushing, urticaria, angioedema and respiratory symptoms.

Non-toxic Reactions

The most common non-toxic adverse food reactions are the carbohydrate malabsorption/intolerance conditions. The most common of these is lactose intolerance due to the relative deficiency of lactase in the gut brush border. This condition is commonly confused with milk allergy, and often patients have completely eliminated milk products from their diets when some amounts of dairy would be easily tolerated. In children, this may occur following a bout of gastroenteritis, but remits in most cases.

In young children, chronic or persistent diarrhea may be due to carbohydrate malabsorption caused by fructose in fruits and fruit juices. When fruit and juice are removed from the diet, the diarrhea, which typically is acidic and may provoke a 'scalded' skin appearance in the perianal area, resolves promptly.

Psychological Reactions

Many individuals have strongly held beliefs about their adverse food reactions or those of their children. Children generally do not believe that they will react to a food unless they have had clear symptoms from food ingestion that they can recall. Sometimes they do develop aversions to foods that have been withheld from the diet for a long time and for which they have never acquired a taste. In addition, children who outgrow their food allergies may continue to have an aversion to the previously proscribed food. In contrast, some children are placed on restricted diets due to parents' strongly held beliefs. Occasionally these diets are so restrictive that they lead to malnutrition. This can reach the point of Munchausen's disease by proxy in which the parents are convinced that a diet change has altered behavior or a subjective symptom.[42]

Evaluation

History

In the evaluation of adverse reactions to food, acquiring a thorough history is crucial to all steps that follow: laboratory testing, food challenges, education and ultimately treatments that are under development. The history must contain sufficient details to be certain that the symptoms are truly due to the putative food, the severity can be assessed, testing can be directed specifically to likely food culprits, and food challenges can be arranged that are likely to reproduce the suspected reaction. The history should include the following: detailed and sequential report of all the symptoms and signs; the timing from ingestion to onset of symptoms; the frequency of occurrence with each suspected food culprit and also the possibility that the particular food has been ingested without provoking symptoms; the quantity of food eliciting the symptoms and if possible a 'threshold' below which no symptoms have occurred; and associated factors such as exercise (food-dependent, exercise-induced anaphylaxis), medication and alcohol consumption. It is also helpful to ascertain whether products with advisory food labeling have been consumed and whether any of these have triggered symptoms.

A history of anaphylaxis increases the need for accurate diagnosis. Records from emergency department visits can be helpful in determining the severity of the reported reaction. In these patients it is crucial to accurately identify the correct food(s) because if the reaction is attributed to the wrong food, life-threatening reactions may recur. In cases of apparent 'idiopathic anaphylaxis', a search for all possible culprits (e.g. spices) may be justified.

Physical Examination

The physical examination of potentially food allergic children may reveal stigmata to support the diagnosis, for example, atopic dermatitis and possibly urticaria in an acute situation. Children with food reactions that trigger GI symptoms often do not have any physical findings when seen for evaluation. If there appears to be malnutrition and failure to thrive, specific testing for other causes should be carried out. Failure to thrive as a symptom of food allergy is very rare unless the child's diet has been severely limited and is nutritionally inadequate.

Respiratory signs may be seen if the food culprit(s) has been ingested recently, but isolated asthma or chronic upper or lower airway symptoms are rarely due to food allergy. When chest symptoms occur as a result of a food reaction, they are often abrupt in onset and accompanied by cutaneous and/or GI symptoms. Rarely, chronic respiratory symptoms are provoked when a food allergen is ingested on a regular basis in the diet.

Laboratory Studies

Skin Testing

Skin testing by the prick/puncture technique is now well established as a cost-effective method of identifying specific IgE antibody to food allergens. Glycerinated extracts are available for many foods as 1:10 or 1:20 weight/volume dilutions. These are placed on the skin accompanied by appropriate positive (histamine) and negative (diluent) controls. The skin is then punctured with one of several devices available for skin testing. Food allergens eliciting wheal diameters at least 3 mm larger than those produced by the negative control are interpreted as positive, while smaller responses are considered negative. The negative predictive accuracies for a few specific food allergens are greater than 95%, so a negative prick skin test (PST) essentially excludes IgE-mediated food hypersensitivity. The converse is not true. The positive predictive accuracy of a positive skin test for many foods is ≤50%, thus indicating the presence of IgE antibody but not confirming a diagnosis of symptomatic food hypersensitivity.[43,44] Several studies suggest that the larger the skin test mean wheal diameter, e.g. >8 mm, the more likely a patient will experience a reaction to that food.[45] When there is a history of a severe or anaphylactic reaction to an isolated food and the skin test is positive, the positive test to the implicated food may be viewed as diagnostic. There *are rare* reports of adverse reactions to PSTs, and most of these are due to aeroallergen extracts.[46] If there is concern about a patient being exquisitely sensitive, the extract can be diluted before applying.

For children less than 3 years of age, the negative predictive accuracy of PSTs is not quite as high (80–85%) as in older children. In this age group, the level of sensitization or reactivity of cutaneous mast cells may be too low to detect by skin testing test. Hill and colleagues have reported that PST wheals ≥8 mm are diagnostic of clinical reactivity in infants and children ≤2 years of age.[45,47] However, skin test results are quite variable since the outcome is dependent upon the reagents utilized (which are not standardized) and the personnel applying and interpreting the test. In a slightly older group of children, Wainstein and colleagues reported that PST wheals >8 mm had a somewhat lower specificity and cautioned that tests may need to be interpreted carefully by practitioners in the context of their own patient population.[48] Kagan and colleagues evaluated a group of 47 children with a positive skin test to a peanut extract (wheal >3 mm), but no known history of peanut ingestion. Only 23 (49%) of the food challenges were positive, confirming that skin tests alone cannot be used to prescribe elimination diets.[49]

The choice of appropriate food extracts to use is based upon the history. It is recommended that only food allergens suspected of provoking symptoms, rather than a 'panel of foods', be utilized in the evaluation. This prevents the common situation of finding numerous positive skin tests in highly atopic children, who tolerate many of the foods to which they may skin test positive.

Some food allergen extracts are more reliable than others. Extracts for peanut, the major tree nuts, egg, milk, and fish can be produced so that they give predictable results in skin testing. Many commercial extracts of fruits and vegetables are not reliable for detecting antibody in the skin. For these foods, use of fresh food is a more reliable means of detecting IgE antibody. The technique is referred to as the 'prick to prick' technique whereby the food is pricked with the skin testing device and then the patient's skin is punctured.

A number of variables must be considered when performing PSTs: (1) commercially prepared extracts frequently lack the labile proteins responsible for IgE-mediated sensitivity to most fruits and vegetables;[50-52] (2) skin testing on skin surfaces that have been treated with topical steroids for atopic dermatitis may induce smaller wheals than tests performed on untreated surfaces; (3) negative PSTs with commercially prepared extracts that do not support convincing histories of food allergic reactions should be repeated with the fresh food prior to concluding that food allergen-specific IgE is absent; and (4) long-term, high-dose systemic corticosteroid therapy may reduce allergen-induced wheal size. Some nuts for which there are no commercially available extracts may be ground with a mortar and pestle and mixed with diluent and then applied to the skin. This same technique may be used for other substances when no commercial extracts are available, e.g. spices. Use of these nonstandardized preparations is most helpful when they are positive. A negative test requires a challenge to exonerate the putative culprit as an offender.

In Vitro Testing

In vitro immunoassays for food allergens have gained wide popularity and usage in the last few years by both allergists and nonspecialists. Radioallergosorbent tests (RAST) that used radioactive reagents have been replaced by various immunoassays that use liquid or solid phase reagents. The Phadia ImmunoCAP® assay has been correlated with blinded food challenges to a few selected foods: peanut, egg, milk, fish, and to some degree tree nuts. These studies have shown a correlation between the level of allergen-specific IgE and the probability of clinical reactivity, but without a history of a suspected allergic reaction, a 'diagnostic' level alone cannot be used to diagnose a food allergy.

In vitro measurements are preferred in a number of situations: (1) patients with extensive dermatographism; (2) patients with extensive skin disease (atopic dermatitis or urticaria); (3) patients who cannot discontinue antihistamines; and more recently (4) use by nonspecialists who do not perform skin testing to evaluate children for potential food allergy. The test measures the quantity of circulating allergen-specific IgE to individual foods and is reported as kilounits of allergen-specific IgE antibody per liter (kU_A/l). (Many laboratories also report 'Class Levels', which are based on the old RAST classification system and have not been correlated with food challenge outcomes.) While the in vitro tests have been considered less sensitive than skin tests, one study comparing serum IgE levels with double-blind, placebo-controlled food challenges (DBPCFCs) found prick-puncture skin tests and immunoassays to have similar sensitivities and specificities.[48]

In two studies (one retrospective and one prospective) utilizing the CAP-System Fluorescent Enzyme Immunoassay™ in children, Sampson used receiver operating characteristic (ROC) curves and first demonstrated that quantification of food-specific

Table 45-2 Predictive Value of Food-Specific IgE

Allergen	Decision Point [kU$_A$/L]	Rechallenge Value
Egg	≥7.0	≤1.5
≤2 yrs old[56]	≥2.0	
Milk	≥15.0	≤7.0
≤2 yrs old[57]	≥5.0	
Peanut	≥14.0	≤5.0
Fish	≥20.0	
Tree nuts[63,64]	≥15.0	<2

Note: Patients with food-specific IgE values less than the listed diagnostic values may experience an allergic reaction following challenge. Unless history strongly suggests tolerance, a physician-supervised food challenge should be performed to determine if the child can ingest the food safely.
Adapted from Sampson HA, Ho DG. Relationship between food-specific IgE concentrations and the risk of positive food challenges in children and adolescents. J Allergy Clin Immunol 1997;100:444–451; Sampson HA. Utility of food-specific IgE concentrations in predicting symptomatic food allergy. J Allergy Clin Immunol 2001;107:891–896.

IgE provided increased positive predictive accuracies for egg, milk, peanut, and fish hypersensitivity compared to PSTs.[53,54] It was concluded that individuals with a history of a food allergic reaction and a serum food allergen-specific IgE level in excess of the '95% decision points' may be considered reactive, and that an oral food challenge would not be needed for further confirmation. A patient with a food allergen-specific IgE less than the 95% predictive value may be reactive, and would require a food challenge to confirm the diagnosis. In addition, recent data suggests that monitoring the allergen-specific IgE values may be useful in predicting when follow-up challenges are likely to be negative, i.e. when patients 'outgrow' their food allergy.[55] For young children, it has been shown that the 'decision points' are lower for milk and egg, but there are important caveats to all these studies that relate to the population under study (Table 45-2).[56,57] In addition, it has been reported that the rate of fall of the serum IgE levels may be a good predictor of when challenges are appropriate. Recent studies have supported the contention that lower levels are associated with earlier resolution of food allergy and that these children may have a 'different' phenotype of food allergy than most children with higher allergen-specific IgE levels.[58-62]

The data above primarily apply to milk, egg, peanut, and to some extent fish allergies, but values for individual fish have not been established. More recently, investigators have found relative diagnostic decision points for tree nuts, which may be useful for establishing appropriate dietary restrictions and food challenges.[63,64] Fleischer's studies suggest that for levels of tree nut allergens below 2 kU$_A$/l, food challenges are reasonable, while levels above 5 kU$_A$/l suggest that reactions are likely enough to consider postponing challenges. Studies suggest that 20% of young peanut allergic patients and about 10% of tree nut allergic children outgrow their allergy, and monitoring allergen-specific IgE may be useful in predicting which children are likely to lose their food allergy. Finally, Knight and colleagues have reported that a combination of skin test size and serum antibody levels to egg white may help clinicians determine the appropriate time for food challenge.[65]

At this time, there are no rigorously controlled studies demonstrating that IgG immunoassays have any clinical utility for diagnosing food allergy. In fact, most individuals make IgG antibodies to the foods they ingest.[66] Serum food-specific IgG levels may be elevated in disorders affecting protein absorption, such as celiac disease and inflammatory bowel disease.

A new line of investigation involves the examination of various epitopes for specific food allergens and their relationships to the persistence or loss of clinical food allergy. It has been found that antibodies to sequential (linear) epitopes are more likely to be associated with persistence of food allergy to specific foods than detection of antibodies to conformational epitopes.[67-73] Peptide microarray technology is being used to characterize patient heterogeneity and possibly more accurately predict clinically significant food allergy as opposed to allergen sensitization without clinical reactivity.[74-77]

Other Tests

Oral Labial Tests

Rance and colleagues have been studying the efficacy of diagnosing food hypersensitivity by applying food extracts to the inner lip of the oral mucosa.[78] However, the predictive accuracy of this approach needs further investigation.

Atopy Patch Test

The atopy patch test is used as a means to identify non-IgE-mediated allergy. Initially it was used for inhalant allergen testing and then expanded for use in conditions involving atopic dermatitis and adverse reactions to foods;[79] see Chapter 49.

Other Laboratory Measurements

Serum tryptase has been proposed for use as a marker of anaphylaxis, and it has proven useful for validating drug and insect sting-induced anaphylactic reactions, but not for food-induced anaphylactic reactions.[80] Vadas and colleagues have looked at platelet-activating factor (PAF) levels and PAF acetylhydrolase activity in peanut allergic patients. Their study suggested that PAF may be an important mediator of severe anaphylaxis in man, primarily due to decreased PAF acetylhydrolyase activity and inadequate PAF inactivation.[81]

Food Challenges

The double-blind, placebo-controlled food challenge (DBPCFC) is recognized as the 'gold standard' for the accurate diagnosis of adverse reactions to food. It may be conducted in various formats to investigate any potential allergic reactions and provides a standard by which to compare other diagnostic tests and determine the efficacy of various treatments. In the clinical setting, the open food challenge, which is less time consuming and costly, is often used to make the diagnosis of food allergy, but care should be taken to assure that the diagnostic accuracy is not being jeopardized for the sake of expediency.

Open Food Challenges

Open food challenges are very useful to exclude food allergy. For example, a young child allergic to milk or egg, who during skin testing is found to have a positive test for peanut even though the child has never knowingly consumed peanut, may be challenged openly under observation so that in the unlikely event of symptoms occurring, they may be treated promptly.[82] In other cases, children may have a vague history of an adverse reaction to a food, but the history or a food diary suggests that the food has been ingested in another food regularly consumed in the

Single-Blind Food Challenges (SBFC)

Single-blind food challenges (SBFCs) are useful in daily clinical allergy practice. They are less time consuming than DBPCFCs and usually provide an excellent diagnostic aid in confirming or refuting histories of adverse reactions to food. In circumstances in which patient opinions or concerns may influence the outcome, the SBFC offers an alternative that will be convincing to most patients and physicians. For immediate symptoms the challenge is administered in a graded fashion over a period of 1 to 2 hours (see below) and then the individual is observed for an additional 2 to 4 hours, depending upon the occurrence of symptoms. The SBFC is especially helpful in shortening a long list of suspected food allergens that are not amenable to open challenge, leaving the DBPCFC for investigating reactions that are more difficult to confirm or refute.

Double-Blind, Placebo-Controlled Food Challenges

The DBPCFC is the 'gold standard' for detecting any suspected permutation of adverse food reactions if the challenge is planned correctly.[83-91] The food challenge is designed to reproduce the individual's history. One approach is to have the active food challenge and the placebo challenge done on separate days. Unfortunately, time constraints and reimbursement policies have rendered this approach less practical in the clinical setting. To decrease the time and number of visits to establish the diagnosis, two food challenges are often administered on the same day. One challenge (active or placebo) is administered in the morning and the other is provided in the afternoon (at least a few hours after the end of the morning challenge). A potential limitation of this approach occurs when a slow or delayed onset of symptoms occurs and may be misinterpreted as a response to the second challenge or missed, making interpretation of the results difficult. In such cases, the challenge must be repeated using separate days for the active food and placebo challenges. When multiple foods are being challenged, some placebo challenges may be omitted if it is found that another suspected food allergen does not elicit symptoms. When evaluating subjective symptoms it may be useful to interchange the active and placebo doses. The process may begin with the first one or two doses being placebos.

The quantity and timing of the challenge doses are determined by the patient history. Some authors recommend that the starting dose be about one half of the amount that is thought to be the minimum quantity likely to elicit the immediate onset of symptoms. Other investigators use a more specific dosing protocol so that every subject receives the same dose at set intervals. The timing of challenges must be arranged so that the interval between each challenge dose is long enough to allow symptoms to occur. This interval is determined from the history. The doses may be doubled at the chosen interval or some other increase in dosing may be chosen. When the challenge is negative with up to 8–10 grams of dried food in a single dose, or 60–100 grams of wet food in a single dose, the challenge is terminated. However, a negative challenge is not considered complete until the food being studied is consumed under observation in usual portions without eliciting symptoms. The ability of the child to ingest the incriminated food(s) without developing symptoms eliminates any concern about the effect of preparation and other variables inherent in the blinded food challenge. Administering an insuf-

ficient quantity of food during the oral challenge is the most likely variable to result in a reaction following a negative blinded challenge. Oral symptoms may be provoked during open feedings if the challenge vehicle prevents sufficient allergen contact with oral tissues. Positive subjective symptoms following a negative blinded challenge also may be due to the subject's strongly held belief that the food will cause symptoms. This is rarely a problem when challenging children.[92-94]

At the present time, many different vehicles are used for administering food challenges. Many of these mask the challenge food rather than completely blinding it; however, for research purposes, the subjects must not be able to discern the contents of the challenge or the results may not be valid. It is possible to hide large quantities of food in various vehicles without the active ingredient being detected. The placebo portion of the challenge may be another food of a similar texture to the challenge food and known to be tolerated by the individual.

For the practitioner wishing to design and carry out food challenges, there are a number of very helpful resources. For more general information, readers may consult Nowak-Wegzryn and colleagues[88] and A Health Professionals Guide to Food Challenges.[95] As noted in these publications, allergists who are equipped to administer allergen immunotherapy and treat systemic reactions are also equipped to treat reactions to food challenges.

Management (see Chapter 52)

In the last few years, a number of treatments for food-allergic individuals have entered clinical trials. Oral treatments include sublingual immunotherapy (SLIT) modeled on the approach being used for pollen allergy. Oral immunotherapy (OIT) has also been around for decades, but only recently, several uncontrolled and two placebo-controlled clinical trials have demonstrated 'desensitization' or partial desensitization to milk, egg and peanut.[96,97,98]

One of the more unusual approaches under investigation is the use of an herbal preparation by Li and colleagues.[99-103] This nine-herb preparation, termed Food Allergy Herbal Formula 2 (FAHF 2) has been shown to eliminate symptoms in a peanut-sensitized mouse model, and a recent phase I trial showed no adverse reactions in man.

Summary Approach

For the clinician evaluating children and adolescents for adverse reactions to food, there are several steps to be followed (Figure 45-1). First and most important is an accurate and detailed history. This allows the categorization of the symptoms into diagnostic categories, especially immediate vs delayed onset of symptoms. Once accomplished, the appropriate diagnostic tests may be chosen. For the specialist, it is recommended that skin testing be undertaken first, with the foods chosen for testing being determined by the history. If the history does not clearly direct the testing, a small panel of skin tests to common food allergens may be used, recognizing that atopic children may have positive skin tests that are not clinically relevant. It should be emphasized to families that skin testing measures the *possibility* more than the probability of clinically relevant food allergy. Serum IgE levels to some food allergens (e.g. egg, milk, peanut, fish, tree nuts) may be useful in further assessing foods provoking positive skin tests since allergen-specific IgE levels have been correlated with the probability of experiencing an allergic reac-

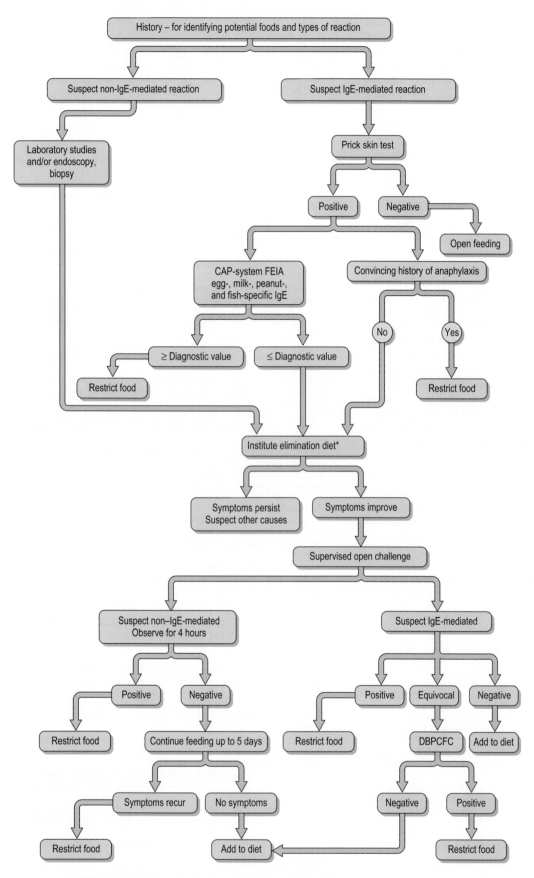

* Up to 2 weeks for IgE-mediated reactions; up to 8 weeks for non–IgE-mediated food hypersensitivity.

Figure 45-1 Algorithm diagnosing food hypersensitivity. *IgE*, immunoglobulin E; *DBPCFC*, double-blind, placebo-controlled food challenge.

tion to a food. Food challenges should then be arranged in cases where the history and laboratory studies do not confirm a diagnosis of food allergy. A program of food allergen avoidance should be outlined for foods that must be restricted. An annual visit to re-evaluate ongoing allergies, reinforce food allergen avoidance precautions, and review the proper use of self-injectable epinephrine is recommended. Periodic food challenges should be arranged based upon the interval history (accidental ingestion without symptoms), changes in skin tests and food-specific IgE levels, and natural history of various food allergies.

The Future

The future holds great promise for more accurate and less cumbersome diagnostic tools for food allergy. A number of promising therapies are in clinical trials and one or more are likely to be successful over time. However, a number of challenges remain to be addressed. Quality of life issues for parents, children and families as a whole have long been neglected. Orderly studies are now underway to develop instruments that may be used by busy clinicians to assess the impact of food allergy on families, which should enable physicians to anticipate and provide appropriate advice to families who may be having problems coping with food allergy issues. Another challenge is the growing practice of utilizing large panels of food allergens in blood tests to screen and diagnose food allergies, which has led to excessively restricted diets and in some cases, malnutrition. Allergists must continue to educate the public about food allergies and the appropriate way to diagnose and manage these disorders.

References

1. May CD. Objective clinical and laboratory studies of immediate hypersensitivity reactions to food in asthmatic children. J Allergy Clin Immunol 1976;58:500–15.
2. Sampson HA. Update on food allergy. J Allergy Clin Immunol 2004;113:805–19.
3. Johansson SG, Bieber T, Dahl R, et al. Revised nomenclature for allergy for global use: report of the nomenclature Review Committee of the World Allergy Organization, Oct 2003. J Allergy Clin Immunol 2004;113:832–6.
4. Eggesbo M, Halvorsen R, Tambs K, et al. Prevalence of parentally perceived adverse reaction to food in young children. Pediatr Allergy Immunol 1999;10:122–32.
5. Bock SA. Prospective appraisal of complaints of adverse reactions to foods in children during the first 3 years of life. Pediatrics 1987;79:683–8.
6. Dean T, Venter C, Pereira B, et al. Patterns of sensitization to food and aeroallergens in the first 3 years of life. J Allergy Clin Immunol 2007;120:1166–71.
7. Ostblom E, Lilja G, Pershagen G, et al. Phenotypes of food hypersensitivity and development of allergic disease during the first 9 years of life. Clin Exptl Allergy 2008;38:1325–32.
8. Venter C, Pereira B, Voigt K, et al. Prevalence and cumulative incidence of food hypersensitivity in the first 3 years of life. Allergy 2008;63:354–9.
9. Venter C, Pereira B, Grundy J, et al. Prevalence of sensitization reported and objectively assessed food hypersensitivity amongst six-year-old children: a population based study. Pediatr Allergy Immunol 2006;17:356–63.
10. Kagan R, Joseph L, Dufresne C, et al. Prevalence of peanut allergy in primary-school children in Montreal, Canada. J Allergy Clin Immunol 2003;112:1223–8.
11. Savage JH, Matsui E, Skripak JM, et al. The natural history of egg allergy. J Allergy Clin Immunol 2007;120:1413–7.
12. Skirpak J, Matsui EC, Mudd K, et al. The natural history of IgE-mediated cow's milk allergy. J Allergy Clin Immunol 2007;120:1172–7.
13. Sicherer SH, Sampson HA. Mini primer on allergic and immunologic diseases: food allergy J Allergy Clin Immunol 2010;123:S116–25.
14. Yocum MW, Butterfield JH, Klein JS, et al. Epidemiology of anaphylaxis in Olmstead County: a population-based study. J Allergy Clin Immunol 1999;104:452–6.
15. Decker WW, Campbell RL, Manivannan V, et al. The etiology and incidence of anaphylaxis in Rochester, Minnesota: a report from the Rochester Epidemiology Project. J Allergy Clin Immunol 2008;122:1161–5.
16. Goodman DL, McDonnell JT, Nelson HS, et al. Chronic urticaria exacerbated by the antioxidant food preservatives, butylated hydroxyanisole (BHA) and butylated hydroxytoluene(BHT). J Allergy Clin Immunol 1990;86:570–5.
17. Sampson HA, McCaskill CM. Food hypersensitivity and atopic dermatitis: evaluation of 113 patients. J Pediatr 1985;107:669–75.
18. Burks AW, Mallory SB, Williams L, et al. Atopic dermatitis: clinical relevance of food hypersensitivity reactions. J Pediatr 1988;113:447–51.
19. Sampson HA. Infantile colic and food allergy: fact or fiction. J Pediatr 1989;115:583–84.
20. Hill DJ, Hudson IL, Sheffield L, et al. A low allergen diet is a significant intervention in infantile colic: results of a community-based study. J Allergy Clin Immunol 1995;96:886–92.
21. Lucassen PLBJ, Assendelft WJJ, Bubbels JW, et al. Infantile colic crying time reduction with a whey hydrolysate: a double-blind randomized placebo-controlled trial. Pediatr 2000;106:1349–54.
22. Hill DJ, Roy N, Heine RG, et al. Effect of a low allergen maternal diet on colic among breastfed infants: a randomized, controlled trial. Pediatr 2005;116:709–15.
23. Iacono G, Cavataio F, Montalto G, et al. Intolerance of cow's milk and chronic constipation in children. N Engl J Med 1998;339:1100–04.
24. Daher S, Tahan S, Sole D, et al. Cow's milk protein intolerance and chronic constipation in children. Pediatr Allergy Immunol 2001;12:339–42.
25. Wang J. Oral allergy syndrome in food allergy, adverse reactions to foods and food additives. In: Metcalfe DD, Sampson HA, Simon RA, editors. Malden MA: Blackwell Publishing; 2008, p. 133–43.
26. Roberts G, Patel N, Levi-Schaffer F, et al. Food allergy as a risk factor for life-threatening asthma in childhood: a case controlled study. J Allergy Clin Immunol 2003;112:168–74.
27. Schroeder A, Kumar R, Pongracic JA, et al. Food allergy is associated with an increased risk of asthma. Clin Exptl Allergy 2009;39:261–70.
28. Bock SA, Munoz-Furlong A, Sampson HA. Fatalities due to anaphylactic reactions to foods. J Allergy Clin Immunol 2001;107:101–3.
29. Bock SA, Munoz-Furlong A, Sampson HA. Further fatalities caused by anaphylactic reactions to foods, 2001–2006. J Allergy Clin Immunol 2007;119:1016–18.
30. Pumphrey RSH, Stanworth SJ. The clinical spectrum of anaphylaxis in north-west England. Clin Exptl Allergy 1996;26:1364–70.
31. Pumphrey RS, Gowland MH. Further fatal allergic reactions to food in the United Kingdom, 199–2006. J Allergy Clin Immunol 2007;119:1018–9.
32. Sampson HA, Munoz-Furlong A, Campbell RL, et al. Second Symposium on the definition and management of anaphylaxis: Summary report – Second National Institute of Allergy and Infectious Disease/Food Allergy and Anaphylaxis Network symposium. J Allergy Clin Immunol 2006;117:391–7.
33. Green PHR, Cellier C. Celiac disease. N Engl J Med 2007;357:1731–43.
34. Guajardo JR, Plotnick LM, Fende JM, et al. Eosinophil-associated gastrointestinal disorders: a world-wide-web based registry. J Pediatr 2002;141:576–81.
35. Blanchard C, Wang N, Stringer KF, et al. Eotaxin-3 and a uniquely conserved gene-expression profile in eosinophilic esophagitis. J Clin Invest 2006;116:536–47.
36. Chehade M, Sampson HA, Morotti RA, et al. Esophagal subepithelial fibrosis in children with eosinophilic esophagitis. J Ped Gastroent Nutr 2007;45:319–28.
37. Kelly KJ, Lasenby AJ, Rowe PC, et al. Eosinophilic esophagitis attributed to gastroesophageal reflux: improvement with an amino acid-based formula. Gastroenterology 1995;109:1503–12.
38. Liacouras CA, Spergel JM, Ruchelli E, et al. Eosinophilic Esophagitis: A 10-year experience in 381 children. Clin Gastroent Hepatol 2005;3:1198–206.
39. Mishra A, Hogan SP, Brandt EB, et al. An etiological role for aeroallergens and eosinophils in experimental esophagitis. J Clin Invest 2001;107:83–90.
40. Sicherer SH. Food protein induced enterocolitis: case presentations and management lessons. J Allergy Clin Immunol 2005;115:149–56.
41. Nowak-Wegrzyn A, Sampson HA, Wood RA, et al. Food protein-induced enterocolitis syndrome caused by solid food proteins. Pediatrics 2003;111:829–35.
42. Roesler TA, Barry PC, Bock SA. Factitious food allergy and failure to thrive. Arch Pediatr Adolesc Med 1994;148:1150–55.
43. Sampson HA. Food allergy. Part 1. Immunopathogenesis and clinical disorders. J Allergy Clin Immunol 1999;103:717–29.
44. Sampson HA. Food allergy. Part 2. Diagnosis and management. J Allergy Clin Immunol 1999;103:981–89.

45. Hill DJ, Heine RG, Hosking CS. The diagnostic value of skin prick testing in children with food allergy. Pediatr Allergy Immunol 2004;15: 435–41.

46. Liccardi G, D'Amato D, Canonica GW, et al. Systemic reactions from skin testing: literature review. J Investig Allergol Clin Immunol 2006;16: 75–8.

47. Hill DJ, Hosking CS, Reyes-Benito MLV. Reducing the need for food allergen challenges in young children: comparison of in vitro with in vivo tests. Clin Exp Allergy 2001;31:1031–5.

48. Wainstein BK, Yee A, Jelley D, et al. Combining skin prick, immediate skin application and specific IgE testing in the diagnosis of peanut allergy in children. Pediatr Allergy Immunol 2007;18:231–9.

49. Kagan R, Hayami D, Lawrence J, et al. The predictive value of a positive prick skin test to peanut in atopic, peanut-naive children. Ann Allergy Asthma Immunol 2003;90;640–45.

50. Ortolani C, Ispano M, Pastorello EA, et al. Comparison of results of skin prick tests (with fresh foods and commercial food extracts) and RAST in 100 patients with oral allergy syndrome. J Allergy Clin Immunol 1989;83:683–90.

51. Pastorello E, Ortolani C, Farioli L, et al. Allergenic cross-reactivity among peach, apricot, plum, and cherry in patients with oral allergy syndrome: an in vivo and in vitro study. J Allergy Clin Immunol 1994;94:699–707.

52. Rance F, Juchet A, Bremont F, et al. Correlations between skin prick tests using commercial extracts and fresh foods, specific IgE, and food challenges. Allergy 1997;52:1031–5.

53. Sampson HA, Ho DG. Relationship between food-specific IgE concentrations and the risk of positive food challenges in children and adolescents. J Allergy Clin Immunol 1997;100:444–51.

54. Sampson HA. Utility of food-specific IgE concentrations in predicting symptomatic food allergy. J Allergy Clin Immunol 2001;107:891–6.

55. Sicherer SH, Sampson HA. Cow's milk protein-specific IgE concentrations in two age groups of milk-allergic children and in children achieving clinical tolerance. Clin Exp Allergy 1999;29:507–12.

56. Boyano-Martinez T, Garcia-Ara C. Diaz-Pena JM, et al. Validity of specific IgE antibodies in children with egg allergy. Clin Exp Allergy 2001;31:1464–69.

57. Garcia-Ara C, Boyano-Martinez T, Diaz-Pena JM, et al. Specific IgE levels in the diagnosis of immediate hypersensitivity to cows' milk protein in the infant. J Allergy Clin Immunol 2001;107:185–90.

58. van der Gugten A, den Otter M, Meijer Y, et al. Usefulness of specific IgE levels in predicting cow's milk allergy. J Allergy Clin Immunol 2008;121:631–3.

59. Shek LPC, Soderstrom L, Ahlstedt S, et al. Determination of food specific IgE levels over time can predict the development of tolerance in cow's milk and hens' egg allergy. J Allergy Clin Immunol 2004;114: 387–91.

60. Rottem M, Shostak D, Foldi S. The predictive value of specific immunoglobulin E on the outcome of milk allergy. Israel Med Assn J 2008;10; 862–64.

61. Perry TT, Matsui EC, Conover-Walker MK, et al. The relationship of allergen specific IgE levels and oral food challenge outcome. J Allergy Clin Immunol 2004;113:144–9.

62. Fleischer DM, Conover-Walker MK, Christie L, et al. The natural progression of peanut allergy resolution and the possibility of recurrence. J Allergy Clin Immunol 2003;112:183–9.

63. Fleischer DM, Conover-Walker MK, Matsui EC, et al. The natural history of tree nut allergy. J Allergy Clin Immunol 2005;116: 1087–93.

64. Maloney JM, Rudengren M, Ahlstedt S, et al. The use of serum-specific IgE measurements for the diagnosis of peanut, tree nut, and seed allergy. J Allergy Clin Immunol 2008;122:145–51.

65. Knight AK, Shreffler WG, Sampson HA, et al. Skin prick test to egg white provides additional diagnositic utility to serum egg white-specific IgE antibody concentration in children. J Allergy Clin Immunol 2006;117: 842–7.

66. Stapel SO, Asero R, Ballmer-Weber BK, et al. Testing for IgG4 against foods is not recommended as a diagnostic tool. EAACI task force report. Allergy 2008;63;793–6.

67. Vila L, Beyer K, Jarvinen K-M, et al. Role of conformational and linear epitopes in the achievement of tolerance in cow's milk allergy. Clin Exptl Allergy 2001;31:1599–606.

68. Chatchatee P, Jarvinen K-M, Bardina L, et al. Identification of IgE-and IgG binding epitopes on αs1-casein: differences in patients with persistent and transient cow's milk allergy. J Allergy Clin Immunol 2001;107: 379–83.

69. Chatchatee P, Jarvinen KM, Bardina L, et al. Identification of IgE and IgG binding epitopes on beta- and kappa-casein in cow's milk allergic patients. Clin Exptl Allergy 2001;31:1256–62.

70. Jarvinen KM, Beyer K, Vila L, et al. B cell epitopes as a screening instrument for persistent cow's milk allergy. J Allergy Clin Immunol 2002;110: 293–7.

71. Cocco RR, Jarvinen K-M, Sampson HA, et al. Mutational analysis of major, sequential IgE-binding epitopes in α s1-casein, a major cow's milk allergen. J Allergy Clin Immunol 2003;112:433–7.

72. Jarvinen K-M, Beyer K, Vila L, et al. Specificity of IgE antibodies to sequential epitopes of hen's egg ovomucoid as a marker for persistence of egg allergy. Allergy 2007;62:758–65.

73. Cocco RR, Marvinen KM, Han N, et al. Mutational analysis of immunoglobulin E-binding epitopes of beta-casein and beta-lactoglobulin showed a heterogeneous pattern of critical amino acids between individual patients and pooled sera. Clin Exptl Allergy 2007;35:831–8.

74. Shreffler WG, Beyer K, Chu T-HT, et al. Microarray immunoassay: association of clinical history, in vitro IgE function, and heterogeneity of allergenic peanut epitopes. J Allergy Clin Immunol 2004:113: 446–82.

75. Shreffler WG, Lencer DA, Bardina L, et al. IgE and IgG4 epitope mapping by microarray immunoassay reveals the diversity of immune response to the peanut allergen, Ara h 2. J Allergy Clin Immunol 2005;116:893–9.

76. Beyer K, Ellman-Grunther L, Jarvinen K-M, et al. Measurement of peptide-specific IgE as an additional tool in identifying patients with clinical reactivity to peanuts. J Allergy Clin Immunol 2003;112:202–7.

77. Cerecedo I, Zamora J, Shreffler WG, et al. Mapping of the IgE and IgG4 sequential epitopes of milk allergens with a peptide microarray-based immunoassay. J Allergy Clin Immunol 2008;122:589–94.

78. Rance F, Dutau G. Labial food challenge in children with food allergy. Ped Allergy Immunol 1997;8:41–4.

79. Turjanmaa K, Darsow U, Niggemann B, et al. EAACI/GA²LEN Position paper: present status of the aopty patch test. Allergy 2006;61:1377–84.

80. Sampson HA, Mendelson L, Rosen JP. Fatal and near-fatal anaphylactic reaction to food in children and adolescents. N Engl J Med 1992;327: 380–4.

81. Vadas P, Gold M, Perelman B, et al. Platelet activating factor, PAF acetyl-hydrolase and severe anaphylaxis. N Engl J Med 2008;358:28–35.

82. Mankad VS, Williams LW, Lee LA, et al. Safety of open food challenges in the office setting. Ann Allergy Asthma Immunol 2008;100:469–74.

83. Niggemann B, Beyer K. Diagnosis of food allergy in children: toward a standardization of food challenge. J Pediatr Gastroenterol Nutr 2007;45:399–404.

84. Niggemann B, Beyer K. Pitfalls in double-blind placebo controlled oral food challenges. Allergy 2007;62;729–32.

85. Chinchilli VM, Fisher L, Craig TJ. Statistical issues in clinical trials that involve the double-blind, placebo-controlled food challenge. J Allergy Clin Immunol 2005;115:592–7.

86. Bock SA, Sampson HA, Atkins FM, et al. Double blind placebo controlled food challenge (DBPCFC) as an office procedure: a manual. J Allergy Clin Immunol 1988;82:986–97.

87. Sicherer SH. Food allergy: when and how to perform oral food challenges. Pediatr Allergy Immunol 1999;10:226–34.

88. Nowak-Wegrzyn A, Assa'ad AH, Bahna SL, et al. Oral food challenge: a working group report. J Allergy Clin Immunol 2009;123;S365–83.

89. Vlieg-Boerstra BJ, Bijleveld CMA, van der Heide S, et al. Development and validation of challenge materials for double-blind, placebo-controlled food challenges in children. J Allergy Clin Immunol 2004;113: 341–6.

90. Vlieg-Boerstra BJ, van der Heide S, Bijleveld CMA, et al. Placebo reactions in double-blind placebo-controlled food challenges in children. Allergy 2007;62:905–12.

91. Huijbers GB, Colen AAM, Jansen JJN, et al. Masking foods for food challenge: practical aspects of masking foods for a double-blind, placebo-controlled food challenge. J Am Dietetic Assn 1994;94:645–9.

92. Bock SA, Atkins FM. Patterns of food hypersensitivity during 16 years of double-blind placebo-controlled food challenges. J Pediatr 1990;117: 561–7.

93. Caffarelli C, Petroccione T. False-negative food challenges in children with suspect food allergy. Lancet 2001;358:1871–2.

94. Sampson HA. Use of food-challenge tests in children. Lancet 2001;358: 1832–3.

95. A Health Professional's Guide to Food Challenges. (Mofedi S & Bock SA eds) 2009 (revised). FairFax, VA: The Food Allergy and Anaphylaxis Network.

96. Enrique E, Pineda F, Malek T, et al. Sublingual immunotherapy for hazelnut food allergy: a randomized double blind placebo controlled study with standardized hazelnut extract. J Allergy Clin Immunol 2005:116:1073–9.

97. Skripak J, Nash SD, Rowley H, et al. A randomized double-blind, placebo controlled study of milk oral immunotherapy for cow's milk allergy. J Allergy Clin Immunol 2008;122:1154–60.

98. Jones SM, Pons L, Roberts JL, et al. Clinical efficacy and immune regulation with peanut oral immunotherapy. J Allergy Clin Immunol 2009;124:292–300 (e97).

99. Li X-M, Zhang T-F, Huang C-K, et al. Food Allergy Herbal Forumla-1 (FAHF-1) blocks peanut induced anaphylaxis in a murine model. J Allergy Clin Immunol 2001;108:639–46.

100. Srivastava KD, Kattan JD, Zou ZM, et al. The Chinese herbal medicine formula FAHF-2 completely blocks anaphylactic reactions in a murine model of peanut allergy. J Allergy Clin Immunol 2005;115:171–8.

101. Qu C, Srivastava K, Ko J, et al. Induction of tolerance after establishment of peanut allergy in the food allergy herbal formula FAHF2 is associated with the up-regulation of interferon-γ. Clin Exptl Allergy 2007;37: 846–55.

102. Kattan JD, Srivastava KD, Zou ZM, et al. Pharmacological and immuno-logical effects of individual herbs in the food allergy herbal formula-2 (FAHF-2) on peanut allergy. Phytother Res 2008;22:651–9.

103. Li X-M, Brown L. Efficacy and mechanisms of action of traditional Chinese medicines for treating asthma and allergy. J Allergy Clin Immunol 2009;123:297–306.

CHAPTER

46

Approach to Feeding Problems in the Infant and Young Child

Arne Høst • Susanne Halken

For the past three decades, an increasing awareness of food allergy has emerged in Western industrialized societies where confirmed food allergy seems to affect around 6% of young children and 3–4% of adults.[1] However, the public perceives food allergy to be much more common.[2,3] Given the public's frequent misperception that various mild symptoms are caused by food-induced allergic reactions, performing a careful evaluation and correct diagnostic procedures is imperative to avoid over-diagnosis, which may lead to malnutrition, eating disorders and psychosocial problems, as well as family disruption.[1-3] In contrast, under-diagnosis may result in unnecessary symptoms, growth failure and physical impairment.

True food allergies (i.e. immune-mediated reactions) are most often immunoglobulin E (IgE)-mediated reactions, which are the most thoroughly investigated type of food allergy. However, recent evidence indicates that non-IgE-mediated reactions may play a major role in delayed reactions.[1] It is evident that a correct classification of an adverse reaction to foods will depend on the extent and the quality of the diagnostic tests and procedures performed. For nonscientific purposes, the diagnosis of an adverse reaction to food will often be based solely on the result of elimination and challenge procedures.

No single laboratory test is diagnostic of food allergy. Therefore, the diagnosis has to be based on strict, well-defined food elimination and challenge procedures, preferably double-blind placebo-controlled food challenges (DBPCFCs) in children older than 2 to 3 years of age.[4,5] In infants, open, controlled challenges have been shown to be reliable when performed under professional observation in a hospital setting or a clinic.[6,7] Food allergy is primarily a problem in infancy and early childhood. Most often the infants develop food allergies in the same order as that in which the foods have been introduced into the diet. Thus the prevalence of reactions to different foods depends in part on the eating habits of a given population.[8]

This review concentrates on gastrointestinal symptoms, which may cause suspicion of food allergy in early childhood, focusing on indications for food allergy evaluation. Specific disease entities, such as enterocolitis, proctocolitis, enteropathies and allergic eosinophilic esophagitis/gastroenterocolitis, are discussed in other chapters (see Chapters 48 and 49).

Frequency

In prospective studies, the incidence of cow's milk protein allergy (CMPA) during the first year of life has been estimated to be about 2–3% based on strict diagnostic criteria, as reviewed by Høst.[9] Other common food allergens in children are egg, peanuts, tree nuts, soy, fish and cereals. The total cumulated incidence of food protein allergy during the first 3 years of life has been found to be about 6%.[10,11] In a recent prospective birth cohort study, the point prevalence of food allergy at 3 years was 2.3%.[3]

Adverse reactions to *food additives* have been demonstrated in school children to affect less than 1% of unselected children when using DBPCFCs.[12] The most common positive reaction was worsening of atopic eczema and urticaria in atopic children. Among children with atopic symptoms referred to hospital allergy clinics,[13] 23% of 335 were suspected of food additive intolerance. However, only 7% reacted to food additive on open challenge and only 2% had reproducible reactions when DBPCFCs were performed. Recent studies indicate that artificial colors and/or preservatives (sodium benzoate) in the diet may result in a dose-dependent increased hyperactivity in 3-year-old and 8- to 9-year-old children in the general population.[14]

In children with symptoms suggestive of food allergy, it has been possible to confirm the diagnosis in only about one third by means of controlled elimination/challenge procedures.[2,9,10]

Age at Onset of Symptoms

The age at which symptoms start depends on the time of introduction of the foods; infants frequently develop food allergies in the same order as that in which the foods have been introduced into the diet. Many prospective studies have demonstrated that symptoms in CMPA develop in early infancy, rarely after 12 months of age.[9] The onset of disease is, in most cases, closely related to the time of introduction of cow's milk-based formula. Allergies against fruit and juice often have a later age of onset.[10] In a Spanish study[8] of 355 children (mean age, 5.4 years), allergy to milk, egg, and fish began predominantly before the second year, demonstrating a clear relationship with the introduction of these foods into the child's diet, whereas allergy to vegetables began after the second year (Table 46-1).

Clinical Features

The clinical features of food allergy in childhood are shown in Table 46-2. In early infancy the most common food allergy is allergy to cow's milk protein. Most infants develop symptoms before 1 month of age, often within 1 week after introduction of

©2010 Elsevier Ltd, Inc, BV
DOI: 10.1016/B978-1-4377-0271-2.00046-8

Table 46-1 Age at Onset of Food Allergy Against Different Foods

Age (yr)	Food
0–1	Milk, egg
1–2	Peanuts, fish in Scandinavian countries
>2	Fruits, legumes, vegetables
>3	Pollen-related cross-reactivities (oral allergy syndrome)

Table 46-2 Clinical Features of Food Allergy in Children

Cutaneous Reactions	
IgE mediated	Atopic dermatitis Urticaria, acute or chronic (rare) Angioedema
Non-IgE mediated	Contact rash (e.g. perioral flare due to benzoic acid in citrus fruits) Atopic dermatitis (some forms?)

Gastrointestinal Reactions	
IgE mediated	Immediate gastrointestinal hypersensitivity (e.g. nausea, vomiting, diarrhea) Oral allergy syndrome Colic
Non-IgE mediated	Allergic eosinophilic esophagitis, gastritis, or gastroenterocolitis Enterocolitis syndrome Dietary protein colitis Dietary protein enteropathy

Respiratory Reactions	
IgE mediated	Rhinoconjunctivitis Asthma (wheezing, cough) Laryngeal edema Food-dependent exercise-induced asthma
Non-IgE mediated	Pulmonary hemosiderosis (Heiner's syndrome [rare])

Systemic Anaphylaxis	
	Anaphylaxis Food dependent exercise-induced anaphylaxis

Other Reactions	
IgE mediated	Otitis media (secondary to allergic rhinitis and eustachian tube dysfunction or an allergic middle ear inflammation)
Unknown mechanisms	Migraine (rare), arthritis (rare), Henoch-Schönlein purpura (rare)

Table 46-3 Common Cross-Reactivities: Food-Pollen Allergy Syndrome (Oral Allergy Syndrome)

Pollen	Fruit/Vegetable
Birch	Apple, hazelnut, carrot, potato, kiwi, celery, cherry, pear, others
Mugwort (artemissia)	Celery, carrot, fennel, parsley, others
Ragweed	Melon, banana
Grass	Potato, tomato, watermelon, kiwi, peanuts?

Serologic cross reactivity is not equivalent to clinical reactivity

classified as delayed reactions. Late reactions may occur after many hours even up to a few days, such as allergic eosinophilic gastroenteritis. Most often delayed reactions are non-IgE mediated. Anaphylaxis has been reported with varying frequencies, reflecting differences in patient selection. It is clear that patterns of reactions to foods may vary due to different exposure levels and different time intervals between exposures as well as different thresholds of reaction.

Immediate IgE-mediated reactions to foods often involve two or more target organs, such as the gastrointestinal tract, the skin, and the lungs, and may result in a variety of symptoms, including life-threatening reactions such as exacerbations of asthma, laryngeal edema, and anaphylaxis with cardiovascular collapse. An exception is the food-pollen allergy, or *oral allergy syndrome* (OAS), a mucosal equivalent of urticaria. The age of onset of 'oral allergy syndrome' is beyond infancy but often before school age. After the ingestion of specific foods (fresh fruits and vegetables), pruritus and swelling in the mouth and oropharynx occurs, which may prompt the child to refuse the offending foods. However, in some cases OAS may progress to more severe reactions.[15,16] OAS is associated with allergic rhinoconjunctivitis and allergy to pollen, especially to birch, grass, ragweed and mugwort. Cross-reactivity occurs when two or more allergens share epitopes and therefore are bound by the same IgE antibodies. Thus patients sensitized to one of the allergens may also react to the other without previous exposure and sensitization. Two major panallergens, profilin and lipid transfer protein (LTP), have been reported to be responsible for a great proportion of clinical reactions to pollen-related food allergens.[17] The most often reported cross-reactivities among pollens, fruits and vegetables are shown in Table 46-3. Other cross-reactivities occcur between natural rubber latex and banana, avocado, peach, kiwi, apricot, grape, passion fruit, pineapple, and chestnut. The diagnosis of OAS is based on a typical history and the demonstration of a positive skin prick test or specific IgE antibodies,[18] and possibly an open challenge.[4]

Gastrointestinal Problems in Early Childhood

Gastrointestinal manifestations of food allergy can be classified as a continuum from clearly IgE-mediated to mixed reactions dominated by eosinophilic granulocytes, to clearly non-IgE-mediated reactions.[19] Immediate gastrointestinal hypersensitivity and oral allergy symptoms are mainly IgE-mediated; allergic eosinophilic esophagitis, allergic eosinophilic gastritis, and allergic eosinophilic gastroenterocolitis are mixed-IgE and non-IgE-mediated reactions, and food protein-induced enterocolitis, proctocolitis and enteropathy, and celiac disease are non-IgE mediated. The most frequent adverse reactions to food in the infant and young child are immediate IgE-mediated reactions with manifestations like nausea, abdominal pain (colic), and

cow's milk-based formula. Similar to other food allergies, the majority have at least two symptoms and symptoms that affect at least two organs. About 50–70% have cutaneous symptoms; 50–60% gastrointestinal symptoms; and about 20–30%, respiratory symptoms.[6] Also, exclusively breast-fed infants may react to food protein in their mother's milk, approximately 0.5%,[9] and in these infants severe atopic eczema is the predominant symptom. CMPA onset after 1 year of age is extremely rare. Symptoms occurring within a few minutes to 2 hours after food exposure (i.e. 'immediate reactions') are mostly IgE mediated, whereas symptoms occurring more than 2 hours after food intake are

Table 46-4 Presenting Gastrointestinal Symptoms in Infants with Cow's Milk Protein Allergy

Symptom	Selected patient samples (%)			Unselected, prospectively followed patients from birth cohorts (%)		
	Goldman et al,[38] 1963[a] (N = 89)	Gerrard et al,[39] 1967[b] (N = 150)	Hill et al,[36] 1986[c] (N = 100)	Gerrard et al,[40] 1973[d] (N = 59)	Jakobsson and Lindberg,[42] 1979[e] (N = 20)	Høst and Halken,[6] 1990[f] (N = 39)
Colic	28	19	14	20	35	46
Vomiting	33	34	34	22	50	38
Diarrhea	37	47	48	41	25	8
Failure to thrive	NG	NG	22	NG	10	8
Diarrhea with blood	NG	NG	4	NG	NG	0
Gastroesophageal reflux	NG	NG	6	NG	NG	NG

NG, Not given.
[a]Age at investigation: Group A median, 6 months (2 weeks to 6 years). Group B median, 10 months (6 weeks to 13 years).
[b]Age at investigation: not given.
[c]Age at investigation: mean, 16 months (3 to 66 months).
[d]Age at investigation: not given, but infants followed 0 to 2 years.
[e]Age at investigation: median, 4 months (3 weeks to 1 year).
[f]Age at investigation: median, 3.5 months (1 to 11 months), infants followed 0 to 3 years.

vomiting within 1 to 2 hours after food intake and diarrhea within 1 to 6 hours. The frequency of presenting gastrointestinal symptoms in infants with CMPA is shown in Table 46-4.

Among non-IgE-mediated disorders, food protein-induced enterocolitis and proctocolitis typically have their onset in early infancy up to 6 to 18 months of age. Mixed IgE- and cell-mediated reactions, allergic eosinophilic esophagitis and allergic eosinophilic gastroenterocolitis may present between early infancy and adolescence. Dietary protein enteropathy and celiac disease occur in early childhood depending on the age of exposure to the antigen involved. The mixed-IgE-and non-IgE-mediated disorders are discussed in detail in other chapters (see Chapters 48 and 49).

The symptoms provoked by immediate gastrointestinal allergy typically develop within minutes to 2 hours after food intake. None of the symptoms are pathognomonic for allergy and may be caused by many other factors or diseases. Symptoms like colic, vomiting and diarrhea may be chronic or intermittent. Frequently, the children have poor appetite, poor weight gain, and intermittent abdominal pain and show failure to thrive. Children who show concomitant symptoms in other organ systems like urticaria or atopic dermatitis or respiratory symptoms may easily be suspected of food allergy. When symptoms from other organ systems are lacking, the cause of the symptoms may remain undiagnosed for prolonged periods. A family history of atopic disease in such cases should give a clue to the diagnosis of possible food allergy. A variety of feeding problems in young infants may be associated with food allergy. Allergic gastrointestinal motility disorders such as gastroesophageal reflux disease (GER), constipation and colic are among the most common disorders in infancy and early childhood. In a subset of infants with these functional disorders, a relation with food allergy has been reported following controlled food elimination and challenge procedures.[20]

Infantile Colic

Infantile colic has often been related to food allergy, especially CMPA, and high frequencies up to 71% of food allergy in children with colic have been reported.[21] In that and another study,[22]

Box 46-1

Symptoms of Gastroesophageal Reflux

Regurgitation

Failure to thrive

Esophagitis

Feeding problems

Signs of pain in particular with meals

Anemia, hematemesis

Stricture symptoms

Respiratory symptoms

Wheezing

Recurrent pneumonia

Apnea, cyanotic episodes

Laryngospasm

Neurologic symptoms

Sandifer's syndrome

the infants with colic due to cow's milk protein only rarely showed other features of CMPA. Although infantile colic is a common symptom of CMPA, it is almost always seen in combination with other features of CMPA.[6,9,23]

Gastroesophageal Reflux

It has been reported that nearly half of the cases of GER in infants less than 1 year of age are not only CMPA associated but also CMPA induced.[24,25] GER is a common disease, affecting up to 10% of infants in the first year of life. It is related to esophagitis but may be present without visible or histologic inflammation of the esophagus. Typical symptoms of GER include vomiting with weight loss and symptoms of esophagitis (dysphagia, vomiting, abdominal pain, sleep disturbance), as well as respiratory symptoms (Box 46-1). Proteins other than cow's milk have been implicated in allergic eosinophilic esophagitis, such as wheat, soy, peanut, and egg, often multiple antigens. Most cases in young infants resolve in less than 1 year. Some studies suggest that a portion of patients have both CMPA and GER, particularly in infants and children with severe GER.[26] Given possible selection bias in previously reported studies, more population-based studies on this subject are warranted to evaluate the significance of this possible causal relationship.

Constipation

Constipation is a common clinical problem affecting up to 10% of infants and children,[27] and in a population-based study from Italy, 1.8% (91/5113) of children up to 12 years fulfilled the criteria for chronic constipation with the highest frequency (3.3%) among children aged 6 months to 6 years.[28] Chronic constipation may cause blood in the stools as well as symptoms of colitis and recurrent abdominal pain in older children. Some reports[29,30,31] describe chronic constipation as a manifestation of CMPA. In a recent study the prevalence of atopy among children with chronic constipation was similar to that in the general population.[28] Thus food allergy should be considered in severe cases of chronic constipation, but constipation does not appear to be a common manifestation of food allergy.

Diarrhea

Diarrhea is often reported as a symptom due to food allergy in young infancy. On the other hand, diarrhea is also a very common symptom due to 'normal reactions' caused by inappropriate or excessive intake of certain foods, such as raisins, carrots, legumes, and other fruit – toddlers' diarrhea. Transient or secondary lactase deficiency may occur in response to gastrointestinal infections, which are very common in infancy. This intolerance to lactose often lasts only a few days, after which there is a complete recovery.

Spitting Up/Vomiting

Symptoms of spitting up and vomiting may be very normal in young infants. The most common cause of vomiting is overfeeding. Such infants show a normal growth and development in contrast to infants with underlying gastrointestinal disease.[19] In some cases nonorganic causes e.g. behavioral causes should be considered.[32]

Failure to Thrive

Failure to thrive may be caused by immediate gastrointestinal food allergy but is more often due to mixed-IgE-and non-IgE-mediated disorders in the gastrointestinal tract causing malabsorption, severe vomiting, or diarrhea.[19] In some children with failure to thrive, organic causes cannot be demonstrated and it may be very difficult to confirm nonorganic causes. A recent report indicated the relevance of 'behavioral causes' such as food refusal, food fixation, abnormal parental feeding practices and onset after a specific trigger.[32]

Differential Diagnoses

The differential diagnostic considerations of possible food-related symptoms are age dependent and include, for example,

---

BOX 46-2

Differential Diagnoses of Food Allergy

Infant

Upper gastrointestinal symptoms

  Infection

  Colic*

  Gastroesophageal reflux*

  Pyloric stenosis (defined age group)

  Hiatal hernia

  Tracheoesophageal fistula

Lower gastrointestinal symptoms

  Enzyme deficiency

  Disaccharidase deficiencies (lactase, sucrase-isomaltase)

  Glucose-galactose malabsorption

  Galactosemia

  Phenylketonuria

  Infection

  Constipation*

  Hirschsprung's disease

Toddler

Infection

Toddler's diarrhea

Gastroesophageal reflux*

Constipation*

Lactose intolerance

Malabsorption (celiac disease, cystic fibrosis)

Bizarre diets

School-age child

Infection

Recurrent abdominal pain

Lactose intolerance

Malabsorption (celiac disease, cystic fibrosis, Schwachman syndrome)

Inflammatory bowel disease

Eosinophilic gastroenteritis*

Other causes (immunodeficiency, Henoch-Schönlein disease)

*Could be caused by food allergy.

---

chronic gastrointestinal infections, nonspecific diarrhea of childhood, irritable bowel syndrome, and recurrent abdominal pain, as described in Box 46-2. Some differential diagnoses of food allergy are mainly related to the upper gastrointestinal tract such as colic, recurrent abdominal pain, gastroesophageal reflux, pyloric stenosis, hiatal hernia, and tracheoesophageal fistula, whereas others are associated with diseases in the lower gastrointestinal tract, such as enzyme deficiencies, malabsorption diseases, constipation, and Hirschsprung's disease.

Nonenteral Infections

Commonly seen in all ages, although most frequent in early infancy, are the nonenteral infections that may cause gastrointestinal upset, regardless of the focus of the infection; 'secondary dyspepsia'. Such sequelae after acute or chronic gastrointestinal infection should always be ruled out before evaluation of food allergy.

Lactose Intolerance

Lactase deficiency is an important differential diagnosis to food allergy, especially cow's milk allergy. Lactose constitutes the majority of the carbohydrate content of human and cow's milk and is an important part of the energy supply for infants in particular. Lactose is degraded in the gastrointestinal mucosa by the enzyme lactase. Lactose intolerance in the newborn is extremely rare and is caused by congenital deficiency of lactase. Acquired or adult-type lactase deficiency usually appears at the age of 3 to 5 years. Adult-type lactase deficiency is very common in those of African and Asian ancestries. It is less common in whites, especially in some groups, such as the Scandinavian populations; in Denmark, only 3% of adults are affected.

Secondary lactase deficiency is temporary and may occur in response to malnutrition or gastrointestinal infections, which cause temporary damage of the villi of the small intestine, where the enzyme lactase is produced. This sensitivity to lactose often lasts only a few days, followed by complete recovery.

Lactose intolerance may be diagnosed by oral lactose challenge tests and measurements of increased H_2 in breath tests, by glucose measurements, or by direct enzyme measurements within a duodenal biopsy. Recently, a genetic test to diagnose the adult type of lactase deficiency has been introduced and found valid, especially in older children.[33]

Adult-type or primary lactase deficiency is a lifelong condition. The treatment of lactose intolerance is to diminish the amount of milk and dairy products with lactose. Avoidance does not need to be complete, such as for children with CMPA. A firm diagnosis of lactose intolerance and the threshold for development of symptoms should be established because the sensitivity to lactose is variable. In many lactose-intolerant individuals, considerable amounts of lactose may be ingested before symptoms develop. Usually the amount of milk product corresponding to one glass of milk during a meal may be ingested without adverse reactions.[34]

Irritable Bowel Syndrome

Irritable bowel syndrome (IBS) or recurrent abdominal pain in children is a clinical syndrome with a variable pathogenic background, including psychosomatic reactions, lactose intolerance, food allergy, and inflammatory conditions such as gastritis or inflammatory bowel disease. It has been concluded that food reactions are unlikely to be major determinants in the pathogenesis of IBS and that double-blind placebo-controlled food challenges are mandatory for investigation of this possible causal relationship.[35]

Toddlers' Diarrhea

To avoid unnecessary investigations for food allergy, it is important to pay attention to this very common 'disorder'. Many infants and young children have a high intake of dietary fiber from enormous amounts of fruits, legumes, vegetables, and raisins and great volumes of fruit juice (instead of water). This is a normal cause of loose stools and diarrhea often resulting in referrals to allergists for investigation of food allergy. There is no reason for such investigations when children have normal growth and development. Laypersons, especially parents, need more information and knowledge about 'normal' reactions to foods in children. The simple advice is to reduce the intake of such foods to normalize the bowel function.

Münchhausen's Syndrome by Proxy

During the past decades, many infants and young children have been investigated for food allergy without a convincing indication for such, often comprehensive, diagnostic procedures. In cases where there is a lack of obvious possible allergic symptoms, physicians should abstain from unnecessary and potentially harmful investigations of healthy children with parent-, often mother-, induced or imaginary symptoms.[36]

Evaluation and Management

In infants and young children, food allergy should be suspected in cases of persistent severe symptoms, especially if there is more than one symptom and if relevant differential diagnoses are excluded (Boxes 46-3 and 46-4).

Gastrointestinal symptoms in food allergy are often chronic or acute vomiting, diarrhea, and colic. Colic appears to be a common symptom,[36] but nearly always in combination with other symptoms.[6,9,23,36] Since most of these gastrointestinal symptoms are nonspecific and may be caused by other conditions, a careful evaluation for other causes is important at an early stage.

None of the symptoms related to immunologically or non-immunologically mediated adverse reactions to foods are

---

BOX 46-3 Key concepts

Characteristics of Food Allergy

- Persistent symptoms
- Symptoms related to food intake
- Allergic predisposition
- Two or more different symptoms
- Symptoms in two or more different organs

BOX 46-4 Therapeutic principles

General Approach to Evaluation of Food Allergy in Children with Gastrointestinal Problems

Consider evaluation in case of

Persistent symptoms in infancy/early childhood with vomiting, diarrhea, colic, or failure to thrive and

Other common differential diagnoses are excluded, especially gastroenteritis and lactose intolerance

Particularly in case of

History of symptoms exacerbated by particular foods or

Other coexisting atopic manifestations, especially

  Atopic eczema/urticaria

  Allergic rhinitis

Initial screen

Careful case history and physical examination

Skin prick test/specific IgE to implicated foods

  Extra suspicion for 'history-positive' foods

  Extra suspicion for common food allergens (milk, hen's egg, wheat, soy, peanut, tree nut, fish, shellfish)

Consider elimination diet for a sufficient period to eliminate symptoms

Consider controlled challenges to exclude/confirm food allergy

pathognomonic, although some characteristics should be suggestive of food allergy (Box 46-3).

No laboratory test is diagnostic of food allergy.[4,7,18] Therefore, the diagnosis has to be based on a careful case history and on strict, well-defined food elimination and challenge procedures establishing a causal relation between the ingestion of a particular food (or food protein) and a subsequent obvious clinical reaction.[4,7,18,19,37] Possible helpful diagnostic tests include skin prick tests or determinations of serum allergen-specific IgE levels, and possibly atopy patch tests. These tests are often useful in choosing the elimination diet and the challenge procedure for the classification of the disorder and for determining the prognosis.

Conclusions

Food allergy is most frequently a problem in infancy and early childhood. Children with food allergy may experience a variety of symptoms affecting different organ systems. The disease manifestations often are localized to the gastrointestinal tract, but food allergy may also cause local symptoms in the skin and the respiratory tract. About 50–70% of allergic infants show cutaneous symptoms; 50–60% gastrointestinal symptoms; and about 20–30% respiratory symptoms. Among young children with cow's milk allergy, the majority have two or more symptoms, and symptoms generally affect two or more organ systems. Mostly, the symptoms occur within a few minutes after food exposure (immediate reactions), but delayed reactions involving the skin, the gastrointestinal tract, and the lungs may also occur. Among children presenting with symptoms suggestive of food allergy, the diagnosis can be confirmed by controlled elimination/challenge procedures in only about one third of individuals.

To avoid unnecessary diets and stigmatization, it is important to rule out 'normal reactions' to foods and relevant differential diagnoses before undertaking specific comprehensive diagnostic procedures for food allergy. To avoid unnecessary diets and the risk of malnutrition, it is important to make the proper diagnosis in case of suspected food allergy.

References

1. Sicherer SH, Leung DY. Advances in allergic skin disease, anaphylaxis, and hypersensitivity reactions to foods, drugs, and insects in 2008. J Allergy Clin Immunol 2009;123:319–27.
2. Rona RJ, Keil T, Summers C, et al. The prevalence of food allergy: a meta-analysis. J Allergy Clin Immunol 2007;120:638–46.
3. Osterballe M, Hansen TK, Mortz CG, et al. The prevalence of food hypersensitivity in an unselected population of children and adults. Pediatr Allergy Immunol 2005;16:567–73.
4. Bindslev-Jensen C, Ballmer-Weber BK, Bengtsson U, et al. Standardization of food challenges in patients with immediate reactions to foods-position paper from the European Academy of Allergology and Clinical Immunology. Allergy 2004;59:690–7.
5. Venter C, Pereira B, Voigt K, et al. Prevalence and cumulative incidence of food hypersensitivity in the first 3 years of life. Allergy 2008;63: 354–9.
6. Høst A, Halken S. A prospective study of cow milk allergy in Danish infants during the first 3 years of life. Clinical course in relation to clinical and immunological type of hypersensitivity reaction. Allergy 1990;45: 587–96.
7. Niggemann B, Beyer K. Diagnosis of food allergy in children: toward a standardization of food challenge. J Pediatr Gastroenterol Nutr 2007;45:399–404.
8. Crespo JF, Pascual C, Burks AW, et al. Frequency of food allergy in a pediatric population from Spain. Pediatr Allergy Immunol 1995;6: 39–43.
9. Host A. Cow's milk protein allergy and intolerance in infancy: some clinical, epidemiological and immunological aspects. Pediatr Allergy Immunol 1994;5(5 Suppl):1–36.
10. Bock SA. Prospective appraisal of complaints of adverse reactions to foods in children during the first 3 years of life. Pediatrics 1987;79: 683–8.
11. Venter C, Pereira B, Voigt K, et al. Prevalence and cumulative incidence of food hypersensitivity in the first 3 years of life. Allergy 2008;63: 354–9.
12. Fuglsang G, Madsen C, Saval P, et al. Prevalence of intolerance to food additives among Danish school children. Pediatr Allergy Immunol 1993;4:123–9.
13. Fuglsang G, Madsen G, Halken S, et al. Adverse reactions to food additives in children with atopic symptoms. Allergy 1994;49:31–7.
14. McCann D, Barrett A, Cooper A, et al. Food additives and hyperactive behaviour in 3-year-old and 8/9-year-old children in the community: a randomised, double-blinded, placebo-controlled trial. Lancet 2007; 370:1560–7.
15. Mari A, Ballmer-Weber BK, Vieths S. The oral allergy syndrome: improved diagnostic and treatment methods. Curr Opin Allergy Clin Immunol 2005;5:267–73.
16. Hansen KS, Ballmer-Weber BK, Sastre J, et al. Component-resolved in vitro diagnosis of hazelnut allergy in Europe. J Allergy Clin Immunol 2009.
17. Asero R, Monsalve R, Barber D. Profilin sensitization detected in the office by skin prick test: a study of prevalence and clinical relevance of profilin as a plant food allergen. Clin Exp Allergy 2008;38: 1033–7.
18. Bruijnzeel-Koomen C, Ortolani C, Aas K, et al. Adverse reactions to food. European Academy of Allergology and Clinical Immunology Subcommittee. Allergy 1995;50:623–35.
19. Sampson HA, Anderson JA. Summary and recommendations: classification of gastrointestinal manifestations due to immunologic reactions to foods in infants and young children. J Pediatr Gastroenterol Nutr 2000;30 (Suppl):S87–S94.
20. Heine RG. Allergic gastrointestinal motility disorders in infancy and early childhood. Pediatr Allergy Immunol 2008;19:383–91.
21. Iacono G, Carroccio A, Montalto G, et al. Severe infantile colic and food intolerance: a long-term prospective study. J Pediatr Gastroenterol Nutr 1991;12:332–5.
22. Lothe L, Lindberg T, Jakobsson I. Cow's milk formula as a cause of infantile colic: a double-blind study. Pediatrics 1982;70:7–10.
23. Hill DJ, Hosking CS. Infantile colic and food hypersensitivity. J Pediatr Gastroenterol Nutr 2000;30(Suppl):S67–S76.
24. Cavataio F, Iacono G, Montalto G, et al. Clinical and pH-metric characteristics of gastro-oesophageal reflux secondary to cows' milk protein allergy. Arch Dis Child 1996;75:51–6.
25. Iacono G, Carroccio A, Cavataio F, et al. Gastroesophageal reflux and cow's milk allergy in infants: a prospective study. J Allergy Clin Immunol 1996;97:822–7.
26. Nielsen RG, Bindslev-Jensen C, Kruse-Andersen S, et al. Severe gastroesophageal reflux disease and cow milk hypersensitivity in infants and children: disease association and evaluation of a new challenge procedure. J Pediatr Gastroenterol Nutr 2004;39:383–91.
27. Clayden GS, Lawson JO. Investigation and management of longstanding chronic constipation in childhood. Arch Dis Child 1976;51: 918–23.
28. Simeone D, Miele E, Boccia G, et al. Prevalence of atopy in children with chronic constipation. Arch Dis Child 2008;93:1044–7.
29. Daher S, Tahan S, Sole D, et al. Cow's milk protein intolerance and chronic constipation in children. Pediatr Allergy Immunol 2001;12: 339–42.
30. Iacono G, Cavataio F, Montalto G, et al. Intolerance of cow's milk and chronic constipation in children. N Engl J Med 1998;339:1100–4.
31. Shah N, Lindley K, Milla P. Cow's milk and chronic constipation in children. N Engl J Med 1999;340:891–2.
32. Levy Y, Levy A, Zangen T, et al. Diagnostic clues for identification of nonorganic vs organic causes of food refusal and poor feeding. J Pediatr Gastroenterol Nutr 2009;48:355–62.
33. Rasinpera H, Savilahti E, Enattah NS, et al. A genetic test which can be used to diagnose adult-type hypolactasia in children. Gut 2004;53: 1571–6.
34. Srinivasan R, Minocha A. When to suspect lactose intolerance: symptomatic, ethnic, and laboratory clues. Postgrad Med 1998;104:109–6, 122.
35. Ortolani C, Bruijnzeel-Koomen C, Bengtsson U, et al. Controversial aspects of adverse reactions to food. European Academy of Allergology and Clinical Immunology (EAACI) Reactions to Food Subcommittee. Allergy 1999;54:27–45.
36. Warner JO, Hathaway MJ. Allergic form of Meadow's syndrome (Munchausen by proxy). Arch Dis Child 1984;59:151–6.
37. Hill DJ, Firer MA, Shelton MJ, et al. Manifestations of milk allergy in infancy: clinical and immunologic findings. J Pediatr 1986;109:270–6.

38. Muraro A, Dreborg S, Halken S, et al. Dietary prevention of allergic diseases in infants and small children. Part II. Evaluation of methods in allergy prevention studies and sensitization markers: definitions and diagnostic criteria of allergic diseases. Pediatr Allergy Immunol 2004;15:196–205.

39. Goldman AS, Anderson Jr DW, Sellers WA, et al. Milk Allergy. I. Oral challenge with milk and isolated milk proteins in allergic children. Pediatrics 1963;32:425–43.

40. Gerrard JW, Lubos MC, Hardy LW, et al. Milk allergy: clinical picture and familial incidence. Can Med Assoc J 1967;97:780–5.

41. Gerrard JW, MacKenzie JW, Goluboff N, et al. Cow's milk allergy: prevalence and manifestations in an unselected series of newborns. Acta Paediatr Scand Suppl 1973;234:1–21.

42. Jakobsson I, Lindberg T. A prospective study of cow's milk protein intolerance in Swedish infants. Acta Paediatr Scand 1979;68: 853–9.

Approach to Feeding Problems in the Infant and Young Child

CHAPTER
47

Prevention and Natural History of Food Allergy

Noah J. Friedman

Although much funding and media attention is focused on new modalities to treat allergic disease, the quest to prevent allergies has continued over the past few decades. The prevention of food allergy in particular, remains a vexing problem and a great opportunity in light of the fact that IgE-mediated sensitivity to ingested substances frequently occurs early in life and is often a harbinger of future atopic disease. Infancy represents a time when an allergic phenotype may be determined. Therefore interventions to prevent food allergies and the development of the atopic phenotype are best made early in life. Numerous factors may be involved in this phenotype determination and are the subject of much current research.

A recent evidence-based position statement summarizing the current knowledge of infant feeding practices for the prevention of allergy has recently been published by the American Academy of Pediatrics (AAP).[1] The conclusions are now very similar to updated recommendations from Europe.[2] However, although lifestyle and dietary manipulation have long been at the center of research, traditional interventions, primarily the restriction of infant diets, have been imperfect, both in terms of results, particularly with regard to long-term allergy prevention, and practicality. Due to logistical barriers inherent in strict dietary avoidance for infants as well as conflicting evidence of the benefit of such diets, other immunomodulatory measures are being evaluated as perhaps a more effective and 'user-friendly' method of primary prevention of food allergy, and atopic disease in general. There has also been developing evidence that early introduction of allergenic foods, rather than their avoidance, might indeed protect against the development of food allergy. Therefore this chapter will concentrate on decades of research on allergy prevention with early dietary intervention, as well as more recent efforts to prevent food allergies through immunomodulation.

Immunomodulation

Immunomodulatory Role of Breast Milk

Studies regarding the effects of breast-feeding and the prevention of allergy remain inconclusive. Even if maternal diets are devoid of allergenic foods, prevention of food allergy in infancy appears to be transient at best. There is now an increasing body of literature to suggest that one reason for this inability to determine a conclusive role for breast-feeding in the prevention of atopy is the complex nature of breast milk itself and its immu-

nostimulatory and immunosuppressive effects on the infant's intestinal milieu (Table 47-1).

Food allergens themselves, passing from the breast milk to the infant, may have either sensitizing or tolerizing effects on the infant's immune system.[3] Secretory IgA (s-IgA) has long been known to be passed to the infant through breast milk, possibly conferring passive protection to the infant's immune system. Past studies have suggested that low levels of colostral s-IgA might be associated with an increased risk of cow's milk allergy in infants.[4] Later studies report that while lower levels of s-IgA to ovalbumin were found in the colostrum and mature milk of allergic as opposed to nonallergic mothers,[5] the presence of these antibodies was not predictive for the development of atopic disease in the infants.[6]

There is some suggestion that cytokine concentration in breast milk differs between allergic and nonallergic mothers, with IL-4, IL-5, and IL-13 being present in higher concentrations in the breast milk of atopic women. These are cytokines known to be intimately involved with IgE production and induction of eosinophils. However, transforming growth factor (TGF)-β and IL-6 are the predominant cytokines in human breast milk.[7] TGF-β has been shown to increase the ability of the infant to produce its own IgA against β-lactoglobulin, casein, ovalbumin, and gliadin.[8] The soluble form of CD14, a cytokine that is thought to be central in the induction of a Th1 response by bacterial antigens,[9] is found in very high concentrations in human breast milk,[10] suggesting that this cytokine may play a role in the protective effect of breast-feeding on the development of allergy.

The composition of polyunsaturated long-chain fatty acids (PUFA) in human breast milk has also been shown to influence the development of atopy in infant. A high arachidonic acid to eicosapentaenoic acid ratio in human breast milk has been shown to increase the risk of allergic disease in the recipient.[6] However, recent studies have called into question the role of n-6 vs n-3 PUFAs in the development of atopy.[11] Others have proposed in studies of both suckling rats and humans[12] that polyamines (including spermine and spermidine) present in breast milk decrease the permeability of the intestinal mucosa and thus are protective against the development of allergic disease in infants. In addition, high levels of eosinophil cationic protein in breast milk have been associated with increased atopic dermatitis and cow's milk allergy in infants.[13]

It is thus clear that breast milk has properties that allow it to be immunostimulatory and immunoprotective. This interplay of factors begins to explain the difficulty in developing a unifying theory of whether breast-feeding is an effective way to prevent food allergies in high-risk infants.

©2010 Elsevier Ltd, Inc, BV
DOI: 10.1016/B978-1-4377-0271-2.00047-X

Table 47-1 Factors in Breast Milk that either Induce or Protect Against Food Allergies

Factors	Inducing	Protective
Antigens	Sensitizing allergens	Tolerizing allergens
Cytokines	IL-4 IL-5 IL-13	TGF-β sCD14
Immunoglobulins		s-IgA to ovalbumin
Polyunsaturated fatty acids	n-3 PUFA	n-3 PUFA
Chemokines	RANTES IL-8	
Polyamines		Spermine Spermidine

IL, Interleukin; *TGF-β*, transforming growth factor-beta; *PUFA*, polyunsaturated fatty acids: *RANTES*, regulated on activation, normal T cell expressed and secreted.

Probiotics

As much of the current thinking in preventing allergic disease led researchers to develop new ways to induce a Th1 phenotype, it became logical to look toward the intestinal microflora. These 1 to 10 billion organisms most likely represent the major source of microbial stimulation of the immune system in the newborn, stimulating the maturation of the reticuloendothelial system. The use of some of these species, called probiotics, is being investigated as a tool in both primary and secondary prevention of food allergy. Lactobacilli have long been known to protect the gut against colonization with pathogens, to be completely nonpathogenic themselves, and to enhance immune responses. Some studies have demonstrated a decrease in the severity of atopic dermatitis in children if they are given probiotics,[14] including demonstration of a significant decrease in atopic dermatitis severity SCORAD scores in a double-blind, placebo-controlled study of probiotic supplemented whey hydrolysate formula.[15] Immunologically, probiotics have been shown to (1) decrease gastrointestinal permeability,[16] (2) decrease soluble CD4 in the serum and eosinophil protein X in the urine of children,[15] (3) decrease effects of bovine casein on lymphocyte proliferation and anti-CD3 antibody induced IL-4 production in vitro,[17] (4) increase TGF-β in breast milk and increase intestinal s-IgA[16] and (5) suppress naturally fed antigen-specific IgE production by stimulation of IL-12 production in mice.[17] Moreover, an orally administered *Lactococcus lactis* strain transfected to secrete IL-10 was recently shown to decrease food-induced anaphylaxis in mice.[18]

Kalliomaki and colleagues[19] reported that infants whose mothers had been given probiotics 4 weeks postpartum and were given either probiotic-supplemented formula, or breast milk from mothers who continued taking probiotics during breast-feeding, had significantly less atopic dermatitis during the first 2 years of life. This was not correlated with a decrease in total serum or food specific IgE. A follow-up study[20] reported a significant increase in the level of TGF-β2 in the breast milk of mothers who had been given probiotics. Conversely, a more recent Australian study[21] of 231 high-risk infants demonstrated no reduction in the risk of atopic dermatitis and an increase in allergic sensitization in those infants given *Lactobacillus acidophilus* supplements as compared to those given placebo. A meta-analysis of 10 studies on the use of probiotics, six of which were prevention studies, concluded that, overall, the literature supports the potential of probiotics in the prevention of pediatric atopic dermatitis, particularly if administered prenatally.[22] However, further research will need to be done to determine the future of this intervention in the prevention of food allergies.

Prebiotics

The ingestion of trans-β-galacto-oligosaccharides or fructo-oligosaccharides also influences gut microflora and thus may have an effect on the development of allergic disease. These oligosaccharides have been dubbed *prebiotics*.[23] Moro and colleagues[24] have demonstrated a decrease in the incidence of atopic dermatitis up to 6 months of age in infants who were given prebiotics for the first 3 to 6 months in comparison to placebo. A follow-up study[25] noted that a decrease in the cumulative incidences for atopic dermatitis, recurrent wheezing and 'allergic urticaria' was still noted in these infants by the age of 2 years. No comment was made about allergic sensitization. On the other hand, Ziegler and colleagues[26] reported no difference in the incidence of eczema in formula-fed infants unselected for high risk for allergies whose diets were supplemented with prebiotics. A meta-analysis of these studies[27] (predating the later Italian study) postulated that the disparity in the findings of the two groups may be attributable to differences in infant risk, prebiotic formulation or the measurement of eczema. It was concluded that there is currently insufficient evidence to determine the role of prebiotic supplementation for the prevention of allergic disease and food hypersensitivity.

'Symbiotics'

A randomized, double-blind, placebo-controlled prospective study reported the effect of a combination of probiotics plus prebiotics, namely symbiotics, during both pregnancy and the first 6 months of life on the development of atopy in the offspring of 1223 pregnant Finnish women.[28] While no statistically significant effect was seen on the development of all allergic diseases by the age of 2 years, they noted a significant decreased cumulative incidence of eczema (both atopic and nonatopic, OR 0.74, 95% CI 0.55–0.98) and atopic dermatitis (associated with IgE only, OR 0.66, 95% CI 0.46–0.95). A recent follow-up study of this group at 5 years of age, reported that continued protection against allergic diseases occurred only in children who had been born by cesarean section.[29] It was speculated that probiotics may be more effective in this group because infants born by cesarean section have been shown to be colonized with bifidobacteria and lactobacilli later than their vaginally born counterparts, perhaps leading to a higher rate of respiratory allergies.[30] Further research is still needed to determine if this combination of supplements will have a role in the prevention of food allergy.

Polyunsaturated Fatty Acids (PUFAs)

It has been theorized that one of the explanations for the recent increase in atopic disease may be due to changes in diet, with increased consumption of n-6 as opposed to n-3 PUFAs. Also, as noted above, the ratio of n6/n3 fatty acids in breast milk has been thought to affect the degree of allergic sensitization in an infant. Over recent years, studies have evaluated the role of altering the intake of these PUFAs in either the pregnant mother or the infant, with regard to the development of atopy. N-3 PUFAs have been thought to have significant antiinflammatory properties. Maternal ingestion of fish oil, rich in n-3 PUFAs, during pregnancy has been shown to subtly affect infant cytokine levels, reducing IL-13 levels in cord blood.[31] It has also been shown to affect the function of antigen presenting cells, in that increased fish oil ingestion during pregnancy led to lower levels of F2-isoprostanes in high-risk infants.[32] IL-5, IL-13, IL-10 and IFN-γ levels were lower in infants whose mothers had been given n-3 PUFA supplements compared to those whose mothers received placebo.[33] These infants were three times less likely to have a positive skin test to egg at 1 year of age (OR 0.34, 95% CI 0.11–1.02). They had a trend towards increased atopic dermatitis (OR 1.88, 95% CI 0.77–4.65) but their atopic dermatitis was much less severe than the placebo group. Conversely, Marks and colleagues[34] reported that a combination of an infant diet with supplemental fish oil high in n-3 PUFA (vs sunflower oil, high in n-6 PUFA) with house dust mite control in high-risk infants had no effect on the development of atopic eczema or asthma in the first 5 years of life. A recent meta-analysis of 10 studies that reported a role of omega 3 or omega 6 oils in the primary prevention of allergic disease demonstrated no statistically significant benefit of the use of these supplements in reduction of the relative risk of asthma, allergic rhinitis or food allergy.[35] Therefore, it is not clear whether the increase of dietary intake of n-3 PUFAs can be recommended as a way of preventing the development of allergies.

Principles of Traditional Allergy Prevention

Dietary Manipulation During Pregnancy

Although in 1980 Michel and colleagues[36] reported specific IgE sensitization to food during gestation, more recent evidence suggests that this is a rare event, occurring in less than 0.3% of monitored pregnancies.[37] In addition, studies that have examined the prophylactic effect of maternal avoidance of highly allergenic foods, such as milk and egg,[38] during pregnancy in high-risk groups showed no beneficial effects in the development of food allergy. The conclusions of a 2006 Cochrane meta-analysis[39] confirmed that 'prescription of an antigen avoidance diet to a high-risk woman during pregnancy is unlikely to reduce substantially her child's risk of atopic disease and that such a diet may adversely affect maternal or fetal nutrition'. It is therefore now widely accepted that maternal avoidance diets during pregnancy should not be recommended as a way to prevent allergic disease. It is important, however, to recommend that smoking mothers discontinue cigarette smoking during pregnancy. While the effect of tobacco smoke on the development of food allergy in infancy is unclear, the deleterious effects of tobacco smoke products in utero on lung function after birth and the reduction in lung function and increase in asthmatic symptoms from second hand smoke during infancy have been clearly documented.[40]

Breast-Feeding

It is a universal axiom that breast-feeding is the best nourishment for infants. It offers the young child numerous nutritional, immunologic, and psychological benefits that cannot be duplicated by formula. The AAP is unequivocal in its advocacy of breast-feeding in the newborn.[41] However, it is also possible that there is a potential immunologic downside to exposing a child at risk of atopy to highly allergenic foodstuffs through breast milk. It has long been known that β-lactoglobulin, casein, and bovine gammaglobulin,[42] three common milk antigens, have been meas-

ured in nanogram concentrations in lactating women who are not specifically avoiding milk during that time. Similarly, egg[43] and wheat[44] antigens have also been detected in breast milk. These substances can be measured as little as 2 to 6 hours after ingestion and can be detected up to 1 to 4 days later. The presence of peanut protein in the breast milk of women 1 to 2 hours after ingestion of peanut has been documented by sandwich enzyme-linked immunosorbent assay (ELISA).[45]

Therefore, the effect of breast-feeding on the development of food allergies has been the source of vigorous debate over the past few decades. Starting with Grulee and Sanford[46] in 1939, who noted in a nonrandomized study of over 20 000 infants that breast-feeding reduced the incidence of eczema 7-fold, numerous studies with a variety of strengths and weaknesses have filled the literature with evidence of both the protective and sensitizing effects of breast-feeding vis-a-vis food allergy. Methodological flaws that make it difficult to directly compare one study to another and draw long-term, clinically relevant conclusions, include insufficient sample size, nonrandomization of study groups, concerns of recall bias or reverse causation, and lack of definitive documentation of food allergy by double-blind, placebo-controlled food challenges. These flaws are present in studies that demonstrate a positive effect of breast-feeding on the prevention of allergies as well as in those that do not support a protective effect. Nevertheless, many important observations have been made.

In 1990 Lucas and colleagues[47] performed the first randomized, prospective study on the effects of breast-feeding on the development of atopic disease, comparing the effects of banked human breast milk versus preterm cow's milk formula for use as the diet for 446 premature neonates. Within the cohort taken as a whole there was no statistically significant difference between the two groups by 18 months of age with regard to the development of allergy, but within the group of children with an atopic family history, the infants who were fed cow's milk formula had a 41% chance of developing an allergic reaction (especially atopic dermatitis) compared to 16% of the breast-fed infants. No skin testing or other confirmatory immunologic data was presented.

More recently, several large studies have also demonstrated a protective effect of breast-feeding with regard to the development of atopy. The German Infant Nutritional Intervention Program,[48] a prospective, randomized interventional study, evaluated > 3900 infants at high-risk for atopy. Infants who received hydrolyzed formula were compared to those who received cow's milk formula. High-risk infants who were exclusively breast-fed had a significantly lower incidence of atopic dermatitis in the first 3 years of life than those who were fed cow's milk formula. A large Swedish prospective birth cohort study[49] demonstrated a lower incidence of asthma at 4 years of age in infants who were breast-fed exclusively for 4 months. A similar Australian study[50] also showed this protective effect at the age of 6 years.

Furthermore, results from both the Swedish and Australian groups suggest that there is benefit to be gained from breast-feeding exclusively for at least 4 months. Earlier, the Swedish group[51] had reported that there was a statistically significant decrease in wheezing (OR 0.78; 95% CI 0.65–0.93), asthma diagnosis (OR 0.66; 95% CI 0.51–0.87), atopic dermatitis (OR 0.8; 95% CI 0.7–1.0) and multiple allergic manifestations (OR 0.66; 95% CI 0.48–0.90) by 2 years of age in infants who were breast-fed for ≥ 4 months compared to those did so for less time. A follow-up study published in 2005[52] reported that the risk of eczema by 4 years of age was also reduced in breast-fed infants (OR 0.78, 95% CI 0.45–0.96). Similarly, Oddy and colleagues[53] reported that the cumulative incidence of asthma was lower in infants who were breast-fed for at least 4 months. The age of asthma diagnosis was also higher in this group in comparison to those who had breast-fed for a shorter period.

Some studies also suggest that breast-feeding had no protective effect on the development of food allergy in comparison to formula feeding. For example, a recent Dutch study of > 2400 infant/mother pairs, who were not specifically high-risk, showed no statistically significant effect of breast-feeding on the incidence of atopic dermatitis in the first year of life.[54]

Conversely, there are also studies that have demonstrated an increased risk of the development of allergic disease in breast-fed children. In the Multicenter Atopy Study,[55] a long term, prospective, observational birth cohort study of 1314 German infants, Bergmann and colleagues reported an increased risk of atopic dermatitis at any point before the age of 7 years in breast-fed infants compared to those who were formula-fed (OR 1.03, 95% CI 1.00–1.06 for each additional month of breast-feeding). However, a clear dose response was not demonstrated, thus raising concerns that a confounding factor, such as reverse causation, may not have been adequately addressed in the multivariate analysis.

In an observational study,[56] Sears and colleagues evaluated approximately 60% of a cohort that had been enrolled in a previous neonatal study. The study suggested that if breast-feeding had been carried out for 4 weeks or longer, an increased risk of asthma between the ages of 9 and 26 years (OR 1.8, 95% CI 1.4–2.5) and an increased incidence of sensitization to environmental allergens at the age of 13 years (OR 1.9 CI 1.4–2.6) were noted. Shortly thereafter, a critique of this study was published,[57] pointing out the concern about recall bias, particularly in the absence of a dose response, and with no correlation to family history. While Sears did concede to some of the suggestions,[58] he noted that recall bias was unlikely to be a concern because the recall of infant feeding practices was corroborated by the records of nurse home visits obtained during the earlier, neonatal study. Potential weaknesses of this study notwithstanding, it is intriguing to note that much can be learned by following a birth cohort into adulthood, particularly if the infant feeding practices of the cohort have been documented from the neonatal period. Further to this point, another Australian study,[59] which followed a cohort of nearly 8600 children into adulthood, found an increased risk of current asthma at the age of 44 years, in people born to atopic mothers if they had been exclusively breast-fed (OR 1.57, 95% CI 1.15–2.14). A lower, but statistically significant risk had also been noted beginning at 14 years of age, reversing a trend of decreased risk of asthma noted at the age of 7 years (OR 0.75, 95% CI 0.58–0.97). These results were also potentially weakened by recall bias, because the history of infant feeding patterns was obtained at the age of 7 years as opposed to being documented in infancy.

A meta-analysis of prospective studies of breast feeding and its effect on the development of atopic dermatitis from 1966 to 2000 was published in 2001, prior to several of the more recent studies noted above.[60] Statistical analysis of these studies revealed a significant protective effect against the development of atopic dermatitis by breast-feeding. The overall odds ratio for this protective effect was 0.68 in all studies combined with an even greater protective effect, an odds ratio of 0.58, in children at risk for atopy. No protective effect was noted in the meta-analysis of the few studies that looked at children with no increased risk for atopy. In a related meta-analysis,[61] the same group demonstrated that exclusive breast-feeding for at least the first 3 months of life also led to a decreased rate of childhood asthma if a positive family history of allergies was present. The protective effect was negligible in children with no family history of atopy.

A review of over 4300 articles evaluated by committee, rather than by meta-analysis was published in 2003.[62] Of these studies, over 90% were discarded as uninformative and only 56 studies were considered sufficiently conclusive to be included in the analysis. The conclusion of the committee was that exclusive breast-feeding reduced the risk of atopic dermatitis in infancy, but that this effect was not seen in later life. The effect was greatest in high-risk children and also protected against the development of cow's milk allergy in this group.

Based on the above data, current guidelines endorse exclusive breast-feeding for at least 4 months in families at high risk for atopic disease. The safety of exclusive breast-feeding for 6 months has been confirmed by meta-analysis.[63] Furthermore, increasing breast-feeding can reduce community-wide infant illness[64] and reduce the cost of health services for the breast-fed infant.[65] There is certainly not enough evidence to the contrary to recommend that high-risk families deny their infant this most natural type of nutrition based purely on their atopic family history.

Breast-Feeding by Asthmatic Mothers

Some have suggested that the presence of maternal asthma could increase the risk of inducing atopy in a breast-fed infant because of potential differences in immunogenicity between the breast milk of asthmatic vs nonasthmatic mothers. It has been noted that IL-4 and IL-8, IgE, RANTES and n6/n3 PUFAs are found in higher concentrations in the breast milk of atopic mothers. In addition, levels TGF-β1 and TGF-β2, which may protect against the development of allergies, are no higher in the breast milk of asthmatic women.[66]

Conflicting results have been noted in several studies over this past decade. As part of the Tucson Children's Respiratory Study, a prospective study of over 1200 newborns, Wright and colleagues[67] noted that exclusively breast-fed babies had a lower incidence of wheezing in the first 2 years of life, irrespective of the presence of maternal asthma. However, after 6 years of age, a higher rate of asthma was noted in atopic children of asthmatic mothers if they had been exclusively breast-fed. A follow-up study[68] noted decreased lung flows at 11 and 16 years of age in children who had been breast-fed by an asthmatic mother for longer than 4 months. On the other hand, in an Australian study of 2600 infants, Oddy and colleagues[69] reported that the presence of maternal asthma led to no statistically significant difference in the incidence of asthma in children who had been breast-fed. Both of these groups, however, noted an overall decrease in the incidence of asthma and atopic disease in early childhood in those children who were breast-fed. Therefore, at this time, breast-feeding should still be recommended regardless of whether or not the mother has asthma.

Dietary Manipulation During Lactation

A possible explanation for the tremendous discrepancy found in the results of these studies examining the role of breast-feeding in the prevention of allergies is that maternal diet was not controlled. As noted above, milk, egg, and peanut allergens have been measured in breast milk and would therefore be expected to be passed on to the young recipient. Whether these food proteins sensitize or act as protective immunomodulators is unclear at this time. Several studies have attempted to determine whether sensitization to highly allergenic foodstuffs could be prevented in high-risk infants if lactating mothers avoided these foods.[38,70,71]

In 1989 Hattevig and colleagues[70] reported the results of a study comparing two groups of high-risk infants. Both groups of infants were fed breast milk and supplemented with hypoallergenic diets, including casein hydrolysate formulas. The mothers of the infants in the study group avoided egg, cow's milk, and fish during the first 3 months of lactation; the mothers of infants in the control group had no such restrictions on their diets. The control group infants had significantly more atopic dermatitis at 3 and 6 months than the children in the study group. No difference was found in the levels of IgE to milk or egg in the two groups after 6 months of age, which was thought to be due to eventual introduction of these foods into the infants' diets. It was also noted that the development of IgG antibodies to ovalbumin in some of the infants did not lead to decreased production of IgE antibodies to egg protein, suggesting that IgG antibodies do not have a protective effect against allergic sensitization. Follow-up at 10 years showed no long-lasting protective effect in the prevention of allergy in the group whose mothers had ingested a hypoallergenic diet during lactation.[71]

In 1996 two studies were published, one a nonrandomized but well-controlled prospective investigation[72] and the other a nonrandomized nested case control study,[73] that contradicted these findings. The former study demonstrated no protective effects on the development of allergic disease in infants if egg and cow's milk were avoided by the mother during 3 months of lactation and solid foods were not introduced until the infant was 3 months old. The latter study actually showed that significantly more eczema and food allergy sensitization was found in the infants whose mothers avoided highly allergenic foods during lactation.

In a prenatally randomized, physician-blinded, parallel-controlled study, the effect of multiple food allergen avoidance in both the lactating mothers and their infants was compared to standard feeding practices in children with a positive family history of allergy.[74] This study found that children whose intake of allergenic foods from pre- and post-natal sources was restricted showed (1) a significantly lower incidence of allergic diseases such as atopic dermatitis at 1 year of age because of a lower incidence of food allergy and (2) lower specific IgE and IgG to cow's milk up to 2 years of age compared with control infants. There was no effect on the occurrence of respiratory allergy or sensitization to environmental allergens from birth to 7 years.[75]

A study published as part of the Avon Longitudinal Study of nearly 16 000 children, demonstrated no correlation between maternal peanut ingestion during pregnancy and the development of peanut allergy. However, it did note a significant increase in peanut allergy in those infants with oozing skin lesions and in those whose mothers used skin care products containing peanut oil.[76] Proof of the principle of IgE sensitization through the skin had already been demonstrated in a murine model,[77] and a subsequent study[78] showed that epicutaneous peanut exposure in mice could prevent the induction of oral tolerance and lead to a strong peanut-specific IL-4 and IgE response. These studies have led to the suggestion that the previous protection thought to be conferred on the infant by maternal peanut avoidance, may have been due to decreased transdermal absorption, rather than decreased oral intake. Furthermore, another recent British study also demonstrated that while peanut consumption during pregnancy and lactation seemed to increase the risk of peanut allergy in children in a statistically related way, the effect became insignificant when adjusted for household peanut exposure, with which a much stronger correlation was noted.[79] A 2006 Cochrane meta-analysis concluded that prescription of an antigen avoidance diet to a high-risk woman during lactation may reduce her child's risk of developing atopic eczema but that better trials are needed.[39]

Soy Formula and Prevention of Allergic Disease

Although a retrospective study in the early 1950s suggested that children at high risk of atopy might have less allergic disease if fed a soy-based formula as opposed to cow's milk formula,[80] studies in the 1960s[81] and 1970s[82] have shown this not to be the case. The latter study, in particular, which was well designed, controlled, randomized, and immunologically supported, showed no difference in the occurrence of atopy in infants fed either soy or cow's milk formula. There is even some evidence that up to 10–15% of children with cow's milk allergy have IgE antibodies to soy. A study of 93 infants with cow's milk allergy (documented by either double-blind, placebo-controlled food challenge or by documentation of cow's milk IgE coupled with a compelling history of anaphylaxis) demonstrated that soy allergy (documented by double-blind, placebo-controlled food challenge) occurred in 13%.[83] A Cochrane meta-analysis in 2006[84] confirmed that there is no evidence that soy formula is effective at preventing either allergic manifestations or food intolerance in high-risk infants. Therefore, soy formula cannot be recommended for primary prevention of allergic disease. It can, however, be recommended as a safe alternative to cow's milk formula in the majority of infants with cow's milk allergy after screening indicates no coexisting soy allergy.

Protein Hydrolysate Formula and Prevention of Allergic Disease

The ideal protein hydrolysate formula should not contain peptides larger than 1.5 kD, should contain no intact proteins, should demonstrate no anaphylaxis in animals, and should reveal protein determinant equivalents less than 1/1 000 000 of the original protein.[85] Most importantly, the formula must be demonstrated safe in milk-allergic infants by both double-blind, placebo-controlled food challenge and by open challenge.

The most hypoallergenic formulas need to be extensively hydrolyzed in order to be composed of small enough peptides to be considered truly safe in children with milk allergy. Three casein hydrolysate formulas, Pregestimil (Mead Johnson Nutritionals, Evansville, IN), Nutramigen (Mead Johnson Nutritionals, Evansville, IN), and Alimentum (Ross Products, Abbott Laboratories, Columbus, OH), are widely available in the USA, fit these criteria, and are considered hypoallergenic.[86] Profylac (ALK, Denmark) is a less extensively hydrolyzed ultrafiltrated formula, unavailable in the USA, which has also been shown to be hypoallergenic.[87] However, although truly hypoallergenic, these formulas are not completely nonallergenic and allergic reactions can occur.[88] Nutramigen has been shown to be hypoimmunogenic by its ability to inhibit the IgG β-lactoglobulin response by an order of more than one log in high risk[89] and normal infants[90] up to 1 year of age.

Neocate (SHS International, Rockville, MD) and EleCare (Ross Products, Abbott Laboratories, Columbus, OH), both amino acid-derived elemental formulas, are safe in most patients who cannot tolerate the protein hydrolysate formulas and are excellent alternatives.[91] Good Start (Nestle, Vevey, Switzerland; called NanHA outside the USA), a partial whey hydrolysate, has numerous peptides of more than 4 kD and can cause allergic reactions in 40–60% of children with IgE-mediated cow's milk allergy and can therefore not be considered a safe alternative for patients with milk allergy.[92]

Numerous prospective, controlled studies to determine the role of protein hydrolysate formulas as either a single intervention or as part of a combined regimen, including a combined maternal/infant avoidance regimen, have been performed.[93,94]

In a particularly well-controlled study, Halken and colleagues[95] demonstrated a degree of cow's milk allergy in infants exclusively fed extensively hydrolyzed formula similar to that of infants who were breast-fed. Exclusive feeding with protein hydrolysate formula appears to be particularly effective if instituted before 6 months of age.[96]

Decreased atopic dermatitis, cow's milk allergy, milk-specific IgE, and asthma have been reported in infants who have been fed extensively and partially hydrolyzed formulas, in comparison with cow's milk or soy formula-fed babies. A greater protective effect was seen, however, with the extensively hydrolyzed formulas. Two prospective, randomized, controlled studies from Scandinavia[97,98] compared extensively hydrolyzed to partially hydrolyzed formulas in primary allergy prevention. In the Swedish study in which mothers and infants avoided cow's milk, egg, and fish, infants fed extensively hydrolyzed formula for 9 months had a significantly lower cumulative incidence of atopic symptoms, eczema, and positive egg skin tests at 9 months as compared to those infants who were fed partially hydrolyzed formula.[97] The Danish study reported that cow's milk allergy, both by parental report as well as documented by food challenge, was significantly reduced from birth to 18 months in children whose breast-feeding was supplemented with an extensively hydrolyzed formula up to 4 months in comparison to those infants who received a partially hydrolyzed formula for the same period of time.[98]

As part of the German Infant Nutrition Initiative,[99] one study demonstrated that while use of an extensively hydrolyzed casein formula was found to be the most effective formula in preventing allergic manifestations in infants with a family history of atopic dermatitis, an extensively hydrolyzed whey formula was found to be inferior to a partially hydrolyzed formula in this regard. When taking into account cost and palatability, this study suggests that partially hydrolyzed formulas could be a reasonable alternative to extensively hydrolyzed formulas for those mothers of infants at high risk for atopy who cannot breast-feed, yet find extensively hydrolyzed formulas impractical. The noted effect was similar when this group was evaluated for atopic dermatitis at 6 years of age.[100] The relative risk between 4 and 6 years of age in infants fed hydrolyzed formulas vs cow's milk formulas was 0.79 for partially hydrolyzed whey formula (95% CI 064–0.97), 0.92 for extensively hydrolyzed whey formula (95% CI, 0.76–1.11) and 0.71 for extensively hydrolyzed casein formula (95% CI, 0.58–0.88). While the prevalence of 'any allergic manifestations' also showed a similar trend in the three groups, such an effect was not noted for any other single allergic manifestation such as asthma or allergic rhinitis.

In 2006, the most recent Cochrane meta-analysis on this topic was published.[101] Among its conclusions was that prolonged feeding with hydrolyzed formula led to a significant reduction in infant allergy in comparison to cow's milk (7 studies, 2514 infants, typical RR 0.79, 95% CI 0.66–0.94). However, there was no reduction in the incidence of infant eczema, childhood eczema incidence or prevalence, childhood allergy, or infant or childhood asthma, rhinitis or food allergy. A reduction in allergy was also noted in infants fed partially hydrolyzed formula vs cow's milk formula (6 studies, 1391 infants, typical RR 0.79, 95% CI 0.65–0.97), and in infants fed extensively hydrolyzed casein vs cow's milk formula (1 study, 431 infants, RR 0.72, 95% CI 0.53–0.97). Extensively hydrolyzed compared with partially hydrolyzed formula led to a significant reduction in food allergy (2 studies, 341 infants, typical RR 0.43, 95% CI 0.19–0.99) but no change in 'all allergy' or other specific allergy. The meta-analysis also reported two trials that compared early, short term hydrolyzed formula to breast milk. No significant effect on infant allergy or cow's milk allergy was noted.

Overall, there is evidence that the use of hydrolysate formulas can have an effect on the development of infant allergy in comparison to to cow's milk formula and can therefore be recommended to families as an option to reduce risk of atopy in their high-risk infant if breast-feeding is impossible or insufficient. Extensively hydrolyzed formula is likely to be superior to partially hydrolyzed formula in this regard. On the other hand, partially hydrolyzed formulas are less expensive and better tasting, and may be considered a reasonable alternative, particularly if cost is an issue. However, partially hydrolyzed formulas cannot be considered a safe alternative for those children with known milk allergy.

Introduction of Solid Foods

Studies that have examined the effect of the early introduction of solid foods to the infant diet on the subsequent development of allergies have also shown conflicting results. A prospective British study of 257 preterm infants[102] demonstrated an increased risk of eczema at 12 months of age in those infants given ≥ 4 solid foods before 17 weeks of age, as opposed to < 4 (OR 3.49, 95% CI 1.51–8.05). Furthermore, low-risk infants (nonatopic parents) who had solid food introduced at < 10 weeks of age, had a higher risk of eczema at 12 months (OR 2.94, 95% CI 1.57–5.52) compared to those who had solid food introduced later. Surprisingly, this effect was not seen in the infants of atopic parents. No confirmatory immunologic data in the infants was reported.

Conversely, a prospective German study of 642 infants[103] showed no evidence of a protective effect of the late introduction of solid foods on the development of wheezing, atopy or eczema. To the contrary, they noted an increased risk of eczema at the age of 5.5 years in all children, irrespective of risk, in whom egg was introduced after 8 months of age as opposed to those in whom egg was introduced earlier (OR 1.6, 95% CI, 1.1–2.4). Similarly, in another ongoing German study of 2612 children,[104] no protective effect on the development of atopic dermatitis or allergic sensitization was noted by delaying the introduction of solid foods past 6 months of age. However, a more diverse diet at the age of 4 months, as opposed to the introduction of various solids after this age, increased the odds of symptomatic atopic dermatitis, although no dose response was noted, making conclusions unclear. In a related report,[105] no association was found between the time of introduction of solids, or the diversity of solids, and eczema in the first 4 years of life. However, in infants who were in a nonintervention group (a generally lower risk group, whose parents were not given any special dietary recommendations), a decreased risk of doctor-diagnosed eczema was observed for avoidance of soybean and nuts for the first year, but an increased risk was seen in infants who avoided egg for the this period. Furthermore, Poole, and colleagues[106] noted an increased risk of wheat allergy if wheat exposure was delayed until after 6 months of age, after adjustment for numerous variables, (OR 3.8, CI 1.18–12.28). An interesting finding was reported by Du Toit and colleagues, noting that Israeli children, who consume large quantities of peanut protein in infancy, had peanut allergy at one tenth the rate of Jewish children in the UK, raising the question of whether this early introduction of peanut protein may be protective against the development of peanut allergy.[107] At this point it is unclear why some studies suggest a tolerizing effect of the introduction of allergenic foods during infancy and others a sensitizing effect. It is possible that the tipping point between sensitization and induction of tolerance lies in the precise timing of the introduction of immunogenic foods, the route of exposure, the amount ingested, the particular allergen, the genetics of the host, or a combination of some or all of these factors.

In summary, the AAP has now concluded that these studies provide no clear evidence that the delayed introduction of solid foods beyond 4 to 6 months helps prevent the development of atopic disease, conforming more to the European position. Some studies suggest that withholding common allergens such as peanut might even increase the risk of food allergy. However, despite the evidence-based conclusion of the AAP, it should be noted that food allergy in a sibling has been reported to be a significant predictor for food allergy in a child.[108] Therefore special care should still be taken before recommending the introduction of highly allergenic foods to a young sibling of a child with significant food allergies.

Natural History of Food Allergy

Food allergy is most commonly acquired during the first year of life, with peak incidence of 6–8% occurring at 1 year of age. The prevalence falls until late childhood, where it plateaus at about 3.5% through adulthood. The prevalence of perceived, but unconfirmed, food allergy or food intolerance, is as high as 25%.[109]

In a Danish study by Host and Halken,[110] 1749 children were followed prospectively from birth to the age of 3 years. Milk allergy was suspected in 117 children (6.7%) and confirmed by milk elimination and oral challenge in 39 (2.2%), with more than half having documented IgE-mediated disease. In a study from the Isle of Wight,[111] all children born over a 1-year period (N = 1456) were followed for the development of peanut and tree nut allergy until 4 years of age. Fifteen (1.2%) of the 981 skin-tested children were found to be sensitized to peanuts or tree nuts. In a large German study,[112] RASTs were performed yearly to the age of 6 years on a birth cohort of 4082 children. Prevalence of sensitization to foods peaked at 10% at 1 year, declining to 3% at 6 years of age. Egg and milk IgE were the most common positives, followed by wheat and soy; no clinical confirmation of food allergy was reported. It appears that prevalence of food allergies has been increasing over recent years. In 2003, Sicherer and colleagues[113] reported that the rate of allergy to a peanut or tree nut, or both, in children, rose from 0.6% to 1.2% between 1997 and 2003, primarily as a result of an increase in the reported allergy to peanuts from 0.4–0.8% over this period. In 2004, the overall prevalence of food allergy in the USA was reported as 6% in young children and 3.7% in adults.[114] The prevalence of milk allergy in children vs adults was 2.5% vs 0.3%, egg 1.3% vs 0.2%, peanut 0.8% vs 0.6%, tree nut 0.2% vs 0.5%, fish 0.1% vs 0.4 % and shellfish 0.1% vs 2.0%.

It had long been established that, whereas milk and egg allergies are most frequently outgrown in childhood, peanut allergy most commonly remains a lifelong issue. Tree nut, fish, and shellfish allergy are also much more likely to continue into adulthood than are egg and cow's milk allergy. Recent studies suggest that milk[115] and egg allergy[116] are more persistent than they were 15 years ago. In addition, the eventual tolerance or persistence of allergy may be predictable by degree of positivity of allergy tests or concomitant allergic conditions. Similar correlations have been reported with peanut allergy. Recently, Ho and colleagues[117]

demonstrated that peanut prick skin test wheal of 6mm or greater (hazard ratio 2.74, 95% CI 1.13–3.79) and specific IgE >3 kU/L (hazard ratio 2.74, 95% CI 1.13–6.61) were predictive of persistent peanut allergy.

Although it had generally been thought that once food allergies have resolved they are unlikely to recur, the unsettling recurrence of peanut[118] and fish[119] allergy has been reported in patients with previously negative food challenges following a history of earlier allergy. Further to this point, in 2003, Fleischer, and colleagues[120] reported that in a group of 84 patients with peanut allergy, 55% of those with peanut IgE levels < 5kU/L were able to pass peanut challenges, while 63% of those with levels < 2kU/L were able to tolerate peanuts. Recurrence of the peanut allergy was reported in 2 patients, both of whom did not ingest peanuts regularly after they had passed their challenges. Two years later,[121] this group also reported that 9% of patients with tree nut allergy could ultimately pass a double-blind, placebo-controlled food challenge to tree nut.

It seems that there are likely different phenotypes of food allergy, whose natural history depends not only on the amount of IgE measured or concomitant allergic conditions but also the specific epitope against which the IgE is directed. Vila and colleagues[122] demonstrated that the specific cow's milk IgE from patients with persistent cow's milk allergy is more likely to bind to the linear (sequential) epitopes of $\alpha 1$- and β-casein as compared to higher levels of IgE to the conformational (native) epitopes in children who had lost their clinical sensitivity to cow's milk as documented by food challenge. Lately, the phenomenon that some children with egg allergy can tolerate heated egg (egg in baked goods) but not whole egg has been studied. Lemon Mulé and colleagues[123] recently reported that a majority of egg-allergic children could tolerate heated egg, particularly those with smaller prick skin test and egg-specific IgE levels. Furthermore, continued ingestion of heated egg led to decreased skin test wheal diameter, ovalbumin-specific IgE and ovalbumin- and ovomucoid-specific IgG4. The authors noted that these immunologic changes parallel those that one would expect to see in clinical tolerance. The same group reported similar immunologic findings in milk-allergic children who could tolerate heated milk products.[124] Seventy five percent of the milk-allergic children were able to tolerate heated milk. The authors postulated that this tolerance could be due to the loss of conformational epitopes that comes from heating. How these findings can be incorporated into clinical practice is still unclear.

Conclusions

A reliable, consistently effective method of preventing food allergies in high-risk children remains elusive. Whereas immunomodulatory measures may be promising as the future of food allergy prevention, they must still be considered experimental and cannot be routinely recommended at this time other than as part of controlled studies. Both European[2] and American[1] analyses of the literature have recently been updated and concur on the best approach to infant feeding with regard to the prevention of atopy. However, despite our best efforts, food allergy continues to rise. Our knowledge continues to evolve. A case in point is that early avoidance of solid foods, which had heretofore been strongly recommended in the USA as part of an allergy prevention program, may actually lead to an increased risk of allergy in some patients and is therefore no longer considered effective. The conclusions of the evidence-based statement for primary prevention of allergy in children by the American Academy of Pediatrics are summarized in Table 47-2. Overall, the best

Table 47-2 Synopsis of Recent AAP Summary of Data, with Regard to Infant Diet and the Primary Prevention of Food Allergy

Interventions	Summary
Pregnancy diet	No evidence of effectiveness
Lactation diet	Maternal antigen avoidance does not prevent atopic disease with the possible exception of atopic dermatitis. More data needed.
Breast-feeding	Evidence exists that exclusive breast-feeding for at least 4 months vs feeding with cow's milk formula decreases cumulative incidence of atopic dermatitis and cow's milk allergy in the first 2 years of life. Evidence exists that exclusive breast-feeding for at least 3 months protects against wheezing in early life, but there is not convincing evidence that exclusive breast-feeding in high-risk infants protects against allergic asthma beyond 6 years of age.
Soy formula	No convincing evidence exists for the use of soy formula for allergy prevention.
Protein hydrolysate formula	Modest evidence exists that atopic dermatitis may be delayed or prevented by the use of an extensively or partially hydrolyzed formula as compared to cow's milk formula in high-risk infants who are not breast-fed exclusively for 4 to 6 months. Not all hydrolyzed formulas have the same protective benefit. Cost must be considered in any decision-making process.
Delayed introduction of solid foods	No convincing current evidence exists that delaying the introduction of solid food, including fish, egg and peanut, beyond 4 to 6 months protects against the development of allergic disease.

From Greer FR, Sicherer SH, Burks AW. Effects of early nutritional interventions on the development of atopic disease in infants and children: the role of maternal dietary restriction, breastfeeding timing of introduction of complementary foods and hydrolyzed formulas. Pediatrics 121:183-191, 2008. Copyright © by the American Academy of Pediatrics, all rights reserved.

BOX 47-1 Key concepts

Prevention and Natural History of Food Allergy

Primary Prevention

Immunomodulation

- Breast milk may be both immunoprotective and immunostimulatory via complex interplay of cytokines and allergen content.
- Probiotics, prebiotics, polyunsaturated fatty acids and vitamin D are still experimental with regard to prevention of food allergy.

Dietary Manipulation

- Dietary manipulation during pregnancy is of no benefit.
- Dietary manipulation during lactation is not recommended.
- Exclusive breast-feeding during first 4 months of life is recommended.
- Soy formula is not recommended in the primary prevention of allergic disease.
- Hydrolysate formulas are recommended in the primary prevention of food allergy for those infants who cannot breast-feed or as a supplement to breast-feeding.

Natural History of Food Allergy

- Peak incidence of food allergy reaches 6–8% at 1 year of age.
- Prevalence plateaus of 1–2% occur during adulthood.
- Egg and cow's milk allergy are frequently 'outgrown', with ≈70% of children with egg allergy and ≈80% of children with milk allergy able to tolerate egg or milk respectively by 16 years of age.
- Peanut allergy and tree nut allergy persist in 80–90% of cases. Resensitization can also occur.
- Ultimate tolerance of allergenic food may be predicted somewhat by degree of positivity of allergy tests, concomitant allergic conditions and specificity of epitope binding.

---

recommendation for families at high risk for allergic disease, who are motivated to do anything they can to reduce their child's risk of atopy, would be breast-feeding for the first 4 months and not smoking. An extensively hydrolyzed formula can be recommended as a supplement, if needed, or as an alternative to nursing if the mother cannot or chooses not to breast-feed. Partially hydrolyzed formula can also be considered if cost or taste is an obstacle. Soy formula is not recommended. Pregnancy or lactation diets are not currently recommended and introduction of solid foods, even 'allergenic' ones, need not be delayed past 4 to 6 months in an effort to prevent food allergies. Probiotics, prebiotics or n-3 PUFA supplements can, similarly, not be recommended at this time for this purpose.

Once food allergies have been diagnosed, skin test and/or serum allergen-specific IgE should be obtained to monitor the degree of sensitization. More sophisticated tests, such as epitope recognition, might also play a role in determining who is most likely to 'outgrow' their food allergies, as well as degree or positivity of allergy tests and concomitant symptoms. Food challenges should be performed to confirm diagnosis and follow clinical course when appropriate (Box 47-1).

Helpful Websites

The Food Allergy and Anaphylaxis Network website (www.foodallergy.org)
Learning early about peanut allergy (leapstudy.co.uk)

Acknowledgement

The author would like to thank Robert S. Zeiger, MD, PhD for his invaluable assistance in the preparation of this manuscript.

References

1. Greer FR, Sicherer SH, Burks AW. Effects of early nutritional interventions on the development of atopic disease in infants and children: the role of maternal dietary restriction, breastfeeding, timing of introduction of complementary foods and hydrolyzed formulas. Pediatrics 2008; 121:183–91.
2. Host A, Halken S, Muraro A, et al. Dietary prevention of allergic disease in infants and small children. Pediatr Allergy Immunol 2008; 19:1–4.
3. Hoppu U, Kalliomaki M, Laiho K, et al. Breast milk: immunomodulatory signals against allergic diseases. Allergy 2001;56:23–6.
4. Taylor B, Wadsworth J, Golding J, et al. Breast feeding, eczema, asthma, and hayfever. J Epidemiol Community Health 1983;37:95–9.
5. Casas R, Bottcher MF, Duchen K, et al. Detection of IgA antibodies to cat, beta-lactoglobulin, and ovalbumin allergens in human milk. J Allergy Clin Immunol 2000;105:1236–40.
6. Duchen K, Casas R, Fageras-Bottcher M, et al. Human milk polyunsaturated long-chain fatty acids and secretory immunoglobulin A antibodies and early childhood allergy. Pediatr Allergy Immunol 2000;11: 29–39.
7. Bottcher MF, Jenmalm MC, Garofalo RP, et al. Cytokines in breast milk from allergic and nonallergic mothers. Pediatr Res 2000;47:157–62.
8. Kalliomaki M, Ouwehand A, Arvilommi H, et al. Transforming growth factor-beta in breast milk: a potential regulator of atopic disease at an early age. J Allergy Clin Immunol 1999;104:1251–7.

501

9. Baldini M, Lohman IC, Halonen M, et al. A polymorphism* in the 5' flanking region of the CD14 gene is associated with circulating soluble CD14 levels and with total serum immunoglobulin E. Am J Respir Cell Mol Biol 1999;20:976–83.

10. Labeta MO, Vidal K, Nores JE, et al. Innate recognition of bacteria in human milk is mediated by a milk-derived highly expressed pattern recognition receptor, soluble CD14. J Exp Med 2000;191:1807–12.

11. Sala-Vila A, Miles EA, Calder PC. Fatty acid composition abnormalities in atopic disease: evidence explored and role in the disease process examined. Clin Exp Allergy 2008;38:1432–11450.

12. Dandrifosse G, Peulen O, El Khefif N, et al. Are milk polyamines preventive agents against food allergy? Proc Nutr Soc 2000;59:81–6.

13. Osterlund P, Smedberg T, Hakulinen H, et al. Eosinophilic cationic protein in human milk is associated with development of cow's milk allergy and atopic eczema in breast-fed infants. Pediatr Res 2004;55:296–301.

14. Majamaa H, Isolauri E. Probiotics: a novel approach in the management of food allergy. J Allergy Clin Immunol 1997;99:179–85.

15. Isolauri E, Arvola T, Sutas Y, et al. Probiotics in the management of atopic eczema. Clin Exp Allergy 2000;30:1604–10.

16. Bodera P, Chcialowski A. Immunomodulatory effect of probiotic bacteria. Recent Pat Inflamm Allergy Drug Discov 2009;3:58–64.

17. Murosaki S, Yamamoto Y, Ito K, et al. Heat-killed Lactobacillus plantarum L-137 suppresses naturally fed antigen-specific IgE production by stimulation of IL-12 production in mice. J Allergy Clin Immunol 1998;102:57–64.

18. Fossard CP, Steidler L, Eigenmann PA. Oral administration of an IL-10-secreting lactococcus lactis strain prevents food-induced IgE sensitization. J Allergy Clin Immunol 2007;119:952–9.

19. Kalliomaki M, Salminen S, Arvilommi H, et al. Probiotics in primary prevention of atopic disease: a randomised placebo-controlled trial. Lancet 2001;357:1076–9.

20. Rautava S, Kalliomaki M, Isolauri E. Probiotics during pregnancy and breast-feeding might confer immunomodulatory protection against atopic disease in the infant. J Allergy Clin Immunol 2002;109:119–21.

21. Taylor AL, Dunstan JA, Prescott SL. Probiotic supplementation for the first 6 months of life fails to reduce the risk of atopic dermatitis and increases the risk of allergen sensitization in high-risk children: a randomized controlled trial. J Allergy Clin Immunol, 2007;119:184–91.

22. Lee, J, Seto D, Bielory L. Meta-analysis of clinical trials of probiotics for prevention and treatment of pediatric atopic dermatitis. J Allergy Clin Immunol, 2008;121:116–21.

23. Miniello VL, Moro GE, Armenio L. Prebiotic in infant formulas: new perspectives. Acta Paediatr Suppl 2003;441:68–76.

24. Moro GE, Arslanoglu S, Stahl B, et al. A mixture of prebiotic oligosaccharides reduces the incidence of atopic dermatitis during the first six months of age. Arch Des Child 2006;91:814–9.

25. Arslanoglu S, Moro GE, Schmitt J. Early dietary intervention with a mixture of prebiotic oligosaccharides reduces the incidence of allergic manifestations and infections during the first two years of life. J Nutr 2008;138:1091–5.

26. Ziegler E, Vanderhoof JA, Petschow B, et al. Term infants fed formula supplemented with selected blends of prebiotics grow normally and have soft stools similar to those reported for breast-fed infants. J Pediatr Gastroenterol Nutr 2007;44:359–64.

27. Osborn DA, Sinn JKH. Probiotics in infants for prevention of allergic disease and food hypersensitivity. Cochrane Database Syst Rev 2007:CD006475.

28. Kukkonen K, Savilhati E, Haahtela T. Probiotics and prebiotic galacto-oligosaccharides in the prevention of allergic diseases: a randomized, double-blind, placebo-controlled trial. J Allergy Clin Immunol 2007;119:192–8.

29. Kuitunen M, Kukkonen K, Juntunen-Backman K, et al. Probiotics prevent IgE-associated allergy until age 5 in cesarean-delivered children but not in the total cohort. J Allergy Clin Immunol 2009;123:335–41.

30. Adlerberth I, Strachan DP, Matricardi PM. Gut microbiota and development of atopic eczema in 3 European cohorts. J Allergy Clin Immunol 2007;120:343–50.

31. Dunstan JA, Mori TA, Barden A, et al. Maternal fish oil supplementation in pregnancy reduces the interleukin-13 levels in cord blood of infants at high risk of atopy. Clin Exp Allergy 2003;33:442–8.

32. Barden AE, Mori TA, Dunstan JA, et al. Fish oil supplementation in pregnancy lowers F2-isoprostanes in neonates at high risk of atopy. Free Radic Res 2004;38:233–9.

33. Dunstan JA, Mori TA, Barden A, et al. Fish oil supplementation in pregnancy modifies neonatal allergen-specific immune responses and clinical outcomes in infants at high risk of atopy: a randomized, controlled trial. J Allergy Clin Immunol 2003;112:1178–84.

34. Marks GB, Mihrshahi S, Kemp AS, et al. Prevention of asthma in the first 5 years of life: a randomized controlled trial. J Allergy Clin Immunol 2006;118:53–71.

35. Anandan C, Nurmatov U, Sheikh A. Omega 3 and 6 oils for primary prevention of allergic disease: systematic review and meta-analysis. Allergy 2009;64:840–8.

36. Michel FB, Bousquet J, Greillier P, et al. Comparison of cord blood immunoglobulin E concentrations and maternal allergy for the prediction of atopic diseases in infancy. J Allergy Clin Immunol 1980;65:422–30.

37. Zeiger RS. Prevention of food allergy in infancy. Ann Allergy 1990;65:430–42.

38. Falth-Magnusson K, Kjellman NI. Development of atopic disease in babies whose mothers were receiving exclusion diet during pregnancy: a randomized study. J Allergy Clin Immunol 1987;80:868–75.

39. Kramer KS, Kakuma R. Maternal dietary antigen avoidance during pregnancy and or lactation for preventing or treating atopic dermatitis in the child. Cochrane Database Syst Rev 2006:CD000133.

40. Carlson K-H, Carlsen KCL. Respiratory effects of tobacco smoking on infants and young children. Paediatric Resp Rev 2008;9:11–20.

41. American Academy of Pediatrics Committee on Nutrition. Hypoallergenic infant formulas. Pediatrics 2000;106:346–9.

42. Stuart CA, Twiselton R, Nicholas MK, et al. Passage of cows' milk protein in breast milk. Clin Allergy 1984;14:533–5.

43. Cant A, Marsden RA, Kilshaw PJ. Egg and cows' milk hypersensitivity in exclusively breast fed infants with eczema, and detection of egg protein in breast milk. Br Med J (Clin Res Ed) 1985;291:932–5.

44. Troncone R, Scarcella A, Donatiello A, et al. Passage of gliadin into human breast milk. Acta Paediatr Scand 1987;76:453–6.

45. Vadas P, Wai Y, Burks W, et al. Detection of peanut allergens in breast milk of lactating women. JAMA 2001;285:1746–8.

46. Grulee CG, Sanford HN. The influence of breast and artificial feeding on infantile eczema. J Pediatr 1939;9:223–5.

47. Lucas A, Brooke OG, Morley R, et al. Early diet of preterm infants and development of allergic or atopic disease: randomised prospective study. Br Med J 1990;300:837–40.

48. Laubereau B, Brockow I, Zirngibl A, et al. Effect of breast-feeding on the development of atopic dermatitis during the first 3 years of life–results from the GINI-birth cohort study. J Pediatr 2004;144:602–7.

49. Kull I, Almqvist C, Lilja G, et al. Breast-feeding reduces the risk of asthma during the first 4 years of life. J Allergy Clin Immunol 2004;114:755–60.

50. Oddy WH, Peat JK, de Klerk NH. Maternal asthma, infant feeding, and the risk of asthma in childhood. J Allergy Clin Immunol 2002;110:65–7.

51. Kull I, Wickman M, Lilja G, et al. Breast feeding and allergic diseases in infants: a prospective birth cohort study. Arch Dis Child 2002;87:478–81.

52. Kull I, Bohme M, Wahlgren CF, et al. Breast-feeding reduces the risk for childhood eczema. J Allergy Clin Immunol 2005;116:657–61.

53. Oddy WH, Holt PG, Sly PD, et al. Association between breast feeding and asthma in 6 year old children: findings of a prospective birth cohort study. Br Med J 1999;319:815–9.

54. Snijders BEP, Thijs C, Kummeling I, et al. Breastfeeding and infant eczema in the first year of life in the KOALA birth cohort study: a risk period-specific analysis. Pediatrics 2007;119:137–41.

55. Bergmann RL, Diepgen TL, Kuss O, et al. Breastfeeding duration is a risk factor for atopic eczema. Clin Exp Allergy 2002;32:205–9.

56. Sears MR, Greene JM, Willan AR, et al. Long-term relation between breastfeeding and development of atopy and asthma in children and young adults: a longitudinal study. Lancet 2002;360:901–7.

57. Peat JK, Allen J, Oddy W, et al. Breastfeeding and asthma: appraising the controversy. Pediatr Pulmonol 2003;35:331–4.

58. Sears MR, Taylor DR, Poulton R. Breastfeeding and asthma: appraising the controversy: a rebuttal. Pediatr Pulmonol 2003;36:366–8.

59. Matheson MC, Erbas B, Balasuriya A, et al. Breast-feeding and atopic disease: a cohort study from childhood to middle age. J Allergy Clin Immunol 2007;120:1051–7.

60. Gdalevich M, Mimouni D, David M, et al. Breast-feeding and the onset of atopic dermatitis in childhood: a systematic review and meta-analysis of prospective studies. J Am Acad Dermatol 2001;45:520–7.

61. Gdalevich M, Mimouni D, Mimouni M. Breast-feeding and the risk of bronchial asthma in childhood: a systematic review with meta-analysis of prospective studies. J Pediatr 2001;139:261–6.

62. van Odjik J, Kull I, Borres MP, et al. Breastfeeding and allergic disease: a multidisciplinary review of the literature (1966–2001) on the mode of early feeding in infancy and its impact on later atopic manifestations. Allergy 2003;58(9):833–43.

63. Kramer MS, Kakuma R. Optimal duration of exclusive breastfeeding (Cochrane Review). Cochrane Database Syst Rev 2002:CD003517.

64. Wright AL, Bauer M, Naylor A, et al. Increasing breastfeeding rates to reduce infant illness at the community level. Pediatrics 1998;101:837–44.

65. Ball TM, Wright AL. Health care costs of formula-feeding in the first year of life. Pediatrics 1999;103:870–6.

66. Duchen K, Casas R, Fageras-Bottcher M, et al. Human milk polyunsaturated longchain fatty acids and secretory immunoglobulin A antibodies and early childhood allergy. Pediatr Allergy Immunol 2000;11:29–39.
67. Wright AL, Holberg CJ, Taussig LM, et al. Factors influencing the relation of infant feeding to asthma and recurrent wheeze in childhood. Thorax 2001;56:192–7.
68. Guilbert TW, Stern DA, Morgan WJ, et al. Effect of breastfeeding on lung function in childhood and modulation by maternal asthma and atopy. Am J Respir Crit Care Med 2007;176:843–8.
69. Oddy WH, Peat JK, de Klerk NH. Maternal asthma, infant feeding, and the risk of asthma in childhood. J Allergy Clin Immunol 2002;110:65–7.
70. Hattevig G, Kjellman B, Sigurs N, et al. Effect of maternal avoidance of eggs, cow's milk and fish during lactation upon allergic manifestations in infants. Clin Exp Allergy 1989;19:27–32.
71. Hattevig G, Sigurs N, Kjellman B. Effects of maternal dietary avoidance during lactation on allergy in children at 10 years of age. Acta Paediatr 1999;88:7–12.
72. Herrmann ME, Dannemann A, Gruters A, et al. Prospective study of the atopy-preventive effect of maternal avoidance of milk and eggs during pregnancy and lactation. Eur J Pediatr 1996;155:770–4.
73. Pollard C, Phil M, Bevin S. Influence of maternal diet during lactation upon allergic manifestation in infants: tolerization or sensitization. J Allergy Clin Immunol 1996;97:240.
74. Zeiger RS, Heller S, Mellon MH, et al. Effect of combined maternal and infant food-allergen avoidance on development of atopy in early infancy: a randomized study. J Allergy Clin Immunol 1989;84:72–89.
75. Zeiger RS, Heller S. The development and prediction of atopy in high-risk children: follow-up at age seven years in a prospective randomized study of combined maternal and infant food allergen avoidance. J Allergy Clin Immunol 1995;95:1179–90.
76. Lack G, Fox D, Northstone K, et al. Factors associated with the development of peanut allergy in childhood. N Engl J Med 2003;348:977–85.
77. Hsieh KY, Tsai CC, Wu CH, et al. Epicutaneous exposure to protein antigen and food allergy. Clin Exp Allergy 2003;33:1067–75.
78. Strid J, Hourihane J, Kimber I, et al. Epicutaneous exposure to peanut protein prevents oral tolerance and enhances allergic sensitization. Clin Exp Allergy 2005;35:757–66.
79. Fox AT, Sasieni P, du Toit G, et al. Household peanut consumption as a risk factor for the development of peanut allergy. J Allergy Clin Immunol 2009;123:417–23.
80. Johnstone DE, Glaser J. Use of soybean milk as an aid in prophylaxis of allergic disease in children. J Allergy 1953;24:434–6.
81. Johnstone DE, Dutton A. The value of hyposensitization therapy for bronchial asthma in children: a 14-year study. Pediatrics 1968;42:793–802.
82. Kjellman NI, Johansson SG. Soy versus cow's milk in infants with a biparental history of atopic disease: development of atopic disease and immunoglobulins from birth to 4 years of age. Clin Allergy 1979;9:347–58.
83. Zeiger RS, Sampson HA, Bock SA, et al. Soy allergy in infants and children with IgE-associated cow's milk allergy. J Pediatr 1999;134:614–22.
84. Osborn DA, Sinn JKH. Soy formula for prevention of allergy and food intolerance in infants. Cochrane Database Syst Rev 2006:CD003741.
85. Oldaeus G, Bradley CK, Bjorksten B, et al. Allergenicity screening of 'hypoallergenic' milk-based formulas. J Allergy Clin Immunol 1992;90:133–5.
86. Sampson HA, Bernhisel-Broadbent J, Yang E, et al. Safety of casein hydrolysate formula in children with cow milk allergy. J Pediatr 1991;118:520–5.
87. Ragno V, Giampietro PG, Bruno G. Allergenicity of milk protein hydrolysate formulae in children with cow's milk allergy. Eur J Pediatr 1993;153:760–2.
88. Lifschitz CH, Hawkins HK, Guerra C, et al. Anaphylactic shock due to cow's milk protein hypersensitivity in a breast-fed infant. J Pediatr Gastroenterol Nutr 1988;7:141–4.
89. Zeiger RS, Heller S, Mellon MH, et al. Genetic and environmental factors affecting the development of atopy through age 4 in children of atopic parents: a prospective randomized study of food allergen avoidance. Pediatr Allergy Immunol 1992;3:110–27.
90. Vaarala O, Saukkonen T, Savilahti E, et al. Development of immune response to cow's milk proteins in infants receiving cow's milk or hydrolyzed formula. J Allergy Clin Immunol 1995;96:917–23.
91. Sampson HA, James JM, Bernhisel-Broadbent J. Safety of an amino acid-derived infant formula in children allergic to cow milk. Pediatrics 1992;90:463–5.
92. Businco L, Cantani A, Longhi MA, et al. Anaphylactic reactions to a cow's milk whey protein hydrolysate (Alfa- Re, Nestle) in infants with cow's milk allergy. Ann Allergy 1989;62:333–5.
93. Vandenplas Y, Hauser B, Van den Borre C, et al. The long-term effect of a partial whey hydrolysate formula on the prophylaxis of atopic disease. Eur J Pediatr 1995;154:488–94.
94. Mallet E, Henocq A. Long-term prevention of allergic diseases by using protein hydrolysate formula in at-risk infants. J Pediatr 1992;121:S95-S100.
95. Halken S, Host A, Hansen LG, et al. Preventive effect of feeding high-risk infants a casein hydrolysate formula or an ultrafiltrated whey hydrolysate formula: a prospective, randomized, comparative clinical study. Pediatr Allergy Immunol 1993;4:173–81.
96. Odelram H, Vanto T, Jacobsen L, et al. Whey hydrolysate compared with cow's milk-based formula for weaning at about 6 months of age in high allergy-risk infants: effects on atopic disease and sensitization. Allergy 1996;51:192–5.
97. Oldaeus G, Anjou K, Bjorksten B, et al. Extensively and partially hydrolysed infant formulas for allergy prophylaxis. Arch Dis Child 1997;77:4–10.
98. Halken S, Hansen KS, Jacobsen HP, et al. Comparison of a partially hydrolyzed infant formula with two extensively hydrolyzed formulas for allergy prevention: a prospective, randomized study. Pediatr Allergy Immunol 2000;11:149–61.
99. von Berg A, Koletzko S, Grubl A, et al. The effect of hydrolyzed cow's milk formula for allergy prevention in the first year of life: the German Infant Nutritional Intervention Study, a randomized double-blind trial. J Allergy Clin Immunol 2003;111:533–40.
100. von Berg A, Filipiak-Pittroff B, Kramer U, et al. Preventive effect of hydrolyzed infant formulas persists until age 6 years: long-term results from the German Infant Nutritional Intervention Study (GINI). J Allergy Clin Immunol 2008;121:1442–7.
101. Osborn DA, Sinn J. Formulas containing hydrolysed protein for prevention of allergy and food intolerance in infants. Cochrane Database Syst Rev 2006:CD003664.
102. Morgan J, Williams P, Norris F, et al. Eczema and early solid feeding in preterm infants. Arch Dis Child 2004;89:309–14.
103. Zutavern A, von Mutius E, Harris J, et al. The introduction of solids in relation to asthma and eczema. Arch Dis Child 2004;89:303–8.
104. Zutavern A, Brockow I, Schaaf B, et al. Timing of solid food introduction in relation to atopic dermatitis and atopic sensitization: results from a prospective birth cohort study. Pediatrics 2006;117:401–11.
105. Filipiak B, Zutavern A, Koletzko I, et al. Solid food introduction in relation to eczema: results from a four-year prospective birth cohort study. J Pediatr 2007;151:352–8.
106. Poole JA, Barriga K, Leung DYM, et al. Timing of initial exposure to cereal grains and the risk of wheat allergy. Pediatrics 2006;117:2175–82.
107. Du Toit G, Katz Y, Sasieni P, et al. Early consumption of peanuts in infancy is associated with a low prevalence of peanut allergy. J Allergy Clin Immunol 2008;122:984–91.
108. Tsai HJ, Kumar R, Pongracic J. Familial aggregation of food allergy and sensitization to food allergens: a family-based study. Clin Exp Allergy 2009;39:101–9.
109. Wood RA. The natural history of food allergy. Pediatrics 2003;111:1631–7.
110. Host A, Halken S. A prospective study of cow milk allergy in Danish infants during the first 3 years of life: clinical course in relation to clinical and immunological type of hypersensitivity reaction. Allergy 1990;45:587–96.
111. Tariq SM, Stevens M, Matthews S, et al. Cohort study of peanut and tree nut sensitisation by age of 4 years. Br Med J 1996;313:514–7.
112. Kulig M, Bergmann R, Klettke U, et al. Natural course of sensitization to food and inhalant allergens during the first 6 years of life. J Allergy Clin Immunol 1999;103:1173–9.
113. Sicherer SH, Munoz-Furlong A, Sampson HA. Prevalence of peanut and tree nut allergy in the United States determined by means of a random digit dial telephone survey: a 5-year follow-up study. J Allergy Clin Immunol 2003;112:1203–7.
114. Sampson HA, Update on food allergy. J Allergy Clin Immunol 2004;113:805–19.
115. Skirpak JM, Matsui EC, Mudd K, et al. The natural history of IgE-mediated cow's milk allergy. J Allergy Clin Immunol 2007;120:1172–7.
116. Savage JH, Matsui EC, Skirpak JM, et al. The natural history of egg allergy. J Allergy Clin Immunol 2007;120:1413–7.
117. Ho MH, Wong WH, Heine RG, et al. Early clinical predictors of remission of peanut allergy. J Allergy Clin Immunol 2008;121:731–6.
118. Busse PJ, Noone SA, Nowak-Wegrzyn AH. Recurrence of peanut allergy. J Allergy Clin Immunol 2002;109:S92.
119. De Frutos C, Zapatero L, Martinez I. Re-sensitization to fish in allergic children after a temporary tolerance period: two case reports. J Allergy Clin Immunol 2002;109:S306.
120. Fleischer DM, Conover-Walker MK, Christie L, et al. The natural progression of peanut allergy: resolution and the possibility of recurrence. J Allergy Clin Immunol 2003;112:183–9.

Prevention and Natural History of Food Allergy

121. Fleischer DM, Conover-Walker MK, Matsui EC, et al. The natural history of tree nut allergy. J Allergy Clin Immunol 2005;116:1087–93.

122. Vila L, Beyer K, Jarvinen KM, et al. Role of conformational and linear epitopes in the achievement of tolerance in cow's milk allergy. Clin Exp Allergy 2001;31:1599–606.

123. Lemon-Mulé H, Sampson HA, Sicherer SH, et al. Immunologic changes in children with egg allergy ingesting extensively heated egg. J Allergy Clin Immunol 2008;122:977–83.

124. Nowak-Wegrzyn A, Bloom KA, Sicherer SH, et al. Tolerance to extensively heated milk in children with cow's milk allergy. J Allergy Clin Immunol 2008;122:342–7.

Enterocolitis, Proctocolitis, and Enteropathies

Scott H. Sicherer

In contrast to intolerances, toxic or pharmacologic responses to foods, food allergies are defined by an adverse immune response to dietary proteins.[1] They are categorized by immunopathophysiology, among disorders with an acute onset following ingestion that are associated with food-specific immunoglobulin E (IgE) antibody (e.g. oral allergy syndrome, anaphylaxis), those that are chronic in nature and sometimes associated with IgE antibody (e.g. eosinophilic gastroenteropathies), and those that are presumed to be cell mediated and not associated with detectable IgE antibody. This chapter focuses upon four non-IgE-mediated food hypersensitivity disorders that affect the gastrointestinal tract: food-protein-induced proctocolits, enterocolitis, enteropathy, and celiac disease.[2] These disorders have overlapping symptoms but are distinguishable clinically and have distinct patterns of symptoms and clinical course.

Epidemiology/Etiology

Dietary Protein Proctocolitis

This disorder of infancy, also known as allergic eosinophilic proctocolitis, is characterized by the presence of mucousy, bloody stools in an otherwise healthy infant. The disorder is attributed to an immune response directed, most commonly, against cow's milk protein. The mean age at diagnosis is approximately 60 days, with a range of 1 day to 6 months.[3,4] The bleeding is often mistakenly attributed to perirectal fissures, although bleeding associated with fissures tends to present with streaks of blood on hard, formed stool rather than mixed in frothy, mucousy stool, which is more typical of proctocolitis. Occasionally there is associated colic or increased frequency of bowel movements, but failure to thrive is absent. About 60% of cases occur in breast-fed infants where the immune response results from maternal ingestion of the food allergen, usually cow's milk, which is passed in immunologically recognizable form into the breast milk. In formula-fed infants, the reaction is associated with cow's milk or, less commonly, soy.[5-7] The disorder has rarely been described in infants fed hypoallergenic, extensively hydrolysed formulas.[8] Associated peripheral blood eosinophilia, hypoalbuminemia or anemia are uncommon.[3-5] Markers of atopy such as atopic dermatitis or a positive family history of atopy are not significantly increased compared with the general population.[3-5] Although described primarily in infants, milk-responsive rectal bleeding and colonic eosinophilia were reported in a series of 16 otherwise healthy 2 to 14-year-old children evaluated in a regional center in Italy.[9] This cohort, described as having protein-induced

proctocolitis presenting in childhood, had disorders other than food allergy largely ruled out; however, these children often had additional gastrointestinal symptoms that may have indicated more widespread inflammation.

Endoscopic examination is usually not needed for diagnostic purposes but, when performed, shows patchy erythema, friability, and a loss of vascularity generally limited to the rectum but sometimes extending throughout the colon.[10] Histologically, high numbers of eosinophils (5 to 20 per high-power field) or eosinophilic abscesses are seen in the lamina propria, crypt epithelium, and muscularis mucosa.[3,11] The eosinophils are frequently associated with lymphoid nodules (lymphonodular hyperplasia).[3,9] However, lymphonodular hyperplasia is not unique to this condition.[3,11] The specific immunologic mechanisms responsible are unknown. Because the disorder is confined to the lower colon and the disorder is most prominent in breast-fed infants, it has been hypothesized that dietary antigens complexed to breast milk IgA may play a part in the activation of eosinophils and the distribution of the inflammatory process.[12]

The frequency of food allergy causing rectal bleeding in infants has not been extensively studied. Xanthakos and colleagues[13] performed colonoscopy and biopsy on 22 infants presenting with rectal bleeding and proved eosinophilic colitis in 14 (64%). The remainder had normal biopsies (23%) or nonspecific colitis (14%). This group recommended dietary elimination for those with eosinophilic colitis and the majority had resolution within 1 to 3 weeks. However, the relationship of cow's milk protein to symptoms was not proven by re-challenge. Arvola and colleagues[14] examined 40 infants presenting with rectal bleeding. Infants were randomized to either avoid cow's milk protein or maintain their current diet. The duration or severity of bleeding was not different between the two groups. During follow-up, cow's milk allergy was diagnosed in 18% of the infants (based upon various criteria including flares of atopic dermatitis and urticaria upon food challenge as well as rectal bleeding) and for these cow's milk allergic infants, there was a reduced length of bleeding if they had been randomized to an elimination diet at study outset. Atopic dermatitis and confirmed inflammation of the colonic mucosa were associated with persistence of cow's milk allergy to the age of 1 year. These studies indicate that food allergy may not be a common cause of rectal bleeding in infants unless there are additional signs of allergy.

Dietary Protein Enterocolitis (Box 48-1)

Dietary protein enterocolitis (also termed *food-protein-induced enterocolitis syndrome* [FPIES]) describes a symptom complex of profuse vomiting and diarrhea usually diagnosed in the first months of life and most commonly attributable to an immune response to cow's milk or soy.[15] Both the small and large bowels are involved in the inflammatory process. When the causal protein remains in the diet, chronic symptoms can include bloody diarrhea, poor growth, anemia, hypoalbuminemia, and fecal leukocytes, and the illness may progress to dehydration and hypotension.[16,17] Removal of the causal protein leads to resolution of symptoms but re-exposure prior to resolution of the allergy results in a characteristic delayed (about 2 hours) onset of vomiting, lethargy, elevation of the peripheral blood polymorphonuclear leukocyte count and possibly reduced temperature, thrombocytosis, hypotension, dehydration, acidemia, and methhemoglobinemia.[18,19] These reactions mimic sepsis.

Powell[20] initially characterized the syndrome. She described nine infants with severe, protracted diarrhea and vomiting. The symptoms developed at 4 to 27 days after birth (mean, 11 days) in infants on a cow's milk-based formula. Switching to a soy-based formula resulted in transient improvement, but symptoms generally recurred in 7 days. Seven of the nine infants were below birth weight, and eight of nine presented with dehydration. Eight of the infants appeared acutely ill and underwent sepsis evaluations that were negative. All infants were noted to have low serum albumin, elevated peripheral blood polymorphonuclear leukocyte counts, and stools that were positive for heme and reducing substances. The hospital course usually involved improvement while on intravenous fluids followed by recurrence of dramatic symptoms with reintroduction of soy- or cow's milk-based formula, including the development of shock in several infants. Follow-up with oral challenges was carried out with cow's milk and soybean formulas at a mean age of 5.5 months, and 14 of the 18 challenges were positive. Ten of 14 challenges resulted in vomiting (onset, 1 to 2.5 hours after ingestion; mean, 2.1 hours) and all experienced diarrhea (onset, 2 to 10 hours; mean, 5 hours) with blood, polymorphonuclear leukocytes and eosinophils, and increased carbohydrate in the stool. There was a rise in peripheral blood polymorphonuclear cell counts in all positive challenges peaking at 6 hours after ingestion, with a mean rise of 9900 cells/mm^3 (range, 5500 to 16 800 cells/mm^3). Only isolated gastrointestinal symptoms were reported.

The results of these studies led Powell[20,21] to propose criteria for a positive oral challenge to diagnose food-protein-induced enterocolitis of infancy.[22] Confirmation of the allergy included a negative search for other causes, improvement when not ingesting the causal protein, and a positive oral challenge resulting in vomiting/diarrhea, evidence of gastrointestinal inflammation through stool examination, and a rise in the peripheral polymor-

phonuclear leukocyte count over 3500 cells/mL. Numerous foods, other than milk and soy, have subsequently been documented as triggers for FPIES, including rice, oat, meats, fish, fruits, vegetables and egg.[19,23-27] The dramatic nature of the presentation often results in evaluations for sepsis or surgical diagnoses,[28] and a delay in final diagnosis until more than one episode occurs.[19]

Since infantile FPIES is a diagnosis that can be made clinically, there are no large series in which biopsies are performed solely in patients fulfilling Powell's criteria. Regarding immunopathology, studies have focused upon the role of T cells and the importance of TNF-α. Heyman and colleagues[29] demonstrated that TNF-α secreted by circulating cow's milk protein-specific T cells increased intestinal permeability, thus possibly contributing to the influx of antigen into the submucosa with further activation of antigen-specific lymphocytes. Fecal TNF-α was also found in increased concentrations after positive milk challenge in patients with cow's milk-induced gastrointestinal reactions.[30,31] Benlounes and colleagues[32] showed that significantly lower doses of intact cow's milk protein stimulated TNF-α secretion from peripheral blood mononuclear cells of patients with active intestinal cow's milk allergy in comparison to either patients whose sensitivity resolved, or those with skin, rather than intestinal, manifestations of cow's milk hypersensitivity. In addition, in vitro kinetic studies differed in these groups, with those having active disease showing two peaks in TNF-α elaboration, the second peak occurring later during culture.[33] Chung and colleagues[34] examined the presence of TNF-α in duodenal biopsy specimens using immunostains in infants with FPIES. Semi-quantitative analyses revealed higher staining for TNF-α in affected infants with villus atrophy compared to those without atrophy and in normal controls. Taken together, these studies support the notion that TNF-α plays a role in the acute and chronic symptoms of FPIES. It is also known that the regulatory cytokine TGF-β1 is involved in the protection of the epithelial barrier of the gut from the penetration of foreign antigens.[35,36] Chung and colleagues[34] demonstrated that the type 1, but not type 2, receptor for TGF-β1 were decreased in duodenal biopsy specimens in patients with FPIES compared to controls. Analysis of humoral features in milk-induced enterocolitis showed milk-protein specific IgA, but very low levels of specific IgG1 and IgG4; this has been theorized to be pathogenic because IgG4 might otherwise block complement fixing antibodies.[37] Specific IgE is sometimes noted as well, and may be a marker of persistence.[18]

Dietary Protein Enteropathy

This disorder is characterized by protracted diarrhea, vomiting, malabsorption, and failure to thrive. Additional features may include abdominal distention, early satiety, edema, hypoproteinemia, and protein-losing enteropathy.[2] Symptoms usually begin in the first several months of life, depending on the time of exposure to the causal proteins. The disorder was described primarily from the 1960s to the 1990s[38-41] and was commonly attributed to cow's milk protein. The diagnosis was made more commonly in infants taking formula, rather than breast-feeding, particularly when such formulas were not commercially processed. A decrease in prevalence was documented in Finland[42] and Spain[43] and attributed to a rise in breast-feeding and/or the use of adapted infant formula. There have been no clear reports of this diagnosis in the past several years, although presentations of eosinophilic gastroenteritis with protein-losing enteropathy share many features with previous descriptions of this disorder.[44,45]

Biopsy reveals variable small bowel villus injury, increased crypt length, intraepithelial lymphocytes, and few eosinophils. The immune mechanisms appear to involve T cell responses[46] and are not associated with IgE antibodies. Cytokine profiles determined from evaluation of lamina propria lymphocytes in affected infants reveal increased interferon (IFN)-γ and interleukin (IL)-4 and less IL-10 production than controls. In addition, IFN-γ-secreting cells were more numerous, indicating an overall predominance of T helper cell type 1-type responses. Kokkonen and colleagues[47] identified an increased density of gamma-delta-positive intraepithelial T cells in children with cow's milk enteropathy compared with controls (but the density was lower than that seen in celiac disease). In some studies, immunohistochemical stains of the mucosa reveal deposition of eosinophil products.[48] Unlike gluten-sensitive enteropathy (celiac disease), this enteropathy generally resolves in 1 to 2 years, and there is no increased threat of future malignancy.[49]

Celiac Disease

Celiac disease, also termed *celiac sprue* or *gluten-sensitive enteropathy*, estimated to affect 1% of the population, is caused by an immune response triggered by wheat gluten or related rye and barley proteins that results in inflammatory injury to the small intestinal mucosa.[50-52] The classic presentation occurs in infants after weaning, at the time when cereals are introduced into the diet. Early (< 4 months of age) or delayed (> 7 months) introduction of wheat may be a risk factor,[53] and breast-feeding may be a related protective factor.[54] Symptoms partly reflect malabsorption, with patients exhibiting failure to thrive, anemia, and muscle wasting. Additional symptoms are varied and include diarrhea, abdominal pain, vomiting, bone pain, and aphthous stomatitis. Subclinical or minimal disease is possible, delaying diagnosis into adulthood. Chronic ingestion of gluten-containing grains in celiac patients is associated with increased risk of enteropathy-associated T cell lymphoma. Celiac disease is associated with autoimmune disorders and IgA deficiency. Another associated disorder is *Dermatitis herpetiformis*,[55] a gluten-responsive dermatitis characterized by pruritic, erythematous papules, and/or vesicles distributed symmetrically on the extensor surfaces of the elbows and knees, and also on the face, buttocks, neck, and trunk. Immunohistologic examination of the skin reveals a deposition of granular IgA at the dermal papillary tips and the disorder is usually (> 85%) associated with celiac disease.

Endoscopy of the small bowel in active celiac disease typically reveals total villous atrophy and extensive cellular infiltrate. The disorder is caused by gliadin-specific T cell responses against deamidated gliadin produced by tissue transglutaminase.[56] Antigen presentation appears to be a central issue in immunopathology because about 95% of patients are HLA DQ2 with the remainder being HLA-DQ8.[50,57] Gliadin is one of the few substrates for tissue transglutaminase, which deamidates specific glutamines within gliadin, creating epitopes that bind efficiently to DQ2 gut-derived T cells.[58] The activation of DQ2 or DQ8-restricted T cells initiates the inflammatory response.[52] Elimination of gliadin from the diet results in a down-regulation of the T cell-induced inflammatory process and normalizing of the mucosal histology.

Differential Diagnosis

Dietary protein-induced proctocolitis, enteropathy, enterocolitis, and celiac disease have in common the pathophysiologic mecha-

nisms of cell-mediated adverse reactions to dietary proteins with symptoms primarily affecting the gastrointestinal tract. Because the gastrointestinal tract has a limited number of responses to inflammatory damage, there is overlap in the symptoms observed with these disorders. Differentiating them from each other requires consideration of key, distinct clinical features, and directed laboratory examinations. Moreover, numerous medical disorders must be considered in the evaluation of patients presenting with gastrointestinal complaints. Some of these disorders include other food hypersensitivities, but food intolerance (non-immune disorders such as lactase deficiency) and toxic reactions (e.g. bacterial poisoning) are potential considerations.

The complete differential diagnosis can encompass virtually any cause of abdominal complaint, including the following categories: infection (viral, bacterial, parasitic), anatomic (pyloric stenosis, anal fissures, motility disorders, lymphangiectasia, Hirschsprung's disease, reflux, intussusception), inflammatory disorders (inflammatory bowel disease), metabolic (disaccharidase deficiencies), malignancy, immunodeficiency, and others. Depending on the constellation of findings, various diagnostic strategies are used that are beyond the scope of this chapter. However, the presence of a number of clinical elements may underscore the possibility of a food allergic disorder. The general approach to the diagnosis of food-allergic disorders affecting the gut is outlined in Figure 48-1. Various features may suggest a differentiation of the disorders described in this chapter from those related to IgE antibody-mediated gastrointestinal allergies (oral allergy, gastrointestinal anaphylaxis) and those that are sometimes associated with IgE antibody (eosinophilic gastroenteropathies and reflux). The chronicity following ingestion of the causal food (acute in IgE antibody-mediated disease), symptoms (isolated vomiting in gastroesophageal reflux disease), and selected test results (biopsy revealing an eosinophilic infiltrate in allergic eosinophilic gastroenteropathy) differentiate these food allergic disorders. The food-related disorders must also be distinguished from a host of disorders that have similar clinical findings but alternative etiologies. Table 48-1 delineates the disorders

Table 48-1 Examples of Clinical Disease that May Overlap Symptoms of Cell-Mediated, Dietary Protein-Induced Disease

Clinical disease	Symptoms
Proctocolitis	Anal fissure Infection Perianal dermatitis Necrotizing enterocolitis Volvulus Hirschsprung's disease Intussusception Coagulation disorders
Enterocolitis	Sepsis/infection Necrotizing enterocolitis Intussusception Lymphangiectasia Volvulus
Enteropathy	Infection Eosinophilic gastroenteropathy Bowel ischemia Inflammatory bowel disease Lymphangiectasia Autoimmune enteropathy Immune deficiency Tropical sprue Malignancy

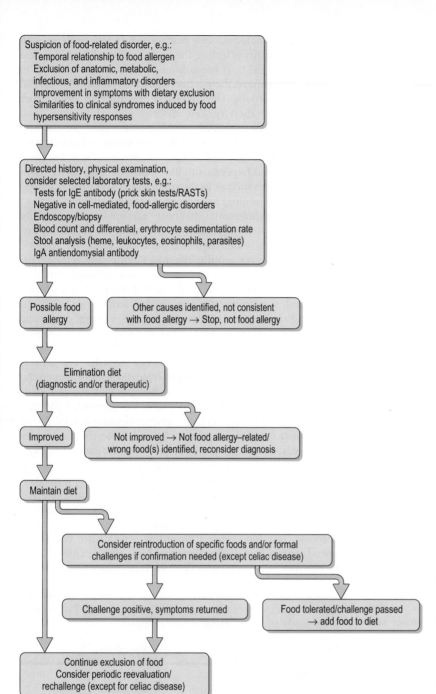

FIGURE 48-1 The evaluation of food allergy requires a simultaneous consideration for alternative diagnoses (infection, anatomic, metabolic, etc.) and disorders caused by food allergy including those described in this chapter and others (i.e. oral allergy syndrome, anaphylaxis, eosinophilic gastroenteropathies, food-related reflux disease) and nonimmune adverse reactions to foods (lactose intolerance). Laboratory tests and decisions for elimination and challenge are based on specific elements of the history and an appreciation for the clinical manifestations and course of the various disorders (see text).

Table 48-2 Clinical Features Helpful to Distinguish Dietary Protein-Induced Proctocolitis, Enteropathy, Enterocolitis, and Celiac Disease

	Vomiting	Diarrhea	Growth	Foods	Other	Onset
Proctocolitis	Absent	Minimal, bloody	Normal	Breast/milk/soy		Days to 6 mo
Enterocolitis	Prominent	Prominent	Poor	Milk/soy/rice/oat	Reexposure: severe, subacute symptoms	Days to 1 yr
Enteropathy	Variable	Moderate	Poor	Milk/soy	Edema	2 to 24 mo
Celiac	Variable	Variable	Poor	Gluten	HLA DQ2–associated	> 4 mo

that may most closely overlap the cell-mediated food allergic disorders.

The distinguishing clinical features of dietary-protein-induced proctocolitis, enteropathy, enterocolitis, and Celiac disease are listed in Table 48-2. Although they may represent a spectrum of disorders with similar etiologies, the treatment and natural course of the diseases vary, making a specific diagnosis imperative. The causal foods, symptoms, and family history usually indicate the likely disorder. In some cases, the diagnosis requires initial confirmation of reactivity/association determined by (1) resolution of symptoms with an elimination diet and (2) recurrence of symptoms after oral challenge. In some cases, specific tests are needed (e.g. serologic tests for IgA endomysial or tissue transglutaminase antibody and small bowel biopsy). The disorders are not IgE antibody-mediated, but if there has been immediate onset of symptoms following ingestion or an association of gastrointestinal allergy with other features of IgE antibody-mediated food allergy (e.g. atopic dermatitis, asthma), screening tests for food-specific IgE antibody (prick skin tests, serum food-specific IgE antibodies) may be helpful in defining the process causing the reactions. A number of tests are of unproved value for the diagnosis of food allergy and should not be used. These include measurement of IgG_4 antibody, provocation-neutralization (drops placed under the tongue or injected to diagnose and treat various symptoms), and applied kinesiology (muscle strength testing).[1]

Evaluation and Management

Dietary Protein Proctocolitis

The diagnosis of dietary protein proctocolitis should be entertained in an infant who is otherwise well and presents with mucousy bloody stools, an absence of symptoms indicating a systemic disease, coagulation defect, or another source of bleeding. The definitive diagnosis requires withdrawal of the presumed allergen with monitoring for resolution of symptoms; however, additional testing and re-feeding of the eliminated protein is advisable after resolution because transient rectal bleeding in infancy is more frequently not related to allergy.[14] A survey of 56 pediatric gastroenterologists showed that 84% prescribe empiric dietary trials.[13] In the absence of biopsy confirmation and especially in the absence of other signs of atopy, re-feeding should be considered soon after resolution of symptoms, given the high rate of spontaneous resolution. In cow's milk- or soy formula-fed infants, substitution with a protein hydrolysate formula can be undertaken. The majority of infants who develop this condition while ingesting protein hydrolysate formulas will experience resolution of bleeding with the substitution of an amino acid-based formula, although follow-up challenges to prove that the formula substitution was required have not been systematically undertaken.[8,59] Management in breast-fed infants requires maternal restriction of cow's milk or possibly soy, egg or other foods.[5] If bleeding is dramatic, monitoring of the red blood cell count is prudent. Progressive bleeding, despite dietary restriction, should prompt reevaluation with consideration for proctocolonoscopy and biopsy.[60] Since there is generally no risk of a severe reaction, the foods can be gradually reintroduced into the diet either as a trial to prove a causal relationship or months afterwards to monitor for resolution of the allergy. However, if there is a suspicion of mild enterocolitis (e.g. vomiting in addition to hematochezia) or a history to suggest IgE-mediated reactions, dietary advancement may require caution with repeated testing (e.g. skin or serum tests for specific IgE to the causal food) and medically supervised oral food challenge.

Enterocolitis

As noted earlier, the diagnosis of dietary protein-induced enterocolitis syndrome rests on clinical and challenge criteria. Most patients would not undergo a formal challenge during infancy because the diagnosis becomes self-evident after elimination of the causal protein, and frequently patients experience inadvertent re-exposure, proving their sensitivity before a diagnostic test feeding. It must be appreciated that chronic ingestion, or re-exposure to the causal food, can result in a clinical picture that is severe and may mimic sepsis. In a review of 17 infants hospitalized with this disorder, Murray and Christie[61] reported 6 infants who presented with acidemia (mean pH 7.03) and methemoglobinemia. Several other clinical features have emerged.[18,19,25,62,63] Based upon studies in the USA and Israel,[25,62,63] approximately half of infants with cow's milk reactions also react to soy and among children reacting to milk/soy, about 25% react to additional proteins such as rice or oat. Sensitivity to milk was lost in 60% and to soy in 25% of the patients after 2 years from the time of presentation. In addition, some patients maintain their allergy beyond the age of 6 years.[64] A retrospective study of 35 children from Australia evaluated over a span of 16 years showed rice (14 children), soy (12) and milk (7) to be the most common triggers and sensitivity was lost by the age of 3 years to rice and soy in about 80%.[19] In a cohort of 23 Korean infants with milk/soy FPIES, resolution rates were 64% for milk and 92% for soy by 10 months of age and all were tolerant by 20 months.[27]

Since there is a high percentage of patients with sensitivity to both cow's milk and soy, switching directly to a casein hydrolysate is recommended. For the rare patients reactive to hydrolysate, an amino acid-based formula is appropriate.[65] Families must be instructed about the careful avoidance of cow's milk and/or soy. Caution and delay is also advised regarding the introduction of common triggers such as rice and oat when milk/soy reactions have already occurred.[15]

Follow-up challenges should be performed at intervals to determine tolerance (approximately every 12 to 24 months, depending on the clinical severity). These challenges should be performed under physician supervision with intravenous fluids and emergency medications immediately available because dramatic reactions, including shock, can occur. Reevaluation for the development of antigen-specific IgE antibody before challenge may be helpful because a few children may convert to IgE-mediated reactions over time.[18] Patch testing was performed in one small study and showed 100% sensitivity and 71% specificity;[66] additional studies are needed to confirm these promising results. In the experience of the author and his colleagues,[18] about half of positive challenges require treatment (usually intravenous fluids). In view of the presumed pathophysiology, corticosteroids have been administered for severe reactions. The role of epinephrine for treatment is not known, but it should be available for severe cardiovascular reactions. Considering the risk for hypotension, the challenge is best performed under physician supervision with consideration for obtaining intravenous access. Food challenges for this non-IgE-mediated syndrome are typically performed with 0.15 to 0.6 g/kg of the causal protein. The challenge protocol and definition of a positive response are shown in Table 48-3.

Dietary Protein Enteropathy and Celiac Disease

There are no specific diagnostic tests for dietary protein-induced enteropathy; therefore, the diagnosis depends on exclusion of alternative diagnoses, biopsy evidence of enteropathy, and proof of sensitivity through dietary elimination and rechallenge. Since the symptoms are not as dramatic as enterocolitis syndrome, observation during dietary ingestion and exclusion of the causal protein must be undertaken to verify the diagnosis. Unlike

Table 48-3 Oral Food Challenges for Food Protein-Induced Enterocolitis Syndrome

Diagnostic Step	Procedures and Assessment
Preparation for challenge	Verify normal weight gain, no gastrointestinal symptoms while off causal protein Obtain baseline stool sample and peripheral blood polymorphonuclear leukocyte count Consider intravenous access Medications ready to treat reaction
Administration of challenge	Administer challenge (typically 0.15–0.6 g/kg) Observe for symptoms (usual onset 1–4 hr) Repeat peripheral blood polymorphonuclear leukocyte count 6 hr after ingestion Collect subsequent stools for 24 hr
Evaluation of positive challenge	Symptoms (vomit, diarrhea) Fecal blood (gross or occult) Fecal leukocytes Fecal eosinophils Rise in peripheral polymorphonuclear leukocyte count (>3500 cells/mm³) Positive challenge: three of five criteria positive Equivocal: two of five criteria positive

From Powell G. Comp Ther 1986;12:28–37; Sicherer SH, Eigenmann PA, Sampson HA. J Pediatr 1998;133:214–219.

dietary protein enteropathy, celiac disease can be evaluated in part through specific in vitro tests. Tests for IgA anti-endomysial antibody (using tissue transglutaminase) are sensitive (85–98%) and specific (94–100%) with excellent positive (91–100%) and negative (80–98%) predictive values.[52,67] If celiac disease is suspected based on a suspicious cadre of findings (family history, steatorrhea, anemia, failure to thrive), serologic tests for IgA endomysial antibody and small bowel biopsy should be undertaken.[51,52] If there is enteropathy, but negative serology, alternative diagnoses (see Tables 48-1 and 48-2) should be reconsidered. If the diagnosis is not strongly suspected, the in vitro tests can be undertaken, and if negative, the diagnosis is generally excluded, but a positive test would warrant confirmation with a biopsy. A gluten-free diet is necessary to treat celiac disease and must be maintained indefinitely. However, enteropathy induced by milk generally resolves in 1 to 2 years, at which time rechallenge is warranted.

Treatment

There are no curative therapies for dietary protein-induced proctocolitis, enteropathy, enterocolitis, or celiac disease; treatment is based solely on dietary elimination. Only patients with dietary protein-induced enterocolitis or some individuals with celiac disease who experience 'celiac crisis' experience severe reactions, so these patients must also be instructed on how to proceed in the event of an accidental exposure. Such patients should report to an emergency department in the event that fluid resuscitation is needed.

Although symptoms may respond to oral steroids, the cornerstone of therapy for these disorders is dietary elimination. Education concerning dietary management is reviewed elsewhere

(Chapter 52). It must be emphasized that education about the details of avoidance is crucial so that dietary elimination trials and therapeutic interventions are accurately undertaken. Often, recurrence of symptoms is caused by poor adherence, possibly from an under-appreciation for the difficulty that strict avoidance poses. Issues of cross-contamination, label reading, restaurant dining, and even the use of medications that may contain causal food proteins make avoidance of major dietary proteins of milk, soy, and gluten very difficult. With celiac disease, oat appears not to be toxic,[52,68] but contamination of oat flour with wheat gluten remains a problem.[69] Support groups and the advice of a knowledgeable dietitian are crucial adjuncts for patients undertaking these nutritionally and socially limiting diets.

Even without performing adjunctive laboratory tests or challenges to confirm a specific disorder, switching among milk, soy, and casein-hydrolysate formulas is commonly undertaken by pediatricians and families as a test of intolerance or allergy. There are no specific guidelines concerning these formula changes. It is helpful to know that only a small proportion of infants with IgE-mediated cow's milk allergy (14%) will react to soy.[70] In contrast, those with FPIES are more likely to be reactive to soy protein. For these infants, a switch to extensively hydrolyzed cow's milk-based formula should be considered. For the few infants with symptoms that persist while taking a casein hydrolysate, amino acid-based formula may be required.[71] Breast-feeding is preferred over commercial formula as the source for infant nutrition, but maternally ingested protein can elicit allergic symptoms in the breast-fed infant.[72] Therefore, maternal dietary manipulation (e.g. avoidance of milk protein) can be undertaken for treatment in breast-fed infants, but with infants who have multiple food allergies this may be difficult, so substitution with infant formulas may be needed in some cases.[73]

Except for celiac disease, resolution of the allergy is expected, so a review of the diet, any accidental exposures, and tests as indicated, are undertaken on a yearly basis with the expectation that proctocolitis will resolve in 1 year and protein-induced enteropathy and enterocolitis would resolve in general in 1 to 3 years. Unfortunately, some patients maintain sensitivity with the latter two disorders later into childhood. It has been hypothesized that some adults with isolated gastrointestinal responses to foods (usually seafood) may also represent patients with a stable form of mild enterocolitis.

Conclusions

Dietary protein-induced proctocolitis, enterocolitis, and enteropathy (including celiac disease) represent well-characterized immunologic responses to dietary proteins (Box 48-2). Although distinct in their clinical presentation, they represent cell-mediated hypersensitivity disorders that are not based on IgE antibody-mediated mechanisms. The symptoms of these disorders generally present in infancy or early childhood and must be differentiated from disorders with similar symptoms, and from each other. A careful clinical history, limited laboratory studies, and directed elimination and challenge can readily disclose the type of disorder and causal foods. Knowledge of the course of these disorders assists in making a plan for long-term therapy: either reintroduction of the food to determine if tolerance has occurred or prolonged dietary elimination. The immunologic mechanisms of these disorders are being elucidated, and these advances are likely to permit improved diagnostic and therapeutic strategies in the future.

References

1. Chapman JA, Bernstein IL, Lee RE, et al. Food allergy: a practice parameter. Ann Allergy Asthma Immunol 2006;96(3 Suppl 2):S1–68.
2. Sampson HA, Anderson JA. Summary and recommendations: classification of gastrointestinal manifestations due to immunologic reactions to foods in infants and young children. J Pediatr Gastroenterol Nutr 2000;30 Suppl:S87–94, 30.
3. Odze RD, Bines J, Leichtner AM, et al. Allergic proctocolitis in infants: a prospective clinicopathologic biopsy study. Hum Pathol 1993;24:668–74.
4. Wilson NW, Self TW, Hamburger RN. Severe cow's milk induced colitis in an exclusively breast-fed neonate: case report and clinical review of cow's milk allergy. Clin Pediatr (Phila) 1990;29:77–80.
5. Lake AM, Whitington PF, Hamilton SR. Dietary protein-induced colitis in breast-fed infants. J Pediatr 1982;101:906–10.
6. Anveden HL, Finkel Y, Sandstedt B, et al. Proctocolitis in exclusively breast-fed infants. Eur J Pediatr 1996;155:464–7.
7. Pittschieler K. Cow's milk protein-induced colitis in the breast-fed infant. J Pediatr Gastroenterol Nutr 1990;10:548–9.
8. Vanderhoof JA, Murray ND, Kaufman SS, et al. Intolerance to protein hydrolysate infant formulas: an underrecognized cause of gastrointestinal symptoms in infants. J Pediatr 1997;131:741–4.
9. Ravelli A, Villanacci V, Chiappa S, et al. Dietary protein-induced proctocolitis in childhood. Am J Gastroenterol 2008;103:2605–12.
10. Jenkins HR, Pincott JR, Soothill JF, et al. Food allergy: the major cause of infantile colitis. Arch Dis Child 1984;59:326–9.
11. Winter HS, Antonioli DA, Fukagawa N, et al. Allergy-related proctocolitis in infants: diagnostic usefulness of rectal biopsy. Mod Pathol 1990;3:5–10.
12. Lake AM. Food-induced eosinophilic proctocolitis. J Pediatr Gastroenterol Nutr 2000;30(Suppl):S58–S60.
13. Xanthakos SA, Schwimmer JB, Melin-Aldana H, et al. Prevalence and outcome of allergic colitis in healthy infants with rectal bleeding: a prospective cohort study. J Pediatr Gastroenterol Nutr 2005;41:16–22.
14. Arvola T, Ruuska T, Keranen J, et al. Rectal bleeding in infancy: clinical, allergological, and microbiological examination. Pediatrics 2006;117:e760–e768.
15. Sicherer SH. Food protein-induced enterocolitis syndrome: case presentations and management lessons. J Allergy Clin Immunol 2005;115:149–56.
16. Hwang JB, Lee SH, Kang YN, et al. Indexes of suspicion of typical cow's milk protein-induced enterocolitis. J Korean Med Sci 2007;22:993–7.
17. Sicherer SH. Food protein-induced enterocolitis syndrome: clinical perspectives. J Pediatr Gastroenterol Nutr 2000;30 Suppl:S45–S49.
18. Sicherer SH, Eigenmann PA, Sampson HA. Clinical features of food protein-induced enterocolitis syndrome. J Pediatr 1998;133:214–9.
19. Mehr S, Kakakios A, Frith K, et al. Food protein-induced enterocolitis syndrome: 16-year experience. Pediatrics 2009;123:e459–e464.
20. Powell GK. Milk- and soy-induced enterocolitis of infancy. J Pediatr 1978;93:553–60.
21. Powell GK. Enterocolitis in low-birth-weight infants associated with milk and soy protein intolerance. J Pediatr 1976;88:840–4.
22. Powell G. Food protein-induced enterocolitis of infancy: differential diagnosis and management. Compr Ther 1986;12:28–37.
23. Bruni F, Peroni DG, Piacentini GL, et al. Fruit proteins: another cause of food protein-induced enterocolitis syndrome. Allergy 2008;63:1645–6.
24. Mehr SS, Kakakios AM, Kemp AS. Rice: a common and severe cause of food protein-induced enterocolitis syndrome. Arch Dis Child 2009;94:220–3.
25. Nowak-Wegrzyn A, Sampson HA, Wood RA, et al. Food protein-induced enterocolitis syndrome caused by solid food proteins. Pediatrics 2003;111(4 Pt 1):829–35.
26. Zapatero RL, Alonso LE, Martin FE, et al. Food-protein-induced enterocolitis syndrome caused by fish. Allergol Immunopathol (Madr) 2005;33:312–6.
27. Hwang JB, Sohn SM, Kim AS. Prospective follow up-oral food challenge in food protein-induced enterocolitis syndrome. Arch Dis Child 2008 [epublication ahead of print].
28. Jayasooriya S, Fox AT, Murch SH. Do not laparotomize food-protein-induced enterocolitis syndrome. Pediatr Emerg Care 2007;23:173–5.
29. Heyman M, Darmon N, Dupont C, et al. Mononuclear cells from infants allergic to cow's milk secrete tumor necrosis factor alpha, altering intestinal function. Gastroenterology 1994;106:1514–23.
30. Kapel N, Matarazzo P, Haouchine D, et al. Fecal tumor necrosis factor alpha, eosinophil cationic protein and IgE levels in infants with cow's milk allergy and gastrointestinal manifestations. Clin Chem Lab Med 1999;37:29–32.
31. Majamaa H, Aittoniemi J, Miettinen A. Increased concentration of fecal alpha1-antitrypsin is associated with cow's milk allergy in infants with atopic eczema. Clin Exp Allergy 2001;31:590–2.
32. Benlounes N, Dupont C, Candalh C, et al. The threshold for immune cell reactivity to milk antigens decreases in cow's milk allergy with intestinal symptoms. J Allergy Clin Immunol 1996;98:781–9.
33. Benlounes N, Candalh C, Matarazzo P, et al. The time-course of milk antigen-induced TNF-alpha secretion differs according to the clinical symptoms in children with cow's milk allergy. J Allergy Clin Immunol 1999;104(4 Pt 1):863–9.
34. Chung HL, Hwang JB, Park JJ, et al. Expression of transforming growth factor beta1, transforming growth factor type I and II receptors, and TNF-alpha in the mucosa of the small intestine in infants with food protein-induced enterocolitis syndrome. J Allergy Clin Immunol 2002;109(1 Pt 1):150–4.
35. Planchon S, Fiocchi C, Takafuji V, et al. Transforming growth factor-beta1 preserves epithelial barrier function: identification of receptors, biochemical intermediates, and cytokine antagonists. J Cell Physiol 1999;181:55–66.
36. Planchon S, Martins C, Guerrant R, et al. Regulation of intestinal epithelial barrier function by TGF-beta 1. J Immunol 1994;153:5730–9.
37. Shek LP, Bardina L, Castro R, et al. Humoral and cellular responses to cow's milk proteins in patients with milk-induced IgE-mediated and non-IgE-mediated disorders. Allergy 2005;60:912–9.
38. Kuitunen P, Visakorpi J, Savilahti E, et al. Malabsorption syndrome with cow's milk intolerance: clinical findings and course in 54 cases. Arch Dis Child 1975;50:351–6.
39. Iyngkaran N, Yadav M, Boey C, et al. Severity and extent of upper small bowel mucosal damage in cow's milk protein-sensitive enteropathy. J Pediatr Gastroenterol Nutr 1988;8:667–74.
40. Yssing M, Jensen H, Jarnum S. Dietary treatment of protein-losing enteropathy. Acta Paediatr Scand 1967;56:173–81.
41. Walker-Smith JA. Food sensitive enteropathies. Clin Gastroenterol 1986;15:55–69.

42. Verkasalo M, Kuitunen P, Savilahti E, et al. Changing pattern of cow's milk intolerance: an analysis of the occurrence and clinical course in the 60s and mid-70s. Acta Paediatr Scand 1981;70:289–95.

43. Vitoria JC, Sojo A, Rodriguez-Soriano J. Changing pattern of cow's milk protein intolerance. Acta Paediatr Scand 1990;79:566–7.

44. Chehade M, Magid MS, Mofidi S, et al. Allergic eosinophilic gastroenteritis with protein-losing enteropathy: intestinal pathology, clinical course, and long-term follow-up. J Pediatr Gastroenterol Nutr 2006;42:516–21.

45. Kondo M, Fukao T, Omoya K, et al. Protein-losing enteropathy associated with egg allergy in a 5-month-old boy. J Investig Allergol Clin Immunol 2008;18:63–6.

46. Hauer AC, Breese EJ, Walker-Smith JA, et al. The frequency of cells secreting interferon-gamma and interleukin-4, - 5, and -10 in the blood and duodenal mucosa of children with cow's milk hypersensitivity. Pediatr Res 1997;42:629–38.

47. Kokkonen J, Haapalahti M, Laurila K, et al. Cow's milk protein-sensitive enteropathy at school age. J Pediatr 2001;139:797–803.

48. Chung HL, Hwang JB, Kwon YD, et al. Deposition of eosinophil-granule major basic protein and expression of intercellular adhesion molecule-1 and vascular cell adhesion molecule-1 in the mucosa of the small intestine in infants with cow's milk- sensitive enteropathy. J Allergy Clin Immunol 1999;103:1195–201.

49. Walker-Smith JA. Cow milk-sensitive enteropathy: predisposing factors and treatment. J Pediatr 1992;121:S111–S115.

50. Sollid LM, Lie BA. Celiac disease genetics: current concepts and practical applications. Clin Gastroenterol Hepatol 2005;3:843–51.

51. Farrell RJ, Kelly CP. Celiac sprue. N Engl J Med 2002;346:180–8.

52. Green PH, Cellier C. Celiac disease. N Engl J Med 2007;357:1731–43.

53. Norris JM, Barriga K, Hoffenberg EJ, et al. Risk of celiac disease autoimmunity and timing of gluten introduction in the diet of infants at increased risk of disease. JAMA 2005;293:2343–51.

54. Ivarsson A, Hernell O, Stenlund H, et al. Breast-feeding protects against celiac disease. Am J Clin Nutr 2002;75:914–21.

55. Egan CA, O'Loughlin S, Gormally S, et al. Dermatitis herpetiformis: a review of fifty-four patients. Ir J Med Sci 1997;166:241–4.

56. Molberg O, McAdam S, Lundin KE, et al. T cells from celiac disease lesions recognize gliadin epitopes deamidated in situ by endogenous tissue transglutaminase. Eur J Immunol 2001;31:1317–23.

57. Johnson TC, Diamond B, Memeo L, et al. Relationship of HLA-DQ8 and severity of celiac disease: comparison of New York and Parisian cohorts. Clin Gastroenterol Hepatol 2004;2:888–94.

58. Anderson RP, Degano P, Godkin AJ, et al. In vivo antigen challenge in celiac disease identifies a single transglutaminase-modified peptide as the dominant A-gliadin T cell epitope. Nat Med 2000;6:337–42.

59. Wyllie R. Cow's milk protein allergy and hypoallergenic formulas [editorial]. Clin Pediatr Phila 1996;35:497–500.

60. Sampson HA, Sicherer SH, Birnbaum AH. AGA technical review on the evaluation of food allergy in gastrointestinal disorders. Gastroenterol 2001;120:1026–40.

61. Murray K, Christie D. Dietary protein intolerance in infants with transient methemoglobinemia and diarrhea. J Pediatr 1993;122:90–2.

62. Burks AW, Casteel HB, Fiedorek SC, et al. Prospective oral food challenge study of two soybean protein isolates in patients with possible milk or soy protein enterocolitis. Pediatr Allergy Immunol 1994;5:40–5.

63. Levy Y, Danon YL. Food protein-induced enterocolitis syndrome: not only due to cow's milk and soy. Pediatr Allergy Immunol 2003;14:325–9.

64. Busse P, Sampson HA, Sicherer SH. Non-reolution of infantile food protein-induced enterocolitis syndrome (FPIES). J Allergy Clin Immunol 2000;105:S129 (abstract).

65. Kelso JM, Sampson HA. Food protein-induced enterocolitis to casein hydrolysate formulas. J Allergy Clin Immunol 1993;92:909–10.

66. Fogg MI, Brown-Whitehorn TA, Pawlowski NA, et al. Atopy patch test for the diagnosis of food protein-induced enterocolitis syndrome. Pediatr Allergy Immunol 2006;17:351–5.

67. Rostom A, Dube C, Cranney A, et al. The diagnostic accuracy of serologic tests for celiac disease: a systematic review. Gastroenterol 2005;128:S38–S46.

68. Hoffenberg EJ, Haas J, Drescher A, et al. A trial of oats in children with newly diagnosed celiac disease. J Pediatr 2000;137:361–6.

69. Thompson T. Oats and the gluten-free diet. J Am Diet Assoc 2003;103:376–9.

70. Zeiger RS, Sampson HA, Bock SA, et al. Soy allergy in infants and children with IgE-associated cow's milk allergy. J Pediatr 1999;134:614–22.

71. Isolauri E, Sutas Y, Makinen KS, et al. Efficacy and safety of hydrolyzed cow milk and amino acid-derived formulas in infants with cow milk allergy. J Pediatr 1995;127:550–7.

72. Jarvinen KM, Makinen-Kiljunen S, Suomalainen H. Cow's milk challenge through human milk evokes immune responses in infants with cow's milk allergy. J Pediatr 1999;135:506–12.

73. Isolauri E, Tahvanainen A, Peltola T, et al. Breast-feeding of allergic infants [see comments]. J Pediatr 1999;134:27–32.

Eosinophilic Esophagitis, Gastroenteritis, and Proctocolitis

Chris A. Liacouras • Jonathan E. Markowitz

The eosinophilic gastroenteropathies are an interesting, yet somewhat poorly defined, set of disorders that by definition include the infiltration of at least one layer of the gastrointestinal (GI) tract with eosinophils. First reported more than 50 years ago, the clinical spectrum of these disorders was defined solely by various case reports. Additional insight into the role of the eosinophil in health and disease has allowed further description of these disorders with respect to the underlying defect that drives the inflammatory response in those afflicted. Perhaps most important to the definition of these disorders has been the understanding of the heterogeneity of the sites affected within the GI tract.

Much as another inflammatory disorder of the GI tract, inflammatory bowel disease (IBD), has been stratified into Crohn's disease and ulcerative colitis based on clinical features including sites of the GI tract affected, the eosinophilic gastroenteropathies can be classified in a similar manner. Within the broad definition of these disorders lie at least three clinical entities that are defined in large part by the presence of abnormal numbers of eosinophils in various GI sites: eosinophilic proctocolitis (EoP), eosinophilic gastroenteritis (EoG), and eosinophilic esophagitis (EoE). In this chapter, we attempt to define these disorders, highlighting their similarities as well as their differences.

Eosinophilic Proctocolitis

EoP, also known as allergic proctocolitis or protein-induced proctocolitis, has been recognized as one of the most common causes of rectal bleeding in infants.[1,2] This disorder is characterized by the onset of rectal bleeding, generally in children younger than 2 months of age.

Epidemiology/Etiology

The GI tract plays a major role in the development of oral tolerance to foods. Through the process of endocytosis by the enterocyte, food antigens are generally degraded into nonantigenic proteins.[3,4] Although the GI tract serves as an efficient barrier to ingested food antigens, this barrier may not be mature for the first few months of life.[5] As a result, ingested antigens may have an increased propensity for being presented intact to the immune system. These intact antigens have the potential for stimulating the immune system and driving an inappropriate response directed at the GI tract. Since the major component of the young infant's diet is milk or formula, it stands to reason that the inciting antigens in EoP are derived from the proteins found in them.

Commercially available infant formulas most commonly utilize cow's milk as the protein source. It is thought that up to 7.5% of the population in developed countries exhibit cow's milk allergy, although there is wide variation in the reported data.[6-8] Soy protein allergy is thought to be less common than cow's milk allergy, with a reported prevalence of approximately 0.5%.[9] However, soy protein intolerance becomes more prominent in individuals who have developed milk protein allergy, with prevalence from 15% to 50% or more in milk protein-sensitized individuals.[10] For this reason, substitution of a soy protein-based formula for a milk protein-based formula in patients with suspected milk protein proctocolitis is often unsuccessful.

Maternal breast milk represents a different challenge to the immune system. Up to 50% of the cases of EoP occur in breast-fed infants, but, rather than developing an allergy to human milk protein, it is thought that the infants are manifesting allergy to antigens ingested by the mother and transferred via the breast milk. The transfer of maternal dietary protein via breast milk was first demonstrated in 1921.[11] Recently, the presence of cow's milk antigens in breast milk has been established.[12-14]

When a problem with antigen handling occurs, whether secondary to increased absorption through an immature GI tract or though a damaged epithelium secondary to gastroenteritis, sensitization results. Once sensitized, the inflammatory response is perpetuated with continued exposure to the inciting antigen. This may explain the reported relationship between early exposures to cow's milk protein or viral gastroenteritis and the development of allergy.[15-17]

Clinical Features

Diarrhea, rectal bleeding, and increased mucus production are the typical symptoms seen in patients who present with EoP.[2,18] In a well-appearing infant, rectal bleeding often begins gradually, initially appearing as small flecks of blood. Usually, increased stool frequency occurs accompanied by water loss or mucus streaks. The development of irritability or straining with stools is also common and can falsely lead to the initial diagnosis of anal fissures. Atopic symptoms, such as eczema and reactive airway disease, may be associated with EoP. Continued exposure to the inciting antigen causes increased bleeding and may, on rare occasions, cause anemia or poor weight gain. Despite the progression of symptoms, the infants generally appear well and rarely appear ill. Other manifestations of GI tract inflammation, such as vomiting, abdominal distention, or weight loss, almost never occur.

Differential Diagnosis

EoP is primarily a clinical diagnosis, although several laboratory parameters and diagnostic procedures may be useful. Initial assessment should be directed at the overall health of the child. A toxic-appearing infant is not consistent with the diagnosis of EoP and should prompt evaluation for other causes of GI bleeding. A complete blood count is useful because the majority of infants with EoP have a normal or, at worst, borderline low hemoglobin count. An elevated serum eosinophil count may be present. Stool studies for bacterial pathogens such as *Salmonella* and *Shigella* should be performed in the setting of rectal bleeding. An assay for *Clostridium difficile* toxins A and B should also be considered, although infants may be asymptomatically colonized with this organism.[19,20] A stool specimen may be analyzed for the presence of white blood cells and specifically for eosinophils. However, the sensitivity of these tests is not well documented, and the absence of a positive finding on these tests does not exclude the diagnosis.[21] Although not always necessary, flexible sigmoidoscopy may be useful to demonstrate the presence of colitis. Visually, one may find erythema, friability, or frank ulceration of the colonic mucosa. Alternatively, the mucosa may appear normal or show evidence of lymphoid hyperplasia.[22,23] Histologic findings typically include increased eosinophils within the lamina propria, with generally preserved crypt architecture. Findings may be patchy, so care should be taken to examine many levels of each biopsy specimen if necessary.[24,25]

Treatment

In a well-appearing patient with a history consistent with EoP, it is acceptable to make an empiric change in the protein source of the formula. Given the propensity of milk-sensitized infants to develop sensitivity to other whole proteins, such as soy, a protein-hydrolysate formula is often the best choice.[16] Resolution of symptoms begins almost immediately after the elimination of the problematic food, and although symptoms may linger for several days to weeks, continued improvement is the rule. If symptoms do not quickly improve or persist beyond 4 to 6 weeks, other antigens should be considered, as well as other potential causes of rectal bleeding. In breast-fed infants, dietary restriction of milk and soy-containing products by the mother may result in improvement; however, care should be taken to ensure that the mother maintains adequate protein and calcium intake from other sources.

Eosinophilic Gastroenteritis

EoG is a general term that describes a constellation of symptoms attributable to the GI tract, in combination with pathologic infiltration by eosinophils. Shaped in large part by case reports and series over the years, there are no strict diagnostic criteria for this disorder. Rather, a combination of GI complaints with supportive histologic findings is sufficient to make the diagnosis. EoG was originally described by Kaijser in 1937.[26] It is a disorder characterized by tissue eosinophilia that can affect different layers of the bowel wall, anywhere from the mouth to the anus.

The gastric antrum and small bowel are frequently affected. In 1970 Klein and colleagues[27] classified EoG into three categories: mucosal, muscular, and serosal forms.

Epidemiology/Etiology

EoG affects patients of all ages, with a slight male predominance. Most commonly, eosinophils infiltrate only the mucosa, leading to symptoms associated with malabsorption, such as growth failure, weight loss, diarrhea, and hypoalbuminemia. Mucosal EoG may affect any portion of the GI tract. A review of the biopsy findings in 38 children with EoG revealed that all patients examined had mucosal eosinophilia of the gastric antrum.[2] Of the patients studied, 79% also demonstrated eosinophilia of the proximal small intestine, with 60% having esophageal involvement and 52% having involvement of the gastric corpus. Those with colonic involvement tended to be under 6 months of age and were ultimately classified as having EoP.

The exact cause of EoG remains unknown. In the past, both immunoglobulin E (IgE)- and non-IgE-mediated sensitivities were thought to be responsible.[28] The association between IgE-mediated inflammatory response (typical allergy) and EoG is supported by the increased likelihood of other allergic disorders such as atopic disease, food allergies, and seasonal allergies.[29,30] Specific foods have been implicated in the cause of EoG.[31,32] In contrast, the role of non-IgE-mediated immune dysfunction, in particular the interplay between lymphocyte-produced cytokines and eosinophils, has also received attention.

Recently, interleukin (IL)-5, a chemoattractant responsible for tissue eosinophilia, has been implicated.[33] Desreumaux and colleagues[34] found that among patients with EoG, the levels of IL-3, IL-5, and granulocyte-macrophage colony-stimulating factor were significantly increased compared with control patients. Once recruited to the tissue, eosinophils may further recruit similar cells through their own production of IL-3 and IL-5, as well as production of leukotrienes.[35] Finally, evidence by Beyer and colleagues[36] suggests that the release of T helper cell type 2 cytokines from patients with milk allergy enteritis occurs on stimulation of milk-sensitive T cells isolated from the GI mucosa. This mixed type of immune dysregulation in EoG has implications for the way this disorder is diagnosed, as well as the way it is treated.

Clinical Features

The most common symptoms of EoG include colicky abdominal pain, bloating, diarrhea, weight loss, dysphagia, and vomiting.[37,38] In addition, up to 50% have a past or family history of atopy.[2] Other features of severe disease include GI bleeding, iron deficiency anemia, protein-losing enteropathy (hypoalbuminemia), and growth failure.[37] Approximately 75% of affected patients have an elevated blood eosinophilia.[39] Males are more commonly affected than females. Rarely, ascites occurs.[39,40]

Differential Diagnosis

EoG should be considered in any patient with a history of chronic symptoms, including vomiting, abdominal pain, diarrhea, anemia, hypoalbuminemia, or poor weight gain in combination with the presence of eosinophils in the GI tract. As identified in Box 49-1, other causes of eosinophilic infiltration of the GI tract include the other disorders of the eosinophilic gastroenteropathy spectrum (EoP, EoE), as well as parasitic infection, IBD, neo-

BOX 49-1

Causes of Gastrointestinal Eosinophilia

Esophagus

Eosinophilic esophagitis

Gastroesophageal reflux

Food allergy

Stomach

Eosinophilic gastroenteritis

Menetrier's disease

Chronic granulomatous disease

Vasculitis

Oral gold therapy

Hyper-IgE syndrome

Idiopathic hypereosinophilic syndrome

Small intestine

Eosinophilic gastroenteritis

Inflammatory bowel disease (Crohn's disease)

Infection (parasites)

Food allergy

Vasculitis

Oral gold therapy

Hyper-IgE syndrome

Idiopathic hypereosinophilic syndrome

Colon

Food allergy

Eosinophilic gastroenteritis

Inflammatory bowel disease (ulcerative colitis)

Infection (parasites)

Vasculitis

---

plasm, chronic granulomatous disease, collagen vascular disease, and the hypereosinophilic syndrome.[41–45]

In an infant, EoG may present in a manner similar to hypertrophic pyloric stenosis, with progressive vomiting, dehydration, electrolyte abnormalities, and thickening of the gastric outlet.[46,47] When an infant presents with this constellation of symptoms in addition to atopic symptoms such as eczema and reactive airway disease, an elevated eosinophil count, and a strong family history of atopic disease, EoG should be considered in the diagnosis before surgical intervention, if possible.

Uncommon presentations of EoG include acute abdomen[48] or colonic obstruction.[49] There also have been reports of serosal infiltration with eosinophils, with associated complaints of abdominal distention, eosinophilic ascites, and bowel perforation.[40,50–54]

Evaluation

When EoG is suspected, there are a number of tests that may aid in the diagnosis, but no single test is pathognomonic. Before EoG can be truly entertained as a diagnosis, the presence of eosinophils in the GI tract must be documented. This is most readily done with biopsies of either the upper GI tract through esophagogastroduodenoscopy or of the lower GI tract through flexible sigmoidoscopy or colonoscopy. A history of atopy is supportive of the diagnosis but is not a necessary feature. Blood evaluation may demonstrate an elevated peripheral eosinophil count or IgE level in approximately 70% of affected individuals.[55] Measures

of absorptive activity such as the *d*-xylose absorption test and lactose hydrogen breath testing may reveal evidence of malabsorption, reflecting small intestine damage. Radiographic contrast studies may demonstrate mucosal irregularities or edema, wall thickening, ulceration, or luminal narrowing. A lacy mucosal pattern of the gastric antrum known as *areae gastricae* is a unique finding that may be present in patients with EoG.[56]

Evaluation of other causes of eosinophilia should be undertaken, including stool analysis for ova and parasites. Signs of intestinal obstruction warrant abdominal imaging. The value of serum food-specific IgE studies, as well as skin testing for environmental antigens, is limited. Skin testing using both traditional prick tests and patch tests may increase the sensitivity for identifying foods responsible for EoG by evaluating both IgE-mediated and T cell-mediated sensitivities.[57]

Treatment

There is as much ambiguity in the treatment of EoG as there is in its diagnosis. This is in large part because the entity of EoG was defined mainly by case series, each of which used their own modes of treatment. Since EoG is a difficult disease to diagnose, randomized trials for its treatment are uncommon, leading to considerable debate as to which treatment is best.

Food allergy is considered one of the underlying causes of EoG, and elimination of pathogenic foods, as identified by any form of allergy testing or by random removal of the most likely antigens, should be a first-line treatment. Unfortunately, this approach results in improvement in only a limited number of patients. In severe cases or when other treatment options have failed, the administration of a strict diet, using an elemental formula, has been shown to be successful.[30,58] In these cases, formulas such as Neocate 1+ or Elecare provided as the sole source of nutrition have been reported to be effective in the resolution of clinical symptoms and tissue eosinophilia.

When the use of a restricted diet fails, corticosteroids are often used due to their high likelihood of success in attaining remission.[38] However, when weaned, the duration of remission is variable and can be short lived, leading to the need for repeated courses or continuous low doses of steroids. In addition, the chronic use of corticosteroids carries an increased likelihood of undesirable side-effects, including cosmetic problems (cushingoid facies, hirsutism, acne), decreased bone density, impaired growth, and personality changes. A response to these side-effects has been to look for substitutes that may act as steroid-sparing agents while still allowing for control of symptoms.

Orally administered cromolyn sodium has been used with some success,[38,59–61] and recent reports have detailed the efficacy of other oral antiinflammatory medications. Montelukast, a selective leukotriene receptor antagonist used to treat asthma, has been reported to successfully treat two patients with EoG.[62,63] Treatment of EoG with inhibition of leukotriene D4, a potent chemotactic factor for eosinophils, relies on the theory that the inflammatory response in EoG is perpetuated by the presence of the eosinophils already present in the mucosa. By interrupting the chemotactic cascade, it is thought that the inflammatory cycle can be broken. Suplatast tosilate, another suppressor of cytokine production, has also been reported as a treatment for EoG.[64]

Given the varied possibilities for treatment of EoG, the combination of therapies incorporating the best chance of success with the smallest likelihood of side-effects should be used. When particular food antigens that may be causing disease can be identified, elimination of those antigens should be first-line therapy. When testing fails to identify potentially pathogenic foods, a systematic elimination of the most commonly involved foods[65] can be made. If this approach fails, total elimination diet with an amino acid-based formula should be considered. Trials of non-steroidal antiinflammatory drugs such as sodium cromolyn, montelukast, and suplatast are a reasonable option, although some might prefer to wait for more definitive studies.

When other treatments fail, corticosteroids remain a reliable treatment for EoG, with attempts at limiting the total dose or the number of treatment courses where possible. Given the diffuse and inconsistent nature of symptoms in this disease, serial endoscopy with biopsy is a useful and important modality for monitoring disease progression.

Eosinophilic Esophagitis

EoE has come to the forefront in individuals previously suspected as having severe, chronic gastroesophageal reflux disease (GERD). EoE is a disease of children and adults characterized by an isolated, severe eosinophilic infiltration of the esophagus manifested by gastroesophageal reflux-like symptoms, such as regurgitation, epigastric and chest pain, vomiting, heartburn, feeding difficulties, and dysphagia unresponsive to acid suppression therapy. In addition, older children and adults often present to physicians or emergency rooms with significant esophageal food impactions.

History

In 1977, Dobbins and colleagues[66] reported one of the first cases of dysphagia associated with EoE. They described a case of a 51-year-old man with asthma and environmental allergies who presented with dysphagia and chest pain. An upper endoscopy demonstrated a severe EoE combined with increased eosinophils in the duodenum. They suggested that the esophageal eosinophilia was part of the larger disease process of EoG. In 1983, Matzinger and Daneman[67] reported dysphagia associated with a significant esophageal eosinophilia in an adolescent. Their patient not only had dysphagia but also displayed food allergies, a peripheral serum eosinophilia, and histologic evidence of eosinophils in his esophagus and stomach. Shortly thereafter, Lee[68] reported on a series of 11 patients with documented EoE consisting of greater than 10 eosinophils per X40 high-power microscopic field (HPF). These patients were initially studied because all 11 presented with dysphagia, symptoms of gastroesophageal reflux, vomiting, and strictures. Although 1 patient improved on antireflux medication, another became asymptomatic after being treated with systemic steroids. No follow-up was conducted for the remaining 9 patients. An allergic disorder was entertained as the cause in many of these patients.

In 1993 Attwood and colleagues[69] were the first to compare patients with EoE with those with GERD. They studied 12 patients who presented with dysphagia and had more than 20 eosinophils per X 40 HPF found by biopsy. These patients had an average of 56 eosinophils per HPF, and their symptoms were unresponsive to acid blockade. Eleven had normal pH probe monitoring; 7 had evidence of systemic allergy including rhinitis, asthma, and eczema; and only 1 had increased antral eosinophils. This group was compared with a group of 90 patients with GERD documented by an abnormal pH probe. All of the patients diagnosed with reflux were responsive to acid blockade, and only 43 had evidence of an esophageal eosinophilia, with a mean number of 3.3 eosinophils per HPF. The patients with severe esophageal eosinophilia did not respond to

acid blockade. Vitellas and colleagues[70] reported on a series of 13 male patients with isolated EoE. Twelve patients demonstrated dysphagia and an increased peripheral eosinophilia, whereas 10 had atopic symptoms and esophageal strictures requiring repeated dilatation. All except 1 patient responded to systemic corticosteroids, and in these patients, esophageal dilatation was no longer required.

Due to the increase in reported cases and the interest in the disorder among gastroenterologists, allergists and pathologists, an international meeting was held in October 2006 among pediatric and adult specialists considered experts in the field of eosinophilic esophagitis. The First International Gastrointestinal Eosinophilic Research Symposium (FIGERS) identified possible etiologies and research studies as well as providing recommendations for the diagnosis, treatment and management of individuals with EoE.[71]

Role of Esophageal Eosinophils

Eosinophils in the GI tract have long been associated with intestinal inflammatory disorders such as EoG, IBD, parasitic infections, and acid-related disorders. In normal, healthy volunteers, eosinophils are commonly visualized in almost all portions of the GI tract (except the esophagus), which often makes the diagnosis of a pathologic process secondary to eosinophilia difficult. In 1996 Bischoff and colleagues[72] suggested that eosinophils released mediators (cationic proteins, leukotrienes, prostaglandins, platelet-activating factor) promote tissue inflammation. They also believed that these cells exert cytotoxic effects by producing oxygen-free radicals and peroxidase. Mast cells were thought to be involved in tissue repair.

In 1982, Winter and colleagues[73] suggested that esophageal intraepithelial eosinophils may be related to tissue injury secondary to gastroesophageal reflux. They postulated that these eosinophils could be used as a new diagnostic criterion for reflux esophagitis. The authors evaluated 46 patients, aged 3 months to 19 years, who had recurrent vomiting, epigastric pain, and other symptoms of GERD including dysphagia, abdominal pain, and regurgitation. Diagnostic testing was performed with pH probes, manometry, and upper endoscopy. These patients were compared with a group of nine asymptomatic control patients. The control group had normal pH probe results, normal esophageal manometry, and no esophageal eosinophils by biopsy. In contrast, in the study group, 18 patients demonstrated esophageal eosinophils on biopsy, with a mean of two eosinophils per HPF. The majority of these patients also had abnormal pH probes and other histologic features of reflux, including basal zone thickening and papillary lengthening. Winter concluded that the presence of intraepithelial eosinophils correlated with delayed esophageal acid clearance. This study was followed by reports from Brown and colleagues[74] and Tummala and colleagues,[75] who performed similar studies in adults and found comparable results. Since then, the finding of intraepithelial esophageal eosinophils has become an accepted feature of gastroesophageal reflux.

Etiology

In the past, the esophageal eosinophil was used as a pathognomonic marker for gastroesophageal reflux. However, in 1995, Kelly and colleagues[76] established that patients with an isolated, severe esophageal eosinophilia unresponsive to measures attempting to control acid, instead responded to a strict elemental diet. They suggested that the cause was specific food allergens. For the next few years, an argument existed among pediatric gastroenterologists and pathologists regarding the etiology of a severe, isolated esophageal eosinophilia.[77-79] The discussion centered on the small numbers of patients who were identified with EoE (most likely because of the belief that esophageal eosinophilia was only considered to be diagnostic of reflux disease) and the lack of controlled trials demonstrating a response of a severe esophageal eosinophilia to the removal of foods. Recently, with the improved knowledge of EoE, including several published reports, EoE is now considered an important cause of esophageal disease.[80-85]

EoE appears to be caused by an abnormal immunologic response to specific food antigens. Although several studies have documented resolution of EoE with the strict avoidance of food antigens, in 1995, Kelly and colleagues[76] published the classic paper on EoE. Because the suspected etiology was an abnormal immunologic response to specific unidentifiable food antigens, each patient was treated with a strict elimination diet that included an amino acid-based formula (Neocate®). Patients were also allowed clear liquids, corn, and apples. Seventeen patients were initially offered a dietary elimination trial, with 10 patients adhering to the protocol. The initial trial was determined by a history of anaphylaxis to specific foods and abnormal skin testing. These patients were subsequently placed on a strict diet consisting of an amino acid-based formula for a median of 17 weeks. Symptomatic improvement was seen within an average of 3 weeks after the introduction of the elemental diet (resolution in eight patients, improvement in two). In addition, all 10 patients demonstrated a significant improvement in esophageal eosinophilia. Subsequently, all patients reverted to previous symptoms on reintroduction of foods. Predietary and postdietary trial evaluations demonstrated a significant improvement in clinical symptoms and almost complete resolution in esophageal eosinophilia, from a mean of 41 eosinophils per HPF to less than 1 per HPF. Open food challenges were then conducted, with a demonstration of a return of symptoms with challenges to milk (7 patients), soy (4), wheat (2), peanuts (2), and egg (1). Although an exact cause was not determined, Kelly[76] suggested an immunologic basis secondary to a delayed hypersensitivity or a cell-mediated hypersensitivity response as the cause for EoE.

A recent report by Spergel and colleagues[57] demonstrated that foods that cause EoE are often not based on an immediate hypersensitivity reaction. By using a combination of traditional skin testing and a newer technique of atopy 'patch testing', he established that a delayed cell-mediated allergic response may be responsible for many cases of EoE. Recently, CD8 lymphocytes have been identified as the predominant T cell within the squamous epithelium of patients diagnosed with EoE.[81] Finally, although other causes of EoE have been suggested, such as aeroallergens or infectious agents, only food antigens have thus far been implicated.[28,80-82,86]

Pathophysiology

Recent research utilizing immunohistochemistry and stereology revealed that the density of activated esophageal tissue eosinophils was 300 times greater among patients with EoE as in those with gastroesophageal reflux or in normal control patients.[87] In addition, T cells, plasma cells and mast cells were also increased in patients with EoE. The investigators hypothesized that in EoE, eosinphils act as effector cells that respond to various antigens and cause epithelial damage. Cytokines, including IL-5, IL-13, and IL-4, are also increased in patients with EoE.[88] In 2007,

Aceves showed significant esophageal remodeling and fibrosis in children with EoE.[89] Esophageal biopsies revealed increased levels of subepithelial fibrosis, elevated TGF-β expression and an increased vascular density and vascular adhesion molecule. These findings suggested a reason for the development of esophageal stricture formation. Finally, micro-array expression analysis performed in patients with EoE revealed the induction of the gene for eotaxin-3, which suggests that genetics may play a vital role in the pathogenesis of EoE.[90]

Clinical Presentation

The presentation of EoE in children is similar to the symptoms associated with gastroesophageal reflux (Table 49-1). Boys appear to develop EoE more frequently than do girls. The typical symptoms include nausea, vomiting, regurgitation, epigastric abdominal pain, and poor eating. Young children may demonstrate food refusal, whereas adolescents often experience dysphagia. Adults present with similar symptoms, but dysphagia occurs much more commonly and can be associated with esophageal strictures. Uncommon symptoms include growth failure, hematemesis, globus, and water brash. The clinical features of EoE may evolve over years. Symptoms such as abdominal pain and heartburn occur regularly; however, patients with vomiting or dysphagia may display these symptoms sporadically, complaining only once or twice a month. Although the use of acid suppression medication often improves the patient's symptoms, it does not eliminate the symptoms or change the abnormal esophageal histology. Approximately 50% of affected children also exhibit other allergic signs and symptoms, including bronchospasm, allergic rhinitis, and eczema. Frequently, there is a strong family history of food allergies or other allergic disorders.

Diagnosis

The diagnosis of EoE can be made only by esophageal biopsy. In 1999 Ruchelli and colleagues[91] studied 102 patients who presented with symptoms of GERD and evidence of esophagitis documented by at least one intraepithelial eosinophil by endoscopy. Once the diagnosis of probable reflux was made, these patients were treated with H_2 blockers and prokinetic agents. If the patients' symptoms persisted after 3 months of therapy with H_2 blockers, a proton pump inhibitor was begun, and the patients were reevaluated 3 months later by endoscopy with biopsy. The treatment response was classified into three categories: clinical improvement (1.1 eosinophils per HPF), relapse of clinical symptoms (6.4 eosinophils per HPF), and failure of medical treatment (24.5 eosinophils per HPF). All except two patients had isolated esophageal involvement. He concluded that the number of esophageal eosinophils predicted whether the patient could be successfully treated with acid suppression medication or whether another cause (allergic disease) was possible.

Although an isolated, severe, esophageal eosinophilia unresponsive to acid blockade is necessary for the diagnosis of EoE, several reports have suggested that the diagnosis of EoE may be made endoscopically without biopsy. Orenstein and colleagues[82,92] reported on a series of children with probable EoE and suggested that the endoscopic appearance (Figure 49-1) revealed a granular, subtle, furrowed, ringed appearance. In addition, a recent report by Teitlebaum and colleagues[81] suggested that in patients successfully treated for EoE, a furrowed, ringed appearance may persist despite normal biopsy results. However, a ringed esophageal appearance can also be

Table 49-1 Comparison Between Eosinophilic Esophagitis and Reflux Esophagitis

	Eosinophilic Esophagitis	Reflux Esophagitis
Symptoms	Nausea, vomiting, epigastric pain, dysphagia	Nausea, dysphagia, vomiting, epigastric pain
Endoscopic findings	Esophageal furrows, rings	Esophageal erythema, ulceration
Histologic findings	Usually >20 eosinophils per HPF	Usually <5 eosinophils per HPF
Esophageal strictures	Midesophageal strictures	Distal esophageal strictures
pH probe results	Normal, except for increased frequency of episodes	Usually abnormal
Peripheral eosinophils	Usually increased	Usually normal
Serum IgE level	Usually increased	Usually normal
Allergic history	Increased incidence of asthma, rhinitis, eczema	Not increased
Family history	Increased incidence of asthma, rhinitis, eczema	Not increased
Acid blockade		
Symptoms	Minimally improved	Significantly improved
Histology	No change in histology	Significantly improved
Fundoplication	Not effective	Effective in severe cases
Corticosteroids	Effective; however, disease recurs when discontinued	Unknown
Dietary therapy	Effective	Not effective

HPF, high-power field.

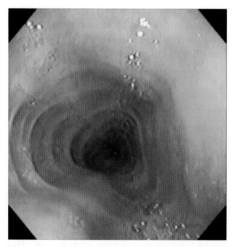

Figure 49-1 Endoscopic photograph of the midesophagus in a 12-year-old patient with eosinophilic esophagitis. Linear furrows and circumferential rings in the mucosa are prominent.

appreciated in patients who have other causes of severe esophagitis.[93,94] Other methods for diagnosis have been attempted, including endoscopic ultrasound.[80,95] Although ultrasound demonstrated that the mucosa-to-submucosa ratio and muscularis propria thickness were greater in EoE patients than a control group, no comparison was made with patients who had esophagitis secondary to other disorders. Finally, EoE can occur in both the mid- and distal portions of the esophagus. Several previous reports in adults have demonstrated mid-esophageal involvement associated with stricture formation.[66,67] In contrast, Liacouras and colleagues[96] established that even in those cases of proximal esophageal involvement, the distal esophagus was also involved. Moreover, peripheral eosinophilia and increased IgE levels have been reported in 20–60% of patients with EoE.[76,81,82,84]

The definitive diagnosis of EoE is made endoscopically in patients who have reflux-like symptoms, who have normal (or borderline normal) pH probes, and who are unresponsive to acid inhibition. This fact underscores the importance of obtaining esophageal biopsy samples whenever questions arise regarding the disease process. The performance of esophageal pH monitoring is also important because significant acid reflux disease can be excluded. In EoE, pH probe findings often reveal frequent, brief reflux episodes but normal esophageal acid clearance and a normal reflux index.[84] The number of esophageal eosinophils per HPF is used to make the diagnosis. A review of recent studies suggests that the vast majority of patients with EoE present with more than 20 eosinophils per HPF.[76,80,82–84,86,91]

Evaluation

Patients with chronic symptoms of vomiting, regurgitation, epigastric abdominal pain, or dysphagia or patients with symptoms of gastroesophageal reflux unresponsive to medical therapy should be evaluated for EoE (Box 49-2). For accurate diagnosis, every evaluation should include a radiographic upper GI series to rule out anatomic abnormalities, a 24-hour pH probe, and an upper endoscopy with biopsy. In a patient with normal anatomy, the presence of an isolated, severe esophageal eosinophilia (>20 eosinophils per HPF), obtained while the patient is receiving adequate gastric acid blockade with a proton pump inhibitor, strongly suggests the diagnosis of EoE (Figure 49-2). Acid disease is excluded with the performance of a 24-hour pH probe. The pH probe should be completed while the patient is off of all acid-suppressing medications. Although the pH probe may reveal frequent, brief reflux episodes (three episodes per hour), the probe should demonstrate normal esophageal acid clearance and a normal reflux index. Patients with severely abnormal pH probe findings should undergo further evaluation for GERD. The

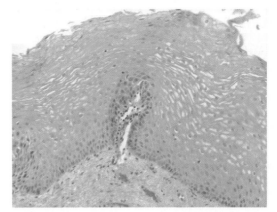

Figure 49-3 Histologic biopsy of squamous esophageal mucosa taken from the distal esophagus of a 10-year-old patient with eosinophilic esophagitis after treatment with a strict elemental diet. Normal stratified epithelium is visualized after treatment.

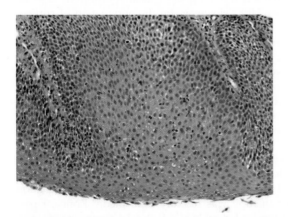

Figure 49-2 Histologic biopsy of squamous esophageal mucosa taken from the distal esophagus of a 10-year-old patient diagnosed with eosinophilic esophagitis before treatment. Numerous eosinophils can be appreciated as well as hyperplasia of the basal layer.

diagnosis of EoE is confirmed on repeat endoscopy with biopsy after treatment (Figure 49-3).

Treatment

The identification and removal of allergic dietary antigens is the mainstay of treatment for EoE. The removal of the offending foods reverses the disease process in patients with EoE, but in many cases, the identification of these foods is extremely difficult. Often, patients with EoE cannot correlate their GI symptoms with the ingestion of a specific food. This occurs because the cause of EoE is most likely based on a delayed hypersensitivity response. Several reports have demonstrated that it takes several days for symptoms to recur following ingestion of antigens that cause EoE.[76,84] Furthermore, allergy testing using skin tests and serum allergen-specific IgE studies provide limited value in the vast majority of patients with EoE.[57] Even when a particular food causing EoE has been isolated, it may take days or weeks for the symptoms to resolve. In addition, although one food may be identified, there may be several other foods (not easily identified) that could also be contributing to EoE. Upper endoscopy with biopsy is the only diagnostic test that has been shown to document resolution of the disease.

Although attempts should be made to identify and eliminate potential food allergens through a careful history, allergy testing and selective elimination diets, because it may be difficult to determine the responsible allergic foods, the administration of a strict diet, using an amino acid-based formula, is often necessary. As established by Kelly and colleagues[76] and Markowitz and colleagues,[97] the use of an elemental diet rapidly improves both clinical symptoms and histology in patients with EoE. Because of poor palatability, the elemental formula is most often provided by continuous nasogastric feeding. The diet may be supplanted by water, one fruit (e.g. apples, grapes), and the corresponding pure fruit juice. The use of this diet not only proves the diagnosis of EoE but also heals the inflamed mucosa. Reversal of symptoms typically occurs within 10 days, with histologic improvement in 4 weeks.[84] Although the strict use of an amino acid-based formula may be difficult for patients (and parents) to comprehend, its benefits outweigh the risks of other treatments. First, only food allergens have thus far been implicated in the etiology of EoE and removal of these allergens cures the disease. In contrast, while the use of other medications, such as corticosteroids, may improve the disease and its symptoms, on their discontinuation, if the offending antigen has not been identified and removed, the disease recurs. Once the esophagus is healed, if allergy testing has not determined the causative foods, foods are reintroduced systematically (Table 49-2). Endoscopy should be used to document an improvement in esophageal histology.

Treatment of EoE with aggressive acid blockade, including medical and surgical therapy, has not been proven to be effective. Several published reports have demonstrated the failure of H$_2$

Table 49-2 Guidelines for Food Reintroduction in Patients with Eosinophilic Esophagitis or Gastroenteritis

Before Food Reintroduction

Diagnosis of eosinophilic esophagitis or gastroenteritis is confirmed by biopsy
Food allergens are identified by skin or patch testing.

If Foods Identified by Allergy Testing

Remove offending foods
    As determined by allergy testing or clinical history
    Alternative option, if no foods identified, is to remove most likely food
        allergens (milk, soy, eggs, wheat, nuts)
Repeat esophageal biopsy in 4 to 6 weeks
If biopsy normal, reintroduce foods (one at a time) every 5 to 7 days
    If symptoms develop, withdraw food; otherwise add two or three additional
        foods
    If no symptoms, a repeat biopsy is necessary to document continued
        resolution of disease
If biopsy abnormal, begin elemental diet (using Neocate 1 +)
    Repeat endoscopic biopsy after 4 weeks to look for disease resolution
    After resolution, reintroduce one new food every 5 to 7 days (see food
        chart)
    If symptoms do not develop, repeat endoscopic biopsy after reintroduction
        of groups of five foods
If positive biopsies recur, remove last introduced foods

Notes:
1. If food has a history of IgE-mediated reaction, initial food reintroduction should be performed as a formal food challenge in a hospital setting.
2. Positive foods, identified by biopsy, allergy testing, or history (and confirmed by biopsy), should be avoided for at least 2 years.

Food chart
(Begin with foods from column A and move to column D and from top to bottom)

A	B	C	D
Vegetables	Citrus fruits	Legumes	Corn
Noncitrus fruits	Tropical fruits	Grains	Peas
	Melons	Meats	Wheat
	Berries	Fish/shellfish	Beef
		Tree nuts	Peanuts
			Soy
			Eggs

Eosinophilic Disorders

- Eosinophilic disorders of the gastrointestinal (GI) tract should be considered in any child who has chronic GI symptoms including abdominal pain, vomiting, nausea, diarrhea, GI bleeding, and failure to thrive.
- These disorders are often difficult to diagnose because they mimic many other GI disorders.
- GI mucosal biopsies are mandatory for the diagnosis of these disorders. Biopsies should be obtained (colonic for eosinophilic proctocolitis and gastroenteritis; esophagus, stomach, and duodenum for eosinophilic esophagitis and gastroenteritis) even when the visual inspection of the mucosa is normal.
- Eosinophilic proctocolitis is typically a disease that occurs in the first year of life and is related to specific food allergies. It usually resolves by the age of 2 years.
- Eosinophilic esophagitis is often mistaken for gastroesophageal reflux disease. Endoscopic biopsy is critical to make the diagnosis. Foods are the causative agent.
- Eosinophilic gastroenteritis is the least understood and most difficult to treat eosinophilic disorder. The cause appears to be an alteration in immunologic function. Treatment options include elemental diets and immunosuppressive medications.

EoE.[68,70] In 1997, Liacouras and colleagues[83] were the first to publish the use of oral corticosteroids in 20 children diagnosed with EoE. These patients were treated with oral methylprednisolone (average dosage, 1.5 mg/kg/day; maximum dosage, 48 mg/day) for 1 month. Symptoms were significantly improved in 19 of 20 patients by an average of 8 days. A repeat endoscopy with biopsy, 4 weeks after the initiation of therapy, demonstrated a significant reduction of esophageal eosinophils, from 34 to 1.5 eosinophils per HPF. However, on discontinuation of corticosteroids, 90% have had recurrence of symptoms.

In 1999, Faubion and colleagues[85] reported that swallowing a metered dose of inhaled corticosteroids was also effective in treating the symptoms of EoE in children. Four patients diagnosed with EoE manifested by epigastric pain, dysphagia, and a severe esophageal eosinophilia unresponsive to aggressive acid blockade, were given fluticasone, four puffs twice a day. Patients were instructed to use inhaled corticosteroids but to immediately swallow after inhalation to deliver the medication to the esophagus. Histologic improvement was not determined. Within 2 months, all four patients responded with an improvement in symptoms. Two patients required repeat use of inhalation therapy. This therapy was recently confirmed.[80] Konikoff performed a randomized, double-blind, placebo-controlled trial utilizing swallowed fluticasone in patients with EoE.[99] The study revealed symptomatic improvement and decreased esophageal eosinophils in those who received the drug compared to those who received placebo. In addition to swallowed fluticasone, Aceves reported an effective alternative by using budesonide mixed with a sucralose suspension.[100] Although this therapy can improve EoE, the side-effects can include esophageal candidiasis and growth failure.[101-102] In addition, symptoms often recur in patients following discontinuation of the therapy.[81]

The mast cell-stabilizing agent cromolyn sodium has also been used to treat children with EoE.[38,103] In a fashion similar to its use for children with EoG, oral cromolyn has been given to patients with a severe esophageal eosinophilia in conjunction with other systemic signs and symptoms of allergic disease. However, no

blocker and proton-pump therapy in patients with EoE.[81,83,91] Although acid blockade may improve clinical symptoms by improving acid reflux that occurs secondary to the underlying inflamed esophageal mucosa, it does not reverse the esophageal histologic abnormality. Furthermore, Liacouras[98] published findings on two patients found to have an isolated eosinophilic infiltration of the esophagus who failed medical therapy and underwent Nissen fundoplication. In both cases, the patients continued to have clinical symptoms and continued evidence of an isolated esophageal eosinophilia by biopsy after fundoplication. Subsequently, each responded to oral corticosteroids with resolution of their clinical symptoms and a return to normal of their esophageal mucosa. In one patient, symptoms recurred on discontinuation of corticosteroids; however, the patient later responded to the introduction of an elemental diet. Similarly, four patients reported by Kelly and colleagues[76] had undergone Nissen fundoplication and continued to have clinical symptoms.

Before 1997, reports suggested that systemic corticosteroids improved the symptoms of EoE in adults identified with a severe

BOX 49-4 Therapeutic principles

Eosinophilic Disorders

Continue Step-Wise Progression if No Improvement in Disease

Eosinophilic Proctocolitis (EoP)

Step 1. Remove milk/soy from diet (and from mother's diet if breast-feeding). Use protein hydrolysate formula.

Step 2. Remove all foods from diet. Use amino acid-based formula.

After resolution of EoP (on above therapy), foods may be reintroduced at 1 year of age. Challenge should be performed in an office setting when the history of symptoms is mild and in a hospital setting if anaphylaxis is a possibility.

Eosinophilic Gastroenteritis (EoG)

Step 1. Administer strict elemental diet using amino acid-based formula.

Step 2. Administer a trial of corticosteroids and cromolyn sodium.

Step 3. Consider other immunosuppressive agents (6-MP, imuran).

Eosinophilic Esophagitis (EoE)

Step 1. Perform endoscopy with biopsy on aggressive acid blockade (omeprazole).

Step 2. Consult allergist; remove suspected foods; repeat endoscopy with biopsy in 4 to 6 weeks.

Step 3. Administer strict amino acid-based formula for 4 weeks followed by repeat endoscopy with biopsy.

Step 4. Reintroduce foods one at a time every 4 to 5 days. Consider repeat endoscopy after every five foods reintroduced unless symptomatic response occurs.

Allergic foods should be avoided.

Corticosteroids should be used only in severe cases to alleviate symptoms until diet restriction can be initiated.

controlled reports have been performed, and efficacy for oral cromolyn in children with EoE has not been established. Finally, the use of montelukast has been reported to provide an improvement in symptoms in patients with eosinophilic disorders of the GI tract.[62]

Conclusions

Eosinophilic disorders of the GI tract are becoming increasingly recognized. Although EoG is rare and difficult to diagnose, EoP and EoE are much more common and easily diagnosed by endoscopic biopsy. EoP is a well-accepted entity, but the diagnosis of EoE has recently been receiving a great deal of attention. Arguments still exist regarding the etiology and treatment of EoE. Further studies are needed to effectively differentiate patients with EoE from those with reflux esophagitis (Boxes 49-3 and 49-4). It appears that significant esophageal eosinophilia (> 20 per HPF) suggests a diagnosis of EoE, whereas esophageal eosinophilia (<15 per HPF) and an improvement with acid blockade suggests GERD. The diagnosis is equivocal when an esophageal biopsy reveals 5 to 20 eosinophils per HPF, thus leading to the question: What is the best way to diagnose and treat patients with EoE?

Future research should focus on clarifying the prevalence and natural history (e.g. the potential development of strictures) and optimizing the diagnostic approach and treatment options of all GI eosinophilic disorders. Many unanswered questions remain. Why have EoG and EoE been reported in some parts of the USA and not at all in others? Can the diagnosis be made using less invasive techniques than endoscopy with biopsy? How can we better identify offending food antigens and allergens other than elemental formulas with a strict protein elimination diet? Do environmental or infectious agents play a role in the disease process? Are there medications that can cure the disease? In addition, biochemical studies need to be pursued so that we can determine a cause of these disorders. Is the eosinophil dysregulation due to an immunologic defect or an allergy? These and other research questions reinforce the limitations of our current understanding of GI eosinophilic disease.

Helpful Websites

The American Partnership for Eosinophilic Disorders website (www.apfed.org)

The Food Allergy and Anaphylaxis Network website (www.foodallergy.org)

References

1. Jenkins HR, Pincott JR, Soothill JF, et al. Food allergy: the major cause of infantile colitis. Arch Dis Child 1984;59:326–9.
2. Goldman H, Proujansky R. Allergic proctitis and gastroenteritis in children. Clinical and mucosal biopsy features in 53 cases. Am J Surg Pathol 1986;10:75–86.
3. Heyman M, Grasset E, Ducroc R, et al. Antigen absorption by the jejunal epithelium of children with cow's milk allergy. Pediatr Res 1988;24: 197–202.
4. Husby S, Host A, Teisner B, et al. Infants and children with cow milk allergy/intolerance. Investigation of the uptake of cow milk protein and activation of the complement system. Allergy 1990;45:547–51.
5. Kerner JA Jr. Formula allergy and intolerance. Gastroenterol Clin North Am 1995;24:1–25.
6. Gerrard JW, MacKenzie JW, Goluboff N, et al. Cow's milk allergy: prevalence and manifestations in an unselected series of newborns. Acta Paediatr Scand Suppl 1973;234:1–21.
7. Host A, Halken S. A prospective study of cow milk allergy in Danish infants during the first 3 years of life. Clinical course in relation to clinical and immunological type of hypersensitivity reaction. Allergy 1990;45: 587–96.
8. Strobel S. Epidemiology of food sensitivity in childhood—with special reference to cow's milk allergy in infancy. Monogr Allergy 1993;31: 119–30.
9. Simpser E. Gastrointestinal Allergy. In: Altschuler SM, Liacouras CA, editors. Clinical pediatric gastroenterology. Philadelphia: Churchill Livingstone; 1998.
10. Eastham EJ. Soy protein allergy. In: Taylor RH, editor. Allergology, immunology, and gastroenterology. New York: Raven Press; 1989.
11. Shannon WR. Demonstration of food proteins in human breast milk by anaphylactic experiments in guinea pig. Am J Dis Child 1921;22:223–5.
12. Makinen-Kiljunen S, Palosuo T. A sensitive enzyme-linked immunosorbent assay for determination of bovine beta-lactoglobulin in infant feeding formulas and in human milk. Allergy 1992;47:347–52.
13. Axelsson I, Jakobsson I, Lindberg T, et al. Bovine beta-lactoglobulin in the human milk. A longitudinal study during the whole lactation period. Acta Paediatr Scand 1986;75:702–7.
14. Pittschieler K. Cow's milk protein-induced colitis in the breast-fed infant. J Pediatr Gastroenterol Nutr 1990;10:548–9.
15. Vandenplas Y, Hauser B, Van den Borre C, et al. Effect of a whey hydrolysate prophylaxis of atopic disease. Ann Allergy 1992;68:419–24.
16. Juvonen P, Mansson M, Jakobsson I. Does early diet have an effect on subsequent macromolecular absorption and serum IgE? J Pediatr Gastroenterol Nutr 1994;18:344–9.
17. Kaczmarski M, Kurzatkowska B. The contribution of some environmental factors to the development of cow's milk and gluten intolerance in children. Rocz Akad Med Bialymst 1988;33–34:151–65.
18. Katz AJ, Twarog FJ, Zeiger RS, et al. Milk-sensitive and eosinophilic gastroenteropathy: similar clinical features with contrasting mechanisms and clinical course. J Allergy Clin Immunol 1984;74:72–8.
19. Donta ST, Myers MG. Clostridium difficile toxin in asymptomatic neonates. J Pediatr 1982;100:431–4.
20. Cooperstock MS, Steffen E, Yolken R, et al. Clostridium difficile in normal infants and sudden infant death syndrome: an association with infant formula feeding. Pediatrics 1982;70:91–5.
21. Hirano K, Shimojo N, Katsuki T, et al. [Eosinophils in stool smear in normal and milk-allergic infants]. Arerugi 1997;46:594–1.
22. Anveden-Hertzberg L, Finkel Y, Sandstedt B, et al. Proctocolitis in exclusively breast-fed infants. Eur J Pediatr 1996;155:464–7.

23. Odze RD, Bines J, Leichtner AM, et al. Allergic proctocolitis in infants: a prospective clinicopathologic biopsy study. Hum Pathol 1993;24:668–74.

24. Machida HM, Catto Smith AG, Gall DG, et al. Allergic colitis in infancy: clinical and pathologic aspects. J Pediatr Gastroenterol Nutr 1994;19:22–6.

25. Goldman H. Allergic disorders. In: Ming S-C, Goldman H, editors. Pathology of the gastrointestinal tract. Philadelphia: WB Saunders; 1992.

26. Kaijser R. Zur Kenntnis der allergischen Affektioner desima Verdeanungaskanal von Standpunkt desmia Chirurgen aus. Arch Klin Chir 1937;188:3664.

27. Klein NC, Hargrove RL, Sleisenger MH, et al. Eosinophilic gastroenteritis. Medicine (Balt) 1970;49:299–319.

28. Spergel JM, Pawlowski NA. Food allergy: mechanisms, diagnosis, and management in children. Pediatr Clin North Am 2002;49:73–96, vi.

29. Park HS, Kim HS, Jang HJ. Eosinophilic gastroenteritis associated with food allergy and bronchial asthma. J Korean Med Sci 1995;10:216–9.

30. Justinich C, Katz A, Gurbindo C, et al. Elemental diet improves steroid-dependent eosinophilic gastroenteritis and reverses growth failure. J Pediatr Gastroenterol Nutr 1996;23:81–5.

31. Leinbach GE, Rubin CE. Eosinophilic gastroenteritis: a simple reaction to food allergens? Gastroenterology 1970;59:874–89.

32. Caldwell JH, Sharma HM, Hurtubise PE, et al. Eosinophilic gastroenteritis in extreme allergy. Immunopathological comparison with nonallergic gastrointestinal disease. Gastroenterology 1979;77:560–4.

33. Kelso A. Cytokines: structure, function and synthesis. Curr Opin Immunol 1989;2:215–25.

34. Desreumaux P, Bloget F, Seguy D, et al. Interleukin 3, granulocyte-macrophage colony-stimulating factor, and interleukin 5 in eosinophilic gastroenteritis. Gastroenterology 1996;110:768–74.

35. Takafuji S, Bischoff SC, De Weck AL, et al. IL-3 and IL-5 prime normal human eosinophils to produce leukotriene C4 in response to soluble agonists. J Immunol 1991;147:3855–61.

36. Beyer K, Castro R, Birnbaum A, et al. Human milk-specific mucosal lymphocytes of the gastrointestinal tract display a TH2 cytokine profile. J Allergy Clin Immunol 2002;109:707–13.

37. Kelly KJ. Eosinophilic gastroenteritis. J Pediatr Gastroenterol Nutr 2000;30:S28-35.

38. Whitington PF, Whitington GL. Eosinophilic gastroenteropathy in childhood. J Pediatr Gastroenterol Nutr 1988;7:379–85.

39. Talley NJ, Shorter RG, Phillips SF, et al. Eosinophilic gastroenteritis: a clinicopathological study of patients with disease of the mucosa, muscle layer, and subserosal tissues. Gut 1990;31:54–8.

40. Santos J, Junquera F, de Torres I, et al. Eosinophilic gastroenteritis presenting as ascites and splenomegaly. Eur J Gastroenterol Hepatol 1995;7:675–8.

41. DeSchryver-Kecskemeti K, Clouse RE. A previously unrecognized subgroup of 'eosinophilic gastroenteritis.' Association with connective tissue diseases. Am J Surg Pathol 1984;8:171–80.

42. Dubucquoi S, Janin A, Klein O, et al. Activated eosinophils and interleukin 5 expression in early recurrence of Crohn's disease. Gut 1995;37:242–6.

43. Levy AM, Yamazaki K, Van Keulen VP, et al. Increased eosinophil infiltration and degranulation in colonic tissue from patients with collagenous colitis. Am J Gastroenterol 2001;96:1522–8.

44. Griscom NT, Kirkpatrick JA Jr, Girdany BR, et al. Gastric antral narrowing in chronic granulomatous disease of childhood. Pediatrics 1974;54:456–60.

45. Harris BH, Boles ET Jr. Intestinal lesions in chronic granulomatous disease of childhood. J Pediatr Surg 1973;8:955–6.

46. Aquino A, Domini M, Rossi C, et al. Pyloric stenosis due to eosinophilic gastroenteritis: presentation of two cases in monoovular twins. Eur J Pediatr 1999;158:172–3.

47. Khan S, Orenstein SR. Eosinophilic gastroenteritis masquerading as pyloric stenosis. Clin Pediatr (Phila) 2000;39:55–7.

48. Redondo-Cerezo E, Cabello MJ, Gonzalez Y, et al. Eosinophilic gastroenteritis: our recent experience: one-year experience of atypical onset of an uncommon disease. Scand J Gastroenterol 2001;36:1358–60.

49. Shweiki E, West JC, Klena JW, et al. Eosinophilic gastroenteritis presenting as an obstructing cecal mass: a case report and review of the literature. Am J Gastroenterol 1999;94:3644–5.

50. Huang FC, Ko SF, Huang SC, et al. Eosinophilic gastroenteritis with perforation mimicking intussusception. J Pediatr Gastroenterol Nutr 2001;33:613–5.

51. Deslandres C, Russo P, Gould P, et al. Perforated duodenal ulcer in a pediatric patient with eosinophilic gastroenteritis. Can J Gastroenterol 1997;11:208–12.

52. Wang CS, Hsueh S, Shih LY, et al. Repeated bowel resections for eosinophilic gastroenteritis with obstruction and perforation. Case report. Acta Chir Scand 1990;156:333–6.

53. Hoefer RA, Ziegler MM, Koop CE, et al. Surgical manifestations of eosinophilic gastroenteritis in the pediatric patient. J Pediatr Surg 1977;12:955–62.

54. Lerza P. A further case of eosinophilic gastroenteritis with ascites. Eur J Gastroenterol Hepatol 1996;8:407.

55. Caldwell JH, Tennenbaum JI, Bronstein HA. Serum IgE in eosinophilic gastroenteritis. Response to intestinal challenge in two cases. N Engl J Med 1975;292:1388–90.

56. Teele RL, Katz AJ, Goldman H, et al. Radiographic features of eosinophilic gastroenteritis (allergic gastroenteropathy) of childhood. AJR Am J Roentgenol 1979;132:575–80.

57. Spergel JM, Beausoleil JL, Mascarenhas M, et al. The use of skin prick tests and patch tests to identify causative foods in eosinophilic esophagitis. J Allergy Clin Immunol 2002;109:363–8.

58. Vandenplas Y, Quenon M, Renders F, et al. Milk-sensitive eosinophilic gastroenteritis in a 10-day-old boy. Eur J Pediatr 1990;149:244–5.

59. Van Dellen RG, Lewis JC. Oral administration of cromolyn in a patient with protein-losing enteropathy, food allergy, and eosinophilic gastroenteritis. Mayo Clin Proc 1994;69:441–4.

60. Moots RJ, Prouse P, Gumpel JM. Near fatal eosinophilic gastroenteritis responding to oral sodium chromoglycate. Gut 1988;29:1282–5.

61. Di Gioacchino M, Pizzicannella G, Fini N, et al. Sodium cromoglycate in the treatment of eosinophilic gastroenteritis. Allergy 1990;45:161–6.

62. Schwartz DA, Pardi DS, Murray JA. Use of montelukast as steroid-sparing agent for recurrent eosinophilic gastroenteritis. Dig Dis Sci 2001;46:1787–90.

63. Neustrom MR, Friesen C. Treatment of eosinophilic gastroenteritis with montelukast. J Allergy Clin Immunol 1999;104:506.

64. Shirai T, Hashimoto D, Suzuki K, et al. Successful treatment of eosinophilic gastroenteritis with suplatast tosilate. J Allergy Clin Immunol 2001;107:924–5.

65. Bengtsson U, Hanson LA, Ahlstedt S. Survey of gastrointestinal reactions to foods in adults in relation to atopy, presence of mucus in the stools, swelling of joints and arthralgia in patients with gastrointestinal reactions to foods. Clin Exp Allergy 1996;26:1387–94,.

66. Dobbins JW, Sheahan DG, Behar J. Eosinophilic gastroenteritis with esophageal involvement. Gastroenterology 1977;72:1312–6.

67. Matzinger MA, Daneman A. Esophageal involvement in eosinophilic gastroenteritis. Pediatr Radiol 1983;13:35–8.

68. Lee RG. Marked eosinophilia in esophageal mucosal biopsies. Am J Surg Pathol 1985;9:475–9.

69. Attwood SE, Smyrk TC, Demeester TR, et al. Esophageal eosinophilia with dysphagia: a distinct clinicopathologic syndrome. Dig Dis Sci 1993;38:109–6.

70. Vitellas KM, Bennett WF, Bova JG, et al. Idiopathic eosinophilic esophagitis. Radiology 1993;186:789–93.

71. Furuta GT, Liacouras CA, Collins MH, et al. Eosinophilic esophagitis in children and adults: A systematic review an consensus recommendations for diagnosis and treatment. Gastroenterology 2007;133(4):1342–63.

72. Bischoff SC, Herrmann A, Manns MP. Prevalence of adverse reactions to food in patients with gastrointestinal disease. Allergy 1996;51:811–8.

73. Winter HS, Madara JL, Stafford RJ, et al. Intraepithelial eosinophils: a new diagnostic criterion for reflux esophagitis. Gastroenterology 1982;83:818–23.

74. Brown LF, Goldman H, Antonioli DA. Intraepithelial eosinophils in endoscopic biopsies of adults with reflux esophagitis. Am J Surg Pathol 1984;8:899–905.

75. Tummala V, Barwick KW, Sontag SJ, et al. The significance of intraepithelial eosinophils in the histologic diagnosis of gastroesophageal reflux. Am J Clin Pathol 1987;87:43–8.

76. Kelly KJ, Lazenby AJ, Rowe PC, et al. Eosinophilic esophagitis attributed to gastroesophageal reflux: improvement with an amino acid-based formula. Gastroenterology 1995;109:1503–12.

77. Sondheimer JM. What are the roles of eosinophils in esophagitis? J Pediatr Gastroenterol Nutr 1998;27:118–9.

78. Hassall E. Macroscopic versus microscopic diagnosis of reflux esophagitis: erosions or eosinophils? J Pediatr Gastroenterol Nutr 1996;22:321–5.

79. Levine MS, Saul SH. Idiopathic eosinophilic esophagitis: how common is it? Radiology 1993;186:631–2.

80. Walsh SV, Antonioli DA, Goldman H, et al. Allergic esophagitis in children: a clinicopathological entity. Am J Surg Pathol 1999;23:390–6.

81. Teitelbaum JE, Fox VL, Twarog FJ, et al. Eosinophilic esophagitis in children: immunopathological analysis and response to fluticasone propionate. Gastroenterology 2002;122:1216–25.

82. Orenstein SR, Shalaby TM, Di Lorenzo C, et al. The spectrum of pediatric eosinophilic esophagitis beyond infancy: a clinical series of 30 children. Am J Gastroenterol 2000;95:1422–30.

83. Liacouras CA, Wenner WJ, Brown K, et al. Primary eosinophilic esophagitis in children: successful treatment with oral corticosteroids. J Pediatr Gastroenterol Nutr 1998;26:380–5.

84. Liacouras CA, Markowitz JE. Eosinophilic esophagitis: A subset of eosinophilic gastroenteritis. Curr Gastroenterol Rep 1999;1:253–8.

85. Faubion WA Jr, Perrault J, Burgart LJ, et al. Treatment of eosinophilic esophagitis with inhaled corticosteroids. J Pediatr Gastroenterol Nutr 1998;27:90–3.

86. Furuta GT. Eosinophilic esophagitis: an emerging clinicopathologic entity. Curr Allergy Asthma Rep 2002;2:67–72.

87. Lucendo AJ, Navarro M, Comas C, et al. Immunophenotypic characterization and quantification of the epithelial inflammatory infiltrate in eosinophilic esophagitis through stereology: an analysis of the cellular mechanisms of the disease and immunologic capacity of the esophagus. Am J Surg Pathol 2007;31:598–606.

88. Yamazaki K, Murray JA, Arora AS, et al. Allergen specific in vitro cytokine production in adult patients with eosinophilic esophagitis. Dig Dis Sci 2006;51:1934–41.

89. Aceves SS, Newbury RO, Dohil R, et al. Esophageal remodeling in pediatric eosinophilic esophagitis. J Clin All Immunol 2007;119:206–12.

90. Blanchard C, Wang N, Stringer KF, et al. Eotaxin-3 and a uniquely conserved gene-expression profile in eosinophilic esophagitis. J Clin Invest 2006;116:536–47.

91. Ruchelli E, Wenner W, Voytek T, et al. Severity of esophageal eosinophilia predicts response to conventional gastroesophageal reflux therapy. Pediatr Dev Pathol 1999;2:15–8.

92. Siafakas CG, Ryan CK, Brown MR, et al. Multiple esophageal rings: an association with eosinophilic esophagitis: case report and review of the literature. Am J Gastroenterol 2000;95:1572–5.

93. Bousvaros A, Antonioli DA, Winter HS. Ringed esophagus: an association with esophagitis. Am J Gastroenterol 1992;87:1187–90.

94. Gupta SK, Fitzgerald JF, Chong SK, et al. Vertical lines in distal esophageal mucosa (VLEM): a true endoscopic manifestation of esophagitis in children? Gastrointest Endosc 1997;45:485–9.

95. Stevoff C, Rao S, Parsons W, et al. EUS and histopathologic correlates in eosinophilic esophagitis. Gastrointest Endosc 2001;54:373–7.

96. Liacouras CA, Spergel JM, Ruchelli E, et al. Eosinophilic esophagitis: a 10-year experience in 381 children. Clin Gastroenterol Hepatol 2005;3:1198–206.

97. Markowitz JE, Spergel JM, Ruchelli E, et al. Elemental diet is an effective treatment for eosinophilic esophagitis in children and adolescents. Am J Gastroenterol 2003 (in press).

98. Liacouras CA. Failed Nissen fundoplication in two patients who had persistent vomiting and eosinophilic esophagitis. J Pediatr Surg 1997;32:1504–6.

99. Konikoff MR, Noel RJ, Blanchard C, et al. A randomized, double blind placebo controlled trial of fluticasone proprionate for pediatric eosinophilic esophagitis. Gastroenterology 2006;131:1381–91.

100. Aceves S, Bastian J, Newbury R, et al. Oral viscous budesonide: a potential new therapy for eosinophilic esophagitis in children. Am J Gastroenterol 2007;102:2271–9.

101. Simon MR, Houser WL, Smith KA, et al. Esophageal candidiasis as a complication of inhaled corticosteroids. Ann Allergy Asthma Immunol 1997;79:333–8.

102. Sharek PJ, Bergman DA. The effect of inhaled steroids on the linear growth of children with asthma: a meta-analysis. Pediatrics 2000;106:E8.

103. Dahl R. Disodium cromoglycate and food allergy. The effect of oral and inhaled disodium cromoglycate in a food allergic patient. Allergy 1978;33:120–4.

Eosinophilic Esophagitis, Gastroenteritis, and Proctocolitis

50

Food Allergy, Respiratory Disease, and Anaphylaxis

John M. James

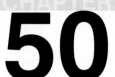

Introduction

While skin and gastrointestinal tract symptoms are commonly observed with allergic reactions to foods, respiratory tract symptoms may also be involved.[1–3] Specific respiratory symptoms that have been attributed to food allergy include nasal congestion, rhinorrhea, sneezing, pruritus of the nose and throat, coughing, wheezing and asthma. In addition, anaphylactic reactions can occur. Exposure is usually through ingestion, but in some cases, inhalation of food allergens may also trigger these reactions.[4] In fact, an increasing number of investigations have highlighted allergic reactions to food allergens that have occurred following inhalation. Food allergy in early childhood does appear to be a good marker for later respiratory allergy including asthma. In addition, studies have demonstrated that food-induced allergic reactions can provoke recurrent episodic or asthmatic responses as well as airway hyperreactivity and persistent asthma. Therefore, evaluation for food allergy should be considered among patients with recalcitrant or otherwise unexplained acute severe asthma exacerbations, asthma triggered following ingestion of particular foods, and in patients with asthma and other manifestations of food allergy (e.g. anaphylaxis, moderate to severe atopic dermatitis). Anaphylactic reactions to foods in children almost always include respiratory tract symptoms. This underscores the importance of observing respiratory tract symptoms as part of a food allergic reaction. Finally, respiratory manifestations of food-induced anaphylaxis, in particular upper or lower airway obstruction, often determine the severity and outcome of the reaction. (Box 50-1)

Epidemiology

Overview

Adverse reactions to foods can provoke clinical signs and symptoms involving the skin, gastrointestinal and respiratory tracts, and in some cases, the cardiovascular system.[1] The two broad groups of immune-mediated reactions include IgE- and non-IgE-mediated mechanisms. The IgE-mediated reactions are usually divided into immediate onset reactions and immediate plus late-phase reactions, which involve an immediate onset of symptoms followed by prolonged or ongoing symptoms. Typical examples of immediate onset, IgE-mediated reactions include allergic reactions following the ingestion of peanuts, tree nuts, shellfish or sesame seeds resulting in laryngeal edema, coughing and/or wheezing. Non-IgE-mediated reactions are typically delayed in onset (i.e. 4 to 48 hours) and most frequently involve the gastrointestinal tract (e.g. celiac disease or gluten-sensitive enteropathy). It is imperative to understand the specific terminology and basic classification of adverse food reactions in order to interpret the scientific studies implicating food allergy in respiratory tract symptoms and anaphylaxis.

Prevalence

There has been an increase in the prevalence of food allergy and its clinical expression over the past 20 years.[1,5] The exact prevalence of respiratory tract symptoms induced by food allergy, however, has been difficult to establish. For many years, there has been a public perception that food allergy-induced asthma is common. This perception has not been substantiated when careful objective investigations, including food challenges, have been undertaken to confirm patient histories.[6,7] The incidence has been estimated to be between 2% and 8% in children and adults with asthma when the specific focus has been on the role of food allergy and respiratory tract manifestations.[8,9] Using a cross-sectional epidemiologic study design in 1141 randomly selected young adults (age: 20–45 years), Australian investigators evaluated the prevalence of IgE-mediated food allergy and the relationships with atopic disease.[10] Those with probable IgE-mediated peanut allergy were more likely to have current asthma, wheeze and a history of eczema, and those with probable IgE-mediated shrimp allergy were also more likely to have current asthma and nasal allergies. No relationships were observed between those subjects with probable IgE-mediated cow's milk, wheat or egg allergy and allergic diseases because of small numbers of subjects with these food allergies in this age group. They concluded that further research, with larger numbers of subjects demonstrating IgE-mediated food allergy, will be required to confirm these results.

A French population study of food allergy was conducted to determine the prevalence, clinical features, specific allergens and risk factors of food allergy.[11] Of the 33 110 persons completing a questionnaire, the overall prevalence of food allergy was estimated to be 3.24%, with rhinitis and asthma documented in 6.5% and 5.7% of respiratory reactions reported, respectively. In addition, the clinical expression of food allergy was dependent on the existence of sensitization to pollens and was typically expressed in the form of rhinitis, asthma and angioedema. Another survey found that 17% of 669 adult respondents in Australia reported food-induced respiratory symptoms[12] While the patients with

DOI: 10.1016/B978-1-4377-0271-2.00050-X

asthma did not report food-related illness more frequently than those respondents without asthma, those reporting respiratory symptoms following food ingestion were more likely to be atopic.

Children with a family history of atopy and sensitization to food proteins in early infancy are at higher risk of developing subsequent respiratory allergic disease.[13] Furthermore, investigators from the Isle of Wight reported that egg allergy in infancy predicts respiratory allergic disease by 4 years of age.[14] In a cohort of 1218 consecutive births followed until 4 years of age, 29 (2.4%) developed egg allergy by 4 years of age. Increased respiratory allergy (e.g. rhinitis, asthma) was associated with egg allergy (OR: 5.0, 95% CI: 1.1–22.3; $p < 0.05$) with a positive predictive value of 55%. Furthermore, the addition of the diagnosis of eczema to egg allergy increased the positive predictive value to 80%. Rhodes and colleagues conducted a prospective cohort study of subjects at risk of asthma and atopy in England.[15] Of 100 babies of atopic parents who were recruited at birth, 73 were followed up at 5 years, 67 at 11 and 63 at 22 years of age. Skin sensitivity to hen's egg, cow's milk or both in the first 5 years of life was predictive of asthma (odds ratio: 10.7; 95% CI, 2.1–55.1; $p = 0.001$, sensitivity 57%; specificity 89%).

Investigators examined the degree of food allergen sensitization to six common foods (e.g. egg, milk, soy, peanut, wheat and fish) in 504 inner-city patients 4 to 9 years (median age 6 years) with asthma enrolled in the National Cooperative Inner City Asthma Study in the USA.[16] Children sensitized to foods had higher rates of asthma hospitalization ($P < 0.01$) and required more steroid medications ($P = 0.25$). In addition, sensitization to foods was correlated with sensitization to more indoor and outdoor aeroallergens ($P < 0.001$). The association of increased asthma morbidity with at least one food sensitization, and findings that patients with sensitization to multiple foods had significantly more asthma morbidity than those with single-food sensitization, suggests that food allergen sensitivity may be a marker for increased asthma severity.

An investigation by Sicherer and colleagues summarized data from a voluntary registry of 5149 individuals (median age: 5 years) with peanut and/or tree nut allergy.[17] The primary objective was to characterize clinical features including respiratory reactions in the registrants. Respiratory reactions, including wheezing, throat tightness and nasal congestion, were reported in 42% and 56% of respondents as part of their initial reactions to peanuts and tree nuts, respectively. One half of the reactions involved more than one system and more than 75% required some form of medical treatment. Interestingly, registrants with asthma were significantly more likely than those without asthma to have severe reactions (33% versus 21%; $P < 0.0001$). A more recent investigation by the same group estimated the prevalence

of seafood allergy in the USA using a nationwide, cross-sectional, random telephone survey and standardized questionnaire. A total of 5529 households completed the survey, representing a census of 14 948 individuals. Fish or shellfish allergy was reported in 5.9% of households. Recurrent reactions were common. Shortness of breath and throat tightness were reported by more than 50% of those surveyed and 16% were treated with epinephrine.[18] (Box 50-2)

Pathogenesis

Mechanisms

Understanding how food allergy induces a significant disruption of normal oral tolerance continues to evolve. Recently, it has become evident that the gut, which is the classic site of sensitization to foods, is only responsible for primary sensitization in a subset of patients. These patients are generally younger and they exhibit their first symptoms shortly after initial feedings to the relevant food. In contrast, a newly recognized route of sensitization for food allergic patients is by initial exposure to aeroallergens through inhalation, with secondary clinical reactions following ingestion of specific cross-reactive foods. In these patients, many years may elapse before the first respiratory symptoms appear. Investigations from Europe suggest that lipid transfer protein (LTP) inhalation may induce significant allergic sensitization through the respiratory tract and this may precede the onset of relevant food allergy.[19,20] For example, inhalation of LTP from specific fruits (e.g. peaches) may lead to allergic sensitization and ultimately allergic reactions following the oral ingestion of these foods.

Allergens

Specific foods are more often implicated in food allergic reactions involving respiratory symptoms and have subsequently been confirmed in well-controlled, blinded food challenges.[6,21–23] These foods include egg, cow's milk, peanut, fish, shellfish and tree nuts (Box 50-3). For example, one group of young children who were allergic to cow's milk was followed from 1 year until 5 years of age.[24] These patients did develop early respiratory symptoms, including nasal symptoms and cough without skin or gastrointestinal symptoms, and 69% of these patients ultimately developed allergic sensitivities to common indoor aeroallergens. In addition, anaphylactic reactions to foods, including significant respiratory symptoms, and rarely fatal anaphylactic reactions, have been reported.[25–28] Some food allergens

Common Food Allergens Implicated in Respiratory Disease

- Chicken egg, cow's milk, peanuts, fish, shellfish and tree nuts have been the main foods responsible for food allergen-induced respiratory reactions.
- Peanuts, tree nuts, sesame seeds and shellfish have most often been responsible for near-fatal and fatal anaphylactic reactions following food ingestion

seem to be more prone to present with respiratory tract symptoms, such as peanuts and tree nuts,[17] fish and shellfish[18] or sesame.[29]

Many food allergens have been implicated as the cause of respiratory tract allergy symptoms following inhalation as opposed to ingestion.[4] For example, studies have implicated and confirmed a wide variety of foods causing allergic symptoms following inhalation, including fish, shellfish, eggs,[30] poppy seed,[31] sunflower seeds,[32] lupine,[33,34] asparagus[35] and soybean.[36]

A high percentage of patients with asthma believe that food additives contribute to worsening of their respiratory symptoms.[37] Several different food additives, including monosodium glutamate (MSG), sulfites and aspartame have been implicated in adverse respiratory reactions,[38] but well-controlled investigations in this area have reported a prevalence rate of less than 5%.[8,21] Focusing on conflicting evidence that some individuals with asthma are more likely to have adverse effects from monosodium glutamate compared to the general population, Woods and co-workers[39] were unable to demonstrate MSG-induced immediate or late asthmatic reactions in 12 adult asthmatics reporting food additive-induced symptoms. In addition, no significant changes in bronchial hyperresponsiveness or soluble inflammatory markers (e.g. eosinophil cationic protein, tryptase) were observed during these challenges. In an investigation utilizing double-blind, placebo-controlled oral MSG challenges in subjects who had histories of adverse reactions to MSG,[40] no specific upper or lower respiratory complaints were observed, but 22 (36.1%) of the 61 enrolled subjects had confirmed adverse reactions to MSG, including headache, muscle tightness, numbness, general weakness and flushing.

Route of Exposure and Subsequent Respiratory Symptoms

Oral Ingestion of Food Allergens

Oral ingestion is the primary route of exposure to food that can cause or exacerbate respiratory symptoms (e.g. laryngeal edema, asthma). The vast majority of published reports, highlighted in this chapter, focus on respiratory tract symptoms following the ingestion of food allergens.

Inhalation of Food Allergens

Some food-allergic individuals may react when exposed to airborne allergens in a seafood restaurant, or when fish, shellfish, or eggs are cooked in a confined area.[30] Seafood allergens aerosolized during food preparation are a source of potential respiratory and contact allergens.[41] A number of reports highlight allergic reactions associated with airborne fish particles,[42,43] including one using air sampling and an immunochemical analytic technique to detect fish allergen in the air of an open-air fish

market.[44] Avoidance of a food allergen, such as fish, should include the prevention of the exposure to aerosolized particles in relevant environments. Finally, an internet-based survey of 51 anaphylactic reactions to foods showed that, while most reactions (40 [78%]) occurred after ingestion, eight (16%) reactions occurred following exclusive skin contact, and three (6%) following inhalation.[45]

Children with IgE-mediated food allergy can develop asthma following inhalational exposure to aerosolized food allergens during the cooking process.[46] Twelve food-allergic children reportedly developed asthma following inhalational exposure to relevant food allergens. Foods implicated included fish, chickpea, milk, egg or buckwheat. Five of nine bronchial challenges were positive with objective clinical features of asthma and two children developed late-phase symptoms with a decrease in lung function. Positive reactions were seen with fish, chickpea and buckwheat. There were no reactions to the seven placebo challenges. These data demonstrate that inhaled food allergens can produce both early- and late-phase asthmatic responses. Finally, Sicherer and colleagues have reported that patients with allergy to peanuts and tree nuts might experience adverse respiratory reactions when they are exposed to them on airline flights serving peanut and tree nut snacks.[47] The exposures can include accidental ingestion or inhalation during commercial flights. Of the allergic reactions reported, some were severe, requiring medications including epinephrine.

Differential Diagnosis of Food-Induced Respiratory Syndromes

Many questions remain when evaluating respiratory manifestations possibly related to foods. Unlike cutaneous symptoms such as urticaria, respiratory manifestations are typically chronic or may be delayed, such as in atopic dermatitis due to the pattern of inflammatory mechanisms involved. This section will review potential manifestations of food allergy in the respiratory tract. (Figure 50-1)

Recurrent or Chronic Rhinitis Induced by Food Allergy

Acute rhinitis accounted for 70% of the overall respiratory symptoms observed in a large group of children undergoing double-blind, placebo-controlled food challenges (DBPCFCs).[48] These symptoms almost uniformly occur in association with other clinical manifestations (i.e. cutaneous and/or gastrointestinal symptoms) during allergic reactions to foods, and rarely occur in isolation.[21,48] Chronic or recurrent rhinitis, mostly in preschool children, is sometimes believed to be due to allergic reactions, mostly to milk. While some patients claim a significant decrease in symptoms after introducing an avoidance diet, a clear association has not been reproduced by double-blind studies.

Recurrent or Chronic Otitis Media Induced by Food Allergy

Serous otitis media has multiple etiologies, with viral upper respiratory tract infections being the most common. Allergic inflammation in the nasal mucosa may cause eustachian tube dysfunction and contribute to subsequent otitis media with effusion. Studies investigating a food allergic mechanism in recurrent serous otitis media are inconclusive.[49,50]

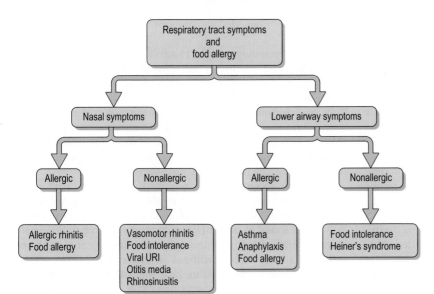

Figure 50-1 Respiratory tract symptoms and food allergy: differential diagnosis. *URI*, upper respiratory tract infection.

Dyspnea Associated with Anemia in Infants

In 1960, Heiner reported a syndrome in infants consisting of recurrent episodes of pneumonia associated with pulmonary infiltrates, hemosiderosis, gastrointestinal blood loss, iron-deficiency anemia and failure to thrive.[51] This syndrome is most often associated with a non-IgE-mediated hypersensitivity to cow's milk proteins. While increased peripheral blood eosinophils and multiple serum precipitins to cow's milk are commonly observed, the specific immunologic mechanisms responsible for this disorder are not known.[52] The diagnosis is suggested by infiltrates on chest X-ray, anemia, hemosiderosis evidenced by bronchioalveolar lavage and the presence of the precipitating antibodies to milk (in most cases). This food-induced syndrome is only very rarely observed even in referral clinics for childhood food allergy.

Eczema within the First 2 Years of Life and Risk of Developing Asthma and Allergic Rhinitis

The presence of persistent eczema in infancy has been identified as an important risk factor for the development of allergic rhinitis and asthma. In one study,[53] children with atopic eczema had a significantly greater risk of asthma (odds ratio [OR] = 3.52, 95% CI = 1.88 –6.59 and allergic rhinitis OR = 2.91, 1.48–5.71). This risk was not observed in the control patients.

Although a family history of atopy and the presence of atopic dermatitis and food allergy appear to contribute to the development of asthma, it is unclear when the airways become involved with the atopic process and whether airway function relates to the atopic characteristics of the infant. In one study of 114 infants (median age 10.7 months; range, 2.6–19.1), atopic status was determined by the presence of specific IgE to foods or aeroallergens and total IgE levels.[54] Exhaled nitric oxide (eNO), forced expiratory flow at 75% exhaled volume (FEF_{75}) and airway reactivity to inhaled methacholine were measured in these infants. Infants sensitized to egg or milk, compared to nonatopic controls, had lower flow rates (FEF_{75}: 336 vs 285 mL/s, P < 0.003) and lower provocative concentration of methacholine to decrease FEF_{75} by 30% (-0.6 vs -1.2, P < 0.02) but no difference in eNO

levels. These data suggest that atopic characteristics of the infant might be important determinants for the development of asthma.

Food Allergy in Infancy and Risk for Wheezing and Hyperactive Airways in Childhood

Children allergic to common food allergens in infancy may be at increased risk of wheezing and bronchial hyperreactivity later in childhood. A case-control study was conducted with 69 children (ages: 7.2–13.3 years) with allergy to egg (N = 60) and/or fish (N = 29) in the first 3 years of life.[55] A control group of 154 children (70 sensitized to inhaled allergens) were recruited with no history of food allergy in the first 3 years of life. Asthma symptoms were reported more frequently in the study group than in the control subjects. Children in the study group showed a significantly increased frequency of positive responses to methacholine challenge compared to the control group. Multivariate logistic regression analysis showed that bronchial hyperresponsiveness, as well as reported current asthma symptoms, were associated with early wheezing and early sensitization to inhaled allergens, but not with atopic dermatitis in infancy or persistence of egg or fish allergy. Therefore, children allergic to egg or fish in infancy may be at increased risk for wheezing illness and hyperactive airways in school age.

Acute Asthma Induced by Food Allergy

The wide use of standardized food challenges has provided a better view of the type and frequency of respiratory reactions in food allergy. Hill and colleagues challenged 100 milk-allergic infants and young children with a mean age of 16.2 months and elicited cough and/or wheeze in 20 patients, rhinitis in 12 patients, and stridor in two patients.[56] Cough and wheezing was more frequent in the groups of patients who initially presented with chronic eczema and recurrent bronchitis, and with urticaria and eczema. Lower respiratory symptoms were only observed in 2/53 patients (4%). In another study of 410 children with a history of asthma, 279 (68%) had a history of food-induced asthma.[57] There were positive food challenges in 168 (60%) of the

279 patients. This investigation documented that 67 (24%) of the 279 children with a history of food-induced asthma had a positive blinded food challenge that included wheezing. The most common foods responsible for these reactions included peanut – 19, cow's milk – 18, egg – 13, and tree nuts – 10. Interestingly, only 5 (2%) of these patients had wheezing as their only objective adverse symptom. In addition, 10 of the group of 188 children without a history of asthma had wheezing elicited by the food challenge, showing a tendency for a bronchial response in the absence of a concomitant asthma.

A total of 320 subjects, presenting primarily with atopic dermatitis, and undergoing blinded food challenges, were monitored for respiratory reactions.[48] The subjects, aged 6 months to 30 years, were highly atopic, had multiple allergic sensitivities to foods, and over one half had a prior diagnosis of asthma. In the 205 (64%) patients with food allergy confirmed by blinded challenges, almost two thirds experienced respiratory reactions during their positive food challenges (e.g. nasal 70%, laryngeal 48%, pulmonary 27%). Overall, 34 (17%) of 205 subjects with positive food challenges developed wheezing as part of their reaction. Furthermore, 88 of these patients were monitored with pulmonary function testing during positive and negative food challenges. Thirteen (15%) developed lower respiratory symptoms, including wheezing in 10 patients, but only 6 patients had a > 20% decrease in FEV1. Wheezing as the sole manifestation of a food-induced respiratory reaction was rare.

In a series of 163 children in which 385 DBPCFCs were performed,[58] 250 challenges (65%), were positive to peanuts (31%), hen's egg (23%) and cow's milk (9%). Cutaneous symptoms were observed in most positive challenges (59%), but respiratory reactions were also frequent (24%). Among the respiratory reactions, oral symptoms (5%), rhinitis and conjunctivitis (6%), and asthma (10%) were observed. Again, isolated asthma was rare, i.e. 2.8% of the challenges. Furthermore, investigations from Italy suggest that asthma and/or rhinitis, as part of the initial presentation of allergy to cow's milk, may be an independent predictor of persistence of this food allergy and a failure to develop oral tolerance.[59]

Food Allergy and Predisposition to Bronchial Hyperreactivity (BHR)

It has been observed in patients with atopic dermatitis and food allergy that the food avoidance diet significantly improved their asthma, despite absence of respiratory symptoms during food challenges. This prompted a series of investigations on bronchial hyperreactivity (BHR) in food allergic patients without acute respiratory symptoms following food ingestion. In one investigation, 26 children with asthma and food allergy were evaluated using methacholine inhalation challenges for changes in their BHR before and after blinded food challenges.[60] Of the 22 positive blinded food challenges, 12 (55%) involved chest symptoms (cough, laryngeal reactions, and/or wheezing). Another 10 (45%) positive food challenges included laryngeal, gastrointestinal and/or skin symptoms without any chest symptoms. Significant increases in BHR were documented several hours after positive food challenges in 7 of the 12 (58%) patients who experienced chest symptoms during these challenges. During the actual food challenges, decreases in FEV1 were not observed in these 7 patients suggesting that significant changes in BHR can occur without significant pulmonary function changes in a preceding food challenge. These data confirmed that food-induced allergic reactions may increase airway reactivity in a subset of patients with moderate to severe

asthma, and may do so without inducing acute asthma symptoms.

In contrast, another study of 11 adult asthmatics, with a history of food-induced wheezing and positive skin tests to the suspected food, concluded that food allergy is an unlikely cause of increased BHR.[61] An equal number of patients had increased BHR, as determined by methacholine inhalation challenges, 24 hours after blinded food challenges to either food allergen or placebo. However, the small number of patients evaluated and the lack of environmental controls prior to the repeat methacholine challenges limit their conclusions.

Two more recent studies indicate that patients with food allergy in the absence of asthma might develop increased BHR. In 35 nonasthmatic patients with food allergy, 10 of 19 patients (53%) were found to have BHR by methacholine inhalation challenges.[62] Similarly, Kivity and colleagues investigated patients with food allergy with or without asthma and/or allergic rhinitis, by spirometry, methacholine challenges and sputum-induced cell analysis.[63] BHR by methacholine challenge was observed in all patients with asthma, and in 40% of patients with food allergy alone. They also found mainly eosinophils in the sputum of patients with asthma, and neutrophils in the patients with food allergy but no asthma. This observation has been confirmed by other investigators who also observed an increased proportion of neutrophils and increased levels of IL-8 in nonasthmatic food allergic patients.[64]

An animal study came to a similar conclusion as mice, sensitized by intraperitoneal injection of ovalbumin in the presence of alum and orally challenged to ovalbumin, had significant airway inflammation for up to 12 days following a single intranasal challenge to ovalbumin.[65] Interestingly, an unrelated antigen, house dust mite, did induce a similar inflammatory response. Taken together, these observations suggest that food sensitization with nonrespiratory manifestations of food allergy may also enhance inflammation in other mucosal tissues. Hence, nonasthmatic patients diagnosed with food allergy should be carefully evaluated for bronchial inflammation in order not to delay appropriate antiinflammatory treatment if necessary.

Respiratory Symptoms Contributing to the Severity of Acute Allergic Reactions to Foods

While the specific cause of anaphylaxis is frequently undetermined, food allergens can be responsible for these severe reactions in a significant number of the cases.[28,66] Until two decades ago, fatal food-induced anaphylaxis had mainly consisted of anecdotal reports of isolated cases. In 1988, Yuninger and colleagues reported a series of seven cases identified over a 16-month period.[26] Five patients reacted to tree nuts or peanuts. Four years later, Sampson and colleagues reported 13 fatal and near fatal anaphylactic reactions in children and adolescents.[25] Again, most patients reacted to tree nuts or peanuts, and all patients had a history of asthma. Moreover, respiratory symptoms were prominent in all patients, and most probably contributed to the outcome of the reaction. More recently Bock and colleagues analyzed the circumstances of 32 fatal cases of food-induced anaphylaxis reported to a national registry.[67] Allergies to peanuts and tree nuts were responsible for most of the fatalities. In addition, all but one patient with adequate information were known to have asthma. These reports highlight an increased risk for severe food-induced anaphylaxis in patients with asthma, in particular those requiring maintenance medications. Follow-up visits in these patients should emphasize the importance of good asthma control, and should assure availability and proper instruction of the use of self-injectable epinephrine. Finally, a 5-year retrospective review from Australia summarized reports of children presenting with anaphylaxis to a local emergency department.[68] There were 123 cases of anaphylaxis in 117 patients; one fatality was reported. Foods were by far the most common trigger (86%) with peanuts and tree nuts leading the list. Respiratory symptoms were the principal presenting symptom (97%).

Patients with Recurrent or Chronic Asthma: Routine Testing for Food Allergy

Food allergy is often suspected in the quest for allergic triggers of recurrent or chronic asthma. A clear link between ingestion of a specific food and worsening of asthma is only rarely reported. In one investigation, 300 consecutive patients with asthma (age range: 7 months to 80 years) were evaluated in a pulmonary clinic.[8] Twenty-five (12%) patients had a history of food allergy suggested by clinical symptoms, and/or positive tests of food-specific IgE antibodies. Food-induced wheezing was documented in 6 (2%) of the cases; all were children aged 4 to 17 years. In another investigation, 140 children, aged 2 to 9 years, with asthma, were screened by clinical history, and testing for food-specific IgE antibodies.[69] Of these children, 32 patients were able to undergo blinded food challenges; 13 (9.2%) had food-induced respiratory symptoms and 8 (5.7%) had specific asthmatic reactions documented during food challenges. Only 1 patient had asthma as the sole symptom during a positive food challenge. Interestingly, the patients with food allergy and asthma were generally younger and had a past medical history of atopic dermatitis.

In a similar investigation, Oehling and co-workers reported that food-induced bronchospasm was present in 8.5% of 284 asthmatic children evaluated.[70] The majority of the allergic sensitizations occurred in the first year of life and was caused by a single food, especially egg. In addition, Businco and colleagues evaluated 42 children (age range: 10 to 76 months) with atopic dermatitis and milk allergy.[71] Eleven (27%) of these patients developed asthmatic symptoms during a positive food challenge. Finally, an investigation from Turkey confirmed that food allergy can elicit asthma in children less than 6 years of age; the incidence was 4%. The most common food allergens implicated were egg and cow's milk.[72]

In order to evaluate food allergy as a risk factor for severe asthma, Roberts and colleagues investigated 19 children with exacerbations of asthma requiring ICU ventilation.[73] When compared to controls, these patients had an increased risk of food allergy (odds ratio, 8.58; 95% CI, 1.85–39.71), multiple allergic diagnoses (4.42; 1.17–16.71) and frequent asthma admissions (14.2; 1.77–113.59). The authors concluded that food allergy and frequent asthma admissions appear to be significant, independent risk factors for life-threatening asthmatic events. As noted earlier, the association of increased asthma morbidity with at least one food sensitization and the increasing morbidity with sensitization to increasing numbers of foods, food allergen sensitivity may be a maker for increased asthma severity.[16] (Box 50-4)

Diagnosis and Management

Medical History

A comprehensive medical history should be obtained in patients suspected of having food allergy-induced respiratory tract symptoms or anaphylaxis.[1,30,74] The history should include questions about the timing of the reaction in relation to food ingestion, the

minimum quantity of food required to provoke symptoms, specific upper and lower respiratory signs and symptoms, the reproducibility of the symptoms and a current or past clinical history of allergy to specific food allergens (e.g. egg). A family history of allergy and/or asthma can be a useful historical point. When there is a history of an unexplained sudden asthma exacerbation, details about preceding food ingestion should be elicited. A history of a severe or anaphylactic reaction following the ingestion of a food may be sufficient to indicate a causal relationship. Finally, documentation of the specific treatment received and its response should be documented.

Physical Examination

In evaluating patients with respiratory complaints that may be induced by food allergy, the physical examination is helpful in assessing overall nutritional status, growth parameters and any signs of allergic disease, especially atopic dermatitis. Moreover, this examination will help rule out other conditions that may mimic food allergy.

Skin Testing for Food Allergy

When used in conjunction with the standard criteria of interpretation, prick skin testing can provide useful information on the sensitization status to suspected food allergens. However, the routine use of large batteries of skin tests for foods in patients presenting with asthma is not appropriate. Of children evaluated in a tertiary care hospital emergency room, 97 patients with asthma or bronchiolitis were skin tested for common foods and aeroallergens. These results were compared to similar testing in 60 control patients without any respiratory disease.[75] Most specific IgE antibody responses among wheezing children were to aeroallergens and the prevalence of specific IgE antibodies to food allergens was low.

Other Testing

Laboratory assessment of food allergy may include the measurement of food-specific IgE antibodies in the serum. When highly

BOX 50-5

Key Points Related to the Evaluation of Food Allergy and Respiratory Symptoms

- The medical history supplemented with appropriate laboratory testing and well-designed food challenges can provide useful information in the work-up of patients with respiratory symptoms that may be induced by food allergy; a diagnosis based solely on history or skin testing/allergen-specific IgE levels is not acceptable.

- If no specific foods are implicated in the history and if skin tests to foods are negative, further work-up for IgE-mediated allergy is not generally indicated.

- With positive skin tests and/or respiratory symptoms associated with specific foods, an elimination diet may be instituted for 7 to 14 days; if symptoms persist, food is not likely to be the problem, except in some cases of atopic dermatitis or chronic asthma.

- Symptoms recurring after a regular diet is resumed should be evaluated with a properly designed food challenge.

sensitive assays are used, the sensitivity and specificity are similar to that of skin tests.[76-78] In contrast, basophil histamine release assays, which are mainly limited to research settings, have not been shown conclusively to be a reproducible, diagnostic test for food allergy.[79]

Food Challenges

When there is a clinical suspicion of a food-induced respiratory tract reaction and the test for specific IgE antibody to the food is positive, an elimination diet may be implemented to see if there is a resolution of clinical symptoms. Food challenges can be very useful confirming this association in patients with food-induced respiratory symptoms. An excellent publication has reviewed the combined clinical experience of six centers doing food challenges.[80] The double-blind, placebo-controlled food challenge (DBPCFC) is the 'gold standard' and should be conducted in a clinic or hospital setting with available personnel and equipment for treating systemic anaphylaxis. If the clinical history does not suggest a high risk of a reaction, oral food challenges can be a practical alternative to DBPCFCs in confirming clinical tolerance to a food. A retrospective medical record review of open food challenges, administered in a university-based pediatric allergy-immunology clinic during a 3-year period, concluded that this type of procedure was safe in the office setting for patients selected based on history and food-specific IgE values.[81] (Box 50-5)

Treatment

Once a food allergy has been confirmed as a cause for respiratory tract symptoms, strict avoidance of the offending food is necessary.[1,21,79] A properly managed elimination diet can lead to resolution of clinical symptoms, such as chronic asthma. Appropriate nutritional counseling is important to ensure that an elimination diet is well-balanced, to provide appropriate substitutes for foods that are eliminated from the diet, and to avoid any anticipated nutritional deficiencies, such as calcium deficiency. Growth parameters should be closely monitored, especially in infants and children on elimination diets.

A written emergency plan should be provided to help patients manage their clinical symptoms caused by accidental ingestion of a relevant food allergen.[25,82] For children, the plan should be given to the appropriate school personnel. Self-injectable epinephrine and antihistamines must be immediately available to treat allergic reactions after accidental ingestions. Epinephrine is the drug of choice to treat acute, severe reactions and to allow time to seek immediate medical attention.

Conclusions

Previous investigations have clearly established the pathogenic role of food allergy in respiratory tract symptoms. These symptoms are typically accompanied by skin and gastrointestinal manifestations and rarely occur in isolation. Specific foods have been implicated in these reactions and a small subset of foods has been associated with severe anaphylactic reactions. Allergic sensitization to foods in infancy predicts the later development of respiratory allergies and asthma. The role of food allergy in otitis media is controversial and probably extremely rare. Likewise, asthmatic reactions to food additives can occur but are uncommon. Food-induced asthma is more common in young pediatric patients, especially those with atopic dermatitis, than in older children and adults, but may be triggered by inhalation of relevant food allergens at any age. Bronchoconstriction induced by food is considered a risk factor for fatal and near-fatal anaphylactic reactions.

Studies have demonstrated that foods can elicit airway hyperreactivity and asthmatic responses; therefore, evaluation for food allergy should be considered among patients with recalcitrant or otherwise unexplained acute severe asthma exacerbations, asthma triggered following ingestion or inhalation of particular foods, and in patients with asthma and other manifestations of food allergy (e.g. anaphylaxis, moderate to severe atopic dermatitis). Practice parameters for the diagnosis and treatment of asthma have recently highlighted the potential role of food allergy in asthma in some patients.[83,84]

References

1. Sicherer SH, Sampson HA. Food allergy. J Allergy Clin Immunology 2006;117:S470–475.
2. Lack G. Clinical practice. Food allergy. N Engl J Med 2008;359:1252–60.
3. Bahna SL. Clinical expressions of food allergy. Ann Allergy Asthma Immunol 2003;90(Suppl. 3):41–4.
4. James JM, Crespo JF. Allergic reactions to foods by inhalation. Curr Allergy Asthma Rep 2007;7:167–74.
5. Nowak-Wegrzyn A, Sampson HA. Adverse reactions to foods. Med Clin N Am 2006;90:97–127.
6. Bock SA. Prospective appraisal of complaints of adverse reactions to foods in children during the first 3 years of life. Pediatr 1987;79:683–8.
7. Jansen JJ, Kardinaal AFM, Huijbers G, et al. Prevalence of food allergy and intolerance in the adult Dutch population. J Allergy Clin Immunol 1994;93:446–56.
8. Onorato J, Merland N, Terral C, et al. Placebo-controlled double-blind food challenges in asthma. J Allergy Clin Immunol 1986;78:1139–46.
9. Nekam KL. Nutritional triggers in asthma. Acta Microbiol Immunol Hung 1998;45:113–7.
10. Woods RK, Thien F, Raven J, et al. Prevalence of food allergies in young adults and their relationship to asthma, nasal allergies and eczema. Ann Allergy Asthma Immunol 2002;88:183–9.
11. Kanny G, Moneret-Vautrin D-A, Flabbee J, et al. Population study of food allergy in France. J Allergy Clin Immunol 2001;108:133–40.
12. Woods RK, Abramson M, Raven JM, et al. Reported food intolerance and respiratory symptoms in young adults. Eur Respir J 1998;11:151–5.
13. Peroni DG, Chatzimichail A, Boner AL. Food allergy: what can be done to prevent progression to asthma? Ann Allergy Asthma Immunol 2002;89:44–51.

14. Tariq SM, Matthews SM, Hakim EA, et al. Egg allergy in infancy predicts respiratory allergic disease by 4 years of age. Pediatr Allergy Immunol 2000;11:162–7.

15. Rhodes HL, Sporik R, Thomas P, et al. Early life risk factors for adult asthma: a birth cohort study of subjects at risk. J Allergy Clin Immunol 2001;108:720–5.

16. Wang J, Visness CM, Sampson HA. Food allergen sensitization in inner-city children with asthma. J Allergy Clin Immunol 2005;115:1076–80.

17. Sicherer SH, Furlong TJ, Munoz-Furlong A, et al. A voluntary registry for peanut and tree nut allergy: characteristics of the first 5149 registrants. J Allergy Clin Immunol 2001;108:128–32.

18. Sicherer SH, Munoz-Furlong A, Sampson HA. Prevalence of seafood allergy in the United States determined by a random telephone survey. J Allergy Clin Immunol 2004;114:159–65.

19. Borghesan F, Mistrello G, Roncarolo D, et al. Respiratory allergy to lipid transfer proteins. Int Arch Allergy Immunol 2008;147:161–5.

20. Fernandez-Rivas C, Gonzalez-Mancebo E, de Durana DA. Allergies to fruits and vegetables. Pediatr Allergy Immunol 2008;19:675–81.

21. Bock SA, Atkins FM. Patterns of food hypersensitivity during sixteen years of double-blind placebo-controlled oral food challenges. J Pediatr 1990;117:561–7.

22. Burks AW, James JM, Hiegel A, et al. Atopic dermatitis and food hypersensitivity reactions. J Pediatr 1998;132:132–6.

23. Sampson HA, McCaskill CM. Food hypersensitivity and atopic dermatitis: evaluation of 113 patients. J Pediatr 1985;107:669–75.

24. Huang SW. Follow-up of children with rhinitis and cough associated with milk allergy. Pediatr Allergy Immunol 2007;18:81–5.

25. Sampson HA, Mendelson L, Rosen JP. Fatal and near-fatal food anaphylaxis reactions in children. N Engl J Med 1992;327:380–4.

26. Yunginger JY, Sweeney KG, Sturner WQ, et al. Fatal food-induced anaphylaxis. J Am Med Assoc 1988;260:1450–2.

27. James JM. Anaphylactic reactions to foods. Immunol Allergy Clin N Am 2001;21:653–67.

28. Wang J, Sampson HA. Food anaphylaxis. Clin Exp Allergy 2007;37: 651–60.

29. Gangur V, Kelly C, Navuluri L. Sesame allergy: a growing food allergy of global proportions? Ann Allergy Asthma Immunol 2005;95:4–11.

30. Sicherer SH. Is food allergy causing your patient's asthma symptoms? J Respir Dis 2000;21:127–36.

31. Keskin O, Sekerel BE. Poppy seed allergy: a case report and review of the literature. Allergy Asthma Proc 2006;27:396–8.

32. Palma-Carlos AG, Palma-Carlos ML, Tengarrinha F. Allergy to sunflower seeds. Eur Ann Allergy Clin Immunol 2005;37:183–6.

33. Crespo JF, Rodriguez J, Vives R, et al. Occupational IgE-mediated allergy after exposure to lupine seed flour. J Allergy Clin Immunol 2001;108: 295–7.

34. Moreno-Ancillo A, Gil-Adrados AC, Doninguez-Noche C, et al. Lupine inhalation induced asthma in a child. Pediatr Allergy Immunol 2005;16: 542–4.

35. Tabar AL, Alvarez-Puebla MJ, Gomez B, et al. Diversity of asparagus allergy: clinical and immunological features. Clin Exp Allergy 2004;34:131–6.

36. Rodrigo MJ, Cruz MJ, Garcia MD, et al. Epidemic asthma in Barcelona: an evaluation of new strategies for the control of soybean dust emission. Int Arch Allergy Immunol 2004;134:158–64.

37. Abramson M, Kutin J, Rosier M, et al. Morbidity, medication and trigger factors in a community sample of adults with asthma. Med J Aust 1995; 162:78–81.

38. Weber RW. Food additives and allergy. Ann Allergy 1993;70: 183–90.

39. Woods RK, Weiner JM, Thien F, et al. The effects of monosodium glutamate in adults with asthma who perceive themselves to be monosodium glutamate-intolerant. J Allergy Clin Immunol 1998;101:762–71.

40. Yang WH, Drouin MA, Herbert M, et al. The monosodium glutamate symptom complex: assessment in a double-blind, placebo-controlled, randomized study. J Allergy Clin Immunol 1997;99:757–62.

41. Goetz DW, Whisman BA. Occupational asthma in a seafood restaurant worker: cross-reactivity of shrimp and scallops. Ann Allergy Asthma Immunol 2000;85:461–6.

42. Crespo JF, Pascual C, Dominguez C, et al. Allergic reactions associated with airborne fish particles in IgE-mediated fish hypersensitive patients. Allergy 1995;50:257–61.

43. Pascual CY, Reche M, Flandor A, et al. Fish allergy in childhood. Pediatr Allergy Immunol 2008;19;573–9.

44. Taylor AV, Swanson MC, Jones RT, et al. Detection and quantification of raw fish aeroallergens from an open-air fish market. J Allergy Clin Immunol 2000;105:166–9.

45. Eigenmann PA, Zamora SA. An internet-based survey on the circumstances of food-induced reactions following the diagnosis of IgE-mediated food allergy. Allergy 2002;57:449–53.

46. Roberts G, Golder N, Lack G. Bronchial challenges with aerosolized food in asthmatic food-allergic children. Allergy 2002;57:713–7.

47. Sicherer SH, Furlong TJ, DeSimone J, et al. Self-reported allergic reactions to peanut on commercial airliners. J Allergy Clin Immunol 1999;104: 186–9.

48. James JM, Bernhisel-Broadbent J, Sampson HA. Respiratory reactions provoked by double-blind food challenges in children. Am J Respir Crit Care Med 1994;149:59–64.

49. Bernstein JM. The role of IgE-mediated hypersensitivity in the development of otitis media with effusion: a review. Otolaryngol Head Neck Surg 1993;109:611–20.

50. Nsouli TM, Nsouli SM, Linde RE, et al. Role of food allergy in serous otitis media. Ann Allergy 1994;73:215–9.

51. Heiner DC, Sears JW. Chronic respiratory disease associated with multiple circulation precipitins to cow's milk. Am J Dis Child 1960;100: 500–2.

52. Heiner DC, Sears JW, Kniker WT. Multiple precipitins to cow's milk in chronic respiratory disease: a syndrome including poor growth, gastrointestinal symptoms, evidence of allergy, iron deficiency anemia and pulmonary hemosiderosis. Am J Dis Child 1962;103:634–54.

53. Lowe AJ, Hosking CS, Bennett CM, et al. Skin prick test can identify eczematous infants at risk of asthma and allergic rhinitis. Clin Exp Allergy 2007;37:1624–31.

54. Tepper RS, Llapur CJ, Jones MH, et al. Expired nitric oxide and airway reactivity in infants at risk for asthma. J Allergy Clin Immunol 2008;122:760–5.

55. Priftis KN, Mermiri D, Papadopoulou A, et al. Asthma symptoms and bronchial reactivity in school children sensitized to food allergens in infancy. J Asthma 2008;45:590–5.

56. Hill DJ, Firer MA, Shelton MJ, et al. Manifestations of milk allergy in infancy: clinical and immunological findings. J Pediatr 1986;109:270–6.

57. Bock SA. Respiratory reactions induced by food challenges in children with pulmonary disease. Pediatr Allergy Immunol 1992;3:188–94.

58. Rance F, Dutau G. Asthma and food allergy: report of 163 cases. Arch Pediatr Suppl 2002;3:402–7.

59. Fiocchi A, Terracciano L, Bouygue GR, et al. Incremental prognostic factors associated with cow's milk allergy outcomes in infant and child referrals: the Milan Cow Milk Allergy Cohort study. Ann Allergy Asthma Immunol 2008;101:166–73.

60. James JM, Eigenmann PA, Eggleston PA, et al. Airway reactivity changes in asthmatic patients undergoing blinded food challenges. Am J Respir Crit Care Med 1996;153:597–603.

61. Zwetchkenbawn JF, Skufca R, Nelson HS. An examination of food hypersensitivity as a cause of increased bronchial responsiveness to inhaled methacholine. J Allergy Clin Immunol 1991;88:360–4.

62. Thaminy A, Lamblin C, Perez T, et al. Increased frequency of asymptomatic bronchial hyperresponsiveness in nonasthmatic patients with food allergy. Eur Respir J 2000;16:1091–4.

63. Kivity S, Fireman E, Sage K. Bronchial hyperactivity, sputum analysis and skin prick test to inhalant allergens in patients with symptomatic food hypersensitivity. Isr Med Assoc J 2005;7:781–4.

64. Wallaert B, Gosset P, Lamblin C, et al. Airway neutrophil inflammation in nonasthmatic patients with food allergy. Allergy 2002;57:405–10.

65. Brandt EB, Scribner TA, Akel HS, et al. Experimental gastrointestinal allergy enhances pulmonary reponses to specific and unrelated allergens. J Allergy Clin Immunol 2006;118:420–7.

66. Webb LM, Lieberman P. Anaphylaxis: a review of 601 cases. J Allergy Clin Immunology 2006;97:39–43.

67. Bock SA, Munoz-Furlong A, Sampson HA. Fatalities due to anaphylactic reactions to foods. J Allergy Clin Immunol 2001;107:191–3.

68. de Silva IL, Hehr SS, Tey D, et al. Paediatric anaphylaxis: a 5 year retrospective review. Allergy 2008;63:1071–6.

69. Novembre E, de Martino M, Vierucci A. Foods and respiratory allergy. J Allergy Clin Immunol 1988;81:1059–65.

70. Oehling A, Baena Cagnani CE. Food allergy and child asthma. Allergol Immunopathol 1980;8:7–14.

71. Businco L, Falconieri P, Giampietro P, et al. Food allergy and asthma. Pediatr Pulmonary Suppl 1995;11:59–60.

72. Yazicioglu M, Baspinar I, Ones U, et al. Egg and milk allergy in asthmatic children: assessment by immulite allergy panel, skin prick tests and double-blind placebo-controlled food challenges. Allergol Immunopathol 1999;27:287–93.

73. Roberts G, Patel N, Levi-Schaffer F, et al. Food allergy as a risk factor for life-threatening asthma in childhood: a case-controlled study. J Allergy Clin Immunol 2003;112:168–74.

74. Sicherer SH, Teuber S. Current approach to the diagnosis and management of adverse reactions to foods. J Allergy Clin Immunol 2004;114: 1146–50.

75. Price GW, Hogan AD, Farris AH, et al. Sensitization (IgE antibody) to food allergens in wheezing infants and children. J Allergy Clin Immunol 1995;96:266–70.

76. Sampson HA, Ho DG. Relationship between food-specific IgE concentrations and the risk of positive food challenges in children and adolescents. J Allergy Clin Immunol 1997;100:444–51.

Food Allergy, Respiratory Disease, and Anaphylaxis

77. Sampson HA. Utility of food specific IgE concentrations in predicting symptomatic food allergy. J Allergy Clin Immunol 2001;107:891-6.

78. Wraith DG, Merret J, Roth A, et al. Recognition of food-allergic patients and their allergens by the RAST technique and clinical investigation. Clin Allergy 1979;9:25-36.

79. James JM, Sampson HA. An overview of food hypersensitivity. Ped Allergy Immunol 1992;3:67-78.

80. Bock SA, Sampson HA, Atkins FM, et al. Double-blind placebo-controlled food challenge (DBPCFC) as an office procedure: A manual. J Allergy Clin Immunol 1988;82:986-97.

81. Mankad VS, Williams LW, Lee LA, et al. Safety of open food challenges in the office setting. Ann Allergy Asthma Immunol 2008;100: 469-74.

82. Hallett R, Teuber SS. Food allergies and sensitivities. Nutr Clin Care 2004;7:122-9.

83. Chapman JA, Bernstein IL, Lee RE, et al. Food allergy: a practice parameter. Ann Allergy Asthma Immuonol 2006;96:S1-S68.

84. Practice Parameters for the Diagnosis and Treatment of Asthma. Spector SL, Nicklas RA, editors. J Allergy Clin Immunol (supplement) 1996;96: 707-869.

CHAPTER

51

Atopic Dermatitis and Food Hypersensitivity

Stacie M. Jones • Wesley Burks

Atopic dermatitis (AD) is a complex, chronic disorder that has been referred to as 'the itch that rashes'. The origin of AD is multifactorial, including many commonly encountered triggers. In 1892 Besnier[1] used the term *neurodermatitis* to describe a chronic, pruritic skin condition seen in patients with a nervous disorder. In the early 1900s, Coca and Cooke[2] noted the occurrence of a similar disorder with asthma and hay fever, and used the term *atopy* to refer to the allergic constellation of these diseases. The term *atopic dermatitis* was then coined by Wise and Sulzberger[3] in 1933 to comprehensively describe this inheritable skin disorder. Since its earliest description, AD has had one primary feature: intense pruritus triggered by a variety of stimuli. In this chapter, we explore how the ingestion of specific foods can trigger the condition of AD.

A strong correlation exists with AD and other atopic conditions and is often the first manifestiation of the atopic march. Approximately 50% of patients with AD will develop it in the first year of life, and as many as 50% to 80% of children with AD will develop allergic respiratory disease later in life.[4] Because of these early historical observations, investigators have explored the role of various allergens as triggers for the pathogenesis of AD (Box 51-1).

Food allergy has been strongly correlated with the development and persistence of AD, especially during infancy and early childhood. The skin is the site that is most often involved in food hypersensitivity reactions. For most skin manifestations of food hypersensitivity, pruritus is a hallmark of the disease.

Pathophysiology

In the early 20th century, Schloss,[5] Talbot,[6] and Blackfan[7] published case reports of patients who had improvement in their AD after avoiding specific foods from their diets. Subsequent conflicting reports spurred controversy related to the role of specific food allergens in the pathogenesis of AD.[8] This controversy has continued into the 21st century, although there now is significant laboratory and clinical evidence that would suggest the debate is no longer valid. Factors important in the pathophysiology of AD include barrier function, innate and adaptive immune responses and genetics, all of which have some relationship to allergen exposure.[9,10] Studies have demonstrated that allergen-induced, IgE-mediated mast cell activation has, as its end product, hypersensitivity reactions characterized by tissue (i.e. skin) infiltration of eosinophils, monocytes and lymphocytes.[9–11] The pattern of cytokine and chemokine expression found in lymphocytes infiltrating acute AD lesions are predominantly those of the T helper cell type 2 (Th2) (interleukin [IL]-4, IL-5, and IL-13).[12,13] In addition, these cytokines promote influx of activated eosinophils and release of eosinophil products.[12–15] Epidermal, myeloid-derived dendritic cells express high-affinity IgE receptors (FcεRI) that bind IgE and are noted in biopsy tissue from inflamed AD skin. These cells take up and present allergens to Th1, Th2 and T regulatory cells, all of which are important in AD.[9] In addition, IgE-bearing Langerhans cells that are up-regulated by cytokines are highly efficient at presenting allergens to T cells, activating a combined Th1/Th2 profile in chronic lesions. Thus it appears that IgE antibody and the Th2 cytokine/chemokine milieu combine to play a major role in AD.

Several articles have speculated on the role of food-specific T cells in the pathophysiology of AD and have used the atopic patch test (APT) to provide further information.[16–20] In some patients who may have a delayed response to foods, authors hypothesize that the reactions may occur via high-affinity IgE receptors expressed on Langerhans and dendritic cells leading to allergen-specific T cell responses capable of promoting IgE production and delayed-type hypersensitivity reactions.

Genetic mutations resulting in clinical disease have provided additional insight into the potential relationship of AD and food allergy. Two disorders provide particularly compelling information. IPEX (immune dysreulation, polyendocrinopathy, enteropathy, X-linked) is a fatal disorder characterized by autoimmune enteropathy, endocrinopathy, severe dermatitis, elevated serum IgE and multiple food allergies.[21] IPEX syndrome results from a mutation in FOXP3, a protein that plays a central role in the generation of regulatory Tcells that are important for balance between oral tolerance and food allergy development. Similarly, mutations in the SPINK5 gene have been associated with Netherton syndrome, an autosomal recessive disorder characterized by an AD-like rash and associated Th2-skewing and increased IgE levels. Japanese investigators have recently found an association of SPINK5 mutations in children with AD and food allergy.[22]

Laboratory Investigation

Several studies support a role for food-specific IgE antibodies in the pathogenesis of AD. Many patients have elevated concentrations of total IgE and food-specific IgE antibodies.[23,24] More than 50 years ago, Wilson and Walzer[25,26] demonstrated that the ingestion of foods would allow antigens to penetrate the gastrointestinal barrier and then be transported in the circulation to IgE-bearing mast cells in the skin. More recent investigations have shown that, in children with food-specific IgE antibodies

DOI: 10.1016/B978-1-4377-0271-2.00051-1

BOX 51-1

Allergic Triggers of Atopic Dermatitis

Food Allergens (Most Common)

Milk

Eggs

Peanuts

Soy

Wheat

Shellfish

Fish

Aeroallergens

Pollen

Mold

Dust mite

Animal dander

Cockroach

Microorganisms

Bacteria

Staphylococcus aureus

Streptococcus species

Fungi/yeasts

Pityrosporum ovale/orbiculare

Trichophytan species

Other yeast species (e.g., *Candida, Malazassia*)

BOX 51-2

Laboratory Investigation of Atopic Dermatitis and Food Hypersensitivity

Positive food challenges produce increases in:

Plasma histamine concentrations

Activation of plasma eosinophils and eosinophil products

Patients ingesting foods to which they are allergic have:

Increased spontaneous basophil histamine release

Histamine-releasing factors that activate basophils from food-sensitive patients

Patients with milk allergy have:

Higher expression of milk-specific activated cutaneous lymphocyte antigen

Patients with milk and peanut allergy (or food allergy?) have:

Differential patterns of expression of IgE binding epitopes that add insight into prognosis

---

undergoing oral food challenges, positive challenges are accompanied by increases in plasma histamine concentration,[27] elaboration of eosinophil products,[28] and activation of plasma eosinophils[29] (Box 51-2).

Children with AD who were chronically ingesting foods to which they were allergic were found to have increased 'spontaneous' basophil histamine release (SBHR) from peripheral blood basophils in vitro compared with children without food allergy or normal subjects.[30] After placement on the appropriate elimination diet, food-allergic children experienced significant clearing of their skin and a significant fall in their SBHR.[30] Other studies have shown that peripheral blood mononuclear cells from food-

allergic patients with high SBHR elaborate specific cytokines termed histamine-releasing factors (HRFs) that activate basophils from food-sensitive, but not food-insensitive, patients. Furthermore, passive sensitization experiments in vitro with basophils from nonatopic donors and IgE from patients allergic to specific foods showed that basophils could be rendered sensitive to HRFs.[30]

Food allergen-specific T cells have been cloned from normal skin and active skin lesions in patients with AD.[31,32] There has been some disagreement in the literature about the validity of in vitro lymphocyte-proliferation responses to specific foods in this disorder. There appears to be an increase in antigen-specific lymphocyte proliferation, but there is considerable overlap in individual responses. Cutaneous lymphocyte-associated antigen (CLA) is a homing molecule that interacts with E-selectin and directs T cells to the skin. A study compared patients with milk-induced AD to control subjects with milk-induced gastrointestinal reactions without AD and with nonatopic control subjects.[31] Casein-reactive T cells from children with milk-induced AD had a significantly higher expression of CLA than *Candida albicans*-reactive T cells from the same patients and either casein or *C. albicans*-reactive T cells from the control groups.[31]

An alternative and emerging paradigm has been championed by several investigators: that sensitization to food allergens can occur via cutaneous exposure to antigen due to poor barrier function in AD skin.[9,33] Lack and colleagues have confirmed peanut allergy in preschool children with AD and increased exposure to peanut-based skin oils.[34] These observations, along with mouse studies demonstrating that epidermal application of ovalbumin results in development of eczematous lesions and ovalubumin-specific IgE production,[35] have lead Lack to hypothesize that environmental exposure to allergens through infants' skin with AD is responsible for allergen sensitivity and allergic disease.[33]

Clinical Studies

Multiple clinical studies have addressed the role of food allergy in AD. Investigators have shown that elimination of the relevant food allergen can lead to improvement in skin symptoms and that repeat challenges can lead to recurrence of symptoms. Several longitudinal studies in high-risk infants have now shown that AD may be delayed or prevented by exclusive breast-feeding, introduction of hydrolyzed infant formulas or prophylactically eliminating highly allergenic foods (e.g. milk, eggs) from the diets of genetically at-risk infants.[36-38]

A number of studies have addressed the therapeutic effect of dietary elimination in the treatment of AD. Atherton and colleagues[39] reported that two thirds of children with AD between the ages of 2 and 8 years showed marked improvement during a double-blind, crossover trial of milk and egg exclusion. However, there were problems in this study, including high dropout and exclusion rates, as well as confounding variables such as environmental factors and other triggers of AD. Another trial by Neild and colleagues[40] was able to demonstrate improvement in some patients during the milk and egg exclusion phase, but no significant difference was seen in 40 patients completing the crossover trial. Another study by Juto and colleagues[41] reported that approximately one third of AD patients had resolution of their rash and that one half improved on a highly restricted diet. The cumulative results of these studies support the role for food allergy in the exacerbation of AD. Certainly, most of the trials failed to control for confounding factors such as other trigger factors, as well as the placebo effect or observer bias.

In one of the original prospective follow-up studies, Sampson and Scanlon[42] studied 34 patients with AD, of whom 17 had food allergy diagnosed by double-blind, placebo-controlled food challenges (DBPCFCs). These patients were placed on appropriate allergen elimination and experienced significant improvement in their clinical symptoms. At 1- to 2-year and 3- to 4-year follow-ups, the subjects were compared with control subjects who did not have food allergy and to children with food allergy who were not compliant with their diet. Food-allergic patients with appropriate dietary restriction demonstrated highly significant improvement in their AD compared with the control groups, and their time frame for outgrowing their food sensitivity was reduced.

Lever and colleagues[43] performed a randomized controlled trial of egg elimination in young children with AD and a positive radioallergosorbent test (RAST) to eggs who presented to their dermatology clinic. At the end of this study, egg allergy was confirmed by oral challenge, and 55 children who were allergic to egg were ultimately identified. There was a significant decrease in the skin area affected, as well as symptom scores in the children avoiding eggs compared with the control subjects (percent involvement, 21.9% to 18.9%; symptom score, 36.7 to 33.5).

Oral food challenges have been used to demonstrate that food allergens can induce symptoms of rash and pruritus in children with food allergy-related AD. Sampson and colleagues,[42,44,45] and Eigenmann and colleagues[46] published a number of articles using DBPCFCs to identify causal food proteins that are involved as trigger factors of AD. In studies during the past 25 years, Sampson and colleagues have conducted more than 4000 oral food challenges with greater than 40% of the challenges resulting in reaction (personal communication). In all of these studies, as well as others to follow, they show that cutaneous reactions occurred in 75% of the positive challenges, generally consisting of pruritic, morbiliform, or macular eruptions in the predilection sites for AD. Isolated skin symptoms were seen in only 30% of the reactions; gastrointestinal (50%) and respiratory (45%) reactions also occurred. Almost all reactions occurred within the first hour of beginning the oral challenges. Clinical reactions to egg, milk, wheat, and soy accounted for almost 75% of the reactions. Some patients had repeated reactions during a series of daily challenges and had increasingly severe AD, further showing that ingestion of the causal food protein can trigger pruritus and scratching with recrudescence of typical lesions of AD.

Subsequent studies confirmed that a limited number of foods cause clinical symptoms in younger patients with AD.[47,48] Milk, eggs, and peanuts generally cause more than 75% of the IgE-mediated reactions. If soy, wheat, fish, and tree nuts are added to this list of foods, more than 98% of the foods that cause clinical symptoms would be identified.

Longitudinal studies have been conducted in general population birth cohorts and cohorts of high-risk infants to determine the role of breast-feeding, maternal diet restriction during pregnancy and lactation, the use of hydrolyzed formulas and delayed food introduction on development of AD and other atopic diseases. These studies have led to new recommendations for early nutritional interventions by the American Academy of Pediatrics in 2008.[49] A recent meta-analysis determined that exclusive breast-feeding during the first 3 months of life is associated with lower incidence rates of AD during childhood in children with a family history of atopy.[50] The authors concluded that breast-feeding should be strongly recommended to mothers of infants with a family history of atopy as a possible means of preventing AD. In two series, infants from atopic families whose mothers excluded eggs, milk, and fish from their diets during lactation (prophylaxis group) had significantly less AD and food allergy compared at 18 months with those infants whose mothers' diets were unrestricted.[51,52] Follow-up at 4 years showed that the prophylaxis group had less AD, but there was no difference in food allergy or respiratory allergy.[52] In a comprehensive, prospective, randomized allergy prevention trial, Zeiger and colleagues[38,53] compared the benefits of maternal and infant food allergen avoidance on the prevention of allergic disease in infants at high risk for allergic disease during a 7-year study period. Breast-feeding was encouraged in both the prophylaxis and control groups. In the prophylaxis group, eggs, cow's milk, and peanuts were restricted from the diets of lactating mothers; a casein hydrolysate formula was used for supplementation or weaning, and solid food introduction was delayed. The control infants received cow's milk formula for supplementation and the American Academy of Pediatrics' recommendations for infant feeding were followed (peanuts, nuts, and fish are not recommended in the first 3 years). The results showed that the prevalence of AD and food allergy in the prophylaxis group was reduced significantly in the first 2 years compared with the control group; however, the period prevalence of AD was no longer significant beyond 2 years. These studies also failed to show that treatment of at-risk infants could modify allergic disease after 2 years of age. In the German Infant Nutritional Intervention Study (GINI),[36] 2252 healthy term infants were randomized to received one of four blinded formulas during the first 4 months of life when breast-feeding was insufficient: partially (PHW) or extensively hydrolyzed whey (EHW), extensively hydrolyzed casein (EHC) or cow's milk (CM). These infants were followed for 6 years for allergic manifestations. The study showed a long-term preventive effect of hydrolyzed infant formulas for AD until age 6 years with the relative risk of a physician diagnosis of AD compared with CM of 0.79 (95% CI, 0.64–0.97) for PHW; 0.92 (95% CI, 0.76–1.11) for EHW; and 0.71 (95% CI, 0.58–0.88) for EHC. Similar findings were noted in a high-risk birth cohort of 120 infants from the Isle of Wight followed for 8 years.[37] In the prophylactic group, infants were either breast-fed with the mother on a low allergen diet or given extensively hydrolyzed formula and placed on an allergen eliminatin diet (egg, milk, soy, wheat, nuts, fish) and dust mite avoidance through age 12 months, and compared to control infants in routine care. Those in the intervention group were noted to have reduced asthma (OR 0.24), AD (OR 0.23), allergic rhinitis (OR 0.42) and atopy (OR 0.13) compared to the controls (p < 0.001). Conversely, several studies in prospective birth cohorts have shown no benefit in delayed dietary introduction of solid foods past 4 months of life on the development of AD and even note that delayed introduction may be associated with highter risk of AD.[54-56]

Recent studies have speculated on the possibility of delayed reactions to food playing a part in exacerbations of AD in certain patients,[16-18,57,58] suggesting that a positive atopy patch test (APT) with T cell infiltration of the skin correlates with clinical late-phase reactions and is associated with T cell-mediated, allergen-specific immune responses.[16] More studies are needed to validate this possibility.

Epidemiology of Food Allergy in Atopic Dermatitis

The prevalence of food allergy in patients with AD varies with the age of the patient and severity of AD. In a study of 2184 Australian infants, investigators found that the earlier the age of onset of AD and the greater the severity of disease, the greater the frequency of associated high levels of food-specific IgE.[59]

Lowe and colleagues also noted that in some infants, sensitization precedes and predicts the development of AD, while in others, AD precedes and predicts the development of sensitization.[60] In a study of children with AD, Burks and colleagues[47,48] diagnosed food allergy in approximately 35% of 165 patients with AD referred to both university allergy and university dermatology clinics. Since many of the patients were referred to an allergist, which might lead to an ascertainment bias favoring food allergic subjects, Eigenmann and colleagues[46] addressed this potential bias by studying 63 unselected children with moderate to severe AD who were referred to a university dermatologist. After an evaluation including oral food challenges, 37% of these patients were diagnosed with food allergy. In another study[61] that evaluated more than 250 children with AD, investigators noted that increased severity of AD in the younger patients was directly correlated with the presence of food allergy. Additional studies in adults with severe AD are relatively limited and have not shown a significant role for food allergy[62] or success in reducing symptoms during trials of elimination diets.[63]

Diagnosis

General Approach

The diagnosis of food allergy in AD is complicated by several factors related to the disease: (1) the immediate response to ingestion of causal foods is down-regulated with repetitive ingestion, making obvious 'cause-and-effect' relations by history difficult to establish; (2) other environmental trigger factors (other allergens, irritants, infection) may play a role in the waxing and waning of the disease, obscuring the effect of dietary changes; and (3) patients have the ability to generate IgE to multiple allergens, many not associated with clinical symptoms, making diagnosis based solely on laboratory testing impossible (Box 51-3).

As outlined in Chapter 45, a careful medical history is essential in the diagnostic work-up (Figure 51-1). For breast-fed infants, a maternal dietary history is also helpful because of the passage of food proteins in breast milk. Selected foods are then evaluated by tests for specific IgE (e.g. prick skin test [PST], food-specific IgE tests), as reviewed in Chapter 45. A small number of foods account for more than 90% of reactions[44,48,64] (Table 51.1). Food additives have been documented to cause flaring of AD but with a much lower prevalence.[65-67]

Patients with AD will often have positive skin tests and/or food-specific IgE tests for several members of a botanical family (e.g. wheat and grass) or animal species (e.g. egg and chicken), more likely indicating immunologic cross-reactivity but not symptomatic intrabotanical or intraspecies cross-reactivity. Therefore, the practice of avoiding all foods within a botanical

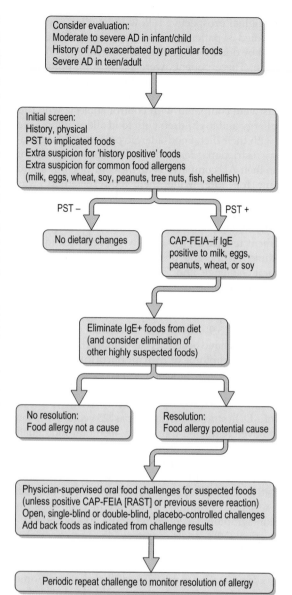

FIGURE 51-1 General approach to evaluation of food allergy in atopic dermatitis (AD). *PST*, Prick skin test. (From Sicherer SH, Sampson HA. J Allergy Clin Immunol 1999;104:S114–S122.)

BOX 51-3

Factors Related to Atopic Dermatitis that Complicate the Diagnosis of Food allergy

- Immediate response to ingestion of causal foods is apparently down-regulated with repetitive ingestion, making obvious 'cause-and-effect' relations by history difficult to establish.

- Other environmental trigger factors (other allergens, irritants, infection) may play a role in the waxing and waning of the disease, obscuring the effect of dietary changes.

- Patients have the ability to generate IgE to multiple allergens, making diagnosis based solely on laboratory testing impossible.

Table 51-1 Foods Responsible for the Majority of Food-Allergic Reactions

Infants	Children	Older Children/ Adults
Cow's milk	Cow's milk	Peanuts
Eggs	Eggs	Tree nuts
Peanuts	Peanuts	Fish
Soy	Soy	Shellfish
	Wheat	
	Tree nuts (walnut, cashew, etc.)	
	Fish	
	Shellfish	

From Sicherer SH, Sampson HA. J Allergy Clin Immunol 1999;104:S114–S122.

Table 51-2 Performance Characteristics of 90% Specificity Diagnostic Decision Points Generated in the Prospective Study in Diagnosing Food Allergy in 100 Consecutive Children and Adolescents Referred for Evaluation of Food Hypersensitivity

Allergen	Decision Point (kU/L)	Sensitivity (%)	Specificity (%)	Efficiency (%)	PPV (%)	NPV (%)
Eggs	7	61	95	68	98	38
Milk	15	57	94	69	95	53
Peanuts	14	57	100	84	100	36
Fish	3	63	91	87	56	93
Soybean	30	44	94	81	73	82
Wheat	26	61	92	84	74	87

From Sampson HA. J Allergy Clin Immunol 2001;107:891–896. *PPV*, positive predictive value; *NPV*, negative predictive value.
Given are PPV and NPV of food-specific IgE concentrations for predicting reactions on oral challenge by using the Pharmacia CAP-RAST System FEIA.
As seen in Table 51-1, the PPVs for eggs, milk, and peanuts on the basis of the 90% specificity values are excellent (i.e. 98–100%) but are less predictive for fish, wheat, and soy (i.e. 56%, 73%, and 74%, respectively).

BOX 51-4

Natural History of Food Hypersensitivity

Food Allergy Often Outgrown by Adolescence

Milk

Eggs

Soy

Wheat

Food Allergy Often not Outgrown by Adolescence

Peanuts

Tree nuts

Fish

Shellfish

---

family when one member is suspected of provoking allergic symptoms generally appears to be unwarranted.

After the laboratory studies are performed, the best initial treatment would be elimination of the suspected food from the diet, followed by a food challenge if indicated (Table 51-2). No further testing or food challenges may be necessary in cases of severe, acute reactions or if dramatic improvement in skin disease occurs. Because symptoms are chronic in AD and often a large number of foods are implicated, it is generally necessary to perform diagnostic oral food challenges.

Oral Food Challenges

As outlined in Chapter 45, oral food challenges are invaluable in the appropriate diagnosis and management of patients with AD and possible food allergy. Oral challenges are also necessary to evaluate the resolution (or development of tolerance) of the specific food allergy and can be performed safely.[68,69] However, oral challenges are contraindicated when there is a clear, recent history of food-induced airway reactivity or anaphylaxis. Additionally, patients should not be instructed to perform home food challenges because of the potential risk of severe allergic reactions.[70]

Management

The elimination of food proteins can often be a difficult task, and incomplete elimination of the offending food can lead to confu-

sion and inconclusive results during an open trial of dietary elimination. For example, in a milk-free diet, patients must be instructed, not only to avoid all milk products, but also to read all food labels to identify 'hidden' sources of cow's milk protein, as reviewed in Chapter 52.

Natural History

Most children outgrow their allergies to milk, eggs, wheat, and soy[71] (Box 51-4); although, recent studies have shown that the rate of resolution of some food allergens (e.g. egg and milk) may be slower than previously described. In one study of the natural history of egg allergy in children followed in a pediatric allergy practice, investigators found the age distribution of resolution of allergy of 4% by age 4 years, 12% by age 6 years, 37% by age 10 years, and 68% by age 16 years.[72] The egg-specific IgE level was predictive of allergy outcome and can be used with skin testing to counsel patients on prognosis.[73] Perry also showed that food-specific IgE levels are helpful in determining the likelihood that a child has outgrown their food allergy.[74] Patients allergic to peanuts, tree nuts, fish, and shellfish are much less likely to lose their clinical reactivity.[75,76] It does appear, however, that approximately 20% of patients who have a reaction to peanuts early in life may outgrow their sensitivity.[76] Only approximately 9% of patients with tree nut allergy will outgrow their allergy.[77] In one study, approximately one third of children with AD and food allergy lost or outgrew their clinical reactivity over 1 to 3 years with strict adherence to dietary elimination, which was believed to have aided in a more timely recovery.[42] Clinical reactivity is lost over time more quickly than the loss of food-specific IgE measured by PST or serum food-specific IgE testing.[74] Certainly, children with food allergy need to be followed at regular intervals with food-specific IgE testing and PST, followed by oral food challenge when indicated, to determine when clinical tolerance is achieved.

Conclusions

The triggers associated with disease pathogenesis and clinical symptoms for patients with AD are vast (Box 51-5). The role of allergens as a trigger factor, particularly food allergens, early in life is clearly very important. A careful history and appropriate diagnostic testing coupled with a comprehensive treatment program can be disease modifying and life altering for patients with AD.

Atopic Dermatitis and Food Hypersensitivity

Food Allergy Pearls

- About one third of children with moderate to severe atopic dermatitis (AD) are affected by food hypersensitivity.

- The younger the child and the more severe the eczema, the more likely the child is affected by food hypersensitivity.

- Egg allergy is the most common food hypersensitivity in children with AD; egg, milk, and peanut allergy account for about 80% of food allergy diagnosed by food challenge in children with AD.

- Appropriate diagnosis of food allergy and elimination of the responsible food allergen lead to significant clearing of the eczematous lesions in the majority of children with AD and food allergy.

- Infants with AD and egg allergy are at high risk for developing respiratory allergy and asthma.

Helpful Website

The Food Allergy and Anaphylaxis Network website (www. foodallergy.org)

References

1. Besnier E. Premiere note et observations preliminaires pour sevir d'introductions a l'etude des prurigos diathesiques. Ann de Dermatol 1892;23:634.
2. Coca A, Cooke R. On the classification of the phenomena of hypersensitiveness. J Immunol 1923;18:163-82.
3. Wise F, Sulzberger M. Eczematous eruptions. In: Year Book of Dermatology and Syphilology. Chicago: Year Book Medical; 1933.
4. Illi S, von Mutius E, Lau S, et al. The natural course of atopic dermatitis from birth to age 7 years and the association with asthma. J Allergy Clin Immunol 2004;113:925-31.
5. Schloss O. Allergy to common foods. Trans Am Pediatr Soc 1915;27: 62-8.
6. Talbot F. Eczema in childhood. Med Clin North Am 1918;985-96.
7. Blackfan K. A consideration of certain aspects of protein hypersensitiveness in children. Am J Med Sci 1920;160:341-50.
8. Hanifin JM. Critical evaluation of food and mite allergy in the management of atopic dermatitis. J Dermatol 1997;24:495-503.
9. Bieber T. Atopic dermatitis. N Engl J Med 2008;358:1483-94.
10. Leung DY, Boguniewicz M, Howell MD, et al. New insights into atopic dermatitis. J Clin Invest 2004;113:651-7.
11. Solley GO, Gleich GJ, Jordon RE, et al. The late phase of the immediate wheal and flare skin reaction: its dependence upon IgE antibodies. J Clin Invest 1976;58:408-20.
12. Hamid Q, Boguniewicz M, Leung DY. Differential in situ cytokine gene expression in acute versus chronic atopic dermatitis. J Clin Invest 1994;94:870-6.
13. Hamid Q, Naseer T, Minshall EM, et al. In vivo expression of IL-12 and IL-13 in atopic dermatitis. J Allergy Clin Immunol 1996;98: 225-31.
14. Tsicopoulos A, Hamid Q, Varney V, et al. Preferential messenger RNA expression of Th1-type cells (IFN-gamma+, IL-2+) in classical delayed-type (tuberculin) hypersensitivity reactions in human skin. J Immunol 1992;148:2058-61.
15. Leiferman KM, Ackerman SJ, Sampson HA, et al. Dermal deposition of eosinophil-granule major basic protein in atopic dermatitis: comparison with onchocerciasis. N Engl J Med 1985;313:282-5.
16. Niggemann B, Reibel S, Wahn U. The atopy patch test (APT): a useful tool for the diagnosis of food allergy in children with atopic dermatitis. Allergy 2000;55:281-5.
17. Niggemann B, Reibel S, Roehr CC, et al. Predictors of positive food challenge outcome in non-IgE-mediated reactions to food in children with atopic dermatitis. J Allergy Clin Immunol 2001;108:1053-8.
18. Kekki OM, Turjanmaa K, Isolauri E. Differences in skin-prick and patch-test reactivity are related to the heterogeneity of atopic eczema in infants. Allergy 1997;52:755-9.
19. Mehl A, Rolinck-Werninghaus C, Staden U, et al. The atopy patch test in the diagnostic workup of suspected food-related symptoms in children. J Allergy Clin Immunol 2006;118:923-9.
20. Devillers AC, de Waard-van der Spek FB, Mulder PG, et al. Delayed- and immediate-type reactions in the atopy patch test with food allergens in young children with atopic dermatitis. Pediatr Allergy Immunol 2009;20:53-8.
21. Torgerson TR, Linane A, Moes N, et al. Severe food allergy as a variant of IPEX syndrome caused by a deletion in a noncoding region of the FOXP3 gene. Gastroenterology 2007;132:1705-17.
22. Kusunoki T, Okafuji I, Yoshioka T, et al. SPINK5 polymorphism is associated with disease severity and food allergy in children with atopic dermatitis. J Allergy Clin Immunol 2005;115:636-8.
23. Johnson EE, Irons JS, Patterson R, et al. Serum IgE concentration in atopic dermatitis: relationship to severity of disease and presence of atopic respiratory disease. J Allergy Clin Immunol 1974;54:94-9.
24. Boguniewicz M, Schmid-Grendelmeier P, Leung DY. Atopic dermatitis. J Allergy Clin Immunol 2006;118:40-3.
25. Walzer M. Studies in absorption of undigested proteins in human beings. I. A simple direct method of studying the absorption of undigested protein. J Immunol 1927;14:143-74.
26. Wilson S, Walzer M. Absorption of undigested proteins in human beings. IV. Absorption of unaltered egg protein in infants. Am J Dis Child 1935;50:49-54.
27. Sampson HA, Jolie PL. Increased plasma histamine concentrations after food challenges in children with atopic dermatitis. N Engl J Med 1984;311:372-6.
28. Suomalainen H, Soppi E, Isolauri E. Evidence for eosinophil activation in cow's milk allergy. Pediatr Allergy Immunol 1994;5:27-31.
29. Magnarin M, Knowles A, Ventura A, et al. A role for eosinophils in the pathogenesis of skin lesions in patients with food-sensitive atopic dermatitis. J Allergy Clin Immunol 1995;96:200-8.
30. Sampson HA, Broadbent KR, Bernhisel-Broadbent J. Spontaneous release of histamine from basophils and histamine-releasing factor in patients with atopic dermatitis and food hypersensitivity. N Engl J Med 1989;321:228-32.
31. Abernathy-Carver KJ, Sampson HA, Picker LJ, et al. Milk-induced eczema is associated with the expansion of T cells expressing cutaneous lymphocyte antigen. J Clin Invest 1995;95:913-8.
32. van Reijsen FC, Bruijnzeel-Koomen CA, Kalthoff FS, et al. Skin-derived aeroallergen-specific T cell clones of Th2 phenotype in patients with atopic dermatitis. J Allergy Clin Immunol 1992;90:184-93.
33. Lack G. Epidemiologic risks for food allergy. J Allergy Clin Immunol 2008;121:1331-6.
34. Lack G, Fox D, Northstone K, et al. Factors associated with the development of peanut allergy in childhood. N Engl J Med 2003;348:977-85.
35. Spergel JM, Mizoguchi E, Brewer JP, et al. Epicutaneous sensitization with protein antigen induces localized allergic dermatitis and hyperresponsiveness to methacholine after single exposure to aerosolized antigen in mice. J Clin Invest 1998;101:1614-22.
36. von Berg A, Filipiak-Pittroff B, Kramer U, et al. Preventive effect of hydrolyzed infant formulas persists until age 6 years: long-term results from the German Infant Nutritional Intervention Study (GINI). J Allergy Clin Immunol 2008;121:1442-7.
37. Arshad SH, Bateman B, Sadeghnejad A, et al. Prevention of allergic disease during childhood by allergen avoidance: the Isle of Wight prevention study. J Allergy Clin Immunol 2007;119:307-13.
38. Zeiger RS, Heller S. The development and prediction of atopy in high-risk children: follow-up at age seven years in a prospective randomized study of combined maternal and infant food allergen avoidance. J Allergy Clin Immunol 1995;95:1179-90.
39. Atherton DJ, Sewell M, Soothill JF, et al. A double-blind controlled crossover trial of an antigen-avoidance diet in atopic eczema. Lancet 1978;1: 401-3.
40. Neild VS, Marsden RA, Bailes JA, et al. Egg and milk exclusion diets in atopic eczema. Br J Dermatol 1986;114:117-23.
41. Juto P, Engberg S, Winberg J. Treatment of infantile atopic dermatitis with a strict elimination diet. Clin Allergy 1978;8:493-500.
42. Sampson HA, Scanlon SM. Natural history of food hypersensitivity in children with atopic dermatitis. J Pediatr 1989;115:23-7.
43. Lever R, MacDonald C, Waugh P, et al. Randomised controlled trial of advice on an egg exclusion diet in young children with atopic eczema and sensitivity to eggs. Pediatr Allergy Immunol 1998;9:13-9.
44. Sampson HA, McCaskill CC. Food hypersensitivity and atopic dermatitis: evaluation of 113 patients. J Pediatr 1985;107:669-75.
45. Sampson HA, Metcalfe DD. Food allergies. JAMA 1992;268:2840-4.
46. Eigenmann PA, Sicherer SH, Borkowski TA, et al. Prevalence of IgE-mediated food allergy among children with atopic dermatitis. Pediatrics 1998;101:E8.
47. Burks AW, Mallory SB, Williams LW, et al. Atopic dermatitis: clinical relevance of food hypersensitivity reactions. J Pediatr 1988;113: 447-51.

48. Burks AW, James JM, Hiegel A, et al. Atopic dermatitis and food hypersensitivity reactions. J Pediatr 1998;132:132-6.

49. Greer FR, Sicherer SH, Burks AW. Effects of early nutritional interventions on the development of atopic disease in infants and children: the role of maternal dietary restriction, breastfeeding, timing of introduction of complementary foods, and hydrolyzed formulas. Pediatrics 2008;121: 183-91.

50. Gdalevich M, Mimouni D, David M, et al. Breast-feeding and the onset of atopic dermatitis in childhood: a systematic review and meta-analysis of prospective studies. J Am Acad Dermatol 2001;45:520-7.

51. Hattevig G, Kjellman B, Sigurs N, et al. Effect of maternal avoidance of eggs, cow's milk and fish during lactation upon allergic manifestations in infants. Clin Exp Allergy 1989;19:27-32.

52. Sigurs N, Hattevig G, Kjellman B. Maternal avoidance of eggs, cow's milk, and fish during lactation: effect on allergic manifestations, skin-prick tests, and specific IgE antibodies in children at age 4 years. Pediatrics 1992;89(4 Pt 2):735-9.

53. Zeiger RS, Heller S, Mellon MH, et al. Effect of combined maternal and infant food-allergen avoidance on development of atopy in early infancy: a randomized study. J Allergy Clin Immunol 1989;84:72-89.

54. Filipiak B, Zutavern A, Koletzko S, et al. Solid food introduction in relation to eczema: results from a four-year prospective birth cohort study. J Pediatr 2007;151:352-8.

55. Snijders BE, Thijs C, van Ree R, et al. Age at first introduction of cow milk products and other food products in relation to infant atopic manifestations in the first 2 years of life: the KOALA Birth Cohort Study. 2008;Pediatrics 122:e115-122.

56. Zutavern A, Brockow I, Schaaf B, et al. Timing of solid food introduction in relation to atopic dermatitis and atopic sensitization: results from a prospective birth cohort study. Pediatrics 2006;117:401-11.

57. Turjanmaa K. 'Atopy patch tests' in the diagnosis of delayed food hypersensitivity. Allerg Immunol (Paris) 2002;34:95-7.

58. Roehr CC, Reibel S, Ziegert M, et al. Atopy patch tests, together with determination of specific IgE levels, reduce the need for oral food challenges in children with atopic dermatitis. J Allergy Clin Immunol 2001;107:548-53.

59. Hill DJ, Hosking CS, de Benedictis FM, et al. Confirmation of the association between high levels of immunoglobulin E food sensitization and eczema in infancy: an international study. Clin Exp Allergy 2008;38: 161-8.

60. Lowe AJ, Abramson MJ, Hosking CS, et al. The temporal sequence of allergic sensitization and onset of infantile eczema. Clin Exp Allergy 2007;37:536-42.

61. Guillet G, Guillet MH. Natural history of sensitizations in atopic dermatitis. A 3-year follow-up in 250 children: food allergy and high risk of respiratory symptoms. Arch Dermatol 1992;128:187-92.

62. de Maat-Bleeker F, Bruijnzeel-Koomen C. Food allergy in adults with atopic dermatitis. Monogr Allergy 1996;32:157-63.

63. Munkvad M, Danielsen L, Hoj L, et al. Antigen-free diet in adult patients with atopic dermatitis: a double-blind controlled study. Acta Derm Venereol 1984;64:524-8.

64. Bock SA, Atkins FM. Patterns of food hypersensitivity during sixteen years of double-blind, placebo-controlled food challenges. J Pediatr 1990;117:561-7.

65. Young E, Patel S, Stoneham M, et al. The prevalence of reaction to food additives in a survey population. J R Coll Physicians Lond 1987;21: 241-7.

66. Fuglsang G, Madsen G, Halken S, et al. Adverse reactions to food additives in children with atopic symptoms. Allergy 1994;49:31-7.

67. Schwartz H. Food allergy: adverse reactions to foods and food additives. In: Asthma and food additives, ed 2, Blackwell Science 1997.

68. Perry TT, Matsui EC, Conover-Walker MK, et al. Risk of oral food challenges. J Allergy Clin Immunol 2004;114:1164-8.

69. Mankad VS, Williams LW, Lee LA, et al. Safety of open food challenges in the office setting. Ann Allergy Asthma Immunol 2008;100:469-74.

70. David TJ. Hazards of challenge tests in atopic dermatitis. Allergy 1989;44(Suppl 9):101-7.

71. Bock SA. The natural history of food sensitivity. J Allergy Clin Immunol 1982;69:173-7.

72. Savage JH, Matsui EC, Skripak JM, et al. The natural history of egg allergy. J Allergy Clin Immunol 2007;120:1413-7.

73. Knight AK, Shreffler WG, Sampson HA, et al. Skin prick test to egg white provides additional diagnostic utility to serum egg white-specific IgE antibody concentration in children. J Allergy Clin Immunol 2006;117: 842-7.

74. Perry TT, Matsui EC, Kay Conover-Walker M, et al. The relationship of allergen-specific IgE levels and oral food challenge outcome. J Allergy Clin Immunol 2004;114:144-9.

75. Skolnick HS, Conover-Walker MK, Koerner CB, et al. The natural history of peanut allergy. J Allergy Clin Immunol 2001;107:367-74.

76. Fleischer DM, Conover-Walker MK, Christie L, et al. The natural progression of peanut allergy: resolution and the possibility of recurrence. J Allergy Clin Immunol 2003;112:183-9.

77. Fleischer DM, Conover-Walker MK, Matsui EC, et al. The natural history of tree nut allergy. J Allergy Clin Immunol 2005;116:1087-93.

CHAPTER

52

Management of Food Allergy

Marion Groetch • Hugh A. Sampson

Overview

The prevalence of food allergy has risen by 18% in children less than 18 years of age in the past decade.[1] The therapeutic management of food allergy currently entails complete dietary avoidance of the identified allergen to prevent chronic and acute food allergic reactions. Although many alternative immunomodulatory approaches are being explored as a means to prevent immunoglobulin E (IgE)-mediated food allergic reactions, dietary avoidance is the only consistently viable treatment option at this time.[2,3]

Allergen elimination diets present great challenges to families and come with potential social, psychological, financial and nutritional burdens.[4] Food is an integral part of social gatherings and without adequate planning, the child and family may feel unable to participate fully in daily activities. Going to parties, eating in friend's homes, even going to school or camp will require planning so that these opportunities can be safely enjoyed. Eating competence is also vitally important to the socialization of the child and children with food allergies may have food aversions and self-limited diets beyond the elimination diet. Anxiety issues may even arise about eating and food in general, which will further impact the child's ability to participate fully in activities. Shopping and meal preparation requires significantly more time when avoiding allergens and specialty allergen-free foods can be more expensive. Lastly, elimination diets may impact nutrient intake and great care must be taken to ensure that the restricted diet continues to provide adequate nutrition for growth and development. Rickets, vitamin and mineral deficiencies, suboptimal growth and failure to thrive have all been associated with food elimination diets.[5-10]

Food allergy management from the dietitian's perspective entails teaching the family how to avoid the allergen, manage the allergy in all areas of daily living, and provide a nutritionally balanced diet within the context of the allergen avoidance diet. The goal of providing extensive education is to reduce the risk of accidental allergen exposure, as well as empowering the family, and eventually the child, to participate in all daily living activities while avoiding the food to which they are allergic. Living with food allergies is a daily challenge but with planning, activities can be safe and manageable, and the allergen avoidance diet nutritionally adequate and enjoyable.

Avoidance Diets – General

Elimination diet education begins with knowing how to identify the allergen in the food supply. The elimination of a single allergen from the diet may seem an easy task. Indeed, if the allergy is to a food that plays a minor role in our food supply, such as cashew nut, the task may be simple enough. On the other hand, if the allergy is to a food that is pervasive in our food supply, such as milk or wheat, avoidance issues become much more complex. Avoidance of a single allergen such as cow's milk necessitates avoidance of many common foods including not only milk, butter, cheese, yogurt and ice cream, but also numerous manufactured products such as crackers, breads, cookies, cereals, cakes, and processed meats and cold cuts that may also contain milk protein as an ingredient. Allergen avoidance sheets are available (*www.foodallergy.org* or *www.faiusa.org*) and are a helpful tool when used as a starting point for allergen avoidance education. Allergen avoidance sheets identify foods and ingredients that typically contain the allergen, in addition to identifying situations that may require special caution. It should be noted that avoidance sheets do not provide the extensive education needed for strict dietary elimination.

Label Reading

The ingredient list provided on the label of packaged foods is an important source of information. The package label must be read each and every time a food item is purchased, even if it has been purchased in the past, as product ingredients may change at any time. In addition to the ingredient list, other information such as advisory statements is provided and those shopping for a family member with food allergies must understand how to read and interpret product labels in order to successfully identify and eliminate food allergens. Food labeling legislation in many countries has undergone some transformation in recent years due to the recognized need for those with food allergies to be able to accurately identify allergenic ingredients on product labels.

In the European Union (EU), clear labeling of 14 identified food allergens on the ingredient label of all packaged foods is required.[11,12] The 14 identified allergens in the EU are:

Milk

Egg

Peanut

©2010 Elsevier Ltd, Inc, BV
DOI: 10.1016/B978-1-4377-0271-2.00052-3

Tree nuts
Fish
Crustacean shell fish
Mollusks
Soybean
Gluten (wheat, rye, barley, oat, spelt, kamut and their hybrid strains)
Celery
Mustard
Sesame
Sulphur dioxide and sulphites at concentrations of more than 10 mg/kg or 10 mg/L expressed as SO2
Lupine

Mollusks and lupine were added as major allergens in the EU effective from 23 December 2008 (Commission Directive 2006/142/EC), in recognition of the fact that these two foods are also commonly associated with food allergic reactions. Lupine is a legume that appears to be commonly allergenic to individuals with peanut allergy.[13] Although only 5% of children with peanut allergy may be clinically reactive to another legume, lupine appears to be the exception. Up to 44% of those with peanut allergy may be clinically reactive to lupine.[13] Lupine is more commonly used as an ingredient in European countries, especially in baked goods where flours made from lupine may be used.

The EU regulations mandate the labeling and full disclosure of ingredients derived from these commonly allergenic foods, even if they are present in small amounts. The EU currently has a '5% rule' that allows some ingredients to be omitted from a product label if those ingredients are part of a defined EU compound (such as jam) and that compound comprises less than 5% of the finished product. This '5% rule', however, does not override the allergen labeling requirement that all intentional sources of the 14 major allergens be identified on a product label regardless of whether or not the ingredient is part of an EU-defined compound.[11,12]

Currently, the European Union Safety Authority has granted exemption for numerous products including highly refined soybean oil; lactilol; distillates made from nuts, whey and cereals; and fish gelatin or isinglass used as a fining agent in wine and beer. To access a full list of the ingredients, which must be included on the product label in European countries as well as those exempt from the labeling law, visit the Official Journal of the European Union at: http://useu.usmission.gov/agri/label.html#Allergen.

In the USA, The Food Allergen Labeling and Consumer Protection Act of 2004, or FALCPA, mandates that food products have labels, in plain English language, that list all ingredients derived from commonly allergenic foods.[14] While allergic reactions may occur to a vast range of food ingredients, eight foods are responsible for 90% of all food allergic reactions.[15] The ingredients identified as the major food allergens, hence subject to the FALCPA, are those derived from these eight major food allergens:

Milk
Egg
Soybean
Wheat
Peanut
Tree nut
Fish
Crustacean shellfish[14]

Additionally, manufacturers must list the specific tree nut (almond, Brazil nut, cashew, hazelnut, pecan, pistachio, walnut, etc.), fish (salmon, tuna, cod, etc.) or crustacean shellfish (crab, lobster, shrimp, etc.) used as an ingredient. Mollusks (clam, muscles, oyster, scallops, etc.) are not considered major food allergens under FALCPA.[14]

The plain language stipulation in this law requires the presence of a major food allergen to be listed on the product label in one of the following ways:

- In parenthesis, following the food protein derivative for example: casein (milk)
- In the ingredient list for example: milk, wheat, peanut
- Immediately below the ingredient list in a 'contains' statement for example: CONTAINS EGG.[11,14]

Additionally, a major food allergen may no longer be omitted from the product label if it is only an incidental ingredient such as in a spice, flavoring, coloring or additive, or used merely as a processing aid in a product.[14] These regulations only apply to ingredients derived from the eight foods that are considered the major allergens. An individual with sensitivity to an ingredient not covered under FALCPA, such as garlic or sesame, would still need to call the manufacturer to ascertain if garlic, sesame or sesame oil was included in a vague ingredient term such as 'spice' or 'natural flavoring' of a product.[14]

Manufactured food products, including those imported for sale in the USA, dietary supplements, medical foods and infant formulas are all required to comply with FALCPA.[14] The only ingredient or derivative of a major allergen that is exempt from FALCPA labeling requirements is 'highly refined oil' from a major food allergen source. The consumption of highly refined oils derived from major food allergens by individuals who are allergic to the source food (soy, peanut), does not appear to be associated with an allergic response. It is general practice, however, to recommend that those with peanut allergy continue to avoid peanut oil as it may be difficult, especially in a restaurant setting, to determine the degree of refinement of the oil. Vegetable oils from allergenic food sources that are not highly refined, such as expelled, expressed, extruded or other crude oils, may contain significant allergenic proteins and therefore may cause an allergic response and are not exempt from FALCPA[11,16,17]

Manufacturers are required to list any intentional allergenic ingredient on the product label, but the presence of ingredients in manufactured foods due to cross-contact are not required to be listed on product labels. Cross-contact occurs when an 'allergen-safe' food unintentionally comes in contact with an allergen during routine methods of growing and harvesting crops, or from the use of shared storage, transportation or production equipment. Cross-contact may lead to significant levels of hidden allergens in a product without identification on the product label. Many manufacturers are addressing the issue of cross-contact with advisory statements such as: 'May contain [allergen]', 'Manufactured in a facility that also manufactures [allergen]' or 'Manufactured on shared equipment with [allergen]'. Those with food allergies should be aware that these statements are currently voluntary and unregulated. Therefore the absence of an advisory statement does not necessarily mean there is no risk of cross-contact. Additionally, as these statements are not regulated, no one statement represents a greater or lesser degree of risk than another.

A 2007 study by Hefle and colleagues evaluated 179 products with peanut advisory labeling. Two different lot numbers of each of these 179 products were analyzed for detectable peanut allergen.[18] The results revealed that 7% (13/179) of the products tested contained detectable levels of peanut in one or both lots and the type of advisory statement used did not reflect the degree of risk. An additional aim of this study was to determine, by survey, if consumers with food allergies or their care-givers were heeding advisory statements. The survey of more than 600 individuals who shop for persons with food allergy indicated that they were more likely to purchase products with advisory labeling in 2006 than in 2003.[18] This may reflect the fact that more and more manufactured products now contain an advisory label. Additionally, consumers were also more likely to purchase products labeled 'Made in a facility with [allergen]' than products labeled 'May contain [allergen]' indicating that consumers are assessing risk based on the label terminology. The FDA is currently working on developing a long-term strategy to assist manufacturers in using allergen advisory labeling that is truthful and not misleading, conveys a clear and uniform message, and adequately informs food allergic consumers and their care-givers of risk. So, while advisory statements may help allergic consumers better assess the safety of a product, if they are applied too broadly, consumers may simply choose to ignore them. Unfortunately, ignoring advisory statements is not without risk and families with food allergies should be advised to continue to avoid products that contain or may contain their child's specific allergens.

The package label provides information to the consumer about the contents of a product and although label ambiguities continue to exist, the newer labeling laws are vastly improved. Consumers should be aware that they may still need to call the manufacturer to ask how a product was made and assess the cross-contact risk before including a product in the diet. Health-care professionals must be prepared to offer extensive education to patients with food allergies so that safe food selections can be made.

Daily Living with Food Allergies

Children with food allergies may be inadvertently exposed to a food allergen in a variety of ways. Poor label reading may lead to an unintentional ingestion of an allergen. Not understanding the risk of cross-contact in a manufactured food product is another risk factor. Consumers with food allergies and their caretakers need to understand that cross-contact may occur outside of the manufacturing industry as well.

Once a food item is purchased and brought into the home, that item must continue to be carefully handled to prevent cross-contact with the identified allergen. Storage of ingredients in the home should be planned to prevent cross-contact. A separate shelf in the refrigerator or cupboard may be reserved for the allergen-free foods. Safe meal preparation to prevent cross-contact in the home is also essential. All food preparation areas, cooking utensils and cooking equipment should be cleansed with warm soapy water and rinsed. Allergen-free foods and meal items can be prepared first, covered, and removed from the area prior to the preparation of other foods for the home.[4]

Families living with food allergies report that avoiding eating in restaurants is the number one cause of decreased quality of life due to the food allergy.[19] Those with food allergies may be especially at risk while dining out since restaurants are not required to list ingredients and the waiting staff are generally ignorant about the ingredients in a dish. These families need guidance on how to minimize risk so they too can enjoy restaurant meals with family and friends.

Planning ahead and communication with restaurant staff is the first key step in obtaining a safe restaurant meal. Calling ahead to ask how a food allergy is accommodated as well as avoiding the restaurant's busiest hours is often helpful. Families should be taught to inform the staff that their child has a food allergy; not to simply ask if a menu item contains their allergen. 'Chef Cards' provide a written list of ingredients to avoid for specific allergens

and are available from websites such as *www.foodallergy.org* or *www.faiusa.org*. In addition to ingredient inquiries, families must learn to inform restaurant staff about cross-contact risk. Cross-contact in a restaurant environment is not uncommon. For example, the same grill might be used to make a cheeseburger that is used for a plain hamburger, or the French fries might have been cooked in the same deep fat fryer as the milk-containing onion rings. The same tongs or mixing bowls may be used to assemble a salad with nuts as is used to assemble a plain green salad. Families should be taught to speak directly to the chef or food service manager to inquire about ingredients and cross-contact risk. It is important to inform the chef that a clean cooking area, cooking equipment and utensils must be used. Ordering single ingredient foods, prepared simply will decrease the risk of hidden ingredients. When the food arrives at the table, families should confirm with the chef that the meal was prepared correctly and not have their child eat the food if there is any doubt as to the safety of the meal.[4] Lastly, as always, emergency medications should be available when eating at home or away from home.[20]

Certain types of eating establishments will present a greater risk of allergen exposure. For example, cafeterias, buffets and salad bars have inherently greater risk of cross-contact due to spillage and shared serving utensils. Asian and other ethnic restaurants may use more allergenic ingredients (soy, peanuts, tree nuts, fish and shell fish) in a wide variety of dishes and the cooking equipment is generally not washed between each meal prepared. Ice cream parlors use the same scooper for all flavors of ice cream. Asking for a clean scooper may not eliminate the risk as previous servings with a contaminated scooper into the vanilla barrel may have already caused cross-contact. For seafood allergies, seafood restaurants may be problematic even if a non-seafood item is ordered because of the greater risk of cross-contact in the kitchen.[20]

Children with food allergies will attend schools just like their nonallergic peers and some planning ahead will help to make the environment safer. Management issues in schools involve informing teachers, nurses, administrators and food service staff about the food allergy. Families should plan to meet with school personnel prior to the start of the school year. Communication with the school about topics such as classroom parties, transportation, supervision in the lunch room if needed, substitute teacher notification, field trips and after school programs will help to plan food allergy management in all areas of the school environment. Labeled and up-to-date emergency medications and food allergy treatment plans prescribed by the physician should be provided by the family and reviewed with school staff.[4]

The Food Allergy Anaphylaxis Network (FAAN) has developed a variety of resources and products including a food allergy treatment plan for physicians and a school food allergy program for schools and a back-to-school tool kit for families. Parents, physicians, school administrators, teachers, school nurses, food service staff, and camp staff will find these resources valuable in the planning required to keep children with food allergies safe (*www.foodallergy.org*).

Nutrition

Overview

Fundamental to the care of any infant or child, including those with food allergies, is the assessment of nutritional status. The child with food allergies does not appear to have altered nutritional needs compared to those without food allergies although a patient with moderate to severe atopic dermatitis may have increased energy and protein needs due to losses through the compromised skin barrier.[21] Children with food allergies are, however, at risk of overall inadequate nutritional intake.[6-8,22] Additionally, feeding problems such as food aversion and a limited acceptance of a variety of foods is common in children with food allergies and may significantly contribute to poor energy and overall nutrient intake. Certain food-allergic disorders such as allergic eosinophilic esophagitis and gastroenteritis are commonly accompanied by poor appetite and early satiety, which may have an impact on overall nutrient intake.[23-25] In general, however, the primary cause of nutritional inadequacies associated with food allergy in children is likely to stem from inadequate substitution of the nutrients inherent in the eliminated food.

The nutritional assessment entails monitoring of growth, physical assessment, biochemical indices and evaluation of the reported dietary intake, which is then compared to the estimation of dietary needs using the Dietary Reference Index (DRI). Additionally, when assessing pediatric nutritional status, eating abilities and competencies must also be determined. Recommending a dietary plan for the nutritional rehabilitation of a child who will not be able to master the foods in the recommended treatment plan will be of little use.

Growth

Several studies have evaluated growth in the pediatric population with food allergy. Christie and colleagues compared height, weight, body mass index and estimates of energy and nutrient intakes in a group of 98 children with food allergy and 99 children without food allergy and found that children with two or more food allergies were shorter, based on height-for-age percentiles than those with no food allergy or only one food allergy.[6] Similarly, Isolauri and colleagues found length and weight-for-length indices in a group of 100 infants with food allergy decreased compared with healthy, age-matched controls.[8] Jensen and colleagues found height for age was significantly reduced in a group of patients living with cow's milk allergy for more than 4 years when compared with height of parents and siblings as well as normal controls.[22]

It is clear that children with food allergies may be at risk for poor growth and as such, growth should be carefully monitored. Growth typically follows predictable increases in length, weight and head circumference and significant changes in growth velocity are not expected. Plotting growth measurements on the appropriate standardized growth chart will allow assessment of growth velocity for that particular child as well as provide a comparison of the growth of the child with the reference population. The Centers for Disease Control and the National Center for Health Statistics (CDC/NCHS) growth charts (*www.cdc.gov/growthchart*) are based on data from 5 US national health examination surveys and five supplemental data sources and described how children from a wide range of social, economic and ethnic backgrounds actually grew.[26] In the US, the CDC growth charts are most commonly used in pediatric practices. If a child's growth measurement (length/height, weight or head circumference) falls below the 5th or above the 95th percentile or it crosses two major growth channels indicating altered growth velocity, that child is considered at nutritional risk.[26]

The World Health Organization growth (WHO) charts (*www.who.int/childgrowth/standards/en/*) are based on a pooled sample from six participating countries used to develop an international standard of normal growth from birth to 5 years under optimal conditions. These growth standards demonstrate that children from across the world's regions living in healthy environments and receiving optimal nutrition attain remarkably similar rates of growth. WHO growth standards for children from birth to 2 years of age were derived from longitudinal data of an infant population that was exclusively breast-fed until 4 to 6 months of age, fed complimentary foods by 6 months of age and that continued breast-feeding until at least 12 months of age. The WHO standards establish the breast-fed child as the normative model for growth and development and, as such, may be more appropriate for those infants in the USA who are exclusively breastfed. The WHO reference standards result in lower estimates of undernutrition except during the first 6 months of life. Using the WHO standard curves, children whose measurements fall below the 2.3 percentile and above the 97.7 percentile are considered at nutritional risk. These international standards can be applied to all children regardless of type of feeding, ethnicity or socioeconomic status.

Plotting a child's growth history (weight, length or height, weight to length or body mass and head circumference) on the appropriate growth chart that is standardized for the population being measured provides a way to follow the typical growth patterns for that child (velocity) and compare those patterns with the reference population. Weight is the most sensitive measure of adequate energy intake and is affected earlier and to a greater extent than linear growth or head circumference by dietary inadequacies. For accuracy, infants should be weighed without clothes or diapers.

Linear growth is determined by recumbent length in the supine position in children less than 2 years of age and in standing height in children older than 3 years of age. Children between 2 and 3 years of age may be measured by either technique although they should be plotted on the appropriate corresponding standard growth chart: 0- to 36-month chart for supine length or 2- to 18-year chart for standing height. Linear growth can be delayed as a result of dietary protein inadequacy or chronic energy deficits.[26]

Body mass index (BMI), defined as weight in kilograms divided by the square of height in meters, may be used after 2 years of age and is helpful as it takes into consideration weight for height.[26] Both the WHO and CDC provide standardized BMI charts. The CDC defines underweight in children as a BMI of less than the 5th percentile. Children are considered to be at risk of overweight when their BMI is greater than the 85th percentile and overweight when their BMI is greater than the 95th percentile.[26]

Dietary Intake Assessment

Dietary intakes can be obtained by 24-hour recall or dietary diary. A 24-hour recall is generally useful when assessing intake in an infant who is predominantly breast- or bottle-fed but may provide limited information for older children, as accuracy of a mixed diet may not be reflected with recall. For older infants and children, a food diary will provide a more accurate estimate of intake. A food diary of at least 3 days (including 1 weekend and 2 weekdays) should include the amount and types of foods ingested and the timing of meals and snacks. A registered dietitian will be able to convert foods from a food diary into nutrients, which can then be compared to estimated needs using the DRI. Even clinicians who are not trained to assess the nutritional intake of a child may glean valuable information from a food diary. For instance, unusual meal patterns such as excessive fruit juice consumption may become apparent from the food diary and may give clues to potential causes of poor growth or nutritional status in a child.

Eating Competence

Eating competence and pediatric nutrition are often discussed side by side because feeding problems are common in childhood, with an estimated 25–35% of otherwise healthy children affected.[27] Eating competence describes a child's ability to eat and enjoy a wide variety of foods of varying flavors and textures that will support adequate nutrition for growth and development.[27]

Eating is a complex, learned process involving the acquisition of physical skills, behaviors, acquired tastes, and attitudes and feelings about eating in general as well as about certain food items in particular.[28] Feeding problems may be mild or severe and may have causes that are developmental in origin, such as oral motor delay/dysfunction or sensory defensiveness or they may be psychosocial in nature. Feeding problems are not uncommon in children with developmental delay or other chronic medical disorders and referral for assessment and management of the feeding problem, generally involving an interdisciplinary approach, is recommended.[29]

Many mild feeding problems or limited eating competencies, not accompanied by developmental delays or medical conditions, are characterized by a tendency to avoid selected food items according to texture, taste, sight, or odor. Even mild, self-selective or 'picky' eating can impact nutritional intake and in combination with an allergen elimination diet, can have serious nutritional implications. Assessment of eating competencies will provide information necessary so that an effective nutrition plan can be devised.

Estimating Nutritional Needs

Energy

The estimated energy requirement (EER) is the average dietary energy intake that is predicted to maintain energy balance. For children, the EER includes the needs associated with the deposition of tissues at rates consistent with good health. There is no established recommended dietary allowance (RDA) for energy because energy intakes exceeding the EER would be expected to result in excessive weight gain. EER can be calculated using the equations provided in the DRI reports (*www.nap.edu*).[30]

Energy is provided in the pediatric diet through three major classes of macronutrients: proteins, carbohydrates and fats. Dietary reference intakes (DRIs) have been established for energy and macronutrients as well as for vitamins and minerals (*www. nap.edu*). Acceptable macronutrient distribution ranges (AMDRs) have also been established for protein, carbohydrates and fats and indicate the range of intake for a particular energy source, expressed as a percentage of total caloric intake that is associated with reduced risk of chronic disease, while providing adequate intakes of essential nutrients.[30]

Protein

Adequate protein in the diet is crucial in all age groups. Many excellent sources of protein are also common allergens including milk, egg, soy, fish, shellfish, peanut and tree nuts. Diets must be carefully planned to meet protein needs when high quality protein sources are eliminated from the diet. Inadequate dietary protein intake may be a contributing factor in the decreased stature reportedly seen in the population of children with food allergies.

Proteins needs may be estimated using the DRI for protein found in Table 52-1.[30] An estimated 65–70% of protein needs should come from sources of high biological value, meaning animal products for the most part, which contain a full complement of indispensable amino acids. Animal products are not necessary to provide optimal protein, but most alternative sources from plants, legumes, grains, nuts, seeds and vegetables do not contain a full complement of indispensable amino acids and therefore greater dietary planning will be required. Additionally, dietary protein recommendations are based on the assumption that energy intake is adequate. If energy intake is insufficient, free amino acids will be oxidized for energy, allowing for less available amino acids for anabolic and synthetic pathways.[30]

Table 52-1 Dietary Reference Intakes for Macronutrients for Children

Nutrient	Age	RDA*/AI g/day (unless otherwise specified)	AMDR % of Total Energy Intake
Protein	0–12 mo	1.5 g/kg/day	ND
	1–3 yr	1.1* g/kg/day	5–20
	4–13 yr	0.95* g/kg/day	10–30
	14–18 yr	0.85* g/kg/day	10–30
Carbohydrates	0–6 mo	60	ND
	7–12 mo	95	ND
	1–18 yr	130*	45–65
Total fat	0–6 mo	31	ND
	7–12 mo	30	ND
	1–3 yr		30–40
	4–18 yr		25–35
n-3 Fatty acids	0–6 mo	0.5	ND
	7–12 mo	0.5	ND
	1–3 yr	0.7	0.6–1.2
	4–8 yr	0.9	0.6–1.2
	Males		
	9–13 yr	1.2	0.6–1.2
	14–18 yr	1.6	0.6–1.2
	Females		
	9–13 yr	1.0	0.6–1.2
	14–18 yr	1.1	0.6–1.2
n-6 Fatty acids	0–6 mo	4.4	ND
	7–12 mo	4.6	ND
	1–3 yr	7	5–10
	4–8 yr	10	5–10
	Males		
	9–13 yr	12	5–10
	14–18 yr	16	5–10
	Females		
	9–13 yr	10	5–10
	14–18 yr	11	5–10

Adapted from the DRI report: Dietary Reference Intakes for Energy, Carbohydrate, Fiber, Fat, Fatty Acids, Cholesterol, Protein, Amino Acids (2002/2006). Available at: www.nap.edu.
*RDA: recommended dietary allowances are set to meet the needs of almost all individuals in a group.
AI: adequate intake is the recommended average daily intake level based on observed or experimentally determined approximations or estimates of nutrient intake by a group (or groups) of apparently healthy people that are assumed to be adequate. The AI is used when an RDA cannot be determined.
AMDR: acceptable macronutrient distribution range is the range of intake for an energy source that is associated with reduced risk of chronic disease while providing adequate intakes of essential nutrients.
ND: not determinable

Fat

Adequate dietary fat is crucial as fats are an important source of concentrated energy, support the transport of fat-soluble vitamins and provide the two fatty acids, omega 3, alpha-linolenic acid (ALA) and omega 6, linoleic acid (LA), which are essential in the human diet. Dietary fat needs may be estimated using the DRI for fats in Table 52.1.[30] Adequate dietary fat is an especially important source of energy and nutrients for rapidly growing infants and toddlers. Dietary fat intakes below 20% of total caloric intake increase risk of energy, vitamin E and essential fatty acid deficient diets.[30] Dietary fat is present in a wide variety of foods, such as dairy products, eggs, meat, fish and poultry, vegetable oils and margarines and many manufactured and processed snack foods, convenience meals and desserts. Children on allergen-restricted diets, who must eliminate not only the allergen but also many processed and manufactured foods, may find it especially difficult to meet dietary fat needs without adding supplemental fats to the diet.

To meet fat recommendations, a balance of saturated, polyunsaturated and monounsaturated dietary fats should be provided. Dietary sources rich in monounsaturated fatty acids (MUFA) include some vegetable oils (canola, olive, high oleic sunflower oil, safflower oil), nuts, seeds and avocado. Polyunsaturated fatty acid (PUFA) sources include vegetable oils (soy and corn oils), nuts and seeds. Most unsaturated fatty acids are naturally present in the *cis* arrangement. Unsaturated fatty acids in the *trans* arrangement are predominantly present in our food supply through hydrogenated oils in stick margarines, crackers, cookies, cakes and other snack foods. Saturated fatty acids are found in full fat dairy products, fatty meats, and tropical oils such as coconut, palm and palm kernel oil. No required role for saturated and *trans* fatty acids have been identified and excessive intakes of these fats may contribute to increased low density lipoprotein levels and decrease high density lipoprotein levels which, are risk factors for heart disease. The Dietary Reference Intake of the National Academy of Sciences recommends keeping saturated and trans fatty acid intake as low as possible while consuming a nutritionally balanced diet.[30] As children with food allergies may find it challenging to meet dietary fat needs, ensuring that total fat intake is sufficient to meet needs is essential. The addition of vegetable oils to the allergen-restricted diet may be required. When it is necessary to supplement the diet with fats, emphasizing the use of predominantly PUFA and MUFA will help to maintain the recommended balance between saturated, polyunsaturated and monounsaturated fat.

Carbohydrates

Carbohydrates make up the remaining energy sources and provide an important supply of numerous vitamins, minerals and trace elements. Carbohydrates should comprise between 45–65% of total caloric intake.[30] Grains, dairy products, legumes, fruits and vegetables provide dietary carbohydrates. Simple sugars and foods with added sugars also contribute carbohydrates and additional energy, but are of little further nutritional benefit and should be limited to no more than 25% of total energy intake. Dietary carbohydrates are an important source of iron, thiamin, niacin, riboflavin and folic acid. Children on wheat avoidance diets should substitute alternative grains to meet the recommended dietary allowance (RDA) for carbohydrate of 130 g/day for adults and children 1 year of age or older.[30]

Macronutrient intake should be considered in the nutritional assessment and modifications made to ensure an appropriate nutritional balance. Meeting the recommended dietary intakes of macronutrients can often be challenging when food groups are eliminated due to food allergies. The acceptable macronutrient distribution range (AMDR) for macronutrients can be found in Table 52-1 and should be used to guide the appropriate intake and distribution of carbohydrates, fats and proteins.[30]

Micronutrients

Variety in the diet contributes to adequacy of nutrients provided. When a food group is eliminated, the nutrients provided by that food group must now be provided by other dietary sources. In 2002, Christie and colleagues found that children with multiple food allergies or cow's milk allergy consumed less dietary calcium than age-specific recommendations compared with children without cow's milk allergy and/or one food allergy.[6] Henricksen and colleagues surveyed a sample of families with young children (31 to 37 months old) with milk allergy and/or egg allergy and assessed dietary intake using a complete 4-day, weighed recording. Children on milk-free diets had significantly lower intake of energy, fat, protein, calcium, riboflavin and niacin.[7]

While it is important to ensure adequate intake of all essential nutrients, certain nutrients will be at greater risk of insufficiency depending on the food allergen and must be adequately replaced by other foods in the diet. When foods are chosen carefully, and appropriate substitutions are made, the diet for a child with food allergies can be nutritionally adequate. When dietary modifications are inadequate to meet vitamin, mineral and trace element needs, appropriate supplementation may be considered. Dietary supplements, however, may pose a risk of contamination with food allergens (even those labeled allergen-free) and they should be chosen carefully, with consideration for safe ingredients as well as risk assessment of potential cross-contact during manufacturing.[21]

The potential consequences of inadequate nutrition in the pediatric population with food allergies warrants closer monitoring of growth by pediatricians since this population is at greater risk of growth failure that may be corrected with dietary intervention by a registered dietitian. As normal growth is not a guarantee of overall nutritional health, it should not be used solely to assess nutritional status in children with food allergies, but rather as a screening tool. Any child with a highly selective repertoire of foods, or a child who cannot or will not accept the nutrient-dense substitutions for the eliminated food, will also benefit from nutritional consultation. Additional signs of nutritional inadequacies may be found in the physical exam, biochemical indices and through the assessment of the dietary intake.

Allergen Elimination Diets – Diagnostic or Therapeutic

Elimination diets may be prescribed short term for diagnostic purposes or long term for treatment of a diagnosed food allergy. When chronic symptoms are present, as in atopic dermatitis, or there are delayed symptoms as in eosinophilic disorders, it may be difficult to determine a cause and effect relationship between the food and the reaction. These allergic disorders may be IgE or non-IgE mediated, so testing as previously described (Chapter 45) may not prove useful. In such cases, manipulation of the diet for a patient with suspected food hypersensitivity may be part of the diagnostic process. Education should be provided to eliminate suspected food allergens from the diet, anticipating reduction or clearance of symptoms. Usually, 7 to 14 days is sufficient to show either remission or significant improvement of symptoms in atopic dermatitis. With allergic eosinophilic disorders, 6 to 8 weeks of allergen elimination may be necessary to achieve remission.[23,31] If symptoms resolve, it is possible that the omitted food is causing the reaction. The food should then be reintroduced under physician supervision and the patient observed for a recurrence of symptoms. Reintroducing an allergenic food after it has been eliminated for 2 to 3 weeks may result in an acute systemic allergic reaction. If multiple foods have been removed for diagnostic purposes they should be added back one at a time while observing for symptoms. If symptoms do not improve with removal of suspected foods, the diet should be reviewed to ensure appropriate avoidance. If symptoms do not clear significantly, even with the most restrictive or elemental diet, it is unlikely that ingested foods are implicated and other etiologies must be considered. The eliminated foods should then be returned to the diet.

Common Allergen Elimination Diets of Early Childhood

The prevalence of food allergy in infants and young children is 6% with the major allergens of early childhood being milk, egg, soy, peanut and wheat.[15,32] Each food or food group eliminated provides essential nutrition that must be replaced by other dietary sources. When initiating any long-term elimination diet, recommending a nutrient dense alternative food source is a crucial preventative measure. Follow-up to ensure that the alternative food source has been accepted and incorporated into the diet is also essential.

Cow's Milk Allergy

Cow's milk allergy (CMA) is the most common food allergy among infants and young children, affecting 2–3% of the population with up to 50% of children with CMA also having adverse reactions to other foods.[15,32,33] CMA affects predominantly the pediatric population, as roughly 80% of children with CMA will develop clinical tolerance. Recent epidemiologic studies indicate that milk allergy may be more persistent with fewer children becoming tolerant to milk in the first few years of life.[34] One large retrospective study from a specialty clinic reported resolution rates in 807 children with CMA and found the rates of resolution were 19% at the age of 4 years, 42% by 8 years, 64% by 12 years, and 79% by 16 years.[34] So while most patients (79%) did eventually develop tolerance, this rate of tolerance was not achieved by 3 to 5 years of age as previously described[15] but rather by 16 years of age, indicating that children with CMA may be required to eliminate milk, a nutrient-dense food source, for longer durations throughout childhood.

The nutritional effect of cow's milk elimination in the pediatric population is great because milk is not only a good source of fat, protein, calcium and vitamin D but is also the primary source for most children. Milk also provides vitamin B12, vitamin A, pantothenic acid, riboflavin and phosphorus. Finding a nutritionally dense substitute for cow's milk in the pediatric diet is essential and parents of children with milk allergy require detailed advice about food choices in order to reduce the risk of low intakes of these nutrients.

The breast-fed infant with CMA may benefit from maternal avoidance of milk protein from the diet, since immunologically recognizable proteins from the maternal diet can be found in breast milk.[35] The nutritional adequacy of the maternal diet may need to be assessed as milk elimination may compromise maternal nutrient intakes, which may in turn have an impact on the composition of the breast milk.[36] While lactation is supported partially by maternal nutritional stores, not all nutrients are preferentially secreted into breast milk. The lactating mother who is avoiding milk and milk products may benefit from continuing on a milk-free vitamin supplement. Vitamin D supplementation from birth is recommended for exclusively breast-fed infants and for formula-fed infants who do not ingest 1000 mL of vitamin D fortified formula. The current recommended dietary allowance (RDA) for vitamin D is 200 IU for infants and children although the American Academy of Pediatrics has recently revised vitamin D guidelines and recommends 400 IU/day for healthy infants, children and adolescents.[37]

For formula-fed infants with CMA, a variety of alternative formulas are available. Although soy formula is not hypoallergenic, many infants (85–90%) with IgE-mediated CMA may tolerate soy formula.[38] For infants with non-IgE-mediated CMA such as proctocolitis or enterocolitis syndrome, the prevalence of hypersensitivity to both soy and milk is greater, with up to 60% of infants reacting to both, so a hypoallergenic formula may be necessary.[35]

Extensively hydrolyzed casein formulas such as Nutramigen (Mead Johnson, Evansville, IN) or Alimentum (Abbott Nutrition, Columbus, OH) and elemental or amino acid-based formulas such as the Elecare (Abbott Nutrition, Columbus, OH) and Neocate lines of formulas (Nutricia, Gaithersburg, MD) are considered to be hypoallergenic.[35] Over 90% of infants with CMA tolerate extensively hydrolyzed infant formulas and for those who continue to exhibit symptoms on the extensively hydrolyzed formulas, an amino acid formula may be warranted. Partially hydrolyzed cow's milk formulas such as Good Start (Nestle) and Gentlease (Enfamil) are not considered hypoallergenic and are not a suitable option for infants with CMA.[38]

Transitioning an infant from a complete formula to a milk product is typically considered around 1 year of age or, ideally, when at least two thirds of the total daily caloric intake comes from a varied solid food diet since a wide variety of foods is more likely to contribute to micronutrient adequacy. However, other criteria for the allergic infant must be considered as a varied dietary intake with multiple food allergies may not be possible. Additionally, the enriched alternative milk source (soy, tree nut or grain-based milks) may not provide comparable nutrition. Alternative mammalian milks, such as goat's or sheep's milk, are also not suitable since up to 92% of individuals with cow's milk protein allergies will also react to goat's milk.[35]

For children with concomitant milk and soy allergy, enriched rice and almond milks may provide a good source of calcium and vitamin D, but they provide essentially no protein and are low in fat. Oat milk contains about 50% less protein than cow's or soy-based milk. Essentially, protein requirements will need to be met entirely through the solid food diet before switching to enriched rice milk. Fat intake will also need to be assessed and additional fat in the form of vegetable oils may be required. Christie and colleagues showed that the risk of consuming inadequate intakes of calcium and vitamin D among children with CMA was decreased if a safe enriched soymilk or commercially prepared infant/toddler formula was provided, suggesting that children with milk allergy should continue to include an adequate, nutrient-dense milk substitute in the diet.[6] It is often the case that a 1-year-old child is not capable of meeting protein and fat needs exclusively through the solid food diet; therefore maintaining the child on a hypoallergenic commercial formula, at least partially through the second year of life or longer, may be warranted.

The nutritional impact of milk allergy is great since milk is an excellent source of protein, calcium, vitamin D, phosphorus,

Table 52-2 Nutrients Provided by Milk and Milk Products and Alternative Dietary Sources

Nutrients in Cow's Milk	Alternative Sources
Macronutrients	
Dietary protein	Commercial formula, meat, fish, poultry, egg, soybean or enriched soy beverage, other legumes, peanut, tree nuts
Dietary fat	Commercial formula, vegetable oils, milk-free margarine, avocado, meats, fish, poultry, peanut, tree nuts, seeds
Micronutrients	
Calcium	Commercial formula, enriched alternative 'milk' beverage (soy, rice, almond, oat, potato), calcium fortified tofu, calcium fortified juice
Vitamin D	Commercial formula, enriched alternative 'milk' beverage, fortified milk-free margarine, fortified eggs, liver, fish liver oils, fatty fish
Vitamin A	Retinol: liver, egg yolk, fortified milk-free margarine Carotene: Dark green leafy vegetables, deep orange fruits and vegetables (broccoli, spinach, carrots, sweet potatoes, pumpkin, apricot, peach, cantaloupe) enriched alternative 'milk' beverage
Pantothenic acid	Meats, vegetables (broccoli, sweet potato, potato, tomato products), egg yolk, whole grains, legumes
Riboflavin (vitamin B2)	Dark green leafy vegetables, enriched and whole grain products
Vitamin B12	Meat, fish, poultry, egg, enriched alternative 'milk' beverage, fortified cereals

Table 52-3 Nutrients Provided by Wheat and Alternative Dietary Sources

Nutrients Provided by Wheat	Alternative Dietary Sources
Macronutrients	
Carbohydrates	Products made with alternative grains: amaranth, buckwheat, corn, millet, oat, rice, sorghum, quinoa; fruits, vegetables, legumes
Fiber	Fruits, vegetables, alternative whole grain products, legumes
Micronutrients	
Thiamin (vitamin B1)	Enriched and whole alternative grain products, nuts, legumes, liver, pork, sunflower seeds
Riboflavin (vitamin B2)	Enriched and whole alternative grain products, milk, dark green leafy vegetables
Niacin (vitamin B3)	Enriched and whole alternative grain products, meat, fish, poultry, liver, peanuts, sunflower seed, legumes
Folic acid	Enriched and whole alternative grain products, beef liver, dark green leafy vegetables, legumes, seeds
Iron	Heme iron: meat, liver, fish, shellfish, poultry Non-heme iron: enriched and whole alternative grain products, legumes and dried fruits

vitamin A, vitamin B12 and riboflavin. Possible alternative dietary sources for these nutrients can be found in Table 52-2.

Wheat Allergy

The child with wheat allergy must avoid all wheat-containing foods, resulting in the elimination of many processed and manufactured products, including bread, cereal, pasta, crackers, cookies, and cakes. Wheat is also commonly used as a minor ingredient in other commercial food products, such as condiments and marinades, cold cuts, soups, soy sauce, some low or nonfat products, hard candies, licorice and jelly beans. Wheat contributes carbohydrates as well as many micronutrients such as thiamin, niacin, riboflavin, iron and folic acid. Whole grain wheat products also contribute fiber to the diet. Alternative dietary sources of these nutrients should be provided. Four servings of wheat-based products, such as whole-grain and enriched cereals or breads, generally provides greater than 50% of the RDA/AI for carbohydrate, iron, thiamin, riboflavin and niacin for children 1 year of age and older, as well as a significant source of vitamin B6 and magnesium. Elimination of wheat products from the diet has great nutritional impact when nutrient-dense alternatives are not provided. Alternative sources for the nutrients found in wheat can be found in Table 52-3.

Many alternative flours are available to patients with wheat allergy, including rice, corn, oat, potato, sorghum, soy, barley, buckwheat, rye, amaranth, millet and quinoa. It has been reported that 20% of individuals with one grain allergy may be clinically reactive to another grain; therefore use of alternative grains should be individualized and based on tolerance as determined by the patient's allergist.[39] Alternative flours (grain, vegetable, legume, seed or nut) may improve the nutritional quality, variety and convenience of the wheat-restricted diet. Many of these flours are commercially available for home use and should be encouraged. There are currently numerous wheat-free and gluten-free products made from these flours as well. As many of these flours or alternative products may not be fortified, those with wheat allergies may choose to substitute fortified infant cereal such as rice or oat cereal, for a portion (up to 25%) of the alternative flour used in baked products for added nutrients such as iron, thiamin, riboflavin, niacin, and zinc.[21]

Egg Allergy

Eggs contribute protein, vitamin B12, riboflavin, pantothenic acid, biotin, and selenium in the diet. Many foods supply the nutrients found in eggs. Egg in the diet does not usually account for a large proportion of daily dietary intake therefore the nutrients lost through egg avoidance are not significant if the allergy stands alone and the diet is otherwise varied.

Egg is a common ingredient in many recipes such as baked goods, casseroles and meat-based dishes, such as meatballs, meatloaf and breaded meats. Learning to replace egg in the diet will help families to continue to enjoy traditional foods. Many commercial egg substitutes actually contain egg protein and therefore are not suitable for those with egg allergy. Egg may be replaced in a recipe using any of the following techniques:

2 tablespoons fruit puree (for binding, not leavening)

1.5 tablespoons water, 1.5 tablespoons oil, 1 teaspoon baking powder

1 teaspoon baking powder, 1 tablespoon liquid, 1 tablespoon vinegar

Potato-based commercial egg replacer (Ener-G foods)

1 packet gelatin, 2 tablespoons warm water – mix when ready to use

1 teaspoon yeast dissolved in a quarter cup of warm water

Soybean Allergy

Soy protein is an ingredient in a surprising variety of manufactured products. The result of eliminating many manufactured foods with soy as an ingredient will have an impact on the variety of manufactured products available to those with soy allergy. Studies show that the vast majority of soy-allergic individuals can tolerate soy oil and soy lecithin.[17] Highly refined soy oil is exempt from allergen labeling in the USA, but soy lecithin is not.[40] Products that contain soy lecithin, with a 'contains soy' statement, may in fact be safe for consumption by many soy-allergic consumers. Families should never assume that a product is safe without first calling the manufacturer to determine if any soy ingredient other than soy lecithin is contained in the product.

While soy itself is a nutritionally dense food, it generally is not a major component of the diet, and therefore the nutrients lost due to soy elimination may easily be replaced. If there are other food allergies or dietary patterns such as vegetarianism, then the child with soy allergy may be at nutritional risk.

Peanut Allergy

Recent studies have indicated that the prevalence of peanut allergy has doubled among children less than 5 years of age in the last decade.[15,41] Avoidance of peanuts and tree nuts in the diet does not necessarily pose any specific nutritional risk when there are no other nutritional risk factors.

Approximately 20% of young children with peanut allergy may eventually develop clinical tolerance.[41] Children with a peanut allergy are at greater risk for tree nut allergies. In fact, about 35% of those allergic to peanut will react to at least one tree nut although these two foods are botanically different, peanut being a legume rather than a nut.[39] Cross-reactivity between peanuts and legumes is rare with only 5% of those with a peanut hypersensitivity reacting to another legume.[39] The legume, lupine, appears to be an exception. Moneraet-Vautrin and colleagues reported that 44% of those allergic to peanut have a positive prick skin test response to lupine.[13] Of those with a positive prick skin test, 7 out of 8 who were challenged were clinically reactive to lupine flour.[13] In recognition of the risk of cross-reactivity with peanut, the EU has included lupine as a major allergen, with products containing lupine or its derivatives requiring full discloser on EU product labels. Lupine is not, however, considered a major allergen in the USA.

Introducing Complementary Foods to Children with Food Allergies

Exclusive breast-feeding is the optimal source of nutrition for infants up to 4 to 6 months of age. Further recommendations on feeding choices in early infancy (4–6 months of age) are discussed in Chapter 47. There is currently no convincing evidence that delaying introduction of complementary solid foods beyond 4 to 6 months of age has a significant protective effect on the development of atopic disease.[38]

Complementary feeding refers to the addition of solid pureed foods to supplement breast- or formula-feeding. An expert panel from the European Academy of Allergology and Clinical Immunology as well as the American Academy of Pediatrics, Committee on Nutrition recommend delayed introduction of complementary, solid pureed foods until 4 to 6 months of age.[38] The timing of introducing solid feedings between 4 to 6 months of age depends on developmental readiness. The infant should have sufficient head, neck and postural strength to be able to sit with assistance. Additionally, infants should be able to indicate their readiness to feed by leaning forward and opening their mouths to accept the spoon as well as indicate satiety or lack of interest by turning the head. Developmental readiness should determine when infants between 4 to 6 months of age begin complementary feedings.

For children with a diagnosed food allergy, a modified schedule of food introduction may be warranted. Single-ingredient foods should be offered first, with 5 to 7 days between each new food introduced to permit association of the new food to any presenting allergic symptom. Selection of foods may be individualized based on the child's allergic history. Generally, infant grains (rice or oat) are a good first choice because fortified infant cereals are a good source of additional iron and infants who are exclusively breastfed may need additional iron sources at this age. Orange vegetables (squash, sweet potato, and carrots) followed by fruits (apple, pear, banana, plum, peach, and apricot) can be introduced next. Green vegetables (spinach, peas, and green beans) may be added, followed by additional grains (barley and wheat) and then meats (lamb, pork, turkey, chicken, and beef). Families should be encouraged to continue to expand the variety of foods offered within the context of the allergen restricted diet.

Eating competence is a skill that must be acquired and exposure to foods of varying tastes and textures will provide valuable learning experiences for the new eater. The early weaning period, from 4 to 7 months of age, is believed to be crucial in determining taste preferences as children who are exposed to foods in this period can acquire a preference after as little as one exposure to the food.[42] However, in later childhood, 10 or more exposures might be necessary for a child to master or accept and enjoy the new food.[43] It appears there may be a window of enhanced acceptance in these early months, when taste preferences are more readily learned.[42,44] Limiting the provision of foods beyond those necessary, due to food allergies for otherwise healthy infants and toddlers, may inadvertently limit these crucial learning experiences.

The ability to eat foods of increased texture (progression from smooth puree to lumpy foods) is dependent on the development of oral motor skills and the experience of chewing.[44] There seems also to be an ideal window for the introduction of lumpy textured foods between the ages of 6 and 10 months as the most marked changes in the efficacy of chewing occurred between these ages, but only if the infant had experience of textured food in the mouth.[42]

For those children who are otherwise healthy, it appears that one key to the prevention of limited food acceptance in early childhood is encouraging a developmentally appropriate variety of flavors and textures. Unfortunately, for many families with a child who has experienced a food-allergic reaction, offering a variety of foods can be frightening and there may be an inclination to limit the selection of foods to those that have been tolerated in the past.

When the diet is limited due to food allergies, encouraging the family to offer whatever variety is available will help the child master basic eating skills and acquire eating competence, which will inevitably lead to improved nutritional status. For instance, an infant with cow's milk allergy can still tolerate a wide variety of fruits, vegetables, meats and grains. Even a child with multiple food allergies can be offered a variety of flavors and textures with some planning. (See Box 52-1.) For instance, a patient allergic to milk, egg, wheat and soy will have many limitations but can still eat a wide range of meats, alternative grains and fruits and vegetables, all served in a variety of ways, in addition to a 'milk' substitute or commercial hypoallergenic formula. Meats can be stewed, broiled, grilled or baked. Homemade meatballs, meatloaf and chicken fingers made with allowed ingredients (alternative flours and egg replacers) are simple to prepare and provide. A variety of items can be made or purchased with alternative grains, such as pasta, pancakes, muffins, cookies, pretzels, breads, and crackers, hot and cold cereals. Offering fruits and vegetables with each meal will help children acquire a taste for their flavors and textures. Encouraging the family to balance the provision of safe foods with a variety of developmentally appropriate foods

will help the child to become a competent eater and allow even a food elimination diet, with appropriate substitutions, to provide adequate nutrition. Delaying the introduction of foods beyond those necessary to avoid due to the allergen restriction may contribute to a limited variety of accepted foods and potentially place the child on a food elimination diet at further nutritional risk.

Oral Food Challenges

A food-allergic child may undergo a food challenge to identify or confirm the presence of reactivity to a suspected food or to determine if clinical tolerance to a particular food has been acquired. An oral food challenge is not always part of the initial diagnostic process and is contraindicated when a recent history of anaphylaxis has occurred.[45,46]

During the physician-supervised oral food challenge, the challenge food or placebo is administered in small incremental doses and gradually increased to the full test dose. The patient is observed for symptoms during the procedure and for a period of time after the full test dose is administered. Although challenges can be open, single-blind, or double-blind, the double-blind, placebo-controlled food challenge (DBPCFC) is the preferred method and is considered to be the 'gold standard' for food allergy testing. Regardless of the type of food challenge, emergency medications should be available and an emergency treatment protocol should be in place.[45,46]

An open challenge involves feeding the challenge food in its usual form without disguise. An open challenge is quick and easy but has the disadvantage of being prone to bias by the clinician, the patient and/or the patient's family. In a single-blind food challenge, the food is disguised for the patient, but not for the clinician. This type of challenge eliminates the possibility of patient bias, but not clinician bias. The DBPCFC removes any bias in the evaluation although it is very labor intensive. In the DBPCFC, both the placebo and the challenge food are disguised and neither the patient nor the clinician administering the test knows which food is the placebo and which is the challenge food. A negative blinded food challenge should be confirmed by an open challenge.[45,46]

In preparation for any food challenge, suspected allergens must be eliminated from the diet for a minimum of 7 to 14 days for IgE-mediated disorders and up to 6 to 8 weeks for eosinophilic disorders.[24] Chronic symptoms of allergic disease, such as asthma or atopic dermatitis, should be under control. The physician should review all medications taken by the patient, as medications such as antihistamines and those with antihistaminic activity have the ability to interfere with or block a reaction. These medications should be discontinued prior to the challenge with sufficient time to allow a normal histamine response. The challenge should be administered in a fasting state or with at least a 2 to 3 hours lapse since the last food or drink.[45,46]

The challenge food may be disguised in a second food, but this challenge vehicle should not be too heavy and should not contain significant fat as it may interfere with the absorption of the challenge protein. The challenge vehicle must also be free of the patient's allergens and without risk of cross-contact with any of the patient's allergens. Challenge vehicles are chosen to mask the taste, odor, texture or color of the challenge food. The choice of vehicle may be limited to what the child is able or willing to eat. Taking into consideration the child's food preferences is important and may determine the successful administration of the challenge.[45] Sample challenge foods and vehicles can be found in Table 52.4.

Table 52-4 Foods and Vehicles Used in the Administration of Challenges

Food	Challenge Substance	Placebo Suggestions	Vehicles
Eggs	Pasteurized dehydrated egg whites	Corn starch, oat flour, white rice flour	Mashed potato, oatmeal, applesauce, milk-free chocolate pudding
Milk	Nonfat dry milk powder or Lactaid milk	Corn starch, white flour, white rice flour	Rice or soy milk, infant formulas, applesauce, milk-free chocolate pudding
Wheat	Arrowhead Mills white or whole-wheat flour	White rice flour, oat flour, barley flour	Applesauce, oatmeal, milk-free chocolate pudding
Soy	Arrowhead Mills soy flour, Isomil formula	White rice flour, corn flour, oat flour, safe formula	Applesauce, oatmeal, milk-free chocolate pudding, safe formula
Peanuts	Peanut flour, peanut butter, crushed peanut (mortar and pestle)	Grain flour, safe tree nut flour or soy nut butter	Oatmeal, tomato-based meatballs or meat patties, home-made chocolate (with added mint extract)
Tree nuts	Crushed suspected nut from the shell	Safe crushed nut from the shell, peanut butter	Peanut butter, milk-free chocolate pudding
Fish	Suspected fish	Safe fish or canned tuna	Safe fish patties, canned tuna
Shellfish	Suspected shellfish	Safe shellfish, canned tuna	Safe fish patties, canned tuna
Corn	Arrowhead Mills corn flour, corn grits	Rice flour, oat flour	Applesauce, oatmeal, milk-free chocolate pudding
Meats	Suspected meat	Safe meat	Meat patties

© 2009. The Food Allergy & Anaphylaxis Network. Used with permission.

The type of food-allergic disorder will determine how the food challenge is conducted. For IgE-mediated food hypersensitivities, 8–10 g of the challenge food or 16–20 g of wet food such as meat or fish will be prepared and mixed in the tolerated vehicle of choice. The challenge is administered with increasing doses of the test food over a 90-minute period. The physician may determine whether the patient may be challenged in the office setting or in the hospital setting. Regardless of the setting, the patient must be evaluated for the development of symptoms throughout the challenge by a board certified physician.[45,46]

For food protein induced enterocolitis syndrome (FPIES), a challenge should only take place in a hospital setting with a heparin lock in place due to the risk of hypotension in about 20% of these reactions. A challenge dose of 0.06–0.6 g of test food protein per kilogram of body weight is provided. The challenge is administered gradually over 30–45 minutes. If no symptoms occur within 3 hours, a full serving size of the challenge food is provided and the patient observed for a subsequent 2 to 3 hours. In the case of FPIES to grains with low protein content such as rice and oat, an age-appropriate serving of the food is measured and one third provided as the initial dose followed by the remaining two thirds of the dose if no reaction occurs within 3 hours.[45,46]

BOX 52-2

Key Food Allergy Management Points

- Provide comprehensive education on the scope of allergen elimination issues such as label reading, avoiding hidden sources of the allergen and cross contact risk. Allergen avoidance sheets are an excellent resource to begin educating families about allergen elimination.
- Provide education to help families manage daily living activities such as going to school or camp, eating in restaurants or friends' homes, shopping and cooking. The goal of education is to reduce the risk of accidental allergen exposure while empowering the family, and eventually the child, to participate in all daily living activities while avoiding the food to which they are allergic.
- Ensure that a nutrient-dense alternative food source is recommended to substitute for the nutrients lost to the elimination diet. Follow-up to ensure the alternative food has been accepted and incorporated into the diet is essential.
- Encourage the family to offer a variety of developmentally appropriate allergen-free foods of varying tastes and textures to help the child develop eating competence and allow even a food elimination diet, with appropriate substitutions, to provide adequate nutrition.
- Use of a complete, commercially available, hypoallergenic formula may be warranted, at least partially through the second year of life in children with milk or milk and soy allergy.
- Monitor growth as it is a sensitive indicator of the provision of adequate energy and protein in the diets of children. Refer for nutrition consultation at the first sign of growth faltering.
- Instruct the family on how to recognize and treat a food allergic reaction.
- Recommend that children with food allergy wear a medical alert bracelet or necklace.
- Instruct families to have their child's epinephrine auto-injector device prescribed by the physician immediately available at all times.
- Instruct families to seek medical help immediately by calling 911 or getting transportation to an emergency room if their child experiences a food allergic reaction, even if epinephrine has already been given.

For eosinophilic disorders, if the test food has never caused an immediate reaction and the patient has no evidence of IgE antibodies to the challenge food, the food may be reintroduced at home and consumed for about 7 days. It may take several days of consumption for symptoms to occur. Again the patient should be observed for symptoms and periodic endoscopy and biopsies are warranted to monitor the histological response to foods being introduced.[45,46]

For a comprehensive guide on physician-supervised food challenges, visit the Food Allergy and Anaphylaxis Network (FAAN) website at *www.foodallergy.org*. An excellent resource entitled, *A Health Professional's Guide to Food Challenges*, is available only to health professionals through this website.

Conclusions

Current treatment of food allergen entails complete dietary avoidance of the identified allergen requiring extensive education. (Box 52.2.) Allergen elimination diets should not be prescribed lightly and the global impact of these diets should be considered. While in theory, elimination of dietary allergens may seem an easy enough task, avoidance issues are complex and accidental ingestions are not uncommon. Hence, food allergy management must also include comprehensive education on how to recognize and treat a food-allergic reaction. This topic is discussed fully in Chapter 45.

References

1. Branum AM LS. Food allergy among U.S. children: trends in prevalence and hospitalizations. NCHS data brief, no 10. Hyattsville, MD: National Center for Health Statistics; 2008.
2. Nowak-Wegrzyn A. Immunotherapy for food allergy. Inflamm Allergy Drug Targets 2006;5:23–34.
3. Enrique E, Cistero-Bahima A. Specific immunotherapy for food allergy: basic principles and clinical aspects. Curr Opin Allergy Clin Immunol 2006;6:466–9.
4. Munoz-Furlong A. Daily coping strategies for patients and their families. Pediatrics 2003;111(6 Pt 3):1654–61.
5. Carvalho NF, Kenney RD, Carrington PH, et al. Severe nutritional deficiencies in toddlers resulting from health food milk alternatives. Pediatrics 2001;107:E46.
6. Christie L, Hine RJ, Parker JG, et al. Food allergies in children affect nutrient intake and growth. J Am Diet Assoc 2002;102:1648–51.
7. Henriksen C, Eggesbo M, Halvorsen R, et al. Nutrient intake among two-year-old children on cows' milk-restricted diets. Acta Paediatr 2000;89:272–8.
8. Isolauri E, Sutas Y, Salo MK, et al. Elimination diet in cow's milk allergy: risk for impaired growth in young children. J Pediatr 1998;132:1004–9.
9. Noimark L, Cox HE. Nutritional problems related to food allergy in childhood. Pediatr Allergy Immunol 2008;19:188–95.
10. Salman S, Christie L, Burks AW. Dietary intakes of children with food allergies: comparison of the Food Guide Pyramid and the Recommended Dietary Allowances, 10th edition. J Allergy Clin Immunol 2002;109:S214.
11. Taylor SL, Hefle SL. Food allergen labeling in the USA and Europe. Curr Opin Allergy Clin Immunol 2006;6:186–90.
12. MacDonald A. Better European food labelling laws to help people with food intolerances. Matern Child Nutr 2005;1:223–4.
13. Moneret-Vautrin DA, Guerin L, Kanny G, et al. Cross-allergenicity of peanut and lupine: the risk of lupine allergy in patients allergic to peanuts. J Allergy Clin Immunol 1999;104(4 Pt 1):883–8.
14. Food Allergen Consumer Protection Act of 2004. Available at: www.cfsan.fda.gov.
15. Sampson HA. Update on food allergy. J Allergy Clin Immunol 2004;113:805–19; quiz 820.
16. Crevel RWR, Kerkhoff MAT, Konig MMG. Allergenicity of refined vegetable oils. Food Chem Toxicol 2000;38:385–93.
17. Taylor SL, Hefle SL, Bindslev-Jensen C, et al. Factors affecting the determination of threshold doses for allergenic foods: how much is too much? J Allergy Clin Immunol 2002;109:24–30.
18. Hefle SL, Furlong TJ, Niemann L, et al. Consumer attitudes and risks associated with packaged foods having advisory labeling regarding the presence of peanuts. J Allergy Clin Immunol 2007;120:171–6.
19. Cohen BL, Noone S, Munoz-Furlong A, et al. Development of a questionnaire to measure quality of life in families with a child with food allergy. J Allergy Clin Immunol 2004;114:1159–63.
20. Furlong TJ, DeSimone J, Sicherer SH. Peanut and tree nut allergic reactions in restaurants and other food establishments. J Allergy Clin Immunol 2001;108:867–70.
21. Mofidi S. Nutritional management of pediatric food hypersensitivity. Pediatrics 2003;111(6 Pt 3):1645–53.
22. Jensen VB, Jorgensen IM, Rasmussen KB, et al. Bone mineral status in children with cow milk allergy. Pediatr Allergy Immunol 2004;15:562–5.
23. Chehade M, Sampson HA. Epidemiology and etiology of eosinophilic esophagitis. Gastrointest Endosc Clin N Am 2008;18:33–44; viii.
24. Spergel JM, Shuker M. Nutritional management of eosinophilic esophagitis. Gastrointest Endosc Clin N Am 2008;18:179–94; xi.
25. Pentiuk SP, Miller CK, Kaul A. Eosinophilic esophagitis in infants and toddlers. Dysphagia 2006; E published 6 Oct.
26. Kuszmarski RJ, Ogden CL, Guo SS, et al. Growth charts for the United States: methods and development. Vital Health Statistics 2002;290:1–190.
27. Fishbein M, Cox S, Swenny C, et al. Food chaining: a systematic approach for the treatment of children with feeding aversion. Nutr Clin Pract 2006;21:182–4.
28. Satter E. Eating competence: definition and evidence for the Satter Eating Competence model. J Nutr Educ Behav 2007;39(5 Suppl):S142–53.
29. Bernard-Bonnin AC. Feeding problems of infants and toddlers. Can Fam Physician 2006;52:1247–51.
30. Trumbo P, Schlicker S, Yates AA, et al. Dietary reference intakes for energy, carbohydrate, fiber, fat, fatty acids, cholesterol, protein and amino acids. J Am Diet Assoc 2002;102:1621–30.
31. Kagalwalla AF, Sentongo TA, Ritz S, et al. Effect of six-food elimination diet on clinical and histologic outcomes in eosinophilic esophagitis. Clin Gastroenterol Hepatol 2006;4:1097–102.
32. Sicherer SH, Sampson HA. 9. Food allergy. J Allergy Clin Immunol 2006;117(2 Suppl Mini-Primer):S470–5.
33. Host A. Frequency of cow's milk allergy in childhood. Ann Allergy Asthma Immunol 2002;89(6 Suppl 1):33–7.
34. Skripak JM, Matsui EC, Mudd K, et al. The natural history of IgE-mediated cow's milk allergy. J Allergy Clin Immunol 2007;120:1172–7.
35. Committee on Nutrition. American Academy of Pediatrics: hypoallergenic infant formulas. Pediatrics 2000;106:346–9.
36. Mannion CA, Gray-Donald K, Johnson-Down L, et al. Lactating women restricting milk are low on select nutrients. J Am Coll Nutr 2007;26:149–55.
37. Wagner CL, Greer FR, American Academy of Pediatrics Section on Breastfeeding, American Academy of Pediatrics Committee on Nutrition. Prevention of rickets and vitamin D deficiency in infants, children, and adolescents. Pediatrics 2008;122:1142–52.
38. Greer FR, Sicherer SH, Burks AW, et al. Effects of early nutritional interventions on the development of atopic disease in infants and children: the role of maternal dietary restriction, breastfeeding, timing of introduction of complementary foods, and hydrolyzed formulas. Pediatrics 2008;121:183–91.
39. Sicherer SH. Clinical implications of cross-reactive food allergens. J Allergy Clin Immunol 2001;108:881–90.
40. Guidance for Industry: Questions and Answers Regarding Food Allergens including the Food Allergen Labeling and Consumer Protection Act of 2004 (Edition 4); Final Guidance. October 2006. www.cfsan.fda.gov/guidance.html.
41. Sicherer SH. Clinical update on peanut allergy. Ann Allergy Asthma Immunol 2002;88:350–61; quiz 361–2, 394.
42. Coulthard H, Harris G, Emmett P. Delayed introduction of lumpy foods to children during the complementary feeding period affects child's food acceptance and feeding at 7 years of age. Matern Child Nutr 2009;5:75–85.
43. Carruth BR, Ziegler PJ, Gordon A, et al. Prevalence of picky eaters among infants and toddlers and their caregivers' decisions about offering a new food. J Am Diet Assoc 2004;104(1 Suppl 1):s57–64.
44. Carruth BR, Skinner JD. Revisiting the picky eater phenomenon: neophobic behaviors of young children. J Am Coll Nutr 2000;19:771–80.
45. A health professional's guide to food challenges; The Food Allergy & Anaphylaxis Network.
46. Nowak-Wegrzyn A, Assa'ad AH, Bahna SL, et al. Work Group report: oral food challenge testing. J Allergy Clin Immunol 2009;123(6 Suppl):S365–83.

53

Role of Barrier Dysfunction and Immune Response in Atopic Dermatitis

Natalija Novak • Donald Y. M. Leung

Atopic dermatitis (AD) is a highly pruritic chronic inflammatory skin disease that commonly presents during early childhood.[1] It is frequently associated with a personal or family history of respiratory allergy, i.e. allergic asthma and/or rhinitis, and can have profound effects on quality of life.[2] Recent interest in AD has been sparked by reports of its increasing prevalence.[3] Management approaches in AD have evolved from our rapidly growing understanding of the mechanisms underlying this skin disease and novel therapeutic avenues.

Epidemiology

AD is a common skin disease with a lifetime prevalence in children of 10–20% in the USA, Northern and Western Europe, Japan, and other westernized countries.[4] A study in Portland found that 17% of school-aged children had AD.[5] This represents the culmination of a 2-fold to 3-fold increase in the prevalence of AD since the 1970s. Interestingly, the prevalence of AD is much lower in countries with large agricultural areas, such as rural China, Eastern Europe, and Africa.

Wide variations in prevalence have been observed among similar ethnic groups of common genetic background, suggesting that environmental factors are critical in determining disease expression.[6] Some of the potential risk factors that have received attention include small family size, increased income and education, migration from rural to urban environments, and increased use of antibiotics, that is, the so-called 'Western Lifestyle'. These observations are supported by studies demonstrating that allergic responses are driven by T helper cell type 2 (Th2) immune responses, whereas infections are induced by Th1 immune responses.[7] Since Th1 responses antagonize the development of Th2 cells, a decreased number of infections or the lack of Th1 polarizing signals (such as endotoxin) during early childhood could predispose to enhanced Th2 allergic responses (see Chapters 1 and 2).

Diagnosis and Differential Diagnosis

Clinical features of AD are listed in Box 53-1.[8] Of the major features, pruritus and chronic or relapsing eczematous dermatitis with typical distribution are essential for diagnosis.[9] Intense pruritus and cutaneous reactivity are cardinal features of AD. Pruritus may be intermittent throughout the day but is usually worse at night. Its consequences are scratching, prurigo papules,

lichenification, and eczematous skin lesions. Patients with AD have a reduced threshold for pruritus. As a result, allergens, reduced humidity, excessive sweating, and low concentrations of irritants (e.g. wool, acrylic, soaps, and detergents) can exacerbate itching and scratching.

During infancy AD is generally more acute with excoriation, vesicles over erythematous skin, and serous exudates. The rash primarily involves the face, scalp, and the extensor surfaces of the extremities (Figure 53-1); the diaper area is usually spared. In older children and in those who have long-standing skin disease, the patient develops chronic AD with lichenification (Figure 53-2) and localization of the rash to the flexural folds of the extremities. AD often subsides as the patient grows older; leaving an adult with skin that is prone to itching and inflammation when exposed to exogenous irritants. At all stages of AD, patients usually have dry, lackluster skin. Chronic hand eczema, the most common form of occupational skin disease, may be the primary manifestation of many adults with AD. Other features, including exogenous allergy or elevated immunoglobulin E (IgE), are variable although commonly seen in AD.

A number of inflammatory skin diseases, immunodeficiencies, skin malignancies, genetic disorders, infectious diseases, and infestations share symptoms and signs with AD. These should be considered and ruled out before a diagnosis of AD is made. Infants presenting in the first year of life with failure to thrive, diarrhea, a generalized scaling erythematous rash, and recurrent cutaneous and/or systemic infections should be evaluated for severe combined immunodeficiency syndrome (see Chapter 9). Wiskott-Aldrich syndrome is an X-linked recessive disorder characterized by thrombocytopenia, abnormalities in humoral and cellular immunity, and recurrent severe bacterial infections. It is associated with cutaneous findings almost indistinguishable from AD. Hyperimmunoglobulin-E syndrome is characterized by elevated serum IgE levels, defective T and B cell function, recurrent deep-seated bacterial infections including cutaneous abscesses caused by *Staphylococcus aureus* (*S. aureus*) and/or pruritic skin disease caused by *S. aureus* pustulosis, or recalcitrant dermatophytosis. Eczema has been reported with human immunodeficiency virus infection. Other conditions that can be confused with AD include psoriasis, ichthyosis, and seborrheic dermatitis.

Adolescents who present with an eczematous dermatitis, with no history of childhood eczema, respiratory allergy, or atopic family history, may have allergic contact dermatitis (see Chapter 56). A contact allergen should be considered in any patient whose AD does not respond to appropriate therapy. Of note, topical

©2010 Elsevier Ltd, Inc, BV
DOI: 10.1016/B978-1-4377-0271-2.00053-5

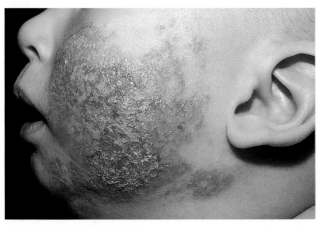

Figure 53-1 Infant with acute atopic dermatitis. Note the oozing and crusting skin lesions. (From Weston WL, Morelli JG, Lane A, eds. Color textbook of pediatric dermatology, 3rd edn. St Louis: Mosby; 2002.)

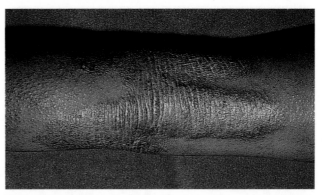

Figure 53-2 Adolescent with lichenification of the popliteal fossa from chronic atopic dermatitis. (From Weston WL, Morelli JG, Lane A, eds. Color textbook of pediatric dermatology, 3rd edn. St Louis: Mosby; 2002.)

BOX 53-1

Clinical Features of Atopic Dermatitis*

Essential Features

- Pruritus
- Facial and extensor eczema in infants and children
- Flexural eczema in adults
- Chronic or relapsing dermatitis

Frequently Associated Features

- Personal or family history of atopic disease
- Xerosis
- Cutaneous infections
- Nonspecific dermatitis of the hands or feet
- Elevated serum IgE levels
- Positive immediate-type allergy skin tests
- Early age of onset

Other Features

- Ichthyosis, palmar hyperlinearity, keratosis pilaris
- Pityriasis alba
- Nipple eczema
- White dermatographism and delayed blanch response
- Anterior subcapsular cataracts, keratoconus
- Dennie-Morgan infraorbital folds, orbital darkening
- Facial erythema or pallor
- Perifollicular accentuation

*Other skin conditions that may mimic atopic dermatitis should be excluded.

---

glucocorticoid contact allergy has been reported increasingly in patients with chronic dermatitis on topical corticosteroid therapy.

Pathogenesis

Interactions between susceptibility genes, the host's environment, and immunologic factors contribute to the pathogenesis of AD. There are two primary disease models: first, AD as a skin disease, which primarily develops from intrinsic defects of epithelial cells and the skin barrier, resulting in numerous abnormalities of the innate and adaptive immunity ('outside-inside'

hypothesis; see Figure 53-3); second, that AD is primarily an immunologic disease with mechanisms related to overactivation of the immune system and Th2-dominated immune responses that impact on skin barrier function secondarily ('inside-outside' hypothesis; see Figure 53-4).[10] It is likely that the combination of a continuous interplay between both hypotheses best explains the complexity of AD.

Genetics

The fact that AD frequently affects more than one family member is consistent with the strong genetic background of this disease.[11,12] Several genetic factors contribute to the complex pathophysiology of AD, indicating that it is not a monogenic but genetically complex disorder.[13,14] It seems most likely that not only AD itself, but different subtypes of AD, such as AD with early onset, childhood AD as compared to adulthood AD, or AD with IgE-mediated allergic reactions, might be based on distinct genetic constellations.[15-19] Therefore, one approach to distinguishing these subtypes could be systematic genetic typing according to variants associated with (1) skin barrier dysfunction, (2) deficient innate immune responses and (3) abnormal adaptive immune reactions in AD.[20]

Genetics and Skin Barrier Dysfunction

Dry skin, mirrored by increased transepidermal water loss, reduced skin hydration, and decreased amounts of natural moisturizing factors, supports a skin barrier impairment in AD.[21,22] A candidate gene region for AD, localized on chromosome 1q21,[13] contains a cluster of genes encoding structural proteins of the epidermal cornification, including S100A proteins, profilaggrin, small proline-rich region proteins (SPRRs) and late envelope proteins (LEP). These form the so-called 'epidermal differentiation complex' (EDC). Filaggrin is a particularly important protein essential to maintaining the formation of the stratum corneum barrier.[23] During the last 2 years, loss-of-function mutations in the filaggrin gene have been shown to be strongly associated with AD. This finding has been replicated and confirmed by a large number of independent studies.[24,25] Moreover, a closer look at the filaggrin loss-of-function carriers within the group of AD patients revealed specific clinical features and subforms of AD that were highly associated. These included AD with early onset and a high level of allergen sensitization.[26,27] Furthermore, specific interactions between genetic predisposition and environmental factors, such as cat exposure at the time of birth, seem to

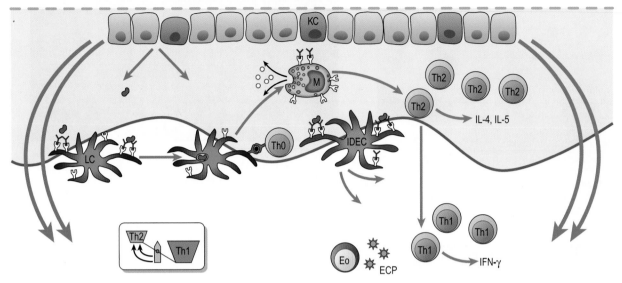

Figure 53-3 The 'outside-inside' paradigm. AD is primarily a skin disease driven by an intrinsic epidermal defect.

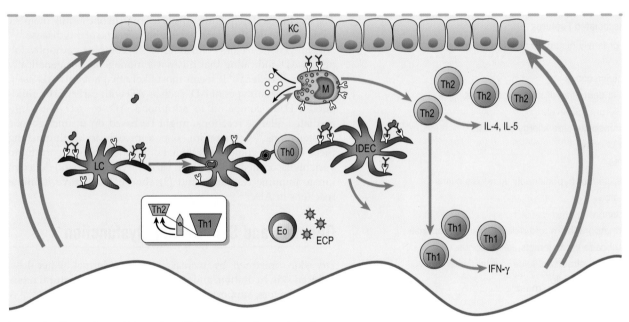

Figure 53-4 The 'inside-outside' paradigm. AD is primarily an immunologic disease.

increase the risk for the manifestation of eczema during the first year of life, especially in children with filaggrin mutations.[28] Interestingly, in the context of genetically mediated skin barrier dysfunction in AD, there have been reports of associations of gene polymorphisms in the SPINK5 gene, which encodes the lymphoepithelial kazal-type related inhibitor (LEKTI), an inhibitor of serine proteases.[29] Studies have also reported associations of gene variants encoding the stratum corneum chymotryptic enzyme (SCCE) with AD, leading to impaired stratum corneum integrity and function.[30] Other studies have reported gene associations for other epidermal components, such as collagen 29 (COL29),[31] or a genetic variant on chromosome 11q13.[32] Aside from these genetically predetermined factors, highly active

endogenous proteases, such as SCCE or mast cell chymase (MCC), as well as exogenous proteases derived from house dust mite allergens or *S. aureus*, cleave corneodesmosomes and accelerate desquamation of corneocytes.[33] Binding of proteinase-activated receptors (PAR)-2 by exogenous proteases delays epithelial regeneration and further contributes to skin barrier impairment in AD.[34]

Genetics and Innate Immunity

First-line host defense by the innate immune system requires intact pattern-recognition receptors (PRR), which sense the environment for invading pathogens.[35,36] Toll-like receptors (TLRs), intracellular nucleotide-binding oligomerization domain (NOD) proteins, or the LPS receptor CD14[37,38] belonging to the PPRs, discriminate between diverse pathogen-associated molecular patterns (PAMP). Deficient maturation of the immune system, as well as reduced responsiveness to PRR stimulation, are postulated to account for a higher prevalence of atopy, and a profound increase in propensity of AD patients to microbial infections.[39] Several studies have focused on the putative association between genetic variations within gene regions encoding components of the innate immune system and AD. A polymorphism within the TLR2 gene has been shown to be associated with severe forms of AD prone to recurrent bacterial infections,[40] and has been linked to functional modifications of TLR2 protein.[41] By contrast, no association of polymorphisms in the TLR2, TLR4 and TLR6 gene with AD could be shown in other studies.[42,43] Moreover, a polymorphism in the TLR9 gene with putative functional effects on TLR9 promoter activity was associated with AD.[44]

Genetics and Adaptive Immunity

Induction of different receptors on effector cells, dendritic cells (DCs), or other cells in the skin after exposure to allergens and microbial pathogens, contributes to various mechanisms involving the adaptive immune system. A wide repertoire of modifications to gene regions encoding components of adaptive immunity has been associated with AD to date.[14,45,46] Soluble factors, such as cytokines and chemokines, which play a crucial role as soluble mediators of the adaptive immune system, show profound variations in AD; it is likely that some of these deviations are already genetically encoded.[47] These comprise genetic variations on chromosome 5q31-33, which cover genes of the Th2 cytokine cluster, such as interleukin (IL)-3; IL-4, IL-5, IL-13, granulocyte-macrophage colony-stimulating factor (GM-CSF),[14,15] functional mutations of the promoter region of RANTES/CCL5 (17q11) and gain-of-function polymorphisms in the IL4RA gene (16q12).[14,15,48,49] Interestingly, polymorphisms in the IL4RA gene region were associated with AD with low IgE serum levels and no allergen sensitization.[48] Beyond this, polymorphisms in the IL18 gene associated with AD might contribute to modified IL-18 production of peripheral blood mononuclear cells (PBMC) of patients with AD after stimulation with microbial components.[50]

A significant association between a specific polymorphism in the mast cell chymase gene and AD has been identified that has no association with asthma or allergic rhinitis.[51] This finding suggests that a genetic variant of mast cell chymase, which is a serine protease secreted by skin mast cells, may have organ-specific effects that contribute to the genetic susceptibility for AD. AD has also been associated with a low-producer of transforming growth factor beta (TGF-β) cytokine genotype.[52] Because TGF-β is an important regulatory gene that down-regulates T cell activation, a low production genotype may contribute to increased skin inflammation. Finally, a genome-wide linkage study[16] suggested linkage for AD on chromosome 3q21, a region that encodes the costimulatory molecules CD80 and CD86.

Systemic Immune Response

Most patients with AD have peripheral blood eosinophilia and increased serum IgE levels.[53] Nearly 80% of children with AD develop allergic rhinitis or asthma. Serum IgE level is strongly associated with the prevalence of asthma, which suggests that allergen sensitization through the skin predisposes the patient to respiratory disease because of its effects on the systemic allergic response.[54] Indeed, when mice are sensitized epicutaneously with protein antigen, it induces allergic dermatitis, elevated serum IgE, airway eosinophilia, and hyperresponsiveness to methacholine. This suggests that epicutaneous exposure to allergen in AD enhances the development of allergic asthma.[55]

An increased frequency of skin-homing T cells producing IL-4, IL-5, and IL-13 but little interferon-gamma (IFN-γ) has been found in the peripheral blood of patients with AD.[56] There is evidence that this predominance of Th2 cells results partially from selective apoptosis of circulating memory/effector Th1 cells.[57] These immunologic alterations are important because IL-4 and IL-13 are the only cytokines that induce germline transcription at the Cε exon, thereby promoting isotype switching to IgE. IL-4 and IL-13 also induce the expression of vascular adhesion molecules, such as vascular cell adhesion molecule-1 involved in eosinophil infiltration, and down-regulate Th1-type cytokine activity. IL-5 plays a key role in the development, activation, and cell survival of eosinophils. In contrast, IFN-γ inhibits IgE synthesis as well as the proliferation of Th2 cells and expression of the IL-4 receptor on T cells. The decreased IFN-γ produced by T cells from AD patients may be the result of reduced production of IL-18.[58] Furthermore, an inverse relationship between skin colonization with *S. aureus* and spontaneous IFN-γ production of CD4+ T cells, as well as induced IFN-γ production of CD8+ T cells, has been observed.[59] Cytotoxic T cells have also been found to be depleted in AD, and an inverse relationship between the SCORAD and the CD4/CD8 ratio has been shown in one study conducted in children with AD.[60,61]

A number of determinants support Th2 cell development in AD. These include the cytokine milieu required for T cell development, pharmacologic factors, the costimulatory signals used during T cell activation, and the antigen-presenting cells (APCs).[54] In this regard, IL-4 promotes Th2 cell development, whereas IL-12, produced by macrophages, dendritic cells, or eosinophils, induces Th1 cells. Mononuclear cells from patients with AD have increased cyclic adenosine monophosphate (cAMP)-phosphodiesterase (PDE) enzyme activity.[62] This cellular abnormality contributes to the increased IgE synthesis by B cells and IL-4 production by T cells in AD as IgE and IL-4 production is decreased in vitro by PDE inhibitors.

Activation of resting T cells following engagement of T cell receptors with the MHC plus peptide complex on APCs requires costimulatory signals, for example, interactions between CD80 or CD86 on APCs and CD28 on T cells. The expression of the costimulatory molecule, CD86, on B cells of AD patients is significantly higher than in normal patients or patients with psoriasis.[63] Importantly, total serum IgE from AD patients and normal subjects correlated significantly with CD86 expression on B cells. Antihuman CD86, but not CD80 mAb, significantly decreased IgE production by peripheral blood mononuclear cells stimulated with IL-4 and anti-CD40 mAb. These data support the concept that CD86 expression in AD promotes IgE synthesis. IL-4 and IL-13 have also been found to induce CD86 expression on B cells, thereby providing an amplification loop for IgE synthesis in AD.

Skin Immunopathology

Pathology

Clinically unaffected skin of AD patients exhibits mild epidermal hyperplasia and a sparse perivascular T cell infiltrate.[64] Increased transepidermal water loss and reduced skin hydration is detectable even in nonlesional AD skin.[65] AD has a biphasic nature characterized by an acute phase, which is predominated by

Th2 cytokines, followed by a chronic phase, featuring Th1 cytokines.[66,67] Acute eczematous skin lesions are characterized by marked intercellular edema (spongiosis) of the epidermis. Dendritic APCs, such as Langerhans cells (LC) and macrophages in lesional, as well as nonlesional, skin of AD patients have surface-bound IgE molecules. Within 24 to 48 hours, a rapid influx of IgE-receptor bearing inflammatory dendritic epidermal cells (IDEC) and up-regulation of the high-affinity IgE receptor (FcεRI) expression after allergen application is detectable in the epidermis of atopy patch test lesions.[68] In the dermis of the acute lesion there is a marked perivenular T cell infiltrate with occasional monocyte-macrophages. The critical role of T cells in AD is suggested by the obligate role of T cells in mouse models of AD.[69] The lymphocytic infiltrate consists predominantly of activated memory T cells bearing CD3, CD4, and CD45RO, suggesting a previous encounter with antigen.

Chronic lichenified lesions are characterized by a hyperplastic epidermis with elongation of the rete ridges, prominent hyperkeratosis, and minimal spongiosis. There is an increased number of IgE-bearing DCs in the epidermis, and macrophages dominate the dermal mononuclear cell infiltrate. Mast cell numbers are increased, but they are typically fully granulated. Increased numbers of eosinophils are observed in chronic AD skin lesions. Eosinophils secrete cytokines and mediators that augment allergic inflammation and induce tissue injury in AD through the production of reactive oxygen intermediates and release of toxic granule proteins.

After topical treatment with calcineurin inhibitors, there is reduced infiltration of T cells and eosinophils, as well as decreased expression of Th2 cytokines.[70,71] Furthermore, surface expression of FcεRI epidermal DCs and the number of epidermal inflammatory DC subtypes decreased, while frequency of LCs increased.[72,73]

Cytokine Expression

Th2- and Th1-type cytokines contribute to the pathogenesis of skin inflammation in AD. Compared with the skin of normal controls, unaffected skin of AD patients has an increased number of cells expressing IL-4 and IL-13, but not IL-5, IL-12, or IFN-γ, mRNA.[64,74] Acute and chronic skin lesions, when compared to normal skin or uninvolved skin of AD patients, have significantly greater numbers of cells that are positive for IL-4, IL-5, and IL-13 mRNA. However, acute AD is not characterized by significant numbers of IFN-γ or IL-12 mRNA-expressing cells.

Chronic AD skin lesions have significantly fewer IL-4 and IL-13 mRNA-expressing cells, but greater numbers of IL-5, granulocyte-macrophage colony-stimulating factor (GM-CSF), IL-12, and IFN-γ mRNA-expressing cells than acute AD. IL-5 and GM-CSF probably contribute to the increased numbers of eosinophils and macrophages. The increased expression of IL-12 in chronic AD skin lesions is of interest because cytokine plays a key role in IFN-γ induction. Its expression in eosinophils and/or macrophages may initiate the switch to Th1 or Th0 cell development in chronic AD.

Activated T cells infiltrating the skin of AD patients have also been found to induce keratinocyte apoptosis, which contributes to the spongiotic process in AD skin lesions.[75] This process is mediated by IFN-γ, which up-regulates Fas on keratinocytes. The lethal hit is delivered to keratinocytes by Fas-ligand expressed on the surface of T cells that invade the epidermis and soluble Fas-ligand released from T cells. Additionally, there is some evidence that caspase-3 cleavage in the spinous epidermal layer contributes to spongiosis as well.[76] The role of regulatory T cell (T regs) subtypes in AD is still unclear. There is some evidence for functional deficiency of resident T regs in the skin,[77] while other studies report increased numbers of local CD4+CD25+Fox p 3+ T regs in patients with AD.[78] In addition, it has been demonstrated that activated CD25 expressing T cells with a phenotype of regulatory T cells, lacking CCR6 expression, promote Th2 immune responses in patients with AD.[79]

Antigen-presenting Cells

AD skin contains an increased number of IgE-bearing LCs, which appear to play an important role in cutaneous allergen presentation to Th2 cells.[80] Binding of IgE to LCs occurs primarily via high-affinity IgE receptors (FcεRI). The clinical importance of these IgE receptors on LCs is supported by the observation that the presence of FcεRI-expressing LCs bearing IgE molecules is required to provoke eczematous skin lesions by application of aeroallergens on uninvolved skin of AD patients. In contrast to mast cells and basophils where the FcεRI is a tetrameric structure constitutively expressed at high levels, this receptor on APCs consists of the α-chain, which binds IgE and γ-chain dimers containing an ITAM (immunoreceptor tyrosine-based activation motif) for downstream signaling, but lacks the classic beta chain.[81] It is thought that allergens which invade the skin are taken up by IgE molecules bound to FcεRI-expressing DCs. In the epidermis, FcεRI expression on DCs is related to the atopic state of the individual with higher expression in AD lesions as compared to nonlesional skin of AD patients or epidermal skin of nonatopic individuals.[82] Different FcεRI-bearing DC subtypes have been identified in lesional AD skin. CD207+/CD1a+, i.e. LCs, as well as CD207−/CD1a+/FcεRI+ DCs are located in the epidermis.[83] CD1c+/FcεRI+ DCs represent the major DC subpopulation of the dermal compartment, while low numbers of CD207+/FcεRI+/CD1a+ DCs are also detectable in the dermis.[84]

Myeloid Dendritic Cells (mDC) Contribute to Allergic Sensitization and Maintenance of Inflammation with Th2-Th1 Switch

LCs bearing FcεRI are the main myeloid DC population present in nonlesional AD skin, while upon allergen challenge and inflammation, FcεRI-bearing myeloid DCs, so called inflammatory dendritic epidermal cells (IDECs), are detectable in the epidermis.[82] After IgE binding and internalization of the allergen, LCs migrate to peripheral lymph nodes, present the processed allergen efficiently to naïve T cells, and initiate a Th2 immune response with sensitization to the antigen. The activated LCs can also present the allergen-derived peptides locally to transiting antigen-specific T cells and induce a T cell-mediated secondary immune response. Aggregation of FcεRI on the surface of LCs in vitro promotes the release of chemotactic factors, which in vivo is thought to contribute to the recruitment of IDECs into the epidermis. IDECs mainly present at inflammatory sites, produce high amounts of proinflammatory cytokines after FcεRI cross-linking, display a high stimulatory capacity towards T cells, and serve as amplifiers of the allergic inflammatory immune response.[85] Moreover, stimulation of FcεRI on the surface of IDEC induces the release of IL-12 and IL-18 and enhances the priming of naïve T cells into IFN-γ producing Th1 or Th0 cells. These mechanisms may contribute to the switch from the initial Th2 immune response in acute phase to the Th1 immune responses in the chronic phase.[85] Additionally, recent data provide evidence for an expression of functional HR4 receptor on IDECs in AD, with down-regulation of CCL2 and IL-12 production upon stimulation of HR4, implying that treatment of AD with HR4 agonists may have beneficial effects on skin inflammation.[86]

Plasmacytoid DC

Human plasmacytoid DCs (PDCs) are the only professional interferon (IFN)-producing cells. They express the IL-3 receptor α-chain (CD123) and the blood dendritic cell antigen (BDCA)-2.[87] Stimulation of PDCs with viral antigens induces the production of IFN-αβ, which is of crucial importance for the defense against viral infections. Human PDCs bear the PRRs TLR7 and TLR9 on their cell surface. Furthermore, they express the high affinity receptor for IgE (FcεRI).[88,89] Based on a close interaction of FcεRI with TLR9, the amount of IFN-α and IFN-β released in response to TLR9 stimulation is profoundly down-regulated in PDCs after FcεRI-aggregation and allergen challenge in vitro.[88,90,91] In view of frequent FcεRI aggregation induced by allergen challenge of PDCs of AD patients, this counterregulation might account for a profoundly reduced release of IFNs after viral antigen stimulation.

Furthermore, as compared to psoriasis, contact dermatitis or lupus erythematosis, the frequency of PDC in the lesional epidermal skin of AD is low,[92] although PDCs are recruited to the dermis during atopy patch test (APT).[67] This might result from Th2 cytokines or IL-10 in the skin micromilieu, leading to apoptosis of PDCs and, together with the counterregulation of FcεRI with TLRs, promote enhanced susceptibility of AD patients to viral skin infections.

Inflammatory Cell Infiltration

Several chemokines have been linked to recruitment of inflammatory cell subtypes such as DCs, T cells, and eosinophils into AD skin including CCL2, CCL3, CCL4, CCL5, CCL11, CCL13, CCL18, CCL20, CCL22, CCL26 and CCL27.[93] Moreover, serum levels of some of these chemokines correlate directly with disease activity[93] and decreased in response to successful topical treatment, as was shown for CCL5 and CCL11 after tacrolimus treatment.[94] A role of CCL18 in the amplification of allergic inflammation by increased homing of memory T cells has also been demonstrated.[95,96] Another chemokine, shown to be selectively up-regulated in AD was CCL1, the ligand to C-C chemokine receptor (CCR)8, which in vitro promoted the recruitment of T cells and Langerhans cell-like DCs.[97] IL-16, a chemoattractant for CD4+ T cells, is increased in acute AD skin lesions.[98,99] The C-C chemokines, RANTES/CCL5, monocyte chemotactic protein-4 (MCP-4/CCL13), and eotaxin/CCL11 have also been found to be increased in AD skin lesions and are likely to contribute to chemotaxis of eosinophils and Th2 lymphocytes into the skin.[100–102] A role for cutaneous T cell-attracting chemokine (CTACK/CCL27) in the preferential attraction of cutaneous lymphocyte antigen bearing (CLA+) T cells to the skin has been reported as well.[103] The chemokine receptor CCR3, which is found on eosinophils and Th2 lymphocytes, can mediate the action of eotaxin, RANTES, and MCP-4. CCR3 also has been reported to be increased in nonlesional and lesional skin of patients with AD.[101] Selective recruitment of CCR4-expressing Th2 cells into AD skin may also be mediated by the monocyte-derived chemokines and thymus- and activation-regulated chemokines, which are increased in AD.[104–106]

IL-31 is a novel cytokine, preferentially expressed by Th2 cells, which signals through a heterodimeric receptor composed of IL-31 receptor A and oncostatin M receptor.[107] Interestingly, up-regulated IL-31 expression has been observed in pruritic AD skin lesions[108] and was inducible by both in vitro staphylococcal enterotoxin B (SEB) stimulation of CLA+ T cells from AD patients, as well as application of SEB to the skin of AD patients in vivo.[107–109] Furthermore, IL-31 induced the expression of the inflammatory chemokines CCL1, CCL17 and CCL22 in keratinocytes.[110] IL-31 induces severe pruritus and dermatitis in transgenic mice[110] and the IL-31 receptor has shown greatest expression in dorsal root ganglia.[107] These findings provide a new link between staphylococcal colonization, subsequent T cell recruitment and activation, and pruritus induction in patients with AD.[107]

In terms of T cells infiltrating inflamed skin, it has been suggested that so-called Th17 cells may be of relevance, not only in psoriasis, but also in AD. Reports from animal models combined with studies using atopy patch tests or microarrays imply that Th17 may be induced in the skin by the topical application of allergens and may therefore promote skin inflammation in AD.[111–113] However, in comparison to psoriasis, Th17 plays most likely a rather minor role in AD skin.[114]

Intrinsic Defect of Keratinocytes in AD

Keratinocytes play an important role in the production of antimicrobial proteins and cytokines in response to stimulation by invading pathogens, mediating both innate and adaptive inflammatory immune reactions. AD keratinocytes also express high levels of the IL-7-like cytokine, thymic stromal lymphopoietin (TSLP), which activates myeloid dendritic cells (DCs) to promote T cell expression of IL-5 and IL-13.[115,116] Skin-specific overexpression of TSLP in a transgenic mouse resulted in an AD-like phenotype, with the development of eczematous lesions containing inflammatory dermal cellular infiltrates, an increase in Th2 CD4+T cells expressing cutaneous homing receptors, and elevated serum levels of IgE,[117] suggesting an important role of TSLP in AD.[118] DCs primed by TSLP may convert to strong inducers of T cell responses of the Th2 type in vitro,[119] so that enhanced TSLP release, triggered by frequent allergen challenge, microbial infections, and inflammation, might initiate and perpetuate Th2 immune responses in AD.

Chronic Skin Inflammation

Chronic AD is linked to the prolonged survival of eosinophils and monocyte-macrophages in atopic skin. IL-5 expression during chronic AD is likely to play a role in prolonging eosinophil survival and enhancement of their function. In chronic AD, the increased GM-CSF expression plays an important role in maintaining the survival and function of monocytes, LCs, and eosinophils.[120] Epidermal keratinocytes from AD patients have significantly higher levels of RANTES expression following stimulation with tumor necrosis factor (TNF)-α and IFN-γ than keratinocytes from psoriasis patients.[121] This may serve as one mechanism by which the TNF-α and IFN-γ production during chronic AD enhances the chronicity and severity of eczema. Mechanical trauma can also induce the release of TNF-α and many other proinflammatory cytokines from epidermal keratinocytes. Thus, chronic scratching plays a role in the perpetuation and elicitation of skin inflammation in AD.

Antimicrobial Peptides

The innate immune system provides a rapid host response to the invasion of microbes. Research results from recent years strongly suggest that impaired innate immune mechanisms might contribute to the susceptibility of AD patients to skin infections. These faulty mechanisms are characterized by a deficiency of antimicrobial peptides (AMPs), such as human cathelicidin LL-37, human beta-defensin (HBD)-2 and HBD-3, and dermicidin-derived antimicrobial proteins in sweat.[122] Defensins are broad-spectrum antibiotics that kill a wide variety of bacterial and fungal pathogens. Antimicrobial activity against viral pathogens is sustained by LL-37.[123] Efficient killing of *S. aureus* is achieved by LL-37 together with HBD2.[124,125] Since inflammatory mediators up-regulate AMP expression, increased amounts of AMP is characteristic of chronic inflammatory skin diseases such as psoriasis or contact dermatitis.[124] Conversely, only weak up-regulation of HBD2, 3 and LL-37 is detectable in both lesional and nonlesional skin of patients with AD.[125] Th2 cytokines, IL-4, IL-13, and IL-10, down-regulate AMP expression in vitro and might account for low AMP in AD skin.[122,126] Moreover, reduced mobilization of human HBD-3 accounts for defective killing of *S. aureus* in AD.[127] In addition to susceptibility to bacterial infections due to low HBD2, 3 and LL-37 expression, cathelicidin deficiency in AD might also predispose to severe viral infections such as eczema vaccinatum caused by orthopox virus[123,128] and eczema herpeticum (EH).[129] In support of this concept, lower levels of cathelicidin are detectable in skin lesions of AD patients with one or more episodes of EH in their history in comparison to AD patients without EH.[128] Dermicidin (DCD) is another recently discovered AMP with antibacterial and antimycotic properties, which is constitutively expressed[130] in human eccrine sweat glands. The amount of several DCD-derived peptides in sweat from AD patients was found to be significantly reduced in those patients with a history of bacterial and viral infections.[131] The low levels of DCD may act as another cause of higher susceptibility of AD patients to microbial infections. Interestingly, both incubation of keratinocytes with Vitamin D3 in vitro, as well as treatment of AD patients with oral Vitamin D3, increases cathelicidin production by keratinocytes, pointing to a novel therapeutic opportunity to improve innate immune responses in AD patients in the near future.[132-135]

Immunologic Triggers

Foods

Well-controlled studies have demonstrated that food allergens induce skin rashes in children with AD.[136] Based on double-blind, placebo-controlled food challenges, approximately 40% of infants and young children with moderate to severe AD have food allergy.[137,138] Food allergies in AD patients induce eczematous dermatitis and contribute to severity of skin disease in some patients,[139] whereas in others, urticarial reactions, contact urticaria, or other noncutaneous symptom complexes are elicited. Removal of food allergens from the patient's diet can lead to significant clinical improvement, but requires a great deal of education because most of the common allergens (e.g. egg, milk, wheat, soy, and peanut) contaminate many foods and are difficult to avoid.[140]

Infants and young children with food allergy generally have positive immediate skin tests or serum IgE directed to various foods. Positive food challenges are accompanied by significant increases in plasma histamine levels and eosinophil activation. Importantly, food allergen-specific T cells have been cloned from the skin lesions of patients with AD, providing direct evidence that foods can contribute to skin inflammation.[141] In mouse models of AD, oral sensitization with foods results in elicitation of eczematous skin lesions on repeat oral food challenges.[142] Immediate skin tests for specific allergens do not always indicate clinical sensitivity in patients. Therefore, clinically relevant food allergy must be verified by controlled food challenges or carefully investigating the effects of a food elimination diet, which is being done in the absence of other exacerbating factors.

Aeroallergens

A number of studies have demonstrated that pruritus and eczematoid skin lesions develop after intranasal or bronchial inhalation challenge with aeroallergens, but not placebo, in AD patients sensitized to inhalant allergens.[143] Epicutaneous application of aeroallergens by patch test techniques on uninvolved atopic skin elicits eczematoid reactions in 30–50% of patients with AD.[106] Positive reactions have been observed to dust mite, weeds, animal dander, and molds. In contrast, patients with respiratory allergy and healthy volunteers rarely have positive allergen patch tests.

Several studies have examined whether avoidance of aeroallergens results in clinical improvement of AD. Most of these reports have involved uncontrolled trials in which patients were placed in mite-free environments; for example, hospital rooms in which acaricides or impermeable mattress covers were used. Such methods have invariably led to improvement in AD. One double-blind, placebo-controlled study using a combination of effective mite-reduction measures, in comparison to no treatment, in the home has reported that a reduction in house dust mites is associated with significantly greater improvement in AD.[144-146]

Laboratory data supporting a role for inhalants include the finding of IgE antibody to specific inhalant allergens in most AD patients. A recent study found that 95% of sera from AD patients had IgE to house dust mites in comparison to 42% of asthmatic subjects.[147] The degree of sensitization to aeroallergens is directly associated with the severity of AD.[148] Isolation from AD skin lesions and allergen patch test sites of T cells that selectively respond to *D. pteronyssinus* (Der p 1) and other aeroallergens provides further evidence that the immune response in AD skin can be elicited by aeroallergens.[149]

Staphylococcus aureus

Patients with AD have an increased tendency to develop bacterial, viral and fungal skin infections. *S. aureus* is found in over 90% of AD skin lesions. The density of *S. aureus* on inflamed AD lesions without clinical superinfection can reach up to 10^7 colony-forming units per cm^2 on lesional skin. Pulsed-field gel electrophoresis of *S. aureus* isolated from families of AD children showed that similar strains are detectable in parents and their children.[150] This finding argues for a high recolonization rate of atopic children.[150] The importance of *S. aureus* is supported by the observation that even AD patients without overt infection show a greater reduction in severity of skin disease when treated with a combination of antistaphylococcal antibiotics and topical corticosteroids in comparison to topical corticosteroids alone.[151]

One strategy by which *S. aureus* exacerbates or maintains skin inflammation in AD is by secreting a group of toxins known to act as superantigens, which stimulate marked activation of T cells and macrophages. The skin lesions of over half of AD patients have *S. aureus* that secrete superantigens such as enterotoxins A, B, and toxic shock syndrome toxin-1.[152,153] An analysis of the peripheral blood skin-homing CLA+ T cells from these patients, as well as T cells in their skin lesions, reveals that they have undergone an expansion of the beta region of the T cell receptor variable chain consistent with superantigenic stimulation.[154,155] Most AD patients make specific IgE antibodies directed against the staphylococcal superantigens found on their skin.[152,153] Basophils from patients with IgE antibodies directed to superantigens release histamine on exposure to the relevant superantigen, but not in response to superantigens to which they have no specific IgE.[152] This raises the interesting possibility that superantigens induce specific IgE and mast cell degranulation in AD patients when the superantigens penetrate their disrupted epidermal barrier. This promotes the itch-scratch cycle critical to the evolution of skin rashes in AD.

A correlation has also been found between the presence of IgE antisuperantigens and severity of AD.[153] The combination of *S. aureus* superantigen plus allergen has been shown to have an additive effect in inducing skin inflammation.[156] Superantigens can also augment allergen-specific IgE synthesis, suggesting that several mechanisms exist by which superantigens could aggravate the severity of AD.[157,158] Fulfilling Koch's postulates, application of the superantigen staphylococcal enterotoxin B (SEB) to the skin can induce skin changes of erythema and induration accompanied by the infiltration of T cells that are selectively expanded in response to SEB.[159,160] In line with this, presence of SEB increased the rate of positive patch test reactions to house dust mite allergens.[161] It is additionally interesting that superantigen profile and production seems to be different in patients with steroid-resistant AD.[162] In a prospective study of patients recovering from toxic shock syndrome, it was found that 14 of 68 patients developed chronic eczematoid dermatitis whereas no patients recovering from Gram-negative sepsis developed eczema.[163] The investigators concluded that superantigens may induce an atopic process in the skin. It is notable that superantigens have been demonstrated to induce T cell expression of the skin-homing receptor via stimulation of IL-12 production.[164]

Increased binding of *S. aureus* to AD skin is likely to be related to underlying atopic skin inflammation. This concept is supported by several lines of investigation. First, it has been found that treatment with topical corticosteroids or tacrolimus will reduce *S. aureus* counts on atopic skin.[165,166] Second, acute inflammatory lesions have more *S. aureus* than chronic AD skin lesions or normal-looking atopic skin. Scratching is likely to enhance *S. aureus* binding by disturbing the skin barrier and exposing extracellular matrix molecules known to act as adhesins for *S. aureus*, for example, fibronectin and collagens. Finally, in studies of *S. aureus* binding to skin lesions of mice undergoing Th1 versus Th2 inflammatory responses, bacterial binding was significantly greater at skin sites with Th2-mediated inflammation.[167] Importantly, the increased bacterial binding did not occur in IL-4 gene knockout mice, indicating that IL-4 plays a crucial role in the enhancement of *S. aureus* binding to skin. IL-4 appears to enhance *S. aureus* binding to the skin by inducing the synthesis of fibronectin, an important *S. aureus* adhesin.

Viral Infections

AD in childhood as well as in adulthood can be complicated by localized or widespread cutaneous viral infections, which are specific for this skin disease. Virus infections observable in AD patients are most often caused by herpes simplex virus (HSV), human papilloma virus (HPV) or molluscipoxvirus. EH is a disseminated HSV-1 or -2 infection with severe systemic illness that occurs in 10–20% of patients with AD. Risk factors for eczema herpeticum (EH) are an early onset of AD, severe and untreated AD, head and neck dermatitis, previous herpes simplex infections and EH, and an elevated serum IgE combined with higher level of specific sensitizations, especially against *Malassezia sympodialis*.[168]

Autoallergens

In the 1920s, several investigators reported that human skin dander could trigger immediate hypersensitivity reactions in the skin of patients with severe AD, suggesting that they made IgE against autoantigens in the skin.[169] The potential molecular basis for these observations was demonstrated by Valenta and colleagues[170] who reported that the majority of sera from patients with severe AD contains IgE antibodies directed against human proteins. One of these IgE-reactive autoantigens has been cloned from a human epithelial cDNA expression library and designated Hom s 1, which is a 55 kDa cytoplasmic protein in skin keratinocytes.[171] Although the autoallergens characterized to date have been mainly intracellular proteins, they have been detected in IgE immune complexes of AD sera, suggesting that release of these autoallergens from damaged tissues could trigger responses mediated by IgE or T cells. This concept is supported by the recent observation that IgE autoallergen titers decreased with resolution of AD.[172] These data suggest that, whereas IgE immune responses are initiated by environmental allergens, allergic inflammation can be maintained by human endogenous antigens, particularly in severe AD.

Currently, the reason for the development of IgE autoreactivity is unclear, but it has been suggested that it might be based on chronic tissue damage due to repeated exposure to allergens in sensitized persons. Several atopy-related autoantigens (ARA), including Hom s 1–5 and DSF 70 have been characterized so far.[173] Strong IgE autoreactivity is detectable in AD patients with high total serum IgE levels, a large amount of sensitizations to food- and aeroallergens, early onset of AD, and severe courses.[174,175] Thus, IgE autoreactivity has been postulated to start in early infancy[174] and to contribute to very severe, therapy-resistant, and chronic courses of disease. Specific IgE against the stress-inducible enzyme, manganese superoxide dismutase (MnSOD), which cross-reacts to the skin-colonizing yeast *Malassezia symdodialis*, correlates with disease activity. MnSOD-specific IgE has been found to induce T cell reactivity in vitro and eczematous reactions in APT in MnSOD-sensitized AD patients.[176]

Conclusions

AD is a common, genetically transmitted, inflammatory skin disease frequently found in association with respiratory allergy (Box 53-2). The keys to management are skin hydration, use of effective topical antiinflammatory agents and avoidance of allergenic triggers and skin irritants. With a better understanding of the immunoregulatory abnormalities underlying AD, new paradigms are emerging to more effectively treat AD and to

---

BOX 53-2 Key concepts

Atopic Dermatitis

- Atopic dermatitis (AD) affects 10–20% of children.
- AD is a genetically transmitted chronic inflammatory allergic skin disease.
- Skin-homing T cells express T helper cell type 2 (Th2) cytokines that induce IgE and eosinophilia.
- Antigen-presenting cells in the skin (e.g. Langerhans cells) express surface-bound IgE molecules.
- Keratinocytes in AD skin have a defective innate immune response.
- Transition from acute to chronic AD is associated with a switch from predominantly Th2 cytokines to a combination of Th1, Th2 and Th17 cytokine gene expression.
- Immunologic triggers include foods, aeroallergens, microbial agents, and autoallergens.

prevent relapses of this skin condition (discussed in more detail in Chapter 54).

References

1. Leung DY, Bieber T. Atopic dermatitis. Lancet 2003;361:151–60.
2. Bieber T. Atopic dermatitis. N Engl J Med 2008;358:1483–94.
3. Stensen L, Thomsen SF, Backer V. Change in prevalence of atopic dermatitis between 1986 and 2001 among children. Allergy Asthma Proc 2008;29:392–6.
4. Williams H, Robertson C, Stewart A, et al. Worldwide variations in the prevalence of symptoms of atopic eczema in the International Study of Asthma and Allergies in Childhood. J Allergy Clin Immunol 1999;103:125–38.
5. Laughter D, Istvan JA, Tofte SJ, et al. The prevalence of atopic dermatitis in Oregon schoolchildren. J Am Acad Dermatol 2000;43:649–55.
6. von Mutius E. The environmental predictors of allergic disease. J Allergy Clin Immunol 2000;105:9–19.
7. Romagnani S. The role of lymphocytes in allergic disease. J Allergy Clin Immunol 2000;105:399–408.
8. Williams HC. Diagnostic criteria for atopic dermatitis: where do we go from here? Arch Dermatol 1999;135:583–6.
9. Akdis CA, Akdis M, Bieber T, et al. Diagnosis and treatment of atopic dermatitis in children and adults: European Academy of Allergology and Clinical Immunology/American Academy of Allergy, Asthma and Immunology/PRACTALL Consensus Report. J Allergy Clin Immunol 2006;118:152–69.
10. Elias PM, Hatano Y, Williams ML. Basis for the barrier abnormality in atopic dermatitis: outside-inside-outside pathogenic mechanisms. J Allergy Clin Immunol 2008;121:1337–43.
11. Schultz Larsen FV, Holm NV. Atopic dermatitis in a population based twin series: concordance rates and heritability estimation. Acta Derm Venereol Suppl (Stockh) 1985;114:159.
12. Larsen FS, Holm NV, Henningsen K. Atopic dermatitis: a genetic-epidemiologic study in a population-based twin sample. J Am Acad Dermatol 1986;15:487–94.
13. Cookson W. The immunogenetics of asthma and eczema: a new focus on the epithelium. Nat Rev Immunol 2004;4:978–88.
14. Hoffjan S, Epplen JT. The genetics of atopic dermatitis: recent findings and future options. J Mol Med 2005;83:682–92.
15. Maintz L, Novak N. Getting more and more complex: the pathophysiology of atopic eczema. Eur J Dermatol 2007;17:267–83.
16. Lee YA, Wahn U, Kehrt R, et al. A major susceptibility locus for atopic dermatitis maps to chromosome 3q21. Nat Genet 2000;26:470–3.
17. Cookson WO, Ubhi B, Lawrence R, et al. Genetic linkage of childhood atopic dermatitis to psoriasis susceptibility loci. Nat Genet 2001;27:372–3.
18. Bradley M, Soderhall C, Luthman H, et al. Susceptibility loci for atopic dermatitis on chromosomes 3, 13, 15, 17 and 18 in a Swedish population. Hum Mol Genet 2002;11:1539–48.
19. Haagerup A, Bjerke T, Schiotz PO, et al. Atopic dermatitis: a total genome-scan for susceptibility genes. Acta Derm Venereol 2004;84:346–52.
20. Novak N. New insights into the mechanism and management of allergic diseases: atopic dermatitis. Allergy 2009;64:265–75.
21. Gupta J, Grube E, Ericksen MB, et al. Intrinsically defective skin barrier function in children with atopic dermatitis correlates with disease severity. J Allergy Clin Immunol 2008;121:725–30.
22. Kezic S, Kemperman PM, Koster ES, et al. Loss-of-function mutations in the filaggrin gene lead to reduced level of natural moisturizing factor in the stratum corneum. J Invest Dermatol 2008;128:2117–9.
23. McGrath JA, Uitto J. The filaggrin story: novel insights into skin-barrier function and disease. Trends Mol Med 2008;14:20–7.
24. Palmer CN, Irvine AD, Terron-Kwiatkowski A, et al. Common loss-of-function variants of the epidermal barrier protein filaggrin are a major predisposing factor for atopic dermatitis. Nat Genet 2006;38:441–6.
25. Baurecht H, Irvine AD, Novak N, et al. Toward a major risk factor for atopic eczema: meta-analysis of filaggrin polymorphism data. J Allergy Clin Immunol 2007;120:1406–12.
26. Weidinger S, Illig T, Baurecht H, et al. Loss-of-function variations within the filaggrin gene predispose for atopic dermatitis with allergic sensitization. J Allergy Clin Immunol 2006;118:214–9.
27. Weidinger S, Rodriguez E, Stahl C, et al. Filaggrin mutations strongly predispose to early-onset and extrinsic atopic dermatitis. J Invest Dermatol 2007;127:504–7.
28. Bisgaard H, Simpson A, Palmer CN, et al. Gene-environment interaction in the onset of eczema in infancy: filaggrin loss-of-function mutations enhanced by neonatal cat exposure. PLoS Med 2008;5:e131.
29. Walley AJ, Chavanas S, Moffatt MF, et al. Gene polymorphism in Netherton and common atopic disease. Nat Genet 2001;29:175–8.
30. Vasilopoulos Y, Cork MJ, Murphy R, et al. Genetic association between an AACC insertion in the 3'UTR of the stratum corneum chymotryptic enzyme gene and atopic dermatitis. J Invest Dermatol 2004;123:62–6.
31. Soderhall C, Marenholz I, Kerscher T, et al. Variants in a novel epidermal collagen gene (COL29A1) are associated with atopic dermatitis. PLoS Biol 2007;5:e242.
32. Esparza-Gordillo J, Weidinger S, Fölster-Holst R, et al. A common variant on chromosome 11q13 is associated with atopic dermatitis. Nat Genet 2009;41:596–601.
33. Cork MJ, Robinson DA, Vasilopoulos Y, et al. New perspectives on epidermal barrier dysfunction in atopic dermatitis: gene-environment interactions. J Allergy Clin Immunol 2006;118:3–21.
34. Jeong SK, Kim HJ, Youm JK, et al. Mite and cockroach allergens activate protease-activated receptor 2 and delay epidermal permeability barrier recovery. J Invest Dermatol 2008;128:1930–9.
35. Medzhitov R, Janeway CA Jr. Decoding the patterns of self and nonself by the innate immune system. Science 2002;296:298–300.
36. Kabelitz D, Medzhitov R. Innate immunity–cross-talk with adaptive immunity through pattern recognition receptors and cytokines. Curr Opin Immunol 2007;19:1–3.
37. Cook DN, Pisetsky DS, Schwartz DA. Toll-like receptors in the pathogenesis of human disease. Nat Immunol 2004;5:975–9.
38. Murray PJ. NOD proteins: an intracellular pathogen-recognition system or signal transduction modifiers? Curr Opin Immunol 2005;17:352–8.
39. Strachan DP. Lifestyle and atopy. Lancet 1999;353:1457–8.
40. Ahmad-Nejad P, Mrabet-Dahbi S, Breuer K, et al. The toll-like receptor 2 R753Q polymorphism defines a subgroup of patients with atopic dermatitis having severe phenotype. J Allergy Clin Immunol 2004;113:565–7.
41. Mrabet-Dahbi S, Dalpke AH, Niebuhr M, et al. The toll-like receptor 2 R753Q mutation modifies cytokine production and Toll-like receptor expression in atopic dermatitis. J Allergy Clin Immunol 2008;121:1013–9.
42. Hoffjan S, Stemmler S, Parwez Q, et al. Evaluation of the toll-like receptor 6 Ser249Pro polymorphism in patients with asthma, atopic dermatitis and chronic obstructive pulmonary disease. BMC Med Genet 2005;28:34.
43. Weidinger S, Novak N, Klopp N, et al. Lack of association between Toll-like receptor 2 and Toll-like receptor 4 polymorphisms and atopic eczema. J Allergy Clin Immunol 2006;118:277–9.
44. Novak N, Yu CF, Bussmann C, et al. Putative association of a TLR9 promoter polymorphism with atopic eczema. Allergy 2007;62:766–72.
45. Novak N, Bieber T, Leung DY. Immune mechanisms leading to atopic dermatitis. J Allergy Clin Immunol 2003;112:S128–39.
46. Steinke JW, Borish L, Rosenwasser LJ. 5. Genetics of hypersensitivity. J Allergy Clin Immunol 2003;111:S495–501.
47. Wollenberg A, Klein E. Current aspects of innate and adaptive immunity in atopic dermatitis. Clin Rev Allergy Immunol 2007;33:35–44.
48. Novak N, Kruse S, Kraft S, et al. Dichotomic nature of atopic dermatitis reflected by combined analysis of monocyte immunophenotyping and single nucleotide polymorphisms of the interleukin-4/interleukin-13 receptor gene: the dichotomy of extrinsic and intrinsic atopic dermatitis. J Invest Dermatol 2002;119:870–5.
49. Weidinger S, Klopp N, Wagenpfeil S, et al. Association of a STAT 6 haplotype with elevated serum IgE levels in a population based cohort of white adults. J Med Genet 2004;41:658–63.
50. Novak N, Kruse S, Potreck J, et al. Single nucleotide polymorphisms of the IL18 gene are associated with atopic eczema. J Allergy Clin Immunol 2005;115:828–33.
51. Mao XQ, Shirakawa T, Yoshikawa T, et al. Association between genetic variants of masT cell chymase and eczema. Lancet 1996;348:581–3.
52. Arkwright PD, Chase JM, Babbage S, et al. Atopic dermatitis is associated with a low-producer transforming growth factor beta(1) cytokine genotype. J Allergy Clin Immunol 2001;108:281–4.
53. Leung DY. Atopic dermatitis: new insights and opportunities for therapeutic intervention. J Allergy Clin Immunol 2000;105:860–76.
54. Beck LA, Leung DY. Allergen sensitization through the skin induces systemic allergic responses. J Allergy Clin Immunol 2000;106:S258–63.
55. Spergel JM, Mizoguchi E, Brewer JP, et al. Epicutaneous sensitization with protein antigen induces localized allergic dermatitis and hyperresponsiveness to methacholine after single exposure to aerosolized antigen in mice. J Clin Invest 1998;101:1614–22.
56. Akdis M, Simon HU, Weigl L, et al. Skin homing (cutaneous lymphocyte-associated antigen-positive) CD8+ T cells respond to superantigen and contribute to eosinophilia and IgE production in atopic dermatitis. J Immunol 1999;163:466–75.
57. Akdis M, Trautmann A, Klunker S, et al. T helper (Th) 2 predominance in atopic diseases is due to preferential apoptosis of circulating memory/effector Th1 cells. FASEB J 2003;17:1026–35.
58. Higashi N, Gesser B, Kawana S, et al. Expression of IL-18 mRNA and secretion of IL-18 are reduced in monocytes from patients with atopic dermatitis. J Allergy Clin Immunol 2001;108:607–14.

59. Machura E, Mazur B, Golemiec E, et al. *Staphylococcus aureus* skin colonization in atopic dermatitis children is associated with decreased IFN-gamma production by peripheral blood CD4+ and CD8+ T cells. Pediatr Allergy Immunol 2008;19:37–45.

60. Leonardi S, Rotolo N, Vitaliti G, et al. IgE values and T lymphocyte subsets in children with atopic eczema/dermatitis syndrome. Allergy Asthma Proc 2007;28:529–34.

61. Ambach A, Bonnekoh B, Gollnick H. Perforin hyperreleasability and depletion in cytotoxic T cells from patients with exacerbated atopic dermatitis and asymptomatic rhinoconjunctivitis allergica. J Allergy Clin Immunol 2001;107:878–86.

62. Hanifin JM, Chan SC, Cheng JB, et al. Type 4 phosphodiesterase inhibitors have clinical and in vitro antiinflammatory effects in atopic dermatitis. J Invest Dermatol 1996;107:51–6.

63. Jirapongsananuruk O, Hofer MF, Trumble AE, et al. Enhanced expression of b7.2 (cd86) in patients with atopic dermatitis: a potential role in the modulation of ige synthesis. J Immunol 1998;160:4622–7.

64. Hamid Q, Boguniewicz M, Leung DY. Differential in situ cytokine gene expression in acute versus chronic atopic dermatitis. J Clin Invest 1994;94:870–6.

65. Proksch E, Folster-Holst R, Jensen JM. Skin barrier function, epidermal proliferation and differentiation in eczema. J Dermatol Sci 2006;43:159–69.

66. Grewe M, Bruijnzeel-Koomen CA, Schopf E, et al. A role for th1 and th2 cells in the immunopathogenesis of atopic dermatitis. Immunol Today 1998;19:359–61.

67. Eyerich K, Huss-Marp J, Darsow U, et al. Pollen grains induce a rapid and biphasic eczematous immune response in atopic eczema patients. Int Arch Allergy Immunol 2008;145:213–23.

68. Kerschenlohr K, Decard S, Przybilla B, et al. Atopy patch test reactions show a rapid influx of inflammatory dendritic epidermal cells in patients with extrinsic atopic dermatitis and patients with intrinsic atopic dermatitis. J Allergy Clin Immunol 2003;111:869–74.

69. Woodward AL, Spergel JM, Alenius H, et al. An obligate role for T cell receptor alphabeta+ T cells but not T cell receptor gammadelta+ T cells, B cells, or CD40/CD40L interactions in a mouse model of atopic dermatitis. J Allergy Clin Immunol 2001;107:359–66.

70. Simon D, Vassina E, Yousefi S, et al. Reduced dermal infiltration of cytokine-expressing inflammatory cells in atopic dermatitis after short-term topical tacrolimus treatment. J Allergy Clin Immunol 2004;114:887–95.

71. Simon D, Vassina E, Yousefi S, et al. Inflammatory cell numbers and cytokine expression in atopic dermatitis after topical pimecrolimus treatment. Allergy 2005;60:944–51.

72. Wollenberg A, Sharma S, Von Bubnoff D, et al. Topical tacrolimus (FK506) leads to profound phenotypic and functional alterations of epidermal antigen-presenting dendritic cells in atopic dermatitis. J Allergy Clin Immunol 2001;107:519–25.

73. Kwiek B, Peng WM, Allam JP, et al. Tacrolimus and TGF-beta act synergistically on the generation of Langerhans cells. J Allergy Clin Immunol 2008;122:126–32.

74. Hamid Q, Naseer T, Minshall EM, et al. In vivo expression of IL-12 and IL-13 in atopic dermatitis. J Allergy Clin Immunol 1996;98:225–31.

75. Trautmann A, Akdis M, Schmid-Grendelmeier P, et al. Targeting keratinocyte apoptosis in the treatment of atopic dermatitis and allergic contact dermatitis. J Allergy Clin Immunol 2001;108:839–46.

76. Simon D, Lindberg RL, Kozlowski E, et al. Epidermal caspase-3 cleavage associated with interferon-gamma-expressing lymphocytes in acute atopic dermatitis lesions. Exp Dermatol 2006;15:441–6.

77. Verhagen J, Akdis M, Traidl-Hoffmann C, et al. Absence of T-regulatory cell expression and function in atopic dermatitis skin. J Allergy Clin Immunol 2006;117:176–83.

78. Szegedi A, Baráth S, Nagy G, et al. Regulatory T cells in atopic dermatitis: epidermal dendritic cell clusters may contribute to their local expansion. Br J Dermatol 2009;160:984–93.

79. Reefer AJ, Satinover SM, Solga MD, et al. Analysis of CD25hiCD4+ 'regulatory' T cell subtypes in atopic dermatitis reveals a novel T(H)2-like population. J Allergy Clin Immunol 2008;121:415–22.

80. Novak N, Peng W, Yu C. Network of myeloid and plasmacytoid dendritic cells in atopic dermatitis. Adv Exp Med Biol 2007;601:97–104.

81. Novak N, Tepel C, Koch S, et al. Evidence for a differential expression of the FcepsilonRIgamma chain in dendritic cells of atopic and nonatopic donors. J Clin Invest 2003;111:1047–56.

82. Wollenberg A, Wen S, Bieber T. Langerhans cell phenotyping: a new tool for differential diagnosis of inflammatory skin diseases [letter]. Lancet 1995;346:1626–7.

83. Wollenberg A, Kraft S, Hanau D, et al. Immunomorphological and ultrastructural characterization of langerhans cells and a novel, inflammatory dendritic epidermal cell (IDEC) population in lesional skin of atopic eczema. J Invest Dermatol 1996;106:446–53.

84. Stary G, Bangert C, Stingl G, et al. Dendritic cells in atopic dermatitis: expression of FcepsilonRI on two distinct inflammation-associated subsets. Int Arch Allergy Immunol 2005;138:278–90.

85. Novak N, Valenta R, Bohle B, et al. FcepsilonRI engagement of Langerhans cell-like dendritic cells and inflammatory dendritic epidermal cell-like dendritic cells induces chemotactic signals and different T cell phenotypes in vitro. J Allergy Clin Immunol 2004;113:949–57.

86. Dijkstra D, Stark H, Chazot PL, et al. Human inflammatory dendritic epidermal cells express a functional histamine H4 receptor. J Invest Dermatol 2008;128:1696–703.

87. Sakurai D, Yamasaki S, Arase K, et al. Fc epsilon RI gamma-ITAM is differentially required for mast cell function in vivo. J Immunol 2004;172:2374–81.

88. Novak N, Allam JP, Hagemann T, et al. Characterization of FcepsilonRI-bearing CD123 blood dendritic cell antigen-2 plasmacytoid dendritic cells in atopic dermatitis. J Allergy Clin Immunol 2004;114:364–70.

89. Nockher WA, Renz H. Neurotrophins in allergic diseases: from neuronal growth factors to intercellular signaling molecules. J Allergy Clin Immunol 2006;117:583–9.

90. Tversky JR, Le TV, Bieneman AP, et al. Human blood dendritic cells from allergic subjects have impaired capacity to produce interferon alpha via Toll-like receptor 9. Clin Exp Allergy 2008;38:781–8.

91. Schroeder JT, Bieneman AP, Xiao H, et al. TLR9- and FcepsilonRI-mediated responses oppose one another in plasmacytoid dendritic cells by down-regulating receptor expression. J Immunol 2005;175:5724–31.

92. Wollenberg A, Wagner M, Gunther S, et al. Plasmacytoid dendritic cells: a new cutaneous dendritic cell subset with distinct role in inflammatory skin diseases. J Invest Dermatol 2002;119:1096–102.

93. Homey B, Steinhoff M, Ruzicka T, et al. Cytokines and chemokines orchestrate atopic skin inflammation. J Allergy Clin Immunol 2006;118:178–89.

94. Park CW, Lee BH, Han HJ, et al. Tacrolimus decreases the expression of eotaxin, CCR3, RANTES and interleukin-5 in atopic dermatitis. Br J Dermatol 2005;152:1173–81.

95. Gunther C, Bello-Fernandez C, Kopp T, et al. CCL18 is expressed in atopic dermatitis and mediates skin homing of human memory T cells. J Immunol 2005;174:1723–8.

96. Pivarcsi A, Gombert M, eu-Nosjean MC, et al. CC chemokine ligand 18, an atopic dermatitis-associated and dendritic cell-derived chemokine, is regulated by staphylococcal products and allergen exposure. J Immunol 2004;173:5810–7.

97. Gombert M, eu-Nosjean MC, Winterberg F, et al. CCL1-CCR8 interactions: an axis mediating the recruitment of T cells and Langerhans-type dendritic cells to sites of atopic skin inflammation. J Immunol 2005;174:5082–91.

98. Laberge S, Ghaffar O, Boguniewicz M, et al. Association of increased CD4+ T cell infiltration with increased IL-16 gene expression in atopic dermatitis. J Allergy Clin Immunol 1998;102:645–50.

99. Reich K, Hugo S, Middel P, et al. Evidence for a role of Langerhans cell-derived IL-16 in atopic dermatitis. J Allergy Clin Immunol 2002;109:681–7.

100. Taha RA, Minshall EM, Leung DY, et al. Evidence for increased expression of eotaxin and monocyte chemotactic protein-4 in atopic dermatitis. J Allergy Clin Immunol 2000;105:1002–7.

101. Yawalkar N, Uguccioni M, Scharer J, et al. Enhanced expression of eotaxin and CCR3 in atopic dermatitis. J Invest Dermatol 1999;113:43–8.

102. Morita E, Kameyoshi Y, Hiragun T, et al. The C-C chemokines, RANTES and eotaxin, in atopic dermatitis. Allergy 2001;56:194–5.

103. Morales J, Homey B, Vicari AP, et al. CTACK, a skin-associated chemokine that preferentially attracts skin-homing memory T cells. Proc Natl Acad Sci USA 1999;96:14470–5.

104. Galli G, Chantry D, Annunziato F, et al. Macrophage-derived chemokine production by activated human T cells in vitro and in vivo: preferential association with the production of type 2 cytokines. Eur J Immunol 2000;30:204–10.

105. Kakinuma T, Nakamura K, Wakugawa M, et al. Thymus and activation-regulated chemokine in atopic dermatitis: serum thymus and activation-regulated chemokine level is closely related with disease activity. J Allergy Clin Immunol 2001;107:535–41.

106. Nakatani T, Kaburagi Y, Shimada Y, et al. CCR4 memory CD4+ T lymphocytes are increased in peripheral blood and lesional skin from patients with atopic dermatitis. J Allergy Clin Immunol 2001;107:353–8.

107. Sonkoly E, Muller A, Lauerma AI, et al. IL-31: a new link between T cells and pruritus in atopic skin inflammation. J Allergy Clin Immunol 2006;117:411–7.

108. Bilsborough J, Leung DY, Maurer M, et al. IL-31 is associated with cutaneous lymphocyte antigen-positive skin homing T cells in patients with atopic dermatitis. J Allergy Clin Immunol 2006;117:418–25.

109. Neis MM, Peters B, Dreuw A, et al. Enhanced expression levels of IL-31 correlate with IL-4 and IL-13 in atopic and allergic contact dermatitis. J Allergy Clin Immunol 2006;118:930-7.

110. Dillon SR, Sprecher C, Hammond A, et al. Interleukin 31, a cytokine produced by activated T cells, induces dermatitis in mice. Nat Immunol 2004;5:752-60.

111. Toda M, Leung DY, Molet S, et al. Polarized in vivo expression of IL-11 and IL-17 between acute and chronic skin lesions. J Allergy Clin Immunol 2003;111:875-81.

112. Eyerich K, Pennino D, Scarponi C, et al. IL-17 in atopic eczema: Linking allergen-specific adaptive and microbial-triggered innate immune response. J Allergy Clin Immunol 2009;123:59-66.

113. He R, Oyoshi MK, Jin H, et al. Epicutaneous antigen exposure induces a Th17 response that drives airway inflammation after inhalation challenge. Proc Natl Acad Sci USA 2007;104:15817-22.

114. Guttman-Yassky E, Lowes MA, Fuentes-Duculan J, et al. Low expression of the IL-23/Th17 pathway in atopic dermatitis compared to psoriasis. J Immunol 2008;181:7420-7.

115. Soumelis V, Reche PA, Kanzler H, et al. Human epithelial cells trigger dendritic cell mediated allergic inflammation by producing TSLP. Nat Immunol 2002;3:673-80.

116. Gilliet M, Soumelis V, Watanabe N, et al. Human dendritic cells activated by TSLP and CD40L induce proallergic cytotoxic T cells. J Exp Med 2003;197:1059-63.

117. Yoo J, Omori M, Gyarmati D, et al. Spontaneous atopic dermatitis in mice expressing an inducible thymic stromal lymphopoietin transgene specifically in the skin. J Exp Med 2005;202:541-9.

118. Esnault S, Rosenthal LA, Wang DS, et al. Thymic stromal lymphopoietin (TSLP) as a bridge between infection and atopy. Int J Clin Exp Pathol 2008;1:325-30.

119. Ebner S, Nguyen VA, Forstner M, et al. Thymic stromal lymphopoietin converts human epidermal Langerhans cells into antigen-presenting cells that induce proallergic T cells. J Allergy Clin Immunol 2007;119:982-90.

120. Bratton DL, Hamid Q, Boguniewicz M, et al. Granulocyte macrophage colony-stimulating factor contributes to enhanced monocyte survival in chronic atopic dermatitis. J Clin Invest 1995;95:211-8.

121. Giustizieri ML, Mascia F, Frezzolini A, et al. Keratinocytes from patients with atopic dermatitis and psoriasis show a distinct chemokine production profile in response to T cell-derived cytokines. J Allergy Clin Immunol 2001;107:871-7.

122. Howell MD. The role of human beta defensins and cathelicidins in atopic dermatitis. Curr Opin Allergy Clin Immunol 2007;7:413-7.

123. Howell MD, Gallo RL, Boguniewicz M, et al. Cytokine milieu of atopic dermatitis skin subverts the innate immune response to vaccinia virus. Immunity 2006;24:341-8.

124. Ong PY, Ohtake T, Brandt C, et al. Endogenous antimicrobial peptides and skin infections in atopic dermatitis. N Engl J Med 2002;347:1151-60.

125. Nomura I, Goleva E, Howell MD, et al. Cytokine milieu of atopic dermatitis, as compared to psoriasis, skin prevents induction of innate immune response genes. J Immunol 2003;171:3262-9.

126. Howell MD, Novak N, Bieber T, et al. Interleukin-10 downregulates anti-microbial peptide expression in atopic dermatitis. J Invest Dermatol 2005;125:738-45.

127. Kisich KO, Carspecken CW, Fieve S, et al. Defective killing of Staphylococcus aureus in atopic dermatitis is associated with reduced mobilization of human beta-defensin-3. J Allergy Clin Immunol 2008;122:62-8.

128. Howell MD, Jones JF, Kisich KO, et al. Selective killing of vaccinia virus by LL-37: implications for eczema vaccinatum. J Immunol 2004;172:1763-7.

129. Howell MD, Wollenberg A, Gallo RL, et al. Cathelicidin deficiency predisposes to eczema herpeticum. J Allergy Clin Immunol 2006;117:836-41.

130. Schittek B, Hipfel R, Sauer B, et al. Dermcidin: a novel human antibiotic peptide secreted by sweat glands. Nat Immunol 2001;2:1133-7.

131. Rieg S, Steffen H, Seeber S, et al. Deficiency of dermcidin-derived antimicrobial peptides in sweat of patients with atopic dermatitis correlates with an impaired innate defense of human skin in vivo. J Immunol 2005;174:8003-10.

132. Hata TR, Kotol P, Jackson M, et al. Administration of oral vitamin D induces cathelicidin production in atopic individuals. J Allergy Clin Immunol 2008;122:829-31.

133. Liu PT, Stenger S, Li H, et al. Toll-like receptor triggering of a vitamin D-mediated human antimicrobial response. Science 2006;311:1770-3.

134. Schauber J, Dorschner RA, Coda AB, et al. Injury enhances TLR2 function and antimicrobial peptide expression through a vitamin D-dependent mechanism. J Clin Invest 2007;117:803-11.

135. Wang TT, Nestel FP, Bourdeau V, et al. Cutting edge: 1,25-dihydroxyvitamin D3 is a direct inducer of antimicrobial peptide gene expression. J Immunol 2004;173:2909-12.

136. Sampson HA. Food allergy. Part 1. Immunopathogenesis and clinical disorders. J Allergy Clin Immunol 1999;103:717-28.

137. Hauk PJ. The role of food allergy in atopic dermatitis. Curr Allergy Asthma Rep 2008;8:188-94.

138. Ramesh S. Food allergy overview in children. Clin Rev Allergy Immunol 2008;34:217-30.

139. Guillet G, Guillet MH. Natural history of sensitizations in atopic dermatitis: a 3-year follow-up in 250 children: food allergy and high risk of respiratory symptoms. Arch Dermatol 1992;128:187-92.

140. Lever R, MacDonald C, Waugh P, et al. Randomised controlled trial of advice on an egg exclusion diet in young children with atopic eczema and sensitivity to eggs. Pediatr Allergy Immunol 1998;9:13-9.

141. van Reijsen FC, Felius A, Wauters EA, et al. T cell reactivity for a peanut-derived epitope in the skin of a young infant with atopic dermatitis. J Allergy Clin Immunol 1998;101:207-9.

142. Li XM, Kleiner G, Huang CK, et al. Murine model of atopic dermatitis associated with food hypersensitivity. J Allergy Clin Immunol 2001;107:693-702.

143. Tupker RA, De Monchy JG, Coenraads PJ, et al. Induction of atopic dermatitis by inhalation of house dust mite. J Allergy Clin Immunol 1996;97:1064-70.

144. Tan BB, Weald D, Strickland I, et al. Double-blind controlled trial of effect of housedust-mite allergen avoidance on atopic dermatitis. Lancet 1996;347:15-8.

145. Gutgesell C, Heise S, Seubert S, et al. Double-blind placebo-controlled house dust mite control measures in adult patients with atopic dermatitis. Br J Dermatol 2001;145:70-4.

146. Holm L, Bengtsson A, Van Hage-Hamsten M, et al. Effectiveness of occlusive bedding in the treatment of atopic dermatitis-a placebo-controlled trial of 12 months' duration. Allergy 2001;56:152-8.

147. Scalabrin DM, Bavbek S, Perzanowski MS, et al. Use of specific IgE in assessing the relevance of fungal and dust mite allergens to atopic dermatitis: a comparison with asthmatic and nonasthmatic control subjects. J Allergy Clin Immunol 1999;104:1273-9.

148. Schafer T, Heinrich J, Wjst M, et al. Association between severity of atopic eczema and degree of sensitization to aeroallergens in schoolchildren. J Allergy Clin Immunol 1999;104:1280-4.

149. Wheatley LM, Platts-Mills TAE. Role of inhalant allergens in atopic dermatitis. In: Leung DYM, Greaves MW, editors. Allergic skin disease: a multi-disciplinary approach. New York: Marcel Dekker; 2000.

150. Bonness S, Szekat C, Novak N, et al. Pulsed-field gel electrophoresis of Staphylococcus aureus isolates from atopic patients revealing presence of similar strains in isolates from children and their parents. J Clin Microbiol 2008;46:456-61.

151. Leyden JJ, Kligman AM. The case for steroid-antibiotic combinations. Br J Dermatol 1977;96:179-87.

152. Leung DY, Harbeck R, Bina P, et al. Presence of IgE antibodies to staphylococcal exotoxins on the skin of patients with atopic dermatitis. Evidence for a new group of allergens. J Clin Invest 1993;92:1374-80.

153. Breuer K, Wittmann M, Bosche B, et al. Severe atopic dermatitis is associated with sensitization to staphylococcal enterotoxin B (SEB). Allergy 2000;55:551-5.

154. Bunikowski R, Mielke ME, Skarabis H, et al. Evidence for a disease-promoting effect of Staphylococcus aureus-derived exotoxins in atopic dermatitis. J Allergy Clin Immunol 2000;105:814-9.

155. Strickland I, Hauk PJ, Trumble AE, et al. Evidence for superantigen involvement in skin homing of T cells in atopic dermatitis. J Invest Dermatol 1999;112:249-53.

156. Herz U, Schnoy N, Borelli S, et al. A human-SCID mouse model for allergic immune response bacterial superantigen enhances skin inflammation and suppresses IgE production. J Invest Dermatol 1998;110:224-31.

157. Hofer MF, Harbeck RJ, Schlievert PM, et al. Staphylococcal toxins augment specific IgE responses by atopic patients exposed to allergen. J Invest Dermatol 1999;112:171-6.

158. Hauk PJ, Hamid QA, Chrousos GP, et al. Induction of corticosteroid insensitivity in human PBMCs by microbial superantigens. J Allergy Clin Immunol 2000;105:782-7.

159. Strange P, Skov L, Lisby S, et al. Staphylococcal enterotoxin B applied on intact normal and intact atopic skin induces dermatitis. Arch Dermatol 1996;132:27-33.

160. Skov L, Olsen JV, Giorno R, et al. Application of Staphylococcal enterotoxin B on normal and atopic skin induces up-regulation of T cells by a superantigen-mediated mechanism. J Allergy Clin Immunol 2000;105:820-6.

161. Langer K, Breuer K, Kapp A, et al. Staphylococcus aureus-derived enterotoxins enhance house dust mite-induced patch test reactions in atopic dermatitis. Exp Dermatol 2007;16:124-9.

162. Schlievert PM, Case LC, Strandberg KL, et al. Superantigen profile of Staphylococcus aureus isolates from patients with steroid-resistant atopic dermatitis. Clin Infect Dis 2008;46:1562-7.

163. Michie CA, Davis T. Atopic dermatitis and staphylococcal superantigens. Lancet 1996;347:324.

164. Leung DY, Gately M, Trumble A, et al. Bacterial superantigens induce T cell expression of the skin-selective homing receptor, the cutaneous lymphocyte-associated antigen, via stimulation of interleukin 12 production. J Exp Med 1995;181:747–53.

165. Nilsson EJ, Henning CG, Magnusson J. Topical corticosteroids and *Staphylococcus aureus* in atopic dermatitis. J Am Acad Dermatol 1992;27: 29–34.

166. Remitz A, Kyllonen H, Granlund H, et al. Tacrolimus ointment reduces staphylococcal colonization of atopic dermatitis lesions. J Allergy Clin Immunol 2001;107:196–7.

167. Cho SH, Strickland I, Tomkinson A, et al. Preferential binding of *Staphylococcus aureus* to skin sites of Th2-mediated inflammation in a murine model. J Invest Dermatol 2001;116:658–63.

168. Peng WM, Jenneck C, Bussmann C, et al. Risk factors of atopic dermatitis patients for eczema herpeticum. J Invest Dermatol 2007;127:1261–3.

169. Valenta R, Mittermann I, Werfel T, et al. Linking allergy to autoimmune disease. Trends Immunol 2009;30:109–16.

170. Valenta R, Seiberler S, Natter S, et al. Autoallergy: a pathogenetic factor in atopic dermatitis? J Allergy Clin Immunol 2000;105:432–7.

171. Valenta R, Natter S, Seiberler S, et al. Molecular characterization of an autoallergen, hom s 1, identified by serum ige from atopic dermatitis patients. J Invest Dermatol 1998;111:1178–83.

172. Kinaciyan T, Natter S, Kraft D, et al. IgE autoantibodies monitored in a patient with atopic dermatitis under cyclosporin A treatment reflect tissue damage. J Allergy Clin Immunol 2002;109:717–9.

173. Seiberler S, Bugajska-Schretter A, Hufnagl P, et al. Characterization of IgE-reactive autoantigens in atopic dermatitis. 1. Subcellular distribution and tissue-specific expression. Int Arch Allergy Immunol 1999;120: 108–16.

174. Mothes N, Niggemann B, Jenneck C, et al. The cradle of IgE autoreactivity in atopic eczema lies in early infancy. J Allergy Clin Immunol 2005;116:706–9.

175. Mittermann I, Reininger R, Zimmermann M, et al. The IgE-reactive autoantigen hom s 2 induces damage of respiratory epithelial cells and keratinocytes via induction of IFN-gamma. J Invest Dermatol 2008;128: 1451–9.

176. Schmid-Grendelmeier P, Fluckiger S, Disch R, et al. IgE-mediated and T cell-mediated autoimmunity against manganese superoxide dismutase in atopic dermatitis. J Allergy Clin Immunol 2005;115: 1068–75.

CHAPTER

54

Management of Atopic Dermatitis

Mark Boguniewicz • Donald Y. M. Leung

Atopic dermatitis (AD) is a common, frequently relapsing inflammatory disease that affects up to 20% of children (see the 'Epidemiology' section of Chapter 53) and has an impact on the quality of life of patients and families in a significant manner. Management approaches in AD have evolved from our understanding of the mechanisms underlying this skin disease. While AD is the most common chronic skin disease of children, it is important to remember the differential diagnosis of a pruritic rash when starting therapy and especially if there are atypical features or response to treatment is suboptimal. Note that while rare, cutaneous T cell lymphoma/mycosis fungoides can occur in adolescents and even children (see Box 54.1). Given the complex nature of the disease and chronic, relapsing course, AD will often require a multipronged approach directed at healing or protecting the skin barrier and addressing the immune dysregulation to improve the likelihood of successful outcomes. This includes proper skin hydration, identification and elimination of flare factors such as irritants, allergens, infectious agents and emotional stressors as well as pharmacologic therapy (Figure 54-1).[1]

Hydration and Skin Barrier Protective Measures

As discussed in the previous chapter, patients with AD have genetic or immune-mediated abnormalities in skin barrier function.[2] Of note, filaggrin contributes not only to barrier integrity, but also to hydration through generation of hygroscopic amino acids that are a key component of natural moisturizing factor (NMF). NMF is also involved in the maintenance of skin pH and regulation of key biochemical events, including protease activity, barrier permeability and cutaneous antimicrobial defense. In addition, filaggrin may also contribute to the acid mantle through acid degradation products. Children with AD have dry skin (xerosis) with microfissures and epidermal defects, which serve as portals of entry for irritants, allergens and skin pathogens. Transepidermal water loss involves even normal appearing skin.

Hydration of the skin can be accomplished through warm (note that lukewarm or tepid are not comfortable temperatures for bathing!) soaking baths for approximately 10 minutes, followed by immediate application of a moisturizer or medication to prevent evaporation and promote healing. Bathing also removes irritants, allergens and skin pathogens and provides symptomatic relief. Bathing should be an enjoyable activity, which can be accomplished by providing appropriate bath toys for younger children that are reserved for tub time or a care-giver may choose to read to them. Older children can read or play

hand-held games that are safe for a tub. It is important that involved areas of eczema are immersed, not just wet. Wet towels can be used to hydrate the head and neck regions, with masks created to make the experience both therapeutic and enjoyable. Young children need to be supervised. Baths can be taken several times per day during eczema flares, while showers may be substituted for milder disease or to accommodate busy schedules, especially in the mornings. Cleansers with minimal defatting activity and a neutral pH can be used as necessary. Preparations that are dye- and fragrance-free formulated for sensitive skin are generally well tolerated. Antibacterial cleansers may be helpful for patients with folliculitis or recurrent skin infections. Patients should be instructed not to scrub with a washcloth while using cleansers. Addition of bleach (sodium hypochlorite) to bath water, especially for patients with methicillin-resistant *Staphylococcus aureus* (MRSA), has been advocated. However, the amount of bleach per volume of water (e.g. an eighth to a half cup per tub of water) and the frequency of such treatments (e.g. 1 to 3 times weekly) have not been well studied and bleach baths can cause significant skin irritation. In a recent controlled study, children with AD were treated with dilute sodium hypochlorite baths (a half cup of 6% bleach added to 40 gallons of water) twice weekly for 5 to 10 minutes, combined with nasal mupirocin twice daily for 5 days each month, over a 3-month period.[3] Patients tolerated the dilute bleach baths although the number of patients colonized with MRSA was low and, despite clinical improvement, patients remained colonized by *S. aureus* even after 3 months of intervention.

Use of an effective moisturizer combined with hydration therapy will help to restore and preserve the stratum corneum barrier.[4] Moisturizers can also improve skin barrier function, reduce susceptibility to irritants, improve clinical parameters of AD and decrease the need for topical corticosteroids.[5,6,7] Ingredients that contribute to effective moisturizers include humectants to attract and hold water in the skin such as glycerol, occlusives such as petrolatum to retard evaporation and emollients such as lanolin to lubricate the stratum corneum.[8]

Moisturizers are available as ointments, creams, lotions and oils. While ointments have the fewest additives and are the most occlusive, in a hot, humid environment they may trap sweat with associated irritation of the skin. Lotions and creams may be irritating due to added preservatives, solubilizers, and fragrances. Lotions contain more water than creams and may be drying due to an evaporative effect. Oils are also less effective moisturizers. Moisturizers should be obtained in the largest size available (one pound jars) since they may need to be applied several times each day on a chronic basis. Vegetable shortening

©2010 Elsevier Ltd, Inc, BV
DOI: 10.1016/B978-1-4377-0271-2.00054-7

(Crisco®) can be used as an inexpensive moisturizer. Of note, patients and care-givers should understand that petroleum jelly (Vaseline®) is an occlusive, not a moisturizer, and thus needs to be applied on damp, not dry skin. Even young children can be taught to apply their moisturizer, allowing them to participate in their skin care. Patients and care-givers need to be instructed to apply moisturizers routinely but not over or immediately prior to topical medications to avoid dilution or interference with medication on skin.

A number of studies suggest that AD is associated with decreased levels of ceramides, contributing not only to a damaged permeability barrier, but also making the stratum corneum susceptible to colonization by *S. aureus*.[9] A ceramide-dominant emollient added to standard therapy in place of moisturizer in children with 'stubborn-to-recalcitrant' AD was shown to result in clinical improvement.[10] Several ceramide-containing creams are available, including Epiceram® which is registered as a medical device and thus available only by prescription. Preliminary data suggest clinical benefit comparable to a topical mid-potency corticosteroid,[11] and in an ongoing study, this ceramide-containing cream is being compared to a low potency topical corticosteroid in children with moderate AD. Other nonsteroidal creams registered as medical devices with unique ingredients include MAS063DP (Atopiclair®)[12] and S236 (Mimyx®).[13] These creams are not FDA-regulated products and have no restrictions on age or length of use. They may be especially attractive to parents who have concerns about using topical corticosteroids and calcineurin inhibitors. However, they are costly and their place in the treatment algorithm for AD has not been definitively established.

Topical Antiinflammatory Therapy

Topical Glucocorticoids

Glucocorticoids have been the cornerstone of antiinflammatory treatment for over 50 years. Because of potential side-effects, topical glucocorticoids are used primarily to control acute exacerbations of AD.[1]

Patients should be carefully instructed in the use of topical glucocorticoids to avoid potential side-effects. The potent fluorinated glucocorticoids should be avoided on the face, the genitalia, and the intertriginous areas. Patients should be instructed to apply topical glucocorticoids to their skin lesions and to use emollients over uninvolved skin. Failure of a patient to respond to topical glucocorticoids is often due to the inadequate amount applied. It is important to remember that it takes approximately 30 g of cream or ointment to cover the entire skin surface of an adult-sized patient for one application. The fingertip unit (FTU) has been proposed as a measure for applying topical corticosteroids and has been studied in children with AD.[14,15] This is the amount of topical medication that extends from the tip to the first joint on the palmar aspect of the index finger. It takes approximately one FTU to cover the hand or groin, 2 FTUs for the face or foot, 3 FTUs for an arm, 6 FTUs for the leg, and 14 FTUs for the trunk. Of note, adequate application of topical corticosteroids has been shown to correlate with clinical improvement.[16] Obtaining medications in larger quantities can result in significant savings for patients.

There are seven classes of topical glucocorticoids, ranked according to their potency based on vasoconstrictor assays from super-potent (class I) to low potent (class VII). Because of their potential side-effects, the super-potent and high-potent glucocorticoids should be used only for short periods of time and in areas that are lichenified, but not on the face or intertriginous areas. The goal is to use moisturizers to enhance skin hydration and lower-potency glucocorticoids or nonsteroidal agents for long-term therapy if needed. Side-effects from topical glucocorticoids are related to the potency ranking of the compound and the length of use as well as the area of the body to which the drug is applied, so it is incumbent on the clinician to balance the need for a more potent steroid with the potential for side-effects. In general, ointments have a greater potential to occlude the epidermis, resulting in enhanced systemic absorption compared to creams. Side-effects from topical glucocorticoids can be divided into local and systemic side-effects. Local side-effects include the development of striae and skin atrophy;[17] systemic side-effects in AD are uncommon unless high-potency steroids are used under occlusion, but adrenal suppression and cataracts have been reported.[18–20] However, disease activity, rather than the use of topical corticosteroids, was shown to be responsible for low basal cortisol values in patients with severe AD.[21] Of note, patients and care-givers continue to use topical corticosteroids suboptimally, primarily due to concerns about their use.[22] This may include delaying application of the medication for a number of days after the start of a flare, which contributes to suboptimal outcomes. An expert consensus from the Dermatology Working

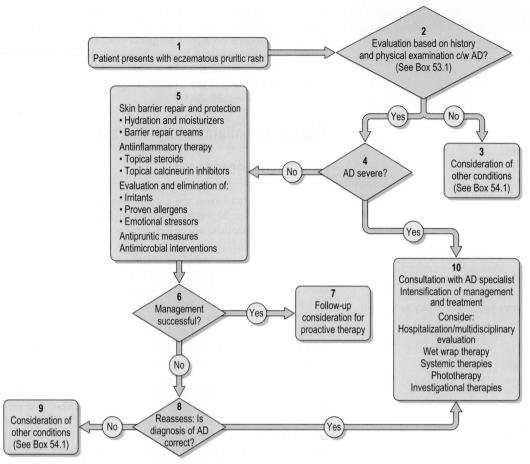

Figure 54-1 Clinical algorithm for diagnosis and management of atopic dermatitis.

Group pointed out that 'in an ideal world, dermatologists, dermatology nurses, … practitioners, … pharmacists would work together to advise and reinforce information about the correct way to apply topical corticosteroids, and to address concerns about the safety of these highly effective agents. But in the real world, expert advice, even when given, is soon forgotten …'.[15] Patients and care-givers need to have a basic understanding of topical corticosteroids, including their risks and benefits. Patients may erroneously assume that the potency of a topical corticosteroid is defined by the percent stated after the compound name (as discussed under 'Education of Patients and Care-givers' later in the chapter). At times, patients may be prescribed a high-potency corticosteroid with instructions to discontinue it within 7 to 14 days without a plan to step down, resulting in rebound flaring of their AD. Of note, only a few topical corticosteroids have been approved for use in very young children. These include desonide and fluticasone cream down to 3 months of age, alclometasone down to 1 year of age and mometasone down to 2 years of age. Indications are typically for up to 3 to 4 weeks.

Patients with AD are often labeled as topical corticosteroid treatment failures. Reasons for this may include inadequate potency of the preparation or insufficient amount dispensed or applied, *S. aureus* superinfection, steroid allergy and possibly corticosteroid insensitivity. A much more common reason for therapeutic failure is nonadherence to the treatment regimen. As with any chronic disease, patients or care-givers often expect quick and lasting benefits and become frustrated with the relapsing nature of AD.[23] These factors need to be considered when faced with a patient not responding to therapy before considering alternative therapy, especially systemic treatment.

Topical Calcineurin Inhibitors

Since their approval by the FDA in 2000 and 2001, respectively, the topical calcineurin inhibitors (TCIs) tacrolimus ointment (Protopic 0.03% and 0.1%) and pimecrolimus cream (Elidel 1%), have become well-established, effective and safe nonsteroidal treatments for pediatric AD.[24] They are currently indicated as second-line treatment for intermittent, noncontinuous use in children aged 2 years and older with moderate-severe AD (tacrolimus ointment 0.03%) and mild-moderate AD (pimecrolimus cream 1%). Tacrolimus ointment 0.1% is indicated for patients 16 years and older. Nevertheless, patients and care-givers frequently misunderstand their place in the treatment algorithm and have concerns about the boxed warning for these drugs. Of note, a Joint Task Force of the American College of Allergy, Asthma and Immunology and the American Academy of Allergy, Asthma and Immunology reviewed the available data and concluded that the risk/benefit ratios of tacrolimus ointment and pimecrolimus cream are similar to those of most conventional therapies for the treatment of chronic relapsing eczema.[25] In addition, a case-control study of a large database that identified a cohort of 293 253 patients with AD found no increased risk of lymphoma with the use of TCIs.[26] Children may be prescribed TCIs to replace topical corticosteroids when the patient is not doing well or during a flare of AD, with unrealistic expectations for this class of drugs. Patients and care-givers may not be instructed about potential side-effects, a common reason for TCIs being discontinued and patients labeled as treatment failures. While several studies have explored the use of TCIs in children under 2 years of age[27] and as early intervention to reduce the incidence of flare and need for topical steroid rescue,[28] they would currently be considered to be off-label therapy.

Proactive Therapy

In patients whose eczema tends to relapse in the same location, an approach that has gained increased attention is that of proactive therapy. After a period of stabilization, topical antiinflammatory therapy is instituted in areas of previously involved, but normal-appearing skin, rather than waiting for a flare of eczema in a traditional reactive approach. Studies with topical corticosteroids[29-32] and TCIs,[33,34] including in pediatric patients,[35,36] have shown clinical benefit with this approach. Of note, it is important to recognize that eczema first needs to be brought under control before a 2 to 3 times weekly, long-term regimen can be instituted. Importantly, proactive therapy is an attempt to control residual disease, since even normal-appearing skin in AD is characterized by immunological abnormalities, not the application of an active drug to nonaffected skin.[37]

Identification and Elimination of Triggering Factors

Patients with AD have hyperreactive skin and a number of different triggers including irritants, allergens, infectious agents and emotional stressors can contribute to cutaneous inflammation and flare of eczema.

Irritants

Patients with AD are more susceptible to irritants than are normal individuals. Thus it is important to identify and eliminate or minimize exposure to irritants such as soaps or detergents, chemicals, smoke, abrasive clothing, and extremes of temperature and humidity. Alcohol and astringents found in toiletries can be drying. Cleansers, ideally formulated for sensitive skin, should be used in place of soaps, especially fragranced ones. Using a liquid rather than powder detergent and adding a second rinse cycle will facilitate removal of the detergent. Recommendations regarding environmental conditions should include temperature and humidity control to avoid problems related to heat, humidity, and perspiration. Every attempt should be made to allow children to be as normally active as possible. Certain sports such as swimming may be better tolerated than other sports involving intense perspiration, physical contact, or heavy clothing and equipment, but chlorine should be rinsed off after swimming with the aid of a cleanser and the skin lubricated. Although ultraviolet light may be beneficial to some patients with AD, sunscreens should be used to avoid sunburn. Sunscreens formulated for the face are often better tolerated.

Specific Allergens

Potential allergens can be identified by taking a careful history and carrying out selective allergy tests. Negative skin tests or serum tests for allergen-specific immunoglobulin E (IgE) have a high predictive value for ruling out suspected allergens. Positive skin or in vitro tests, particularly to foods, often do not correlate with clinical symptoms and should be confirmed with controlled food challenges and, if indicated, trials of specific elimination diets. Avoidance of foods implicated in controlled challenges has

been shown to result in clinical improvement.[38] Infants who do not improve on formulas containing hydrolyzed proteins can be tried on amino acid formulas.[39] However, these can add a significant financial burden for the family. Extensive elimination diets which, in some cases, can be nutritionally deficient, are rarely if ever required, because even with multiple positive allergy tests, the majority of children will react to three or fewer foods on controlled challenge. Unfortunately, patients with multiple positive allergy tests are often labeled as multiple food-allergic with no attempts to prove clinical relevance. Food challenges after getting the eczema under control and establishing a baseline for immediate, and less frequently delayed, reactions can be of immense value in managing the patient and helping the family with this stressful issue. In addition, consultation with a dietician familiar with food allergies can be extremely helpful to ensure a nutritionally sound diet for the child and suggest practical advice to caregivers.[40] The Food Allergy and Anaphylaxis Network (*www.foodallergy.org*) is an especially useful resource for patients and families with food allergy (see also Chapter 52 on food allergy).

In patients allergic to dust mites, prolonged avoidance of dust mites has been found to result in improvement of AD.[41-44] Avoidance measures include: using dust mite-proof casings on pillows, mattresses, and box springs; washing bedding in hot water weekly; removing bedroom carpeting; and decreasing indoor humidity levels with air conditioning. Because there are many triggers contributing to the flare of AD, attention should be focused on identifying and controlling the flare factors that are important to the individual patient. In addition, allergic contact dermatitis may be overlooked in children and patch testing should be considered in children with AD.[45] In a recent study to determine the frequency of positive and relevant patch tests in children referred for patch testing in North America, of the children with a relevant positive reaction, 34.0% had a diagnosis of AD.[46]

Emotional Stressors

AD patients often respond to frustration, embarrassment and other stressful events with increased pruritus and scratching. In some instances, scratching is simply habitual and less commonly associated with secondary gain. Psychologic evaluation or counseling should be considered in patients who have difficulty with emotional triggers or psychologic problems contributing to difficulty in managing their disease. Relaxation, behavioral modification, or biofeedback may be helpful in patients who scratch habitually.[47]

Infectious Agents

Children with AD often are colonized or infected with various microbial organisms including bacteria, especially *Staphylococcus aureus* (Figure 54-2), viruses including Herpes simplex virus, and occasionally yeast or fungi. Methicillin-resistant *S. aureus* (MRSA) is becoming an increasingly important pathogen in patients with AD. Antistaphylococcal antibiotics are helpful in the treatment of patients who are heavily colonized or infected with *S. aureus*.[48] Cephalosporins or penicillinase-resistant penicillins are usually beneficial for patients who are not colonized with resistant *S. aureus* strains. Erythromycin and other macrolide antibiotics are usually of limited utility due to increasing frequency of erythromycin-resistant *S. aureus*. Topical mupirocin is useful for the treatment of localized impetiginized lesions; however, in patients with extensive skin infection, a course of systemic antibiotics is more practical. A newer topical antibiotic, retapamulin ointment

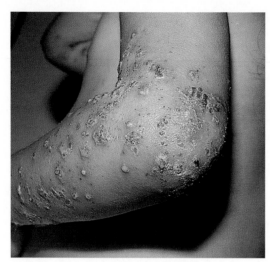

Figure 54-2 Patient with atopic dermatitis who is secondarily infected with *Staphylococcus aureus*. Note multiple pustules and areas of crusting. (From Weston WL, Morelli JG, Lane A, eds. Color textbook of pediatric dermatology, 3rd edn. St Louis: Mosby; 2002.)

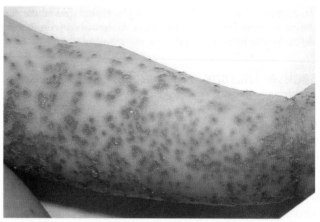

Figure 54-3 Eczema herpeticum, the primary skin maifestation of herpes simplex in atopic dermatitis. (From Fireman P, Slavin R, eds. Atlas of allergies, 2nd edn. London: Mosby-Wolfe; 1996.)

1%, used twice daily for 5 days was shown to be as effective as oral cephalexin twice daily for 10 days in the treatment of patients with secondarily infected dermatitis and was well tolerated.[49] Use of topical neomycin, on the other hand, can result in development of allergic contact dermatitis as neomycin is among the more common allergens causing contact dermatitis.[50] Treatment for nasal carriage with an intranasal antibiotic may lead to clinical improvement of AD.[51] MRSA may require culture and sensitivity testing to assist in appropriate antibiotic selection. However, patients and care-givers need to be instructed that the best defense against microbes is an intact skin barrier and basic skin care principles as discussed above should be emphasized. Of note, antiinflammatory therapy alone, with either a topical corticosteroid or topical calcineurin inhibitor, has been shown to improve AD and reduce *S. aureus* colonization of the skin.[52]

Although antibacterial cleansers have been shown to be effective in reducing bacterial skin flora,[53] they may be too irritating to use on inflamed skin in AD. Baths with dilute sodium hypochlorite (bleach) may also be of benefit to AD patients, especially those with recurrent MRSA as discussed above under 'Hydration and Skin Barrier Protective Measures', although they can be irritating. Of note, a recent controlled study, while showing clinical benefit, did not demonstrate decreased skin colonization by *S. aureus* even with combined nasal treatment with mupirocin and after 3 months of treatment.[3] Use of antimicrobial clothing is another potential antimicrobial therapy for patients with AD. One study compared the efficacy of an antimicrobial silk fabric (DermaSilk) with that of a topical corticosteroid in the treatment of AD.[54] Other studies have shown that silver-impregnated clothing reduced staphylococcal colonization, improved clinical parameters and reduced topical corticosteroid use in AD.[55]

AD can be complicated by disseminated herpes simplex virus infection, resulting in Kaposi's varicelliform eruption or eczema herpeticum (Figure 54-3). Vesicular lesions are umbilicated, tend to crop, and often become hemorrhagic and crusted. These lesions may coalesce to large, denuded, and bleeding areas that can extend over the entire body. Herpes simplex can provoke recurrent dermatitis and may be misdiagnosed as impetigo, although herpetic lesions can become superinfected by *S. aureus*.[56] The presence of punched-out erosions, vesicles, and/or infected skin lesions that fail to respond to oral antibiotics should initiate a search for herpes simplex. This can be diagnosed by a Giemsa-stained Tzanck smear of cells scraped from the vesicle base or by viral culture or PCR. Test results may be falsely negative if the samples are inadequate. Ideally, vesicle fluid should be obtained by unroofing one or more intact vesicles. Treatment may be with oral acyclovir for less severe infections or intravenous acyclovir for widely disseminated disease or toxic-appearing patients at 30 mg/kg/day divided every 8 hours (for patients < 1 year old) or 1500 mg/m^2/day divided every 8 hours (for patients > 1 year old) for 7 to 21 days, depending on the clinical course.[57] Lumbar puncture should be considered if meningitis is suspected, but the presence of infected lesions over the lumbar areas should preclude this procedure. Ophthalmology consultation should be obtained for patients with periocular or suspected eye involvement. Acyclovir prophylaxis may be necessary for patients with recurrent eczema herpeticum.

In patients with AD, smallpox vaccination, or even exposure to vaccinated individuals, may cause a severe widespread skin rash called eczema vaccinatum similar in appearance to eczema herpeticum.[58] An increased risk of fatalities resulting from eczema vaccinatum has been reported in AD. Even if not fatal, eczema vaccinatum is often associated with severe scarring and lifelong complications following recovery from this illness.

Fungi may play a role in chronic inflammation of AD. There has been particular interest in the role of Malassezia (Pityrosporum) in AD. *Malassezia sympodialis* is a lipophilic yeast commonly present in the seborrheic areas of the skin. IgE antibodies against *M. sympodialis* are found in AD patients, most frequently in patients with a head and neck distribution of dermatitis. The potential importance of *M. sympodialis* as well as other dermatophyte infections is further supported by the reduction of AD skin severity in patients treated with antifungal agents.[59] However, even patients with IgE antibodies to *M. sympodialis* often respond better to topical steroids than to topical antifungal therapy and systemic antifungal therapy may benefit AD patients through antiinflammatory properties.[60]

Control of Pruritus

The treatment of pruritus in AD should be directed primarily at the underlying causes. Reduction of skin inflammation and dryness with topical glucocorticoids and skin hydration, respectively, will often symptomatically reduce pruritus. Inhaled and ingested allergens should be eliminated if documented to contribute to eczema. Systemic antihistamines act primarily by blocking the H1 receptors in the dermis and thereby ameliorating histamine-induced pruritus. However, histamine is only one of many mediators that can induce pruritus of the skin, minimizing benefit from antihistamine therapy. Some antihistamines have anxiolytic agents and may offer symptomatic relief through their tranquilizing and sedative effects. Studies of newer nonsedating antihistamines have shown variable results in the effectiveness of controlling pruritus in AD patients although they may be useful in the subset of AD patients with concomitant urticaria.[61] Because pruritus is usually worse at night, sedating antihistamines such as hydroxyzine or diphenhydramine may offer an advantage with their soporific side-effects when used at bedtime. Doxepin hydrochloride has both tricyclic antidepressant and H1- and H2-histamine receptor blocking effects. Thus, it may be useful in treating children and adolescents who do not respond to H1 sedating antihistamines. If nocturnal pruritus remains severe, short-term use of a sedative to allow adequate rest may be appropriate. Treatment of AD with topical antihistamines or topical anesthetics is not recommended because of potential cutaneous sensitization.

Other Treatments

Tar Preparations

Coal tar preparations may have antipruritic and antiinflammatory effects on the skin.[62] The antiinflammatory properties of tars, however, are not well characterized and are usually not as pronounced as those of topical glucocorticoids. Tar shampoos can be beneficial for scalp dermatitis. Tar preparations should not be used on acutely inflamed skin because this can result in skin irritation. Side-effects associated with tars include folliculitis and photosensitivity.

Phototherapy

Natural sunlight in moderation may be beneficial to patients with AD; however, if the sunlight occurs in the setting of high heat or humidity, triggering sweating and pruritus, it may be deleterious. Broad-band ultraviolet B, broad-band ultraviolet A, narrow-band ultraviolet B (311 nm), UVA-1 (340 to 400 nm), and combined UVAB phototherapy can be useful adjuncts in the treatment of AD. Studies in children are limited and in general, UV therapy should be restricted to adolescents, except in exceptional cases.[1] Short-term adverse effects with phototherapy may include erythema, pain, pruritus, and pigmentation; long-term adverse effects include premature skin aging and cutaneous malignancies.

Systemic Therapy

Systemic Glucocorticoids

The use of systemic glucocorticoids, such as oral prednisone, is rarely indicated in the treatment of chronic AD.[1] The dramatic clinical improvement that may occur with systemic glucocorticoids is frequently associated with a severe rebound flare of AD following the discontinuation of systemic glucocorticoids. Short courses of oral glucocorticoids may be appropriate for an acute exacerbation of AD while other treatment measures are being instituted. If a short course of oral glucocorticoids is given, it is important to taper the dosage and begin intensified skin care, particularly with topical glucocorticoids and frequent bathing

followed by application of emollients, in order to prevent rebound flaring of AD. Patients who are oral steroid-dependent AD, or treated with frequent courses of systemic steroids, need to be evaluated for corticosteroid side-effects, including adrenal suppression, osteoporosis, cataracts and muscle weakness, and switched to other therapy.

Cyclosporin A

Cyclosporin A (CsA) is a potent immunosuppressive drug that acts primarily on T cells by suppressing cytokine transcription. Studies, including in children have demonstrated that patients with severe AD, refractory to conventional treatment, can benefit from short-term CsA treatment with reduced skin disease and improved quality of life.[63] A 1-year study of CsA (5 mg/kg/day) in a pediatric population using either intermittent or continuous treatment showed no significant differences between these two approaches with respect to efficacy or safety parameters, and a subset of patients remained in remission after treatment was stopped.[64] In addition, children as young as 22 months of age were shown to respond to low-dose (2.5 mg/kg/day) CsA.[65] Nevertheless, risks must be weighed against benefits and lab parameters, especially serum creatinine and blood pressure monitored.

Azathioprine

Azathioprine is a purine analogue with antiinflammatory and antiproliferative effects; it has been used for severe AD, including in children, although no controlled trials have been reported.[66] Myelosuppression is a significant adverse effect, although thiopurine methyl transferase levels may predict individuals at risk.[1]

Mycophenolate Mofetil

Mycophenolate mofetil (MMF), a purine biosynthesis inhibitor used as an immunosuppressant in organ transplantation, has been used for treatment of refractory inflammatory skin disorders.[67] The drug has generally been well tolerated with the exception of one patient developing herpes retinitis that may have been secondary to this immunosuppressive agent. Dose-related bone marrow suppression has also been observed. A retrospective analysis of children treated with MMF as systemic monotherapy for severe, recalcitrant AD found that of 14 patients, 4 achieved complete clearance, 4 had > 90% improvement, 5 had 60–90% improvement and 1 failed to respond.[68] Initial responses occurred within 8 weeks (mean 4 weeks), and maximal effects were attained after 8 to 12 weeks at MMF doses of 40–50 mg/kg/day in younger children and 30–40 mg kg/day in adolescents. MMF was well tolerated in all patients, with no infectious complications or significant lab abnormalities.

Education of Patients and Care-givers

Education is a critical component of AD management, especially when the disease is severe or relapsing. Important components include teaching about the chronic or relapsing nature of AD, exacerbating factors and therapeutic options with risks versus benefits and prognosis. Strategies include one-on-one communication, direct demonstration with reinforcement, group discussions, classroom teaching, and written materials including an AD Home Care or Action Plan. Observing the patient's or caregiver's method of treatment will often reveal fundamental errors which may explain why a patient is not experiencing the expected therapeutic response. Patients or care-givers are often observed applying inadequate amounts of topical medications, layering therapy, thus diluting or blocking specific drugs and misunderstanding the potency of topical corticosteroids based on the misperception that corticosteroid potency is based on the percent value (e.g. 2.5% vs 0.05%), rather than on the specific corticosteroid preparation (e.g. mometasone vs hydrocortisone). AD Home Care or Action Plans are integral to the management of children with AD, as without them, patients or care-givers may forget or confuse skin care recommendations.[47] These plans should fit the child's and family's needs and should be reviewed and modified at all follow-up visits.

Providing patients and care-givers with appropriate educational resources is an important component of management. Educational brochures and videos can be obtained from the National Eczema Association (800-818-7546 or *www.nationaleczema.org*). Information, instruction sheets and brochures including the comprehensive booklet, *Understanding Atopic Dermatitis,* are available from National Jewish Health Lung Line (800 222-LUNG or *www.njc.org*) as well as from national organizations such as the American Academy of Allergy, Asthma and Immunology (*www.aaaai.org*) or the American Academy of Dermatology (*www.aad.org*).

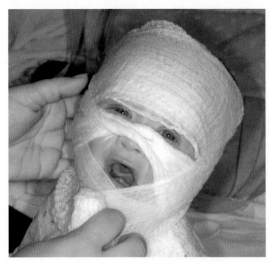

Figure 54-4 Facial eczema treated with wet, followed by dry, gauze, and secured with a dressing such as surgical Spandage®. (Reprinted from Boguniewicz M, Nicol N, Kelsay K, et al. A multidisciplinary approach to evaluation and treatment of atopic dermatitis. Semin Cutan Med Surg 2008;27:115–27, with permission from Elsevier.)

Wet Wrap Therapy

Wet wrap therapy has been used successfully as part of a step-up therapy regimen for treating severe or recalcitrant AD for over two decades.[69] This therapeutic intervention can improve penetration of topical medications, reduce pruritus and inflammation and act as a barrier against trauma from scratching.[70] A recent study of wet wraps demonstrated recovery of the epidermal barrier with clinical improvement associated with release of lamellar body and restoration of intercellular lipid lamellar structure.[71] Of note, 1 week after discontinuation of wet wraps, increased water content and decreased transepidermal water loss (TEWL) was still maintained. Wet wrap therapy has been shown to benefit patients during acute flares of AD.[72] This study points to the usefulness of this intervention in acute AD flares and suggests that the time for topical corticosteroid application may be shortened. One form of this treatment modality involves using tubular bandages applied over diluted topical corticosteroids. Children with severe AD showed significant clinical improvement after 1 week of treatment.[73] Of note, there was no significant difference noted using several dilutions of the mid-potency topical corticosteroid. This would suggest that clinical benefit can be obtained with this treatment in more severe patients even with the use of lower-potency corticosteroids. A different technique used successfully at National Jewish Health in Denver employs clothing, such as long underwear and cotton socks, selectively wet based on distribution of the patient's eczema, applied over an undiluted layer of topical corticosteroids with a dry layer of clothing on top.[69,47,70] Treating facial eczema requires nursing skills with wet, followed by dry, gauze expertly applied with eyes and mouth carefully cut out and secured with a dressing such as surgical Spandage® (Figure 54-4). A DVD demonstrating wrap therapy can be purchased through the Professional Education Department at National Jewish Health (*www.nationaljewish.org*). Wraps may be removed when they dry out (approximately 2 hours), however, it is often practical to apply them at bedtime and most children are able to sleep with them on. Overuse of wet wraps may result in chilling or maceration of the skin and may be complicated by secondary infection. However, a controlled study of wet wrap therapy with topical corticosteroids found that *S. aureus* colonization was

decreased with this intervention.[74] While use of wet wrap therapy over topical calcineurin inhibitors is not indicated on current package labeling, this approach is used 'off-label' by clinicians. Wet wrap therapy should be thought of as an acute crisis intervention, not as part of maintenance therapy, although occasionally it can be used on a more chronic basis to select areas of resistant dermatitis with appropriate monitoring. An evidence-based critical review of wet wrap therapy in children concluded, with a grade C recommendation, that: (i) wet wrap therapy using cream or ointment and a double layer of cotton bandages, with a moist first layer and a dry second layer, is an efficacious short-term intervention treatment in children with severe and/or refractory AD; (ii) the use of wet wrap dressings with diluted topical corticosteroids is a more efficacious short-term intervention treatment in children with severe and/or refractory AD than wet wrap dressings with emollients only; (iii) the use of wet wrap dressings with diluted topical corticosteroids for up to 14 days is a safe intervention treatment in children with severe and/or refractory AD, with temporary systemic bioactivity of the corticosteroids as the only reported serious side-effect; (iv) lowering the absolute amount of applied topical corticosteroid to once daily application and further dilution of the product can reduce the risk of systemic bioactivity.[75]

Multidisciplinary Approach to Atopic Dermatitis

Given the complex nature of AD, its relapsing course and incompletely understood pathogenesis, a significant number of patients have suboptimal outcomes with their prescribed treatment regimens. In addition, there is a significant impact on the quality of life of patients and families that leads to frustration and often a search for alternative therapies, which may not be in the best interest of the child. While children with AD of all severities could benefit from a multidisciplinary approach, those who especially should be considered candidates include those failing conventional therapy, those with recurrent skin infections, those diagnosed with multiple food allergies, those whose disease is having a significant impact on their or their family's quality of life, those with concerns about medication side-effects, and those with need for in-depth education. The significant and sustained clinical improvement often seen in patients treated with a multidisciplinary approach may be due, in large part, to in depth, hands-on education, along with changes in environmental exposures, reduction in stressors, and assurance of adherence with therapy. Of note, a high percentage of these patients experience significant improvement, even when treated with medications that previously were believed to be ineffective, when the treatment is integrated into a comprehensive and individualized management program.

The Atopic Dermatitis Program (ADP) at National Jewish Health in Denver, Colorado consists of a team of pediatric allergist-immunologists with extensive experience in basic and clinical research in AD, a nurse practitioner/dermatology clinical specialist, pediatric psychiatrist, child psychologists, allergy-immunology fellows-in-training, physician assistants, nurse educators, child life specialists, creative art therapist, social workers, dietitians and rehabilitation therapists.[47] Dermatologists are available for consultation if the diagnosis of AD is in question or phototherapy is being considered. Patients undergo comprehensive evaluation and treatment that is tailored to their needs and the goals of the family. Our ADP provides single day consultations, multi-day out-patient clinic visits, rarely in-patient hospitalization or a day program for more extensive evaluation, education and treatment typically over 5 to 14 days. In the controlled environment of the day program, patients and care-givers interact with members of the multidisciplinary team, and importantly, with other patients and families in group meetings and informal settings. In addition, sleep disturbance and response to interventions can be evaluated with overnight observation.[76]

Investigational or Unproven Therapy

Intravenous Immunoglobulin

High-dose intravenous immunoglobulin (IVIG) could have immunomodulatory effects in AD and in addition, IVIG could interact directly with microbes or toxins involved in the pathogenesis of AD. IVIG has been shown to contain high concentrations of staphylococcal toxin-specific antibodies that inhibit the in vitro activation of T cells by staphylococcal toxins.[77]

Treatment of severe refractory AD with IVIG has yielded conflicting results. Studies have not been controlled and have involved small numbers of patients.[78,79] Children appear to have a better response than adults, including to IVIG, as monotherapy and the duration of response was also shown to be more prolonged in children. However, additional controlled studies are needed to answer the question of efficacy in a more definitive manner.

Interferon-γ

IFN-γ is known to suppress IgE responses and down-regulate Th2 cell proliferation and function. Several studies of patients with AD, including a multicenter, double-blinded, placebo-controlled trial, have demonstrated that treatment with recombinant IFN-γ results in clinical improvement.[80] Reduction in clinical severity of AD was correlated with the ability of IFN-γ to decrease total circulating eosinophil counts. Influenza-like symptoms are commonly observed side-effects seen early in the treatment course.

Probiotics

Data from one meta-analysis suggests a modest role for probiotics in children with moderately severe disease in reducing the Scoring of Atopic Dermatitis Severity Index score (mean change from baseline, -3.01; 95% confidence interval, -5.36 to -0.66; $P = 0.01$).[81] Duration of probiotic administration, age, and type of probiotic used did not affect outcome. Another meta-analysis found that current evidence is more convincing for probiotic' efficacy in prevention rather than treatment of pediatric AD.[82] On the other hand, supplementation with Lactobacillus GG during pregnancy and early infancy neither reduced the incidence of AD nor altered the severity of AD in affected children, but was associated with an increased rate of recurrent episodes of wheezing bronchitis.[83] A recent Cochrane review concluded that probiotics are not an effective treatment for eczema in children and that probiotic treatment carries a small risk of adverse events.[84]

Vitamin D

Vitamin D deficiency is being increasingly recognized in the US population and may play a role in various allergic illnesses.[85] Of interest, vitamin D may play an important role in regulation of antimicrobial peptides in keratinocytes as discussed in Chapter 53.[86] A trial with oral vitamin D supports this hypothesis.[87] In one small pediatric study, children with AD were treated with oral vitamin D in a randomized, controlled trial. Investigator Global Assessment (IGA) score improved by 1 IGA category in four of five subjects treated with vitamin D versus one of six on placebo. Similar improvements were seen for change in the EASI score.[88] Larger trials with vitamin D in AD are ongoing.

Omalizumab

Anecdotal reports suggest clinical benefit in some patients with AD including children treated for their asthma with monoclonal anti-IgE (omalizumab) subcutaneous injections.[89] Treatment of adult patients with severe AD and significantly elevated serum IgE levels did not show benefit when omalizumab was used as monotherapy.[90] In contrast, significant improvement in three adolescent patients was observed when omalizumab was added to the usual therapy.[91] Specific markers have not been found to identify potential responders and at present, use of this monoclonal antibody is not indicated for AD.

Allergen Immunotherapy

Unlike allergic rhinitis and extrinsic asthma, specific immunotherapy with aeroallergens has not been proven to be efficacious in the treatment of AD. There are anecdotal reports of disease improvement, but also exacerbation. A study of specific immunotherapy over 12 months in adults with AD sensitized to dust mite allergen showed clinical improvement as well as reduction in topical steroid use,[92] although these results may not be applicable to pediatric AD. Well-controlled studies in children with AD are still required to determine the role for specific immunotherapy in this disease. In addition, preliminary studies with sublingual immunotherapy suggest a role for a subset of children with AD sensitized to dust mite allergen,[93] but again, this data needs to be reproduced in a larger pediatric population, especially in light of the natural history of AD.

BOX 54-2 Therapeutic principles

Atopic Dermatitis

- Proper skin hydration and moisturizers needed to repair and help preserve skin barrier function.
- Topical antiinflammatory therapy can be used for both treatment of acute flares and prevention of relapses.
- Avoidance of proven food and inhalant allergens may prevent or lessen flares.
- Measures to decrease microbial colonization can improve atopic dermatitis.
- Sedating antihistamines may provide symptomatic relief through sedating side-effects.
- Addressing psychosocial aspects of a chronic, relapsing illness and providing education with written skin care instructions can lead to improved outcomes.

Conclusions

AD is a common genetically transmitted inflammatory skin disease frequently found in association with respiratory allergy. Key management concepts include protection of the skin barrier, skin hydration, avoidance of irritants and proven allergic triggers and effective use of topical antiinflammatory agents (Box 54-2). Education of patients and care-givers is an essential part of treating AD patients of all levels of severity and a multi-disciplinary approach to management may be the best approach for a number of patients. Better understanding of the complex genetic and immunoregulatory abnormalities underlying AD may allow for development of more specific treatments and suggest new paradigms for managing this disease.

Helpful Websites

National Jewish Health (www.nationaljewish.org)

The National Eczema Association (www.nationaleczema.org)

The American Academy of Allergy, Asthma, and Immunology (www.aaaai.org)

The American Academy of Dermatology (www.aad.org)

References

1. Akdis CA, Akdis M, Bieber T, et al. Diagnosis and treatment of atopic dermatitis in children and adults: European Academy of Allergology and Clinical Immunology/American Academy of Allergy, Asthma and Immunology/PRACTALL Consensus Report. J Allergy Clin Immunol 2006;118:152–69.
2. O'Regan GM, Sandilands A, McLean WH, et al. Filaggrin in atopic dermatitis. J Allergy Clin Immunol 2008;122:689–93.
3. Huang JT, Abrams M, Tlougan B, et al. Treatment of *Staphylococcus aureus* colonization in atopic dermatitis decreases disease severity. Pediatrics 2009;123:e808–814.
4. Loden M. Biophysical properties of dry atopic and normal skin with special reference to effects of skin care products. Acta Derm Venereol Suppl (Stockh) 1995;192:1–48.
5. Loden M, Andersson AC, Lindberg M. Improvement in skin barrier function in patients with atopic dermatitis after treatment with a moisturizing cream (Canoderm). Br J Dermatol 1999;140:264–7.
6. Hanifin JM, Hebertt AA, Mays SR. Effects of a low-potency corticosteroid lotion plus a moisturizing regimen in the treatment of atopic dermatitis. Curr Ther Res 1998;59:227–33.
7. Lucky AW, Leach AD, Laskarzewski P, et al. Use of an emollient as a steroid-sparing agent in the treatment of mild to moderate atopic dermatitis in children. Pediatr Dermatol 1997;14:321–4.
8. Johnson AW. Overview: fundamental skin care–protecting the barrier. Dermatol Ther 2004;17(Suppl 1):1–5.
9. Macheleidt O, Kaiser HW, Sandhoff K. Deficiency of epidermal protein-bound omega-hydroxyceramides in atopic dermatitis. J Invest Dermatol 2002;119:166–73.
10. Chamlin SL, Kao J, Frieden IJ, et al. Ceramide-dominant barrier repair lipids alleviate childhood atopic dermatitis: changes in barrier function provide a sensitive indicator of disease activity. J Am Acad Dermatol 2002;47:198–208.
11. Elias PM, Hatano Y, Williams ML. Basis for the barrier abnormality in atopic dermatitis: outside-inside-outside pathogenic mechanisms. J Allergy Clin Immunol 2008;121:1337–43.
12. Boguniewicz M, Zeichner JA, Eichenfield LF, et al. MAS063DP is effective monotherapy for mild to moderate atopic dermatitis in infants and children: a multicenter, randomized, vehicle-controlled study. J Pediatr 2008;152:854–9.
13. Eberlein B, Eicke C, Reinhardt HW, et al. Adjuvant treatment of atopic eczema: assessment of an emollient containing N-palmitoylethanolamine (ATOPA study). J Eur Acad Dermatol Venereol 2008;22:73–82.
14. Long CC, Mills CM, Finlay AY. A practical guide to topical therapy in children. Br J Dermatol 1998;138:293–6.
15. Bewley A. Expert consensus: time for a change in the way we advise our patients to use topical corticosteroids. Br J Dermatol 2008;158:917–20.
16. Niemeier V, Kupfer J, Schill WB, et al. Atopic dermatitis – topical therapy: do patients apply much too little? J Dermatolog Treat 2005;16:95–101.
17. Luger TA, Lahfa M, Folster-Holst R, et al. Long-term safety and tolerability of pimecrolimus cream 1% and topical corticosteroids in adults with moderate to severe atopic dermatitis. J Dermatolog Treat 2004;15:169–78.
18. Gilbertson EO, Spellman MC, Piacquadio DJ, et al. Super potent topical corticosteroid use associated with adrenal suppression: clinical considerations. J Am Acad Dermatol 1998;38:318–21.
19. Ellison JA, Patel L, Ray DW, et al. Hypothalamic-pituitary-adrenal function and glucocorticoid sensitivity in atopic dermatitis. Pediatrics 2000;105:794–9.
20. Kane D, Barnes L, Fitzgerald O. Topical corticosteroid treatment: systemic side-effects. Br J Dermatol 2003;149:417.
21. Haeck IM, Timmer-de Mik L, Lentjes EG, et al. Low basal serum cortisol in patients with severe atopic dermatitis: potent topical corticosteroids wrongfully accused. Br J Dermatol 2007;156:979–85.
22. Charman CR, Morris AD, Williams HC. Topical corticosteroid phobia in patients with atopic eczema. Br J Dermatol 2000;142:931–6.
23. Zuberbier T, Orlow SJ, Paller AS, et al. Patient perspectives on the management of atopic dermatitis. J Allergy Clin Immunol 2006;118:226–32.
24. Orlow SJ. Topical calcineurin inhibitors in pediatric atopic dermatitis: a critical analysis of current issues. Paediatr Drugs 2007;9:289–99.
25. Fonacier L, Spergel J, Charlesworth EN, et al. Report of the Topical Calcineurin Inhibitor Task Force of the American College of Allergy, Asthma and Immunology and the American Academy of Allergy, Asthma and Immunology. J Allergy Clin Immunol 2005;115:1249–53.
26. Arellano FM, Wentworth CE, Arana A, et al. Risk of lymphoma following exposure to calcineurin inhibitors and topical steroids in patients with atopic dermatitis. J Invest Dermatol 2007;127:808–16.
27. Kapp A, Papp K, Bingham A, et al. Long-term management of atopic dermatitis in infants with topical pimecrolimus, a nonsteroid antiinflammatory drug. J Allergy Clin Immunol 2002;110:277–84.
28. Boguniewicz M, Eichenfield LF, Hultsch T. Current management of atopic dermatitis and interruption of the atopic march. J Allergy Clin Immunol 2003;112:S140–150.
29. Van Der Meer JB, Glazenburg EJ, Mulder PG, et al. The management of moderate to severe atopic dermatitis in adults with topical fluticasone propionate. The Netherlands Adult Atopic DermatitisStudy Group. Br J Dermatol 1999;140:1114–21.
30. Hanifin J, Gupta AK, Rajagopalan R. Intermittent dosing of fluticasone propionate cream for reducing the risk of relapse in atopic dermatitis patients. Br J Dermatol 2002;147:528–37.
31. Berth-Jones J, Damstra RJ, Golsch S, et al. Twice weekly fluticasone propionate added to emollient maintenance treatment to reduce risk of relapse in atopic dermatitis: randomised, double blind, parallel group study. BMJ 2003;326:1367.
32. Peserico A, Stadtler G, Sebastian M, et al. Reduction of relapses of atopic dermatitis with methylprednisolone aceponate cream twice weekly in addition to maintenance treatment with emollient: a multicentre, randomized, double-blind, controlled study. Br J Dermatol 2008;158:801–7.
33. Wollenberg A, Reitamo S, Girolomoni G, et al. Proactive treatment of atopic dermatitis in adults with 0.1% tacrolimus ointment. Allergy 2008;63:742–50.
34. Breneman D, Fleischer AB Jr, Abramovits W, et al. Intermittent therapy for flare prevention and long-term disease control in stabilized atopic dermatitis: a randomized comparison of 3-times-weekly applications of tacrolimus ointment versus vehicle. J Am Acad Dermatol 2008;58:990–9.

35. Thaci D, Reitamo S, Gonzalez Ensenat MA, et al. Proactive disease management with 0.03% tacrolimus ointment for children with atopic dermatitis: results of a randomized, multicentre, comparative study. Br J Dermatol 2008;159:1348–56.

36. Paller AS, Eichenfield LF, Kirsner RS, et al. Three times weekly tacrolimus ointment reduces relapse in stabilized atopic dermatitis: a new paradigm for use. Pediatrics 2008;122:e1210–1218.

37. Wollenberg A, Bieber T. Proactive therapy of atopic dermatitis: an emerging concept. Allergy 2009;64:276–8.

38. Sicherer SH, Sampson HA. 9. Food allergy. J Allergy Clin Immunol 2006;117:S470–475.

39. Woodmansee DP, Christiansen SC. Improvement in atopic dermatitis in infants with the introduction of an elemental formula. J Allergy Clin Immunol 2001;108:309.

40. Boguniewicz M, Moore N, Paranto K. Allergic diseases, quality of life and the role of the dietician. Nutr Today 2008;43:6–10.

41. Tan BB, Weald D, Strickland I, et al. Double-blind controlled trial of effect of housedust-mite allergen avoidance on atopic dermatitis. Lancet 1996;347:15–8.

42. Ricci G, Patrizi A, Specchia F, et al. Effect of house dust mite avoidance measures in children with atopic dermatitis. Br J Dermatol 2000;143:379–84.

43. Holm L, Bengtsson A, van Hage-Hamsten M, et al. Effectiveness of occlusive bedding in the treatment of atopic dermatitis: a placebo-controlled trial of 12 months' duration. Allergy 2001;56:152–8.

44. Arlian LG, Platts-Mills TA. The biology of dust mites and the remediation of mite allergens in allergic disease. J Allergy Clin Immunol 2001;107:S406–13.

45. Mailhol C, Lauwers-Cances V, Rance F, et al. Prevalence and risk factors for allergic contact dermatitis to topical treatment in atopic dermatitis: a study in 641 children. Allergy 2009;64:801–6.

46. Zug KA, McGinley-Smith D, Warshaw EM, et al. Contact allergy in children referred for patch testing: North American Contact Dermatitis Group data, 2001–2004. Arch Dermatol 2008;144:1329–36.

47. Boguniewicz M, Nicol N, Kelsay K, et al. A multidisciplinary approach to evaluation and treatment of atopic dermatitis. Semin Cutan Med Surg 2008;27:115–27.

48. Boguniewicz M, Sampson H, Leung SB, et al. Effects of cefuroxime axetil on Staphylococcus aureus colonization and superantigen production in atopic dermatitis. J Allergy Clin Immunol 2001;108:651–2.

49. Parish LC, Jorizzo JL, Breton JJ, et al. Topical retapamulin ointment (1%, wt/wt) twice daily for 5 days versus oral cephalexin twice daily for 10 days in the treatment of secondarily infected dermatitis: results of a randomized controlled trial. J Am Acad Dermatol 2006;55:1003–13.

50. Albert MR, Gonzalez S, Gonzalez E. Patch testing reactions to a standard series in 608 patients tested from 1990 to 1997 at Massachusetts General Hospital. Am J Contact Dermat 1998;9:207–11.

51. Luber H, Amornsiripanitch S, Lucky AW. Mupirocin and the eradication of Staphylococcus aureus in atopic dermatitis. Arch Dermatol 1988;124:853–4.

52. Hung SH, Lin YT, Chu CY, et al. Staphylococcus colonization in atopic dermatitis treated with fluticasone or tacrolimus with or without antibiotics. Ann Allergy Asthma Immunol 2007;98:51–6.

53. Stalder JF, Fleury M, Sourisse M, et al. Comparative effects of two topical antiseptics (chlorhexidine vs KMn04) on bacterial skin flora in atopic dermatitis. Acta Derm Venereol Suppl (Stockh) 1992;176:132–4.

54. Senti G, Steinmann LS, Fischer B, et al. Antimicrobial silk clothing in the treatment of atopic dermatitis proves comparable to topical corticosteroid treatment. Dermatology 2006;213:228–33.

55. Gauger A, Fischer S, Mempel M, et al. Efficacy and functionality of silver-coated textiles in patients with atopic eczema. J Eur Acad Dermatol Venereol 2006;20:534–41.

56. Bork K, Brauninger W. Increasing incidence of eczema herpeticum: analysis of seventy-five cases. J Am Acad Dermatol 1988;19:1024–9.

57. Wollenberg A, Wetzel S, Burgdorf WH, et al. Viral infections in atopic dermatitis: pathogenic aspects and clinical management. J Allergy Clin Immunol 2003;112:667–74.

58. Vora S, Damon I, Fulginiti V, et al. Severe eczema vaccinatum in a household contact of a smallpox vaccinee. Clin Infect Dis 2008;46:1555–61.

59. Back O, Scheynius A, Johansson SG. Ketoconazole in atopic dermatitis: therapeutic response is correlated with decrease in serum IgE. Arch Dermatol Res 1995;287:448–51.

60. Boguniewicz M, Schmid-Grendelmeier P, Leung DY. Atopic dermatitis. J Allergy Clin Immunol 2006;118:40–3.

61. Simons FE. Prevention of acute urticaria in young children with atopic dermatitis. J Allergy Clin Immunol 2001;107:703–6.

62. Langeveld-Wildschut EG, Riedl H, Thepen T, et al. Modulation of the atopy patch test reaction by topical corticosteroids and tar. J Allergy Clin Immunol 2000;106:737–43.

63. Berth-Jones J, Finlay AY, Zaki I, et al. Cyclosporine in severe childhood atopic dermatitis: a multicenter study. J Am Acad Dermatol 1996;34:1016–21.

64. Harper JI, Ahmed I, Barclay G, et al. Cyclosporin for severe childhood atopic dermatitis: short course versus continuous therapy. Br J Dermatol 2000;142:52–8.

65. Bunikowski R, Staab D, Kussebi F, et al. Low-dose cyclosporin A microemulsion in children with severe atopic dermatitis: clinical and immunological effects. Pediatr Allergy Immunol 2001;12:216–23.

66. Murphy LA, Atherton DJ. Azathioprine as a treatment for severe atopic eczema in children with a partial thiopurine methyl transferase (TPMT) deficiency. Pediatr Dermatol 2003;20:531–4.

67. Grundmann-Kollmann M, Podda M, Ochsendorf F, et al. Mycophenolate mofetil is effective in the treatment of atopic dermatitis. Arch Dermatol 2001;137:870–3.

68. Heller M, Shin HT, Orlow SJ, et al. Mycophenolate mofetil for severe childhood atopic dermatitis: experience in 14 patients. Br J Dermatol 2007;157:127–32.

69. Nicol NH. Atopic dermatitis: the (wet) wrap-up. Am J Nurs 1987;87:1560–3.

70. Nicol NH, Boguniewicz M. Successful strategies in atopic dermatitis management. Dermatol Nurs 2008:(Suppl):3–18.

71. Lee JH, Lee SJ, Kim D, et al. The effect of wet-wrap dressing on epidermal barrier in patients with atopic dermatitis. J Eur Acad Dermatol Venereol 2007;21:1360–8.

72. Foelster-Holst R, Nagel F, Zoellner P, et al. Efficacy of crisis intervention treatment with topical corticosteroid prednicarbat with and without partial wet-wrap dressing in atopic dermatitis. Dermatology 2006;212:66–9.

73. Wolkerstorfer A, Visser RL, De Waard van der Spek FB, et al. Efficacy and safety of wet-wrap dressings in children with severe atopic dermatitis: influence of corticosteroid dilution. Br J Dermatol 2000;143:999–1004.

74. Schnopp C, Holtmann C, Stock S, et al. Topical steroids under wet-wrap dressings in atopic dermatitis: a vehicle-controlled trial. Dermatology 2002;204:56–9.

75. Devillers AC, Oranje AP. Efficacy and safety of 'wet-wrap' dressings as an intervention treatment in children with severe and/or refractory atopic dermatitis: a critical review of the literature. Br J Dermatol 2006;154:579–85.

76. Bender BG, Ballard R, Canono B, et al. Disease severity, scratching, and sleep quality in patients with atopic dermatitis. J Am Acad Dermatol 2008;58:415–20.

77. Takei S, Arora YK, Walker SM. Intravenous immunoglobulin contains specific antibodies inhibitory to activation of T cells by staphylococcal toxin superantigens [see comment]. J Clin Invest 1993;91:602–7.

78. Wakim M, Alazard M, Yajima A, et al. High dose intravenous immunoglobulin in atopic dermatitis and hyper-IgE syndrome. Ann Allergy Asthma Immunol 1998;81:153–8.

79. Jolles S. A review of high-dose intravenous immunoglobulin treatment for atopic dermatitis. Clin Exp Dermatol 2002;27:3–7.

80. Hanifin JM, Schneider LC, Leung DY, et al. Recombinant interferon gamma therapy for atopic dermatitis. J Am Acad Dermatol 1993;28:189–97.

81. Michail SK, Stolfi A, Johnson T, et al. Efficacy of probiotics in the treatment of pediatric atopic dermatitis: a meta-analysis of randomized controlled trials. Ann Allergy Asthma Immunol 2008;101:508–16.

82. Lee J, Seto D, Bielory L. Meta-analysis of clinical trials of probiotics for prevention and treatment of pediatric atopic dermatitis. J Allergy Clin Immunol 2008;121:116–21 e111.

83. Kopp MV, Hennemuth I, Heinzmann A, et al. Randomized, double-blind, placebo-controlled trial of probiotics for primary prevention: no clinical effects of Lactobacillus GG supplementation. Pediatrics 2008;121:e850–6.

84. Boyle RJ, Bath-Hextall FJ, Leonardi-Bee J, et al. Probiotics for treating eczema. Cochrane Database Syst Rev 2008:CD006135.

85. Oren E, Banerji A, Camargo CA Jr. Vitamin D and atopic disorders in an obese population screened for vitamin D deficiency. J Allergy Clin Immunol 2008;121:533–4.

86. Schauber J, Gallo RL. Antimicrobial peptides and the skin immune defense system. J Allergy Clin Immunol 2008;122:261–6.

87. Hata TR, Kotol P, Jackson M, et al. Administration of oral vitamin D induces cathelicidin production in atopic individuals. J Allergy Clin Immunol 2008;122:829–31.

88. Sidbury R, Sullivan AF, Thadhani RI, et al. Randomized controlled trial of vitamin D supplementation for winter-related atopic dermatitis in Boston: a pilot study. Br J Dermatol 2008;159:245–7.

89. Vigo PG, Girgis KR, Pfuetze BL, et al. Efficacy of anti-IgE therapy in patients with atopic dermatitis. J Am Acad Dermatol 2006;55:168–70.

90. Krathen RA, Hsu S. Failure of omalizumab for treatment of severe adult atopic dermatitis. J Am Acad Dermatol 2005;53:338–40.

91. Lane JE, Cheyney JM, Lane TN, et al. Treatment of recalcitrant atopic dermatitis with omalizumab. J Am Acad Dermatol 2006;54:68–72.

92. Werfel T, Breuer K, Rueff F, et al. Usefulness of specific immunotherapy in patients with atopic dermatitis and allergic sensitization to house dust mites: a multi-centre, randomized, dose-response study. Allergy 2006;61: 202–5.

93. Pajno GB, Caminiti L, Vita D, et al. Sublingual immunotherapy in mite-sensitized children with atopic dermatitis: a randomized, double-blind, placebo-controlled study. J Allergy Clin Immunol 2007;120: 164–70.

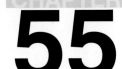

CHAPTER

55

Urticaria and Angioedema

Bruce L. Zuraw

Urticaria (hives) typically present as a pruritic generalized eruption with erythematous circumscribed borders and pale, slightly elevated centers (Figure 55-1A). Angioedema is characterized by an asymmetric nondependent swelling that is generally not pruritic (see Figure 55-1B). The pathophysiology of urticaria and angioedema is similar, resulting from increased vascular permeability with leakage of plasma into the superficial skin in urticaria and into the deeper skin layers in angioedema. Recognition of urticaria and angioedema is generally obvious, and often made by the patient or the patient's family. In contrast, these disorders are often frustratingly difficult to treat and their cause is elusive. Affected patients may manifest symptoms that range from transient and mildly annoying hives to severe and potentially fatal angioedema. Quality of life has been reported to be moderately to severely impaired in patients with chronic urticaria.[1] An efficient and cost-effective approach to the management of urticaria and angioedema depends on a careful assessment of the characteristics and likely cause of the swelling. This chapter provides a framework to differentiate the various types of urticaria and angioedema, then outlines a directed evaluation and treatment plan based on the etiology (Box 55-1).

Epidemiology/Etiology

Epidemiology

Urticaria and angioedema are commonly encountered in the general population.[2] Most of the information about their epidemiology is based on observations made in adult patients.[3] Urticaria/angioedema is conventionally classified as either *acute* or *chronic,* defined as the continuous or frequent occurrence of lesions for longer than 6 weeks.[4] Although arbitrary, this distinction has significant implications regarding the cause, course, and treatment of the swelling. The majority of patients with urticaria or angioedema experience acute swelling, and this is thought to be particularly true in children. Approximately 50% of affected patients have both urticaria and angioedema, 40% only urticaria, and 10% only angioedema.[5] Surveys have indicated that 15–23% of the populace experience urticaria at least once during their lifetime.[2] The prevalence of chronic urticaria is estimated to range from 0.5% to 5%.[6] Atopic individuals are at increased risk for acute urticaria/angioedema and some forms of physical urticaria; however, most patients with chronic urticaria/angioedema are not atopic.

Etiology

Most urticaria/angioedema is caused by mast cell degranulation with release of histamine, which is the primary mediator of the immediate wheal and flare.[7] A delayed inflammatory response resulting from mast cell degranulation, termed the *late-phase cutaneous response*, consists of variable amounts of erythema and induration that begin in 1 to 2 hours, peak at 6 to 12 hours, and persist for up to 24 hours after degranulation.[8] The late-phase cutaneous response is mediated by a variety of mast cell mediators (including cytokines, chemokines, and leukotrienes) that recruit inflammatory cells into the site of degranulation. Taken together, these observations have been interpreted to suggest that mast cell degranulation is a final common pathway linking most of the diverse types of urticaria/angioedema. Immunoglobulin E (IgE)-mediated mast cell degranulation in response to allergens is responsible for many cases of acute urticaria/angioedema in children. The most common sources of allergen that trigger IgE-mediated urticaria or angioedema are drugs and foods.

A significant proportion of acute urticaria/angioedema cases, as well as the vast majority of cases of *chronic* urticaria or angioedema, cannot be linked to IgE-mediated allergy. In these cases, nonimmunologic mechanisms or immune processes not involving IgE may also feed into the final common pathway of mast cell stimulation, histamine release, and resultant urticaria/angioedema. A variety of non-IgE stimuli can lead to mast cell degranulation and manifestation of acute or chronic urticaria/angioedema, including direct mast cell degranulators, viral infections, anaphylatoxins, various peptides/proteins, and several types of physical stimuli. In the pediatric population, viral infections are the most common cause of acute urticaria.[9,10] A form of acute urticaria resembling erythema multiforme, called urticaria multiforme (or acute annular urticarial hypersensitivity), is distinguished by transient annular urticarial lesions often accompanied by angioedema, that respond to antihistamines.[11]

The underlying cause of mast cell degranulation in the majority of patients with chronic urticaria/angioedema cannot be determined, and these patients are said to have chronic idiopathic urticaria/angioedema.[3] Understanding the cause of chronic idiopathic urticaria remains a particular challenge. The skin of these patients demonstrates a nonnecrotizing mononuclear cell infiltrate around small venules,[7,12] with increased numbers of basophils, eosinophils, and T helper cells. Approximately 40% of patients with chronic urticaria have been found to possess circulating autoantibodies with specificity for IgE or

©2010 Elsevier Ltd, Inc, BV
DOI: 10.1016/B978-1-4377-0271-2.00055-9

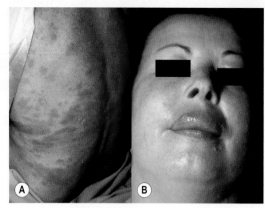

Figure 55-1 Typical examples of swelling. **(A)** Diffuse urticaria with areas of confluence. **(B)** Angioedema of the upper lip and face.

BOX 55-1 Key concepts

Urticaria and Angioedema

- The distinction between acute and chronic urticaria/angioedema has important diagnostic and therapeutic implications.

- The most common type of swelling in children is acute urticaria/angioedema.

- Cause of acute urticaria can usually be determined and is most likely to involve IgE-mediated reactions, viral infections, or bites and stings.

- Cause of chronic urticaria/angioedema is typically idiopathic; however, physical stimuli often contribute to the symptoms.

- Chronic urticaria/angioedema must be distinguished from urticarial vasculitis.

- Recurrent angioedema without urticaria suggests the possibility of hereditary angioedema.

- Most cases of chronic urticaria/angioedema resolve within 3 to 4 years.

---

the high-affinity FcεR.[13-15] Skin testing with autologous serum or plasma may be useful for screening patients for these antibodies.[16] Basophil degranulation has also been implicated in chronic urticaria and angioedema, but ex vivo basophil histamine tests have been less sensitive than autologous plasma skin testing in detecting autoantibodies. Approximately 30% of children with chronic idiopathic urticaria had positive autologous serum skin tests.[17,18] The functional and prognostic significance of these autoantibodies remains unclear.

Some, but not all, studies have found an increased prevalence of thyroid antimicrosomal and antithyroglobulin antibodies in adult and pediatric urticaria/angioedema patients, with about half of these patients having goiters or abnormal thyroid function.[19-22] Despite the lack of a demonstrable causal relationship, treatment with levothyroxine in order to decrease the thyroid-stimulating hormone level below 2.0 mU/L has been recommended in patients with chronic urticaria, even in the absence of known thyroid disease or antithyroid antibodies.[23] Additionally, an increased cumulative prevalence of urticaria/angioedema has been found in thyroid disease patients with antimicrosomal and antithyroglobulin antibodies (primarily Hashimoto's thyroiditis) but not in patients with other types of thyroid disease.[24] An association between urticaria and a variety of other autoimmune diseases, including Still's disease, insulin-dependent diabetes mellitus, and SLE, has also been described,[25] although patients with chronic idiopathic urticaria do not appear to be at higher risk of developing a systemic autoimmune disease.[26] An association between celiac disease and severe chronic urticaria has been described in children, with improvement of the urticaria in some patients following institution of a gluten-free diet.[27] Activation of thrombin with subsequent generation of C5a has also been suggested as a potential underlying mechanism in chronic urticaria.[28]

Rare cases of severe urticaria/angioedema associated with marked weight gain, pronounced leukocytosis, and striking eosinophilia have been described and the syndrome has become known as the *Gleich syndrome*.[29] These patients have increased serum levels of cytokines (including IL-5) during attacks,[30] and respond favorably to treatment with corticosteroids. Other cases of urticaria/angioedema have been reported in association with parathyroid disease, polycythemia vera, hemolytic uremic syndrome, Schnitzler syndrome (chronic urticaria, monoclonal IgM, arthralgia, fever and adenopathy), and pregnancy. Genetic causes of swelling are transmitted as autosomal dominant traits, and include: hereditary angioedema (HAE); Muckle-Wells syndrome (urticaria, deafness, and amyloidosis); vibratory angioedema; familial cold autoinflammatory syndrome (formally called *familial cold urticaria);* familial localized heat urticaria of delayed type; erythropoietic protoporphyria with solar urticaria; C3 inactivator deficiency with urticaria; and serum carboxypeptidase N deficiency with angioedema. With the exception of HAE, these genetic diseases are very rare.

HAE has a prevalence thought to range between 1 per 30000 to 1:80000, and presents as recurrent angioedema in the absence of urticaria. It is caused by a functional deficiency of the plasma protein C1 inhibitor (C1 INH). Most HAE patients begin to manifest angioedema symptoms in childhood, often by the age of 2 to 3 years. Symptoms typically increase around puberty then persist throughout life. Two major types of HAE have been described:[31] type I HAE comprises 85% of cases and is characterized by low C1 INH antigenic and functional levels; type II HAE comprises the other 15% of cases and is characterized by normal C1 INH antigenic levels with low C1 INH functional activity due to secretion of a dysfunctional protein. Type I and type II HAE are caused by mutations in the C1 INH gene, resulting in increased plasma kallikrein activity and generation of the vasoactive mediator bradykinin.[31]

A novel familial form of recurrent angioedema has also been described and is called type III HAE. Clinically, this syndrome closely resembles type I and type II HAE; however, type III HAE primarily affects females and is characterized by normal C1 INH function.[32,33] In many of these patients, attacks of angioedema are temporally related to states of increased estrogen levels, whether endogenous (such as pregnancy) or exogenous (such as birth control pills or hormonal replacement therapy). A gain-of-function mutation in Hageman factor (coagulation factor XII) has been found in a minority of type III HAE kindreds;[34] however, the underlying cause of type III HAE remains unclear. C1 INH deficiency may also be acquired; however, this occurs primarily in older adults and has not been reported in children.

Familial cold autoinflammatory syndrome and Muckle-Wells syndrome have recently been shown to be associated with mutations in a newly described gene that encodes cryopyrin.[35] It has become clear that these belong to a family of autoinflammatory urticarial syndromes that can be referred to as cryopyrinopathies. Neonatal-onset multisystem inflammatory disease (NOMID) is a particularly severe form of a cryopyrinopathy. Based on the elevated IL-1 levels found in these patients, the IL-1 receptor antagonist anakinra has been successfully used to prevent attacks.[36]

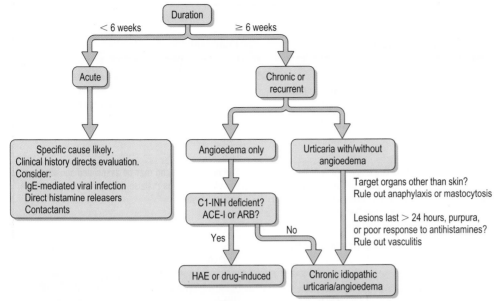

Figure 55-2 Diagnostic algorithm for urticaria/angioedema. *ACE-I*, angiotensin-converting enzyme inhibitor; *ARB*, angiotensin II receptor blocker; *HAE*, hereditary angioedema.

Differential Diagnosis

Recognition of urticaria and angioedema is generally obvious on examination. The single most important step in the differential diagnosis is to visualize the lesions during swelling. Individual urticarial lesions seldom last for more than a few hours (up to 24 hours), which distinguishes it from almost all other skin diseases. In addition, urticarial lesions blanch with pressure and new hives frequently develop as the older ones fade. If the lesions do not itch, the diagnosis should be reconsidered. Angioedema is not dependent and is typically not symmetrical. Figure 55-2 presents an algorithm for the approach to the differential diagnosis.

Acute Urticaria/Angioedema

A cause of acute urticaria/angioedema can frequently be determined. Most cases in children will be secondary to IgE-mediated reactions or viral infections. Drugs that frequently cause urticaria or angioedema on an IgE-mediated basis include penicillin and other antibiotics. The most common foods associated with IgE-mediated urticaria or angioedema depend, in large part, on the age of the patient. In younger children, egg, milk, soy, peanut, and wheat are the most common allergens, whereas fish, seafood, nuts, and peanuts are common offenders in older children.[37] Acute urticaria can also be triggered by ingestion of fish containing high levels of bioactive amines in the absence of specific IgE (scromboid poisoning).[38] Urticaria and angioedema are the most common manifestations of anaphylactic reactions to insect stings and bites. Immunologic reactions to the saliva of bedbugs, fleas, or mites can cause papular urticaria, especially on the legs of children.

Mast cell degranulation and urticaria/angioedema can also result from exposure to direct mast cell degranulators (such as strawberries, narcotic drugs, polymyxin antibiotics, D-tubocurarine, or dextran volume expanders), penetrating substances (such as nettles, Portuguese man-of-war, other forms of sea life, moth and butterfly scales, tarantula hairs, or caterpillar foot processes), or substances that can produce urticaria on contact with intact skin (such as latex, industrial chemicals, benzoic acid, sorbic acid, and numerous other agents that can produce either nonimmunologically or immunologically mediated reactions).[39]

Chronic Urticaria/Angioedema

This is a diagnosis of exclusion, based on history, examination, and carefully selected testing. No clear relationships have been found between chronic urticaria and food allergy, ingestion of food additives, or focal infections.[40,41] Some parasitic infestations may be associated with urticaria/angioedema; however, this association is suggested by finding substantial eosinophilia, elevated IgE level, abdominal symptoms, or a history of recent foreign travel. *Helicobacter pylori* infection has also been suggested as a link to chronic urticaria.[42-44]

The physical urticarias involve mast cell degranulation precipitated by discrete physical stimuli (Table 55-1). Physical urticaria is typically encountered in the setting of chronic idiopathic urticaria/angioedema. The percentage of children with chronic urticaria who also have a physical component ranges from 1% to >10%.[3] A variety of provoking stimuli have been described, including mechanical (pressure or stroking), thermal (heat or cold), solar, and aquagenic. In its mildest form, dermographism may occur in up to 2–5% of the general population; however, symptomatic dermographism (Figure 55-3A) can account for the majority of hives in some patients with chronic urticaria.[2] Delayed pressure urticaria is more angioedematous than urticarial and causes significant morbidity.[1] Primary and secondary acquired forms of cold urticaria have been described.[45] Primary acquired cold urticaria is often seen in children and is frequently associated with asthma, allergic rhinitis, and progression to frank anaphylaxis.[46] The physician should be aware that patients with acquired cold urticaria have drowned when exposed to cold water, and must be warned to avoid cold water and never to swim alone.

Familial cold autoinflammatory syndrome is marked by cold-induced erythematous rash, fever, arthralgias, leukocytosis and conjunctivitis.[35] Cholinergic urticaria (Figure 55-3B) is relatively common in children, may be confused with exercise-induced

Table 55-1 Major Physical Urticaria Syndromes

Type	Provoking Stimuli	Diagnostic Test	Comment
Mechanically Provoked			
Dermographism (urticaria factitia)	Rubbing or scratching of skin causes linear wheals	Stroking the skin (especially the back) elicits linear wheal	Primary (idiopathic or allergic) or secondary (urticaria pigmentosa or transient following virus or drug reaction)
Delayed dermographism	Same	Same	Rare
Delayed-pressure urticaria	At least 2 hr after pressure is applied to the skin, deep, painful swelling develops, especially involving the palms, soles, and buttocks	Attach two sandbags or jugs of fluid (5–15 lbs) to either end of a strap and apply over the shoulder or thigh for 10 to 15 min. A positive test exhibits linear wheals or swelling after several hours	Can be disabling and may be associated constitutional symptoms such as malaise, fever, arthralgia, headache, and leukocytosis
Immediate-pressure urticaria	Hives develop within 1 to 2 min of pressure	Several minutes of pressure elicit hives	Rare; seen in conjunction with hypereosinophilic syndrome
Thermally Provoked			
Acquired cold urticaria	Change in skin temperature rapidly provokes urticaria	Place ice cube on extremity for 3 to 5 min, then observe for pruritic welt and surrounding erythema as the skin rewarms over subsequent 5 to 15 min	Relatively common, may occur transiently with exposure to drugs or with infections; other rare cases may be associated with cryoproteins or may be transferable by serum
Familial cold autoinflammatory syndrome	Intermittent episodes of rash, arthralgia, fever, and conjunctivitis occur after generalized exposure to cold	Symptoms occur 2 to 4 hr after exposure to cold blowing air	Autosomal-dominant inflammatory disorder previously called familial cold 'urticaria'; results from mutation of CIAS1 gene, coding for cryopyrin
Cholinergic urticaria	Heat, exertion, or emotional upsets cause small punctate wheals with prominent erythematous flare. May be related more to sweating than to heat per se	Methacholine cutaneous challenge is sometimes helpful; better to reproduce the lesions by exercising in a warm environment or while wearing a wet suit or plastic occlusive suit	Differs from exercise-induced anaphylaxis in that it features smaller wheals and is induced by heat as well as by exercise but does not generally cause patients to collapse. Relatively common in patients with chronic urticaria; can be passively transferred by plasma in some patients
Localized heat urticaria	Urtication occurs at sites of contact with a warm stimulus	Hold a test tube containing warm water against the skin for 5 min	Rare
Miscellaneous Provoked			
Solar urticaria	Urticaria develops in areas of skin exposed to sunlight	Controlled exposure to light; can be divided depending on the wavelength of light eliciting the lesions	Types include genetic abnormality in protoporphyrin IX metabolism as well as types that can be passively transferred by IgE in serum
Aquagenic urticaria	Tiny perifollicular urticarial lesions develop after contact with water of any temperature	Apply towel soaked in 37°C water to the skin for 30 min	Rare; systemic symptoms can occur; females affected more than males; familial form has been described

anaphylaxis, and can be associated with angioedema, wheezing, or even syncope.[47] Persistent cholinergic erythema, a variant of cholinergic urticaria, can be mistaken for a drug eruption or cutaneous mastocytosis.[48] Successful treatment of severe cholinergic urticaria with danazol or anti-IgE has been described.[49,50] Many patients have combinations of different physical urticarias, such as cold and cholinergic urticaria, cold and localized heat urticaria, or dermographism with cold urticaria.

Mast cell degranulation and whealing may also occur because of mastocytosis, a primary disorder of mast cell proliferation. Mastocytosis in adults is not infrequently associated with somatic mutations in *c-kit*, a tyrosine kinase membrane receptor for stem cell factor that regulates mast cell proliferation.[51] Mutations in c-kit in pediatric mastocytosis are uncommon. The most common forms of mastocytosis in children are solitary mastocytomas or cutaneous mastocytosis (urticaria pigmentosa), usually presenting within the first year of life and resolving by adolescence.[52,53] Urtication of affected skin following stroking (Darier's sign) is a cardinal sign of cutaneous mastocytosis; however, diffuse urticaria is not part of mastocytosis. Cutaneous mastocytosis can be associated with systemic symptoms such as shortness of breath, hypotension, or gastrointestinal upset. Systemic mastocytosis (in which mast cells infiltrate other organs, including the bone marrow, spleen, bone, liver or lymph nodes) is uncommon in the pediatric population.

Idiopathic anaphylaxis is not caused by any external allergen and often includes a prominent component of urticaria and/or angioedema.[54] Some idiopathic anaphylaxis patients have systemic symptoms such as diarrhea, wheezing, hypotension, and generalized flushing, whereas others may have only recurrent life-threatening angioedema. Idiopathic anaphylaxis that presents with purely cutaneous symptoms can be indistinguishable from severe recurrent angioedema. The angioedema of idiopathic anaphylaxis can also resemble HAE; however, a positive family history as well as complement abnormalities will clearly identify HAE.

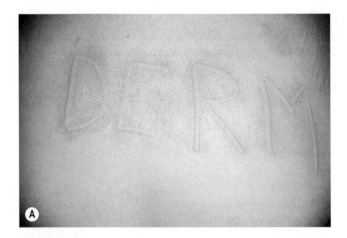

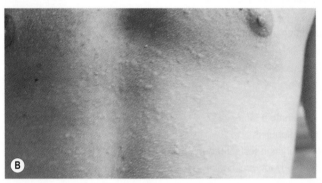

Figure 55-3 Examples of physical urticaria. **(A)** Dermatographism. (From Weston WL, Morelli JG, Lane A, eds. Color textbook of pediatric dermatology, 3rd edn. St Louis: Mosby; 2002.). **(B)** Cholingergic urticaria. (From Fireman P, Slavin R, eds. Atlas of allergies, 2nd edn. London: Mosby-Wolfe; 1996.)

Although not common in children, urticarial vasculitis must be distinguished from chronic idiopathic urticaria/angioedema. When flagrant, urticarial vasculitis is characterized by palpable purpura and bruising or discoloration that persists after the hive disappears. Persistence of individual urticarial lesions for >24 hours or a poor response to antihistamine therapy may suggest the possibility of urticarial vasculitis.[55] Urticarial vasculitis ranges from relatively benign cutaneous hypersensitivity vasculitis to the hypocomplementemic urticarial vasculitis syndrome.[56] In children, most cases of cutaneous vasculitis represent Henoch-Schonlein purpura or hypersensitivity vasculitis.[57] Adults may manifest urticarial vasculitis as part of an underlying connective tissue disease such as systemic lupus erythematosus, Sjögren's syndrome, essential mixed cryoglobulinemia, or polymyositis. The hypocomplementemic urticarial vasculitis syndrome is rarely seen in children.[58]

Angioedema

Angioedema is usually associated with urticaria, nondependent, asymmetric, and associated with little or no itching. When occurring with urticaria, the diagnosis and etiology of angioedema is based on the parameters described above for urticaria. Recurrent angioedema without urticaria (including recurrent unexplained abdominal pain) should suggest a possible diagnosis of HAE. This is particularly important to recognize and treat because of its potential morbidity and mortality. Unfortunately, delays in diagnosis are the rule rather than the exception, and repeated surveys have shown a 10- to 20-year interval between onset of symptoms and establishment of the correct diagnosis.[59]

Angioedema may also occur during the treatment of hypertension with angiotensin-converting enzyme (ACE) inhibitors or, less commonly, with angiotensin II receptor blockers.[60] ACE is a peptidase that degrades bradykinin (among other peptides), and the mechanism of ACE inhibitor-associated angioedema is suspected to be due to diminished catabolism of bradykinin.[61] There are also several forms of facial edema that can be confused with angioedema, including the granulomatous cheilitis accompanying Crohn's disease and the Melkersson-Rosenthal syndrome (a rare syndrome of recurrent orofacial swelling, relapsing facial paralysis, and fissured tongue).

Evaluation and Management

History

A discerning history is the most important diagnostic procedure in the evaluation of urticaria/angioedema, and dictates which, if any, of the large number of etiologic possibilities should be pursued. First, one should determine: whether the urticaria/angioedema is acute or chronic, the duration of the individual lesions, and the presence of pruritus (a defining symptom for urticaria). Other important information includes: *when* lesions occur, *where* the patient is when lesions occur, and *what* has the patient suspected? Specific inquiry should be made about drugs (including over-the-counter products), foreign sera, foods, food additives, herbal or homeopathic treatments, psychologic factors, inhalants, bites and stings, direct contact of skin with various agents, connective tissue diseases, and exposure to physical agents. It is important to assess the duration of individual lesions as well as response to prior therapy. Associated respiratory, gastrointestinal, or musculoskeletal symptoms should be inquired about.

The history should elicit information about factors that may influence the severity of urticaria/angioedema. In many patients, the disease is aggravated by vasodilating stimuli, such as heat, exercise, emotional stress, alcoholic drinks, fever, and hyperthyroidism. Premenstrual exacerbations also are common. Aspirin and other cyclooxygenase (COX)-1 inhibiting nonsteroidal anti-inflammatory drugs (NSAIDs) can cause acute urticaria. They can also lead to exacerbations of chronic urticaria or angioedema in up to 30% of patients, but hives generally continue even when aspirin is assiduously avoided. Urticaria/angioedema has also been reported in patients taking COX-2 inhibitors;[62] however, COX-2 inhibitors and acetaminophen typically do not trigger urticaria or angioedema.[63] A retrospective random review of 1007 charts of atopic children revealed that 41 (4.07%) had experienced NSAID-induced facial angioedema.[64] Intermittent use of NSAIDS was associated with a higher rate of angioedema than chronic regular use.[65] Angioedema occurring during the treatment of hypertension by ACE inhibitors may be related to the kininase activity of this enzyme.

Patients with HAE manifest a unique set of symptoms.[59] Attacks of swelling in HAE typically last 72 or more hours. Many HAE attacks appear to be triggered by minor trauma or stress. Although the precipitating stimulus is usually obscure, attacks are frequently preceded by a prodromal syndrome, often including a nonpruritic erythematous rash that may have a serpentine shape. HAE often shows a striking periodicity with attacks of angioedema followed by several weeks or more during which the patient does not swell. Daily episodes of angioedema suggest a diagnosis other than HAE. The swelling in HAE most commonly affects the extremities, face, gastrointestinal tract, or upper airway. Virtually all HAE patients experience extremity and gastrointestinal attacks during their lifetime, and the frequency of attacks in these two locations are similar. Abdominal attacks can be severe, and may resemble a surgical abdomen. Recurrent school absences because of abdominal pain may be a presenting symptom of HAE because of angioedema of the abdominal wall. It is not unusual to obtain a history of a normal exploratory laparotomy for presumed appendicitis. Laryngeal attacks are considerably less common, although over 50% of HAE patients will experience a laryngeal attack at some point in their life. Angioedema of the larynx in HAE can result in closure of the airway with asphyxiation. Prior to the time when most patients had an accurate diagnosis and access to treatment, over 30% of HAE patients died from airway attacks.[59] Even today, however, HAE patients continue to die from their disease, albeit at a much lower rate.

A positive family history of angioedema can often be elicited; however, up to 20% of HAE patients have de novo mutations.[66] HAE typically presents around puberty, although symptoms may begin in younger children and then worsen at puberty. It is often very helpful to ask whether the patient has ever been treated for the angioedema with antihistamines, corticosteroids, or epinephrine as these medications do not have significant benefit for the angioedema in HAE.

Physical Examination

A complete physical examination is important, especially in cases of chronic urticaria and angioedema, to rule out an underlying condition such as a connective tissue, viral, or endocrine disease. Urticarial lesions typically are generalized and may involve any part of the body, and individual lesions often coalesce into large lesions. Angioedema is usually asymmetric and typically involves loose connective tissue such as the face or mucous membranes involving the lips or tongue. Occasionally, the appearance of the lesions gives a clue as to the type of urticaria being encountered: linear wheals suggest dermographism; small wheals surrounded by large areas of erythema suggest cholinergic urticaria; wheals limited to exposed areas suggest solar or cold urticaria; and wheals mainly on the lower extremities suggest papular urticaria or urticarial vasculitis.

Diagnostic Procedures

The laboratory evaluation of patients with urticaria or angioedema must be tailored to the clinical situation. In most cases no specific etiology can be established, and the diagnostic approach should therefore be carefully selected and cost effective. If the history or examination provide clues to the cause of the urticaria/angioedema, the evaluation should be pursued using the appropriate tests (e.g. skin testing to confirm IgE-mediated food or drug allergy). In the absence of a specific likely cause, the laboratory evaluation should be minimal. Box 55-2 summarizes a limited laboratory evaluation that could be performed in patients with chronic urticaria/angioedema to exclude important underlying disease. Because the cause of chronic urticaria or angioedema is not related to extrinsic allergen exposure in the vast majority of cases, routine skin testing is not cost effective and typically only increases the frustration of both the patient and physician when no culprit is identified.[67] Patients with a suggestive history of physical urticaria may be challenged to confirm the diagnosis (see Table 55-1). Patients with recurrent angioedema without urticaria should be evaluated for HAE (Table 55-2).

BOX 55-2

Suggested Testing for Chronic Urticaria/Angioedema of Unknown Etiology

Basic Tests

Routine screening:
  CBC with differential
  ESR or CRP
  Urinalysis
Optional tests:
  Liver function tests
  Thyroid function and autoantibodies
  Anti-FcεR or anti-IgE antibodies
  Stool for ova and parasites
  Physical challenges

Discretionary Tests Based on Evaluation

If vasculitis is suspected:
  Antinuclear antibody
  Skin biopsy
  CH_{50}
  Rheumatoid factor
  Cryoglobulins
If liver function tests abnormal:
  Serology for viral hepatitis

Treatment

Reassurance is an important aspect of therapy for urticaria/angioedema. Skin lesions are often more frightening in appearance than the generally favorable prognosis warrants and are self-limited. Patients and their families should be reassured that most urticaria/angioedema spontaneously remits without any irreversible damage to one's health. Patients should, however, be made aware of the need for an emergency room visit if laryngeal edema occurs. If the patient has experienced laryngeal edema, many physicians would prescribe and instruct the patient in the use of self-injectable epinephrine. However, one should avoid generating undue anxiety about laryngeal edema because the only known fatalities from this cause have been in patients with HAE, angiotensin-converting enzyme inhibitor-associated angioedema, or anaphylactic reactions.

Guidelines for treating patients with urticaria/angioedema are summarized in Box 55-3. Obviously the preferred treatment is avoidance of causative agents when these can be identified. This generally is the case when allergy to drugs, foods, inhalants, insects, or contactants is involved. An explanation of the disease process and its triggers should also be helpful for patients with physical urticaria such as dermographism, cholinergic urticaria, and delayed-pressure urticaria. Common sense avoidance measures should be reviewed with patients afflicted with cold or solar urticaria. Treatment of any discovered underlying disease is imperative, and genetic counseling should be provided to families with hereditary forms of these conditions. In addition, patients should avoid, to the extent feasible, potentiating factors such as alcoholic drinks, heat, exertion, and aspirin.

Antihistamines are the mainstay of treatment for acute or chronic urticaria/angioedema (Figure 55-4). Used at a sufficient dose, they alleviate pruritus and suppress hive formation. Corticosteroids should not be used except in extraordinary circumstances such as hypocomplementemic urticarial vasculitis or

Table 55-2 Complement Evaluation of Patients with Recurrent Angioedema

Assay	Idiopathic Angioedema	Type I HAE	Type II HAE	Acquired C1 INH Deficiency	Vasculitis
C4	nl	Low	Low	Low	Low or nl
C4d/C4 ratio	nl	High	High	High	High or nl
C1 INH level	nl	Low	nl	Low	nl
C1 INH function	nl	Low	Low	Low	nl
C1q	nl	nl	nl	Low	Low or nl
C3	nl	nl	nl	nl	Low or nl

HAE, hereditary angioedema; *INH,* inhibitor; *nl,* normal.

BOX 55-3 Therapeutic principles

Treatment of Urticaria/Angioedema

Avoidance of known provoking stimuli can greatly improve treatment outcomes.

H_1 antihistamines are the mainstay of treatment, and second-generation H_1 antihistamines are preferred because they have fewer side-effects.

Difficult cases may require treatment with various combinations of second-generation H_1 antihistamines, first-generation H_1 antihistamines, H_2 antihistamines, and leukotriene receptor antagonists.

Delayed-pressure urticaria does not generally respond well to antihistamines.

Corticosteroids should be avoided whenever possible and in particular for the treatment of chronic urticaria/angioedema without delayed-pressure urticaria.

The angioedema of hereditary angioedema does not respond to antihistamines, corticosteroids, or epinephrine; oropharyngeal attacks of hereditary angioedema must be treated as a medical emergency.

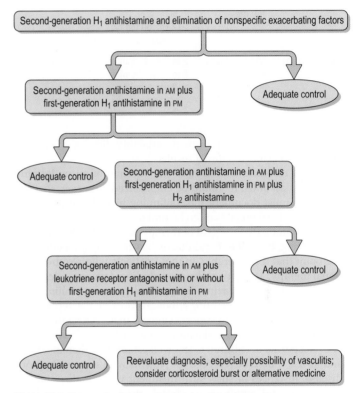

Figure 55-4 Therapeutic algorithm for chronic urticaria/angioedema.

---

delayed-pressure urticaria (which typically does not respond to antihistamines). Most first-generation H_1 antihistamines are effective in urticaria. Among the commonly employed drugs of this type, hydroxyzine and doxepin have the greatest potency. Common side-effects of the first-generation H_1 antihistamines (particularly drowsiness and anticholinergic effects) are a substantial issue, and have limited the usefulness of these drugs.[68] In addition, children may experience either sedation or a paradoxical agitation response to first generation H_1 antihistamines.[69]

Second-generation H_1 antagonists cross the blood-brain barrier poorly, producing much less central drowsiness or agitation and have much less anticholinergic effect. Second generation H_1 antagonists have thus become the preferred drugs for the first-line treatment of urticaria/angioedema.[70] In instances where the pruritus interferes with sleep, use of a sedating antihistamine at bedtime may be preferred. The most commonly used second-generation H1 antihistamines in the USA are cetirizine, loratadine, desloratadine, and fexofenadine. Each of these has been shown to be well tolerated and effective for the treatment of urticaria/angioedema.[71] The recommended doses for the pediatric population is shown in Table 55-3.

If a second-generation H_1 antihistamine does not provide adequate relief, combination therapy may be tried. A sedating H1 antihistamine given at bedtime can be used in conjunction with

a second-generation H_1 antihistamine in the morning. Because the cutaneous vasculature expresses H_2 as well as the more abundant H_1 receptors, the addition of an H_2 antihistamine (e.g. cimetidine or ranitidine) may provide significant benefit for patients who are refractory to H_1 antihistamines alone. Leukotriene receptor antagonists have shown some promise in the treatment of urticaria/angioedema, particularly in combination with an antihistamine regimen;[72] however, clear evidence of benefit from randomized, double-blinded studies is lacking.[73] The addition of ephedrine or terbutaline is another option but is generally not effective and is often associated with significant side-effects. Cyproheptadine is thought to be particularly effective for the treatment of cold urticaria.[74] Ketotifen, and leukotriene receptor antagonists have also been shown to be helpful in severe cases of cold urticaria.[75,76] Delayed pressure urticaria is a particularly difficult problem, as it typically does not respond well to any antihistamine. Although some patients appear to be helped by cetirizine.[77] some patients with delayed pressure urticaria require systemic corticosteroids. While almost all patients will respond

Table 55-3 Dosing of Second Generation H1 Antihistamines in the Pediatric Population

Drug	Supplied As	Dosage	Earliest Approved Age
Cetirizine	Tablets: 5, 10 mg Syrup: 5 mg/tspn	6 mo to 5 yr: 2.5 mg/d or 0.25 mg/kg/d 6 to 11 yr: 5 mg/d ≥12 yr: 10 mg/d	6 mo
Loratadine	Tablets/reditabs: 10 mg Syrup: 5 mg/tspn	2 to 6 yr: 5 mg/d ≥6 yr: 10 mg/d	
Fexofenadine	Tablets: 30, 60, 180 mg	6 to 11 yr: 30 mg bid ≥12 yrs: 60 mg bid or 180 mg/d	6 mo
Desloratadine	Tablets/reditabs: 5 mg	2 to 5 yr: 1.25 mg/d 6 to 11 yr: 2.5 mg/d ≥12 yrs: 5 mg/d	6 mo

Table 55-4 Drugs Used for Long-Term Prophylaxis of HAE in Children

Drug Class and Name	Usual Pediatric Dose (Typical Range of Doses)	Side-Effects
Antifibrinolytic Agents		
Epsilon aminocaproic acid	0.05 g/kg BID (0.025 g/kg BID – 0.1 g/kg BID)	*Common*: nausea, vertigo, diarrhea, postural hypotension, fatigue, muscle cramps with increased muscle enzymes *Uncommon*: thrombisis
Tranexemic acid	20 mg/kg BID (10 mg/kg BID – 25 mg/kg TID)	
17α-Alkylated Androgens		
Danazol	50 mg/d (50 mg/wk – 200 mg/d)	*Common*: weight gain, virilization, acne, altered libido, muscle pain/cramps, headache, depression, fatigue, nausea, constipation, menstrual abnormalities, increase in liver enzymes, hypertension, altered lipid profile *Uncommon*: decreased rate of growth in children, masculinization of female fetus, cholestatic jaundice, peliosis hepatis, hepatocellular adenoma
Stanozolol	0.5 – 1 mg/day for children <6 yr; up to 2 mg/d for children ≥6 yr	
Oxandrolone	0.1 mg/kg/d	

to antihistamine therapy, patient variability dictates an empiric approach to achieve optimal results.

Lack of response should raise the question of an underlying urticarial vasculitis. It should be emphasized, however, that the physician must document the continuing hives by direct observation. Furthermore, it is often helpful to counsel the patient and patient's family that the goal of therapy is not to totally suppress the swelling, but rather to minimize the urticaria/angioedema to the point that it is tolerable. In those patients who require additional therapy, a variety of drugs (including dapsone, colchicine, methotrexate, sulfasalazine, intravenous gammaglobulin) have been reported to be helpful, although most of the reports are anecdotal. A number of reports suggest that cyclosporine may be safely used to treat resistant chronic urticaria.[78,79] The safety of cyclosporine in children is less well established than in adults, and its use should be reserved for patients with severe refractory disease. Instances of successful treatment with omalizumab for cholinergic and autoimmune chronic urticaria have also been reported.[50,80]

Parenteral corticosteroids are often effective in controlling severe urticaria/angioedema as well as urticarial vasculitis;[81] however, the potential side-effects from chronic use of corticosteroids mandates that they be used at the lowest possible dose for the shortest period of time.[82,83] Urticarial vasculitis has been reported to respond favorably to hydroxychloroquine, which has a superior safety profile compared to that of corticosteroids.[84]

The treatment of HAE is entirely distinct from that of allergic or idiopathic angioedema. Treatment of HAE is best considered as three separate goals: long-term prophylaxis, short-term prophylaxis, and treatment of acute attacks. Long-term prophylaxis may be required to decrease the frequency and/or severity of swelling in patients with frequent severe attacks or with a history of serious attacks involving the upper airway. Long-term prophylaxis with synthetic 17α-alkylated androgens or antifibrinolytic drugs (Table 55-4) reduce the number and severity of attacks,[31] however, potential side-effects limit their use in children.[85,86] If used, these drugs should be titrated down to the lowest effective dose that provides adequate control of the HAE based on clinical responses. Plasma-derived C1 INH was recently approved in the USA for use as long-term prophylaxis of HAE.

While many children with HAE do not require long-term prophylactic therapy, plasma-derived C1 INH replacement therapy is the treatment of choice for children with HAE who require long-term prophylaxis.

Short-term prophylaxis for HAE is indicated before expected trauma, such as surgery or dental procedures. Patients can be given either C1 INH replacment therapy (with plasma-derived C1 INH concentrate or fresh frozen plasma if the concentrate is not available) 1 to 12 hours prior to the procedure or high-dose anabolic androgen therapy (e.g. danazol 200 mg three times daily) begun 7 to 10 days before the procedure, for protection.[31,87]

Until recently, there was no medication approved for use in the USA that will reliably treat acute HAE attacks. Fresh frozen plasma has been used by many physicians to treat acute attacks of HAE. While generally effective, occasional patients respond to fresh frozen plasma with a rapid and substantial worsening of the swelling.[31] Thus, the management of acute attacks was primarily concerned with symptomatic control of the swelling, and was quite suboptimal. Abdominal attacks require aggressive intravenous replacement of the fluid loss that occurs because of third spacing, as well as control of pain and nausea with parenteral narcotic and antiemetic drugs. Oropharyngeal attacks may lead to death secondary to asphyxiation, and therefore require hospitalization for careful monitoring of airway patency. Acute angioedema of the extremities is typically not treated at all, even though it may lead to significant absentiism from school or work.

Replacement therapy with purified C1 INH has been repeatedly shown to work extremely well to treat acute episodes of HAE.[88] Three successful randomized, double-blind, placebo-controlled studies of C1 INH replacement in acute attacks of

HAE have recently been completed in the USA resulting in the approval of C1 INH for treatment of acute attacks. Additionally, two drugs that specifically focus on bradykinin (the plasma kallikrein inhibitor ecallantide and the B2 bradykinin receptor antagonist icatibant) have recently undergone randomized, double-blind, placebo-controlled trials for the acute treatment of HAE resulting in the approval of ecallantide for treatment of acute attacks.

Conclusions

Urticaria and angioedema are common clinical problems whose manifestations range from trivial and intermittent to life threatening. To minimize spending time and money unnecessarily on complicated workups, while simultaneously not overlooking important diagnoses, the clinician must be able to characterize urticaria/angioedema by chronicity, type, and increasingly, by pathogenesis. With careful detective work, the cause of acute urticaria/angioedema can often be determined and appropriate interventions can be instituted that should lead to prompt resolution of the problem. A discrete cause of chronic urticaria, by contrast, is rarely established, forcing the clinician into the role of suppressing symptoms but not curing the problem. Although frequently frustrating for both the patient and the physician, the treatment of chronic urticaria can almost always achieve adequate results until the swelling disorder spontaneously remits. Hereditary angioedema is a rare but important cause of recurrent angioedema, and timely screening for HAE is the key to protect these patients from potentially severe morbidity and mortality.

Helpful Websites

The American Contact Dermatitis Society website (www.contactderm.org/)
The American Academy of Dermatology website (www.aad.org/)
The American Academy of Allergy, Asthma, and Immunology website (www.aaaai.org)
The Hereditary Angioedema (HAE) Association website (www.hereditaryangioedema.com)

References

1. Poon E, Seed PT, Greaves MW, et al. The extent and nature of disability in different urticarial conditions. Br J Dermatol 1999;140:667–71.
2. Mathews KP. Urticaria and angioedema. J Allergy Clin Immunol 1983;72:1–14.
3. Greaves MW. Chronic urticaria in childhood. Allergy 2000;55:309–20.
4. Vonakis BM, Saini SS. New concepts in chronic urticaria. Curr Opin Immunol 2008;20:709–16.
5. Champion RH, Roberts S, Carpenter RG, et al. Urticaria and angioedema: a review of 554 patients. Br J Derm 1969;81:588–97.
6. Kasperska-Zajac A, Brzoza Z, Rogala B. Sex hormones and urticaria. J Dermatol Sci 2008;52:79–86.
7. Hennino A, Berard F, Guillot I, et al. Pathophysiology of urticaria. Clin Rev Allergy Immunol 2006;30:3–11.
8. Atkins PC, Zweiman B. The IgE-mediated late-phase skin response: unraveling the enigma. J Allergy Clin Immunol 1987;79:12–5.
9. Novembre E, Cianferoni A, Mori F, et al. Urticaria and urticaria related skin condition/disease in children. Eur Ann Allergy Clin Immunol 2008;40:5–13.
10. Sackesen C, Sekerel BE, Orhan F, et al. The etiology of different forms of urticaria in childhood. Pediatr Dermatol 2004;21:102–8.
11. Shah KN, Honig PJ, Yan AC. 'Urticaria multiforme': a case series and review of acute annular urticarial hypersensitivity syndromes in children. Pediatrics 2007;119:e1177–83.
12. Ying S, Kikuchi Y, Meng Q, et al. TH1/TH2 cytokines and inflammatory cells in skin biopsy specimens from patients with chronic idiopathic urticaria: comparison with the allergen-induced late-phase cutaneous reaction. J Allergy Clin Immunol 2002;109:694–700.
13. Hide M, Francis DM, Grattan CE, et al. Autoantibodies against the high-affinity IgE receptor as a cause of histamine release in chronic urticaria. N Engl J Med 1993;328:1599–604.
14. Sabroe RA, Greaves MW. Chronic idiopathic urticaria with functional autoantibodies: 12 years on. Br J Dermatol 2006;154:813–9.
15. Soundararajan S, Kikuchi Y, Joseph K, et al. Functional assessment of pathogenic IgG subclasses in chronic autoimmune urticaria. J Allergy Clin Immunol 2005;115:815–21.
16. Asero R, Tedeschi A, Riboldi P, et al. Plasma of patients with chronic urticaria shows signs of thrombin generation, and its intradermal injection causes wheal-and-flare reactions much more frequently than autologous serum. J Allergy Clin Immunol 2006;117:1113–7.
17. Brunetti L, Francavilla R, Miniello VL, et al. High prevalence of autoimmune urticaria in children with chronic urticaria. J Allergy Clin Immunol 2004;114:922–7.
18. Du Toit G, Prescott R, Lawrence P, et al. Autoantibodies to the high-affinity IgE receptor in children with chronic urticaria. Ann Allergy Asthma Immunol 2006;96:341–4.
19. Leznoff A, Sussman GL. Syndrome of idiopathic chronic urticaria and angioedema with thyroid autoimmunity: a study of 90 patients. J Allergy Clin Immunol 1989;84:66–71.
20. Rumbyrt JS, Katz JL, Schocket AL. Resolution of chronic urticaria in patients with thyroid autoimmunity. J Allergy Clin Immunol 1995;96:901–5.
21. Verneuil L, Leconte C, Ballet JJ, et al. Association between chronic urticaria and thyroid autoimmunity: a prospective study involving 99 patients. Dermatology 2004;208:98–103.
22. Levy Y, Segal N, Weintrob N, et al. Chronic urticaria: association with thyroid autoimmunity. Arch Dis Child 2003;88:517–9.
23. Monge C, Demarco P, Burman KD, et al. Autoimmune thyroid disease and chronic urticaria. Clin Endocrinol (Oxf) 2007;67:473–5.
24. Lanigan SW, Short P, Moult P. The association of chronic urticaria and thyroid autoimmunity. Clin Exp Derm 1987;12:335–8.
25. Criado RF, Criado PR, Vasconcellos C, et al. Urticaria as a cutaneous sign of adult-onset Still's disease. J Cutan Med Surg 2006;10:99–103.
26. Ryhal B, DeMera RS, Shoenfeld Y, et al. Are autoantibodies present in patients with subacute and chronic urticaria? J Investig Allergol Clin Immunol 2001;11:16–20.
27. Caminiti L, Passalacqua G, Magazzu G, et al. Chronic urticaria and associated coeliac disease in children: a case-control study. Pediatr Allergy Immunol 2005;16:428–32.
28. Asero R, Tedeschi A, Riboldi P, et al. Severe chronic urticaria is associated with elevated plasma levels of D-dimer. Allergy 2008;63:176–80.
29. Gleich GJ, Schroeter AL, Marcoux JP, et al. Episodic angioedema associated with eosinophilia. N Engl J Med 1984;310:1621–6.
30. Butterfield JH, Leiferman KM, Abrams J, et al. Elevated serum levels of interleukin-5 in patients with the syndrome of episodic angioedema and eosinophilia. Blood 1992;79:688–92.
31. Zuraw BL. Clinical practice. Hereditary angioedema. N Engl J Med 2008;359:1027–36.
32. Binkley KE, Davis 3rd A. Clinical, biochemical, and genetic characterization of a novel estrogen-dependent inherited form of angioedema. J Allergy Clin Immunol 2000;106:546–50.
33. Bork K, Barnstedt SE, Koch P, et al. Hereditary angioedema with normal C1-inhibitor activity in women. Lancet 2000;356:213–7.
34. Dewald G, Bork K. Missense mutations in the coagulation factor XII (Hageman factor) gene in hereditary angioedema with normal C1 inhibitor. Biochem Biophys Res Commun 2006;343:1286–9.
35. Hoffman HM, Mueller JL, Broide DH, et al. Mutation of a new gene encoding a putative pyrin-like protein causes familial cold autoinflammatory syndrome and Muckle-Wells syndrome. Nat Genet 2001;29:301–5.
36. Hoffman HM, Rosengren S, Boyle DL, et al. Prevention of cold-associated acute inflammation in familial cold autoinflammatory syndrome by interleukin-1 receptor antagonist. Lancet 2004;364:1779–85.
37. Baxi S, Dinakar C. Urticaria and angioedema. Immunol Allergy Clin North Am 2005;25:353–67, vii.
38. Chegini S, Metcalfe DD. Contemporary issues in food allergy: seafood toxin-induced disease in the differential diagnosis of allergic reactions. Allergy Asthma Proc 2005;26:183–90.
39. Burdick AE, Mathias C. The contact urticaria syndrome. Derm Clin 1985;3:71–84.
40. Simon RA. Additive-induced urticaria: experience with monosodium glutamate (MSG). J Nutr 2000;130:1063S–6S.
41. Rorsman H. Basophilic leukopenia in different forms of urticaria. Acta Allergol 1962;17:168–84.
42. Greaves MW. Pathophysiology of chronic urticaria. Int Arch Allergy Immunol 2002;127:3–9.

43. Sadighha A, Shirali R, Zahed GM. Relationship between *Helicobacter pylori* and chronic urticaria. J Eur Acad Dermatol Venereol 2009;23: 198-9.

44. Yadav MK, Rishi JP, Nijawan S. Chronic urticaria and *Helicobacter pylori*. Indian J Med Sci 2008;62:157-62.

45. Wanderer AA, Grandel KE, Wasserman SI, et al. Clinical characteristics of cold-induced systemic reactions in acquired cold urticaria syndromes: recommendations for prevention of this complication and a proposal for a diagnostic classification of cold urticaria. J Allergy Clin Immunol 1986;78:417-23.

46. Alangari AA, Twarog FJ, Shih MC, et al. Clinical features and anaphylaxis in children with cold urticaria. Pediatrics 2004;113: e313-7.

47. Lawrence CM, Jorizzo JL, Kobza-Black A, et al. Cholinergic urticaria with associated angio-oedema. Br J Dermatol 1981;105:543-50.

48. Black AK. Unusual urticarias. J Dermatol 2001;28:632-4.

49. La Shell MS, England RW. Severe refractory cholinergic urticaria treated with danazol. J Drugs Dermatol 2006;5:664-7.

50. Metz M, Bergmann P, Zuberbier T, et al. Successful treatment of cholinergic urticaria with anti-immunoglobulin E therapy. Allergy 2008;63: 247-9.

51. Metcalfe DD, Akin C. Mastocytosis: molecular mechanisms and clinical disease heterogeneity. Leuk Res 2001;25:577-82.

52. Ben-Amitai D, Metzker A, Cohen HA. Pediatric cutaneous mastocytosis: a review of 180 patients. Isr Med Assoc J 2005;7:320-2.

53. Briley LD, Phillips CM. Cutaneous mastocytosis: a review focusing on the pediatric population. Clin Pediatr (Phila) 2008;47:757-61.

54. Hogan MB, Kelly MA, Wilson NW. Idiopathic anaphylaxis in children. Ann Allergy Asthma Immunol 1998;81:140-2.

55. Tosoni C, Lodi-Rizzini F, Cinquini M, et al. A reassessment of diagnostic criteria and treatment of idiopathic urticarial vasculitis: a retrospective study of 47 patients. Clin Exp Dermatol 2009;34:166-70.

56. Wisnieski JJ. Urticarial vasculitis. Curr Opin Rheumatol 2000;12: 24-31.

57. Blanco R, Martinez-Taboada VM, Rodriguez-Valverde V, et al. Cutaneous vasculitis in children and adults: associated diseases and etiologic factors in 303 patients. Medicine (Baltimore) 1998;77: 403-18.

58. Cadnapaphornchai MA, Saulsbury FT, Norwood VF. Hypocomplementemic urticarial vasculitis: report of a pediatric case. Pediatr Nephrol 2000;14:328-31.

59. Frank MM, Gelfand JA, Atkinson JP. Hereditary angioedema: the clinical syndrome and its management. Ann Intern Med 1976;84: 586-93.

60. Warner KK, Visconti JA, Tschampel MM. Angiotensin II receptor blockers in patients with ACE inhibitor-induced angioedema. Ann Pharmacother 2000;34:526-8.

61. Byrd JB, Adam A, Brown NJ. Angiotensin-converting enzyme inhibitor-associated angioedema. Immunol Allergy Clin North Am 2006;26: 725-37.

62. Kelkar PS, Butterfield JH, Teaford HG. Urticaria and angioedema from cyclooxygenase-2 inhibitors. J Rheumatol 2001;28:2553-4.

63. Grattan CE. Aspirin sensitivity and urticaria. Clin Exp Dermatol 2003;28: 123-7.

64. Capriles-Behrens E, Caplin J, Sanchez-Borges M. NSAID facial angioedema in a selected pediatric atopic population. J Investig Allergol Clin Immunol 2000;10:277-9.

65. Settipane RA, Constantine HP, Settipane GA. Aspirin intolerance and recurrent urticaria in normal adults and children. Epidemiology and review. Allergy 1980;35:149-54.

66. Pappalardo E, Cicardi M, Duponchel C, et al. Frequent de novo mutations and exon deletions in the C1 inhibitor gene of patients with angioedema. J Allergy Clin Immunol 2000;106:1147-54.

67. The diagnosis and management of urticaria: a practice parameter. Part I: acute urticaria/angioedema. Part II: chronic urticaria/angioedema. Joint Task Force on Practice Parameters. Ann Allergy Asthma Immunol 2000;85:521-44.

68. Qidwai JC, Watson GS, Weiler JM. Sedation, cognition, and antihistamines. Curr Allergy Asthma Rep 2002;2:216-22.

69. Simons FE, Simons KJ. The pharmacology and use of H1-receptor-antagonist drugs. N Engl J Med 1994;330:1663-70.

70. Zuberbier T, Bindslev-Jensen C, Canonica W, et al. EAACI/GA2LEN/ EDF guideline: management of urticaria. Allergy 2006;61:321-31.

71. Wedi B, Kapp A. Evidence-based therapy of chronic urticaria. J Dtsch Dermatol Ges 2007;5:146-57.

72. Bagenstose SE, Levin L, Bernstein JA. The addition of zafirlukast to cetirizine improves the treatment of chronic urticaria in patients with positive autologous serum skin test results. J Allergy Clin Immunol 2004;113:134-40.

73. McBayne TO, Siddall OM. Montelukast treatment of urticaria. Ann Pharmacother 2006;40:939-42.

74. Wanderer AA. Essential acquired cold urticaria. J Allergy Clin Immunol 1990;85:531-2.

75. Hani N, Hartmann K, Casper C, et al. Improvement of cold urticaria by treatment with the leukotriene receptor antagonist montelukast. Acta Derm Venereol 2000;80:229.

76. St-Pierre JP, Kobric M, Rackham A. Effect of ketotifen treatment on cold-induced urticaria. Ann Allergy 1985;55:840-3.

77. Kontou-Fili K, Maniatakou G, Paleologos G, et al. Cetirizine inhibits delayed pressure urticaria. Part 2. Skin biopsy findings. Ann Allergy 1990;65:520-2.

78. Grattan CE, O'Donnell BF, Francis DM, et al. Randomized double-blind study of cyclosporin in chronic 'idiopathic' urticaria. Br J Dermatol 2000;143:365-72.

79. Vena GA, Cassano N, Colombo D, et al. Cyclosporine in chronic idiopathic urticaria: a double-blind, randomized, placebo-controlled trial. J Am Acad Dermatol 2006;55:705-9.

80. Spector SL, Tan RA. Effect of omalizumab on patients with chronic urticaria. Ann Allergy Asthma Immunol 2007;99:190-3.

81. Poon M, Reid C. Do steroids help children with acute urticaria? Arch Dis Child 2004;89:85-6.

82. Zuberbier T, Maurer M. Urticaria: current opinions about etiology, diagnosis and therapy. Acta Derm Venereol 2007;87:196-205.

83. Grattan CE, Humphreys F. Guidelines for evaluation and management of urticaria in adults and children. Br J Dermatol 2007;157:1116-23.

84. Lopez LR, Davis KC, Kohler PF, et al. The hypocomplementemic urticarial-vasculitis syndrome: therapeutic response to hydroxychloroquine. J Allergy Clin Immunol 1984;73:600-3.

85. Gompels MM, Lock RJ, Abinun M, et al. C1 inhibitor deficiency: consensus document. Clin Exp Immunol 2005;139:379-94.

86. Farkas H, Varga L, Szeplaki G, et al. Management of hereditary angioedema in pediatric patients. Pediatrics 2007;120:e713-22.

87. Bowen T, Cicardi M, Bork K, et al. Hereditary angiodema: a current state-of-the-art review, VII: Canadian Hungarian 2007 International Consensus Algorithm for the Diagnosis, Therapy, and Management of Hereditary Angioedema. Ann Allergy Asthma Immunol 2008;100: S30-40.

88. Waytes AT, Rosen FS, Frank MM. Treatment of hereditary angioedema with a vapor-heated C1 inhibitor concentrate. N Engl J Med 1996;334: 1630-4.

CHAPTER

56

Contact Dermatitis

Luz Fonacier • Mark Boguniewicz

Contact dermatitis (CD) includes a spectrum of inflammatory skin reactions induced by exposure to external agents. Clinically, CD most commonly manifests as a dermatitis or eczema, but it can present as urticaria, erythroderma, phototoxic or photoallergic reactions, hypopigmentation or hyperpigmentation, and even acneiform. The more common type of CD results from tissue damage caused by contact with irritants (irritant CD), whereas contact with allergens causes allergic contact dermatitis (ACD). The former is seen commonly in infants as diaper dermatitis, whereas nickel and poison ivy are more frequent causes of ACD in the pediatric population.[1]

An estimated 85000 chemicals exist in the world, and the majority of these agents, when applied to the skin, induce an irritant CD. Approximately 2800 substances have been identified as contact allergens.[2] The majority of these agents, when applied to the skin can induce an irritant CD.[3] Identifying the responsible agent is essential for the appropriate management of patients with CD. The diagnosis is usually inferred by the clinical presentation, which must then be supported by a history of exposure to the offending agent. It is only when the implicated agent is identified and strictly avoided that resolution occurs.

Epidemiology

While ACD has been considered to occur less frequently in children, possibly because of reduced exposure to contact allergens or because the immune system in children may be less susceptible to contact allergens, recent studies show that ACD may affect as many as 20% of the pediatric population.[4] In some general population based US studies, positive patch testing (PT) was seen in 13–24% and the relevance rate reported in one study was 7%.[5] A cross-sectional study of 1501 children aged 12 to 16 years using questionnaires, examination, and patch testing found that the point prevalence of contact allergy was 15.2% (girls [19.4%] > boys [10.3%]; $P < 0.001$), and present or past ACD was found in 7.2% (girls [11.3%] > boys [2.5%]).[6] In other studies looking specifically at pediatric populations, up to 52% showed positive reactions on patch testing.[7-18] ACD is considered rare in the first few months of life but has been reported as early as 1 week of age from a hospital ID bracelet.[19] The prevalence increases with increasing age and by 10 years of age, the incidence reaches that seen in adults. Subsequently, variations for some allergens depend on the patterns of exposure. With advancing age, ACD diminishes in severity and in the loss of allergic response in previously sensitized individuals.[20]

In patients suspected of having ACD and referred for patch testing, the positive patch test rates ranging from 14% to 70% and 56% to 93% were of current relevance. In a study by Seidenari and colleagues[21] in Italian children, the highest percentage of positive responses was found in children less than 3 years of age, suggesting a higher sensitization rate in small children. In a study designed to look specifically at infants and young children, Bruckner and colleagues[22] found that 24.5% of asymptomatic children aged 6 months to 5 years were sensitized to one or more contact allergens. Approximately one half of the sensitized children were younger than 18 months. In the adolescent age group, females have significantly higher rates of ACD on the face. This is likely to be explained by increased exposure to nickel in piercing and to preservative and fragrance in cosmetic products. A US-based study showed nickel, fragrance, cobalt, thimerosal, Balsam of Peru, potassium dichromate, neomycin, lanolin, thiuram mix and p-phenylenediamine (PPD) to be common allergens in children.[5] Less common, but emerging allergens include cocamidopropyl betaine in 'no tears' shampoos, baby washes and cleansers and disperse dyes in clothing materials. In a different study looking at age-related specific allergens, thiomerosal (19%),mercury (19%) and thiuram mix (7%) were most common in patients between 0 and 5 years of age, thimerosal (22%), mercury (18%) and nickel sulfate (12%) in patients between 6 and 10 years of age, and nickel (28%), thimerosal (21%) and mercury (18%) in children between 11 and 15 years of age, showing that with increasing age, nickel takes the place of mercurials as the principal allergen.[23] The distribution between males and females was equal. With respect to race, in a large study of more than 9000 individuals, De Leo and colleagues[24] found no difference in the overall response rate to allergens on patch testing between white and black patients, although reactivity to specific allergens differed, likely reflecting differences in exposures rather than a genetic basis.

Pathogenesis

Irritant Contact Dermatitis

Irritant CD results from contact with agents that abrade or irritate the skin. Irritation is usually a cytotoxic event produced by a wide variety of chemicals, detergents, solvents, alcohol, creams, lotions, ointments, and powders and by environmental factors such as wetting, drying, perspiration, and temperature extremes. A major finding after exposure to skin irritants is perturbation of the skin barrier with an associated increase in

DOI: 10.1016/B978-1-4377-0271-2.00056-0

transepidermal water loss. The mechanism associated with this barrier perturbation may include disorganization of the lipid bilayers in the epidermis.[25] In addition, these changes can stimulate an array of proinflammatory cytokine production in the epidermis.[26]

Although allergens are not implicated in irritant CD, the skin-associated immune system is clearly involved, and historically few differences were noted when irritant and ACD were compared immunohistopathologically.[27] An important difference between the two forms of CD is that the irritant form does not require prior sensitization and immunologic memory is not involved in the clinical manifestation. The cellular infiltrate includes CD4[+] T cells with a T helper cell type 1 (Th1)-type profile.[28] A number of studies have identified the epidermal keratinocyte as a key effector cell in the initiation and propagation of contact irritancy. Keratinocytes, which make up the majority of cells in the epidermis, can release both preformed and newly synthesized cytokines, as well as up-regulate major histocompatibility complex (MHC) class II molecules and induce adhesion molecules in response to irritants.[29] These mediators can cause direct tissue damage, activating the underlying mast cells, which in turn release their proinflammatory mediators. This is recognized by the increase in dermal mast cell density, and their mediators are thought to be largely responsible for the vasodilation that occurs in the early stages of acute irritant dermatitis. Other mast cell pleiotropic proinflammatory cytokines are thought to stimulate leukocyte recruitment and activation in the acute inflammatory responses. The 'final' cellular damage results from inflammatory mediators released by activated, nonsensitized T cells. The inflammatory response is dose and time dependent. Any impairment to the epidermal barrier layer (e.g. fissuring, overhydration) renders the skin more susceptible to an irritant effect. The clinical presentation of irritant CD is usually restricted to the skin site directly in contact with the offending agents, with little or no extension beyond the site of contact. The evolution and resolution of irritant CD are less predictable than those of ACD.

Allergic Contact Dermatitis

ACD is recognized as the prototypic cutaneous cell-mediated hypersensitivity reaction in which a distinct type of dendritic cell, the epidermal Langerhans cells, plays a pivotal role.[30] The offending agent, acting as an antigen, initiates the immunologic reaction at the site of contact with the skin. Most environmental allergens are haptens (>500 daltons) that bind to carrier proteins to form complete antigens before they can cause sensitization. The thickness and integrity of the skin influence the allergic response. Thus thinner sites such as the eyelids, earlobes, and genital skin are most vulnerable, whereas the thicker palms and soles are more resistant. Exposure patterns determine the clinical appearance and course of the dermatitis. Recently, an association of filaggrin gene (*FGN*) mutations with contact sensitization to nickel and contact sensitization to nickel combined with intolerance to fashion jewelry, but not with other contact allergens, was demonstrated.[31] Thus, *FLG* deficiency may represent a risk factor for contact sensitization to allergens.

The immune response of ACD requires completion of both an afferent and an efferent limb. The afferent limb consists of the hapten gaining entrance to the epidermis, activating keratinocytes to release inflammatory cytokines and chemokines including tumor necrosis factor (TNF)-α, GM-CSF, interleukin (IL)-1β, IL-10, and macrophage inflammatory protein (MIP)-2. The latter in turn activate Langerhans cells, other dendritic cells, and

endothelial cells, leading to an accumulation of even more dendritic cells at the site of antigen contact. In addition, the release of IL-1β by epidermal Langerhans cells promotes their egress from the epidermis. After the uptake of antigen, Langerhans cells process it while migrating to regional lymph nodes, where they present it to naïve T cells. An important property of Langerhans cells and dendritic cells is their ability to present exogenous antigens on both MHC class I and class II molecules. This cross-priming leads to the activation of both CD4[+] and CD8[+] hapten-specific T cells.[32] Although classic delayed-type hypersensitivity reactions are mediated primarily by CD4[+] cells, CD to haptens is mediated primarily by CD8[+] cells with a Th1-type cytokine profile.[33,34]

On subsequent contact of the skin with a hapten, that is, during the elicitation phase of ACD, other antigen-presenting cells (APCs), including macrophages and dermal dendritic cells may stimulate antigen-specific memory T cells and contribute to the initiation of the local inflammatory response (the dermatitis reaction). The sensitized T cells home in on the hapten-provoked skin site, releasing their inflammatory mediators, which results in epidermal spongiosis ('eczema'). Secondary or subsequent hapten exposure shortens the period of latency from contact to appearance of the rash.

Of interest, recent evidence suggests that a significant number of nickel-specific T cells isolated from allergic subjects can be directly activated by the metal in the absence of professional APCs.[35] T-T nickel presentation was MHC class II restricted, independent of CD28 triggering, and was followed by CD25, CD80, CD86 up-regulation, cytokine release, and cell proliferation. The results demonstrate that the epitopes recognized by APC-independent T cell clones do not require processing. Thus in T-T presentation the epitopes were generated by a direct interaction of the hapten with MHC class II molecules expressed on T cells. Nevertheless, not all of the processing-independent clones belonged to the APC-independent subtype, suggesting that independence from APC processing was necessary but not sufficient for T-T presentation. It is likely that fewer epitopes are generated by T cells on interaction with nickel, whereas professional APCs may display a broader spectrum of nickel epitopes. These data suggest that in the efferent phase of ACD, T lymphocytes can simultaneously act as effector cells and APCs. In particular, the subset of APC-independent lymphocytes may play a role in the initiation and rapid amplification of the cutaneous allergic reaction, representing a subset of nickel-reactive T cells not requiring professional APCs for complete functional activation.

Keratinocyte Apoptosis and Eczema

Spongiosis is a well-established histologic hallmark of the epidermis in eczema. It is characterized by the diminution and rounding of keratinocytes (condensation), and widening of intercellular spaces resulting in a spongelike appearance of the epidermis that progresses sometimes to the formation of small intraepidermal vesicles. The function and integrity of the epidermis are dependent on specific cell surface adhesion molecules. Trautmann and colleagues[36] made the important observation that activated T cells infiltrating the skin in eczematous dermatoses induced keratinocyte apoptosis, resulting in spongiosis. They investigated the effects of immunomodulatory agents on an in vitro model of eczematous dermatitis using keratinocyte/T cell cocultures. In addition, these authors performed in vivo studies in ACD, demonstrating resolution of epidermal spongiosis and cellular infiltrate in skin successfully treated with both topical corticosteroids and tacrolimus 0.1% ointment.[37]

T Cell Recruitment in Allergic Contact Dermatitis

The recruitment of T cells into the skin is regulated by the expression of the specific skin homing receptor, cutaneous lymphocyte-associated antigen (CLA), which mediates rolling of T cells over activated endothelial cells expressing E-selectin.[38] In addition, chemokine receptors have been proposed as important regulators of the tissue targeting of T cells. In this respect, CLA+ T cells co-express the chemokine receptor CCR4, the ligand for thymus and activation-regulated chemokine TARC (CCL17) and macrophage-derived chemokine (CCL22). CCR4 triggered by TARC exposed on the endothelial cell surface during inflammatory skin disorders is thought to augment integrin-dependent firm adhesion of T cells to endothelial intercellular adhesion molecule (ICAM)-1.[39] T cell migration into peripheral tissues mostly depends on their chemokine receptor profiles. Th1-type cells express high levels of CCR5 and CXCR3, interacting with MIP-1β (CCL4) and interferon gamma (IFN-γ)-inducible protein 10 (CXCL10), respectively, whereas Th2-type cells express primarily CCR3, CCR4, and CCR8 and interact with eotaxin (CCL11), TARC and MDC, and I-309 (CCL1).[40]

Epidermal keratinocytes have been shown to be an important source of inflammatory mediators for the initiation and amplification of skin immune responses. Treatment with IFN-γ or IFN-γ plus TNF-α induces keratinocytes to express ICAM-1 and MHC class II molecules and to release a number of chemokines and cytokines, including IL-1, TNF-α, and GM-CSF.[41] IL-17, modulates many of the effects induced by IFN-γ. Of note, IL-4, a Th2 cytokine, acts synergistically with the Th1 cytokine IFN-γ to enhance keratinocyte ICAM-1 expression and release of the CXCR3 agonistic chemokines, IP-10, monokines induced by IFN-γ (Mig; CXCL9), and IFN-inducible T cell α-chemoattractant (I-TAC; CXCL11), thus augmenting both recruitment and retention of Th1-type cells in lesional skin.[42]

Effector T Cells in Allergic Contact Dermatitis

Both CD4 and CD8 T cells participate in ACD, with CD8 T cells predominating in effector mechanisms of tissue damage.[43] Budinger and colleagues[44] demonstrated that nickel-responsive peripheral T cells from patients with nickel-induced CD showed a significant overexpression of T cell receptor (TCR)-Vβ17, and the frequency of TCR-Vβ17+ T cells correlated significantly with the in vitro reactivity of peripheral blood mononuclear cells to nickel. In addition, the cutaneous infiltrate of nickel-induced patch test reactions consisted primarily of Vβ17+ T cells, suggesting that T cells with a restricted TCR-Vβ repertoire predominate in nickel-induced CD and may be crucial in the effector phase of nickel hypersensitivity. Of note, these nickel-specific T cells produced IL-5 but not IFN-γ, consistent with a Th2-type cytokine profile. Other studies have shown nickel-specific T cells with a Th1-type profile;[45] in addition, nickel-specific CD4+ Th1-type cells have been shown to be cytotoxic (along with CD8+ T cells) against keratinocytes, whereas Th2-type nickel-reactive T cells were not.[46] More recently, IL-17-producing TH17 cells have been shown to play a role in the immunopathology of ACD, including in both innate and adaptive immune responses to nickel.[47]

Regulatory T Cells in Allergic Contact Dermatitis

Cavani and colleagues[48] described nickel-specific CD4+ T cells from nickel-allergic subjects that secrete predominantly IL-10,

---

BOX 56-1

Differential Diagnosis of Contact Dermatitis

Other Eczematous Dermatoses

Seborrheic dermatitis

Atopic dermatitis

Nummular eczema

Neurodermatitis (lichen simplex chronicus)

Acrodermatitis enteropathica

Psoriasis

Noneczematous Dermatoses

Dermatophytosis

Bullous impetigo

Vesicular viral eruptions

Urticarial vasculitis

Mycosis fungoides

Erythroderma related to adverse drug reaction, Sezary syndrome, psoriasis (generalized contact dermatitis)

---

which blocks the maturation of dendritic cells including IL-12 release, thus impairing their capacity to activate specific T effector lymphocytes. Thus regulatory T cells may limit excessive tissue damage and participate in the resolution of ACD.

Evaluation and Management

Differential Diagnosis

A number of both eczematous and noneczematous dermatoses should be considered in the evaluation of a child with suspected CD (Box 56-1). Seborrheic and atopic dermatitis occur commonly, whereas psoriasis and zinc deficiency are less common.

Spectrum of Contact Dermatitis

Contact dermatitis could be allergic (20%) or irritant (80%). The innate allergenicity or irritancy of the allergen, the site of contact, the degree of contact, the exposure time to contactants, the thickness and integrity of the skin involved, the environmental conditions, the immunocompetency of the patient and genetics affect the type, severity and location of the CD. However, there is frequent overlap between ACD and irritant CD because many allergens at high enough concentrations can also act as irritants. Impairment to the epidermal barrier layer such as fissuring may increase allergen entry into the epidermis.

Diagnosis of Contact Dermatitis

History

A careful, thorough, and comprehensive, age-appropriate history should include possible contact exposure of the child such as diapers, hygiene products, perfume-containing products, moisturizers, cosmetics, sun blocks, tattoos, body piercing, textiles with dyes and fire retardant, medications, pets and pet products, school projects, recreational exposure sports, work, etc. Irritant CD may be the cause of the dermatitis or an aggravating factor. The frequent hand-washing, use of water, and soaps, detergents and cleansers used, should be noted. The evolution of the skin reaction is influenced by many factors, including the patient's skin, age, color, ambient conditions, the use of topical or other oral medication and response to all prior treatment. Because the majority of contact reactions present as eczematous eruptions, it is essential to note clinical evolution from acute vesiculation to chronic lichenification.

Unfortunately, although history can strongly suggest the cause of CD, relying solely on the history, other than with obvious nickel reactions and a few other allergens, may confirm sensitization in only 10–20% of patients with ACD. At times, CD may be superimposed on atopic dermatitis. The impaired epidermal barrier layer of all atopics, with or without active dermatitis, subjects them to a greater risk for both allergic sensitization and irritation.

Physical Examination

The diagnosis of ACD is suspected from the clinical presentation of the rash and the possible exposure to a contact allergen. The objective findings found on physical exam include the appropriate identification of all the primary and secondary skin lesions. CD can be described as acute, subacute, or chronic. Acute dermatitis can present with erythematous papules, vesicles, and even bullae. Chronic CD is generally pruritic, erythematous and may be associated with crusting, scaling, fissuring, excoriations and lichenification. Irritant CD is usually confined to the area of the skin in direct contact with the offending agents, with little or no extension beyond the site of contact (Figure 56-1). Less common

clinical presentations of CD that may be overlooked include urticaria, acneiform, and pigmentary changes. A broader spectrum of irritant CD, including *acute, acute delayed, cumulative, traumatic,* and *subjective,* has been described.[49]

Regional Considerations in Children

Hand Dermatitis

Hand dermatitis deserves special consideration not only because it is extremely common but also because the differential diagnosis can be challenging. Because the palmar skin is much thicker than the dorsum of the hands, ACD rarely involves the palms, occurring most often on the thinner skin between the fingers and the dorsum of the hands (Figure 56-2).

Hand dermatitis may be due to irritant CD or ACD, atopic dermatitis, dyshidrosis and psoriasis. Because of significant overlap, it may be difficult to distinguish the etiology of the hand dermatitis. Common causes of irritant CD of the hands include water, detergents, and solvents. Patch tests in patients with hand eczema showed relevant allergens including nickel sulfate (17.6%), potassium dichromate (7.2%), rubber elements including thiuram mix, carba mix, p-phenylenediamine and MBT (19.6%) and cobalt chloride (6.4%).[50,51] A Swedish study of 5700 patients showed that specific allergens correlated with eczema localized to different sites on the hand.[52] Patients whose entire hands were involved were more likely to react to thiuram mix, p-phenylenediamine, chromate and Balsam of Peru, while those with involvement of the fingers and interdigital spaces or palm were more likely to react to nickel, cobalt, and 5-chloro-2-methyl-4-isothiazolin-3-one/2-methyl-4-isothiazolin-3-one.

The prevalence of hand eczema in patients with atopic dermatitis is 2- to 10-fold higher than in nonatopic individuals. Certain morphologic features can help distinguish the different contributing factors to hand eczema. Involvement of the dorsal aspect of the hand and fingers, combined with volar wrist involvement, suggests atopic dermatitis as a contributing etiologic factor. Irritant CD commonly presents as a localized dermatitis without vesicles over webs of fingers extending onto the dorsal and ventral surfaces ('apron' pattern), dorsum of the hands, palms and ball of the thumb. In contrast, ACD is often associated with vesicles and tends to favor the fingertips, nail folds, dorsum of the hands and, less commonly, involves the palms. Since irritant CD of the hands can precede ACD, pattern changes such as increasing dermatitis from web spaces to fingertips or from palms to dorsal surfaces should prompt patch testing.[53]

PATCH TEST SCORING

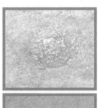
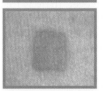
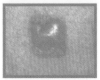

?	**Doubtful**
	· Faint macular
	· Homogeneous erythema
	· No infiltration
+	**Weak positive**
	· Erythema
	· Infiltration
	· Papules
++	**Strong positive**
	· Erythema
	· Infiltration
	· Papules
	· Discrete vesicles
+++	**Extreme positive**
	· Bullous
	· Ulcerative
IR	**Irritant reaction**
	· Discrete patchy erythema without infiltration

Figure 56-1 Patch test grading.

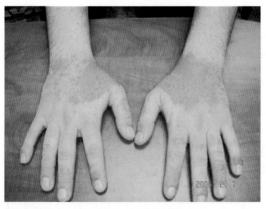

Figure 56-2 Allergic contact dermatitis of the hand.

Face and Eyelid Dermatitis

Eyelid dermatitis may be due to ACD (55–63.5%), irritant CD (15%), atopic dermatitis (<10%) and seborrheic dermatitis (4%).[54] The eyelid is susceptible to ACD because of higher exposure to allergens, greater sensitivity to allergens including aeroallergens, and easy accessibility to touch, facilitating the transfer of chemicals applied to other areas of the body (e.g. nails, scalp) to the eyelid. Although CD is considered to be the most common cause of eyelid dermatitis, it is believed that 25% of patients with atopic dermatitis may have chronic eyelid dermatitis. In evaluating patients with eyelid dermatitis, one must note if other areas of the body are involved. Pure eyelid dermatitis may be distinct from those with other areas of involvement.[55] Common allergens causing eyelid dermatitis are fragrances (facial tissues, cosmetics), preservatives, nickel (eyelash curlers), thiuram (rubber sponges, masks, balloons, toys), cocamidopropyl betaine and amidoamine (shampoos), tosylamide formaldehyde resin (nail polish) and gold.[56] Facial tissues may contain fragrances, formaldehyde, or benzalkonium chloride. Shampoos, conditioners, hair sprays, gels, and mousses may cause eyelid dermatitis without causing scalp or forehead lesions. Paraphenylenediamine (PPD) and ammonium persulfate can cause urticaria and/or eyelid edema.

Similar to eyelid dermatitis, facial dermatitis may occur secondary to allergens transferred to the face from other regions of the body. Most commercially available cosmetics are virtually free of sensitizing components, but ACD in response to moisturizers, sunscreens, foundations, and powders does occur and usually produces a symmetric dermatitis. Rubber-sensitive individuals may react to rubber sponges, masks, balloons, children's toys, and other products that are in contact with the face.

The scalp skin is relatively resistant to allergens in shampoos and hair dyes, and the dermatitis may be manifest on the face or eyelids. Severe burns of the scalp and hair can be caused by the misuse of hair straighteners and relaxers. The manufacturers of hair dyes recommend patch testing with the product before each application.

Oral Mucous Membranes, Perioral Dermatitis and Cheilitis

Perioral dermatitis and cheilitis are common in children and are associated with lip licking, lip chewing, thumb sucking, or excessive drooling. Objectively, changes may be barely visible or may vary from a mild erythema to a fiery red color, with or without edema. Juices of foods and even chewing gum ingredients may contribute to skin irritation of these areas. Cinnamon flavorings and peppermint are the most common causes of allergic cheilitis from toothpastes.[57] Other buccal mucosal diseases include the burning mouth syndrome, stomatitis, oral lichenoid lesions and gingivitis.

Contact allergy of the mucous membrane is rare and use of patch testing to evaluate patients with mucosal involvement is controversial. In a series of 331 patients with different oral diseases (burning mouth syndrome, cheilitis, gingivitis, orofacial granulomatosis, perioral dermatitis, lichenoid tissue reaction and recurrent aphthous stomatitis), metals (nickel and gold) were most frequently positive on patch testing.[58] Metals, including mercury, chromate, nickel, gold, cobalt, beryllium, and palladium have been used in orthodontic materials and are important allergens in patients with dental implants or orthodontic devices presenting with oral lichenoid lesions. Other allergens with a high percentage of positive reactions on patch testing include flavorings and preservatives. Fragrance mix is used as a flavoring in food products, skin care products, and dentifrices. Balsam of Peru is found in dentifrice, mouthwash, lipstick, and food. Dodecyl gallate is a preservative used to extend the shelf life of oil-based foods such as peanut butter, soups, and pastries. Toothpaste, fluoride mouth washes, chewing gum and other foods may contain cinnamic aldehyde, flavorings and peppermint, which are common causes of allergic cheilitis. Thus, an oral antigen screening series should include not only metals but also flavorings, preservatives, medications and dental acrylates. In patients with cheilitis, patch test should include an even more comprehensive panel of flavorings and preservatives. The usefulness of patch testing in the evaluation orofacial granulomatosis and recurrent aphthous stomatitis is questionable.[58]

Flexural Areas of Neck and Axillary Dermatitis

The thin intertriginous skin of the neck is vulnerable to irritant reactions from 'perms', hair dyes, shampoos, and conditioners. 'Berloque' dermatitis from certain perfumes or nail polish presents as localized areas of eczema. Nickel-sensitive individuals may react to wearing a necklace or to zippers.

ACD can be caused by deodorants but not antiperspirants. These agents generally cause a dermatitis involving the entire axillary vault, whereas textile ACD spares the apex of the vault. Irritant CD can occur from shaving and depilating agents. However, sweat and perspiration may cause increased deodorant allergen in the periphery giving a dermatitis that is less intense in the apex of the axillae.

Diaper Dermatitis

Eruptions in the diaper area are the most common dermatologic disorder of infancy.[59] Friction, occlusion, maceration and increased exposure to water, moisture, urine and feces[60] contribute to irritant CD, and are probably the most common causes of diaper dermatitis. The prevalence of diaper dermatitis, an irritant CD, in infants has been estimated to be 7–35% with a peak incidence between ages 9 and 12 months.[61] However, a more recent large-scale study in Great Britain demonstrated an incidence of 25% in the first 4 weeks of life alone.[62]

ACD to rubber chemicals (mercaptobenzothiazole, cyclohexyl thiophathalimide) or glues (p-tertiary butyl phenol-formaldehyde resin) has been reported and called 'Lucky Luke' CD.[63] The characteristic dermatitis is predominantly located on the outer buttocks and hips in toddlers ('gun holster' pattern) and is caused by the elastic bands that hold tightly on the thighs to prevent leaking. Treatment usually involves increasing the frequency of diaper changes, using superabsorbent disposable diapers and applying topical agents such as low-potency corticosteroids and barrier ointments or creams. When secondary *Candida albicans* infection is present, a topical antifungal agent is beneficial. There has been a definite decrease in the incidence of diaper dermatitis due to the availability of newer and improved diapers, including those with superabsorbent gel.[64]

Medication, douches, spermicides, sprays, and cleaners can cause CD in the genital area. Fragrances found in liners, toilet paper, soap, and bubble baths can cause a reaction in sensitized patients. Contraceptive devices can affect rubber and latex-sensitive individuals. Ammonia and/or the acidity of urine may cause an irritant dermatitis, especially in incontinent patients. The ingestion of spices, antibiotics, or laxatives may cause anal itching.

Leg Dermatitis

Shaving agents, moisturizers, and rubber in the elastic of socks can cause allergic reactions in children. Local absorption of the

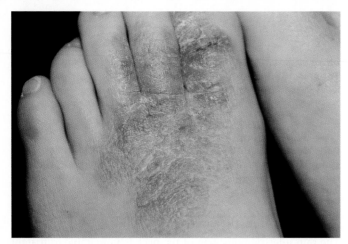

Figure 56-3 Chronic dermatitis on dorsa of feet and toes caused by potassium dichromate allergy from chronic exposure to leather tennis shoes. (From Weston WL, Lane AT, Morelli JG. Dermatitis. In: Color Textbook of Pediatric Dermatology, 4th edn. 2007, Mosby.)

Table 56-1 Reported Causes of Systemic Allergic Contact Dermatitis

Contact Sensitizer	Systemic Reaction to
Glucocorticoids	Oral hydrocortisone
Benadryl cream	Oral Benadryl
Neomycin	Oral neomycin
Penicillin	Oral penicillin
Sulfonamide	Para-amino sulfonamide hypoglycemics (tolbutamide, chlorpropamide)
Thiuram	Antabuse
Colophony, Balsam of Peru, Fragrance mix	Spices: clove, nutmeg, cinnamon, cayenne pepper
Ethylenediamine	Aminophylline (Alternative: oral theophylline, IV theophylline) Piperazine and ethanolamine (Atarax, Antivert) (Alternatives: diphenhydramine, chlorpheniramine, fexofenadine)
Nickel	Nickel in tap water, utensils and food
Chromate	Inhaled chromium: oral potassium dichromate

topical medication has also been noted to produce an 'autosensitization', resulting in a generalized 'id' reaction.

Foot Dermatitis

In their evaluation of CD in children, Romaguera and Vilaplana[7] found that foot eczema was the most frequent localization. Irritant dermatitis of the feet may occur in children because of excessive perspiration or the use of synthetic footwear. More commonly, children can also develop allergic sensitization to rubber accelerators (MBT mix, thiuram mix, carba mix, and PPD mix), dichromates (Figure 56-3), or cements used in the manufacture of shoes. Other chemicals in footwear (e.g. leather, adhesives, glues, and dyes) or in topical medications (e.g. creams, ointments, and antiperspirants) can cause ACD. Chemical agents, such as chrome used in the tanning and dyeing processes of leather, and colophony used in glues in soles and insoles, may be sensitizing. Reactions to nickel sulfate were also frequent with metal present in footwear buckles, eyelets and ornaments.[65] The dorsal aspect of the foot and toes, especially the hallux is more commonly involved in ACD. The interdigital areas are rarely involved. Irritant dermatitis can involve either the dorsum or the sole. The majority of patients with CD of the feet also have hyperhidrosis. 'Sweaty sock' dermatitis needs to be distinguished from CD, atopic dermatitis, and tinea pedis. Patients should be encouraged to wear cotton socks and to change them frequently, along with breathable footwear. Occasionally, a dusting powder (Zea-SORB) may be needed. Other causes of foot dermatitis are tinea pedis, AD, psoriasis, dyshidrosis, and nummular eczema.

Generalized Dermatitis

Dermatitis with scattered generalized distribution is a difficult diagnostic and therapeutic challenge because it lacks the characteristic distribution that gives a clue as to the possible diagnosis of ACD. The frequency of positive and relevant patch testing is unknown. Zug and colleagues[66] examined the yield of patch testing, relevant allergens and allergen sources in patients with scattered generalized dermatitis referred for patch testing. Approximately 15% of the patients patch tested had scattered generalized dermatitis only and approximately half (49%) had a positive patch test deemed at least possibly relevant to their dermatitis. The prevalence of scattered generalized dermatitis was higher in patients with a history of atopic dermatitis. The two most common allergens identified were nickel and balsam of Peru.[67] Hjorth reported two children who were patch test positive to balsam of Peru whose eczema flared after oral intake of naturally occurring balsams. Other relevant positive patch test reactions in this patient population include preservatives (formaldehyde, quaternium 15, methyldibromoglutaronitrile/phenoxyethanol, diazolidinyl urea, 2-bromo-2-nitropropane-1,3-diol, imidazolidinyl urea, and DMDM hydantoin) and propylene glycol. Dyes such as Disperse Blue 106 in synthetic fibers in children's garments have also been implicated.[21]

Advising patients to use skin care products without the most frequent, relevant allergens (formaldehyde-releasing preservatives, fragrances, and propylene glycol) is one strategy that may be helpful while awaiting definitive patch testing results. However, 8–10% of patients with scattered generalized dermatitis remain in the unclassified eczema category.[66]

Systemic ACD is a localized or generalized inflammatory skin disease that occurs in sensitized individuals when they are exposed to the specific allergen orally, transcutaneously, intravenously or by inhalation. It can manifest as a reactivation of a previous dermatitis, reactivation of a previously positive patch test or a systemic inflammatory skin disease, such as the 'baboon syndrome'.[68-72] Patients allergic to ethylenediamine may react to systemic aminophylline and antihistamines of the piperazine or ethanolamine families. Similar reactions have been reported to glucocorticoids, diphenhydramine, neomycin, penicillin, sulfonamides (reaction to oral hypoglycemics such as tolbutamide, chlorpropamide), thiuram (reaction to oral Antabuse), colophony, Balsam of Peru, fragrance mix (reaction to spices such as cloves, nutmeg, cinnamon, cayenne pepper). Nickel-sensitive patients may develop systemic reactions from the ingestion of nickel in tap water or foods cooked in nickel utensils and from eating canned foods (Table 56-1).

Patch Testing

Unfortunately, even with an extensive history and physical exam, only about 10–20% of patients with ACD can be diagnosed

BOX 56-2 Key concepts

Evaluation and Management of Contact Dermatitis

- Irritant contact dermatitis is much more common than allergic contact dermatitis.
- Response to a contactant is influenced by factors related to the agent, the host, the exposure, and the environment.
- The higher the index of suspicion for allergic contact dermatitis, the more frequent the correct diagnosis.
- The greatest abuse of patch testing is lack of use.
- Patch testing is indicated for any persistent eczematous eruption on the dorsum of the hands but rarely for palmar rashes.
- Patients with a suggestive history or physical findings but negative results on Thin-layer Rapid-Use Epicutaneous Test should be considered for further evaluation in a patch testing clinic.

BOX 56-3 Key concepts

Approach to Patch Testing in Allergic Contact Dermatitis

- Understand the underlying pathophysiology.
- Select the proper patient to test.
- Never test with an unknown substance.
- Apply the patches properly, and instruct the patient or family in proper care.
- Interpret the patch test results correctly.
- Determine the relevance of the results.
- Counsel the patient and/or family.

accurately without a patch test. Patch testing should be considered for any patient with a chronic, pruritic, or recurrent eczematous dermatitis, especially those with eyelid or hand involvement.[73]

Virtually any eczematous lesion could be caused or aggravated by a contactant (Box 56-2). Patch testing is needed to identify the responsible allergens, is helpful in young children suspected of ACD and remains the gold standard for confirming ACD. The paradox of patch testing lies in its deceptive simplicity. Although the application of antigens for patch testing is rather simple, antigen selection and patch test interpretation require an experienced clinician (Box 56-3).

Selection of Appropriate Subjects to Test

The higher the index of suspicion, the more frequent the diagnosis of ACD. Indeed, the observation that the greatest abuse of patch testing is its lack of use holds true even for the pediatric population. Most recently, the North American Contact Dermatitis Group (NACDG) sought to determine the frequency of positive and relevant patch tests in children referred for patch testing in North America. In addition, they compared results of patch testing children and adults, as well as results with international data on contact allergy in children. No significant difference in the overall frequency of at least one relevant positive patch test reaction was noted in children (51.2%) compared with adults (54.1%).[74] The most frequent positive reactions in children were to nickel (28.3%), cobalt chloride (17.9%), thimerosal (15.3%), neomycin sulfate (8.0%), gold sodium thiosulfate (7.7%), and

fragrance mix (5.1%). For children aged 0 to 18 years, the most frequent relevant positive reactions were to nickel sulfate (26.0%), cobalt (12.4%), neomycin (4.4%), fragrance mix (4.1%), gold (3.6%), and quaternium 15 (3.6%).

34.0% of the children with a relevant positive reaction had atopic dermatitis. Of note, 15% and 39% of children had relevant allergens not included in the NACDG series or T.R.U.E. TEST® (thin-layer rapid use epicutaneous test, Allerderm), respectively. It is important for the clinician to remember that the majority of patients will be allergic to a single allergen or a single group of allergens and that there is a risk of false-positive patch test results. Some patients may benefit more from direct therapeutic intervention (i.e. allergen avoidance) than from patch testing. Ideally, one needs to know the value of all the clinical data before patch testing, in predicting a clinically relevant response to any of the allergens tested. Immunocompromised patients, including those on oral steroids or those on cancer chemotherapy or immunosuppressive drugs, are not appropriate candidates for patch testing. Ideally, the dermatitis should be quiescent. The skin site where the patch tests are to be applied should have had no potent steroid applied for 5 to 7 days before testing. Patients should avoid sun or ultraviolet light exposure for 96 hours. Systemic antihistamines have no effect on patch test results.

Sources of Allergens

Commercially available standardized patch test allergens have been calibrated with respect to nonirritant concentrations and compatibility with the test vehicle. Test systems currently available in the USA are the T.R.U.E. TEST® and the standardized allergens loaded in Finn chambers or allergEAZE patch test chambers. Individual chambers are filled with contactants, applied to the skin and held in place by hypoallergenic tape. Certain screening panels such as the NACD Series with a range from 65 to 70 allergens are not FDA-approved but conform to standards of care recommended by CD experts. Commercial sources of customized patch test materials include Smart Practice Canada (1.866.903.2671), Hermal Pharmaceutical Laboratories, Inc. (1.800.HERMAL-1), Dormer Laboratories, Inc. and Trolab Allergens.

Allergens

The ideal number of patch tests to be applied depends on the patient and the usefulness of patch testing is enhanced with the number of allergens tested. Allergens not found on commercially available screening series in the USA frequently give relevant reactions, and personal products are a useful supplement especially in facial or periorbital dermatitis.

The T.R.U.E. TEST® consists of a standard battery of 28 allergens and a negative control on three panels (Table 56-2). The allergens in the T.R.U.E. TEST® are in a vehicle attached to an adhesive backing. Comparative results of the T.R.U.E. TEST® and Finn Chamber method have shown a 64–98% concordance in results, depending on the allergen. However, a further study suggested that false-negative results may occur with the T.R.U.E. TEST®, particularly with fragrance mix and rubber additives (thiuram and carba mix).[75] In addition, the T.R.U.E. TEST® has higher false-negative reactions to neomycin, cobalt and lanolin. Allergens including gold, bacitracin, MDGN/PE (methyldibromoglutaronitrile/phenoxyethanol), propylene glycol, bromonitropropane, cinnamic aldehyde, DMDM hydantoin, ethylene urea/melamine formaldehyde have a prevalence of more than

Table 56-2 Thin-layer Rapid Use Epicutaneous Test (T.R.U.E. TEST®) Antigens

Antigen	Common Exposures
Panel 1.1	
Nickel sulfate	Snaps, jewelry
Wool alcohols (lanolin)	Cosmetics, soaps, topical medications, moisturizers
Neomycin sulfate	Topical antibiotics
Potassium dichromate	Chrome-tanned leather, cement
Caine mix	Topical anesthetics
Fragrance mix	Fragrances, scented household products
Colophony	Cosmetics, adhesives, household products
Paraben mix	Preservative in topical formulations, cosmetics
Balsam of Peru	Foods, cosmetics, fragrances, topical medications
Ethylenediamine dihydrochloride	Topical medications, eyedrops
Cobalt dichloride	Metal-plated objects, paints
Panel 2.1	
p-tert-Butylphenol formaldehyde resin	Fabrics, waterproof glues
Epoxy resin	Two-part adhesives
Carba mix	Rubber products, shampoos, disinfectants
Black rubber mix	All black rubber products, some hair dyes
CL+ ME– Isothiazolinone (MCI/MI)	Cosmetics, skin care products, topical medications
Quaternium-15	Preservative in cosmetics and skin care products
Mercaptobenzothiazole	Rubber products, adhesives
p-Phenylenediamine	Permanent or semipermanent hair dyes, cosmetics, printing ink
Formaldehyde	Fabric finishes, cosmetics
Mercapto mix	Rubber products, glues for leather and plastics
Thimerosal	Preservative in contact lens solutions, cosmetics, injectable drugs
Thiuram mix	Rubber products, adhesives
Panel 3.1	
Diazolidinyl urea	Products for personal care, hygiene, and haircare; cosmetics; pet shampoos
Imidazolidinyl urea	Products for personal care, hygiene, and haircare; cosmetics; liquid soaps; moisturizers
Budesonide	Nasal corticosteroid spray; asthma controller medication in inhaler, nebulized suspension and dry powder forms; creams, lotions and ointments
Tixocortol-21-pivalate	Antiinflammatory preparations
Quinoline mix	Paste bandages; prescription and non prescription topical antibiotics and antifungal creams, lotions, ointments; animal food

2% in the NACDG 2004 but are not included in the current T.R.U.E. TEST®. A number of other standardized allergens can be tested individually with the Finn Chamber attached to the back with Scanpor tape or an alternative patch testing system (allergEAZE, SmartPractice Canada). Clinicians need to be aware of the limitations of each system of patch testing for individual allergens.[76] Caution should be exercised when testing for non-standardized antigens to avoid adverse effects and false-positive or negative responses. Ideally, at least two control subjects should be tested with any nonstandardized allergen. 'Leave-on' cosmetics (make-up, perfume, moisturizer, nail polish), clothing and most foods are tested 'as is', whereas 'wash-off' cosmetics (soap, shampoo) are tested at 1:10-1:100 dilution.

Patch testing should never be performed with an unknown substance. Photopatch tests should be performed by a clinician with expertise in ultraviolet radiation if photocontact dermatitis is suspected. Additional guidelines for patch testing including strength of recommendations and quality of evidence have been recently published by the British Association of Dermatologists Therapy Guidelines and Audit Subcommittee.[77] The T.R.U.E. TEST® may serve as triage or a screening tool in an allergists' practice but occupational exposures may benefit from early referral for supplemental testing.

Selection of Allergens in Children

Available data show that the sensitization profile of children does not differ significantly from that of adults. Thimerosal, neomycin sulfate, nickel sulfate, mercury, amide chloride, cobalt chloride, fragrance mix, bufexamac, Compositae mix, propylene glycol and turpentine are the substances with the highest sensitization rates in childhood.[78] It has been suggested that in very young children, allergens such as formaldehyde, formaldehyde-releasing preservatives, mercaptobenzothiazole and thiuram be diluted 50%, and potassium dichromate 25% in petrolatum, to avoid irritant false positive reactions.[79,80] However, most studies to date suggest that the same test concentrations as in adults can be used.[81]

Due to the limited surface available for testing and the potential risk of active sensitization, the German Contact Dermatitis Research Group[78] recommends a panel of 12 contact allergens as a standard series in children from 6 to 12 years of age. Based on their frequency and clinical relevance, the allergens included are nickel sulfate, thiuram mix, colophony, mercaptobenzothiazole, fragrance mix I, fragrance mix II, mercapto mix, bufexamac, dibromdicyanobutane, chlormethylisothiazolinone, neomycin, and compositae mix. When history suggests exposure to shoe allergens, p-tert-butylphenol-formaldehyde resin and potassium dichromate are added. Wool alcohols/lanolin 30% is added when there is exposure to skin care products, Disperse blue if clothing dermatitis is suspected and paraphenylenediamine if there is exposure to henna, tattoos and hair dyes. Children under the age of 6 years should be tested if there is a high degree of suspicion and only selectively with the suspected contact allergens. Children older than 12 years and adolescents can be tested in the same manner as adults.

Patch Testing Procedure

Standardized criteria for patch testing have been set by the Task Force on Contact Dermatitis of the American Academy of Dermatology. All results are dependent on the recommended protocol for application, removal, and interpretation of results.

Table 56-3 Patch Test Interpretation

Grade	Patch Test Grading	CLINICAL Interpretation of Grading
0	No reaction	No evidence for contact allergy
+/−	Mild erythema only	Doubtful for contact allergy
1+	50% of patch test site erythematous with edema	Possible (versus false-positive) contact allergy
2+	50% of patch test site with erythematous papules	Probable contact allergy
3+	50% of patch test site with vesicles or bullae	Definite contact allergy

Patch tests are typically applied to the upper- or mid-back areas (2.5 lateral to a mid-spinal reference point) which must be free of dermatitis and hair and kept in place for 48 hours. After securing the patches with hypoallergenic tape, patients are instructed to keep the area dry and avoid activities that will cause excessive sweating or excessive movement that may cause displacement of the patches. In infants and small children, the patch tests can be covered with fabric adhesive tape or a stockinet vest. Patch tests are removed after 48 hours and read 30 minutes after to allow resolution of erythema and irritative effect from the tape and/or chamber if present. A second reading should be done 3 to 5 days after the initial application. 30% of relevant allergens negative at the 48-hour reading become positive in 96 hours. Irritant reactions tend to disappear by 96 hours. Metals (gold, potassium dichromate, nickel, cobalt), topical antibiotics (neomycin, bacitracin), topical corticosteroids and PPD may become positive after 7 days. More than 50% of positive patch test to gold was delayed for about 1 week.

The American Contact Dermatitis Society has established a grading system that is almost universally recognized (Table 56-3). Alternative grading with the T.R.U.E. TEST® is shown in Figure 56-1. Relevance of positive reactions to the clinical presentation needs to be carefully evaluated. Conversely, patients with negative results may need to be referred for more complete testing to a patch test clinic.

Determining Clinical Relevance

The relevance of positive reactions to clinical ACD can only be established by carefully correlating the history, including exposure to the allergen. A positive patch test reaction may be relevant to present or previous dermatitis; multiple true-positives can occur and mild responses may still represent allergic reaction. Thus, understanding the sources of antigen in the patient's environment is required to be able to advise the patient adequately regarding avoidance and alternatives in ACD. A positive patch test is considered to be a 'definite' reaction of ACD if the result of a 'use test' with the suspected item was positive or the reaction of the patch test with the object or product was positive. It would be 'probable' if the antigen could be verified as present in known skin contactants and the clinical presentation was consistent; and 'possible' if the patient is exposed to circumstances in which skin contact with materials known to contain allergen was likely. Multiple sensitivities are possible if different allergens are present in different products used simultaneously, or concomitant sensitization occurs if allergens are present in the same products and both induce sensitization. Cross-sensitization

can also occur. Common combinations of a positive patch test are: PPD and benzocaine (cross-sensitizer); thiuram mix, carba mix and mercapto mix (rubber products); quarternium 15 and paraben, (quarternium-15, a formaldehyde releaser and formaldehyde are preservatives that are frequently combined and cosensitize); cobalt and nickel (cobalt is used in alloys with nickel and chromium and cosensitize). Poly sensitization is common in children. Children with and without atopic dermatitis have the same rate of positive patch test.

The repeat open application test (ROAT) or exaggerated use test may be done to confirm the presence or absence of ACD. The suspected allergen (for 'leave-on' but not 'wash-off' products) is applied to the antecubital fossa twice daily for 7 days, and observed for dermatitis. The absence of a reaction makes CD unlikely. If eyelid dermatitis is considered, ROAT can be carried out on the back of the ear.

Additional tests used less frequently in the diagnosis of CD include skin biopsy to differentiate from other diseases (listed in Box 56-1). Prick or intradermal testing may be helpful, especially in the evaluation of contact urticaria. Contact urticaria can also be evaluated with an 'open' patch test as an alternative to the prick or intradermal test. Potassium hydroxide preparation for fungal hyphae or cultures may be needed to identify fungal disease.

Allergens of Particular Importance in Children

Nickel

Nickel is a more common cause of ACD than all other metals combined, even in children. Of 391 children aged 18 years or less who were patch tested between 2001 and 2004 by the North American Contact Dermatitis Group, 28% had a positive patch test to nickel, and 26% were deemed to have a nickel allergy of either current or past relevance.[82] In 2008, the American Contact Dermatitis Society selected it as the 'contact allergen of the year', pointing to its rise in incidence and high sensitization rate in children. It is more common in adolescents, girls more than boys, and ear piercing is the most important predisposing factor. The prevalence of nickel allergy among those children with pierced ears was 13% compared to 1% among those without pierced ears.[83] The risk of sensitization to nickel appears higher when earlobes are pierced before the age of 20 years (p < 0.05)[84] and is increased with the number of piercings.[85] Thus, some authors recommend that ear piercing be delayed until after 10 years of age, presumably to allow for the development of immune tolerance.[86]

Nearly 5 million people in the USA and Canada undergo orthodontic treatment. In patients with contact allergy to orthodontics, nickel is the most common allergen. Nickel is commonly used in orthodontics but stainless steel, which contains about 8% nickel that is not normally biologically available, is generally considered safe in nickel-allergic patients. However, recent studies suggest that certain flexible titanium-nickel arch wires used in orthodontics release increased amounts of nickel compared to stainless steel and may need to be avoided in patients with known nickel sensitivity.[87] A Finnish study of adolescents and the effect of age, gender, onset, duration and specific orthodontic treatment, and age of ear piercing on the incidence of nickel sensitization, found that 35% of the girls who had their ears pierced prior to orthodontic treatment were nickel-allergic versus none of the girls who had orthodontic treatment prior to ear piercing.[88] The mechanism responsible was suggested to be oral tolerance.[89] In females, nickel sensitivity may increase the risk of developing hand eczema.[90] The presence of releasable nickel from the surface of any object can be detected using the di-methylglyoxime spot test; a pink color indicates the presence of releasable nickel. Despite some studies suggesting benefit,[91,92] the evidence for dietary avoidance of nickel is not strong (quality of evidence IV, strength of recommendation C).[77]

Chromate

Chromate is found in leather, especially shoes, where chromium salts are used in the tanning process. Metallic chromium is not an allergen. Chromate sensitivity can be associated with hand or foot dermatitis, which can persist even after chromate avoidance.

Thimerosal

Thimerosal is a mercuric derivative of thiosalicylic acid that has been used as a preservative in vaccines, cosmetics, tattoo inks, eye drops, and contact lens solutions as well as a disinfectant (e.g. merthiolate).[93,94] It may cross-react with mercury, which is used as preservative material in shoe manufacturing and in some antiseptic solutions. Although many children react to it on patch testing, these are rarely of clinical significance and individuals reacting to thimerosal typically have no reactions when given vaccines containing this preservative.[5,95-97] Data from the North American Contact Dermatitis Group reported thimerosal as the fifth most common allergen, inducing allergic reactions in 11% of patch-tested patients.[98] However, in only 17% of patients with sensitivity to thimerosal was the patch test result considered clinically relevant to their dermatitis, ranking thimerosal last in relevance among the 50 allergens tested. Thimerosal was named the contact (non)allergen of the year in 2002 with recommendations for removal from the allergy patch testing screening tray.[99] Because of its potential toxicity and allergenicity in children, precautionary measures are underway to remove thiomerosal from vaccines.[100] Systemic reactions manifesting as an exanthem that preferentially involves the buttocks and flexural aspects of extremities, and known as the baboon syndrome, have been observed in children, mainly after exposure to metallic mercury vapors.[68] Aside from thimerosal, reactions to adjuvants (e.g. aluminum hydroxide), stabilizers (e.g. gelatin), preservatives, and antibiotics (e.g. neomycin) in vaccines have been reported.

Aluminum

Aluminum may cause cutaneous granulomas in response to vaccines containing aluminum hydroxide. These tend to resolve spontaneously, although children subsequently have positive patch tests to metallic aluminum or their salts.[101] The aluminum sensitivity appears to be lost with time as it occurs rarely in adults.

Rubber Chemicals

Rubber chemicals, including thiuram mix, mercaptobenzothiazole, and mercapto mix are used in the manufacturing of rubber products, including dipped (e.g. balloons, gloves) and molded (e.g. pacifiers, handle bars) products. Mixed dialkyl thioureas (MDTU), a mixture of two thiourea chemicals used for rubber acceleration and as antioxidants in the manufacturing of neoprene, was designated as the 'contact allergen of the year for

2009' by the American Contact Dermatitis Society. Large quantities of thioureas have been shown to leach from neoprene compounds and the levels were found to be sufficient to elicit ACD.[102] This allergen mixture has been found to have one of the highest relevancy rates in the NACDG database. ACD from the allergens in neoprene include cases caused by orthopedic braces, prostheses, splints, and foot supports; athletic shoes; rubber masks, swim goggles and wet suits; computer wrist rests; neoprene gloves; and rubber-based materials in automobiles.

Special Considerations

Plant Dermatitis (Phytodermatoses)

A number of plants can cause irritant reactions through mechanical or chemical injury. Most mechanical injury from plants is trivial, although inoculation of cactus hairs can give rise to pruritus. Implanted cacti spines can be removed by applying sticky tape to the skin and gently peeling it off. 'Itching powder' from rose hip hairs has caused maculopapular, and sometimes pustular, eruptions at sites of contact. Chemical irritants caused by oxalate crystals results from contact with mustard, horseradish, and capsaicinoids in chili peppers. Contact with stinging nettles injects a mixture of inflammatory mediators, including histamine, causing a hive, and an unidentified neurotoxin that causes localized numbness and tingling.

Plants of the *Toxicodendron* group, including poison ivy and poison oak, are the most common causes of allergic plant dermatitis in children in the USA. Even newborns can be sensitized to the oleoresin (urushiol). Because this is a potent antigen, the clinical reaction typically results in vesicles and bullae, often with a characteristic linear appearance. Of note, the fluid content of vesicles is not antigenic. On the other hand, the oleoresin can be transferred by handling exposed animals, clothing, or sports equipment, even pet dander. Soap and water inactivate the antigen. Urishiol is also found in cashew nut trees, Japanese lacquer, Ginkgo biloba, and mango skin, and the ingestion of cashews or contact with mango skin can cause a similar rash. Rhus patch testing is not recommended because it has a significant sensitizing capacity.

The Compositae family (Asteraceae), the second largest plant family, represents approximately 10% of the world's flowering plants. ACD to compositae may manifest as acute or chronic dermatitis of exposed sites. Although typically seen in florists, farmers, and professional gardeners, recent studies indicate that ACD to compositae may be more common in children than previously believed. Positive patch test reactions on screening with two different Compositae mixes detected 4.2% and 2.6% positives among children and adolescent, with significantly higher positive results in children with atopic dermatitis reported.[103] The dermatitis has an airborne contact pattern distribution in the exposed areas of the hands and face with symptoms worse in late spring or summer and worse after picking daisies, dandelions or playing outdoors. Belloni Fortina and colleagues[104] suggested adding Compositae mix to the pediatric screening series when investigating dermatitis of air-exposed areas in children with atopic dermatitis; however, this carries the risk of false positive results or sensitization. Cross-reactivity between fragrance terpenes and Compositae plant extracts may be a cause of false positive patch test to Compositae.[105] In summary, ACD to Compositae should be suspected in children with a family or personal history of atopy, summer-related or -exacerbated dermatitis, and a history of plant exposure.

Ambrosia species, which include ragweed, can cause allergic plant dermatitis when pollinating, in both atopic and nonatopic individuals. Repeated contact with ornamental cut flowers, including *Alstromeria* (the lily and tulip family of plants), can result in an ACD that presents with a fissured dermatitis of the fingertips. Finally, plants that contain furocoumarins (psoralens), including parsley, parsnips, and wild carrots, can cause phytotoxic reactions, especially in summer when psoralens are most abundant in the plants where children are playing. These reactions occur when the skin, contaminated with psoralens, is exposed to ultraviolet A light. They occur typically during the summer months, when psoralens are most abundant in wild garden plants and children are playing outdoors.

Dermatitis from Topical Medications

The topical application of anesthetics, antihistamines, antibiotics, and even antiinflammatory drugs along with preservatives or fragrances has been implicated in sensitization and contact reactions. Neomycin is a frequent and potent sensitizer in children, as is diphenhydramine in topical form. Contact allergy to topical corticosteroids can be difficult to diagnose.[106] It should be suspected in any patient whose skin condition worsens with the application of a corticosteroid. There have been a number of reports of contact allergy in the nasal mucosa to budesonide nasal spray and stomatitis with budesonide for oral inhalation.[107] Patch testing to corticosteroids is not standardized, is complicated by the concurrent antiinflammatory actions of the medication, and should be performed by clinicians familiar with this problem. Corticosteroids representative of different groupings typically used in patch testing include tixocortol, triamcinolone, dexamethasone, and budesonide. Sensitized patients must be instructed to avoid the systemic use of those drugs.

Contact Dermatitis to Cosmetics

An average adult applies 12 personal hygiene products daily and in the course of using these products, is exposed to 168 discrete chemicals. Children, and especially adolescents, may be exposed to similar numbers. Exposure to multiple potential allergens occurs repeatedly with the use of cosmetics and it is not unusual for these products to manifest as contact allergy distant from the sites on which the agent is applied. This phenomenon is termed *ectopic contact dermatitis* and requires diligent evaluation to elucidate the cause of the eruption.

Fragrances are one of the most common causes of ACD from the use of cosmetics in the USA. They can be found in cosmetics and personal hygiene products such as shampoo/shower gels, detergents, diapers, moisturizers, and even scented toys, either overtly to add an appealing scent or to mask unpleasant odors.

The term *unscented* can erroneously suggest that a product does not contain fragrance when, in fact, a masking fragrance can be present. *Fragrance-free* products are typically free of classic fragrance ingredients and generally acceptable for the allergic patient. However, if a fragrance-based chemical is added to a product for a purpose other than to act as a fragrance (such as the preservative benzyl alcohol), the product can still claim that it is fragrance-free. The addition of botanical and natural chemicals can also alter the smell of the product. Diagnosing fragrance allergy is essential for appropriate avoidance. The fragrance mix that is popularly used for patch testing contains eight different fragrances and will diagnose approximately 85% of fragrance-allergic individuals.

Table 56-4 Cosmetic Preservatives

Formaldehyde Releaser	Non Formaldehyde Releaser
Quarternium 15	MCI/MI
Diazolidinyl urea	Parabens
Imidazolidinyl urea	Chloroxylenol
Bromonitropropane DMDM hydantoin	Iodopropynylbutylcarbamate Benzalkorium chloride Thimerosal

Note: Paraben, quarternium-15 and formaldehyde preservatives are frequently combined and cosensitize.

Preservatives are present in most aqueous-based cosmetics and personal hygiene products to prevent rancidity. These preservatives are grouped into two broad categories: formaldehyde releasers and nonformaldehyde releaser (Table 56-4). Individuals who are allergic to formaldehyde cannot use any of the formaldehyde releasers. Common sensitizers that are formaldehyde releasers include quaternium-15, whereas thimerosal, benzalkonium chloride, and parabens are nonformaldehyde releasers. Paraben is the most commonly used preservatives in cosmetic, pharmaceutical and industrial products because of its broad spectrum of activity against yeasts, molds, and bacteria.

Excipients, including propylene glycol, ethylenediamine, and lanolin are inert substances that make up the base of a product and serve to solubilize, sequester, thicken, foam, or lubricate the active component in a product. They can cause ACD or, in higher concentrations, can act as irritants. Lanolin is a common component of consumer products. Unfortunately, its composition has not been fully characterized. Medicaments containing lanolin are more sensitizing than lanolin-containing cosmetics. Lanolin is a weak sensitizer when applied on normal skin but a stronger sensitizer on damaged skin.

Hair products are second only to skin care products as the most common cause of cosmetic allergy. In addition to routine hair care products, intermittent cosmetic hair products such as permanent or semi-permanent hair dye and permanent wave solutions are commonly used.

p-Phenylenediamine (PPD)

New trends in permanent and temporary tattoos have emerged in our adolescent population. The use of black henna mixtures, containing indigo, henna and PPD and/or diaminotoluens to temporarily paint the skin is even used in some cultures primarily before major events. The addition of PPD to give henna (auburn to red color) a darker shade of brown to black is increasingly used in body painting and the need for a policy for use in children has been suggested.[108] Adolescents working in hair salons may be exposed to PPD, the most common allergen affecting hairdressers. A number of chemicals may cross-react with PPD (Table 56-5).[109]

Glycerol thioglycolate is the active ingredient in permanent wave solutions. Cocamidopropyl betaine, amphoteric surfactant in shampoos, bath products and cleansers can also cause ACD from hair products.

Nail cosmetics and glues have become increasingly popular and fashionable. There are several varieties of sculpting nails and the currently marketed products contain various methacrylate ester monomers, dimethacrylates, and trimethacrylates as well as cyanoacrylate-based glues. Clinical allergy to acrylics in nails

Table 56-5 Chemicals that May Cross-React with p-Phenylenediamine

Product Class	Chemicals
Sunscreens	PABA and padimate O
Antiinfective	Sulfonamides and p-aminosalicylic acid
Diuretics	Thiazides
Anesthetics	Benzocaine and related 'caines'
Textile dyes	Azo dyes
Antidiabetic	Sulfonylureas
COX-2 inhibitors	Celecoxib
Rubber accelerators	N-isopropyl-N'-phenyl-p-phenylenediamine
Black rubber mix	

can present locally at the distal digit or ectopically on the eyelids and face. Patch testing to a variety of acrylates and nail polish resin may be necessary to delineate the causative agent.

Sunscreens are frequently present in cosmetics such as moisturizers, lip preparations, and foundations. As a group they are the most common cause of photoallergic CD. *Chemical-free* sun blocks use physical blocking agents instead of photoactive chemicals and include titanium dioxide and zinc oxide, which are rarely sensitizers.

Contact Dermatitis in Athletes

The skin of athletes is exposed to repeated trauma, heat, moisture, and numerous allergens and chemicals and is predisposed to irritant CD or ACD. Early recognition can facilitate appropriate therapy and prevention.[110]

In swimmers, chemicals used to disinfect swimming pools such as chlorine can cause both irritant CD and ACD. In such cases, the dermatitis may spare the area of the skin under the swimwear. However, swimwear and equipment including goggles, nose plugs, nose clips, ear plugs, fins and swim caps may also cause CD. Although ACD from swimming goggles usually presents with well-demarcated, bilateral periorbital edema and erythema with varying degrees of pruritus, exudate, and scaling, conjunctival injection and hypopigmentation have been reported.[111,112] Patch testing to rubber products should ideally include a piece of material taken from the offending goggles. Allergens include rubber and chemicals used in manufacturing; neoprene, benzoyl peroxide, phenol-formaldehyde resin, thioureas, and antioxidants are frequently used in rubber production.

'Jogger's nipples' are painful, erythematous, and crusted erosions and represent irritant dermatitis caused by friction from the running shirt.[113] Other skin and nail problems are associated with irritant CD and ACD from the shoes, shirts and topical medications. Contact allergens include components of rubber, leather, glues, or dyes used in the manufacture of running shoes. Sweat helps leach out the chemicals from the shoes responsible for causing ACD. Rubber insoles from tennis shoes containing mercaptobenzothiazole and dibenzothiazyl disulfide have been reported to cause recurrent eczematous eruptions of the feet and can be prevented by switching to new innersoles such as polyurethane.[114] Analgesic sprays, topical salicylates, and antiinflammatory creams and gels have also caused ACD in athletes. In a large case series of student athletes, benzocaine and lanolin (found in topical anesthetics and massage creams) were the most prevalent allergens responsible for CD in runners.[115]

CD in soccer or football players is usually caused by equipment or chemicals used on the field. 'Cement burns' presenting as erythematous, edematous plaques, bullae, and erosions on the upper inner thighs are due to the lime component used in field markings. The characteristic rash, a history of exposure to wet field lines, and worsening of symptoms after taking a hot shower, point to the diagnosis. Patch testing performed on a few of the athletes has been negative. Treatment includes removing contaminated clothing, cleaning the areas with water and applying topical antibiotics or petroleum jelly. Urea-formaldehyde resin in shin pads has caused ACD in soccer players.

Like runners, soccer players may develop ACD from topical anesthetic creams, epoxy resins, nickel in certain athletic shoes and tincture of benzoin used in conjunction with athletic tape.[110]

Ball handling in baseball and basketball can cause both irritant CD and ACD. 'Basketball pebble fingers' manifesting as small petechiae and abrasions on a shiny denuded surface of the fingertips and pads is an irritant CD resulting from mechanical irritation from the ball's pebbled surface. An eczematous rash on both palms, the palmar fingertips and base of the thumbs may be due to rubber allergy.[116] Protective knee padding and adhesives in athletic tape contain rubber accelerators and formaldehyde resins.

Tennis players can develop irritant CD due to friction of the medial thighs and this manifests as erythematous eruptions over the opposing areas. ACD can be caused by isophorone diamine and epoxy resin used in the manufacture of tennis rackets, neoprene splints to prevent or relieve tennis elbow, squash balls with N-isopropyl-N-phenylparaphenylenediamine and rubber and medications and anesthetic sprays with ethyl chloride.

Fiberglass in hockey sticks, epoxy resin adhesives in a face mask and dyes used in the manufacture of hockey gloves have caused ACD.[64,117] Weightlifters have developed ACD to the nickel and palladium found in weights or bars[118] and the chalk used to achieve a better grip.[119] In summary, the young athlete is constantly exposed to allergens in clothing, equipment, environment and medications. The unique presentation of the rash, a careful sports-directed history and allergen-directed patch testing enhances the ability to diagnose and care for the young athlete with dermatitis.

Treatment and Prevention

The identification of the allergen to improve avoidance of contact to the allergen and education of patients and/or families is the mainstay of treatment for ACD. All other measures are palliative and temporary. Compliance with allergen avoidance is frequently difficult.

Once the offending agent is identified, patients and/or caregivers must be educated regarding the nature of the dermatitis, triggering agents, and irritant factors. A list of potential exposure alternatives and substitutes to cosmetics should be offered to the patient to increase compliance. (usually listed in textbooks, such as Fisher's *Contact Dermatitis*[120] or Marks and DeLeo's *Contact and Occupational Dermatitis*[121]). The American Contact Dermatitis Society maintains a topical skin care product database called the Contact Allergen Replacement Database (CARD). After patch testing, patients can be provided with a comprehensive list of skin care products that are free of their identified allergens.

After removal of the offending agent, topical therapy may be used. Topical antiinflammatory agents, primarily corticosteroids (CSs), are most effective when treating localized dermatitis.

Topical CS is the first-line treatment for ACD. The formulation of topical CS prescribed will depend on the location and extent of the dermatitis. Low-potency CSs are recommended for the thinner skin of the face and flexural areas, and high-potency CSs are indicated for thickened, lichenified lesions. Ointments are generally more potent, more occlusive and contain fewer sensitizing preservatives than creams and lotions. Patients with sensitivity to preservatives can use preservative-free CSs such as fluocinolone (Synalar®) ointment, triamcinolone (Aristocort®) ointment or betamethasone dipropionate (Diprosone®) ointment. Of note, high-potency CSs should not be used for diaper dermatitis, yet the results of one survey revealed that a combination antifungal-corticosteroid product containing betamethasone dipropionate was used in 6% of encounters.[122]

Cool compresses are usually soothing and mildly antipruritic. The addition of aluminum subacetate (Burrow's solution), calamine, or colloidal oatmeal may help acute, oozing lesions. In chronic eruptions, emollients, lubricants, and moisturizers may be used, but they should be nonsensitizing and fragrance-free. Excessive hand washing should be discouraged in patients with hand dermatitis and nonirritating or sensitizing moisturizers must be used after washing. Soaps and nonalkaline cleansers should be avoided. Rarely, antibiotics may be needed for secondary infection.

For extensive and severe CD, systemic corticosteroids may offer relief within 12 to 24 hours.

Topical calcineurin inhibitors, approved for intermittent use in children with atopic dermatitis 2 years of age and older, have been used in both animal models and patients with ACD.[123,124] These immunomodulatory agents do not induce skin atrophy and may be especially valuable in treating facial or eyelid dermatitis, although use in ACD or irritant CD would be off-label at the present time. Burning or stinging has been the primary adverse reaction seen with these agents.

Antihistamines may offer some benefit in contact urticaria. Sedating antihistamines may offer some relief from pruritus. Oral diphenhydramine should not be used in patients with ACD to diphenhydramine in a calamine base (Caladryl®) or hydroxyzine hydrochloride (Atarax®) in ethylenediamine-sensitive patients. Other treatments include ultraviolet light as well as immunomodulating agents such as methotrexate, azathioprine and mycophenolate mofetil.

Whereas mechanical barriers against contact, such as protective gloves, clothing, and barrier creams, are helpful in some cases (nickel allergy), results are often disappointing. For nickel-allergic patients, barriers such as gloves, covers for metal buttons and identification of nickel by the dimethyl-gloxime test can be prescribed but results can be disappointing.[125]

For diaper dermatitis, allergic, irritant and infectious causes have to be considered. Frequency of diaper changes using improved product design features, such as superabsorbent disposable diapers, are believed to explain the decline in diaper dermatitis among infants.[126] Low-potency CSs and barrier ointments or creams can be used for a limited period of time.[127] When secondary *C. albicans* infection is present, a topical antifungal agent should be used. Possible treatments include minimizing diaper use and using disposable diapers, barrier creams, mild topical cortisones, and antifungal agents. A gentle cleansing routine, frequent diaper changes, and a thick barrier cream help control this condition.[128]

Patient education regarding the nature of the dermatitis, triggering agents, irritant factors plus instruction for avoidance, and appropriate substitutes will not only aid in clearing the dermatitis but also prevent or minimize recurrences. At present, hyposensitization of patients with ACD is not a viable therapy.[129]

Conclusions

CD includes irritant and allergic forms and can affect patients of any age. Identification and avoidance of the allergen is key to the successful treatment of ACD. Patch testing remains the gold standard for diagnosis of ACD, and negative results in the face of a convincing clinical presentation should prompt consideration for further evaluation by a specialist in CD. A limited number of interventions effectively prevent or treat irritant and allergic CD, but well-controlled, outcome-blinded studies, particularly in the area of ACD prevention, are needed.[130] New insights into the immune mechanisms involved may lead to better treatment strategies, including induction of tolerance, especially with difficult-to-avoid allergens.

Summary and Recommendations

The following may decrease risk of developing allergic and irritant CD:

1. Use mild detergents in children.
2. Use products generally free of fragrances and preservatives.
3. Limit the use of topical antibiotics to decrease sensitization and the development of resistance strains.
4. Delay ear piercing possibly until after 10 years of age.
5. 'Natural' herbal supplements are not necessarily safe and without adverse effects.
6. Start strategies of avoidance of allergen exposure as early as possible.
7. There is good and fair-quality evidence that barrier creams containing dimethicone or perfluoropolyethers, short-term use of high-lipid content moisturizers, use of cotton liners if occlusive gloves are worn, and use of softened fabrics, can prevent the development of ICD.
8. There is good- and fair-quality evidence that lipid-rich moisturizers can effectively treat ICD.

Helpful Websites

American Contact Dermatitis Society website includes 'Find a Physician' for Patch Testing (www.contactderm.org)
The American Academy of Dermatology website (www.aad.org)
T.R.U.E. TEST® website (www.truetest.com)

References

1. Mortz CG, Andersen KE. Allergic contact dermatitis in children and adolescents. Contact Dermatitis 1999;41:121–30.
2. Beltrani VS, Beltrani VP. Contact dermatitis. Ann Allergy Asthma Immunol 1997;78:160–73;quiz 174–6.
3. De Groot AC. Patch testing: test concentrations and vehicles for 3700 chemicals. 2nd ed. Amsterdam, the Netherlands: Elsevier; 1994.
4. Militello G, Jacob SE, Crawford GH. Allergic contact dermatitis in children. Curr Opin Pediatr 2006;18:385–90.
5. Jacob SE, Brod B, Crawford GH. Clinically relevant patch test reactions in children: a United states Based Study. Pediatric Dermatol 2008;25:520–7.
6. Mortz CG, Lauritsen JM, Bindslev-Jensen C, et al. Prevalence of atopic dermatitis, asthma, allergic rhinitis, and hand and contact dermatitis in adolescents. The Odense Adolescence Cohort Study on Atopic Diseases and Dermatitis. Br J Dermatol 2001;144:523–32.
7. Romaguera C, Vilaplana J. Contact dermatitis in children: 6 years experience (1992–1997). Contact Dermatitis 1998;39:277–80.
8. Manzini BM, Ferdani G, Simonetti V, et al. Contact sensitization in children. Pediatr Dermatol 1998;15:12–7.
9. Shah M, Lewis FM, Gawkrodger DJ. Patch testing in children and adolescents: five years' experience and follow-up. J Am Acad Dermatol 1997;37:964–8.

10. Stables GI, Forsyth A, Lever RS. Patch testing in children. Contact Dermatitis 1996;34:341–4.

11. Wilkowska A, Grubska-Suchanek E, Karwacka I, et al. Contact allergy in children. Cutis 1996;58:176–80.

12. Rudzki E, Rebandel P. Contact dermatitis in children. Contact Dermatitis 1996;34:66–7.

13. Katsarou A, Koufou V, Armenaka M, et al. Patch tests in children: a review of 14 years experience. Contact Dermatitis 1996;34:70–1.

14. Wantke F, Hemmer W, Jarisch R, et al. Patch test reactions in children, adults and the elderly: a comparative study in patients with suspected allergic contact dermatitis. Contact Dermatitis 1996;34:316–9.

15. Sevila A, Romaguera C, Vilaplana J, et al. Contact dermatitis in children. Contact Dermatitis 1994;30:292–4.

16. Goncalo S, Goncalo M, Azenha A, et al. Allergic contact dermatitis in children: a multicenter study of the Portuguese Contact Dermatitis Group (GPEDC). Contact Dermatitis 1992;26:112–5.

17. Rademaker M, Forsyth A. Contact dermatitis in children. Contact Dermatitis 1989;20:104–7.

18. Balato N, Lembo G, Patruno C, et al. Patch testing in children. Contact Dermatitis 1989;20:305–7.

19. Fisher AA. Allergic contact dermatitis in early infancy. Cutis 1994;54:300–2.

20. Kwangsukstith C, Maibach HI. Effect of age and sex on the induction and elicitation of allergic contact dermatitis. Contact dermatitis 1995;33:289–98.

21. Seidenari S, Giusti F, Pepe P, et al. Contact sensitization in 1094 children undergoing patch testing over a 7 year period. Pediatr Dermatol 2005;22:1–5.

22. Bruckner AL, Weston WL, Morelli JG. Does sensitization to contact allergens begin in infancy? Pediatrics 2000;105:e3.

23. Fernandez Vozmediano JM, Armario Hita. Allergic contact dermatitis in children. Dermatol Venereol 2005;19:42–6.

24. DeLeo VA, Taylor SC, Belsito DV, et al. The effect of race and ethnicity on patch test results. J Am Acad Dermatol 2002;46:S107–12.

25. Fartasch M, Schnetz E, Diepgen TL. Characterization of detergent-induced barrier alterations: effect of barrier cream on irritation. J Invest Dermatol Symp Proc 1998;3:121–7.

26. Wood LC, Jackson SM, Elias PM, et al. Cutaneous barrier perturbation stimulates cytokine production in the epidermis of mice. J Clin Invest 1992;90:482–7.

27. Brasch J, Burgard J, Sterry W. Common pathogenetic pathways in allergic and irritant contact dermatitis. J Invest Dermatol 1992;98:166–70.

28. Hoefakker S, Caubo M, van't Erve EH, et al. In vivo cytokine profiles in allergic and irritant contact dermatitis. Contact Dermatitis 1995;33:258–66.

29. Lisby S, Baadsgaard O. Mechanisms of irritant contact dermatitis. In: Rycroft RJG, Menne T, Frosch PJ, et al., editors. Textbook of contact dermatitis. London: Springer-Verlag; 2001.

30. Novak N, Bieber T. The skin as a target for allergic diseases. Allergy 2000;55:103–7.

31. Novak N, Baurecht H, Schafer T, et al. Loss-of-function mutations in the filaggrin gene and allergic contact sensitization to nickel. J Invest Dermatol 2008;128:1430–5.

32. Krasteva M, Kehren J, Horand F, et al. Dual role of dendritic cells in the induction and down-regulation of antigen-specific cutaneous inflammation. J Immunol 1998;160:1181–90.

33. Grabbe S, Schwarz T. Immunoregulatory mechanisms involved in elicitation of allergic contact hypersensitivity. Immunol Today 1998;19:37–44.

34. Xu H, DiIulio NA, Fairchild RL. T cell populations primed by hapten sensitization in contact sensitivity are distinguished by polarized patterns of cytokine production: interferon gamma-producing (Tc1) effector CD8+ T cells and interleukin (Il) 4/Il-10-producing (Th2) negative regulatory CD4+ T cells. J Exp Med 1996;183:1001–12.

35. Nasorri F, Sebastiani S, Mariani V, et al. Activation of nickel-specific CD4+ T lymphocytes in the absence of professional antigen-presenting cells. J Invest Dermatol 2002;118:172–9.

36. Trautmann A, Akdis M, Kleemann D, et al. T cell-mediated Fas-induced keratinocyte apoptosis plays a key pathogenetic role in eczematous dermatitis. J Clin Invest 2000;106:25–35.

37. Trautmann A, Akdis M, Schmid-Grendelmeier P, et al. Targeting keratinocyte apoptosis in the treatment of atopic dermatitis and allergic contact dermatitis. J Allergy Clin Immunol 2001;108:839–46.

38. Robert C, Kupper TS. Inflammatory skin diseases, T cells, and immune surveillance. N Engl J Med 1999;341:1817–28.

39. Campbell JJ, Haraldsen G, Pan J, et al. The chemokine receptor CCR4 in vascular recognition by cutaneous but not intestinal memory T cells. Nature 1999;400:776–80.

40. Sallusto F, Mackay CR, Lanzavecchia A. The role of chemokine receptors in primary, effector, and memory immune responses. Annu Rev Immunol 2000;18:593–620.

41. Albanesi C, Scarponi C, Cavani A, et al. Interleukin-17 is produced by both Th1 and Th2 lymphocytes, and modulates interferongamma- and interleukin-4-induced activation of human keratinocytes. Invest Dermatol 2000;115:81–7.

42. Cavani A, Albanesi C, Traidl C, et al. Effector and regulatory T cells in allergic contact dermatitis. Trends Immunol 2001;22:118–20.

43. Martin S, Lappin MB, Kohler J, et al. Peptide immunization indicates that CD8+ T cells are the dominant effector cells in trinitrophenyl-specific contact hypersensitivity. J Invest Dermatol 2000;115:260–6.

44. Budinger L, Neuser N, Totzke U, et al. Preferential usage of TCR-Vbeta17 by peripheral and cutaneous T cells in nickel-induced contact dermatitis. J Immunol 2001;167:6038–44.

45. Kapsenberg ML, Wierenga EA, Stiekema FE, et al. Th1 lymphokine production profiles of nickel-specific CD4+T lymphocyte clones from nickel contact allergic and non-allergic individuals. J Invest Dermatol 1992;98:59–63.

46. Cavani A, Mei D, Guerra E, et al. Patients with allergic contact dermatitis to nickel and nonallergic individuals display different nickel-specific T cell responses: evidence for the presence of effector CD8+ and regulatory CD4+ T cells. J Invest Dermatol 1998;111:621–8.

47. Larsen JM, Bonefeld CM, Poulsen SS. IL-23 and TH17-mediated inflammation in human allergic contact dermatitis. J Allergy Clin Immunol 2009;123:486–92.

48. Cavani A, Nasorri F, Prezzi C, et al. Human CD4+ T lymphocytes with remarkable regulatory functions on dendritic cells and nickel-specific Th1 immune responses. J Invest Dermatol 2000;114:295–302.

49. Iliev D, Elsner P. Clinical irritant contact dermatitis syndromes. Immunol Allergy Clin North Am 1997;17:365–75.

50. Duarte I, Terumi Nakano J, Lazzarini R. Hand eczema: evaluation of 250 patients. Am J of Contact Derm 1998;9:216–23.

51. Warshaw EM, Ahmed RL, Belsito DV, et al. Contact dermatitis of the hands: cross-sectional analyses of North American Contact Dermatitis Group Data, 1994–2004. J Am Acad Dermatol 2007;57:301–14.

52. Edman B. Statistical relations between hand eczema and contact allergens. In: Menne T, Maibach HI, editors. Hand eczema. 2nd ed. Boca Raton (LA): CRC Press; 2000:75–83.

53. Warshaw E, Lee G, Storrs FJ. Hand dermatitis: a review of clinical features, therapeutic options, and long-term outcomes. Dermatitis 2003;14:119–28.

54. Ayala F, Fabbrocini G, Bacchilega R, et al. Eyelid dermatitis: an evaluation of 447 patients. Dermatitis 2003;14:69–74.

55. Guin JD. Eyelid dermatitis: experience in 203 cases. J Am Acad Dermatol 2002;47:755–65.

56. Rietschel RL, Warshaw EM, Sasseville D, et al. Common contact allergens associated with eyelid dermatitis: data from the North American Contact Dermatitis Group 2003–2004 Study Period. Dermatitis 2007;18:78–81.

57. Sainio EL, Kanerva L. Contact allergens in toothpastes and a review of their hypersensitivity. Contact Dermatitis 1995;33:100–5.

58. Torgerson RR, Davis MDP, Bruce AJ, et al. Contact allergy in oral disease. J Am Acad Dermatol Aug 2007;57:315–21.

59. Jordon WE, Lawson KD, Berg RW, et al. Diaper dermatitis: frequency and severity among a general infant population. Pediatr Dermatol 1986;3:198–207.

60. Bonifazi E. Napkin dermatitis-causative factors. In: Harper J, Oranje A, Prose N, editors. Textbook of pediatric dermatology. London: Blackwell Scientific Publications; 2000.

61. Scheinfeld, N. Diaper dermatitis: a review and brief survey of eruptions of the diaper area: therapy in practice. Am J Clin Dermatol 2005;6(5):273–81.

62. Philipp R, Hughes A, Golding J. Getting to the bottom of nappy rash. ALSPAC Survey Team. Avon Longitudinal Study of Pregnancy and Childhood. Br J Gen Pract 1997;47:493–7.

63. Belhadjali H, Giordano-Labadie F, Rance F, et al. 'Lucky Luke'contact dermatitis from diapers: a new allergen? Contact Dermatitis 2001; 44:248.

64. Reid CM, van Grutten M, Rycroft RJ. Allergic contact dermatitis from ethylbutylthiourea in neoprene. Contact Dermatitis 1993;n28:193.

65. Lazzarini R, Duarte I, Marzagao C. Contact dermatitis of the feet: a study of 53 cases. Dermatitis September 2004;15:125–30.

66. Zug KA, Rietschel RL, Warshaw EM, et al. The value of patch testing patients with a scattered generalized distribution of dermatitis: retrospective cross-sectional analyses of North American Contact Dermatitis Group data, 2001 to 2004. J Am Acad Dermatol 2008;59:426–31.

67. Hjorth N. Eczematous allergy to balsams, allied perfumes and flavoring agents. Copenhagen: Munkgaard; 1961. p. 134.

68. Moreno-Ramirez D, Garcia-Bravo B, Pichardo AR, et al. Baboon syndrome in childhood: easy to avoid, easy to diagnose, but the problem continues. Pediatr Dermatol 2004;21:250–3.

69. Goossens C, Sass U, Song M. Baboon syndrome. Dermatology 1997;194:421–22.

70. Audicana M, Bernedo N, Gonzalez I, et al. An unusual case of baboon syndrome due to mercury present in a homeopathic medicine. Contact Dermatitis 2001;45:185.

71. Alegre M, Pujol RM, Alomar A. A generalized itchy flexural eruption in a 7-year-old boy. Arch Dermatol 2000;136:1055–60.

72. Bartolome B, Cordoba S, Sanchez-Perez J, et al. Baboon syndrome of unusual origin. Contact Dermatitis 2000;43:113.

73. Beattie PE, Green C, Lowe G, et al. Which children should we patch test? Clin Exp Dermatol 2007;32:6–11.

74. Zug KA, McGinley-Smith D, Warshaw EM, et al. Contact allergy in children referred for patch testing: North American Contact Dermatitis Group data, 2001–2004. Arch Dermatol 2008;144:1329–36.

75. Sherertz EF, Fransway AF, Belsito DV, et al. Patch testing discordance alert: false-negative findings with rubber additives and fragrances. J Am Acad Dermatol 2001;45:313–4.

76. Suneja T, Belsito DV. Comparative study of Finn Chambers and T.R.U.E. test methodologies in detecting the relevant allergens inducing contact dermatitis. J Am Acad Dermatol 2001;45:836–9.

77. Bourke J, Coulson I, English J, et al. Guidelines for the management of contact dermatitis: an update. Br J Dermatol 2009;60:946–54.

78. Heine G, Schnuch A, Uter W, et al. Frequency of contact allergy in German children and adolescents patch tested between 1995 and 2002: results from the Information Network of Departments of Dermatology and the German Contact Dermatitis Research Group. Contact Dermatitis 2004;51:111–7.

79. Fisher AA. Allergic contact dermatitis in early infancy. Cutis 1994;54:387–8.

80. Carder KR. Hypersensitivity reactions in neonates and infants. Dermatol Ther 2005;18:160–75.

81. Weston WL, Weston JA, Kinoshita J, et al. Prevalence of positive epicutaneous tests among infants, children, and adolescents. Pediatrics 1986;78:1070–4.

82. Kornik R, Zug KA. Nickel. Dermatitis 2008;19:3–8.

83. Larsson-Stymne B, Widstrom L. Ear piercing: a cause of nickel allergy in schoolgirls. Contact Dermatitis 1985;3:289–93.

84. Rystedt I, Fischer T. Relationship between nickel and cobalt sensitization in hard metal workers. Contact Dermatitis 1983;9:95–200.

85. Dotterud LK, Falk ES. Metal allergy in north Norwegian schoolchildren and its relationship with ear piercing and atopy. Contact Dermatitis 1994;31:308–13.

86. Kütting B, Brehler R, Traupe H. Allergic contact dermatitis in children: strategies of prevention and risk management. Eur J Dermatol 2004;14:80–5.

87. Rahilly G, Price N. Nickel allergy and orthodontics. J Orthod 2003;30:171–4.

88. Kerosuo H, Kullaa A, Kerosuo E, et al. Nickel allergy in adolescents in relation to orthodontic treatment and piercing of ears. Am J Orthod Dentofacial Orthop 1996;109:148–54.

89. White JM, Goon AT, Jowsey IR, et al. Oral tolerance to contact allergens: a common occurrence? A review. Contact Dermatitis 2007;56:247–54.

90. Christensen OB, Moller H. Nickel allergy and hand eczema. Contact Dermatitis 1975;1:129–35.

91. Veien NK, Hattel T, Laurberg G. Low nickel diet: an open, prospective trial. J Am Acad Dermatol 1993;29:1002–7.

92. Antico A, Soana R. Chronic allergic-like dermatopathies in nickel sensitive patients: results of dietary restrictions and challenge with nickel salts. Allergy Asthma Proc 1999;20:235–42.

93. Breithaupt A, Jacob SE. Thimerosal and the relevance of patch-test reactions in children. Dermatitis 2008;19:275–7.

94. Gon Valo M, Figueiredo A, Gon Valo S. Hypertensivity to thiomersal: the sensitizing moiety. Contact Dermatitis 1996;34:201–03.

95. Wantke F, Demmer CM, Gotz M, et al. Contact dermatitis from thimerosal: 2 years' experience with ethylmercuric chloride in patch testing thimerosal-sensitive patients. Contact Dermatitis 1994;30:115–7.

96. Suneja T, Belsito D. Thiomersal in the detection of clinically relevant allergic contact reactions. J Am Acad Dermatol 2001;45:23–7.

97. Osawa J, Kitamura K, Ikezawa Z, et al. A probable role for vaccines containing thiomersal in thiomersal hypersensitivity. Contact Dermatitis 1991;24:178–82.

98. Marks JG Jr, Belsito DV, DeLeo VA, et al. North American Contact Dermatitis Group patch-test results, 1996–1998. Arch Dermatol 2000;136:272–3.

99. Belsito DV. Thimerosal: contact (non)allergen of the year. Am J Contact Dermat 2002;13:1–2.

100. Van't Veen AJ. Vaccines without thiomersal: why so necessary, why so long coming? Drugs 2001;61:565–72.

101. Kaaber K, Nielsen AO, Veien NK. Vaccination granulomas and aluminum allergy: course and prognostic factors. Contact Dermatitis 1992;26:304–6.

102 Anderson BE. Mixed dialkyl thioureas. Dermatitis 2009;20:3–5.

103. Paulsen E, Otkjaer A, Andersen KE. Sesquiterpene lactone dermatitis in the young: is atopy a risk factor? Contact Dermatitis 2008;59:1–6.

104. Fortina AB, Romano I, Peserico A. Contact sensitization to compositae mix in children. J Am Acad Dermatol 2005;53:877–80.

105. Paulsen E, Andersen KE. Colophonium and Compositae mix as markers of fragrance allergy: cross reactivity between fragrance terpenes, colophonium and compositae plant extracts. Contact Dermatitis 2005;53:285–91.

106. Matura M, Goossens A. Contact allergy to corticosteroids. Allergy 2000;55:698–704.

107. Gonzalo Garijo MA, Bobadilla Gonzalez P. Cutaneous-mucosal allergic contact reaction due to topical corticosteroids. Allergy 1995;50:833–6.

108. Jacob SE, Zapolanski T, Chayavichitsilp P, et al. p-Phenylenediamine in black henna tattoos: a practice in need of policy in children. Arch Pediatr Adolesc Med 2008;162:790–2.

109. De Leo V. p-Phephenylenediamine. Dermatitis 2006;17:53–5.

110. Kockentiet B, Adams BB. Contact dermatitis in athletes. J Am Acad Dermatol 2007;56:1048–55.

111. Goette DK. Raccoon-like periorbital leukoderma from contact with swim goggles. Contact Dermatitis 1984;10:129–31.

112. Vaswani SK, Collins DD, Pass CJ. Severe allergic contact eyelid dermatitis caused by swimming goggles. Ann Allergy Asthma Immunol 2003;90:672–3.

113. Mailler EA, Adams BB. The wear and tear of 26.2: dermatological injuries reported on marathon day. Br J Sports Med 2004;38:498–501.

114. Jung JH, McLaughlin JL, Stannard J, et al. Isolation, via activity-directed fractionation, of mercaptobenzothiazole and dibenzothiazyl disulfide as 2 allergens responsible for tennis shoe dermatitis. Contact Dermatitis 1988;19:254–9.

115. Ventura MT, Dagnello M, Matino MG, et al. Contact dermatitis in students practicing sports: incidence of rubber sensitisation. Br J Sports Med 2001;35:100–2.

116. Rodriguez-Serna M, Molinero J, Febrer I, et al. Persistent hand eczema in a child. Am J Contact Dermat 2002;13:35–6.

117. Helm TN, Bergfeld WF. Sports dermatology. Clin Dermatol 1998;16:159–65.

118. Guerra L, Misciali C, Borrello P, et al. Sensitization to palladium. Contact Dermatitis 1988;19:306–7.

119. Scott MJ Jr, Scott NI, Scott LM. Dermatologic stigmata in sports: weightlifting. Cutis 1992;50:141–5.

120. Fisher AA, editors. Contact dermatitis. Philadelphia: Lea & Febiger; 1986.

121. Marks JG Jr, DeLeo VA. Contact and occupational dermatology. St Louis: Mosby; 1992.

122. Ward DB, Fleischer AB Jr, Feldman SR, et al. Characterization of diaper dermatitis in the United States. Arch Pediatr Adolesc Med 2000;154:943–6.

123. Queille-Roussel C, Graeber M, Thurston M, et al. SDZ ASM 981 is the first non-steroid that suppresses established nickel contact dermatitis elicited by allergen challenge. Contact Dermatitis 2000;42:349–50.

124. Gupta AK, Adamiak A, Chow M. Tacrolimus: a review of its use for the management of dermatoses. J Eur Acad Dermatol Venereol 2002;16:100–14.

125. Marks JG Jr, Elsner P, DeLeo VA. Contact and occupational dermatology. 3rd ed. Mosby Inc; 2002.

126. Runeman B. Skin interaction with absorbent hygiene roducts. Clin Dermatol 2008;26:45–51.

127. Atherton DJ. A review of the pathophysiology, prevention and treatment of irritant diaper dermatitis. Curr Med Res Opin 2004;20:645–9.

128. Shin HT. Diaper dermatitis that does not quit. Dermatol Ther 2005;18:124–35.

129. Marks JG Jr, Trautlein JJ, Epstein WL, et al. Oral hyposensitization to poison ivy and poison oak. Arch Dermatol 1987;123:476–8.

130. Saary J, Qureshi R, Palda V, et al. A systematic review of contact dermatitis treatment and prevention. J Am Acad Dermatol 2005;53:845.

57

Allergic and Immunologic Eye Disease

Leonard Bielory • Catherine Origlieri • Rudolph S. Wagner

Allergic disease affects as many as 25% of the pediatric population. The direct costs of upper airway allergies are approximately $5.9 billion, with children (< 12 years) accounting for 38% ($2.3 billion) of the total.[1] In a study of 5000 allergic children, ocular allergy was reported in 32% as the single manifestation of their allergies.[2] Although frequent, ocular allergy is rarely the sole culprit of the pediatric red eye, which requires the clinician to be able to distinguish an allergic response from nonallergic inflammatory responses of anterior surface of the eye. This chapter provides an overview of pediatric allergic eye disease and an approach to proper diagnosis and management.

Eye Anatomy, Histology, and Immune Function

The eye is a common target of local and systemic inflammatory disorders and due to its considerable vascularization and vessel sensitivity, particularly in the conjunctiva, ocular inflammation can be quite pronounced. Besides alarming the parents of affected children, ocular inflammation can pose a formidable diagnostic challenge to clinicians, and thus a solid understanding of the eye's anatomy, histology, and immune function is essential.

The eye is essentially constructed of four layers that are predominantly involved in immunologic reactions (Figure 57-1):

1. The anterior portion, consisting of the eyelids, conjunctiva (palbepral and bulbar), and tear fluid layer, providing the eye's primary barrier against environmental aeroallergens, chemicals, and infectious agents
2. The collagenous sclera, involved in autoimmune disorders
3. The highly vascular uvea, involved in systemic inflammatory reactions associated with circulating immune complexes and cell-mediated hypersensitivity reactions
4. The retina, an extension of the central nervous system.

The eye is immunologically distinctive because it lacks formed lymph nodes in the orbit, lacrimal gland, eyelids, and conjunctiva, while having a distinctive and a unique anterior chamber immune system. Interestingly, the spleen appears to function as the primary lymphoid organ for intraocular reactions. Immunologic hypersensitivity reactions involving the eye incorporate the spectrum of classic Gell and Coombs classification.[3] (Table 57-1).

Eyelids

Designed to protect, moisten, and cleanse the ocular surface, the eyelids are the first line of defense for the eye. The palpebral skin is extremely thin compared to the dermal thickness elsewhere on the human body (0.55 mm compared to the thickness of the 2 mm integument of the face), which explains the common extensive involvement of the eyelid in minor inflammatory insults.

Conjunctiva

The conjunctiva is the most immunologically active tissue and consists of a thin mucous membrane that extends from the lid margin of the eyelid to the limbus of the eye. Anatomically, the conjunctiva is divided into three parts: (1) the palpebral conjunctiva which lines the inner surface of the eyelids; (2) the bulbar conjunctiva which covers the anterior portion of the sclera; and (3) the fornix or conjunctival sac bounded by the bulbar and palpebral conjunctiva. Histologically, the conjunctiva consists of two distinct layers: the epithelium and the substantia propria. The epithelial layer is composed of two to five cells of stratified columnar cells, whereas the lamina propria is composed of loose connective tissue.

Inflammatory cells such as mast cells, eosinophils, and basophils normally do not reside in the ocular epithelium, but are found in the substantia propria. Mast cells at a concentration of up to 6000/mm^3 are present in this layer with the predominance (> 95%) of connective tissue type (MC$_{TC}$) containing both chymase and tryptase.[4-6] However, in chronic forms of allergic conjunctivitis there is an increase in mucosal type mast cells (MC$_T$), which contain tryptase that can migrate to the epithelial layer.[5] Epithelial cells have also been found to have an extensive proinflammatory capability in the production of various cytokines, e.g. tumor necrosis factor alpha (TNF-α), interleukin (IL)-6, IL-10 as well as various adhesion molecules, such as intracellular adhesion molecules (ICAM-1).

Various mononuclear cells, including Langerhans cells, CD3$^+$ lymphocytes, and CD4$^+$/CD8$^+$ lymphocytes are also an active component of the anterior surface immune response that are primarily found in the epithelial layer. Langerhans' cells, which serve as antigen-presenting cells in the skin, have a similar role in the eye.[4] The primary lymphoid organ for intraocular reactions is the spleen. Although lymphatics do drain from the lateral conjunctiva to the preauricular nodes (e.g. parotid node) just anterior to the tragus of the ear, the nasal conjunctival lymphatics drain to the submandibular nodes. It is generally believed that activated conjunctival lymphocytes travel first to these regional lymph nodes, then to the spleen, and ultimately back to the conjunctiva.

©2010 Elsevier Ltd, Inc, BV
DOI: 10.1016/B978-1-4377-0271-2.00057-2

Table 57-1 Categories of Pediatric Ocular Inflammation

Category	Recognition Component	Soluble Mediators	Time Course	Cellular Response	Clinical Example
IgE/mast cell	IgE	Leukotrienes Arachadonates Histamine	Seconds Minutes	Eosinophils Neutrophils Basophils	Allergic conjunctivitis Anaphylaxis Vernal keratoconjunctivitis
Cytotoxic antibody	IgG IgM	Complement	Hours Days	Neutrophils Macrophages	Mooren's ulcer Pemphigus Pemphigoid
Immune complex	IgG IgM	Complement	Hours Days	Neutrophils Eosinophils Lymphocytes	Serum sickness uveitis Corneal immune rings Lens-induced uveitis Behçet's syndrome Kawasaki's disease Vasculitis
Delayed hypersensivity	Lymphocytes Monocytes	Lymphokines Monokines	Days Weeks	Lymphocytes Monocytes Eosinophils Basophils	Corneal allograft rejection Sympathetic ophthalmia Sarcoid-induced uveitis

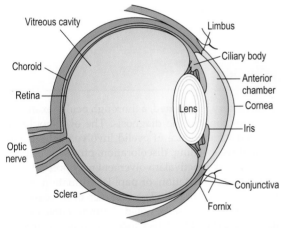

Figure 57-1 Cross-section of the eye. Sagittal cross-sectional view of the human eye revealing the parts commonly involved in immunologic reactions: eyelids (blepharitis and dermatitis); conjunctiva (conjunctivitis); cornea (keratitis); sclera (episcleritis and scleritis); optic nerve (neuritis); iris (iritis); vitreous (vitreitis); choroids (choroiditis); and retina (retinitis). The last four parts involve the inner portion of the eye (the uveal tract) and are classified as forms of uveitis.

Tear Film

The conjunctival surface is bathed in a thin layer of tear film that appears at approximately 2 to 4 weeks after birth. Traditionally the tear film has been described as simply containing an outer lipid layer, a middle aqueous layer, and an inner mucoprotein layer. A more recent model of tear film structure describes an aqueous layer with a gradient of mucin that decreases from the ocular surface to the overlying lipid layer.[7] Goblet cells distributed along the conjunctival surface produce this mucin, which decreases the surface tension of the tear film, thus maintaining a moist hydrophobic corneal surface. The outermost lipid component of the tear film decreases the evaporation rate of the aqueous tears. The aqueous portion of the tear film contains a variety of solutes, including electrolytes, carbohydrates, ureas, amino acids, lipids, enzymes, tear-specific prealbumin, and immunologically active proteins, including immunoglobulin A (IgA), IgG, IgM, IgE, tryptase, histamine, lysozyme, lactoferrin, ceruloplasmin, vitronectin, and cytokines.

Uveal Tract

The uveal tract is comprised of the iris, ciliary body, and choroid, each of which possesses a rich vascular architecture and pigment. The pigment acts as a filtering system and the ciliary body is involved in the production of aqueous humor and is a common site for the deposition of immune complexes. In addition, disturbances in the production or outflow of aqueous humor may lead to increased intraocular pressure (IOP; i.e. glaucoma). There are congenital forms of glaucoma that are not specifically associated with immunologic disorders but must be considered in the differential diagnosis of pediatric conjunctivitis ('pink eye' or 'red eye').

Differential Diagnosis

The differential diagnosis of the pediatric red eye can be broadly divided into four categories: allergic, infectious, immunologic, and nonspecific (Figure 57-2). Each category possesses distinct signs and symptoms.[8] These indicators are summarized in Table 57-2 and can be used as a guide to delineate pediatric red eye.

History

A detailed and accurate history is the most important element in distinguishing allergic from nonallergic causes of pediatric conjunctivitis. Generally, this information is obtained from the parents or guardian, yet an astute clinician must not overlook input from the verbal child. Not only may the child's information prove clinically insightful, but this interaction helps to establish good rapport with the child, which will be beneficial during the eye exam.

When evaluating a newborn, a full prenatal history, including developmental delays and maternal infections (e.g. herpes simplex virus, *Chlamydia*, or human immunodeficiency virus [HIV]), needs to be obtained. Ocular trauma from forceps or vacuum delivery has been known to occur. In addition, ocular medications such as silver nitrate and erythromycin given at childbirth may cause chemical irritation. In the older child, recent exposure to individuals with conjunctivitis or upper respiratory

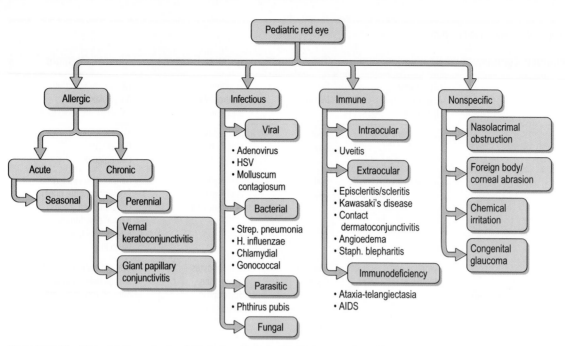

Figure 57-2 The differential diagnosis of pediatric 'red eye' includes infectious agents (e.g. chlamydial disease, adenovirus), allergic conditions (e.g. SAC, PAC, GPC, VKC), immunologic disorders (e.g. Kawasaki's disease, uveitis, ataxia-telangiectasia) and nonspecific causes (e.g. foreign body, chemical irritation, nasolacrimal obstruction).

tract infection, either within the family or at school, may suggest exposure to adenovirus infection in an endemic area. The conjunctivitis-otitis media syndrome, occurring frequently in preschool children, is usually caused by nontypable *Haemophilus influenzae* or *Streptococcus pneumoniae*.[9,10] Family history is particularly important when inherited disorders are suspected. Accidental trauma resulting in corneal abrasions or ocular foreign bodies may also occur, especially in the curious and mobile toddler. Yet, while accidents occur frequently, child abuse must also be considered; in these circumstances a thorough social history is merited. In teenagers, a sexual history may suggest a chlamydial or neisserial infection. Patient use and abuse of over-the-counter topical medications (e.g. vasoconstrictors, artificial tears, cosmetics, or contact lens wear) has the potential to produce inflammation (conjunctivitis medicamentosa or toxic keratopathy). As with all allergies, environmental factors and time of onset must be addressed, including seasonal variation and exposure to smoking, cleaning supplies, pets, air-conditioning, carpets, and other sources of irritants.

Many of the signs and symptoms of allergic conjunctivitis are nonspecific as they involve the four classical signs of inflammation (calor, dolor, rubor, and tumor), originally recorded by the Roman encyclopedist Celsus in the 1st century A.D. and include heat, pain, redness, swelling, tearing, irritation, stinging, burning, and photophobia. Symptoms tend to improve with cool, rainy weather and are exacerbated by warm, dry weather. The true hallmark of allergic conjunctivitis is itching. Pruritus can be mild or prominent and may last from hours to days. A stringy or ropy discharge is also characteristic of a persistent ocular allergy, and may range from serous to purulent. While a purulent discharge may be present, morning crusting and difficulty opening the lids are more characteristic of bacterial causes, especially Gram-negative organisms (e.g. *Neisseria* and *Haemophilus*). Environmental allergens affect both eyes at once, although a unilateral reaction may result if one eye is inoculated with animal hair or dander. Ocular pain is not typically associated with allergic conjunctivitis and suggests an extraocular process such as a corneal abrasion, scleritis or foreign body, or an intraocular process such as uveitis.

Eye Examination

Once a complete history is obtained, a thorough ocular examination is necessary to confirm the diagnosis. The eye should be carefully examined for evidence of eyelid involvement such as blepharitis, dermatitis, swelling, discoloration, ptosis, or blepharospasm (Table 57-3). Conjunctival involvement may present with chemosis, hyperemia, cicatrisation, or papillae formation on the palpebral and bulbar membranes. The presence of increased or abnormal secretions should also be noted. A fundoscopic examination should be performed to detect such conditions as uveitis (often associated with autoimmune disorders) and cataracts (associated with atopic disorders and chronic steroid use).

The examination starts with a simple inspection of the face and area surrounding the eye. A horizontal skin crease on the nose (nasal salute) suggests a history of allergic rhinitis. Allergic shiners are ecchymotic-looking areas beneath the eyes thought to result from impaired venous return from the subcutaneous tissues (Figure 57-3). Angioedema commonly involves the conjunctiva, but it more commonly affects periorbital space and more prominently around the lower lids secondary to gravity. Nonallergic indicators may also be present. Eyelid or nasal vesicular eruptions are often seen in ophthalmic zoster, but can also reflect recurrent bacterial infections associated staphylococcal blepharoconjunctivitis due to constant rubbing of the eyelids. Scratches and scars on the face or eyelid suggest ocular injury. In addition, palpation of the sinuses and the preauricular and cervical chain lymph nodes are of diagnostic importance.

Next, the conjunctiva should be thoroughly inspected with the bulbar conjunctiva examination performed by looking directly at the eye and asking the patient to look up and then down, while gently retracting the opposite lid. Examine the palpebral (tarsal) conjunctiva by grasping the upper lid at its base with a cotton swab on the superior portion of the lid while gently pulling the lid out and up as the patient looks down. To return the lid to its normal position, have the patient look up. The lower tarsal conjunctiva is examined by placing a finger near the lid margins,

Table 57-2 Differential Diagnosis of Pediatric Conjunctivitis

	Predominant Cell Type	Chemosis	Lymph Node	Cobblestoning	Discharge	Lid Involvement	Pruritus	Gritty Sensation	Pain	Seasonal Variation
Allergic										
AC	Mast cell EOS	+	-	-	Clear mucoid	-	+	+/-	-	+
VKC	Lymph EOS	+/-	-	++	Stringy mucoid	+	++	+/-	+/- if cornea is involved	+
GPC	Lymph EOS	+/-	-	++	Clear white	-	++	+	-	+/-
Infectious										
Bacterial	PMN	+/-	+	-	++ Mucopurulent	-	-	+	+/-	+/-
Viral	PMN Monolymph	+/-	++	+/-	Clear mucoid	-	-	+	+/-	+/-
Chlamydial	Monolymph	+/-	+/-	+	++ Mucopurulent	-	-	+	+/-	+/-
Immunologic										
Kawasaki's disease	PMN, lymph	+/-	++	-	Serous mucoid	-	-	+/-	+/-	-
Uveitis	Lymph	-	-	-	-	-	-	-	++	-
Sarcoidosis	Lymph	-	-	-	-	Grey flat papules	-	-	+/-	-
JRA	Lymph	-	-	-	-	-	-	-	+/-	-
Episcleritis	Lymph	-	-	-	-	-	-	-	++	-
Contact dermatoconjunctivitis	Lymph	-	-	-	+/-	++	+	-	+/- if cornea is involved	-
Angioedema	Mast cell	++	-	-	-	+++	+/-	-	-	-
Ataxia-telangiectasia	-	-	-	-	-	-	-	-	-	-
Staphlococcal blepharitis	Monolymph	+/-	-	-	++ mucopurulent	++	+	++	+/- if cornea is involved	-
Nonspecific										
Congenital entropion epiblepharon	-	-	-	-	Serous watery	++	-	+	+++	-
Congenital glaucoma	-	-	-	-	Serous	+/-	-	+/-	+++	-
Corneal abrasion	-	-	-	-	Serous watery	+	-	+/-	+++	-
Chemical	-	-	-	-	Serous mucoid	++	-	+/-	+++	-
Nasolacrimal obstruction	PMN If secondary infection	-	-	-	Mucopurulent	+	-	+/-	+/-	-

AC, allergic conjunctivitis; EOS, eosinophils; VKC, vernal keratoconjunctivitis; GPC, giant papillary conjunctivitis; PMN, polymorphonuclear leukocytes; JRA, juvenile rheumatoid arthritis.

Table 57-3 Ocular Clinical Signs

Disorder	Description
Blepharitis	Inflammation of the eyelids; sometimes associated with the loss of eyelashes (madarosis)
Chalazion	A chronic, granulomatous inflammation of the meibomian gland
Chemosis	Edema of the conjunctiva due to transudate leaking through fenestrated conjunctival capillaries
Epiphora	Excessive tearing; may be due to increased tear production or more commonly congenital obstruction of the nasolacrimal drainage system. This may occur in as many as 20% of infants, but resolves spontaneously in most cases before 1 year of age.[86] Children with chronic sinusitis and/or rhinitis may have intermittent nasolacrimal duct obstruction since the distal nasolacrimal duct drains below the inferior meatus. Congenital glaucoma may also present with epiphora. but has other characteristic findings (e.g. corneal enlargement. photophobia and eventually corneal edema presenting as a corneal haze) usually within the first year of life*
Hordeolum	Synonymous with a sty
Keratitis	Inflammation and infection of the corneal surface, stroma, and endothelium, with numerous causes
Leukocoria	A white pupil; seen in patients with Chédiak-Hegashi syndrome (a neutrophil defect), retinoblastoma, cataracts and retrolental fibroplasia
Papillae	Large, hard, polygonal, flat-topped excrescences of the conjunctiva seen in many inflammatory and allergic ocular conditions
Phlyctenule	The formation of a small, gray, circumscribed lesion at the corneal limbus that has been associated with staphylococcal sensitivity, tuberculosis and malnutrition
Proptosis	Forward protrusion of the eye or eyes
Ptosis	Drooping of the eyelid, which may have neurogenic, muscular, or congenital causes. Conditions specific to the eyelid that may cause a ptotic lid include chalazia, tumors, and preseptal cellulitis
Scleritis	Inflammation of the tunic that surrounds the ocular globe. Episcleritis presents as a red, somewhat painful eye in which the inflammatory reaction is located below the conjunctiva and only over the globe of the eye. The presence of scleritis should prompt a search for other systemic immune-mediated disorders
Trichiasis	In-turned eyelashes; usually results from the softening of the tarsal plate within the eyelid
Trantas' dots	Pale, grayish-red, uneven nodules with a gelatinous composition seen at the limbal conjunctiva in vernal conjunctivitis

*Data from Seidman DJ, Nelson LB, Calhoun JH, et al. Pediatrics 1986; 77:399–404.

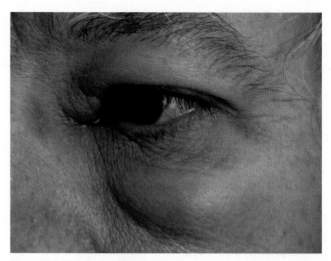

Figure 57-3 Patient with allergic shiner.

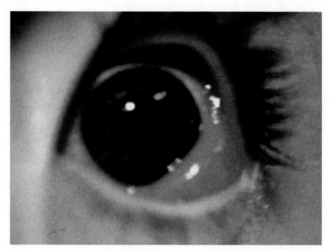

Figure 57-4 Conjunctival edema or chemosis with milky appearance obscuring conjunctival vessels in an acute allergic reaction.

everting the lower eyelid and drawing downward. A 'milky' appearance of the conjunctiva is characteristic of allergy and is the result of the obscuring of blood vessels by conjunctival edema (Figure 57-4). In contrast, a velvety, beefy-red conjunctiva with purulent discharge suggests a viral or bacterial etiology while follicular or papillary hyperplasia of the conjunctival surface reflects a more persistent or chronic inflammatory condition. Follicles appear as grayish, clear, or yellow bumps varying in

diameter from a pinpoint to 2 mm, with conjunctival vessels on their surface, while papillae contain a centrally located tuft of vessels. Although a fine papillary reaction is nonspecific, giant papillae (greater than 1 mm) on the upper tarsal conjunctiva indicate an allergic source. Papillae are generally not seen in active viral or bacterial conjunctivitis. However, the presence of follicles, a lymphocytic response in the conjunctiva, is a specific finding that occurs primarily in viral and chlamydial infections, but is also seen in chronic and persistent forms of ocular allergy.

The cornea is best examined with a slit lamp biomicroscope, although many important clinical features can be seen with the naked eye or with the use of an ophthalmoscope. The cornea should be perfectly smooth and transparent. Dusting of the cornea may indicate punctate epithelial keratitis. A localized corneal defect may suggest erosion or a larger ulcer that could be related to major basic protein deposition. Surface lesions can best be demonstrated by applying fluorescein dye to the eye, preferably following the instillation of a topical anesthetic drop (Figure 57-5). The end of the fluorescein strip is touched to the marginal tear meniscus. When the patient blinks the dye is dispersed throughout the ocular surface and stains wherever an epithelial defect exists as in a corneal or conjunctival abrasion. A light utilizing a cobalt filter found on most modern ophthalmoscopes will best demonstrate the abnormal accumulations of the

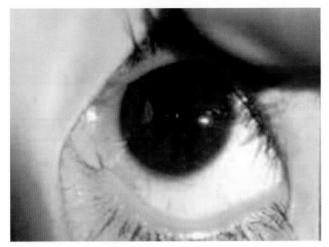

Figure 57-5 Triangular corneal abrasion highlighted with fluorescein dye.

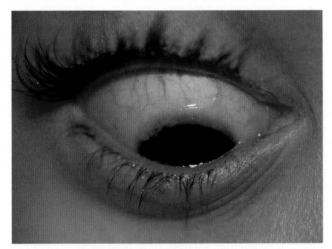

Figure 57-6 Limbal conjunctivitis (a form of vernal conjunctivitis).

dye. Mucus adhering to the corneal or conjunctival surfaces is considered pathologic.

The limbus is the zone immediately surrounding the cornea that becomes intensely inflamed with a deep pink coloration in cases of anterior uveitis or iritis, the so-called ciliary flush. Discrete swellings with small white dots are indicative of degenerating cellular debris, which is commonly seen in vernal conjunctivitis (Fig. 57-6). The anterior chamber is examined for clearness or cloudiness of the aqueous humor and for the presence of blood, either diffuse or settled out (i.e. hyphema) or the settling out of pus (i.e. hypopyon). A shallow anterior chamber suggests narrow-angle glaucoma and is a contraindication for the use of mydriatic agents. An estimation of the anterior chamber depth can be made by illuminating it from the side with a pen light; if the iris creates a shadow on the far side from the light, then there is a high index of suspicion for increased IOP (i.e. glaucoma).

Allergic Disorders

Conjunctivitis caused by IgE-mast cell-mediated reactions is the most common hypersensitivity response of the eye. An estimated 50 million mast cells reside at the interface of the conjunctiva. Direct exposure of the ocular mucosal surface to the environment stimulates these mast cells, clinically producing the acute- and late-phase signs and symptoms of allergic conjunctivitis.[11,12] In

addition, the conjunctiva is infiltrated with inflammatory cells such as neutrophils, eosinophils, lymphocytes, and macrophages. Interestingly, acute forms of allergic conjunctivitis lack an eosinophilic predominance, as seen in asthma. However, eosinophils and other immunologically active cells are prevalent in the more chronic forms.

Seasonal Allergic Conjunctivitis

Seasonal allergic conjunctivitis (SAC) is the most common allergic conjunctivitis, representing over half of all cases. As its name implies, SAC is characterized by symptoms that are seasonal and related to specific aeroallergens. Symptoms predominate in the spring and in some areas during the fall (Indian summer). Grass pollen is thought to produce the most ocular symptoms. Commonly associated with nasal or pharyngeal symptoms, patients report itchy eyes and/or a burning sensation with watery discharge. A white exudate may be present that turns stringy in the chronic form of the condition. The conjunctiva appears milky or pale pink and is accompanied by vascular congestion, which may progress to conjunctival swelling (chemosis). Symptoms are usually bilateral but not always symmetric in degree of involvement. SAC rarely results in permanent visual impairment but can interfere greatly with daily activities.

Perennial Allergic Conjunctivitis

Perennial allergic conjunctivitis (PAC) is actually considered a variant of SAC that persists throughout the year. Dust mites, animal dander, and feathers are the most common allergens. Symptoms are analogous to SAC and 79% of PAC patients have seasonal exacerbations. In addition, both PAC and SAC are similar in distribution of age, sex, and associated symptoms of asthma or eczema. The prevalence of PAC has been reported to be lower than that of SAC (3.5:10 000) although subjectively more severe,[13] but with the increasing prevalence of the allergies as reported in the International Study of Asthma and Allergies in Childhood this may be clearly underrepresented and in fact perennial forms of ocular allergy may be more common than pure seasonal forms.

Vernal Keratoconjunctivitis

Vernal keratoconjunctivitis (VKC) is a severe, bilateral, recurrent, chronic ocular inflammatory process of the upper tarsal conjunctival surface. It has a marked seasonal incidence, and its frequent onset in the spring has led to use of the term *vernal catarrh*. It occurs most frequently in children and young adults who have a history of seasonal allergy, asthma, and eczema. The age of onset for VKC is usually before puberty, with boys being affected twice as often as girls. After puberty it becomes equally distributed between the sexes and 'burns out' by the third decade of life (about 4 to 10 years after onset). VKC may threaten sight if the cornea is involved and is more common in persons of Asian or African origin.

Symptoms of VKC include intense pruritus exacerbated by time and exposure to wind, dust, bright light, hot weather, or physical exertion associated with sweating. Associated symptoms involving the cornea include photophobia, foreign body sensation, and lacrimation. Signs include: conjunctival hyperemia with papillary hypertrophy ('cobblestoning') reaching 7 to 8 mm in diameter in the upper tarsal plate; a thin, copious milk-white fibrinous secretion composed of eosinophils, epithelial

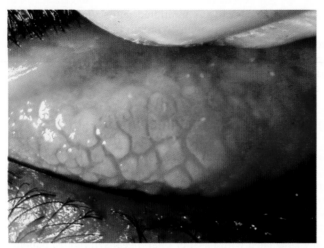

Figure 57-7 Conjunctival hyperemia with papillary hypertrophy (cobblestoning) on an everted palpebral conjunctiva of the upper eyelid in a patient with vernal conjunctivitis.

cells, and Charcot-Leyden granules; limbal or conjunctival 'yellowish-white points' (Horner's points and Trantas' dots) lasting 2 to 7 days; an extra lower eyelid crease (Dennie's line); corneal ulcers infiltrated with Charcot-Leyden crystals; or pseudomembrane formation of the upper lid when everted and exposed to heat (Maxwell-Lyon's sign; Figure 57-7). Although VKC is a bilateral disease, it may affect one eye more than the other.

VKC is characterized by conjunctival infiltration by eosinophils, degranulated mast cells, basophils, plasma cells, lymphocytes, and macrophages. Degranulated eosinophils and their toxic enzymes (e.g. major basic proteins) have been found in the conjunctiva and in the periphery of corneal ulcers, a fact that may suggest their etiopathogenic role in many of the problems associated with VKC.[12,13] MC_T cells are increased in the conjunctiva of these patients.[6] Tears from VKC patients have been found to contain higher levels of leukotrienes and histamine (16 ng/mL) when compared to controls (5 ng/mL).[14] Tears from VKC patients also contain major basic protein, Charcot-Leyden crystals, basophils, IgE and IgG specific for aeroallergens (e.g. ragweed pollen) and eosinophils (in 90% of cases).[15] The tear-specific IgE does not correlate with the positive immediate skin tests that VKC patients may have, thus reflecting that it represents more than a chronic allergic response as reflected in a study that suggested that exposure to house dust mite allergen aggravates VKC symptoms.[16]

Giant Papillary Conjunctivitis

Giant papillary conjunctivitis (GPC) is associated with the infiltration of basophils, eosinophils, plasma cells, and lymphocytes. GPC has been directly linked to the continued use of contact lenses with a seasonal increase of symptoms during spring pollen season, including itching; signs include a white or clear exudate upon awakening that chronically becomes thick and stringy. Patients may develop Trantas' dots, limbal infiltration, and bulbar conjunctival hyperemia and edema. Upper tarsal papillary hypertrophy ('cobblestoning') has been described in 5–10% of soft and 3–4% of hard contact lens wearers. The contact lens polymer, the preservative (thimerosal), and proteinaceous deposits on the surface of the lens have been implicated in GPC, but this remains controversial. Analysis of the glycoprotein deposits on disposable soft contact lenses has revealed that the higher the water content, the higher the protein integration

(lysozyme, tear-specific prealbumin, and the heavy chain components of IgG) into the lens.[17]

Immunologic Disorders

Kawasaki's Disease

Kawasaki's disease (KD) (*mucocutaneous lymph node syndrome*) is an acute exanthematous illness that almost exclusively affects children with 50% of cases occuring in males < 2 years of age, and with an increased prevalence in individuals of Japanese ancestry. Five of the following six criteria must be present for diagnosis: (1) fever, (2) bilateral conjunctival injection, (3) changes in upper respiratory tract mucous membrane, (4) changes in skin and nails, (5) maculopapular cutaneous eruptions, and (6) cervical lymphadenopathy. The cutaneous eruption characteristically involves the extremities and desquamates in the later stages. The disease may occur in cyclic epidemics, supporting an infectious hypothesis (with *Rickettsia*-like organisms being demonstrated by electron microscopy) causing a hypersensitivity response. KD is usually benign and self-limited, although 2% of Japanese KD cases (nearly all male) experience sudden cardiac death[18] due to an acute thrombosis of aneurysmally dilated coronary arteries secondary to direct vasculitic involvement.

The most typical ocular finding is bilateral nonexudative conjunctival vasodilatation, typically involving the bulbar conjunctiva. Anterior uveitis is seen in 66% of patients, and is usually mild, bilateral and symmetric;[19] superficial punctate keratitis is seen in 12% of patients. Vitreous opacifications and papilledema have been reported. Choroiditis has been reported in a case of infantile periarteritis nodosa, which may be indistinguishable from KD. On magnetic resonance imaging of the brain, deep white matter lesions, typical of the vasculopathic lesions of systemic vasculitis, as opposed to the periventricular lesions more characteristic of multiple sclerosis, have been seen.

Uveitis

Uveitis may be anatomically classified as anterior, intermediate, posterior, or diffuse. Patients typically complain of diminished or hazy vision accompanied by black floating spots. Severe pain, photophobia, and blurred vision occur in cases of acute iritis or iridocyclitis. The major signs of anterior uveitis are pupillary miosis and ciliary/perilimbal flush (a peculiar injection seen adjacent to the limbus) that can be easily confused as conjunctivitis. Vitreal cells and cellular aggregates are characteristic of intermediate uveitis that can be seen with the direct ophthalmoscope. Cells, flare, keratic precipitates on the corneal endothelium, and exudates with membranes covering the ciliary body can be visualized with the slit lamp and indirect ophthalmoscopy.

Anterior uveitis may be confused with conjunctivitis because its primary manifestations are a red eye and tearing; ocular pain and photophobia are also present. Anterior uveitis may be an isolated phenomenon that presents to an ophthalmologist or may be associated with a systemic autoimmune disorder that presents to a general practitioner. It is found in approximately 50% of cases of HLA-linked spondyloarthropathies (HLA-B27 e.g. ankylosing spondylitis (sacroileitis), Reiter's syndrome), infections, such as Klebsiella bowel infections (resulting from molecular mimicry), brucellosis, syphilis, and tuberculosis; HLA B5, Bw22, A29, and D5 genotypes as well as inflammatory bowel diseases (e.g. Crohn's disease). The inflammatory response in the anterior chamber of the eye results in an increased concentration of proteins (flare [i.e. Tyndall effect]), a constricted pupil (miosis) with afferent pupillary defect (a poor response to illumination), or cells in the aqueous humor. White cells can pool in the anterior chamber forming a hypopyon or stick to the endothelial surface of the cornea, forming keratic precipitates. The sequelae of anterior uveitis may be acute, which may result in synechia (adhesions of the posterior iris to the anterior capsule of the lens), angle-closure glaucoma (blockage of the drainage of the aqueous humor), and cataract formation.

Posterior uveitis commonly presents with inflammatory cells in the vitreous, retinal vasculitis, and macular edema, which threatens vision. Posterior uveitis caused by toxoplasmosis occurs as a result of congenital transmission. Serologic assays for toxoplasmosis (enzyme-linked immunosorbent assay or immunofluorescent antibody) assist in the diagnosis.[20]

Panuveitis is the involvement of all three portions of the uveal track, including the anterior, intermediate (pars plana), and posterior sections. In an Israeli study it was clearly linked (over 95% of cases) to a systemic autoimmune disorder, such as Behçet's disease.[21]

Sarcoidosis

Sarcoidosis is rare in children with 50–80% having ocular involvement associated with anterior, intermediate, posterior, or diffuse nongranulomatous uveitis. Classically, noncaseating granulomas appear as 'mutton fat precipitates', obstructive glaucoma, Koeppe nodules at the pupillary margin, or sheathing of vessels ('candle wax drippings'). The ocular inflammatory response may occur independently of any evidence of systemic involvement. Diagnostic tests include biopsy of the conjunctival or lacrimal granulomas, serum angiotensin-converting enzyme and lysozyme, chest radiograph for hilar adenopathy, and gallium scan. Biopsy of the lacrimal gland, the conjunctiva, or the periocular skin is only useful when direct visualization reveals a nodule. Other granulomatous processes involving the eye include toxocariasis, tuberculosis, and histoplasmosis, which may occur months to years after the primary infection.

Juvenile Rheumatoid Arthritis

Juvenile rheumatoid arthritis (JRA), accounting for 70% of chronic arthritis in children, exists as three subtypes: (1) systemic JRA (10–20%) that is usually characterized by a febrile onset, lymphadenopathy, and evanescent rash; (2) polyarticular JRA (30–40%) characterized by involvement of multiple (>4) joints with few systemic manifestations; and (3) pauciarticular JRA (40–50%) characterized by no more than four joints involved, usually larger joints and a positive antinuclear antibody (≈75%). Anterior uveitis can develop in all types although it is seen most often in pauciarticular JRA (≈25%). JRA is associated with chronic bilateral iridocyclitis and Russell bodies (large crystalline deposits of immunoglobulin in the iris). Ocular manifestations do not parallel the patient's arthritis; instead, onset generally occurs within 7 years after joint inflammation, so frequent screening and early detection is crucial to decrease vision loss.

Blepharitis

Blepharitis is defined as an inflammation of the eyelids, sometimes associated with the loss of eyelashes (madarosis). It is one of the most common causes of pediatric red eye and is often misdiagnosed as an ocular allergy. In children, the two most common forms of blepharitis include staphylococcal blepharitis and meibomian gland obstruction.

Staphylococcal blepharitis is characterized by colonization of the lid margin by *Staphylococcus aureus*. Antigenic products, such as staphylococcal superantigens, appear to have a primary role (not actual infection) in the induction of chronic eyelid eczema as reflected by relatively normal tear concentrations of antiinfection proteins (lysozyme, lactoferrin), IgA and IgG antibodies.[22] Patients typically complain of persistent burning, itching, tearing, and a feeling of 'dryness'. These symptoms tend to be more severe in the morning and an exudative crust may be present leading to a child's eye becoming 'glued shut'. The signs of staphylococcal blepharitis include conjunctival injection, dilated blood vessels, erythema, scales, collarettes of exudative material around the eyelash bases, foamy exudates in the tear film and even a form of chronic papillary conjunctivitis. In addition, corneal immune deposits may cause severe photophobia. Treatment is directed towards eyelid hygiene with detergents (baby shampoo) and steroid ointments applied to the lid margin. Within several weeks to months, the patient usually improves and becomes asymptomatic.

Meibomian gland obstruction may result in an acute infection (internal hordeolum or stye) but more commonly produces a chalazion. A chalazion is a localized granulomatous inflammation caused by an accumulation of lipids and waxes within the meibomian gland. Clinically, this results in edema, erythema, and burning of the eyelid, which over time may evolve into a firm, painless nodule. Bilateral eye involvement and conjunctivitis may also be present, which further contribute to allergic mimicry; once again, eyelid hygiene is the mainstay of therapy.

Phthirus pubis, the pubic or crab louse, has a predilection for eyelash infestation[23] and may also cause blepharitis. Often the lice may be visualized with direct inspection. Involvement of the eyelashes in prepubertal children should raise the suspicion of sexual abuse.

Ocular rosacea is a rare cause of blepharitis in children, although it is believed to be underdiagnosed due to its typically mild symptoms.[24,25] The majority of cases are unilateral and present with a chronic red eye or recurrent chalazia with a female:male ratio of 3:1. Conjunctival phlyctenules that appear as clear vesicles are pathognomonic for this condition, and are thought to arise from inflammation directed against the bacterial flora of the eyelids. Treatment with lid hygiene, antibiotics, topical corticosteroids, and topical cyclosporine may prevent serious complications including corneal involvement.

Episcleritis

Inflammation of the scleral surface is termed *episcleritis*. It occurs mainly in adolescents and young adults, presenting as a localized injection of the conjunctiva around the lateral rectus muscle insertion (Figure 57-8). Typically, the inflammation is bilateral and accompanied by ocular pain. The presence of pain and absence of pruritus distinguishes episcleritis from allergic conjunctivitis. Episcleritis is self-limited and usually not associated with systemic disease.

Contact Dermatoconjunctivitis

Contact dermatitis involving the eyelids frequently causes the patient to seek medical attention for a cutaneous reaction that elsewhere on the skin would be of less concern. The eyelid skin, being soft, pliable, and thin, increases the eyelid susceptibility to

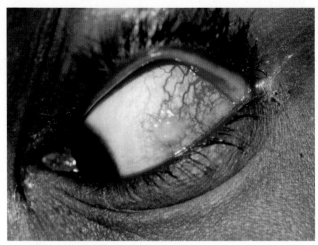

Figure 57-8 Localized bulbar conjunctival vascular injection in a patient with nodular episcleritis.

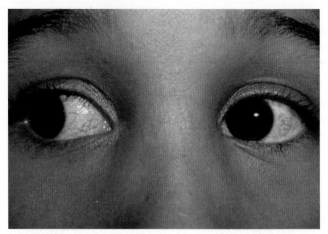

Figure 57-9 Tortuous conjunctival vessels on the bulbar conjunctiva in a patient with ataxia-telangiectasia.

contact dermatitis. The eyelid skin is capable of developing significant swelling and redness with minor degrees of inflammation; cosmetics are a major offender. Ironically, contact dermatitis of the lids or periorbital area is more often caused by cosmetics applied to the hair, face, or fingernails than by cosmetics applied to the eye area. In addition, preservatives such as thimerosal, which are found in contact lens cleaning solutions and other topical agents, have been shown by patch tests to be among the culprits. Because of the high incidence of irritant false-positive reactions, patch testing is generally used as a confirmatory tool, not as the first line of investigation. As of yet, no diagnostic test exists for irritant contact dermatitis.

Angioedema

Angioedema is the swelling of the dermis, of which the conjunctiva is one of the most commonly involved sites in a variety of systemic hypersensitivity reactions. A documented local IgE-mast cell sensitization has been reported to papain enzyme in contact lens cleaning solution in which serum specific IgE to papain and chymopapain were detected.[26] The anatomy of the eyelid consists of loose epidermal tissue that provides an extensive reservoir for edema to even minor allergic reactions, but should also include the differential diagnosis of periorbital cellulitis which may be life-threatening.

Ataxia-Telangiectasia

Louis-Bar's Syndrome

Ataxia-telangiectasia presents with large tortuous vessels on the bulbar conjunctiva, most prominent in the exposed canthal regions,[27] (Figure 57-9) that typically become evident between 1 and 6 years of age and progress with time. There are no other signs or symptoms of conjunctivitis. These children eventually develop ataxia, hypogammaglobulinemia (with absent or deficient IgA) and recurrent sinopulmonary infections.[28]

Acquired Immunodeficiency Syndrome

Children stricken with acquired immunodeficiency syndrome (AIDS) rarely have eye involvement. Cytomegalovirus retinitis

is the most frequently encountered disorder, affecting approximately 7% of children with AIDS, and can lead to permanent vision loss if untreated. It is characterized by regions of intraretinal hemorrhage and white areas of edematous retina. HIV cotton-wool spots retinitis, herpes zoster retinitis, and toxoplasmosis retinitis have also been documented in children.

Treatment

Once an allergic etiology is identified, treatment is approached in a step-wise fashion. Treatment can be divided into primary, secondary, and tertiary interventions (Table 57-4), as well as by acute (seasonal) versus chronic (persistent).

Current treatment is primarily aimed at restoring the patient's quality of life and may require at least 2 weeks of therapy.

Primary Intervention

Nonpharmacologic interventions are commonly the first line of treatment to be considered. Interventions include minimizing environmental allergens or avoidance of them, application of cool compresses to the eye, lubrication and use of disposable contact lenses, and the use of preservative-free lubricants.[29,30]

Environmental Control

Avoidance of allergens remains the first option in the management of any ocular disorder.

Cold Compresses

Cold compresses provide considerable symptomatic relief, especially from ocular pruritus. In general, all ocular medications provide additional subjective relief when refrigerated and immediately applied in a cold state.

Lubrication

Tear substitutes consist of saline combined with a wetting and viscosity agent, such as methylcellulose or polyvinyl alcohol. Artificial tears can be applied topically 2 to 4 times daily as necessary. This primarily assists in the direct removal and dilution of allergens that may come in contact with the ocular surface. Ocular lubricants also vary by class, osmolarity, and electrolyte composition; no product has yet emerged as a clear favorite. Parents should be given the name of one or two brands from

Table 57-4 Overview for the Treatment of Pediatric Ocular Allergic Disorders in a Step-Wise Format

Therapeutic Intervention	Clinical Rationale	Pharmaceutic Agents	Comments
Primary			
Avoidance	Effective, simple in theory, typically difficult in practice		>30% symptom improvement
Cold compresses	Decrease nerve c-fiber stimulation, reduce superficial vasodilation		Effective for mild-moderate symptoms
Preservative-free tears	Lavage, dilutional effect	Artificial tears	Extremely soothing, recommend refrigeration to improve symptomatic relief, inexpensive OTC, safe for all ages, comfortable, use as needed
Secondary			
Topical antihistamine and decongestants	Antihistamine relieves pruritus, vasoconstrictor relieves injection	Antazoline naphazoline, pheniramine naphazoline	No prescription required, quick onset, more effective than systemic antihistamines, limited duration of action, frequent dosing required
Topical antihistamine and mast cell stabilizer (plus other mechanisms)	Single agent with multiple actions, has immediate and prophylactic activity, eliminates need for 2-drug therapy, comfort enhances patient compliance	Olopatadine (Patanol), ketotifen (Zaditor), azelastine (Optivar), bepotastine (Bepreve)	Twice daily dosing, dual acting agents, antihistamine, mast cell stabilizer, inhibitor of inflammatory mediators, more effective at relieving symptoms than other classes of agents, longer duration of action, safe and effective for 3 years and older
Topical mast cell stabilizers	Safe and effective for allergic diseases specially those associated with corneal changes	Cromolyn (Crolom), lodoxamide (Alomide), nedocromil (Alocril), pemirolast (Alamast)	Cromolyn relives mild-to-moderate symptoms of vernal keratoconjunctivitis, vernal conjunctivitis, vernal keratitis. Lodoxamide is highly potent
Topical antihistamines	Relieves signs and symptoms of pruritus and erythema	Levocabastine (Livostin), emedastine (Emadine)	Dosing 1–4 times daily, safe and effective for 3 years and older
Topical NSAIDs	Relieves pruritus	Ketorolac (Acular)	Stinging and/or burning on instillation experienced up to 40% of patients
Tertiary			
Topical corticosteroids	Relieves all facets of the inflammatory response including erythema, edema and pruritus	Loteprednol (Lotemax, Alrex), rimexolone (Vexol), fluorometholone (FML)	Appropriate for short-term use only, contraindicated in patients with viral infections
Immunotherapy	Identify and modulate allergen sensitivity		Adjunctive, although may be considered in secondary treatment in conjunction with allergic rhinitis
Ancillary			
Oral antihistamines	Mildly effective for pruritus	Loratadine, fexofenadine, cetirizine	May cause dry eyes, worsening allergy symptoms, may not effectively resolve the ocular signs and symptoms of allergy

NSAID, nonsteroidal antiinflammatory drug; *OTC,* over the counter.

each class of lubricant to try until a suitable product or combination of products is found.

Contact Lenses

In general, adolescent patients who have seasonal allergy should avoid contact lens use during seasonal flare-ups. The need for clean lenses with minimal deposit build-up must be stressed, and the use of daily wear lenses with rigid disinfecting and cleaning techniques is recommended. Alternatively, daily disposable lenses should be used.[31,32] When such individuals wear contact lenses (CLs), a special set of circumstances arises that increases the risk of ocular infection. The risk is greatest if the lenses are soft and, therefore, provide for little tear exchange beneath their surface. Under such circumstances, limited tear flow allows for a greater build-up of lens deposits and metabolic wastes, while permitting increased tear evaporation from the lens surface.[33]

In a study evaluating the impact of daily disposable lenses versus patient's standard chronic wear lenses, 67% reported that the 1-day disposable lenses provided improved comfort in comparison to the lenses they wore prior to the study. This compared with 18% agreeing that the new pair of habitual lenses provided improved comfort, suggesting that the use of 1-day disposable lenses may be an effective strategy for managing allergy-suffering contact lens wearers.[34] Overall, the newer soft silicone with increased gas permeability have had a higher satisfaction rate of comfort (56%) than the rigid gas permeable lens (14%), while 63% of nonatopic and only 47% of atopic subjects described their lenses as very comfortable to wear.[35,36]

Secondary Intervention

The development of therapeutic agents in the treatment of ocular allergy is ongoing to specifically address the various signs and symptoms of allergic inflammation of the conjunctival surface. The increase in ocular allergy drug development correlates with the recognition of its increasing prevalence in the industrialized countries of the USA and the European Union, leading to an upsurge of research into the pathophysiologic and immunologic inflammatory processes associated with ocular allergy. In the search for more effective medications for ocular allergy, the Conjunctival Allergen Challenge (CAC), also known as the Conjunctival Provocation Test (CPT), has been critical as a standardized model for the assessment of efficacy and duration of effect that new agents have on the allergy signs and symptoms of erythema (redness), pruritus (itching), epiphora (tearing), lid swelling and conjunctival swelling (chemosis). Many of the newer agents are also being evaluated for their potential treatment of the more chronic ocular allergy-associated disorders, such as atopic keratoconjunctivitis, or the potential to treat both ocular and nasal symptoms as the medication does drain down the nasolacrimal duct onto the nasal mucosa.

Decongestants

Topical decongestants act primarily as vasoconstrictors that are highly effective in reducing erythema and are widely used in combination with topical antihistamines. The decongestants are applied topically 2 to 4 times daily as necessary. They have no effect in diminishing the allergic inflammatory response. Vasocon-A is the only antihistamine/decongestant proven to be effective in treating the signs and symptoms (itch and redness) of allergic conjunctivitis. The usual dose is 1 to 2 drops per eye every 2 hours, up to four times daily. The primary contraindication is narrow-angle glaucoma. Excessive use of these agents has been associated with an increased conjunctival hyperemia known as the rebound phenomenon (a form of conjunctivitis medicamentosa).[37]

Antihistamines

Initially, oral antihistamines were extensively employed to systemically control the symptoms of allergic rhinoconjunctivitis, although with an obvious delayed onset of action on the ocular domain when compared to topical antihistamine agents. However, the oral antihistamine appears to have a longer biological half-life and this can have a longer-lasting effect. Information on oral antihistamine use in the treatment of allergic conjunctivitis is commonly buried within studies on allergic rhinitis instead of *rhinoconjunctivitis*. Oral antihistamines, especially the older generation (e.g. chlorpheniramine) appear to have an effect on excessive tearing (lacrimation and epiphora).[38] Another assessment tool has been ocular challenge testing (OCT), which has shown that oral antihistamines, such as terfenadine or loratadine, can increase the tolerance to a dose of specific allergen treatment in children and adults several-fold.[39,40] Oral antihistamines can offer relief from the symptoms of ocular allergy but have a delayed onset of action. Newer, second-generation H_1 receptor (nonsedating) antagonists are less likely to cause unwanted sedative or anticholinergic (dry eye) effects compared to earlier compounds.[41] It has, therefore, been suggested that the concomitant use of an eye drop may treat ocular allergic symptoms more effectively.[42]

H_1 stimulation principally mediates the symptom of conjunctival pruritus whereas the H_2 receptor appears to be clinically involved in vasodilation.[43-46] Although topical antihistamines can be used alone to treat allergic conjunctivitis, they have been shown to have a synergistic effect when used in combination with a vasoconstrictor or when the agents themselves have been shown to have effects on other mediators of allergic inflammation. Dosing is 1 to 4 times daily and is safe for children 3 years and older.

In general, the older topical antihistamines are known to be irritating to the eye, especially with prolonged use, and may be associated with ciliary muscle paralysis, mydriasis, angle-closure glaucoma and photophobia, especially those that are nonselective and block muscarinic receptors. Interestingly, this effect is more pronounced in patients with lighter irides and has not been reported with the newer topical agents.

The newer topical antihistamines have also been found to have other potential antiinflammatory actions, such as mast cell stabilization, cytokine expression or interleukin release (discussed later in the chapter).

Antihistamines with Multiple-Antiinflammatory Activities (Table 57-5)
Olopatadine

Olopatadine 0.01% (Patanol™ and Pataday™) possesses antihistaminic activity and mast cell stabilizing effects. Olopatadine was approximately 10 times more potent as an inhibitor of cytokine secretion (50% inhibitory concentration 1.7 to 5.5 nmol/L) than predicted from binding data whereas antazoline and pheniramine were far less potent (20 to 140 times) in functional assays, including TNF-α mediator release from human conjunctival mast cells. It has been shown to be significantly more effective than placebo in relieving itching and redness for up to 8 hours.[47] In a comparison study with another multiple-action agent, ketotifen, olopatadine fared only slightly better over 2 weeks.[48] In a reformulated form it has been approved for once a day treatment of ocular allergy (Pataday™).[49]

Epinastine

Epinastine 0.05% (Elestat™) is another topical antihistamine with other antiinflammatory properties that include H_2-receptor antagonism, masT cell stabilization, and inhibition of cytokine production. Pre-treatment by epinastine differentially reduced histamine, TNF-α and β, IL-5, IL-8, and IL-10. In vivo, epinastine and olopatadine pretreatment significantly reduced the clinical scores and eosinophil numbers while epinastine also reduced neutrophils (P < 0.02) reflecting that there are different patterns of inhibition of inflammation.[50] The role of the histamine H1, H2 and H3 receptor affinities is unclear in the actual treatment, but from past clinical experience it would appear that having such multiple binding would be beneficial. In an animal model of histamine-induced vascular leakage epinastine, azelastine and ketotifen had a shorter duration of effect than olopatadine.[51] In CAC placebo trials, multiple signs and symptoms (ocular itching, eyelid swelling conjunctival and episcleral hyperemia, and chemosis) of allergic conjunctivitis were significantly reduced by instillation of epinastine compared with vehicle.[52]

Bepotastine

Bepotastine 1.5% (Bepreve™) is the newest of the FDA-approved ophthalmic antihistamines with evidence for multiple antiinflammatory properties that include H_1-receptor antagonism, masT cell stabilization, and inhibition of cytokine production including IL-5.[47,53,54] Pretreatment by bepotastine differentially reduced IL-5 as well as itching associated with LTB-4 injection in an animal model.[54,55] The agent also appears to have the highest selectivity for H1.[56] Bepotastine besilate was originally developed in Japan by Tanabe in conjunction with Ube Industries and was approved in Japan as an oral preparation (Talion®) in July 2000 for the treatment of allergic rhinitis and subsequently approved for the treatment of pruritus/itching accompanying urticaria and other skin conditions (in Jan 2002). Since bepotast-

Table 57-5 Topical Multiple Action Agent Treatments for Ocular Allergy

	Azelastine HCl 0.05% (Optivar™)	Epinastine HCl 0.05% (Elestat™)	Ketotifen Fumarate 0.25% (Zaditor™)*	Olopatadine HCl 0.2% (Pataday™)	Bepotastine Besilate 1.5% (Bepreve™)
Indication	Relief of itching associated with allergic conjunctivitis	Relief of itching associated with allergic conjunctivitis	Temporary prevention of itching of the eye caused by allergies	Relief of itching associated with allergic conjunctivitis	Treatment of itching associated with allergic conjunctivitis
Dosage	1 drop in each affected eye twice a day	1 drop in each affected eye twice a day (age 3 yrs and older)	1 drop in each affected eye every 8 to 12 hr	1 drop in each affected eye once a day	1 drop in each affected eye twice a day (age 2 yrs and up)
Adverse event	Transient sting (≈30%) Headache (≈15%) Bitter taste (≈10%)	Cold symptoms (≈10%) URI (≈10%)	Headache (≈10–25%) Conjunctival injection (≈10–25%) Rhinitis (≈10–25%)	Cold syndrome (≈10%) Pharyngitis (≈10%)	Taste (≈25%)

*Ketotifen (Zaditor™) is now available over-the-counter in the USA.

ine relieves antihistamine-resistant pruritus, it is possible that mechanisms of action other than H1 histamine receptor antagonism are also responsible for the antipruritic effects of this agent. In CAC placebo trials, multiple signs and symptoms (ocular itching, eyelid swelling, tearing, total nonocular symptoms score, nasal congestion and rhinorrhea) of allergic conjunctivitis were significantly reduced by instillation of Bepotastine compared with vehicle.[57]

Ketotifen

Ketotifen 0.025% (Zaditor™) is a benzocycloheptathiophene that has been shown to display several antimediator properties, including strong H_1 receptor antagonism and inhibition of leukotriene formation.[58,59] Ketotifen has also been shown to have pronounced antihistaminic and antianaphylactic properties that result in moderate to marked symptom improvement in the majority of patients with asthma, atopic dermatitis, seasonal or perennial rhinitis, allergic conjunctivitis, chronic or acute urticaria, and food allergy. It has been reported in several studies to have a mild stinging effect on the conjunctival surface. Ketotifen is distinguished from the cromones, sodium cromolyn and nedocromil by a conjoint mast cell stabilizing, several antimediator properties including strong H1 receptor antagonism and inhibition of leukotriene formation.[60] This is now available as an over-the-counter therapy for ocular allergy.

Azelastine

Azelastine 0.05% (Optivar™) is a second-generation H_1 receptor antagonist that has demonstrated in a pediatric SAC study that the response rate to azelastine eye drops group (74%) was significantly higher than that in the placebo group (39%) and comparable with that in the levocabastine group.[61] Apart from the ability to inhibit histamine release from mast cells and to prevent the activation of inflammatory cells, it is likely that the antiallergic potency of azelastine is partially the result of down-regulation of ICAM-1 expression during the early- and late-phase components of ocular allergic response that probably leads to a reduction of inflammatory cell adhesion to epithelial cells confirming the prophylactic properties of azelastine.[62] It is safe to use in children 3 years and older.

Mast Cell Stabilizers

Cromolyn

Cromolyn 4% (Crolom™) is the prototypic mast cell stabilizer. The efficacy of this medication appears to be dependent on the concentration of the solution used (i.e. 1% solution – no effect; 2% solution – possible effect; and 4% solution – probable effect).[30,63] Sodium cromolyn was originally approved for more severe forms of conjunctivitis (e.g. GPC, VKC) but many physicians have used it for the treatment of allergic conjunctivitis with an excellent safety record, although the original studies reflecting its clinical efficacy were marginal for allergic conjunctivitis when compared to placebo[40,43] and in some animal models.[64] Cromolyn sodium 4% ophthalmic solution is applied 4 to 6 times daily with the dosage being decreased incrementally to twice daily as symptoms permit. It is approved for children 3 years and older. The major adverse effect is burning and stinging, which has been reported in 13–77% of patients treated.

Lodoxamide

Lodoxamide 0.1% (Alomide™) is a mast cell stabilizer that is approximately 2500 times more potent than cromolyn in the prevention of histamine release in several animal models.[65] Lodoxamide is effective in reducing tryptase and histamine levels and the recruitment of inflammatory cells in the tear fluid after allergen challenge,[43,44] as well as tear eosinophil cationic protein[66] and leukotrienes (BLT and $CysLT_1$) when compared to cromolyn. In early clinical trials lodoxamide (0.1%) was shown to deliver greater and earlier relief in patients with more chronic forms, such as VKC, including upper tarsal papillae, limbal signs (papillae, hyperemia, and Trantas' dots), and conjunctival discharge, and to improve epithelial defects seen in the chronic forms of conjunctivitis (VKC, GPC) than cromolyn.[67] In patients with allergic conjunctivitis, it is approved for the treatment of VKC at a concentration of 0.1% four times daily. Lodoxamide may be used continuously for 3 months in children older than 2 years of age.

Pemirolast

Pemirolast potassium 0.1 % (Alamast™) is a mast cell stabilizer for the prevention and relief of ocular manifestations of allergic conjunctivitis. It was originally marketed for the treatment of bronchial asthma and allergic rhinitis and then registered in Japan as an ophthalmic formulation for the treatment of allergic and vernal conjunctivitis.[68] It has been studied in children as young as 2 years of age, with no reports of serious adverse events. In various animal and in vitro studies it was found to be superior and, in others, equivalent to cromolyn.[69] The usual regimen is 1 to 2 drops four times daily for each eye.

Nedocromil

Nedocromil 2% (Alocril) is a pyranoquinoline that inhibits various activities on multiple cells involved in allergic inflammation including eosinophils, neutrophils, macrophages, mast cells, monocytes, and platelets. Nedocromil inhibits activation and release of inflammatory mediators such as histamine, prostaglandin D2 and leukotrienes c4 from eosinophils. The mechanism of action of nedocromil may be due partly to inhibition of axon reflexes and release of sensory neuropeptides, such as substance P, neurokinin A, and calcitonin-gene related peptides. Nedocromil does not possess any antihistamine or corticosteroid activity.[70] Nedocromil has been shown to improve clinical symptoms in the control of ocular pruritus and irritation in the treatment of SAC.[71-78] Its safety profile is similar to that of sodium cromolyn, but it is more potent and can be given just twice daily. The results of several placebo-controlled studies have shown that nedocromil is effective in alleviating the signs and symptoms of SAC and provides relief in approximately 80% of patients.[72] In a comparative study, nedocromil sodium eye drops (2%) were more efficacious than sodium cromolyn for hyperemia, keratitis, papillae, and pannus and took less time to have an effect for itching, grittiness, hyperemia, and keratitis.[73]

Nonsteroidal Antiinflammatory Drugs

Topically applied inhibitors of the cyclooxygenase system (1% Suprofen)[74] have been used in the treatment of VKC.[73,74] Ocufen (diclofenac) is one of three topical nonsteroidal antiinflammatory drugs (NSAIDs) approved for the treatment of intraocular inflammatory disorders. Another topically applied NSAID (0.03% flurbiprofen) has been examined for the treatment of allergic conjunctivitis and was found to decrease conjunctival, ciliary, and episcleral hyperemia and ocular pruritus when compared to the control (vehicle-treated eyes). Pruritus is associated with prostaglandin release. It has been shown that prostaglandins can lower the threshold of human skin to histamine-induced pruritus, which may also be the primary benefit of these medications in the eye.

Ketorolac Tromethamine

Ketorolac tromethamine (Acular™, Allergan) was approved for the treatment of SAC with a primary mechanism of action on the inhibition of cyclooxygenase, thus blocking the production of prostaglandins but not the formation of leukotrienes. Clinical studies have shown that prostanoids are associated with ocular itching and conjunctival hyperemia and thus inhibitors can interfere with ocular itch and hyperemia produced by antigen-induced and SAC.[75-77] NSAIDs (e.g. ketorolac) do not mask ocular infections, affect wound healing, increase IOP, or contribute to cataract formation, unlike topical corticosteroids. A recent study compared diclofenac sodium with ketorolac tromethamine with the results for both agents being similar.[78] Treatment group differences were observed for the pain/soreness score with an advantage observed for the diclofenac sodium group over ketorolac tromethamine (20.7% versus 3.2%). This agent and other NSAIDs are classically associated with a low-to-moderate incidence of burning and stinging upon installation into the eye.

Tertiary Intervention

Topical Corticosteroids

When topically administered medications such as antihistamines, vasoconstrictors, cromolyn sodium, and other multiple-action agents are ineffective, mild topical steroids are a consideration. Topical corticosteroids are highly effective in the treatment of acute and chronic forms of allergic conjunctivitis and are even required for control of some of the more severe variants of conjunctivitis including VKC and GPC. However, the local administrations of these medications are not without possible localized ocular complications including increased IOP (e.g. in glaucoma), viral infections, and cataract formation. Topically or systemically administered steroids will produce a transient rise in IOP in susceptible individuals; this trait is thought to be genetically influenced.[77,79-81] Unlike efficacy, which varies among the steroid esters, IOP effects are consistent among the different esters of the same corticosteroid base.

Loteprednol

Loteprednol 0.2% (Alrex™) is an ophthalmic suspension approved for the treatment of ocular allergy. One of its unique features is its claim to be a site-specific steroid (i.e. the active drug resides at the target tissue long enough to render a therapeutic effect but rarely long enough to cause secondary effects such as increased IOP and posterior subcapsular cataract development). The higher dose Loteprednol (0.5%) formulation has been shown to be effective in reducing the signs and symptoms of GPC, acute anterior uveitis, and inflammation following cataract extraction with intraocular lens implantation,[77] as prophylactic treatment for the ocular signs and symptoms of SAC administered 6-weeks before the onset of the allergy.[79]

It is recommended that only patients with more chronic forms of allergic conjunctivitis use topical steroids in a routine manner. Ophthalmologic consultation should be obtained for any patient using ocular steroids for more than 2 weeks to assess cataract formation or increased IOP. Consultation is also merited for any persistent ocular complaint or if the use of strong topical steroids or systemic steroids is being considered.

Immunotherapy

The efficacy of allergen immunotherapy is well established, although it appears that allergic rhinitis may respond better to treatment than allergic conjunctivitis.[82] Similarly, for allergic patients who had asthma and rhinoconjunctivitis when exposed to animal dander (Fel d-I allergen), immunotherapy clearly improved the overall symptoms of rhinoconjunctivitis, decreased the use of allergy medications, and required a 10-fold increase in the dose of allergen to induce a positive OCT reaction after 1 year of immunotherapy with the specific cat allergen.[83] Symptom assessment post challenge for ragweed-sensitive patients treated for at least 2 years with specific ragweed immunotherapy revealed that nasal symptoms responded more than ocular symptoms when compared with controls.[84] The effect of immunotherapy specific for Japanese cedar (*Cryptomeria japonica*) pollinosis had reduced the daily total symptom medication score, not only in cedar, but also in the cross-allergenic Japanese cypress (*Chamaecyparis obtusa*) pollination season, but not significantly.[85] Thus immunotherapy plays more of an important role in the 'long-term' control of rhinoconjunctivitis.

New Directions and Future Developments

Cyclosporine, a fungal antimetabolite that has known antiinflammatory properties, was FDA approved in 2002 as an ophthalmic solution to increase tear production in patients with tear film dysfunction. The safety and efficacy of ophthalmic cyclosporine, however, has not been established in patients under 16 years of age. This agent acts on IL-2, which has an immunomodulatory effect on the activation of T lymphocytes. Studies and reports on the use of topical cyclosporine in cases of VKC have demonstrated marked and lasting improvement in symptoms.[86] Likewise, tacrolimus has been shown to improve the signs and symptoms of VKC when administered as an ophthalmic solution or ointment, with results occurring in as little as one week.[87,88] Tacrolimus is a macrolide antibiotic that acts primarily on T lymphocytes by inhibiting the production of lymphokines, particularly IL-2. It has been effective in the treatment of immune-mediated ocular diseases such as corneal graft rejection, keratitis, scleritis, ocular pemphigoid, and uveitis. The drug is approximately 100 times as potent as cyclosporine. Both tacrolimus and cyclosporine have been shown in vitro to inhibit histamine release.[89]

Alternative delivery systems for topical agents are also under investigation. A liposomal drug delivery system is currently being developed that provides increased therapeutic activity with decreased toxicity. Liposomal-encased compounds have been shown to have a greater penetrating effect into the cornea, aqueous humor, vitreous humor, and conjunctiva. Immunization approaches using 'naked plasmid' DNA (pDNA) are being pursued as well. This approach induces an altered antiallergic immune state in which there is a preference for the T helper cell type 1 response, producing primarily IgG2a whereas allergens would normally induce an IgG1 and IgE response.[89,90] Additional areas of future research include cytokine antagonists and anti-IgE therapy.[12]

Sublingual immunotherapy has been approved for use in Europe and appears to have potential for patients with single allergen-induced symptoms. The impact of this therapy on ocular symptoms appears limited and it is undergoing multiple clinical studies for its efficacy and cost effectiveness in studies in the USA.[90-92]

Recent studies have demonstrated the potential of the positive impact of intranasal treatment (intranasal steroids and possibly intranasal antihistamines) on allergic rhinitis and its associated ocular allergy symptoms.[93,94] It appears that this treatment would be best for mild to moderate cases, such as in seasonal allergic conjunctivitis (more than in perennial allergic conjunctivitis). Such patients would still benefit the most from topical allergy medications.

Complementary and alternative medicine (CAM) represents another realm of therapy that may be effective, particularly in the treatment of allergic conjunctivitis. Evidence shows herbal remedies (e.g. butterbur, *Urtica dioica*, citrus unshiu powder), dietary products (e.g. *Spirulina*, cellulose powder), Indian Ayurvedic medicine, and Traditional Chinese medicine to have an effect on the symptoms of allergic rhinoconjunctivitis.[95,96] Randomized, placebo-controlled trials are needed to evaluate the safety and efficacy of CAM in both children and adults alike, particularly as interest in CAM gains popularity among the general population.

Conclusions

Ocular allergies in children encompass a spectrum of clinical disorders. A basic understanding of the eye's immune response coupled with a step-wise diagnostic approach facilitates proper diagnosis and treatment (Boxes 57-1 and 57-2). As we develop a greater understanding of the biomolecular mechanisms of these disease states, treatment will continue to progress from symptomatic relief to more directed therapeutic interventions.

BOX 57-1 Key concepts

Allergic Eye Disease

- Conjunctivitis caused by IgE mast cell-mediated reactions are the most common hypersensitivity responses of the eye.
- Seasonal allergic conjunctivitis is the most common allergic conjunctivitis, representing over half of all cases.
- Grass pollen, dust mites, animal dander, and feathers are the most common allergens.
- Most environmental allergens affect both eyes at once.
- The hallmark of allergic conjunctivitis is pruritus.
- A stringy or ropy discharge may also be characteristic of allergy.
- A detailed history is the cornerstone to proper diagnosis.
- Eye examination: simple observation alone may be diagnostic.
- Ocular inflammation caused by systemic immunologic diseases are frequently observed in children.
- Immunologic disorders of the eye commonly affect the interior portion of the visual tract and are associated with visual disturbances.

BOX 57-2 Therapeutic principles

Allergic Eye Disease

- Approached in a step-wise fashion:
  Primary: avoidance, cold compresses, artificial tears
  Secondary: topical antihistamines, decongestants, mast cell stabilizers, nonsteroidal antiinflammatory drugs, multiple action agents
  Tertiary: Topical corticosteroids, immunotherapy (immunotherapy may be considered in the secondary category for some cases)
- Novel approaches: cyclosporine, tacrolimus, liposomal drug delivery systems, cytokine antagonists, anti-IgE therapy, complementary and alternative medicine
- Ophthalmology consultation is merited for any persistent ocular complaint or if the use of strong topical steroids or systemic steroids is being considered

---

References

1. Ray NF, Baraniuk JN, Thamer M, et al. Direct expenditures for the treatment of allergic rhinoconjunctivitis in 1996, including the contributions of related airway illnesses. J Allergy Clin Immunol 1999;103(3 Pt 1):401-7.
2. Marrache F, Brunet D, Frandeboeuf J, et al. The role of ocular manifestations in childhood allergy syndromes. Rev Fr Allergol Immunol Clin 1978;18:151-5.
3. Bielory L. Allergic and immunologic disorders of the eye. Part I. Immunology of the eye. J Allergy Clin Immunol 2000;106:805-16.
4. Gillette TE, Chandler JW, Greiner JV. Langerhans cells of the ocular surface. Ophthalmology 1982;89:700-11.
5. Irani AA. Ocular Mast Cells and Mediators. In: Bielory L, editor. Ocular allergy. New York: W.B. Saunders; 1997, p. 1-17.
6. Irani AM, Butrus SI, Tabbara KF, et al. Human conjunctival mast cells: distribution of MCT and MCTC in vernal conjunctivitis and giant papillary conjunctivitis. J Allergy Clin Immunol 1990;86:34-40.
7. Lemp MA. Advances in understanding and managing dry eye disease. Am J Ophthalmol 2008;146:350-6.
8. Bielory L. Differential diagnoses of conjunctivitis for clinical allergist-immunologists. Ann Allergy Asthma Immunol 2007;98:105-14; quiz 14-7, 52.

9. Wald ER, Greenberg D, Hoberman A. Short term oral cefixime therapy for treatment of bacterial conjunctivitis. Pediatr Infect Dis J 2001;20:1039-42.

10. Murphy TF, Faden H, Bakaletz LO, et al. Nontypeable Haemophilus influenzae as a pathogen in children. Pediatr Infect Dis J 2009;28:43-8.

11. Choi SH, Bielory L. Late-phase reaction in ocular allergy. Curr Opin Allergy Clin Immunol 2008;8:438-44.

12. Bielory L. Allergic and immunologic disorders of the eye. Part II. Ocular allergy. J Allergy Clin Immunol 2000;106:1019-32.

13. Dart JK, Buckley RJ, Monnickendan M, et al. Perennial allergic conjunctivitis: definition, clinical characteristics and prevalence. A comparison with seasonal allergic conjunctivitis. Trans Ophthalmol Soc U K 1986;105(Pt 5):513-20.

14. Abelson MB, Baird RS, Allansmith MR. Tear histamine levels in vernal conjunctivitis and other ocular inflammations. Ophthalmology 1980;87:812-4.

15. Udell IJ, Gleich GJ, Allansmith MR, et al. Eosinophil granule major basic protein and Charcot-Leyden crystal protein in human tears. Am J Ophthalmol 1981;92:824-8.

16. Mumcuoglu YK, Zavaro A, Samra Z, et al. House dust mites and vernal keratoconjunctivitis. Ophthalmologica 1988;196:175-81.

17. Tripathi PC, Tripathi RC. Analysis of glycoprotein deposits on disposable soft contact lenses. Invest Ophthalmol Vis Sci 1992;33:121-5.

18. Dreborg S, Agrell B, Foucard T, et al. A double-blind, multicenter immunotherapy trial in children, using a purified and standardized *Cladosporium herbarum* preparation. I. Clinical results. Allergy 1986;41:131-40.

19. Bligard CA. Kawasaki disease and its diagnosis. Pediatr Dermatol 1987;4:75-84.

20. Rosenbaum JT. An algorithm for the systemic evaluation of patients with uveitis: guidelines for the consultant. Semin Arthritis Rheum 1990;19:248-57.

21. Weiner A, BenEzra D. Clinical patterns and associated conditions in chronic uveitis. Am J Ophthalmol 1991;112:151-8.

22. Dougherty JM, McCulley JP. Tear lysozyme measurements in chronic blepharitis. Ann Ophthalmol 1985;17:53-7.

23. Hogan DJ, Schachner L, Tanglertsampan C. Diagnosis and treatment of childhood scabies and pediculosis. Pediatr Clin North Am 1991;38:941-57.

24. Donaldson KE, Karp CL, Dunbar MT. Evaluation and treatment of children with ocular rosacea. Cornea 2007;26:42-6.

25. Doan S, Chang P, Hoang-Xuan T. Conjunctival and lid inflammation in children. Contemporary Ophthalmology 2009;8:1-8.

26. Bernstein DI, Gallagher JS, Grad M, et al. Local ocular anaphylaxis to papain enzyme contained in a contact lens cleansing solution. J Allergy Clin Immunol 1984;74(3 Pt 1):258-60.

27. Boder E, Sedgwick RP. Ataxia-telangiectasia: a familial syndrome of progressive cerebellar ataxia, oculocutaneous telangiectasia and frequent pulmonary infection. Pediatrics 1958;21:526-54.

28. Harley RD, Baird HW, Craven EM. Ataxia-telangiectasia. Report of seven cases. Arch Ophthalmol 1967;77:582-92.

29. Bielory L. Update on ocular allergy treatment. Expert Opin Pharmacother 2002;3:541-53.

30. Bielory L. Ocular allergy guidelines: a practical treatment algorithm. Drugs 2002;62:1611-34.

31. Lemp MA. Contact lenses and associated anterior segment disorders: dry eye, blepharitis, and allergy. Ophthalmol Clin North Am 2003;16:463-9.

32. Lemp MA, Bielory L. Contact lenses and associated anterior segment disorders: dry eye disease, blepharitis, and allergy. Immunol Allergy Clin North Am 2008;28:105-17.

33. Lemp MA. Is the dry eye contact lens wearer at risk? Yes. Cornea 1990;9(Suppl 1):S48-50; discussion S4.

34. Hayes VY, Schnider CM, Veys J. An evaluation of 1-day disposable contact lens wear in a population of allergy sufferers. Cont Lens Anterior Eye 2003;26:85-93.

35. Kari O, Haahtela T. Is atopy a risk factor for the use of contact lenses? Allergy 1992;47(4 Pt 1):295-8.

36. Kari O, Teir H, Huuskonen R, et al. Tolerance to different kinds of contact lenses in young atopic and non-atopic wearers. Clao J 2001;27:151-4.

37. Spector SL, Raizman MB. Conjunctivitis medicamentosa. J Allergy Clin Immunol 1994;94:134-6.

38. Bielory L. Role of antihistamines in ocular allergy. Am J Med 2002;113(Suppl 9A):34S-7S.

39. Ciprandi G, Buscaglia S, Pesce GP, et al. Protective effect of loratadine on specific conjunctival provocation test. Int Arch Allergy Appl Immunol 1991;96:344-7.

40. Kjellman NI, Andersson B. Terfenadine reduces skin and conjunctival reactivity in grass pollen allergic children. Clin Allergy 1986;16:441-9.

41. Hingorani M, Lightman S. Therapeutic options in ocular allergic disease. Drugs 1995;50:208-21.

42. Butrus S, Portela R. Ocular allergy: diagnosis and treatment. Ophthalmol Clin North Am 2005;18:485-92, v.

43. Abelson MB, Udell IJ. H2-receptors in the human ocular surface. Arch Ophthalmol 1981;99:302-4.

44. Jaanus SD. Oral and topical antihistamines: pharmacologic properties and therapeutic potential in ocular allergic disease. J Am Optom Assoc 1998;69:77-87.

45. Sharif NA, Wiernas TK, Griffin BW, et al. Pharmacology of [3H]-pyrilamine binding and of the histamine-induced inositol phosphates generation, intracellular Ca^{2+} -mobilization and cytokine release from human corneal epithelial cells. Br J Pharmacol 1998;125:1336-44.

46. Yanni JM, Sharif NA, Gamache DA, et al. A current appreciation of sites for pharmacological intervention in allergic conjunctivitis: effects of new topical ocular drugs. Acta Ophthalmol Scand 1999;228(Suppl):33-7.

47. Tashiro M, Duan X, Kato M, et al. Brain histamine H1 receptor occupancy of orally administered antihistamines, bepotastine and diphenhydramine, measured by PET with 11C-doxepin. Br J Clin Pharmacol 2008;65:811-821.

48. Aguilar AJ. Comparative study of clinical efficacy and tolerance in seasonal allergic conjunctivitis management with 0.1% olopatadine hydrochloride versus 0.05% ketotifen fumarate. Acta Ophthalmol Scand 2000;78(Suppl 230):52-5.

49. Scoper SV, Berdy GJ, Lichtenstein SJ, et al. Perception and quality of life associated with the use of olopatadine 0.2% (Pataday) in patients with active allergic conjunctivitis. Adv Ther 2007;24:1221-32.

50. Galatowicz G, Ajayi Y, Stern ME, et al. Ocular anti-allergic compounds selectively inhibit human mast cell cytokines in vitro and conjunctival cell infiltration in vivo. Clin Exp Allergy 2007;37:1648-56.

51. Beauregard C, Stephens D, Roberts L, et al. Duration of action of topical antiallergy drugs in a guinea pig model of histamine-induced conjunctival vascular permeability. J Ocul Pharmacol Ther 2007;23:315-20.

52. Abelson MB, Gomes P, Crampton HJ, et al. Efficacy and tolerability of ophthalmic epinastine assessed using the conjunctival antigen challenge model in patients with a history of allergic conjunctivitis. Clin Ther 2004;26:35-47.

53. Kobayashi M, Kabashima K, Nakamura M, et al. Downmodulatory effects of the antihistaminic drug bepotastine on cytokine/chemokine production and CD54 expression in human keratinocytes. Skin Pharmacol Physiol. 2009;22:45-48.

54. Andoh T, Kuraishi Y. Suppression by bepotastine besilate of substance P-induced itch-associated responses through the inhibition of the leukotriene B4 action in mice. Eur J Pharmacol Oct 10 2006;547:59-64.

55. Kaminuma O, Ogawa K, Kikkawa H, et al. A novel anti-allergic drug, betotastine besilate, suppresses interleukin-5 production by human peripheral blood mononuclear cells. Biol Pharm Bull 1998;21:411-3.

56. Kato M, Nishida A, Aga Y, et al. Pharmacokinetic and pharmacodynamic evaluation of central effect of the novel antiallergic agent betotastine besilate. Arzneimittelforschung 1997;47:1116-24.

57. Abelson MB, Torkildsen GL, Williams JI, et al. Time to onset and duration of action of the antihistamine bepotastine besilate ophthalmic solutions 1.0% and 1.5% in allergic conjunctivitis: a phase III, single-center, prospective, randomized, double-masked, placebo-controlled, conjunctival allergen challenge assessment in adults and children. Clin Ther 2009;31:1908-21.

58. Tomioka H, Yoshida S, Tanaka M, et al. Inhibition of chemical mediator release from human leukocytes by a new antiasthma drug, HC 20-511 (ketotifen). Monogr Allergy 1979;14:313-7.

59. Nishimura N, Ito K, Tomioka H, et al. Inhibition of chemical mediator release from human leukocytes and lung in vitro by a novel antiallergic agent, KB-2413. Immunopharmacol Immunotoxicol 1987;9:511-21.

60. Grant SM, Goa KL, Fitton A, et al. Ketotifen. A review of its pharmacodynamic and pharmacokinetic properties, and therapeutic use in asthma and allergic disorders. Drugs 1990;40:412-48.

61. Sabbah A, Marzetto M. Azelastine eye drops in the treatment of seasonal allergic conjunctivitis or rhinoconjunctivitis in young children. Curr Med Res Opin 1998;14:161-70.

62. Ciprandi G, Buscaglia S, Pesce G, et al. Allergic subjects express intercellular adhesion molecule–1 (ICAM-1 or CD54) on epithelial cells of conjunctiva after allergen challenge. J Allergy Clin Immunol 1993;91:783-92.

63. Friday GA, Biglan AW, Hiles DA, et al. Treatment of ragweed allergic conjunctivitis with cromolyn sodium 4% ophthalmic solution. Am J Ophthalmol 1983;95:169-74.

64. Kamei C, Izushi K, Tasaka K. Inhibitory effect of levocabastine on experimental allergic conjunctivitis in guinea pigs. J Pharmacobiodyn 1991;14:467-73.

65. Johnson HG, White GJ. Development of new antiallergic drugs (cromolyn sodium, lodoxamide tromethamine). What is the role of cholinergic stimulation in the biphasic dose response? Monogr Allergy 1979;14:299-306.

66. Leonardi A, Borghesan F, Avarello A, et al. Effect of lodoxamide and disodium cromoglycate on tear eosinophil cationic protein in vernal keratoconjunctivitis. Br J Ophthalmol 1997;81:23-6.

67. Santos CI, Huang AJ, Abelson MB, et al. Efficacy of lodoxamide 0.1% ophthalmic solution in resolving corneal epitheliopathy associated with vernal keratoconjunctivitis. Am J Ophthalmol 1994;117:488-97.

68. Nakagawa Y, Jikuhara Y, Higasida M, et al. [Suppression of conjunctival provocation by 0.1% pemirolast potassium ophthalmic solution in VKC]. Arerugi 1994;43:1405-8.

69. Yanni JM, Miller ST, Gamache DA, et al. Comparative effects of topical ocular anti-allergy drugs on human conjunctival mast cells. Ann Allergy Asthma Immunol 1997;79:541-5.

70. Gonzalez JP, Brogden RN. Nedocromil sodium: a preliminary review of its pharmacodynamic and pharmacokinetic properties, and therapeutic efficacy in the treatment of reversible obstructive airways disease. Drugs 1987;34:560-77.

71. Leino M, Carlson C, Jaanio E, et al. Double-blind group comparative study of 2% nedocromil sodium eye drops with placebo eye drops in the treatment of seasonal allergic conjunctivitis. Ann Allergy 1990;64: 398-402.

72. Verin P. Treating severe eye allergy. Clin Exp Allergy 1998;28(Suppl 6):44-8.

73. Verin PH, Dicker ID, Mortemousque B. Nedocromil sodium eye drops are more effective than sodium cromoglycate eye drops for the long-term management of vernal keratoconjunctivitis. Clin Exp Allergy 1999;29: 529-36.

74. Wood TS, Stewart RH, Bowman RW, et al. Suprofen treatment of contact lens-associated giant papillary conjunctivitis. Ophthalmology 1988;95: 822-6.

75. Abelson MB, Butrus SI, Weston JH. Aspirin therapy in vernal conjunctivitis. Am J Ophthalmol 1983;95:502-5.

76. Meyer E, Kraus E, Zonis S. Efficacy of antiprostaglandin therapy in vernal conjunctivitis. Br J Ophthalmol 1987;71:497-9.

77. Howes JF. Loteprednol etabonate: a review of ophthalmic clinical studies. Pharmazie 2000;55:178-83.

78. Tauber J, Raizman MB, Ostrov CS, et al. A multicenter comparison of the ocular efficacy and safety of diclofenac 0.1% solution with that of ketorolac 0.5% solution in patients with acute seasonal allergic conjunctivitis. J Ocul Pharmacol Ther 1998;14:137-45.

79. Dell SJ, Shulman DG, Lowry GM, et al. A controlled evaluation of the efficacy and safety of loteprednol etabonate in the prophylactic treatment of seasonal allergic conjunctivitis. Loteprednol Allergic Conjunctivitis Study Group. Am J Ophthalmol 1997;123:791-7.

80. Dell SJ, Lowry GM, Northcutt JA, et al. A randomized, double-masked, placebo-controlled parallel study of 0.2% loteprednol etabonate in patients with seasonal allergic conjunctivitis. J Allergy Clin Immunol 1998;102:251-5.

81. Friedlaender MH, Howes J. A double-masked, placebo-controlled evaluation of the efficacy and safety of loteprednol etabonate in the treatment of giant papillary conjunctivitis. The Loteprednol Etabonate Giant Papillary Conjunctivitis Study Group I. Am J Ophthalmol 1997;123: 455-64.

82. Bielory L, Mongia A. Current opinion of immunotherapy for ocular allergy. Curr Opin Allergy Clin Immunol 2002;2:447-52.

83. Alvarez-Cuesta E, Cuesta-Herranz J, Puyana-Ruiz J, et al. Monoclonal antibody-standardized cat extract immunotherapy: risk-benefit effects from a double-blind placebo study. J Allergy Clin Immunol 1994;93: 556-66.

84. Donovan JP, Buckeridge DL, Briscoe MP, et al. Efficacy of immunotherapy to ragweed antigen tested by controlled antigen exposure. Ann Allergy Asthma Immunol 1996;77:74-80.

85. Ito Y, Takahashi Y, Fujita T, et al. Clinical effects of immunotherapy on Japanese cedar pollinosis in the season of cedar and cypress pollination. Auris Nasus Larynx 1997;24:163-70.

86. Mendicute J, Aranzasti C, Eder F, et al. Topical cyclosporin A 2% in the treatment of vernal keratoconjunctivitis. Eye 1997;11(Pt 1):75-8.

87. Talymus Ophthalmic Suspension 0.1%, ClinicalStudyResults.org. 2009 [cited 2009 May 20]; Available from: http://www.clinicalstudyresults. org/drugdetails/viewfile.php?study_name=FJ-506D-AC09+Summary& file=%2Fdocuments%2Fcompany-study_8768_0.pdf

88. Vichyanond P, Tantimongkolsuk C, Dumrongkigchaiporn P, et al. Vernal keratoconjunctivitis: result of a novel therapy with 0.1% topical ophthalmic FK-506 ointment. J Allergy Clin Immunol 2004;113:355-8.

89. Sperr WR, Agis H, Semper H, et al. Inhibition of allergen-induced histamine release from human basophils by cyclosporine A and FK-506. Int Arch Allergy Immunol 1997;114:68-73.

90. Agostinis F, Foglia C, Landi M, et al. The safety of sublingual immunotherapy with one or multiple pollen allergens in children. Allergy 2008;63:1637-9.

91. Seasonal allergic rhinitis: limited effectiveness of treatments. Prescrire Int 2008;17:28-32.

92. Durham SR, Riis B. Grass allergen tablet immunotherapy relieves individual seasonal eye and nasal symptoms, including nasal blockage. Allergy 2007;62:954-7.

93. Bielory L. Ocular symptom reduction in patients with seasonal allergic rhinitis treated with the intranasal corticosteroid mometasone furoate. Ann Allergy Asthma Immunol 2008;100:272-9.

94. Origlieri C, Bielory L. Intranasal corticosteroids and allergic rhinoconjunctivitis. Curr Opin Allergy Clin Immunol 2008;8:450-6.

95. Mainardi T, Kapoor S, Bielory L. Complementary and alternative medicine: herbs, phytochemicals and vitamins and their immunologic effects. J Allergy Clin Immunol 2009;123:283-94; quiz 95-6.

96. Bielory L, Heimall J. Review of complementary and alternative medicine in treatment of ocular allergies. Curr Opin Allergy Clin Immunol 2003;3:395-9.

58

Drug Allergy

Roland Solensky • Louis M. Mendelson

The clinician is frequently confronted with patients who have histories of various medication allergies. In the pediatric population, antibiotics are by far the most commonly implicated medications in allergic reactions. This chapter will concentrate on the clinical management of pediatric patients who present with a history of drug allergy, and basic science will only be included as it relates to diagnosis and treatment. Due to space limitations, the entire wide spectrum of all drug hypersensitivity disorders cannot be addressed (Box 58-1) and for that discussion, the reader is referred to other texts.[1,2] Instead, our discussion will focus on the most clinically relevant reactions – to antibiotics, aspirin (acetylsalicylic acid [ASA]) and other nonsteroidal antiinflammatory drugs (NSAIDs), and local anesthetics.

Etiology/Epidemiology

Patients and physicians commonly refer to all adverse drug reactions (ADRs) as being 'allergic', but the term drug allergy, or drug hypersensitivity, should be applied only to those reactions that are known (or presumed) to be mediated by an immunologic mechanism. ADRs are broadly divided into predictable and unpredictable reactions (Table 58-1). The majority of ADRs are predictable in nature, and examples of these reactions include medication side effects (such as β-agonist-associated tremor) and drug-drug interactions (such as cardiac arrhythmia from the combination of terfenadine and erythromycin). Allergic reactions are a type of unpredictable reaction and they are thought to account for less than 10% of all ADRs.

The overall incidence of allergic drug reactions is difficult to estimate accurately due to the wide spectrum of disorders they encompass and a lack of accurate diagnostic tests. Additionally, most studies on incidence of allergic drug reactions include only adult subjects. There are limited epidemiological data for specific types of hypersensitivity disorders in pediatric patients. For example, the incidence of anaphylaxis in children and adolescents who received intramuscular injections of penicillin G was 1.23[3] and 2.17[4] per 10000 injections. In a large pediatric practice, 7.3% of children developed cutaneous eruptions due to oral antibiotics (although no testing or challenges were performed to confirm an allergy).[5]

While true drug allergy is relatively uncommon, many more children are labeled as being 'allergic' to various medications, particularly antibiotics such as penicillins, and end up carrying the label into adulthood. These patients are more likely to be treated with alternate antibiotics, which may be less effective, more toxic, more expensive and lead to the development and spread of certain types of drug resistant bacteria.[6–9] For example, vancomycin and fluoroquinolones are much more likely to be prescribed for patients who report a history of penicillin allergy.[10–12] Hence, an important and often underappreciated aspect of drug allergy is the morbidity, mortality and economic cost associated with the unnecessary withholding of indicated therapy.

Risk factors for the development of drug allergy are poorly understood and most of the limited data come from studies on penicillin allergy in adult subjects. The presence of atopy is not a risk factor for drug allergy,[13] although patients with asthma may be more prone to having severe reactions (as is the case with food allergies[14,15]). The parental route of administration and repeated courses of the same or cross-reacting antibiotic appear to favor the development of immediate-type drug allergy.[16] Genetic susceptibility has been described for several types of drug allergy.[17–19] Patients with 'multiple drug allergy syndrome' have an inherent predilection to develop hypersensitivity reactions to more than one noncross-reacting medication.[20–23]

There is no single classification scheme that is able to account for all allergic drug reactions. The widely used Gell and Coombs classification scheme of type I to type IV hypersensitivity reactions can be applied to some drug-induced allergic reactions (Table 58-2). Recently, type IV reactions have been subdivided into four types according to the effector cell involved: IVa (macrophages), IVb (eosinophils), IVc (T cells), IVd (neutrophils).[24] (Table 58-3). Certain reactions cannot be categorized into any classification scheme despite the fact that we have insight into their underlying mechanism. In other instances, reactions cannot be classified because the mechanism responsible for their elicitation is not understood.

Most medications, due to their relatively small size, are unable to elicit an immune response independently. Drugs must first covalently bind to larger carrier molecules such as tissue or serum proteins to act as complete multivalent antigens. This process is called haptenation and the drugs act as haptens. The elicited immune response may be humoral (with the production of specific antibodies), cellular (with the generation of specific T cells), or both. Most drugs are not reactive in their native state and must be converted (either enzymatically or via spontaneous degradation) to reactive intermediates in order to bind to proteins. Frequently, the identity of the intermediates is not known, making it impossible to develop accurate diagnostic tests for drug allergy.

The p-i concept (pharmacological interaction with immune receptors) is a recently described mechanism of drug allergy and it is an exception to the hapten hypothesis described above, since

BOX 58-1

Partial List of Pediatric Drug Hypersensitivity Disorders

Multisystem

Anaphylaxis

Serum-sickness and serum sickness-like reactions

Drug fever

Hypersensitivity syndrome

Vasculitis

Lupus erythematosus-like syndrome

Generalized lymphadenopathy

Skin

Urticaria/angioedema

Stevens-Johnson syndrome

Toxic epidermal necrolysis

Fixed drug eruption

Maculopapular or morbilliform rashes

Contact dermatitis

Photosensitivity

Erythema nodosum

Bone Marrow

Hemolytic anemia

Thrombocytopenia

Neutropenia

Aplastic anemia

Eosinophilia

Lung

Bronchospasm

Pneumonitis

Pulmonary edema

Pulmonary infiltrates with eosinophilia

Kidney

Interstitial nephritis

Nephrotic syndrome

Liver

Hepatitis

Cholestasis

Heart

Myocarditis

Table 58-1 Classification of Adverse Drug Reactions

Predictable reactions occur in otherwise normal patients, are generally dose-dependent, and are related to the known pharmacologic actions of the drug. Unpredictable reactions occur only in susceptible individuals, are dose-independent, and are not related to the pharmacologic actions of the drug.

Reactions	Example
Predictable	
Overdosage	Acetaminophen – hepatic necrosis
Side-effect	Albuterol – tremor
Secondary effect	Clindamycin – *Clostridium difficile* pseudomembranous colitis
Drug-drug interaction	Terfenadine/erythromycin – torsade de pointes arrhythmia
Unpredictable	
Intolerance	Aspirin – tinnitus (at usual dose)
Idiosyncratic	Chloroquine – hemolytic anemia in G6PD-deficient patient
Allergic	Penicillin – anaphylaxis
Pseudoallergic	Radiocontrast material – anaphylactoid reaction

---

Table 58-2 Gell and Coombs Classification Scheme for Allergic Reactions

Type	Mechanism	Example
Type I	IgE antibodies leading to mast cell/basophil degranulation	Penicillin – anaphylaxis
Type II	IgG/IgM-mediated cytotoxic reaction against cell surface	Quinidine – hemolytic anemia
Type III	Immune complex deposition reaction	Cephalexin – serum sickness
Type IV	Delayed T cell-mediated reaction	Neomycin – contact dermatitis

---

Table 58-3 Subclassification of Gell and Coombs Type IV Allergic Reactions

Type	Mechanism	Example
Type IVa	T_H1 cells activate macrophages/monocytes by secreting interferon-γ	Tuberculin reaction
Type IVb	T_H2 cells secrete IL-4, IL-5 and IL-13 which leads to eosinophilic activation	Maculopapular eruption with eosinophilia
Type IVc	Cytotoxic T cells (both CD4 and CD8) emigrate to tissues and result in cell death	Maculopapular and bullous eruptions
Type IVd	T cell-dependent neutrophilic inflammatory response	Acute generalized exanthematous pustulosis (AGEP)

---

it requires neither haptenation nor formation of reactive intermediates. In this scheme, a drug binds noncovalently to a T cell receptor, which leads to an immune response via interaction with a major histocompatibility complex (MHC) receptor.[24,25] No sensitization is required, since there is direct stimulation of memory and effector T cells, analogous to the concept of superantigens. It is not clear what proportion of allergic reactions to drugs, such as antibiotics, occur via the p-i mechanism vs the hapten mechanism.

Diagnostic Tests

This section will familiarize the reader with the available diagnostic tests for antibiotic allergy. A full discussion of how to apply these tests in clinical situations follows in the Evaluation and Management section. ASA/NSAIDs and local anesthetics, which are diagnosed by provocative challenges rather than

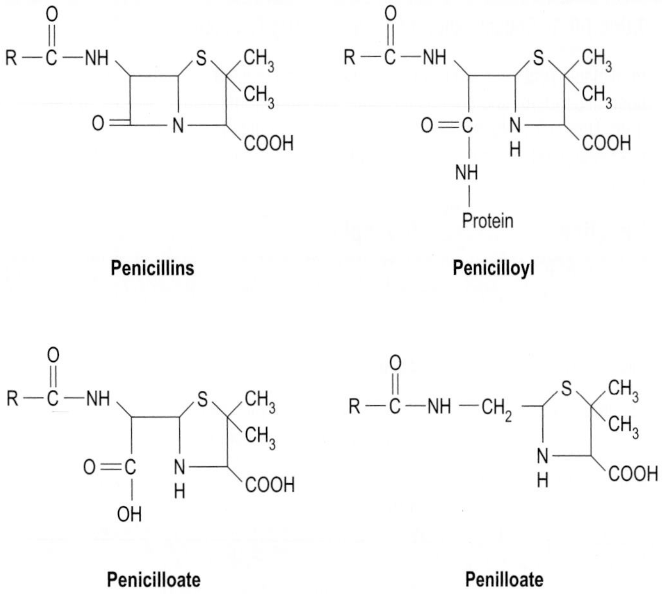

Figure 58-1 Structures of major and minor penicillin antigenic determinants. The R-group side chain determines the specific penicillin.

testing, are discussed only in the section on 'Evaluation and Management'.

Penicillins

The immunochemistry of penicillin, as it relates to immunoglobulin E (IgE)-mediated reactions, was elucidated in the 1960s,[26–28] allowing for the development of validated diagnostic skin test reagents. Under physiologic conditions, 95% of penicillin spontaneously degrades to penicilloyl – also called the major antigenic determinant (Figure 58-1). The remaining portion of penicillin degrades mainly to penicilloate and penilloate, which, along with penicillin, are called the minor antigenic determinants (see Figure 58-1). Penicilloyl was commercially available for skin testing as Pre-Pen from 1974 until 2004, but since then it has been commercially unavailable in the USA (at the time of writing, Pre-Pen is expected to return to the market in late 2009). Penicillin G is available in an aqueous intravenous preparation. Penicilloate and penilloate, which are often produced in a mixture (minor determinant mixture [MDM]), are not commercially available in the USA. Nevertheless, many allergists have access to MDM,[29] presumably from local medical centers.

Penicillin skin testing is particularly useful because of its high negative predictive value. In large series that used both major and minor determinants, only 1–3% of skin test-negative patients experienced mild, self-limited reactions when challenged with penicillins.[13,30,31] Approximately 10–20% of penicillin skin test-positive individuals are positive only to MDM (not Pre-Pen or penicillin G),[13,30,32] therefore skin testing with Pre-Pen and penicillin G alone (without MDM) may fail to detect about 10–20% of truly allergic patients. Since about 10% of patients who report a penicillin allergy are truly allergic, omitting MDM from skin testing may fail to detect about 1–2% (10–20% of 10%) of 'all comers' who are labeled penicillin allergic.

Over the last two decades, a subset of patients who are able to tolerate penicillin but develop allergic reactions to amoxicillin or ampicillin has been recognized.[33] For unclear reasons, this type of selective allergy seems to be less common among patients in the USA[32,34] (Louis Mendelson, personal communication) and much more common in patients from Southern Europe.[35,36]

Table 58-4 Commonly Used Penicillin Skin Testing Reagents

Reagent	Concentration	Comment
Penicilloyl-polylysine	6×10^{-5} M	Not commercially available presently
Penicillin G	10 000 units/ml	Commercially available
Penicilloate/penilloate	0.01 M	Not commercially available presently
Ampicillin (intravenous)	1–25 mg/mL	Commercially available
Amoxicillin (intravenous)	1–25 mg/mL	Not commercially available in the USA

Patients selectively allergic to amoxicillin or ampicillin do not mount an immune response to the core β-lactam portion of the molecule, but rather form IgE antibodies directed against particular R group side chains (see Figure 58-1).[33] Skin testing with major and minor penicillin determinants is negative, whereas nonirritating concentrations of the culprit aminopenicillin produce a positive response. For amoxicillin and ampicillin, concentrations up to 25 mg/mL have been reported to be nonirritating for intradermal testing.[33,37] While the predictive value of such testing is not well established, a positive response is suggestive of an immediate-type allergy. Hence, for patients who reacted to amoxicillin or ampicillin, skin testing should be performed with this antibiotic in addition to the major and minor determinants. Table 58-4 summarizes the commonly used penicillin skin test reagents.

Immediate-type penicillin skin testing should be performed only by experienced personnel in a setting prepared to treat possible allergic reactions. Epicutaneous testing should precede intradermal tests, and appropriate positive (histamine) and negative (normal saline) controls should be used. When carried out in this manner, penicillin skin testing is safe.[13,30,31] A positive response to both prick and intradermal testing is defined by the diameter of the wheal, which should be 3 mm or greater than that of the negative control.[1]

There are no validated tests for penicillin-induced delayed maculopapular eruptions. Delayed intradermal skin tests and patch tests have been found to be positive in some patients by European investigators,[38,39] but these findings have not been reproduced in the USA[40] (and the authors' unpublished observations in 50 patients).

In vitro ELISA-type assays are commercially available for IgE directed at penicilloyl, penicillin, amoxicillin and ampicillin; however, their predictive values have not been defined. When performed in academic settings, the sensitivity of in vitro tests for penicilloyl-specific IgE was as low as 45%.[41] Commercial assays have not been similarly analyzed. Additionally, there is no in vitro test for the minor penicillin determinants. A positive in vitro IgE test for penicillin suggests the presence of allergy, but a negative test does not reliably rule out an immediate-type allergy. The basophil activation test is another, more recently developed, in vitro test for penicillin and other β-lactam allergies. a Limited number of publications using the basophil activation test for penicillin allergy indicates it is inferior to penicillin skin testing.[42,43]

Non-Penicillin Antibiotics

Unfortunately, for antibiotics other than penicillin, we generally lack insight into the relevant allergenic determinants that are produced by metabolism or degradation. As a result, there is no available validated skin testing for these antibiotics. Skin testing with the native antibiotic can be helpful, since a positive response using a concentration that is known to be nonirritating suggests the presence of drug-specific IgE antibodies.[1] A negative response, however, does not rule out an allergy. To determine a nonirritating concentration for a given antibiotic, one can refer to previous reports or skin test several nonallergic volunteers. A helpful reference is a recent report of nonirritating concentrations of 16 commonly used antibiotics, as determined in 25 healthy subjects (Table 58-5).[44] The skin testing procedure, precautions, and interpretation for non-penicillins are identical to those outlined for penicillin earlier.

Evaluation and Management

When Penicillin Skin Testing is Unavailable

As discussed earlier, Pre-Pen is presently commercially unavailable and without it, penicillin skin testing is not recommended. Also, in remote areas, physicians may not have access to an allergist/immunologist to perform penicillin skin testing even if appropriate reagents are available. In these situations, elective evaluation of penicillin allergy is not recommended; instead, evaluation should be limited to patients who require treatment with penicillins. In the absence of penicillin skin testing, tests for serum penicillin-specific IgE may be utilized and, if positive, penicillins should be avoided or administered via rapid desensitization. A negative in vitro test lacks sufficient negative predictive value to rule out an allergy, therefore, depending on the history, penicillin should be administered either via graded challenge or rapid desensitization (see the section on 'Treatment Options'). For example, if a patient reports a non-life-threatening reaction to penicillin more than 10 years ago, it is less likely that the patient is allergic, and penicillin may be administered via cautious graded challenge, particularly if it is given orally. (Figure 58-2.) For more recent and/or severe reactions, penicillin should be administered via rapid desensitization. (Figure 58-2.) Also, more caution needs to be exercised in patients being treated via the parenteral route. Patients who report reactions consistent with severe non-IgE-mediated reactions (such as Stevens Johnson syndrome [SJS], toxic epidermal necrolysis [TEN], interstitial nephritis, or hepatitis) are not candidates for graded challenge or desensitization.

When Penicillin Skin Testing is Available

When penicillin skin testing is available, the ideal time to perform skin testing for evaluation of penicillin allergy in children is

Table 58-5 Nonirritating Concentrations of Commonly Used Antibiotics*

Antibiotic	Full-Strength Concentration (mg/mL)	Nonirritating Concentration (Dilution from Full Strength)
Cefotaxime	100	10-fold
Cefuroxime	100	10-fold
Cefazolin	330	10-fold
Ceftazidime	100	10-fold
Ceftriaxone	100	10-fold
Tobramycin	40	10-fold
Ticarcillin	200	10-fold
Clindamycin	150	10-fold
Trimethoprim-sulfa	80 (sulfa component)	100-fold
Gentamycin	40	100-fold
Aztreonam	50	1000-fold
Levofloxacin	25	1000-fold
Erythromycin	50	1000-fold
Nafcillin	250	10 000-fold
Vancomycin	50	10 000-fold
Azithromycin	100	10 000-fold

Data from Empedrad RB, Earl HS, Gruchalla RS. J Allergy Clin Immunol 2003; 112:629–630.
*Skin testing was performed intradermally with intravenous formulations of the antibiotics.

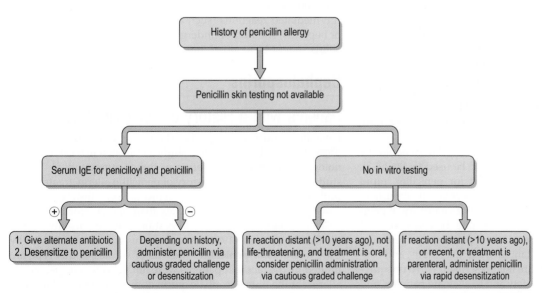

Figure 58-2 Management of pediatric patients with a history of penicillin allergy without availability of penicillin skin testing. Evaluation should be limited to situations when treatment with penicillin is anticipated.

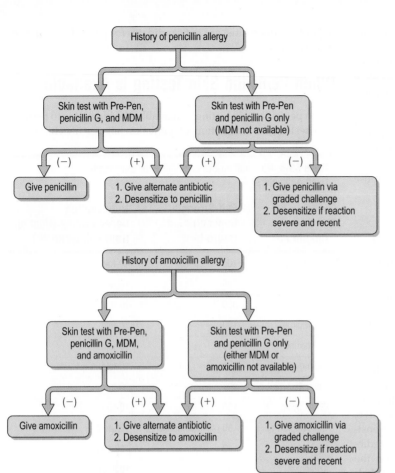

Figure 58-3 Management of pediatric patients with a history of penicillin or amoxicillin allergy when penicillin skin testing is available. Ideally, skin testing is performed electively, not in situations of acute need.

when they are well and not in immediate need of the antibiotic.[45] Testing in acute situations, when children are sick, is often difficult if not impossible to accomplish. Patient reaction history alone, without skin testing, cannot reliably rule out an allergy to penicillin;[46,47] therefore, even patients with vague reaction histories are candidates for penicillin skin testing. Up to 10% of patients carry a label of penicillin allergy, but about 90% of them lack penicillin-specific IgE and are able to receive penicillins safely.[13,45,48,49] These children are commonly denied access, not only to penicillins but also to other β-lactams, which leaves the clinician with few acceptable antibiotic choices. Often, once a label of penicillin allergy is made, it is carried indefinitely into adulthood. Patients with a history of penicillin allergy are frequently treated with broad-spectrum antibiotics,[8,9,12] the use of which contributes to the development of multiple-drug-resistant bacteria.[7,50] It is known that more judicious use of broad-spectrum antibiotics can help reduce the spread of antibiotic resistance.[51,52] One way to achieve this goal is to identify, via 'elective' skin testing, the numerous children and adolescents who are mistakenly labeled as 'penicillin allergic'.

If penicillin skin testing is positive, penicillins should be avoided and alternative antibiotics should be used (Figure 58-3). If the patient develops an absolute need for penicillin, rapid desensitization can be performed (see the section on 'Treatment Options'). In the vast majority of children with a history of penicillin allergy, skin testing is negative. Despite the test's excellent negative predictive value, patients, their parents, and referring physicians are frequently reluctant to 'trust' the results, and consequently β-lactam antibiotics are not prescribed.[53,54] To unequivocally prove the medication's safety and to alleviate patients' and physicians' concerns, an oral challenge with the identical antibiotic that caused the previous reaction should be performed.

In the past, there was theoretical concern that patients might become re-sensitized (or redevelop their allergy) as a result of a course of penicillin, placing them at risk of an immediate reaction during subsequent exposure. However, evidence does not suggest that children are at increased risk of becoming re-sensitized. Mendelson and colleagues[45] reported that among 240 history-positive/skin test-negative children and adolescents, only 1% converted to a positive skin test following a course of penicillin. These findings have been confirmed in an additional 1500 pediatric patients by the authors (unpublished observations).

Patients whose histories are clearly consistent with severe non-IgE-mediated reactions (such as SJS, TEN, interstitial nephritis, or hepatitis) should not undergo penicillin skin testing and penicillins should be avoided indefinitely.

Cephalosporins

Patients with a History of Penicillin Allergy

Penicillins and cephalosporins share a common β-lactam ring (Figure 58-4) and early in vitro studies indicated extensive immunologic cross-reactivity between these compounds.[55] Recent studies of patients with a history of penicillin allergy treated with cephalosporins (without prior penicillin skin testing) demonstrated much lower reaction rates than ones performed in the 1970s (see Table 58-6). This observation may be partially due to the fact that, prior to 1980, cephalosporins were contaminated by trace amounts of penicillin.[56] Results of studies of this type are limited by the fact that patients were not proven to be penicillin-allergic at the time of cephalosporin administration, and the vast majority likely lacked penicillin-specific IgE at the time of treatment with cephalosporins. More informative clinical studies are

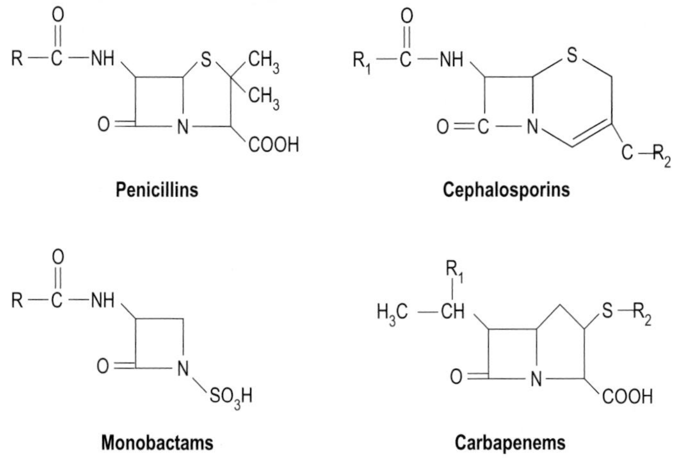

Figure 58-4 Structures of β-lactam antibiotics, all of which share a common four-member β-lactam ring.

those in which patients with positive penicillin skin tests are challenged with cephalosporins (Table 58-7), and overall, only 3.4% of patients reacted to cephalosporins. Patients who are selectively allergic to aminopenicillins, based on limited data, exhibit higher rates of cross-reactivity with cephalosporins that share an identical R-group side chain (such as amoxicillin and cefadroxil).[37,57] Therefore, more caution should be exercised in patients who are selectively allergic to aminopenicillins when they are treated with cephalosporins that contain identical R-group side chains. Tables 58-8 and 58-9 list groups of β-lactam antibiotics that share identical R1 or R2 group side chains.

Figure 58-5 outlines the clinical approach to children with a history of penicillin allergy who require treatment with cephalosporins. When penicillin skin testing is available, ideally children should be tested when they are well and not in immediate need of antibiotic therapy (to optimize choice of antibiotic therapy, as discussed previously). Since 90% or more will be penicillin skin test-negative, they are not at increased risk of

Table 58-6 Summary of Reports in Which Cephalosporins Were Administered to Patients with a History of Penicillin Allergy (No Skin Testing Performed)

Reference (year)	Cephalosporin Reaction Rate		Comments
	History of Penicillin Allergy	**No History of Penicillin Allergy**	
Dash (1975)[96]	7.7% (25/324)	0.8% (140/17 216)	No reaction details
Petz (1978)[97]	8.1% (57/701)	1.9% (285/15 007)	No reaction details
Goodman et al (2001)[98]	0.33% (1/300)	0.04% (1/2431)	Reaction questionable
Daulat et al (2004)[99]	0.17% (1/606)	0.06% (15/22 664)	Reaction = eczema
Fonacier et al (2005)[100]	8.4% (7/83)	N/A	Reactions convincing

Table 58-7 Summary of Reports in Which Cephalosporins Were Administered to Patients with Positive Penicillin Skin Tests*

Reference	No. of Patients	No. of Reactions (%)	Reaction(s) to Cephalosporin	Skin Test
Girard[45]	23	2 (8.7)	Cephaloridine	No
Assem and Vickers[46]	3	3 (100)	Cephaloridine	No
Warrington et al[101]	3	0		Yes
Solley et al[102]	27	0		No
Saxon et al[103]	62	1 (1.6)	Not noted	No
Blanca et al[104]	17	2 (11.8)	Cefamandole	No
Shepherd and Burton[105]	9	0		No
Audicana et al[106]	12	0		Yes
Pichichero[107]	39	2 (5.1%)	Cefaclor and ?	No
Novalbos et al[108]	23	0		Yes
Macy[34]	42	1 (2.4%)	Cefixime	No
Romano[58]	75	0		Yes
Greenberger and Klemens[109]	6	0		No
Park[49]	37	2 (5.4%)	Not noted	No
TOTAL	377	13 (3.4%)		

*All patients had positive skin test responses to Pre-Pen, Penicillin G, and/or minor determinant mixture. Patients negative to the major and minor penicillin determinants but positive to amoxicillin or ampicillin are not included.

Table 58-8 Groups of β-Lactam Antibiotics that Share Identical R₁-Group Side Chains. Each Column Represents a Group with Identical R₁ Side Chains. Brand Names Are Included for Commercially Available β-Lactams

Amoxicillin (Amoxil)	Ampicillin (Principen)	Ceftriaxone (Rocephin)	Cefoxitin (Mefoxin)	Cefamandole (Mandol)	Ceftazidime (Ceftaz, Fortaz)
Cefadroxil (Duracef)	Cefaclor (Ceclor)	Cefotaxime (Claforan)	Cephaloridine	Cefonicid (Monocid)	Aztreonam (Azactam)
Cefprozil (Cefzil)	Cephalexin (Keflex)	Cefpodoxime (Vantin)	Cephalothin		
Cefatrizine	Cephradine (Velosef)	Cefditoren (Spectracef)			
	Cephaloglycin	Ceftizoxime (Cefizox)			
	Loracarbef (Lorabid)	Cefmenoxime (Cefmax)			

Table 58-9 Groups of β-Lactam Antibiotics that Share Identical R₂-Group Side Chains. Each Column Represents a Group with Identical R₂ Side Chains. Brand Names Are Included for Commercially Available β-Lactams.

Cephalexin (Keflex)	Cefotaxime (Claforan)	Cefuroxime (Ceftin)	Cefotetan (Cefotan)	Cefaclor (Ceclor)	Ceftibuten (Cedax)
Cefadroxil (Duricef)	Cephalothin	Cefoxitin (Mefoxin)	Cefamandole (Mandol)	Loracarbef (Lorabid)	Ceftizoxime (Cefizox)
Cephradine (Velosef)	Cephaloglycin		Cefmetazole		
	Cephapirin (Cefadyl)		Cefpiramide		

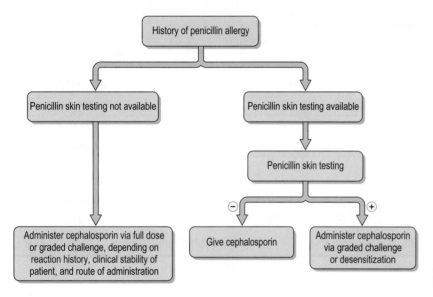

Figure 58-5 Administration of cephalosporins to pediatric patients with a history of penicillin allergy.

having allergic reactions to cephalosporins and therefore can receive them safely. If skin testing is positive, the clinician has the option of administering the cephalosporin via graded challenge or rapid desensitization (see Figure 58-5). Under most circumstances, we recommend a graded challenge (see the section on 'Treatment Options'), given that the likelihood of reacting is only about 2–3% (Table 58-6). If penicillin skin testing is unavailable, depending on the reaction history, the likelihood that the patient is penicillin-allergic, the clinical stability of the patient, and the route of administration (oral vs parenteral), cephalosporins may be administered via either full dose or graded challenge.[1] Skin testing with cephalosporins (using a nonirritating concentration) prior to administering them to patients with a history of penicillin allergy may be considered, based on limited data.[58]

Patients with a History of Cephalosporin Allergy

The evaluation of patients with a history of cephalosporin allergy who require the same or another cephalosporin is limited by lack of standardized validated cephalosporin skin test reagents (see Figure 58-6). Skin testing with nonirritating concentrations of native cephalosporins can be of some value, especially if it is positive, but its negative predictive value is uncertain. Additionally, there are no definitive data on the extent of cross-reactivity among different cephalosporins, and hence, the safety of administering a given cephalosporin to a patient who has previously experienced an allergic reaction to another cephalosporin is not known. The general belief is that the allergic response to cephalosporins is directed at the R group side chains, rather than the β-lactam portion of the molecule and that patients who have reacted to one cephalosporin can tolerate other cephalosporins with dissimilar side chains. Recent investigations into potential allergic cross-reactivity among cephalosporins using cephalosporin skin testing or in vitro IgE testing places some doubt on this theory.[59–62] Collectively, approximately half of the 95 subjects demonstrated a positive test only to the cephalosporin that caused their reaction, whereas the other half showed positive tests to more than one cephalosporin, including ones with dissimilar R-group side

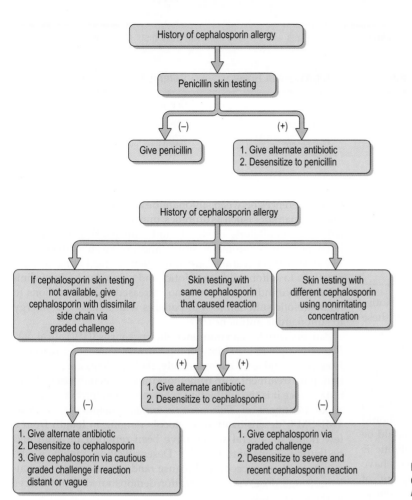

Figure 58-6 Management of pediatric patients with a history of cephalosporin allergy. (From Bernstein IL, Gruchalla RS, Lee RE, et al. Ann Allergy Asthma Immunol 1999;83:665–700.)

chains.[59-62] The results suggest that some cephalosporin-allergic patients form cross-reacting IgE antibodies, but none of the patients were challenged to confirm this suspicion. Additionally, there are no published series of patients allergic to a given cephalosporin challenged with alternate cephalosporins.

Other β-Lactam Antibiotics

Monobactams

Monobactams differ from other β-lactams by their monocyclic ring structure (see Figure 58-4), and aztreonam is the prototype drug in this class. In vitro studies showed no immunologic cross-reactivity between aztreonam and either penicillin or cephalosporins, with the exception of ceftazidime, which shares an R group side chain identical with aztreonam.[63] Lack of clinical cross-reactivity has been confirmed in numerous penicillin skin test-positive subjects who were challenged and tolerated aztreonam.[64,65] Therefore, patients who are allergic to penicillins or cephalosporins (except for ceftazidime) can safely receive aztreonam. Conversely, patients who have reacted to aztreonam can safely receive penicillins and cephalosporins (except for ceftazidime).

Carbapenems

Allergic cross-reactivity between penicillin and carbapenems has been studied via retrospective evaluation of hospitalized patients with a history of penicillin allergy who were treated with imipenem or meropenem. (see Table 58-10). Most of these reports demonstrated somewhat increased rates of reactions to carbap-

Table 58-10 Summary of Reports in Which Carbapenems Were Administered to Patients with a History of Penicillin Allergy (No Skin Testing Performed)

Reference	Carbapenem Reaction Rate		
	History of Penicillin Allergy	No History of Penicillin Allergy	P value
McConnell et al[110]	6.3% (4/63)	N/A	N/A
Prescott et al[111]	11% (11/100)	2.7% (3/111)	0.024
Sodhi et al[112]	9.2% (15/163)	3.9% (4/103)	0.164
Cunha et al[113]	0% (0/110)	N/A	N/A

enems in patients with a history of penicillin allergy compared to those without a history. However, none of these patients underwent penicillin skin testing to indicate whether the patient was allergic at the time of treatment with carbapenbems and it is highly likely that the vast majority were not penicillin-allergic. Carbapenem challenges in penicillin skin test-positive patients have been reported in three recent studies (see Table 58-11).[66-68] Combining the results, 317 penicillin skin test-positive patients tolerated carbapenems (and each was also carbapenem skin test-negative), whereas 3 patients had positive skin tests to carbapenems and were not challenged. Hence, the data on allergic cross-reactivity between penicillin and carbapenems is very similar to that for penicillin/cephalosporins. Therefore, the

Table 58-11 Summary of Reports in Which Carbapenems Were Administered to Patients with Positive Penicillin Skin Tests (All Patients Were Also Skin Tested with Carbapenems)

Reference	No. of Patients	No. of Reactions	Carbapenem Given	Comment
Romano A[66]	110	0	Imipenem	One patient imipenem skin test-positive
Romano A[67]	103	0	Meropenem	One patient meropenem skin test-positive
Atanaskovic[68]	107	0	Meropenem	One patient meropenem skin test-positive

clinical approach to carbapenem administration in patients with a history of penicillin allergy is analogous to what was described for cephalosporins.

Non-β-Lactam Antibiotics

The lack of reliable diagnostic tests for non-β-lactam antibiotics makes evaluation of children who have reacted to one of these medications more challenging. As discussed earlier, some information can be gleaned from skin testing with nonirritating concentrations of the native antibiotics, but an immediate-type allergy cannot be ruled out. Consequently, unlike penicillin allergy, it is not practical to evaluate these patients on an elective basis. Unless the previous reaction was clearly predictable in nature, such as emesis from erythromycin, the medication should be avoided in the future. Evaluation with skin testing should be performed only if readministration of the culprit antibiotic is being considered. This commonly occurs in patients who have reacted to several different antibiotics and are 'running out' of antibiotic choices. If skin testing with a nonirritating concentration of the antibiotic is positive, the medication should be avoided. If such a patient develops an absolute need for the antibiotic, acute desensitization should be performed. If skin testing is negative, either desensitization or a graded challenge can be performed, depending on the 'strength' of the history of the previous reaction. The total dose of the antibiotic used in skin testing can be used as a starting point for desensitization or graded challenge (see the section on 'Treatment Options'). Patients who previously experienced SJS, TEN, or other serious non-IgE-mediated reactions, should not be given the same antibiotic.

Aside from the β-lactams, the two most commonly used antibiotics in children are macrolides and sulfonamides; a brief discussion of these antibiotics follows.

Sulfonamides

Sulfonamide drugs are those that contain an SO_2-NH_2 moiety. The majority of adverse reactions to sulfonamide antibiotics are non-IgE-mediated delayed cutaneous reactions.[69] They vary from benign, self-limited maculopapular/morbilliform eruptions to severe, potentially life-threatening reactions such as SJS and TEN. Metabolism of sulfonamides produces a number of reactive intermediates that appear to play a pivotal role in various allergic reactions.[69] Despite this knowledge, there are no in vitro or in vivo tests that can predict a patient's risk of developing an adverse reaction to sulfonamides. A provocative challenge with a sulfonamide remains the only way to determine whether a patient is truly allergic, but this should be reserved for cases in which alternate antibiotics cannot be substituted and if the previous reaction was not severe. Due to the propensity of sulfonamides to cause severe cutaneous reactions such as SJS and TEN, most children who have reacted to a member of the family should simply avoid all sulfonamide antibiotics. There are structural differences between sulfonamide antibiotics and nonantibiotic sulfonamides (such as diuretics, oral hypoglycemics, carbonic anhydrase inhibitors, celecoxib and sumatriptan), in that the latter lack an N_4 aromatic amine and an N_1 substituted ring. These structural features are important in mediating allergic reactions to sulfonamide antibiotics and a growing body of clinical evidence indicates there is no increased risk of reactions to nonantibiotic sulfonamides in patients with a history of allergy to sulfonamide antibiotics.[23,70]

Patients with human immunodeficiency virus (HIV) are at particularly high risk of developing various cutaneous reactions from sulfonamides.[69] Unfortunately, these patients are also likely to require treatment with trimethoprim-sulfamethoxazole (TMP-SMX), since it is the antibiotic of choice for both prophylaxis and acute treatment of *Pneumocystis carinii* pneumonia. Various TMP-SMX 'desensitization' protocols ranging in length from a few hours to several weeks have been reported in adult and pediatric patients with HIV.[71-73] 'Desensitization' may be a misnomer for these procedures because randomized trials of rechallenge (single dose) vs desensitization demonstrated no differences in the success rates.[74,75]

Macrolides

Hypersensitivity reactions to macrolides, particularly IgE-mediated ones, appear to be less common compared to β-lactam and sulfonamide antibiotics. While there are no published studies addressing the degree of allergic cross-reactivity among the different macrolides, our clinical experience is that it is low. This observation may partly be due to the structural difference between azithromycin (which is an azalide) and erythromycin or clarithromycin. Furthermore, it is possible that passage of time between the initial macrolide reaction and when a patient is treated with another macrolide resulted in resolution of the allergy. There is evidence for waning of allergy to macrolides from studies in which patients with suspected macrolide were challenged with the same antibiotic to which they reacted previously. Of 209 adult patients with a convincing history of immediate-type allergy to macrolides, only 22 (10.5%) reacted to the same macrolide antibiotic during a supervised graded challenge.[76,77] Therefore, in children who have reacted to a given macrolide antibiotic, it is reasonable to evaluate the safety of another macrolide when treatment is anticipated. This can be done via skin testing (using a nonirritating concentration of the native antibiotic) followed by graded challenge, assuming testing is negative. If testing is positive and there is an absolute need to treat the patient with a macrolide, rapid desensitization can be performed.

Local Anesthetics

True hypersensitivity reactions to local anesthetics in children are uncommon and usually consist of a delayed contact dermatitis;

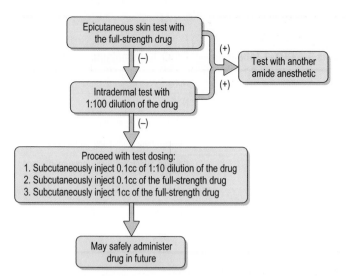

Figure 58-7 Management of pediatric patients with previous reactions to local anesthetics. Intervals between steps are 15 minutes. Generally, an amide is used because the benzoate esters cross-react immunologically whereas the amides do not, and frequently patients do not know which drug they reacted to previously. (Data from Patterson R, DeSwarte RD, Greenberger PA, et al. Allergy Proc 1994; 15:239–264.)

anaphylaxis from local anesthetics occurs very rarely, if ever.[78] Most adverse reactions are vasovagal, anxiety or toxic reactions, or predictable side-effects of epinephrine. Unfortunately, patients who experience any adverse reaction are frequently labeled as being 'allergic' and told to avoid all 'caines' in the future. Evaluation of children with a supposed allergy to local anesthetics serves to alleviate dentists' and physicians' concerns and may prevent these patients from being subjected to the increased risk of general anesthesia. Figure 58-7 summarizes the approach to children with previous reactions to local anesthetics. Data from patch testing suggest there is cross-reactivity among the benzoate esters but not among the amides (Table 58-12).[78] While these findings may have no significance on immediate-type reactions, it is generally recommended that if a patient previously reacted to an ester, an amide should be used in evaluation for re-administration. If the identity of the previous local anesthetic is not known or if it was an amide, another amide can be used. Additionally, during skin testing and challenge, one should attempt to employ the same agent that will subsequently be used by the dentist or physician.

Aspirin and Other Nonsteroidal Antiinflammatory Drugs

Aspirin (acetylsalicylic acid [ASA]) and other NSAIDs have been associated with five types of allergic and pseudo-allergic reactions (Table 58-13).[79] Reactions that are caused by modifying effects on arachidonic acid metabolism – namely respiratory reactions (in patients with aspirin-exacerbated respiratory disease [AERD]) and urticarial reactions (in patients with underlying chronic idiopathic urticaria) show cross-reactivity with other NSAIDs, as one would expect. Patients with AERD, however, can safely receive tartrazine, azo and nonazo dyes, sulfites, monosodium glutamate, and usual doses of acetaminophen (although a minority of patients experiences mild reactions above 1000 mg).[79,80] Recently, drugs that selectively block the cyclooxygenase-2 (COX-2) enzyme, such as celecoxib, have also been found to be safe in patients with AERD[81] and virtually all aspirin-sensitive patients with chronic idiopathic urticaria.[82]

Table 58-12 Benzoate Esters and Amides Constituting the Two Major Classes of Local Anesthetics*

Generic Name	Available Forms	Examples of Trade Names
Benzoate Esters		
Benzocaine	Topical	Orajel, Hurricane, Lanacaine, many others
Butamben picrate	Topical	Butesin
Chloroprocaine	Injectable	Nesacaine
Cocaine	Topical	Cocaine
Procaine	Injectable	Novocain
Proparacaine	Ophthalmic	Alcaine, Opthcaine, Opthetic
Tetracaine	Injectable, topical, ophthalmic	Pontocaine
Amides		
Bupivacaine	Injectable	Marcaine, Sensorcaine
Dibucaine	Topical	Nupercaine
Etidocaine	Injectable	Duranest, Durnest MPF
Lidocaine	Injectable, topical	Xylocaine, Dilocaine, Nervocaine, many others
Mepivacaine	Injectable	Carbocaine, Polocaine, Isocaine
Prilocaine	Injectable	Citanest
Ropivacaine	Injectable	Naropin
Combination		
Lidocaine/Prilocaine	Topical	EMLA

*Patch testing data indicate there is cross-reactivity among the esters but not the amides.

Unlike respiratory reactions, acute urticarial or anaphylactic reactions in otherwise normal individuals are medication specific (Table 58-13). Hence it is reasonable to perform graded challenges in these individuals with another NSAID to identify an agent that can be safely used in the future. Not uncommonly, patients with acute urticarial reactions are mistakenly told to avoid all NSAIDs indefinitely.

With the exception of respiratory reactions in asthmatics, there are no data on the incidences of these reactions in children; however, clinical experience suggests that it is low. This observation may be partly the result of the infrequent use of ASA caused by concerns of Reye's syndrome in children. The incidence of ASA sensitivity in children with asthma has been investigated in six prospective studies in which blinded oral challenges were performed.[83–88] The rate of positive challenges varied from 0% to 28%, and there was a trend for more respiratory reactions in adolescents compared to younger children. Overall, the data indicate that ASA sensitivity in asthmatic children under the age of 10 years is rare, but thereafter it begins to approach the reported incidence in adults.

Patients with AERD, whose nasal disease or asthma is poorly controlled with use of medications, are candidates for ASA desensitization. This procedure, unlike the one described for antibiotic desensitization in the Treatment Options section below, involves administration of ASA in order to cautiously induce a respiratory reaction, following which patients enter a refractory phase that can be maintained with continued administration of ASA. Long-term studies of patients maintained on chronic ASA

Table 58-13 Major Types of Hypersensitivity Reactions to ASA and Other NSAIDs

Reaction Type	Underlying Disease	Cross-Reactions	COX-1 Inhibition	Other Immunologic Mechanisms
Cross-reacting respiratory	Asthma, rhinitis, polyposis	ASA/NSAIDs	Yes	None
Cross-reacting urticaria	Chronic urticaria	ASA/NSAIDs	Yes	None
Urticaria/anaphylaxis	None	None	No	IgE-mediated (presumed)
Aseptic meningitis (only NSAIDs)	None	None	No	Delayed hypersensitivity (presumed)
Hypersensitivity pneumonitis (only NSAIDs)	None	None	No	Delayed hypersensitivity (presumed)

Modified from Stevenson DD. Immunol Allergy Clin North Am 1998;18:773–798.
ASA, acetylsalicylic acid (aspirin); *NSAIDs*, nonsteroidal antiinflammatory drugs; *COX*, cyclooxygenase; *IgE*, immunoglobulin E.

Table 58-14 Penicillin Oral Desensitization Protocol

Step*	Penicillin (mg/mL)	Amount (mL)	Dose Given (mg)	Cumulative Dose (mg)
1	0.5	0.1	0.05	0.05
2	0.5	0.2	0.1	0.15
3	0.5	0.4	0.2	0.35
4	0.5	0.8	0.4	0.75
5	0.5	1.6	0.8	1.55
6	0.5	3.2	1.6	3.15
7	0.5	6.4	3.2	6.35
8	5	1.2	6	12.35
9	5	2.4	12	24.35
10	5	5	25	49.35
11	50	1	50	100
12	50	2	100	200
13	50	4	200	400
14	50	8	400	800

Observe patient for 30 minutes, then give full therapeutic dose by the desired route.
*Interval between doses is 15 minutes.
Modified from Sullivan TJ. Drug allergy. In: Middleton E, Reed CE, Ellis EF, et al, eds. Allergy: principles and practice, 4th edn. St Louis: Mosby; 1993.

desensitization demonstrated improved clinical outcomes for both upper and lower respiratory diseases.[89-91] ASA desensitization is rarely performed in children, because severe, poorly controlled AERD is encountered very infrequently in the pediatric population. Full discussion of ASA desensitization is beyond the scope of this chapter and the reader is referred to other texts.[1,79]

Treatment Options

Desensitization

Rapid desensitization to an antibiotic should be considered in children who have an IgE-mediated allergy, and no acceptable alternative treatment is available. Desensitization is an induction of temporary tolerance, which converts a child who is highly allergic to a drug to a state in which the child can tolerate treatment with the medication. Although most published desensitization protocols involve penicillin, the principle has been applied successfully to other antibiotics, including cephalosporins,

sulfonamides, vancomycin, macrolides, quinolones, aminoglycosides, pentamidine, and antituberculin agents.[72] Rapid desensitization is thought to somehow render mast cells unresponsive to the drug used in the procedure, but the exact immunologic mechanism is unknown. Desensitization can be performed either by the oral or intravenous route. Tables 58-14 and 58-15 list representative protocols for penicillin desensitization, and these can be modified and used for other classes of antibiotics.

Several principles of management have been derived from studies on penicillin desensitization,[92-95] and presumably they hold true for other antibiotics also. First, the amount of drug the patient tolerated during skin testing determines a safe initial dose for desensitization, which generally translates to 1/10000 or less of the full therapeutic dose. Second, doubling the dose every 15 minutes until the recommended dose is reached is effective in nearly all instances. Mild reactions occur in about a third of patients, but no fatal or life-threatening reactions have been reported. Third, desensitization does not prevent non-IgE reactions such as serum sickness, hemolytic anemia, or interstitial nephritis from occurring. Fourth, for the patient to remain in a

Table 58-15 Penicillin Intravenous Desensitization Protocol Using a Continuous Infusion Pump

Step*	Penicillin (mg/mL)	Amount (mL)	Dose Given (mg)	Cumulative Dose (mg)
1	0.001	4	0.001	0.001
2	0.001	8	0.002	0.003
3	0.001	16	0.004	0.007
4	0.001	32	0.008	0.015
5	0.001	60	0.015	0.03
6	0.001	120	0.03	0.06
7	0.001	240	0.06	0.12
8	0.1	5	0.125	0.245
9	0.1	10	0.25	0.495
10	0.1	20	0.5	1
11	0.1	40	1	2
12	0.1	80	2	4
13	0.1	160	4	8
14	10	3	7.5	15
15	10	6	15	30
16	10	12	30	60
17	10	25	62.5	123
18	10	50	125	250
19	10	100	250	500
20	10	200	500	1000

Observe patient for 30 minutes, then give full therapeutic dose by the desired route.
*Interval between doses is 15 minutes.

desensitized state, it is necessary to continue treatment with the antibiotic. If treatment is stopped, the patient reverts back to being allergic and is again at risk of developing anaphylaxis and desensitization would need to be repeated.

Rapid desensitization should be performed only by a physician experienced in the procedure, in a monitored setting (inpatient or outpatient), with intravenous access and necessary medications and equipment to treat anaphylaxis. Pharmacy staff should be consulted prior to the procedure to assist with preparation of the required drug dilutions. Generally, oral desensitization is preferred because it is assumed to be safer, but taste may be an issue in younger children or some medications may not be available in an oral form, in which case the intravenous route can be used. Patients should not be pretreated with corticosteroids or antihistamines because they may mask early signs of an allergic reaction. Treatment with β-adrenergic blocking medications should temporarily be withheld before desensitization. Patients should be continually observed for the presence of IgE-mediated allergic symptoms, along with regular monitoring of vital signs and peak expiratory flow values. Before the procedure, patients with asthma or other pulmonary disease should be optimally controlled. If mild reactions occur, they should be treated and the dose not be advanced until they have resolved.

Graded Challenge

Graded challenge, also known as test dosing, refers to cautious administration of a medication to a patient who is unlikely to be truly allergic to it.[1] Unlike desensitization, test dosing does not modify the immune response to a drug. Graded challenges are most commonly undertaken with medications for which testing cannot adequately rule out an allergy. Examples include non-penicillin antibiotics, penicillins (when Pre-Pen or MDM is not available) and cephalosporin administration in penicillin-allergic patients. Children who previously experienced severe reactions or who are suspected to be allergic to a medication should undergo desensitization rather than graded challenge.

Most graded challenges can be safely carried out in an office without intravenous access but with preparedness to treat potential allergic reactions including anaphylaxis. The pace of the challenge and degree of caution exercised depend on the likelihood that the patient may be allergic and the physician's experience and comfort level with the procedure. Generally, the starting dose is 1/10 to 1/100 of the full dose and approximately 5- to 10-fold increasing doses are administered every 30 to 60 minutes until the full therapeutic dose is reached. At the first sign of any allergic reaction, the procedure should be abandoned and the patient should be treated appropriately. If at a later point the patient requires the medication, it should be administered via desensitization.

Conclusions

Children commonly experience adverse reactions to medications, many of which are falsely labeled as being allergic and subsequently avoided due to a fear of causing a severe life-

Drug Allergy

- Children are commonly labeled as being allergic to various medications and a thorough allergy evaluation can help determine which patients are truly at risk of a severe reaction.

- The majority of children labeled as allergic to medications, particularly antibiotics, can take them without fear of a severe reaction.

- The ideal time to evaluate drug allergy in children is when they are well and not in acute need of treatment.

BOX 58-3 Therapeutic principles

1. Penicillin allergy

   a. About 10% of children are labeled as being 'penicillin allergic'.

   b. The vast majority of children with the label of penicillin allergy can safely take all β-lactam antibiotics without fear of an allergic reaction.

   c. The ideal way to determine whether a child has an IgE-mediated allergy to penicillin is by skin testing with the appropriate penicillin reagents, followed by an oral challenge (assuming the test is negative).

   d. When penicillin skin testing is possible, the ideal time to evaluate penicillin allergy in children is when they are well and not in immediate need of antibiotic treatment.

   e. When penicillin skin testing is not possible, evaluation of penicillin allergy should be limited to children who are likely to require treatment with it.

   f. Physicians should make an effort to evaluate penicillin allergy in children and not allow them to unnecessarily carry the label into adulthood.

2. Allergy to nonpenicillin antibiotics

   a. There are no validated skin testing reagents to accurately rule out an IgE-mediated allergy.

   b. Skin testing with nonirritating concentrations of antibiotics can assist the clinician in evaluating a possible allergy.

   c. Graded challenge or desensitization can be used in situations where need for an antibiotic arises.

3. Allergy to local anesthetics

   a. True immediate-type allergic reactions to local anesthetics are very rare.

   b. Skin testing followed by graded challenge rules out an allergy to local anesthetics in virtually all children.

4. Aspirin (acetylsalicylic acid [ASA])/nonsteroidal antiinflammatory drug (NSAID) allergy

   a. Reactions to ASA and NSAIDs are less frequent in children than they are in adults.

   b. Reactions in patients with underlying asthma or chronic urticaria are cross-reactive among all NSAIDs.

   c. Reactions in patients without underlying asthma or chronic urticaria, including anaphylaxis/angioedema/urticaria, are medication specific.

threatening reaction (Box 58-2). If a child has reacted to several different medications, such as antibiotics, physicians are often at their 'wit's end' about how to approach future inevitable treatment courses. Likewise, parents of patients are apprehensive and concerned that their child may 'die' because of a lack of safe medications. Using the tools (Box 58-3) discussed in this chapter, physicians can play an important role in helping to sort out which medications a child can safely receive, and in many cases prevent them from needlessly being labeled as allergic for the rest of their lives.

References

1. Solensky R, Khan D, Bloomberg GR, et al. Drug hypersensitivity: an updated practice parameter. Ann Allergy Asthma Immunol 2009; in press.
2. Volcheck GW, Hagan JB, Li JT, editors. Drug hypersensitivity. Immunol Allergy Clin North Am 2004;23:345-543.
3. International Rheumatic Fever Study Group. Allergic reactions to long-term benzathine penicillin prophylaxis for rheumatic fever. Lancet 1991;337:1308-10.
4. Napoli DC, Neeno TA. Anaphylaxis to benzathine penicillin G. Pediatr Asthma Allergy Immunol 2000;14:329-32.
5. Ibia EO, Schwartz RH, Wiederman BL. Antibiotic rashes in children: a survey in a private practice setting. Arch Dermatol 2000;136:849-54.
6. MacLaughlin EJ, Saseen JJ, Malone DC. Costs of beta-lactam allergies: selection and costs of antibiotics for patients with a reported beta-lactam allergy. Arch Fam Med 2000;9:722-6.
7. Martinez JA, Ruthazer R, Hansjosten K, et al. Role of environmental contamination as a risk factor for acquisition of vancomycin-resistant enterococci in patients treated in a medical intestive care unit. Arch Intern Med 2003;163:1905-12.
8. Puchner TC, Zacharisen MC. A survey of antibiotic prescribing and knowledge of penicillin allergy. Ann Allergy Asthma Immunol 2002: 24-9.
9. Solensky R, Earl HS, Gruchalla RS. Clinical approach to penicillin allergic patients: a survey. Ann Allergy Asthma Immunol 2000;84:329-33.
10. Cieslak PR, Strausbaugh LJ, Fleming DW, et al. Vancomycin in Oregon: who's using it and why. Infect Control Hosp Epidemiol 1999;20:557-60.
11. Kwan T, Lin F, Ngai B, et al. Vancomycin use in 2 Ontario tertiary care hospitals: a survey. Clin Invest Med 1999;22:256-64.
12. Lee CE, Zembower TR, Fotis MA, et al. The incidence of antimicrobial allergies in hospitalized patients: implications regarding prescribing patterns and emerging bacterial resistance. Arch Intern Med 2000;160: 2819-22.
13. Gadde J, Spence M, Wheeler B, et al. Clinical experience with penicillin skin testing in a large inner-city STD Clinic. JAMA 1993;270: 2456-63.
14. Bock SA, Munoz-Furlong A, Sampson HA. Fatalities due to anaphylactic reactions to foods. J Allergy Clin Immunol 2001;107:191-3.
15. Bock SA, Munoz-Furlong A, Sampson HA. Further fatalities caused by anaphylactic reactions to food, 2001-2006. J Allergy Clin Immunol 2007;119:1016-8.
16. Adkinson NF. Risk factors for drug allergy. J Allergy Clin Immunol 1984;74:567-72.
17. Roujeau JC, Huynh TN, Bracq C, et al. Genetic susceptibility to toxic epidermal necrolysis. Arch Dermatol 1987;123:1171-3.
18. Yang CW, Hung SI, Juo CG, et al. HLA-B*1502-bound peptides: implications for the pathogenesis of carbamazepine-induced Stevens-Johnson syndrome. J Allergy Clin Immunol 2007;120:870-7.
19. Yang J, Qiao H, Zhang Y, et al. HLA-DRB genotype and specific IgE responses in patients with allergies to penicillins. Chin Med J 2006;119:458-66.
20. Asero R. Detection of patients with multiple drug allergy syndrome by elective tolerance tests. Ann Allergy Asthma Immunol 1998;80: 185-8.
21. Kamada MM, Twarog F, Leung DYM. Multiple antibiotic sensitivity in a pediatric population. Allergy Proc 1991;12:347-50.
22. Moseley EK, Sullivan TJ. Allergic reactions to antimicrobial drugs in patients with a history of prior drug allergy (abstract). J Allergy Clin Immunol 1991;87:226.
23. Strom BL, Schinnar R, Apter AJ, et al. Absence of cross-reactivity between sulfonamide antibiotics and sulfonamide nonantibiotics. N Engl J Med 2003;349:1628-35.
24. Pichler WJ. Delayed drug hypersensitivity reactions. Ann Intern Med 2003;139:683-93.
25. Schmid DA, Depta JP, Luthi M, et al. Transfection of drug-specific T cell receptors into hybridoma cells: tools to monitor drug interaction with T cell receptors and evaluate cross-reactivity to related compounds. Mol Pharmacol 2006;70:356-65.
26. Levine BB, Ovary Z. Studies on the mechanism of the formation of the penicillin antigen. III. The N-(D-alpha-benzyl-penicilloyl) group as an antigenic determinant responsible for hypersensitivity to penicillin G. J Exp Med 1961;114:875-904.

27. Levine BB, Redmond AP. Minor haptenic determinant-specific reagins of penicillin hypersensitivity in man. Int Arch Allergy Appl Immunol 1969;35:445-55.

28. Parker CW, deWeck AL, Kern M, et al. The preparation and some properties of penicillenic acid derivatives relevant to penicillin hypersensitivity. J Exp Med 1962;115:803-19.

29. Wickern GM, Nish WA, Bitner AS, et al. Allergy to beta-lactams: a survey of current practices. J Allergy Clin Immunol 1994;94:725-31.

30. Sogn DD, Evans R, Shepherd GM, et al. Results of the National Institute of Allergy and Infectious Diseases collaborative clinical trial to test the predictive value of skin testing with major and minor penicillin derivatives in hospitalized adults. Arch Intern Med 1992;152:1025-32.

31. Sullivan TJ, Wedner HJ, Shatz GS, et al. Skin testing to detect penicillin allergy. J Allergy Clin Immunol 1981;68:171-80.

32. Macy E, Richter PK, Falkoff R, et al. Skin testing with penicilloate and penilloate prepared by an improved method: amoxicillin oral challenge in patients with negative skin test responses to penicillin reagents. J Allergy Clin Immunol 1997;100:586-91.

33. Blanca M, Vega JM, Garcia J, et al. Allergy to penicillin with good tolerance to other penicillins: study of the incidence in subjects allergic to betalactams. Clin Exp Allergy 1990;20:475-81.

34. Macy E, Burchette R. Oral antibiotic adverse reactions after penicillin skin testing: multi-year follow-up. Allergy 2002;57:1151-8.

35. Blanca M, Mayorga C, Torres MJ, et al. Clinical evaluation of Pharmacia CAP System RAST FEIA amoxicilloyl and benzylpenicilloyl in patients with penicillin allergy. Allergy 2001;56:862-70.

36. Bousquet PJ, Co-Minh HB, Arnoux B, et al. Importance of mixture of minor determinants and benzylpenicilloyl poly-L-lysine skin testing in the diagnosis of beta-lactam allergy. J Allergy Clin Immunol 2005;115:1314-6.

37. Sastre J, Quijano LD, Novalbos A, et al. Clinical cross-reactivity between amoxicillin and cephadroxil in patients allergic to amoxicillin and with good tolerance of penicillin. Allergy 1996;51:383-6.

38. Romano A, Quaratino D, DiFonso M, et al. A diagnostic protocol for evaluating nonimmediate reactions to aminopenicillins. J Allergy Clin Immunol 1999;103:1186-90.

39. Romano A, Quaratino D, Papa G, et al. Aminopenicillin allergy. Arch Dis Child 1997;76:513-7.

40. Primeau MN, Hamilton RG, Whitmore E, et al. Negative patch tests and skin tests in patients with delayed cutaneous to penicillins (abstract). J Allergy Clin Immunol 2002;109:S267.

41. Romano A, Di Fonso M, Papa G, et al. Evaluation of adverse cutaneous reactins to aminopenicillins with emphasis on those manifested by maculopapular rashes. Allergy 1995;50:113-8.

42. Sanz ML, Gamboa PM, Antepara I, et al. Flow cytometric basophil activation test by detection of CD63 expression in patients with immediate-type reactions to betalactam antibiotics. Clin Exp Allergy 2002;32:277-86.

43. Torres MJ, Padial A, Mayorga C, et al. The diagnostic interpretation of basophil activation test in immediate allergic reactions to betalactams. Clin Exp Allergy 2004;34:1768-75.

44. Empedrad R, Darter AL, Earl HS, et al. Nonirritating intradermal skin test concentrations for commonly prescribed antibiotics. J Allergy Clin Immunol 2003;112:629-30.

45. Mendelson LM, Ressler C, Rosen JP, et al. Routine elective penicillin allergy skin testing in children and adolescents: study of sensitization. J Allergy Clin Immunol 1984;73:76-81.

46. Solensky R, Earl HS, Gruchalla RS. Penicillin allergy: prevalence of vague history in skin test-positive patients. Ann Allergy Asthma Immunol 2000;85:195-9.

47. Wong BBL, Keith PK, Waserman S. Clinical history as a predictor of penicillin skin test outcome. Ann Allergy Asthma Immunol 2006;97.

48. Jost BC, Wedner HJ, Bloomberg GR. Elective penicillin skin testing in a pediatric outpatient setting. Ann Allergy Asthma Immunol 2006;97:807-12.

49. Park M, Markus P, Matesic D, et al. Safety and effectiveness of a preoperative allergy clinic in decreasing vancomycin use in patients with a history of penicillin allergy. Ann Allergy Asthma Immunol 2006;97:681-7.

50. Murray BE. Vancomycin-resistant enterococcal infections. N Engl J Med 2000;342:710-21.

51. Hospital Infection Control Practices Advisory Committee Hospital. Recommendations for preventing the spread of vancomycin resistance. MMWR 1995;44(RR-12):1-13.

52. Rao GG. Risk factors for the spread of antibiotic-resistant bacteria. Drugs 1998;55:323-30.

53. Lacuesta GA, Moote DW, Payton K, et al. Follow-up of patients with negative skin tests to penicillin (abstract). J Allergy Clin Immunol 2002;109:S143.

54. Warrington RJ, Burton R, Tsai E. The value of routine penicillin allergy skin testing in an outpatient population. Allergy Asthma Proc 2003;24:199-202.

55. Abraham GN, Petz LD, Fudenberg HH. Immunohaematological cross-allergenicity between penicillin and cephalothin in humans. Clin Exp Immunol 1968;3:343-57.

56. Pedersen-Bjergaard J. Specific hyposensitization of patients with penicillin allergy. Acta Allergol 1969;24:333-61.

57. Miranda A, Blanca M, Vega JM, et al. Cross-reactivity between a penicillin and a cephalosporin with the same side chain. J Allergy Clin Immunol 1996;98:671-7.

58. Romano A, Gueant-Rodriguez RM, Viola M, et al. Cross-reactivity and tolerability of cephalosporins in patients with immediate hypersensitivity to penicillins. Ann Intern Med 2004;141:16-22.

59. Antunez C, Blanca-Lopez N, Torres MJ, et al. Immediate allergic reactions to cephalosporins: evaluation of cross-reactivity with a panel of penicillins and cephalosporins. J Allergy Clin Immunol 2006;117:404-10.

60. Romano A, Gueant-Rodriguez RM, Viola M, et al. Diagnosing immediate reactions to cephalosporins. Clin Exp Allergy 2005;35:1234-42.

61. Romano A, Mayorga C, Torres MJ, et al. Immediate allergic reactions to cephalosporins: cross reactivity and selective responses. J Allergy Clin Immunol 2000;106:1177-83.

62. Romano A, Quaratino D, Aimone-Gastin I, et al. Cephalosporin allergy: characterization of unique and cross-reacting cephalosporin antigens. Int J Immunopathol Pharmacol 1997;10:187-91.

63. Saxon A, Swabb EA, Adkinson NF. Investigation into the immunologic cross-reactivity of aztreonam with other beta-lactam antibiotics. Am J Med 1985;78(Suppl 2A):19-26.

64. Adkinson NF. Immunogenicity and cross-allergenicity of aztreonam. Am J Med 1990;88(Suppl 3C):S3-14.

65. Vega JM, Blanca M, Garcia JJ, et al. Tolerance to aztreonam in patients allergic to betalactam antibiotics. Allergy 1991;46:196-202.

66. Atanaskovic-Markovic M, Gaeta F, Medjo B, et al. Tolerability of meropenem in children with IgE-mediated hypersensitivity to penicillins. Allergy 2008;63:237-40.

67. Romano A, Viola M, Gueant-Rodriguez RM, et al. Tolerability of meropenem in patients with IgE-mediated hypersensitivity to penicillins. Ann Intern Med 2007;146:266-9.

68. Romano A, Viola M, Gueant-Rodriquez RA, et al. Imipenem in patients with immediate hypersensitivity to penicillins. N Engl J Med 2006;354:2835-7.

69. Dibbern DA, Montanaro A. Allergies to sulfonamide antibiotics and sulfu-containing drugs. Ann Allergy Asthma Immunol 2008;100:91-100.

70. Patterson R, Bello AE, Lefkowith F. Immunologic tolerability profile of celecoxib. Clin Ther 1999;21:2065-79.

71. Demoly P, Messaad D, Sahla H, et al. Six-hour trimethoprim-sulfamethoxazole-graded challenge in HIV-infected patients. J Allergy Clin Immunol 1998;102:1033-6.

72. Solensky R. Drug desensitization. Immunol Allergy Clin N Am 2004;24:425-43.

73. Yango MC, Kim K, Evans R. Oral desensitization to trimethoprim-sulfamethoxazole in pediatric patients. Immunol Allergy Practice 1992;56:17-24.

74. Bonfanti P, Pusterla L, Parazzini F, et al. The effectiveness of desensitization versus rechallenge treatment in HIV-positive patients with previous hypersensitivity to TMP-SMX: a randomized multicentric study. Biomed Pharmacother 2000;54:45-9.

75. Leoung GS, Stanford JF, Giordano MF, et al. Trimethoprim-sulfamethoxazole (TMP-SMZ) dose escalation versus direct rechallenge for Pneumocystis carinii pneumonia prophylaxis in human immunodeficiency virus-infected patients with previous adverse reaction to TMP-SMZ. J Infect Dis 2001;184:992-7.

76. Benahmed S, Scaramuzza C, Messaad D, et al. The accuracy of the diagnosis of suspected macrolide antibiotic hypersensitivity: results of a single-blinded trial. Allergy 2004;59:1130-3.

77. Messaad D, Sahla H, Benahmed S, et al. Drug provocation tests in patients with a history suggesting an immediate drug hypersensitivity reaction. Ann Intern Med 2004;140:1001-6.

78. Soto-Aguilar MC, deSchazo RD, Dawson ES. Approach to the patient with suspected local anesthetic sensitivity. Immunol Allergy Clin N Am 1998;18:851-65.

79. Stevenson DD. Aspirin and NSAID sensitivity. Immunol Allergy Clin N Am 2004;24:491-505.

80. Settipane RA, Shrank PJ, Simon RA, et al. Prevalence of cross-sensitivity with acetaminophen in aspirin-sensitive asthmatic subjects. J Allergy Clin Immunol 1995;96:480-5.

81. Woessner K, Simon RA, Stevenson DD. The safety of celecoxib in aspirin exacerbated respiratory disease. Arthritis Rheum 2002;46:2201-6.

82. Viola M, Quaratino D, Gaeta F, et al. Celecoxib tolerability in patients with hypersensitivity (mainly cutaneous reactions) to nonsteroidal anti-inflammatory drugs. Int Arch Allergy Immunol 2005;137:145-50.

83. Debley JS, Carter ER, Gibson RL, et al. The prevalence of ibuprofen-sensitive asthma in children: a randomized controlled bronchoprovocation challenge study. J Pediatr 2005;47:233-88.

84. Fisher TJ, Guilfoile TD, Kesarwala HH, et al. Adverse pulmonary responses to aspirin and acetaminophen in chronic childhood asthma. Pediatrics 1983;71:313-8.

85. Rachelefsky GS, Coulson A, Siegel SC, et al. Aspirin intolerance in chronic childhood asthma: detected by oral challenge. Pediatrics 1975;56:443-8.

86. Schuhl JF, Pereyra JG. Oral acetylsalicylic acid (aspirin) challenge in asthmatic children. Clin Allergy 1979;9:83-8.

87. Towns SJ, Mellis CM. Role of acetyl salicylic acid and sodium metabisulfite in chronic childhood asthma. Pediatrics 1984;73:631-7.

88. Vedanthan PK, Menon MM, Bell TD, et al. Aspirin and tartrazine oral challenge: incidence of adverse response in chronic childhood asthma. J Allergy Clin Immunol 1977;60:8-13.

89. Berges-Gimeno MP, Simon RA, Stevenson DD. Long-term treatment with aspirin desensitization in asthmatic patients with aspirin-exacerbated respiratory disease. J Allergy Clin Immunol 2003;111:180-6.

90. Stevenson DD, Hankammer MA, Mathison DA, et al. Aspirin desensitization treatment of aspirin-sensitive patients with rhinosinusitis-asthma: long-term outcomes. J Allergy Clin Immunol 1996;98:751-8.

91. Sweet JM, Stevenson DD, Simon RA, et al. Long-term effects of aspirin desensitization-treatment for aspirin-sensitive rhinosinusitis-asthma. J Allergy Clin Immunol 1990;85:59-65.

92. Borish L, Tamir R, Rosenwasser LJ. Intravenous desensitization to beta-lactam antibiotics. J Allergy Clin Immunol 1987;80:314-9.

93. Stark BJ, Earl HS, Gross GN, et al. Acute and chronic desensitization of penicillin-allergic patients using oral penicillin. J Allergy Clin Immunol 1987;79:523-32.

94. Sullivan TJ, Yecies LD, Shatz GS, et al. Desensitization of patients allergic to penicillin using orally administered beta-lactam antibiotics. J Allergy Clin Immunol 1982;69:275-82.

95. Wendel GD, Stark BJ, Jamison RB, et al. Penicillin allergy and desensitization in serious infections during pregnancy. N Engl J Med 1985;312:1229-32.

96. Dash CH. Penicillin allergy and the cephalosporins. J Antimicrob Chemother 1975;1(Suppl):107-18.

97. Petz LD. Immunologic cross-reactivity between penicillins and cephalosporins: a review. J Infect Dis 1978;137(Suppl):S74-9.

98. Goodman EJ, Morgan MJ, Johnson PA, et al. Cephalosporins can be given to penicillin-allergic patients who do not exhibit an anaphylactic response. J Clin Anesth 2001;13:561-4.

99. Daulat SB, Solensky R, Earl HS, et al. Safety of cephalosporin administration to patients with histories of penicillin allergy. J Allergy Clin Immunol 2004;113:1220-2.

100. Fonacier L, Hirschberg R, Gerson S. Adverse drug reactions to cephalosporins in hospitalized patients with a history of penicillin allergy. Allergy and Asthma Proc 2005;26:135-41.

101. Warrington RJ, Simons FER, Ho HW, et al. Diagnosis of penicillin allergy by skin testing: the Manitoba experience. Can Med Assoc J 1978;118:787-91.

102. Solley GO, Gleich GJ, Dellen RGV. Penicillin allergy: clinical experience with a battery of skin-test reagents. J Allergy Clin Immunol 1982;69:238-44.

103. Saxon A, Beall GN, Rohr AS, et al. Immediate hypersensitivity reactions to beta-lactam antibiotics. Ann Intern Med 1987;107:204-15.

104. Blanca M, Fernandez J, Miranda A, et al. Cross reactivity between penicillins and cephalosporins: clinical and immunologic studies. J Allergy Clin Immunol 1989;83:381-5.

105. Shepherd GM, Burton DA. Administration of cephalosporin antibiotics to patients with a history of penicillin allergy (abstract). J Allergy Clin Immunol 1993;91:262.

106. Audicana M, Bernaola G, Urrutia I, et al. Allergic reactions to beta-lactams: studies in a group of patients allergic to penicillin and evaluation of cross-reactivity with cephalosporin. Allergy 1994;49:108-13.

107. Pichichero ME, Pichichero DM. Diagnosis of penicillin, amoxicillin, and cephalosporin allergy: reliability of examination by skin testing and oral challenge. J Pediatr 1998;132:137-43.

108. Novalbos A, Sastre J, Cuesta J, et al. Lack of allergic cross-reactivity to cephalosporins among patients allergic to penicillins. Clin Exp Allergy 2001;31:438-43.

109 Greenberger PA, Klemens JC. Utility of penicillin major and minor determinants for identification of allergic reactions to cephalosporins. J Allergy Clin Immunol 2005;115:S182.

110. McConnell SA, Penzak SR, Warmack TS, et al. Incidence of imipenem hypersensitivity reactions in febrile neutropenic marrow transplant patients with a history of penicillin allergy. Clin Infect Dis 2000;31:1512-4.

111. Prescott WA, DePestel DD, Ellis JJ, et al. Incidence of carbapenem-associated allergic-type reactions among patients with versus patients without a reported penicillin allergy. Clin Infect Dis 2004;38:1102-7.

112. Sodhi M, Axtell SS, Callahan J, et al. Is it safe to use carbapenems in patients with a history of allergy to penicillin? J Antimicrob Chemother 2004;54:1155-7.

113. Cunha BA, Hamid NS, Krol V, et al. Safety of meropenem in patients reporting penicilliin allergy: lack of allergic cross reactions. J Chemother 2008;20:233-7.

59

Latex Allergy

Kevin J. Kelly

Introduction

Nearly 30 years have passed since a worldwide epidemic of immunoglobulin E (IgE)-mediated allergy to natural rubber latex (referred to as NRL or latex) occurred. Introduction of health-care standard precautions resulting in a marked increase in personal exposure to latex, and manufacturing changes in latex production may have resulted in sensitization to protein allergens retained in finished products. This chapter reviews the clinical presentation of latex allergy (LA), production and manufacturing, patterns of latex use in the context of clinical symptoms, allergens, diagnosis, clinical and laboratory cross-reactivity with foods and pollens, and treatment options.

Clinical Manifestations – Initial Observations

The clinical circumstances in patients who develop LA are highly variable and may not be readily recognized by patients. This requires clinicians to have a high index of suspicion and astute diagnostic skills.

In 1927, a single case of chronic urticaria from contact with rubber prosthetics was reported in the German literature.[1] It was not until 1979 that the first clear case of LA was reported in a homemaker.[2] The diagnosis was confirmed by a medical history of intense pruritus and atopic dermatitis after the use of rubber gloves, with confirmation by patch test and prick-test-induced hives from a latex glove. The clinical spectrum of LA was broadened by the first report of latex exposure in a health-care worker causing urticaria, rhinitis and ocular symptoms.[3] After the introduction of standard precautions, an exponential rise in latex exam glove use paralleled a rise in reporting of LA (Figure 59-1). A 1987 prevalence study confirmed the presence of LA in 15/512 (2.9%) hospital employees screened by prick test to latex.[4] A subset of individuals (operating room personnel) had the highest prevalence at 6.2%. Atopy was found to be a strong contributing factor to LA development with 10/15 (66.7%) of subjects having environmental allergies. In 1987, Axelsson reported five individuals with systemic reactions to latex gloves; only one was a health-care worker.[5] Seaton completed the medical literature spectrum of latex allergy manifestations a decade after the first modern publication, when a case of occupational asthma caused by latex gloves was confirmed, and suggested that latex exposure came from airborne allergen.[6] Previous mucosal reactions of conjunctivitis and rhinitis were believed to have come from direct allergen transfer by hand contact. This report moved the medical community toward an understanding that the environment could be contaminated by allergen-carrying glove powder.

After these earliest observations, specific risk groups emerged with common exposures. Throughout the first decade of reporting this disorder, women, health-care workers and atopic individuals were identified as being at risk. Reports identified individuals undergoing surgical operations having severe allergic reactions during anesthesia. Two children with spina bifida suffered anaphylactic reactions when undergoing anesthesia with two completely different clinical scenarios. One child experienced systemic symptoms within 15 minutes of anesthesia induction and prior to surgical incision while the other child's reaction occurred at the time of closure of the surgical incision. These reactions were characterized by generalized flushing, expiratory wheezing, marked increase in airway pressure needed to mechanically ventilate, and severe hypotension requiring epinephrine for symptom reversal. These observations were confirmed in the next 3 years by multiple clinical observations of allergic reactions in spina bifida patients undergoing surgery.[7-9]

Spina Bifida

Children with spinal bifida (SB) emerged in the early 1990s as the highest risk group for developing LA.[10] Recurrent exposure to latex products in their daily care, multiple surgeries, atopic disposition and epigenetic factors may all contribute to this response. Patients with SB seem exceptionally capable of mounting an IgE response to latex proteins, with subjects undergoing surgery in a prior year having a 68% prevalence of NRL sensitization. Alarmingly, one of every eight patients in one hospital with SB, prior to the use of latex avoidance precautions in the operating room, developed systemic allergic reactions during anesthesia, representing a 500-fold higher rate of anaphylaxis than expected during general anesthesia and surgery. Two case series reported anaphylaxis occurring 40 to 220 minutes into surgery with direct mucosal glove contact, while another series noted anaphylaxis within 30 minutes of the induction of anesthesia.[9,10] One case series compared differences between SB patients who developed intraoperative anaphylaxis and those SB patients who did not, while a second case series compared SB to atopic and nonatopic control groups. SB groups developed LA more frequently than atopic subjects (40.5% vs 11.4%) and at > 20 times the rate of healthy controls (40.5% vs 1.9%). Other case series without control groups suggest that atopy, >5 surgeries, high antilatex IgE (>3.5 kU/L), and skin test reactivity to foods (kiwi, pear or tomato) are important factors.[11-15]

DOI: 10.1016/B978-1-4377-0271-2.00059-6

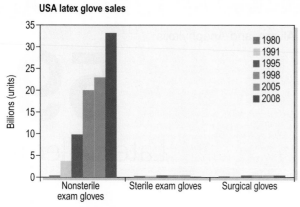

USA latex glove sales

Figure 59-1 This graph of latex examination glove sales in the USA since 1980 demonstrates that the dramatic increase in use of gloves is with nonsterile examination gloves and may represent one of the major contributing causes of the epidemic of latex allergy seen in the 1980s and 1990s. In 1980, examination glove sales were less than 300 million but exceeded 33 billion in 2008, or nearly a 100-fold rise in sales. Surgical glove use nearly doubled during that same time frame.

Latex Allergy in Patients with Urologic or Neurologic Defects

In addition to patients with SB, patients with cloacal anomalies, chronic renal failure or bladder anomalies were at risk for latex anaphylaxis. Two studies published in the same year reached opposite conclusions about the risk of LA or sensitization in patients with spinal cord injuries. Konz performed a cross-sectional study of 36 SB patients, 50 patients with spinal cord injury, 10 patients with cerebrovascular accidents, and 10 healthy controls.[16] While 72% of the SB subjects had clinical histories and confirming tests compatible with LA, no positive histories were identified in either of the other two groups with neural disease. Antilatex IgE was noted in 4% of spinal cord injured patients despite no history of latex-induced reactions. Vogel reported only 2/67 spinal cord injured patients with a clinical history of latex reactions, but 10 (15%) with evidence of latex sensitization, a historically higher rate than the general population.[17] Regardless, there appear to be significant differences between neurologically injured patients and patients with SB.

Health-Care Workers

Although an extensive review of LA in this group will not be reported, the clinical manifestations of health-care workers' (HCW) disease are quite different.[18-22] While most children with LA do not have irritant dermatitis or contact dermatitis, the majority of latex-allergic health-care workers show evidence of dermatitis, with the irritant type being the most prevalent. Dermatitis often heralds the development of IgE-mediated symptoms of urticaria, angioedema, occupational asthma, rhinoconjunctivitis and anaphylaxis, but is not a prerequisite for the development of LA. The prevalence of HCW disease has ranged from 5% to 17% with > 50% having latex-induced asthma. Several reasons for LA development in this group include frequent use of latex gloves, manufacturing changes that lead to higher allergen content of gloves, processing changes, or manufacturing changes.

Surgery

Multiple reports suggest that surgical intervention increases LA risk.[12,23] In addition, children with cerebral palsy, esophageal atresia, gastroschisis, and omphalocoele may be at higher risk. Since these diseases are confounded by frequent latex glove use and multiple surgeries, the contribution of each variable is unclear.

Latex Allergy in the General Population

Multiple reports and clinical experience have shown that individuals with no apparent risk factors of exposure, SB, health-care work or surgery may develop LA. The symptoms in these individuals are usually predicted by the route of exposure; rhinitis, conjunctivitis and asthma occur after inhalation, while anaphylaxis occurs after abdominal mucosa or intravenous exposure. The most dramatic presentations were the first cases of anaphylaxis seen after rectal mucosal surface exposure to latex balloons, latex glove or condom materials. In the 1980s, air contrast barium enema procedures used a catheter that was inflated to help retain the air and barium in the colon.[24,25] Rectal manometry with a balloon-tipped catheter or covered by condom material was common. Case series described severe anaphylaxis, including death, associated with these procedures. Only in retrospect were these cases identified as LA, with most occurring in non-health-care workers, although some were atopic or had had prior surgery. One particular catheter was implicated in the barium enema induced anaphylaxis (E-Z-Em Company) with as many as 148 episodes of anaphylaxis and 9 deaths. Since most of these subjects were not from identified risk groups, it raises significant concern about the risk in the general population.

Two large studies[23,26] showed a prevalence of LA in children of 0.7–1.1%, well below the reported prevalence in children with SB and health-care workers. These observations were contrasted by serologic studies from blood donors, non-health-care workers, and consecutive emergency department patients, demonstrating antilatex IgE presence in the blood of 4–8% of these subjects.[26-31] Whether this represents a predictable rate of false-positive tests in low-prevalence populations, or accurate results in subjects at risk of latex-allergic reactions following future exposures, is unclear.

Fruit Allergy and Concurrent Latex Allergy

Clinical observations raised the question of pan-allergens and clinical cross-reactivity of fruit and latex. Multiple clinical reactions to bananas, kiwi, avocado, mango, chestnut, papaya and stone fruits such as cherries or peaches have been published in known latex-allergic subjects.[31-38] In addition, individuals with primary food allergy have had clinical reactions to latex, but much less frequently than might have been expected from the initial frequency of in vitro allergen cross-reactions. This syndrome has been coined the 'latex-fruit syndrome' and was extended to the 'latex-vegetable syndrome' when cross-reactions were found between a number of vegetables and latex proteins.

Over 50% of individuals with LA may have clinical reactions to fruit (Table 59-1) due to specific cross-reacting allergens.[28] A common tertiary structure of Hev b 6 (hevein) is shared with two banana proteins, avocado and chestnut. Kiwi has significant homology with Hev b 5.[39-41] While Hev b 7 has structural similarity to patatin from potato, the clinical relevance may be minor. Hev b 8, a profilin, may cross-react with other plant profilins. Hev b 2 is a pathogen-related protein β-1,3-glucan with cross-reactive homology. Hev b 12 is a lipid transfer protein that has been a common protein type to cause clinical reactions to vegetables and fruit in patients who are pollen reactive.

Latex-fruit syndrome was investigated from the perspective of whether individuals with primary fruit allergy have concurrent

Table 59-1 Foods that Cross-React with *Hevea brasiliensis* Latex

Primary Food Allergies Causing Latex Reactions	Clinical Cross-Reacting Foods
Bananas	Avocados
Melons	Bananas
Peaches	Chestnuts
	Kiwi
	Papaya
	Potato

Foods with In Vitro Cross-Reactivity but Uncommon In Vivo Symptoms in Latex Allergy	
Apple	Passion fruit
Bell pepper	Pear
Celery	Pineapple
Cherry	Tomato
Fig	Turnip
Mango	Wheat

LA. Of 57 subjects with primary fruit allergy, 49 (86%) had IgE reactivity in serum and/or skin test. Only 6 (12.2%) reported prior symptoms from latex exposure; however, fruit allergy symptoms preceded these.[42]

The concern of hidden food allergen has been brought to light by multiple reports of transfer of allergen to food (a bagel, cheese, lettuce, and doughnut) by handlers wearing latex gloves.[43,44]

Diabetes and Latex Allergy

The development of LA in patients with type 1 diabetes was unexpected.[45] In 1995, anaphylaxis was reported during surgery and was presumed to be from latex contamination of injectable medication drawn from a latex rubber top bottle during anesthesia. A series of case reports[46–48] and a prevalence study investigating the risk of LA in individuals who require insulin injection were subsequently reported. Local allergic reactions at the site of insulin injection occurred after the needle used to draw up the insulin was inserted through a rubber-stopped bottle containing latex. Removal of the latex top and subsequent drawing up of the insulin into the syringe did not produce allergic reactions in any of these cases. These observations suggest that the latex stopper does not contaminate the medication vial, but does contaminate the needle during insertion. One report in the pharmacy literature found that multiple needle punctures of multi-dose vials did not elute allergen in enough quantity to result in allergic reactions. Serum samples from children with type 1 diabetes demonstrate that latex-specific IgE was detectable only in atopic diabetic children, but was not more prevalent than in nondiabetic atopic subjects. In this study, 7/112 (6%) of subjects had IgE antibody and were all derived from the atopic group of 42 subjects (17%). In contrast, none (0/70) of the nonatopic subjects had antilatex IgE antibody detected in the serum.[49]

Latex Production

Produced by nearly 2000 lactiferous plants and trees, the polymer cis-1, 4 polyisoprene has been exploited for broad commercial use from the tree *Hevea brasiliensis* and recently from other lactiferous plants such as guayule latex.[50–54] Commercial use of latex from *Hevea brasiliensis* dates back to the 19th century, although

evidence of NRL materials found at archeological excavations reveal that rubber materials were being produced as long ago as 1600 BC. Charles Goodyear's critical discovery of sulphur heat vulcanization, a method that effectively cross-links the rubber polyisoprene while reducing the tackiness and sensitivity to temperature change of latex, catapulted NRL use into one of the most important industries in the world. Worldwide latex consumption has increased dramatically, even in the last decade, with nearly 6 million tons/year produced in 1995 and over 8.79 million tons/year utilized in 2005, mainly due to China's spectacular economic growth. Latex demand for NRL in Japan, Europe and North American has remained stable. Whether a new epidemic of LA will emerge in China is unknown but is very concerning.

Rubber hydrocarbon (cis-1,4 polyisoprene) makes up the majority of the latex suspension while protein, carbohydrate, lipids, inorganic constituents and amino acids are a minor percentage of the mix. Despite proteins being a minor portion of NRL, the retention of these proteins in finished products is the cause of IgE-mediated reactions in humans. During the manufacturing of latex products, over 200 different chemicals have been utilized and fall into broad categories of accelerators of cross-linking, antioxidants, antiozonates, biocides, colorants, epoxies and plasticizers. It is the accelerator class of chemicals, including thiurams, thiazoles and carbamates, which most frequently cause type IV cell-mediated contact dermatitis of the skin from latex. Synthetic rubber materials and alternative medical glove materials may retain these same chemicals, resulting in contact dermatitis. Gloves made of either polyvinyl chloride, styrene butadiene rubber, or Tactylon® (styrene ethylene butylene styrene) do not contain these accelerators.

Latex Collection

NRL flows through a circulation system of the tree and is collected when bark is shaved off just short of the cambium layer. Latex is treated with a stabilizer such as sodium sulfite, formaldehyde, ammonia (0.05–0.2%), or ammonia with a 1:1 mixture of zinc oxide and tetramethylthiuram disulfide (TMTD). A number of chemicals can be used to enhance the yield of latex. Such chemicals (e.g. 2-chloroethylphosphonic acid or ethepon) may enhance the quantity and type of allergenic proteins. Demand to produce more medical-grade latex with the advent of standard precautions in the 1980s resulted in more frequent tapping of trees and reduced storage time of latex. As many allergenic proteins are defense proteins, this production may have been enhanced. Failure to destroy proteins through reduced storage times may have enhanced the allergen content of finished products as well.

Latex Product Manufacturing

Approximately 88% or more of the world's harvested latex is acid coagulated, prepared as dry raw rubber in sheets or crumbs of technically specified rubber and dried at 60°C or higher temperature. Allergic IgE reactions have been rarely reported from this type of rubber but delayed hypersensitivity contact reactions may be seen.

The other 10–12% of NRL is produced in a latex concentrate by centrifugation or creaming to make products such as gloves and condoms from a dipping method. Most latex is concentrated to 60% isoprene, stabilized in either a high concentration of ammonia (0.7%) or low ammonia (0.2%) with TMTD and zinc oxide, stored in tanks for at least 2 to 3 weeks and often longer, before being shipped to manufacturers. After shipping, the latex is prepared by the manufacturer with proprietary methods, for dipping of forms (e.g. gloves) coated with a surface coagulant, into latex slurry. The latex adheres to the former, is wet leached, heat vulcanized, dried and various methods are used to prevent the latex products from sticking to each other. In the past, the most common agent used to prevent sticking was highly cross-linked cornstarch powder or talc. Given its ability to act as a carrier of latex allergen, cornstarch powder has fallen out of favor. Talc was found to induce granulomatous inflammation and decrease wound healing and has mostly been abandoned in medical-grade gloves. Halogenation or surface coating with a synthetic polymer has been useful in replacing donning powder.

Latex Allergens

Field latex varies its protein content by clonal origin of the rubber plant, climatic factors, soil types, fertilizers and yield enhancers used for the rubber cultivation. Latex-producing trees are susceptible to invasion by a variety of microorganisms, especially fungi, and insects that can injure and kill the tree. NRL contains numerous defense-related proteins and enzymes that are integral in the protection of the plant, biosynthesis of polyisoprene and coagulation of latex, but which cause allergic sensitization and clinical reactions in susceptible hosts. Proteins present in freshly harvested latex are detected in finished latex products, either in their natural configuration or an altered configuration, which may lead to the formation of neo-antigens.[50] Based on their IgE-binding properties, the Allergen Nomenclature Subcommittee of IUIS has accepted 13 proteins as latex allergens (http://www.allergen.org).

Immunologic Properties

The immunologic properties of individual latex allergens have been evaluated by immune responses in either health-care workers or patients with SB since those individuals make up the majority of subjects found to have clinical disease. The allergens that the general population reacts to are likely to parallel these current observations (Table 59-2).

Functional Properties of Latex Allergens

Latex proteins are involved in rubber biosynthesis (Hev b 1, 3, 6, 7), plant defense (Hev b 2, 4, 6.01–6.03, 7, 11, 12, 13), enzyme actions and structural formation (Hev b 5, 8, 9). Some of these proteins have multiple functions and have variable IgE responses in humans who contact them.[41,51]

Immune Responses to Rubber Biosynthesis Proteins

The four allergens most involved in rubber biosynthesis include Hev b 1, Hev b 3, Hev b 6.01–6.03 and Hev b 7. What is most interesting is the dichotomy of reactions seen between health-care workers and SB patients to this particular group of allergens. SB patients react more frequently to Hev b 1 and Hev b 3 than other risk groups, possibly due to genetic differences, surgical exposure, timing or route of exposure to the allergens.

Hev b 1 (Rubber Elongation Factor or REF)

A tetramer with a molecular mass of 58 kDa and tightly bound on large rubber particles (>350 nm in diameter), Hev b 1 is a major allergen, inducing IgE reactions in 13–32% of latex sensitive health-care workers and 52–100% of SB patients. This very important allergen must be present in sufficient quantity for diagnosis in patients with SB.[55-57]

Hev b 3 (REF Homolog)

This protein, with strong IgE binding reactivity in patients with SB and LA, is associated with the small rubber particles (< 75 nm) in latex. Clinical and immunologic reactivity of Hev b 3 with serum IgE in health-care workers is less frequent and weaker than in SB patients. The amino acid sequence homology is 47% when compared to Hev b 1. Pre-incubated latex-allergic sera with Hev b 1 shows > 80% enzyme linked immunosorbent assays (ELISA) inhibition to solid phase Hev b 3, indicating the presence of similar conformational allergens in these proteins.[56-58]

Hev b 7 (Patatin-Like Protein)

An important potato storage protein allergen (Sol t 1), Hev b 7, a 46 kD protein with patatin storage protein homology, inhibits rubber biosynthesis, but also has defense hydrolase and esterase activity which inhibits the growth of invertebrate pests. IgE-binding reactivity occurs with 23% health-care workers with LA, but has not been demonstrated to be a major allergen for patients with SB.[59]

Hev b 6.01–6.03

Hev b 6.01–6.03 has latex coagulation activity, but will be presented under defense-related proteins.

Immune Responses to Plant Defense-Related Proteins

The Hevea latex allergens that have defense-related functions include Hev b 2, 4, 6.01–6.03, 7 (see above), 11, 12, and 13. Most latex-allergic patients recognize one or more of these allergens and their potential cross-reactions with fruit proteins account for the serious allergic reactions after ingestion of a food with such proteins. In addition, hevamine, a common protein that is not officially accepted as an allergen, is also a defense-related protein that some individuals develop IgE antibody against.[34,35,38-40,59-61]

Higher plants have a defense system of proteins that are compared frequently to the immune system of animals, but in reality are significantly different. Static defense proteins (e.g. storage proteins) may exert antifungal activity (e.g. lectins) or antimicrobial activity. Pathogenesis-related proteins (PR-proteins) are encoded by the host plant but are induced only in pathological situations (e.g. tapping of a latex tree). There are 14 identified families of PR-proteins with defense functions and many are associated with food allergy cross-reactions in pollen-induced food allergy and the latex-fruit syndrome. Thus it is important to understand the type of defense proteins that are allergens in NRL in order to predict which fruit and environmental allergens will cause clinical cross-reactivity.

Hev b 2

This basic β-1,3-glucanase exhibits significant IgE binding with latex-sensitized SB and health-care workers.[60] IgE reactivity may range from 20 to 61% of patients with clinical symptoms from latex allergen content. Foods such as banana, potato and tomato may contain β-1,3-glucanase activity, but it is not clear if this is truly the protein resulting in cross-reactions.[62,63]

Table 59-2 *Hevea brasiliensis* Latex Allergens

Allergens	Allergen Name	Molecular Weight kDa	Function	Significance as Allergens
Hev b 1	Elongation factor **Tetramer**	14.6 58	Rubber biosynthesis	Major
Hev b 2	1,3-glucanase	34/36	Defense protein	Major
Hev b 3	Elongation factor	23	Rubber biosynthesis	Major
Hev b 4	Microhelix complex **Dimer**	50–57 100–115	Defense protein	Major
Hev b 5		16	Enzyme	Major
Hev b 6.01	Prohevein	20	Defense protein	Major
Hev b 6.02	Hevein	4.7	Defense protein	Major
Hev b 6.03	C-terminal hevein	14	Defense protein	Major
Hev b 7	Patatin homologue	42.9	Defense protein Inhibit rubber biosynthesis	Minor
Hev b 8	Latex profiling	14	Structural protein	Minor
Hev b 9	Latex enolase	51	Enzyme	Minor
Hev b 10	Mn superoxide dismutase	26	Enzyme	Minor
Hev b 11	Class 1 chitinase	33	Defense protein	Minor
Hev b 12	Lipid transfer protein	9.3	Defense protein	Major
Hev b 13	Latex esterase	42	Enzyme	Major

Hev b 4

This microhelix component of latex is an acidic protein (50–57 kDa) with 65% of health-care workers found to have IgE against this component. However, only 14% of these patients showed peripheral blood mononuclear cell (PBMC) stimulation to Hev b 4.

Hev b 6 (Prohevein)

Hev b 6.01, one of the most abundant latex proteins, has two distinct domains; a 4.7 kD C-terminal domain (Hev b 6.02) and an N-terminal 14 kD peptide (Hev b 6.03).[38-41] Prohevein has strong reactivity with IgE from health-care workers and SB patients with LA. The 43 amino acid long N-domain exhibits IgE binding with a significantly higher number of latex-sensitized patients when compared to the 144 amino acid long C-domain of Hev b 6. Skin test reactions correlate well with the in vitro IgE to latex allergens. Epitope mapping of the prohevein molecule revealed more IgE-binding regions near the N-terminal end of the protein.

Hev b 11 (Endochitinase)

The class 1 chitinase shares homology with N-terminal hevein domain (resulting in cross-reactivity and the latex fruit syndrome) and also shares epitopes with chitinases from avocado, chestnut, and banana. They appear to be minor contributors to disease.[35,37,38]

Hev b 12 (Lipid Transfer Protein):

Lipid transfer proteins with antifungal and antibacterial activity are named for their ability to transfer phospholipids from liposomes to mitochondria, and are widely distributed in the plant kingdom.[64] This class of proteins is the most important allergen in the Prunoideae fruits such as peach, cherry, apricot and plum, which may help explain the cross-reactivity seen in stone fruits in latex-allergic health-care workers.

Hev b 13 (Latex Esterase)

The biologic role of this protein is not as well defined, but it is one of the major allergens found in natural and finished latex products that health-care workers react to. This important allergen correlates well with the allergenic content of finished latex gloves and has been proposed to be one of four allergens used in a standard to measure immunologic allergenic content of manufactured products.[65]

Immune Responses to Common Enzymes and Structural Proteins

Hev b 5

A proline-rich protein with a 46% amino acid sequence homology to an 18.9 kDa acidic protein from kiwi, Hev b 5 has been cloned and expressed with a molecular mass of 16 kDa.[65,66] It is presumed to be partially responsible for clinical reactions to kiwi in LA patients. This protein is a major allergen with strong IgE-binding reactivity with both health-care workers (92%) and SB (56%) patients.

Hev b 8 (Profilin)

Profilin, an actin binding protein, is involved in the formation of the actin network of plant exoskeleton. The purified latex profilin, when used in skin prick testing, showed positive reactions in 100% (24/24) SB patients and 6/17 health-care workers with LA, but its role in the clinical induction of symptoms is unclear, due to carbohydrate binding in vitro.[67-70]

Algorithm for Diagnosed Immediate Hypersensitivity in Latex Allergy

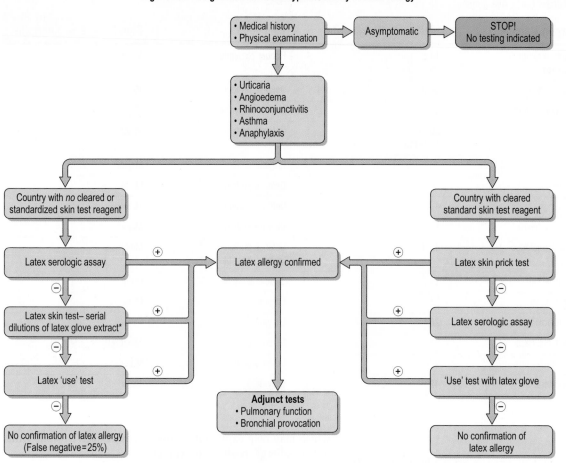

* Latex skin tests and latex 'use' tests, especially with unstandardized latex, may result in anaphylaxis

Figure 59-2 This algorithm outlines the common decision analysis for the diagnosis of latex allergy. Countries that lack an FDA cleared skin test reagent, such as the USA, are significantly hindered from making a diagnosis, especially with a 25% rate of false negative serological assays. Patients with histories and physical examinations inconsistent with latex allergy should not undergo testing. This is due to the high rate of false positive serological assays in populations with a low prevalence of disease.

Hev b 9 (Enolase)

A high degree of cross-reactivity can be expected because of the homology of enolases present in different organisms. However, unpublished work from our laboratory on sera from 26 health-care workers with LA failed to demonstrate any IgE binding with the recombinant latex Hev b 9 and fungal enolases.

Hev b 10 (Manganese Superoxide Dismutase)

This highly conserved enzyme (MnSOD) has been reported from a number of fungi and bacteria, as well as from human beings, but its role in cross-reactive allergenicity is unclear.[34,35,38,61]

Diagnosis of Latex Allergy

The diagnosis of LA in a patient requires a medical provider to take a complete medical history, perform a physical examination, and then supplement the clinical conclusions with appropriate testing. An algorithm that outlines one method of approaching the diagnosis is included in Figure 59-2. Epicutaneous skin testing or serologic testing for antilatex IgE in the absence of a clinical history and physical exam are inadequate for an accurate diagnosis of LA, since each of those tests has variable sensitivity, specificity, positive predictive values, and negative predictive

values. Testing for LA has been hindered in the USA by lack of a standard reagent clearance through USFDA.

Skin Testing

Skin testing has been the most sensitive and predictive test for confirming a diagnosis.[11,71-74] Achieving the highest sensitivity has required the use of more than one source material for latex (e.g. natural latex nonammoniated and a latex glove extract).[11,72] In one series, the sensitivity of using two source materials was 100%, specificity of 99%, and a negative test having 100% predictive value in concluding that a patient was not allergic to latex.[11] Failure of a skin test reagent to be approved in the USA may relate to the frequency of adverse reactions to epicutaneous testing with latex allergen.[11,71,75] Early information demonstrated that skin testing resulted in a high rate of systemic reactions not seen with other allergens approved for skin testing. This high rate of reaction was confirmed in a comparative retrospective study from the Mayo Clinic where the rate of systemic reactions to latex was 228/100000 latex skin tests, while the rate of reactions of this nature to other allergens was 72/100000 penicillin skin tests and 23/100000 aeroallergen tests.[75] This represents a 10-fold elevated risk of systemic reactions to latex skin testing in comparison to aeroallergen tests. Even the multicenter skin test study with cloned latex resulted in 16% of subjects having systemic, albeit mild, reactions to skin testing.[71] Comparisons of latex extracts made using different techniques indicated that the protein content obtained from a latex glove can vary widely, depending on the extraction method.[72] In addition, the stability of the different latex antigens is variable. Since the antigen content of gloves can vary several 100-fold, nonstandardized extracts may contain vastly different amounts of latex protein. Some of the risk associated with latex skin tests can be attributed to uncharacterized extracts. Although the algorithm in Figure 59-2 recommends skin testing, it may be safest to perform such tests with a commercial latex standardized reagent, such as the Stallergenes S.A. (Marseilles, France) used in Europe.

In Vitro Testing for LA

Detection of antilatex IgE in serum of patients has been the most widely accepted testing method in the USA.[73,75-80] These include research laboratory prepared enzyme linked immunosorbent assays (ELISA) or commercial tests from Pharmacia, UniCAP FEIA (Pharmacia, Peapack, NJ), AlaSTAT (Diagnostic Products Corporation, Los Angeles, CA), and Hycor HYTECH (Hycor Biomedical, Inc., Garden Grove, CA) systems.

Comparative performance of the three commercially available serologic assays for latex-specific IgE was studied in 117 clinically allergic individuals and 195 clinically nonallergic controls. When compared to skin test, both the Pharmacia CAP and AlaSTAT had similar sensitivities of 76% and 73% respectively with 97% specificity. Unfortunately, 25% of the latex-sensitized cases had false negative results. HyTECH had a significantly lower specificity of 73% which indicates that 27% of the positive results are erroneous.[76] Thus, screening studies for LA in a population with a low prevalence of disease, may result in a significant number of false positive reactions. In addition, 25% of patients with disease may have a false negative test. These characteristics make these tests undesirable for screening without a follow-up definitive test.

Other in vitro methods of diagnosing LA have included basophil histamine release, CD 63 activation of basophils and lymphocyte proliferation methods.[81-83] These assays are more specific but lack sensitivity. Their most useful activity has been to identify specific IgE epitopes and T cell epitopes. These tests have not become useful clinical tools although genetic altering of strongly allergenic epitopes may be useful in down-regulating and inducing tolerance by immunotherapy in latex allergic subjects.[84]

In Vivo Provocation Testing

In addition to using serologic testing or skin prick testing in diagnosing LA, it is sometimes necessary to understand whether a specific allergen or latex product reported by the clinical history is truly responsible for the symptoms, or to clarify discordant serum and skin test results. Provocation tests for diagnosing LA have included 'glove use tests', utilizing standardized gloves as described in the multi-center latex skin test study.[78] In addition, multiple investigations have used a 'latex glove wearing' test with or without a coupled inhalation test. The critical value of the provocation test is making certain that objective measurable or observable reactions are measured.[85] These may include such things as urticaria, angioedema or pulmonary function changes.

Some investigators have used inhalation provocation challenges alone or mucous membrane allergen contact. These have been progressive, graded challenges and are currently only standardized in research settings. Assuring standard allergen content in the provocation may be helped by the LEAP© assay or equivalent.[86]

Prevention and Treatment of the Patient with Latex Allergy

Prevention of LA has focused on avoidance strategies for children who have SB, individuals who require multiple surgeries, as well as health-care workers and other occupations that require contact with natural rubber latex gloves.[87-93] The prototype patient for prevention of LA is the infant born with SB. These measures include complete abstinence of latex materials used in the care of these patients from birth. This means preventing contact with latex gloves, catheters, dressings, tape or other medical devices that contain latex in the hospital and home setting. Given the level of disability and the vast number of surgeries in these subjects, an opinion article to vastly change care and prevent LA was published in 1996. Given that over 40 000 devices and materials contained natural rubber latex as a component, stopping all use of latex-containing materials became impractical. Avoiding the use of latex materials that were made by a dipping process with short vulcanization times and low heat

---

BOX 59-1 Key concepts

Latex Allergy

- Natural rubber latex (NRL) is contained in thousands of consumer and medical products and is responsible for an epidemic of IgE-mediated latex allergy in the past three decades.

- Products made by a dipping method (e.g. gloves, condoms) have the highest content of allergenic protein that may result in urticaria, angioedema, asthma, rhinoconjunctivitis and anaphylaxis.

- Latex finished products contain multiple chemicals that may induce cell-mediated contact dermatitis, although this is uncommon in pediatrics.

- Latex proteins may have clinical cross-reactivity with multiple foods leading to clinical allergic responses, especially to banana, avocado and/or kiwi, in nearly 50% of latex-allergic subjects.

- A small subset of patients with fruit and vegetable allergies may develop allergic reactions from cross-reactions to latex but in less than 15% of patients.

- Patients with spina bifida are at highest risk of developing latex allergy.

- Occupational asthma is a common problem seen in adult workers exposed to latex materials that use a cornstarch donning powder, which may carry latex protein into the ambient environment.

- Diagnosis is best achieved by performance of a history, physical examination, and allergy tests using skin test, serologic tests and provocation tests, although standard reagents are lacking.

- Serologic tests may produce false positive results by a variety of mechanisms while up to 25% of serologic tests may be falsely negative.

- Avoidance of latex through 'latex safe precautions' is essential for the treatment of latex allergy.

- Immunotherapy is promising but adverse reactions are very high and not recommended at this time.

was the most likely strategy to prevent allergic reactions. Indeed, the concept of 'latex safe' environments vs 'latex-free' environments turned out to be safe, practical and ideal for patients with LA.

Further observations in Canada, Europe and the USA noted that airborne latex was created by cornstarch donning powder from latex gloves which continued to sensitize and cause allergic reactions, not only in patients, but health-care workers.[89–93] This has led to a change in manufacturing and possibly in the prevalence of LA in health-care workers through powder-free glove use, reduced airborne latex exposure and reduction in product allergen content.

The care of the patient with LA requires that individuals avoid personal contact of the skin and mucous membranes with latex materials. In addition, they should only enter areas where airborne latex allergen is controlled by use of nonpowdered latex products. If the individuals are health-care workers, they should use nonlatex gloves and only work in areas where either powder-free latex gloves are used routinely or nonlatex gloves are used.

Rarely, immunotherapy is a consideration for the cure of LA. However, the side-effects of such therapy, length of time to achieve tolerance, and lack of a standardized reagent make this therapy relatively futile.[94,95] The promise of modified allergens to make immunotherapy safer and more effective is on the horizon.[84]

References

1. Stern G. Uberempfindlichkeit gegen Kautschuk als ursache von Urticaria und Quinckeschem Ödem. Klin Wochenschr 1927;6:1096–7.
2. Nutter AF. Contact urticaria to rubber. Br J Dermatol 1979;101:597–8.
3. Forstrom L. Contact urticaria from latex surgical gloves. Contact Dermatitis 1980;16:33–4.
4. Turjanmaa, K. Incidence of immediate allergy to latex gloves in hospital personnel. Contact Dermatitis 1987;17:270–5.
5. Axelsson JGK, Johansson SGO, Wrangsjo K. IgE-mediated anaphylactoid reactions to rubber. Allergy 1987;42:46–50.
6. Seaton A, Cherrie B. Rubber glove asthma. Br Med J 1988;296:531–2.
7. Slater J. Rubber Anaphylaxis. N Eng J Med 1989;320:1126–30.
8. Kelly KJ, Setlock M, Davis JP. Anaphylactic reactions during general anesthesia among pediatric patients. MMWR 1991;40:437.
9. Gold M, Swartz J, Braude B, et al. Intraoperative anaphylaxis: an association with latex sensitivity. J Allergy Clin Immunol 1991;87:662–6.
10. Kelly KJ, Pearson ML, Kurup VP, et al. A cluster of anaphylactic reactions in children with spina bifida during general anesthesia: epidemiologic features, risk factors, and latex hypersensitivity. J Allergy Clin Immunol 1994;94:53–61.
11. Kelly KJ, Kurup V, Zacharisen M, et al. Skin and serologic testing in the diagnosis of latex allergy. J Allergy Clin Immunol 1993;91:1140–5.
12. Hourihane JO, Allard MN, Wade AM, et al. Impact of repeated surgical procedures on the incidence and prevalence of latex allergy: a prospective study of 1263 children. J Pediatr 2002;140:479–82.
13. Nieto A, Extornell F, Mazon A, et al. Allergy to latex in spina bifida: a multivariatae study of associated factors in 100 consecutive patients. J Allergy Clin Immunol 1996;98:501–7.
14. Cremer R, Hoppe A, Korsch E, et al. Natural rubber latex allergy: prevalence and risk factors in patients with spina bifida compared with atopic children and controls. Eur J Pediatr 1998;157:13–6.
15. Bernardini R, Novembre E, Lombardi E, et al. Risk factors for latex allergy in patients with spina bifida and latex sensitization. Clin Exp Allergy 1999;29:681–6.
16. Konz KR, Chia JK, Kurup VP, et al. Comparison of latex hypersensitivity among patients with neurologic defects. J Allergy Clin Immunol 1995;95:950–4.
17. Vogel LC, Schrader T, Lubicky JP. Latex allergy in children and adolescents with spinal cord injuries. J Pediatr Orthop 1995;15:517–20.
18. Tarlo S, Sussman G, Holness D. Latex sensitivity in dental students and staff: a cross-sectional study. J Allergy Clin Immunol 1997;99:396–401.
19. Kelly KJ, Walsh-Kelly CM. Latex allergy: a patient and health care system emergency. Ann Emerg Med 1998;32:723–29.
20. Liss GM, Sussman GL, Deal K, et al. Latex allergy: epidemiological study of 1351 hospital workers. Occup Environ Med 1997;54:335–42.
21. Lagier F, Vervloet D, Lhermet I, et al. Prevalence of latex allergy in operating room nurses. J Allergy Clin Immunol 1993;90:319–22.
22. Yassin MS, Lierl MB, Fischer TJ, et al. Latex allergy in hospital employees. Ann Allergy 1994;72:245–9.
23. Ylitalo L, Turjanmaa K, Palosuo T, et al. Natural rubber latex allergy in children who had not undergone surgery and children who had undergone multiple operations. J Allergy Clin Immunol 1997;100:606–12.
24. Ownby DR, Tomlanovich M, Sammons N, et al. Anaphylaxis associated with latex allergy during barium enema examinations. Am J Radiol 1991;156:903–8.
25. Schwartz EE, Glick SN, Foggs MB, et al. Hypersensitivity reactions after barium enema examination. AJR Am J Roentgenol 1984;143:103–4.
26. Bernardini R, Novembre E, Ingargiola A, et al. Prevalence and risk factors of latex sensitization in an unselected pediatric population. J Allergy Clin Immun 1998;101:621–5.
27. Levenbom-Mansour MH, Oesterle JR, Ownby DR, et al. The incidence of latex sensitivity in ambulatory surgical patients: a correlation of historical factors with positive serum IgE levels. Anesth Analg 1997;85:44–9.
28. Reinheimer G, Ownby DR. Prevalence of latex-specific IgE antibodies in patients being evaluated for allergy. Ann Allergy Asthma Immunol 1995;74:184–7.
29. Ownby DR, Ownby HEB, McCullough JA, et al. The prevalence of anti-latex IgE antibodies to natural rubber latex in 1000 volunteer blood donors. J Allergy Clin Immunol 1996;97:1188–92.
30. Grzybowski M, Ownby DR, Rivers EP, et al. The prevalence of latex-specific IgE in patients presenting to an urban emergency department. Ann Emerg Med 2002;40:411–9.
31. Liss GM, Sussman GL. Latex sensitization: occupational versus general population prevalence rates. Am J Ind Med 1999;35:196–200.
32. Blanco C, Carrillo T, Castillo R, et al. Latex allergy: clinical features and cross reactivity with fruits. Ann Allergy 1994;73:309–14.
33. Kurup VP, Kelly T, Elms N, et al. Cross reactivity of food allergens in latex allergy. Allergy Proceedings 1994;15:211–6.
34. Yagami T. Defense-related proteins as families of cross-reactive plant allergens. Recent Res Devel Allergy & Clin Immunol 2000;1:41–64.
35. Brehler R, Theissen U, Mohr C, et al. 'Latex fruit syndrome' frequency of cross-reacting IgE antibodies. Allergy 1997;52:404–10.
36. Beezhold DH, Sussman GL, Liss GM, et al. Latex allergy can induce clinical reactions to specific foods. Clin Exp Immunol 1996;26:416–22.
37. Ahlroth M, Alenius H, Turjanmaa K, et al. Cross-reacting allergens in natural rubber latex and avocado. J Allergy Clin Immunol 1995;96:167–73.
38. Breiteneder H, Ebner C. Molecular and biochemical classification of plant-derived food allergens. J Allergy Clin Immunol 2000;106:27–36.
39. Alenius H, Kalkkinen N, Reunala T, et al. The main IgE binding epitopes of a major latex allergen, prohevein is present in its 43 amino acid fragment hevein. J Immunol 1996;156:1618–25.
40. Banerjee B, Wang X, Kelly KJ, et al. IgE from latex-allergic patients binds to cloned and expressed B cell epitopes of prohevein. J Immunol 1997;159:5724–32.
41. Breiteneder H. The allergens of *Hevea brasiliensis*. ACI International 1998;10:101–9.
42. Garcia Ortiz JC, Moyano JC, Alvarez M, et al. Latex allergy in fruit allergic patients. Allergy 1998;53:532–6.
43. Schwartz HJ. Latex: a potential hidden 'food' allergen in fast food restaurants. J Allergy Clin Immunol 1995;95:139–40.
44. Beezhold DH, Reschke JE, Allen JH, et al. Latex protein: a hidden 'food' allergen. Allergy Asthma Proc 2000;21:301–6.
45. Vassallo SA, Thurston TA, Kim SH, et al. Allergic reaction to latex from stopper of a medication vial. Anesth Analg 1995;80:1057–8.
46. Towse A, O'Brien M, Twarog FJ, et al. Local reaction secondary to insulin injection: a potential role for latex antigens in insulin vials and syringes. Diabetes Care 1995;18:1195–7.
47. Roest MA, Shaw S, Orton DI. Insulin-injection-site reactions associated with type I latex allergy. N Engl J Med 2003;348:265–6.
48. Thomsen DJ, Burke TG. Lack of latex allergen contamination of solutions withdrawn from vials with natural rubber stoppers. Am J Health-Syst Pharm 2000;57:44–7.
49. Danne T, Niggermann B, Weber B, et al. Prevalence of latex specific IgE antibodies in atopic and nonatopic children with type 1 diabetes. Diabetes Care 1997;20:476–8.
50. Makinen-Kiljunen S, Turjanmaa K, Palosuo T, et al. Characterization of latex antigens and allergens in surgical gloves and natural rubber by immunoelectrophoretic methods. J Allergy Clin Immunol 1992;90:230–5.
51. Subramaniam A. The chemistry of natural rubber latex. In: Fink JN, editor. Immunology and allergy clinics of North America. Philadelphia: W.B. Saunders; 1995, p. 1–20.
52. http://www.madehow.com/Volume-3/Latex.html (accessed 20 May 2007).
53. Burger K. The changing outlook for natural rubber. In: Natural rubber (Newsletter of the Rubber Foundation Information Center for Natural Rubber) 2005;40:1–2.

54. Ownby DR. A history of latex allergy. J Allergy Clin Immunol 2002;110:S27–32.

55. Chen ZP, Cremer R, Posch A, et al. On the allergenicity of Hev b 1 among health care workers and patients with spina bifida allergic to natural rubber latex. J Allergy Clin Immunol 1997;100:684–93.

56. Kurup VP, Yeang HY, Sussman GL, et al. Detection of immunoglobulin antibodies in the sera of patients using purified latex allergens. Clin Exp Allergy 1999;30:359–69.

57. Alenius H, Palosuo T, Kelly K, et al. IgE reactivity to 14-kD and 27-kD natural rubber proteins in latex-allergic children with spina bifida and other congential anomalies. Int Arch Allergy Immunol 1993;102:61–6.

58. Banerjee B, Kanitpong K, Fink JN, et al. Unique and shared IgE epitopes of Hev b 1 and Hev v 3 in latex allergy. Mol Immunol 2000;37:789–98.

59. Beezhold DH, Sussman GL, Kostyal DA, et al. Identification of a 46-kD latex protein allergen in health care workers. Clin Exp Immunol 1994;98:408–13.

60. Breton F, Coupe M, Sanier C, et al. Demonstration of beta-1,3-glucanase activities in lutoids of Hevea brasiliensis latex. J Nat Rubb Res 1995;10:37–45.

61. Yagami T, Sato M, Nakamura A, et al. Plant defense-related enzymes as latex antigens. J Allergy Clin Immunol 1998;101:379–85.

62. Johnson BD, Kurup VP, Sussman GL, et al. Purified and recombinant latex proteins stimulate peripheral blood lymphocytes of latex allergic patients. Int Arch Allergy Immunol 1999;120:270–9.

63. Wagner S, Radauer C, Hafner C, et al. Characterization of cross-reactive bell pepper allergens involved in the latex-fruit syndrome. Clin Exp Allergy 2004;34:1739–46.

64. Fernández-Rivas M, Benito C, González-Mancebo E, et al. Allergies to fruits and vegetables. Pediatr Allergy Immunol 2008;19:675–81.

65. Yeang H, Arif SAM, Raoulf-Heimsouth M, et al. Hev b 5 and Hev b 13 as allergen markers to estimate the allergenic potency of latex gloves. J Allergy Clin Immunol 2004;114:593–8.

66. Slater JE, Vedvick T, Arthur-Smith A, et al. Identification, cloning, and sequence of a major allergen (Hev b 5) from natural rubber latex (Hevea brasiliensis). J Biol Chem 1996;271:25394–9.

67. Yagami A, Nakazawa Y, Suzuki K, et al. Curry spice allergy associated with pollen-food allergy syndrome and latex fruit-syndrome. J Dermatol 2009;36:45–9.

68. Raulf-Heimsoth M, Kespohl S, Crespo JF, et al. Natural rubber latex and chestnut allergy: cross-reactivity or co-sensitization? Allergy 2007;62:1277–81.

69. Ebo DG, Hagendorens MM, Bridts CH, et al. Sensitization to cross-reactive carbohydrate determinants and the ubiquitous protein profilin: mimickers of allergy. Clin Exp Allergy 2004;34:137–44.

70. Nieto A, Mazon A, Boquete M, et al. Assessment of profilin as an allergen for latex-sensitized patients. Allergy 2002;57:776–84.

71. Hamilton RG, Adkinson F, and the Multicenter Latex Skin Testing Study Task Force. Diagnosis of natural rubber latex allergy: multicenter latex skin testing efficacy study. J Allergy Clin Immunol 1998;102:482–90.

72. Fink JN, Kelly KJ, Elms N, et al. Comparative studies of latex extracts used in skin testing. Ann Allergy Asthma Immunol 1996;76:149–52.

73. Kelly K, Kurup V, Reijula K, et al. The diagnosis of natural rubber latex allergy. J Allergy Clin Immunol 1994;93:813–6.

74. Hamilton R, Peterson E, Ownby D. Clinical and laboratory-based methods in the diagnosis of natural rubber latex allergy. J Allergy Clin Immunol 2002:110:S47–56.

75. Valyasevi MA, Maddox DE, Li JT. Systemic reactions to allergy skin tests. Ann Allergy Asthma Immunol 1999;83:132–6.

76. Hamilton RG, Biagini RE, Krieg EF. Multi-Center Latex Skin Testing Study Task Force. Diagnostic performance of FDA-cleared serological assays for natural rubber latex-specific IgE antibody. J Allergy Clin Immunol 1999;103:925–30.

77. Ownby D, McCullough J. Testing for latex allergy. J Clin Immunoassay 1993;16:109–13.

78. Biagini R, Krieg E, Pinkerton L, et al. Receiver operating characteristics analyses of Food and Drug Administration-cleared serological assays for natural rubber latex-specific immunoglobulin E antibody. Clin Diagn Lab Immunol 2001:8;1145–9.

79. Lundberg M, Chen Z, Rihs HP, et al. Recombinant spiked allergen extracts. Allergy 2001;56:794–95.

80. Ownby D, Magera B, Williams P. A blinded, multi-center evaluation of two commercial in vitro tests for latex-specific IgE antibodies. Ann Allergy Asthma Immunol 2000:84:193–6.

81. Turjanmaa K, Rasanen L, Lehto M, et al. Basophil histamine release and lymphocyte proliferation tests in latex contact urticaria. Allergy 1989:44:181–6.

82. Ebo D, Lechkar B, Schuerwegh A, et al. Validaton of a two-color flow cytometric assay detecting in vitro basophil activation for the diagnosis of IgE- mediated natural rubber latex allergy. Allergy 2002;57:706–12.

83. Murali P, Kelly K, Fink J, et al. Investigations into the cellular immune responses in latex allergy. J Lab Clin Med 1994;124:638–43.

84. Karisola P, Mikkola J, Kalkkinen N, et al. Construction of hevein (Hev b 6.02) with reduced allergenicity for immunotherapy of latex allergy by comutation of six amino acid residues on the conformational IgE epitopes. J Immunol 2004 Feb 15;172:2621–8.

85. Kurtz KM, Hamilton RG, Schaefer JA, et al. A hooded exposure chamber method for semi-quantitative latex aeroallergen challenge. J Allergy Clin Immunol 2001;107:178–84.

86. Beezhold D. LEAP: Latex ELISA for Antigenic Proteins ©* preliminary report. Guthrie Journal 1992:61;77–81.

87. Kelly KJ, Sussman G, Fink JN. Stop the sensitization. J Allergy Clin Immunol 1996;98:857–58.

88. Committee Report: Task Force on Allergic Reactions to Latex. J Allergy Clin Immunol 1993;92(1, Part 1):16–8. (Committee Members: Slater J, Abramson S, Graft D, Honsinger R, Kelly K, Kwittken P, Ownby D, Virant F.).

89. Baur X, Ammon J, Chen Z, et al. Health risk in hospitals through airborne allergens for patients presensitised to latex. Lancet 1993:342:1148–9.

90. Tarlo S, Sussman G, Contala A, et al. Control of airborne latex by use of powder-free latex gloves. J Allergy Clin Immunol 1994;93:985–9.

91. Kelly KJ. Management of the latex allergy patient. In: Fink JN, editor. Immunology and allergy clinics of North America. Philadelphia: W.B. Saunders; 1995, p. 139–57.

92. Baur X, Chen Z, Allmers H. Can a threshold limit value for natural rubber latex airborne allergens be defined? J Allergy Clin Immunol 1998:101(1, Part 1):24–7.

93. Allmers H, Schmengler J, Skudlik C. Primary prevention of natural rubber latex allergy in the German health care system through education and intervention. J Allergy Clin Immunol 2002:110:318–23.

94. Nettis E, Colanardi MC, Soccio AL, et al. Double-blind, placebo-control-led study of sublingual immunotherapy in patients with latex-induced urticaria: a 12-month study. Br J Dermatol 2007;156:674–81.

95. Sastre J, Fernandez-Nieto M, Rico P, et al. Specific immunotherapy with a standardized latex extract in allergic workers: a double-blind, placebo-controlled study. J Allergy Clin Immunol 2003;111:985–94.

60

Insect Sting Anaphylaxis

Robert E. Reisman

Stinging insect allergy is a relatively common medical problem, estimated to affect at least 0.3% to 3% of the population, and responsible for at least 40 deaths per year in the USA[1] and considerable anxiety in lifestyle. During the past 30 years, the pathogenesis, diagnosis, and treatment of allergic reactions caused by insect stings have been clarified, and reliable guidelines have been established for the assessment of this allergic disease. The availability of purified insect venoms and the clinical application of measurements of venom-specific immunoglobulin E (IgE) (skin test, venom-specific IgE), and serum venom-specific IgG provide the appropriate tools to understand and modulate this disease process. Criteria have been established for the use of venom as a diagnostic skin test reagent, correlating with the presence of potential clinical insect sting allergy. Insect venom immunotherapy (VIT) is remarkably effective in individuals at potential risk of insect sting anaphylaxis, inducing a permanent 'cure' in many individuals.

There remain pertinent unresolved issues, including the identification of individuals who may be at risk for initial insect sting anaphylaxis, further insight into factors that affect the natural history of venom allergy, and objective criteria with which to define the adequate duration of VIT. Other observations that require resolution are the rare occurrence of sting reactions in people with negative venom skin tests[2,3] and elevation of baseline serum tryptase levels in some people who have more severe allergic reactions.[4] This chapter reviews the general concepts relating to insect sting allergy and, in particular, addresses those aspects that are more relevant to children.

Epidemiology/Etiology

Development of Insect Sting Allergy

At present, no predictive criteria identify individuals at risk of acquiring an insect sting allergy. The majority of people who have had insect sting anaphylaxis have tolerated prior stings without reaction. In general, no time relationship exists between the last uneventful sting and the subsequent sting that leads to an allergic reaction.[5] A further confusing observation is the occurrence of initial insect sting anaphylaxis after the first known insect sting, primarily in children, raising the issue of the cause of sensitization or the pathogenesis of this initial reaction.[6] As insect stings always cause pain, in contrast to insect bites, the history in this regard seems reliable.

In the past, there has been a common misconception that large local reactions after insect stings, particularly those that were increasing in size with each sting, might precede an anaphylactic reaction. These large local reactions are defined as reactions extending from the sting site, often peaking in 24 to 48 hours and lasting up to 1 week. For example, the swelling from a sting on the finger may extend to the wrist or elbow. Clinical observations in recent years indicate that these large local reactions tend to be repetitive with a very low incidence, perhaps less than 5%, of subsequent systemic allergic reactions.[7]

Venoms are potent sensitizing substances. For example, individuals who collect snake venoms often develop inhalant-type allergy to venom. The occurrence of many simultaneous stings, such as 100 to 200 stings, can sensitize individuals for subsequent single-sting anaphylaxis. This potential problem is now recognized more often because of the increasing spread of the 'killer bees', which may inflict several hundred stings at one time.[8]

Demographic Studies

Demographic studies suggest that the incidence of insect sting allergy in the general population ranges between 0.4% and 3%. Approximately 33–40% of individuals who have insect sting anaphylaxis are atopic. There is a 2:1 male/female ratio that is probably a reflection of exposure rather than any specific sex predilection. The majority of reactions that do occur are in younger individuals, although the fatality rate is greater in adults.[9-12] It is estimated that 40 to 50 deaths per year occur in the USA as the result of insect sting anaphylaxis. Most individuals had no warning or indication of their allergies and had tolerated prior stings with no difficulty.

The Insects

Insects that sting are members of the order Hymenoptera of the class Insecta. There are two major subgroups: vespids, which include the yellow jacket, hornet, and wasp; and aphids, which include the honeybee and bumblebee (Figure 60-1). In most parts of the USA, yellow jackets are the principal cause of allergic reactions. These insects nest in the ground or in the walls of homes and are frequently disturbed by lawn mowing, gardening, or other outdoor activities. Yellow jackets feed on substances containing sugar and are commonly attracted to food and garbage. Hornets nest in shrubs and trees and are disturbed by activities such as trimming hedges. Wasps are more prevalent early in the summer season. In some areas of the country, such as Texas, they are the most frequent cause of sting reactions. Honeybees and bumblebees are docile and sting only when provoked. People

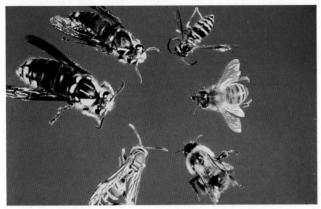

FIGURE 60-1 The Common stinging insects. Shown clockwise from the top right portion of the figure are a yellow jacket, honeybee, bumblebee, Polistes wasp, and two hornets. (From Reisman RE. Insect stings. N Engl J Med 1994; 331:523–527.Copyright 1994 Massachusetts Medical Society. All rights reserved.)

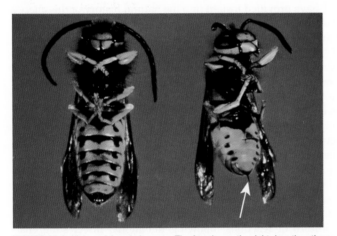

FIGURE 60-2 Male and female hornets. The female, on the right, has the stinger which protrudes from the abdomen (arrow). (From Reisman RE. Insect stings. N Engl J Med 1994; 331:523–527.Copyright 1994 Massachusetts Medical Society. All rights reserved.)

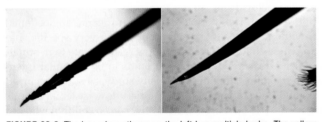

FIGURE 60-3 The honeybee stinger on the left has multiple barbs. The yellow jacket stinger on the right is smooth.

have received multiple stings from honeybees when their hives, which contain thousands of insects, were threatened.

The stinging apparatus originates in the abdomen of the female insect (Figure 60-2). It consists of a sac containing venom attached to a barbed stinger. The honeybee's stinger has multiple barbs, which usually cause the stinging apparatus to detach from the insect, leading to its death. In contrast, the stingers of vespids have few barbs and these insects can inflict multiple stings (Figure 60-3).

Africanized honeybees, or 'killer bees', have received much publicity.[8] They entered the USA in south Texas and are now present in Arizona and California. They were introduced into Brazil from Africa in 1956 for the purpose of more productive

pollination and have gradually spread north. The venom components of the Africanized honeybees and the domesticated European honeybees that are found throughout the USA are similar. The venom of the Africanized honeybee is no more allergic or toxic than that of the European honeybee. However, African honeybees are much more aggressive. Massive stinging incidents have occurred, leading to death from venom toxicity. Africanized honeybees are expected to continue to move northward, although they do not survive well in colder climates.

The fire ant, *Solenopsis invicta*, is a nonwinged Hymenopteran. This insect is found in the southeastern and south central USA, especially along the Gulf Coast. They have now spread to California. The fire ant attaches itself to a person by biting with its jaws. It then pivots around its head and stings at multiple sites in a circular pattern. The stinger is located on the abdomen. Within 24 hours a sterile pustule develops, which is diagnostic of the fire ant's sting. Allergic reactions to fire ant stings are becoming increasingly common in the southern USA.[13,14]

Unlike insect stings, insect bites rarely cause anaphylaxis. Biting insects, such as mosquitoes, deposit salivary gland secretions that have no relation to venom allergens. Anaphylaxis has been described after the bites of deer flies, bed bugs and black flies. Large local reactions, however, are much more common, and recent studies suggest that the reactions to mosquito bites may be associated with IgE and perhaps IgG antibodies.

These large local reactions from mosquito bites are more common in young children. Over time and with repeated exposure, the reactions become less intense and are less frequent problems in adolescents and adults. Elevated titers of salivary gland-specific IgE and IgG correlate with the intensity of the local reactions and appear to be the responsible immunologic mediators of the reactions.[15]

Differential Diagnosis: Reaction to Insect Stings

Normal Reaction

The usual or normal reaction to an insect sting consists of localized pain, swelling, and erythema at the site of the sting. This reaction usually subsides within several hours. Little treatment is needed other than analgesics and cold compresses.

Large Local Reactions

More extensive local reactions are common. Swelling extends from a sting site over a large area, often peaking at 48 hours and lasting as long as 7 days. Fatigue and nausea may develop. The cause of these large local reactions has not been established, although they may be mediated by IgE antibodies. After a large local reaction occurs, most people, including children, have positive skin tests to venom, suggesting the possibility of an allergic pathogenesis.[7,16] Medical treatment usually consists of aspirin or antihistamines. If the swelling is extensive and disabling, systemic steroids, such as prednisone, 40 mg/day taken orally for 2 or 3 days, are beneficial.

On occasion, large local reactions are confused with cellulitis. However, cellulitis rarely develops after an insect sting; the author has never seen this occur. A common therapeutic error, particularly in emergency department settings, is to treat with antibiotics. In addition, tetanus prophylaxis is unnecessary.

In people who have had large local reactions from stings, the risk for subsequent anaphylaxis is very low. In our study of a large series of individuals, the risk of anaphylaxis was about 5%.[7] In one study of children, the risk of anaphylaxis was only 2%.[16] In this latter study, most children had positive skin tests, which became less reactive over time.

People who have had large local reactions do not require venom skin tests and they generally are not candidates for VIT. Also, in our study the occurrence of subsequent large local reactions was not affected by VIT.[7] However, one recent case report indicated that VIT could have been helpful in reducing the large local reaction in a patient who was repeatedly exposed to insect stings.[17] A subsequent follow-up study with placebo controls also suggested that VIT reduced the size and duration of large local reactions.[18]

There is one report showing that sublingual immunotherapy with honeybee venom reduced the extent of large local reactions from honeybee stings, with a good safety profile.[19] Further studies will be needed to verify these results and, more importantly, determine whether the sublingual immunotherapy is an appropriate substitution for the extremely effective traditional venom immunotherapy used for treatment of systemic reactors, discussed below.

Toxic Reactions

Toxic reactions to constituents of venom may occur after many simultaneous stings (50 to 100). The reaction has the same clinical characteristics as anaphylaxis. Exposure to large amounts of insect venom frequently stimulates production of IgE antibodies. People may have positive venom skin tests after toxic reactions. If they do, they are at potential risk for allergic reactions to subsequent single stings.

Unusual Reactions

There have been rare reports of vasculitis, nephrosis, neuritis, encephalitis, and serum sickness occurring in a temporal relationship to insect stings.[20] Sometimes anaphylaxis has preceded these reactions. The symptoms usually start several days to several weeks after the sting and may last for a long period.

Serum sickness, characterized by urticaria, joint pain, and fever, may occur approximately 7 to 10 days after an insect sting.[21] An immune pathogenesis is suggested by consistent findings of venom-specific IgE and, on occasion, venom-specific IgG. People who have had venom-induced serum sickness may be at risk for acute anaphylaxis after subsequent insect stings and may therefore be candidates for VIT, which provides protection from subsequent sting reactions.

Anaphylaxis

Other than a prior reaction, no clinical criteria or predictors identify people at potential risk for anaphylaxis from insect stings. The clinical features of anaphylaxis from an insect sting are the same as those from anaphylaxis from any other cause. The most common symptoms are dermal: generalized urticaria, flushing, and angioedema. Life-threatening symptoms include edema of the upper airways, circulatory collapse with shock and hypotension, and bronchospasm. The symptoms usually start within 10 to 15 minutes after a sting; on occasion, reactions have occurred as long as 72 hours later. Compared with adults, children have a higher incidence of dermal (hives, angioedema) reactions only and a lower incidence of more severe anaphylactic symptoms.[22]

Severe anaphylaxis, however, may occur at any age, but most deaths from anaphylaxis have occurred in adults. In our study[23] of 158 patients with severe anaphylaxis, there was a fairly uniform age distribution. Of the reactions, 21% occurred in children younger than 10 years old, and an additional 19% occurred in individuals between the ages of 11 and 20. There were 45 patients who had the most severe reactions as defined by loss of consciousness. This reaction was more common in adults; 24% of those were younger than 20 years.

Evaluation and Management

Natural History of Insect Sting Anaphylaxis

To assess appropriate intervention, it is necessary to understand the natural history of any disease process. This is particularly true of insect sting allergy. Observations of individuals who have had allergic reactions from insect stings and who did not receive VIT have provided insight into the natural history of this allergy and suggest that insect sting allergy is a self-limiting process for many people. In the initial study[24] that documented the efficacy of VIT, 40% of people treated with either placebo or whole body extracts failed to react to subsequent stings. These observations were extended in a study of a large number of people who had insect sting reactions and were observed without treatment.[5] Overall, the incidence of field reactions was higher in adults than in children but averaged about 60%. There was no relationship between the time interval between the sting reaction and subsequent reactions. The severity of the anaphylactic symptoms was an important criterion. The individuals with more severe reactions had a higher incidence of re-sting reactions. Finally, when a subsequent reaction did occur, the symptoms were generally similar to those that had occurred previously.

Studies of reactions following intentional insect sting challenges in individuals who had prior reactions and positive skin tests have shown similar results. Reaction rates to these intentional re-stings have varied from 25% to 60%.[25-27] Unfortunately, no immunologic criteria, such as skin test reactivity or titers of serum venom-specific IgE or IgG, distinguish or identify sting challenge reactors from nonreactors.

Children who have dermal reactions (urticaria, angioedema) only, without other allergic symptoms, are a very specific subgroup. These children have a very low reaction rate to re-stings, and when a reaction does occur, it tends to be of similar intensity.[28] In the Johns Hopkins University study, 84 stings occurred in 36 children receiving VIT with a very low systemic allergic reaction rate (1.2%). There were 196 stings in 86 children who did not receive VIT with 18 reactions, a reaction rate of 18.6% per patient and 9.2% per sting. Of the reactions that did occur, 16 were milder and 2 were similar in severity. None were more severe. In the large study of field stings,[5] 64 children had dermal symptoms only with the initial reaction; 30% had repeat reactions, of which 2 were of moderate intensity and 1 was of severe intensity. Thus 3 children had more severe symptoms with a re-sting. Overall these data suggest that children who have dermal reactions only have a very benign prognosis and generally do not retain their allergic sensitivity.

The prevalence and natural history of imported fire ant venom allergy has not been as well studied as winged Hymenoptera venom allergy. A recent study by Partridge and colleagues[29] examined 183 children living in an imported fire ant endemic area. Exposure to venom was assessed by measurement of imported fire ant venom (IFAV) specific IgG and sensitization by measurement of IFAV-specific IgE along with a questionnaire regarding sting histories. The prevalence of IFAV-specific IgG increased from 11.9% in children aged less than 1 year to 97.5% in those aged 11 to 30 years. Serum IFAV-specific IgE was detected in 7.1% of children less than 1 year, 57.1% of those aged 2 to 5 years and 64.4% of those aged 6 to 10 years. There was a significant correlation between the presence of IFAV-specific IgG and IgE. Despite the high rate of sensitization, as defined by the presence of IFAV-specific IgE, the number of anaphylactic reactions to imported fire ant stings was low. This dichotomy between clinical sensitivity and immunologic reactivity has been described in studies of reactions to other stinging insects.

In a small follow-up study of 12 children who had had generalized cutaneous reactions, and 8 children who had had large local reactions from IFA stings, none had more severe reactions from re-stings up to 20 years later.[30] Most reactions are described as small to large local swelling at the sting site. These limited data suggest a benign prognosis for children who have had large local or generalized cutaneous reactions only from IFA stings, again analogous to experience with winged Hymenoptera.

Diagnosis and Detection of Venom-Specific IgE

Venom Skin Tests

The diagnosis of potential venom allergy is dependent on the history of insect sting anaphylaxis and the presence of venom-specific IgE, usually detected by the immediate skin test reaction. Both of these components are necessary to document the diagnosis of insect sting allergy and the possibility of administering VIT.

A positive venom skin test without a history of an allergic reaction does not indicate a risk for venom anaphylaxis. The majority of people who have had large local insect sting reactions do have positive venom skin tests but, as noted earlier, have a small risk of anaphylaxis. Some individuals who experience a 'normal' insect sting will have a transient positive skin test.

Five commercial venoms (honeybee, yellow jacket, Polistes wasp, yellow hornet, and white-faced hornet) are available for testing and treatment. People suspected of having insect sting allergy are usually tested with all five venoms. Intradermal skin tests are performed starting with venom doses usually around 0.001 μg/mL and testing up to a concentration of 1 μg/mL.[31] Greater venom concentrations may cause irritative reactions that are not immunologically specific.

Skin tests with extracts prepared from whole bodies of fire ants appear to be reliable in identifying allergic individuals with few false-positive reactions in nonallergic controls.[13,14] Fire ant venom, which is not commercially available at present, has been collected and compared with fire ant whole body extract. The results of skin tests and in vitro tests show that venom is a better diagnostic antigen. However, whole body extracts can be prepared that apparently contain sufficient allergen and are reliable for skin test diagnosis. These results suggest that the allergens responsible for reactions can be preserved in the preparation of these whole body extracts, but future availability of fire ant venom may provide a more potent, reliable material.

In Vitro Measurement of Venom-Specific IgE

Venom-specific IgE can also be measured in the serum by in vitro tests (FEIA; fluorescene-enzyme immunoassays). In general, the skin test is a more sensitive test for the detection of venom-specific IgE than the in vitro test. In addition, the sensitivity of the FEIA may vary from laboratory to laboratory. The skin test remains a preferred test for the diagnosis of venom allergy. When skin tests cannot be performed or reliably interpreted, such as in people with dermatographism, or when they give equivocal results in the presence of a highly suspect history, measurement of serum venom-specific IgE may be helpful.

Chipps and colleagues[32] reported 44 children (mean age, 9.6 years) who had experienced allergic reactions to an insect sting and positive venom skin tests. Venom-specific IgE was detected in 77% of the children. In our studies[23] of people with serious anaphylaxis, 144 of 149 individuals had positive venom skin tests. Five individuals had negative skin tests up to a venom testing concentration of 0.1 μg/mL; three of these people had positive FEIAs and one had a borderline FEIA. The one person with negative skin tests (0.1 μg/mL) and a negative FEIA was tested 10 years after the sting reaction.

People have been described who had a history of venom anaphylaxis, had negative venom skin tests, and reacted again to a subsequent intentional sting challenge.[2] This observation has raised the issue of the accuracy or reliability of the venom skin test. These individuals represent a very small percentage of people who have had allergic reactions to insect stings.

Although the issue of the approach to the negative skin test reactor who has had moderate to severe sting anaphylaxis is still under review, the current recommendation is to perform an FEIA. If the FEIA is positive, VIT would be indicated. If the FEIA is negative, skin tests should be repeated in 3 to 6 months. Individuals with a history of a moderately severe reaction should be advised about the potential sensitivity and to carry emergency medication.[2,3]

Baseline serum tryptase levels have been found to be elevated in some people who had insect sting anaphylaxis, particularly in individuals who have had more severe symptoms. This has led to a search for mast cell disease in these people. The venom skin test may be reactive or nonreactive. It is postulated that with an increased number of mast cells, venom may release mediators on either an immunologic or a nonimmunologic basis and lead to more severe symptoms. These people may require more intensive VIT, as discussed later.[4]

Therapy

Acute Reaction

The medical treatment for acute anaphylaxis is the same as that for anaphylaxis from any cause and is detailed in Chapter 61. Epinephrine is the drug of choice and should be administered as soon as possible, even if symptoms are mild. The use of other medications depends on the symptom complex and includes antihistamines, steroids, oxygen, and vasopressors. Specific attention should be directed at the airway patency because upper airway swelling has been a major cause of death.

If the insect stinger remains in the skin, which most frequently occurs after a honeybee sting, it should be gently flicked off. Care should be taken to avoid squeezing the sac, which could inject more venom. Since the venom is deposited very quickly after the sting, this procedure may not be very helpful unless it is done immediately after the sting.

Prophylaxis

Individuals at risk of an allergic reaction are advised to use precautions to avoid subsequent stings. When outside, especially when involved in activities that might increase insect exposure such as gardening, these individuals should wear slacks, long-sleeve shirts, and shoes. Cosmetics, perfumes and hair sprays, which attract insects, should be avoided. Light-colored clothing is less likely to attract insects. Particular care should be taken outside around food and garbage, which especially attracts yellow jackets. Individuals at risk are advised to carry epinephrine, available in preloaded syringes for self-administration. As mentioned earlier, epinephrine should be administered at the earliest sign of an acute allergic reaction from an insect sting. Studies comparing individuals who have had fatal allergic reactions with individuals who have had serious nonfatal reactions suggest that the use of epinephrine may be the decisive factor in determining the outcome.[33]

Venom Immunotherapy

Insect venom extracts for diagnosis and therapy have been available for approximately 30 years. Although some questions remain, the concepts of the treatment have been fairly well established. This therapy is remarkably effective, preventing subsequent allergic reactions in more than 98% of treated patients and, in many instances, providing a permanent 'cure'. Major remaining issues relate to the refining of the selection process for people requiring VIT and refining criteria for duration of treatment.

Treatment: Venom Immunotherapy

Patient Selection

Potential candidates for VIT are people who have had an allergic reaction from an insect sting and have a positive venom skin test or elevated levels of serum venom-specific IgE (Table 60-1). As noted, studies of the natural history of insect sting allergy have shown that only approximately 60% or less of these individuals will have a subsequent reaction when re-stung.[5] The incidence of these sting reactions is influenced by age and the nature of the initial anaphylactic symptoms. Adults are more likely to have re-sting reactions than children, and the more severe the symptoms, the more likely it is that the reaction will recur. These

Table 60-1 Indications for Venom Immunotherapy in Patients with Positive Venom Skin Tests or Elevated Titers of Venom-Specific IgE (FEIA)*

Insect Sting Reaction	Venom Immunotherapy
'Normal' transient pain, swelling	No
Extensive local swelling	No[†]
Anaphylaxis	
Severe	Yes
Moderate	Yes
Mild, dermal only	
Children	No
Adults	Yes[‡]
Serum sickness	Yes
Toxic	Yes

*Venom immunotherapy is not indicated for individuals with negative venom skin tests and negative fluorescent enzyme-linked immunoassay (FEIA).
†Venom immunotherapy might be effective and a trial might be advisable if sting risk is high (see text).
‡Patients in this group might be managed without venom (see text).

observations influence the decision regarding patient selection for immunotherapy. Children with dermal (hives, angioedema) reactions only have a very benign prognosis, do not require immunotherapy,[5,28] and can be managed with availability of epinephrine. An obvious problem is how long to keep epinephrine available; at this time, no clear-cut answer to that question is available. This recommendation for availability of epinephrine is not a benign recommendation. Patients and families are often concerned about having it available in all situations, including school, work and home, and as indicated in a recent study, must be continually re-educated regarding its use.[34] Currently, the author recommends a negative skin test as a criterion to indicate loss of clinical sensitivity and to advise patients and families that continued availability of epinephrine is no longer necessary. Children are retested about every 2 to 3 years.

Individuals of any age, including very young children who have had severe allergic reactions should be advised to receive VIT; this is particularly true of people who have had loss of consciousness. Current recommendations are to administer VIT to adults who have had mild to moderate allergic sting reactions. This decision may require evaluation of other risk factors such as coexisting medical problems, concomitant medication use, patient lifestyle, and risk of sting exposure. People who have had serum sickness-like reactions are also candidates for VIT. If these individuals are re-exposed to venom, they are at potential risk for acute anaphylaxis.

A diagnostic sting challenge has been suggested as a criterion for initiating VIT. This approach has been suggested because of the repeated observations that only 60% or less of individuals thought to be at risk for a sting reaction because of a history of a prior reaction and the presence of a positive skin test do react when re-stung. The problems with the sting challenge relate to its safety, reliability and practicality. Observations of both field stings and intentional sting challenges have shown similar results. Approximately 20% of individuals who initially tolerate a re-sting with no difficulty react after another subsequent sting.[5,35] More important, this diagnostic sting challenge raises serious medical and ethical issues. Life-threatening reactions have occurred following intentional sting challenges in patients who did not receive VIT. It is the author's opinion that patients who have a high risk of serious anaphylaxis, such as adults who have had prior severe reactions, should not be intentionally rechallenged and should be given immunotherapy on the basis of their history and skin test reactivity, recognizing that some of these patients may not need therapy. Furthermore, in the USA it is highly impractical to have sufficient referral centers for diagnostic challenge studies.

Hauk and colleagues[36] conducted sting challenges in 113 children with histories of sting anaphylaxis; children who had had life-threatening anaphylaxis were omitted. Two challenges were performed at 2- to 6-week intervals. The authors concluded that the dual sting challenge was the best predictor of reactions to subsequent stings and need for VIT. They also stated that these challenge procedures were not recommended for adults because of increased risk.

Venom Selection

The commercial venom product brochure recommends treatment with all venoms to which there are positive skin tests. As a result, many people are treated with multiple venoms, despite the history of a single-sting reaction. The basic issue is really whether multiple skin test reactions represent specific venom allergy or cross-reactivity among different venoms. Extensive studies of venom cross-reactivity can be summarized as follows.[37-40]

- Extensive cross-reactivity exists between the two major North American hornet venoms, yellow hornet and bald-faced hornet.
- Extensive cross-reactivity exists between yellow jacket and hornet venoms.
- Limited cross-reactivity exists between yellow jacket and Polistes venoms.
- A more complex relationship exists between honeybee and vespid venoms. There may be no cross-reaction, extensive cross-reaction, or reaction to a major allergen in one venom cross-reacting with a minor allergen in the other venom.

The practical application of these data suggest that almost all people who have had allergic reactions to yellow jacket or hornet stings should be expected to have positive skin test reactions to both of these venoms. In this situation, VIT with one venom, more commonly yellow jacket, provides adequate protection.[41] Approximately 50% of people who have had yellow jacket or hornet sting reactions also have positive skin test reactions to Polistes venom. Polistes VIT is not necessary. The converse is also true, with half of the people who have had Polistes sting reactions having positive skin tests to yellow jacket or hornet venom and requiring treatment with Polistes venom only.

People who have had positive skin tests to both yellow jacket and honeybee venoms are more difficult to treat with single venoms, unless the history of the offending insect is clear.

The implications of these observations for therapy are clear. If the offending insect can be identified accurately or if there is a significant difference in the degree of skin test reactivity, knowledge of these cross-reactions should lead to single-venom therapy whenever possible, despite the presence of multiple positive skin test reactions. This is particularly true in children in whom the administration of a single venom is much better tolerated than the administration of three or four venoms.

Bumblebees, which are solitary bees, are rare causes of insect sting reactions. Recently, however, exposure to bumblebees has become a potential occupational hazard because of their use in greenhouses for pollination. Bumblebee venom is not commercially available at the present for diagnosis and treatment. People who have had allergic reactions to bumblebee stings should be tested with honeybee venom but may not react because of sensitivity to an allergen specific to the bumblebee venom.[42] If skin test reactions to honeybee venom are positive, it can be used for immunotherapy. In an excellent review, deGrout[43] has postulated that there are two categories of patients with bumblebee venom sensitivity. There are people initially sensitized to honeybee venom who then react to bumblebee venom due to cross-reactive allergens. Honeybee venom should be effective immunotherapy. The second group consists of people primarily sensitized to bumblebee venom as the result of frequent exposure and stings. Immunotherapy with honeybee venom is not effective; bumblebee venom is needed.

Immunotherapy with whole body fire ant extract appears to be quite effective. Since this extract is a good diagnostic agent, a good therapeutic response could be anticipated. One study that compared the results of fire ant re-stings in whole body extract-treated patients and untreated patients confirmed the effectiveness of treatment.[44] In the treatment group, there were 47 re-stings with one systemic reaction in contrast to the 11 untreated control patients, in whom 11 re-stings in 6 patients all resulted in systemic reactions.

Allergic reactions to fire ant stings are more common in children and have been reported in children as young as 15 to 39 months old.[45] As mentioned earlier,[30] little data are available for children who have had cutaneous allergic reactions only, but what there is does suggest that they could be managed with the availability of emergency medication.

Dosing Schedule

VIT is administered in a manner similar to other forms of immunotherapy (Tables 60-2 and 60-3). Treatment is initiated in small doses, usually from 0.01 to 0.1 µg, and incremental doses are given until the maintenance dose is reached, traditionally 100 µg. The selection of a starting dose is really based on the intensity of the skin test reaction rather than on the nature of the allergic symptoms. A number of dosing regimens have been suggested. A commonly used schedule suggests the use of two or three injections during weekly build-up phases with doses doubled or tripled at 30-minute intervals. Maintenance doses can then be reached in 4 to 6 weeks. Rush desensitization therapy has also been given with multiple doses administered, often in a hospital setting, over a period of 2 or 3 days to 1 week. The more rapid schedules appear to be accompanied by a more rapid increase in venom-specific IgG. A slower schedule used for other types of allergen immunotherapy is the weekly administration of a single-venom dose. Reported immunotherapy reaction rates with both rapid and slower schedules vary but are not significantly different. The critical issue is to reach the top maintenance dose.

Once the top maintenance dose is reached, it can be administered every 4 weeks during the first year. The maintenance interval can then be extended to 6 weeks after the first year and to 8 weeks after the second year. This has been done with no loss of clinical effectiveness or increase in reaction rate. Further studies indicate that the interval can be extended to 3 months with no difficulty,[46] but a 6-month dosing interval does not provide adequate protection.[47] The top maintenance dose for a single venom is 100 µg; 50 µg has been given as the top dose with good results.[41] A mixed vespid venom preparation that contains the two hornet venoms and yellow jacket venom is available for therapy. The top dose of this preparation is 300 µg.

Venom Immunotherapy Reactions

VIT may cause reactions similar to those induced by other types of allergenic extracts. These reactions may pose a more difficult clinical problem because to ensure protection, it is necessary to

Table 60-2 General Venom Immunotherapy Dosing Guidelines

Initial dose	Dose of 0.01 to 0.1 µg, depending on degree of skin test reaction
Incremental doses	Schedules vary from 'rush' therapy, administering multiple venom injections over several days, usually in a hospital setting, to traditional once-weekly injections (see Table 60-3)
Maintenance dose	Doses of 50 to 100 µg of single venoms, 300 µg of mixed vespid venom
Maintenance interval	4 wks 1st yr 6 wks 2nd yr 8 wks 3rd yr Can be extended after 3rd year (see text)
Duration of therapy	Stop if skin test becomes negative and serum venom specific IgE is undetectable (FEIA) or if the finite time, 3 to 5 years, has been reached (see text)

Table 60-3 Representative Examples of Venom Immunotherapy Dosing Schedules*

	Traditional	Modified Rush	Rush
Day			
1	0.1	0.1	0.1[†]
		0.3	0.3
		0.6	0.6
			1.0
			3.0
			6.0
			15.0
2			30.0
			50.0[‡]
			75.0
3			100.0
Week			
1	0.3	1.0	
		3.0	
		6.0	
2	0.6	10.0	100
		15.0	Repeat every 4 wks
3	1.0	30.0	
4	3.0	40.0	
5	6.0	50.0[‡]	
6	15.0	65.0	
7	30.0	80.0	
8	50.0[‡]	100.0	
9	65.0		
10	80.0	100.0	
11	100.0	Repeat every 4 wks	
12			
13	100.0		
	Repeat every 4 wks		

*Starting dose may vary depending on patient's skin test sensitivity. Subsequent doses modified by local or systemic reactions. Doses expressed in micrograms.
[†]Sequential venom doses administered on same day at 20- to 30-minute intervals.
[‡]Fifty micrograms may be used as top dose.

administer maximum venom doses. Reduction of doses, as done with other forms of allergenic extracts, may not be clinically effective. Fortunately, reactions to VIT are uncommon, and the majority of individuals are able to reach maintenance doses.

Large Local Reactions

Venoms are intrinsically irritating and cause pain at the injection site. Local swelling may occur and can cause considerable morbidity. Several approaches are available to minimize these reactions. The venom dose can be split into two injections, thus limiting the amount of venom delivered at one site. The addition of a small amount of epinephrine with the venom may minimize the immediate local swelling. If the swelling is extensive and particularly delayed in onset, the addition of a small amount of steroid with the venom usually effectively inhibits this large local reaction. Administration of an antihistamine 30 to 60 minutes before the venom injection may also be beneficial.

Systemic Reactions

Systemic reactions to VIT are unusual and much less common than those induced by pollen immunotherapy. After a reaction, the next dose is usually reduced approximately 25%, and subsequent doses are slowly increased. If individuals are receiving multiple venoms, it might be advisable to administer single venoms on separate days.

The concomitant administration of β-adrenergic blocking drugs can increase the severity of anaphylaxis. For this reason, allergen immunotherapy, which always has a risk of causing anaphylaxis, should not be given to people taking beta blockers. Venom allergy is a more complex issue as VIT is a remarkably effective treatment for prevention of anaphylaxis. A study by Müller and Haeberli addressed this concern.[48] The systemic allergic reaction rate from VIT was compared in patients with cardiovascular disease who were receiving beta blockers with patients who were not taking beta blockers. No difference was found. These findings support the clinical impression that if beta blocker treatment is needed and cannot be discontinued, VIT can be safely administered. A slower build-up dosing schedule and longer observation period after venom injections are prudent.

ACE inhibitors also have been suggested as potentially exacerbating the severity of allergic reactions[49] and one report has recommended that patients omit their ACE inhibitor medications for 24 hours before receiving VIT. The author does not believe that current evidence supports stopping or withholding these medications.

Pretreatment with H1 antihistamines did reduce the systemic allergic side-effects from the honeybee venom immunotherapy administered in an ultra rush regimen.[50] The study was done in adults. An increased efficacy of antihistamine pretreatment as measured by sting challenges was not found, although potentially beneficial immunologic responses were found in the antihistamine pretreatment patients. Honeybee venom as compared to vespid venoms and the ultra rush regimen as compared to the modified rush regimen, are associated with a higher incidence of systemic reactions during the build-up phase. The author does not recommend routine pretreatment with antihistamines, but for selected patients with more extreme side effects, antihistamine pretreatment could be considered.

Generalized Fatigue

Another reaction occasionally noted after injections of other allergenic extracts such as mold and dust, but more frequently venom, is the occurrence of generalized fatigue and aching, sometimes associated with large local swelling. Successful treatment of this reaction is usually accomplished with the administration of aspirin approximately 30 minutes before the injection and every 4 hours thereafter for 1 to 2 days, if needed. If symptoms are severe, steroids such as prednisone administered daily for several days can be helpful.

Other Reactions

There have been no identified adverse reactions caused by long-term VIT. Injections appear to be safe during pregnancy with no effect on the pregnancy or the fetus.

Monitoring of Venom Immunotherapy

VIT is associated initially with increasing titers of serum venom-specific IgG, occasionally increasing and subsequently decreasing titers of serum venom-specific IgE, and a highly successful clinical response. A minority of individuals will develop negative venom skin tests while receiving VIT. As described later, this is one criterion for stopping treatment. Repeat venom skin tests approximately every 2 years are recommended. In a study of 62 children,[51] 28 developed a negative venom skin test to one or more venoms after 3 years of VIT. However, only two children converted to negative tests with all treatment venoms.

Stimulation of venom-specific IgG has been associated with clinical immunity to insect stings. For individual patients, however, there is no absolute titer that is directly related to successful treatment. In my opinion, the overall success rate of VIT and review of relative data do not support the routine measurement of venom-specific IgG.[52,53]

Results

VIT is highly effective in preventing subsequent anaphylaxis in individuals at risk. Repeat anaphylaxis occurs in only about 2–5% of people treated following re-stings.[54] In the author's experience with children and adults,[41] 258 re-stings in 108 people led to three systemic reactions (2.7% per patient, 1.2% per re-sting). Graft and colleagues[55] reported that during a 3- to 6-year period, 200 re-stings in 49 VIT-treated children resulted in only four mild systemic reactions (98% efficacy). Another study of children receiving bee VIT reported five reactors in 55 children after field re-stings.[56]

VIT treatment significantly improves quality-of-life issues for patients and family compared with recommended treatment with epinephrine availability only.[57]

Patients with systemic mastocytosis are at risk for more severe anaphylaxis. Venom immunotherapy is very effective treatment for people with systemic mastocytosis who have had allergic reactions from insect stings and have detectable venom specific IgE.[58] VIT is not recommended in the absence of venom specific IgE.

Treatment Failures

VIT is very effective, protecting approximately 98% of treated people. If a re-sting reaction does occur, it is initially advisable to determine whether the appropriate venom has been administered. Culprit insect identification is important and repeat testing may be necessary to verify specific venom sensitivity. If the specific treatment is correct, then the venom dose should be increased by 50% to 100%. For example, if the maintenance dose is 100 μg, it should be increased to 150 or 200 μg. Increasing the venom dose has been shown to be highly effective, preventing subsequent re-sting reactions.[59]

Duration of Therapy

The question of duration of treatment or when it is safe to discontinue VIT has been a persistent issue (Box 60-1). Several criteria have been suggested as reliable guidelines: these include conversion to a negative venom skin test, a fall in serum venom-specific IgE to undetectable levels, and a finite period of treatment (3 to 5 years), regardless of the persistence of skin test reactivity or serum antibody.

BOX 60-1

Venom Immunotherapy: When to Stop

Suggested criteria for stopping venom immunotherapy

Conversion to a negative venom skin test and undetectable serum venom specific IgE

Persistence of positive venom skin test: 3 to 5 years of therapy

Factors that may influence decision to stop therapy

Severe anaphylactic symptoms, such as loss of consciousness, caused by insect sting

Systemic reactions to venom immunotherapy

Unchanged venom skin test sensitivity during venom immunotherapy

Honeybee venom allergy (compared with vespid venom allergy)

Presence of significant medical problems, such as cardiovascular disease

Access to emergency medical care

A position statement from the Insect Committee of the American Academy of Allergy, Asthma and Immunology has addressed this issue,[60] and these conclusions are supported by published studies.[61-63] These data strongly suggest that conversion to a negative venom skin test and absence of detectable venom-specific IgE are an absolute criterion for stopping VIT.[62-64] However, there have been several anecdotal reports of people who continue to have allergic reactions to insect stings, apparently despite the presence of negative venom skin tests, which suggest the need for continuous monitoring of this guideline.

It appears that 3 to 5 years of VIT is adequate for the large majority of individuals who have had mild to moderate anaphylactic reactions, despite the persistence of a positive skin test.[60-64] The re-sting reaction rate after cessation of VIT is low, generally in the range of 5–10%. People who have had severe anaphylactic symptoms such as hypotension, laryngeal edema, or loss of consciousness have a higher risk of repeated severe systemic reactions if therapy is discontinued. For this reason, the author currently recommends that individuals who have had severe symptoms and retain positive venom skin tests receive VIT indefinitely, which at this point, can be administered every 8 to 12 weeks. Other suggested risk factors that have been associated with the occurrence of re-sting reactions after cessation of VIT include systemic reactions to VIT, persistence of significant skin test reactivity, and honeybee venom allergy compared with vespid venom allergy. These decisions regarding the cessation of therapy also should include consideration of other medical problems, concomitant medication, patient lifestyle and patient preference.

Conclusions

Insect sting anaphylaxis is a relatively common problem, estimated to affect at least 0.3–3% of the population and responsible for at least 40 deaths per year in the USA (see Boxes 60-2 and 60-3). The allergic reactions are mediated by IgE antibodies directed at constituents in insect venoms. In addition, increasing numbers of reactions occur from fire ant stings and nonwinged Hymenopterans present in the southeastern USA and slowly extending westward. Anaphylactic symptoms are typical of those occurring from any cause. The majority of reactions in children are mild and frequently only dermal (hives, angioedema).

BOX 60-2 Key concepts

Differential Diagnoses: Reaction to Insect Stings

- Insect stings always cause pain at the sting site associated with some swelling and erythema.
- Large local reactions from insect stings tend to recur after subsequent re-stings, with little risk of developing anaphylaxis.
- Many simultaneous stings (50 to 100) may sensitize a person for risk of subsequent single sting-induced anaphylaxis.
- Unusual reactions, usually involving neurologic or vascular pathology, have occurred in a temporal relationship to insect stings.
- No absolute criteria predict the occurrence of initial venom-induced anaphylaxis. Serious anaphylactic reactions may occur at any age; fatalities are more common in adults.

BOX 60-3 Key concepts

Evaluation and Management

- Approximately 60% or less of people who have had an anaphylactic reaction from an insect sting and have positive venom skin tests will have another reaction to a subsequent resting.
- The risk of a resting reaction is related to age and severity of the initial reaction. Resting reactions are more likely to occur in adults than in children and in people who have had more severe reactions.
- The venom skin test is the preferred diagnostic test to detect potential insect sting allergy. The fluorescent-enzyme-linked immunoassay (FEIA), for measurement of serum venom-specific IgE, is indicated when the skin test cannot be done or the reaction is equivocal.
- People at risk for insect sting anaphylaxis should (1) be educated regarding measures to avoid stings, (2) carry emergency medication, particularly epinephrine, and (3) be advised to receive venom immunotherapy.

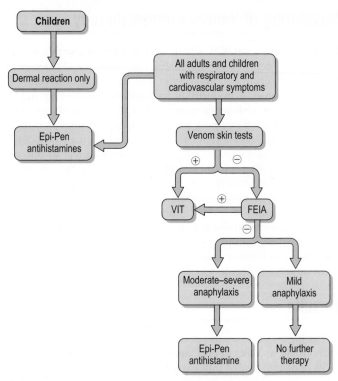

FIGURE 60-4 Evaluation and management of the history of insect sting anaphylaxis. *VIT*, venom immunotherapy; *FEIA*, radioallergosorbent test.

The more severe reactions, such as shock and loss of consciousness, can occur at any age but are relatively more common in adults. Following insect sting anaphylaxis, about 50% of unselected individuals will continue to have allergic reactions to subsequent stings. The natural history of the disease process is influenced by the severity of the anaphylactic symptoms. Children with dermal reactions have only a benign course and are unlikely to have recurrent reactions. (Figure 60-4 illustrates a clinical algorithm of evaluation and management of insect sting anaphylaxis.) Individuals with more severe reactions are more likely to have recurrent anaphylaxis. Individuals with a history of insect sting anaphylaxis and positive venom skin tests should have epinephrine available and are candidates for subsequent VIT, which provides almost 100% protection against subsequent re-sting reactions. Recommendations for the duration of VIT are still evolving. VIT therapy can be stopped if skin test reactions become negative and serum venom specific IgE is undetectable. For most individuals, 3 to 5 years of therapy appears adequate despite the persistence of these positive tests. Individuals who have had life-threatening reactions, such as loss of consciousness, and retain positive venom skin tests should receive VIT indefinitely.

References

1. Barnard JH. Studies of 400 Hymenoptera sting deaths in the United States. J Allergy Clin Immunol 1973;52:259-64.
2. Golden DB, Kagey-Sobotka A, Norman PS, et al. Insect sting allergy with negative venom skin test responses. J Allergy Clin Immunol 2001;107:897-901.
3. Reisman RE. Insect sting allergy: the dilemma of the negative skin test reactor. J Allergy Clin Immunol 2001;107:781-2.
4. Ludolph-Hauser D, Rueff F, Fries C, et al. Constitutively raised serum concentrations of masT cell tryptase and severe anaphylactic reactions to Hymenoptera stings. Lancet 2001;357:361-2.
5. Reisman RE. Natural history of insect sting allergy: relationship of severity of symptoms of initial sting anaphylaxis to resting reactions. J Allergy Clin Immunol 1992;90:335-9.
6. Reisman RE, Osur SL. Allergic reactions following first insect sting exposure. Ann Allergy 1987;59:429-32.
7. Mauriello PM, Barde SH, Georgitis JW, et al. Natural history of large local reactions from stinging insects. J Allergy Clin Immunol 1984;74:494-8.
8. McKenna WR. Killer bees: what the allergist should know. Pediatr Asthma Allergy Immunol 1992;4:275-85.
9. Chaffee FH. The prevalence of bee sting allergy in an allergic population. Acta Allergol 1970;25:292-3.
10. Settipane GA, Boyd GK. Prevalence of bee sting allergy in 4,992 boy scouts. Acta Allergol 1970;25:286-91.
11. Golden DB. Epidemiology of allergy to insect venoms and stings. Allergy Proc 1989;10:103-7.
12. Lockey RF, Turkeltaub PC, Baird-Warren IA, et al. The Hymenoptera venom study, I, 1979-82: demographics and history-sting data. J Allergy Clin Immunol 1988;82:370-381.
13. Kemp SF, deShazo RD, Moffitt JE, et al. Expanding habitat of the imported fire ant (*Solenopsis invicta*): a public health concern. J Allergy Clin Immunol 2000;105:683-91.
14. Stafford CT. Hypersensitivity to fire ant venom. Ann Allergy Asthma Immunol 1996;77:87-95.
15. Simons F, Simons R, Peng Z. Mosquito allergy in monograph on Insect allergy. American Academy of Allergy Asthma and Immunology. Levine MI, Lockey RF, editors. Pittsburgh: Dave Lambert Associates; 2003.
16. Graft DF, Schuberth KC, Kagey-Sobotka A, et al. A prospective study of the natural history of large local reactions after Hymenoptera stings in children. J Pediatr 1984;104:664-8.

17. Hamilton RG, Golden DB, Kagey-Sobotka A, et al. Case report of venom immunotherapy for a patient with large local reactions. Ann Allergy Asthma Immunol 2001;87:134-7.

18. Golden DBK, Kelly D, Hamilton RG, et al. Venom immunotherapy reduces large local reactions to insect stings. J Allergy Clin Immunol 2009;123:1371-5.

19. Severino MG, Cortellini GC, Bonadonna P, et al. Sublingual immunotherapy for large local reactions caused by honeybee sting: a double-blind, placebo controlled trial. J Allergy Clin Immunol 2008;122:44-8.

20. Light WC, Reisman RE, Shimizu M, et al. Unusual reactions following insect stings: clinical features and immunologic analysis. J Allergy Clin Immunol 1977;59:391-7.

21. Reisman RE, Livingston A. Late-onset allergic reactions, including serum sickness, after insect stings. J Allergy Clin Immunol 1989;84:331-7.

22. Golden DBK, Lichtenstein LM. Insect sting allergy. In: Kaplan AP, editor. Allergy. New York: Churchill Livingstone; 1985.

23. Lantner R, Reisman RE. Clinical and immunologic features and subsequent course of patients with severe insect-sting anaphylaxis. J Allergy Clin Immunol 1989;84:900-6.

24. Hunt KJ, Valentine MD, Sobotka AK, et al. A controlled trial of immunotherapy in insect hypersensitivity. N Engl J Med 1978;299:157-61.

25. Blaauw PJ, Smithuis LO. The evaluation of the common diagnostic methods of hypersensitivity for bee and yellow jacket venom by means of an in-hospital insect sting. J Allergy Clin Immunol 1985;75:556-62.

26. Parker JL, Santrach PJ, Dahlberg MJ, et al. Evaluation of Hymenoptera-sting sensitivity with deliberate sting challenges: inadequacy of present diagnostic methods. J Allergy Clin Immunol 1982;69:200-7.

27. van der Linden PW, Hack CE, Struyvenberg A, et al. Insect-sting challenge in 324 subjects with a previous anaphylactic reaction: current criteria for insect-venom hypersensitivity do not predict the occurrence and the severity of anaphylaxis. J Allergy Clin Immunol 1994;94:151-9.

28. Valentine MD, Schuberth KC, Kagey-Sobotka A, et al. The value of immunotherapy with venom in children with allergy to insect stings. N Engl J Med 1990;323:1601-3.

29. Partridge ME, Blackwood W, Hamilton RG, et al. Prevalence of allergic sensitization to imported fire ants in children living in an endemic region of the southeastern United States. Ann Allergy Asthma Immunol 2008;100:54-8.

30. Nguyen SA, Napoli DC. Natural history of large local and generalized cutaneous reactions to imported fire ant stings in children. Ann Allergy Asthma Immunol 2005;94:387-90.

31. Hunt KJ, Valentine MD, Sobotka AK, et al. Diagnosis of allergy to stinging insects by skin testing with Hymenoptera venoms. Ann Intern Med 1976;85:56-9.

32. Chipps BE, Valentine MD, Kagey-Sobotka A, et al. Diagnosis and treatment of anaphylactic reactions to Hymenoptera stings in children. J Pediatr 1980;97:177-84.

33. Barnard JH. Nonfatal results in third-degree anaphylaxis from Hymenoptera stings. J Allergy 1970;45:92-6.

34. Goldberg A, Confino-Cohen R. Insect sting-inflicted systemic reactions: attitudes of patients with insect venom allergy regarding after-sting behavior and proper administration of epinephrine. J Allergy Clin Immunol 2000;106:1184-9.

35. Franken HH, Dubois AE, Minkema HJ, et al. Lack of reproducibility of a single negative sting challenge response in the assessment of anaphylactic risk in patients with suspected yellow jacket hypersensitivity. J Allergy Clin Immunol 1994;93:431-6.

36. Hauk P, Friedl K, Kaufmehl K, et al. Subsequent insect stings in children with hypersensitivity to Hymenoptera. J Pediatr 1995;126:185-90.

37. Mueller U, Elliott W, Reisman RE, et al. Comparison of biochemical and immunologic properties of venoms from the four hornet species. J Allergy Clin Immunol 1981;67:290-8.

38. Reisman RE, Mueller U, Wypych J, et al. Comparison of the allergenicity and antigenicity of yellow jacket and hornet venoms. J Allergy Clin Immunol 1982;69:268-74.

39. Reisman RE, Wypych JI, Mueller UR, et al. Comparison of the allergenicity and antigenicity of Polistes venom and other vespid venoms. J Allergy Clin Immunol 1982;70:281-7.

40. Reisman RE, Muller UR, Wypych JI, et al. Studies of coexisting honeybee and vespid-venom sensitivity. J Allergy Clin Immunol 1984;73:246-52.

41. Reisman RE, Livingston A. Venom immunotherapy: 10 years of experience with administration of single venoms and 50 micrograms maintenance doses. J Allergy Clin Immunol 1992;89:1189-95.

42. Hoffman DR, El-Choufani SE, Smith MM, et al. Occupational allergy to bumblebees: allergens of *Bombus terrestris*. J Allergy Clin Immunol 2001;108:855-60.

43. deGrout H. Allergy to bumblebees. Curr Opin Allergy Clin Immunol 2006;6:294-7.

44. Freeman TM, Hylander R, Ortiz A, et al. Imported fire ant immunotherapy: effectiveness of whole body extracts. J Allergy Clin Immunol 1992;90:210-5.

45. Bahna SL, Strimas JH, Reed MA, et al. Imported fire ant allergy in young children: skin reactivity and serum IgE antibodies to venom and whole body extract. J Allergy Clin Immunol 1988;82:419-24.

46. Goldberg A, Confino-Cohen R. Maintenance venom immunotherapy administered at 3-month intervals is both safe and efficacious. J Allergy Clin Immunol 2001;107:902-6.

47. Goldberg A, Confino-Cohen R. Effectiveness of maintenance bee venom immunotherapy administered at 6-month intervals. Ann Allergy Asthma Immunol 2007;99:352-7.

48. Müller UR, Haeberli G. Use of β-blockers during immunotherapy for Hymenoptera venom allergy. J Allergy Clin Immunol 2005;115:606-10.

49. Ober AI, MacLean JH, Hannaway PJ. Life-threatening anaphylaxis to venom immunotherapy in a patient taking an angiotensin-converting enzyme inhibitor. J Allergy Clin Immunol 2003;112:1008-9.

50. Müller UR, Jutel M, Reimers A, et al. Clinical and immunologic effects of H1 antihistamine preventative medication during honeybee venom immunotherapy. J Allergy Clin Immunol 2008;122:1001-7.

51. Graft DF, Schuberth KC, Kagey-Sobotka A, et al. The development of negative skin tests in children treated with venom immunotherapy. J Allergy Clin Immunol 1984;73:61-8.

52. Golden DB, Lawrence ID, Hamilton RH, et al. Clinical correlation of the venom-specific IgG antibody level during maintenance venom immunotherapy. J Allergy Clin Immunol 1992;90:386-93.

53. Reisman RE. Should routine measurements of serum venom-specific IgG be a standard of practice in patients receiving venom immunotherapy? J Allergy Clin Immunol 1992;90:282-4.

54. Mueller UR. Insect sting allergy. New York: Gustav Fischer Verlag; 1990.

55. Graft DF, Schuberth KC, Kagey-Sobotka A, et al. Assessment of prolonged venom immunotherapy in children. J Allergy Clin Immunol 1987;80:162-9.

56. Gold SG. A six year review of bee venom immunotherapy in children (abstract). J Allergy Clin Immunol 2002;109:S202.

57. Elberink HO, Munchy JD, Guyatt A, et al. Insect venom allergy and the burden of the treatment (BoT): Epipen vs venom immunotherapy (VIT) (abstract). J Allergy Clin Immunol 2002;109:S80.

58. deOlano OG, Alvarez-Twose I, Estaban-Lopez MI, et al. Safety and effectiveness of immunotherapy in patients with indolent systemic mastocytosis presenting with Hymenoptera venom anaphylaxis. J Allergy Clin Immunol 2008;121:519-426.

59. Rueff F, Wenderoth A, Przybilla B. Patients still reacting to a sting challenge while receiving conventional Hymenoptera venom immunotherapy are protected by increased venom doses. J Allergy Clin Immunol 2001;108:1027-32.

60. American Academy of Allergy, Asthma and Immunology Position Statement. The discontinuation of Hymenoptera venom immunotherapy: report from the Committee on Insects. J Allergy Clin Immunol 1998;101:573-5.

61. Golden DB, Kwiterovich KA, Kagey-Sobotka A, et al. Discontinuing venom immunotherapy: extended observations. J Allergy Clin Immunol 1998;101:298-305.

62. Lerch E, Muller UR. Long-term protection after stopping venom immunotherapy: results of restings in 200 patients. J Allergy Clin Immunol 1998;101:606-12.

63. van Halteren HK, van der Linden PW, Burgers JA, et al. Discontinuation of yellow jacket venom immunotherapy: follow-up of 75 patients by means of deliberate sting challenge. J Allergy Clin Immunol 1997;100:767-70.

64. Reisman RE. Duration of venom immunotherapy: relationship to the severity of symptoms of initial insect sting anaphylaxis. J Allergy Clin Immunol 1993;92:831-6.

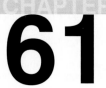

CHAPTER

61

Anaphylaxis: an Overview of Assessment and Management

F. Estelle R. Simons

Introduction

In this chapter, a general overview of anaphylaxis in infants, children and teens, is presented. The areas covered include: epidemiology, mechanisms and triggers, clinical diagnosis, risk assessment, long-term risk reduction in the community, and prevention and management of acute anaphylaxis in the physician's office.[1-4]

Anaphylaxis is currently defined as a serious allergic reaction that is rapid in onset and may cause death.[5] In all age groups, it is considered to be highly likely when any one of three clinical criteria are fulfilled[5] (Box 61-1). Initial signs and symptoms in infants and children with anaphylaxis, even ultimately fatal anaphylaxis, are more likely to involve respiratory distress than circulatory collapse. The presence of reduced blood pressure or shock is not required in order to make the diagnosis. The term anaphylactoid is no longer recommended for use.[1-3,5]

The diagnosis of anaphylaxis potentially leads to disrupted activities, impaired quality of life, psychosocial burdens, and anxiety.[6-10] The impact of anaphylaxis on infants, children, and teens and their families is variable, as assessed by validated instruments that include general health-related quality-of-life questionnaires, age group-specific food- or venom-specific quality-of-life questionnaires, and expectation-of-outcome questionnaires. It ranges from death, the ultimate impact … through severe impact that occasionally leads to referral to a psychologist or a psychiatrist[9] … through moderate or minimal impact … to complete absence of impact if the anaphylaxis is unrecognized or undiagnosed, or if despite accurate diagnosis, there is denial of the possibility of recurrence of anaphylaxis (Figure 61-1).

The impact of anaphylaxis can be reduced by appropriate risk assessment and appropriate long-term risk reduction measures.[6-10] The aim of these measures is to achieve a state of minimal impact for patients and care-givers, in which they are aware of the risk of anaphylaxis, but confident that they are using appropriate risk reduction measures and that they are prepared to manage an anaphylaxis episode if preventive measures fail.

Epidemiology of Anaphylaxis

The true rate of occurrence of anaphylaxis from all triggers in the general pediatric population is unknown. Population-based estimates of anaphylaxis in the community are difficult to evaluate because of use of different anaphylaxis case definitions and different measures of occurrence, such as incidence or prevalence; however, the rate of occurrence of anaphylaxis appears to be increasing, especially in the first two decades of life.[11-17] In a retrospective, population-based study, the incidence rate of anaphylaxis doubled from 21 per 100000 person years in the 1980s to 49.8 per 100000 person years in the 1990s.[13] The highest incidence rate (70 per 100000 person years) was reported in those who were 0.8 to 19 years of age. Similar results have been reported in other studies.[15-17] In addition, most of the case series of anaphylaxis fatalities in the general population include teens, children, and infants.[17-21]

Mechanisms of Anaphylaxis

In the pediatric population, the underlying pathologic mechanism in anaphylaxis usually involves immunoglobulin E (IgE), high-affinity IgE receptors (FcεR1 receptors), mast cells, basophils, and release of cytokines, chemokines, and chemical mediators of inflammation such as histamine and tryptase[1-3,22] (Figure 61-2). Less commonly other immunologic mechanisms are implicated.[2] IgG-mediated anaphylaxis has been reported in humans after administration of dextran or monoclonal antibodies such as infliximab.[23] Activation of the contact system through the prekallikrein-kallikrein pathway, leading to generation of the potent vasoactive mediator bradykinin, and activation of the complement cascade, leading to generation of the anaphylatoxins C3a and C5a have also been reported.[24] Nonimmunologic activation of mast cells by physical factors such as exercise, or exposure to cold air or cold water, or ingestion of medications such as opioids may also trigger anaphylaxis.[1,2,22]

Regardless of the mechanism, mast cells and basophils play an important role in initiating and amplifying the acute response. Activation of tyrosine kinases and calcium influx results in rapid release of granule-associated preformed mediators such as histamine, tryptase, and carboxypeptidase A3. Activation of phospholipase A2, cyclo-oxygenases, and lipoxygenases leads to production of arachidonic acid metabolites, including prostaglandins and leukotrienes, and to synthesis of platelet-activating factor. In addition, numerous cytokines and chemokines are synthesized and released.[22]

©2010 Elsevier Ltd, Inc, BV
DOI: 10.1016/B978-1-4377-0271-2.00061-4

Clinical Criteria for Anaphylaxis

Anaphylaxis is highly likely when any *one* of the following three criteria is fulfilled:

1. Acute onset of an illness (minutes to several hours) with involvement of the skin, mucosal tissue, or both (e.g. generalized hives, pruritus or flushing, swollen lips-tongue-uvula)

   And at least one of the following:

   – Respiratory compromise (e.g. dyspnea, wheeze-bronchospasm, stridor, reduced PEF, hypoxemia)

   – Reduced BP* or associated symptoms of end-organ dysfunction (e.g. hypotonia [collapse], syncope, incontinence)

2. Two or more of the following that occur rapidly after exposure to a *likely allergen for that patient* (minutes to several hours):

   – Involvement of the skin-mucosal tissue (e.g. generalized hives, itch-flush, swollen lips-tongue-uvula)

   – Respiratory compromise (e.g. dyspnea, wheeze-bronchospasm, stridor, reduced PEF, hypoxemia)

   – Reduced BP* or associated symptoms (e.g. hypotonia [collapse], syncope, incontinence)

   – Persistent gastrointestinal symptoms (e.g. crampy abdominal pain, vomiting)

3. Reduced BP* after exposure to *known allergen for that patient* (minutes to several hours):

   – Infants and children: low systolic BP* (age-specific) or > 30% decrease in systolic BP*

   – Adults: systolic BP* of <90 mm Hg or >30% decrease from that person's baseline

---

PEF, peak expiratory flow; *BP*, blood pressure.
*Low systolic blood pressure for children is defined as less than 70 mm Hg from 1 month to 1 year, and less than (70 mm Hg + [2 × age in years]) from 1 to 10 years.
(Adapted from Sampson HA, Munoz-Furlong A, Campbell RL, et al. J Allergy Clin Immunol 2006;117:391–397.)

Triggers of Anaphylaxis

In the pediatric population, based on surveys[4,25] and surveillance studies, food is by far the most common trigger of anaphylaxis. Peanut, tree nuts, shellfish, finned fish, milk, and egg, are the predominant food triggers in many countries, however, there are important geographic variations; for example, sesame or peach are predominant triggers in some countries. Potential food triggers include: substituted, cross-reacting, or cross-contacting foods; additives such as spices and colorants; foods previously unrecognized as allergens; contaminants such as storage mites in flour; and food parasites such as the nematode *Anisakis simplex* in fish[1,25–35] (Box 61-2, Figure 61-2).

Other triggers include venom from stinging insects such as bees, yellow jackets, wasps, hornets, and fire ants, and rarely, saliva from biting insects such as mosquitoes and caterpillars.[25–30,36–38] Medication triggers include antibiotics such as penicillins and cephalosporins, nonsteroidal antiinflammatory drugs (NSAIDs) such as ibuprofen, antineoplastic agents such as L-asparaginase, and newly recognized triggers such as loperamide and oversulfated chondroitin sulfate contaminants in heparin.[25–30,39–42] Anaphylaxis in the perioperative period is most commonly triggered by suxamethonium and other neuromuscular blockers/muscle relaxants, but any inhaled, injected, or topically applied agent can be implicated in this setting.[26–31,43] Although natural rubber latex in medical equipment and supplies is now a less commonly reported trigger than it was in the 1990s,[25] latex-triggered anaphylaxis still occurs in perioperative and other health-care settings, and natural rubber latex found in pacifiers, bottle nipples, toys, balls, balloons, and condoms remains a risk factor in community settings.[25–30,44]

Biologic agents, including monoclonal antibodies such as infliximab and omalizumab,[45,46] and allergens used in skin tests, especially intradermal tests, allergen challenge/provocation tests or allergen-specific immunotherapy by any route,[47,48] are potential anaphylaxis triggers.

Vaccines that protect against infectious diseases seldom trigger anaphylaxis, as documented in the Vaccine Adverse Event Reporting System (VAERS)[23,26–30,49,50] (Box 61-2). If they do, the culprit is not usually the microbial content. Rather, it is likely to be an excipient such as: gelatin, yeast, dextran, polysorbate-80;

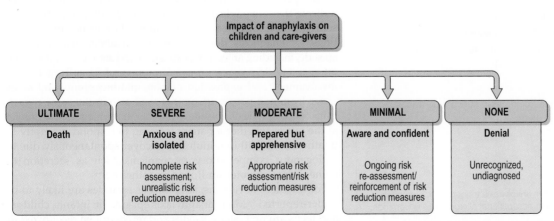

Figure 61-1 The impact of a previous episode of anaphylaxis on infants, children, teens, and their care-givers ranges from the ultimate impact, death, to no impact at all. Careful risk assessment, and implementation of appropriate risk reduction measures helps to minimize the impact of anaphylaxis on children and their care-givers. Risk assessment measures include confirmation of the diagnosis and the trigger(s). Risk reduction measures to prevent anaphylaxis recurrences include avoidance of confirmed triggers, and immunomodulation where appropriate, e.g. venom immunotherapy to prevent stinging insect-triggered anaphylaxis. Emergency preparedness measures include availability of an epinephrine auto-injector at all times, an anaphylaxis emergency action plan, and appropriate medical identification.

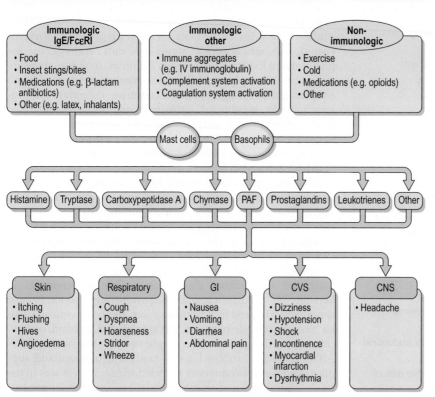

ANAPHYLAXIS PATHOGENESIS

Figure 61-2 Summary of the pathogenesis of anaphylaxis. Details about mechanisms, triggers, key cells and mediators are found in the text. Two or more target organ systems are usually involved concurrently in anaphylaxis. The rare exception, especially in the pediatric population, is isolated hypotension after exposure to a known trigger. (Adapted from Simons FER. J Allergy Clin Immunol 2008; 121:S402–407.)

BOX 61-2

Anaphylaxis Triggers in the Community

Allergen Triggers (IgE-Dependent Immunologic Mechanism)*

Foods, e.g. peanut, tree nut, shellfish, fish, milk, egg

Food additives, e.g. spices, colorants, vegetable gums, and contaminants

Stinging insects: *Hymenoptera* species, e.g. bees, yellow jackets, wasps, hornets, and fire ants

Medications, e.g. beta-lactam antibiotics, ibuprofen

Biologic agents, e.g. monoclonal antibodies (infliximab, omalizumab) and allergens (challenge tests, specific immunotherapy)

Natural rubber latex

Vaccines to prevent infectious diseases

Inhalants (rare), e.g. horse or hamster dander, grass pollen

Previously unrecognized allergens (foods, venoms, biting insect saliva, medications, biologic agents)

Nonimmune Triggers

Physical factors, e.g. exercise,† cold, heat, sunlight/ultraviolet radiation

Medications, e.g. opioids

Ethanol

Idiopathic*

*In the pediatric population, some anaphylaxis triggers, e.g. hormones (progesterone), seminal fluid, and occupational allergens are uncommon, as is idiopathic anaphylaxis.

†Exercise with or without a co-trigger, such as a food or medication, cold air or cold water.

(Adapted from references 1–3 and 31–52.)

---

egg, found in influenza or yellow fever vaccines; or an antimicrobial such as neomycin or polymyxin B.[23,49]

In exercise-induced anaphylaxis, food is a common co-trigger; food-sensitized immune cells may be relatively innocuous until they are redistributed from gut-associated circulatory depots during exercise. Medication such as an NSAID may also be a co-trigger. Concurrent exposure to cold air or cold water can be co-triggers with exercise, or can trigger anaphylaxis independently of exercise.[26–31,51,52]

Clinical Diagnosis of the Acute Anaphylaxis Episode

In the pediatric population, surveys and surveillance studies indicate that anaphylaxis occurs most frequently in community settings, especially in the home, rather than in health-care settings.[25–30] Diagnosis depends on a meticulous history of the episode, including antecedent exposures and activities, and sudden onset and rapid progression of symptoms and signs. Target organ involvement and expression of potential symptoms and signs differ from one person to another, and also in the same person from one anaphylaxis episode to another. It is impossible to predict at the outset whether a patient is going to respond promptly to treatment, die within minutes, or recover spontaneously due to endogenous compensatory mechanisms such as secretion of epinephrine, angiotensin II, and endothelin I.[2,3]

For a variety of reasons, anaphylaxis episodes are likely to be under-reported.[14] Many anaphylaxis episodes in infants, children and teens are first-ever episodes and might not be recognized as such, especially if symptoms are mild and/or transient. Patients who are dyspneic, dysphonic or in shock might not be able to describe their symptoms. Skin symptoms such as itching, and signs such as flushing, urticaria, or angioedema, are helpful in the diagnosis; however, cutaneous involvement is absent or unrecognized in 10–20% of anaphylaxis episodes,[25–30] and it can be missed if itching is not described, or if the patient's skin is not fully examined. Hypotension sometimes goes undocumented if no suitable-size blood pressure cuff is available, or if the initial blood pressure measurement is made after epinephrine administration.

Care-givers might fail to recognize an anaphylaxis episode in a child because they have a neurologic or psychiatric disorder, or because they have ingested medications or chemicals such as ethanol that impair cognition and judgment. Anaphylaxis in a known asthmatic with acute respiratory symptoms might not be recognized if accompanying symptoms such as itching or hives, or dizziness suggestive of impending shock are missed.[3]

Diagnostic dilemmas often involve acute generalized hives, acute asthma, syncope (faint), anxiety/panic attack, and aspiration of a foreign body.[2] Peanuts and tree nuts, in addition to being common triggers of anaphylaxis, account for one third of foreign body aspirations. The differential diagnosis of anaphylaxis also includes excess histamine syndromes, e.g. systemic mastocytosis, urticaria pigmentosa, or clonal mast cell disorder; restaurant (postprandial) syndromes, e.g. scombroid poisoning and monosodium glutamate or sulfite sensitivity; and nonorganic diseases, e.g. vocal cord dysfunction, Munchausen syndrome or Munchausen syndrome by proxy. The so-called flush syndromes are rare in the pediatric age group. The possibility of nonallergic red man syndrome, seizure, stroke, or other forms of shock (hypovolemic, cardiogenic, or septic) should be considered.

Recognition and diagnosis of anaphylaxis presents unique challenges in infants, who cannot describe their symptoms and may have signs that are potentially difficult to interpret because they also occur in healthy infants[53] (Table 61-1). The differential diagnosis of anaphylaxis in infants includes age-related entities such as congenital malformations leading to acute symptoms of obstruction in the respiratory and/or gastrointestinal tracts, and apparent life-threatening event/sudden infant death syndrome[53] (Box 61-3).

Minimal Role of Laboratory Tests in Diagnosing Anaphylaxis in the Pediatric Population

No optimal rapid, sensitive, specific, diagnostic test is available for diagnosing acute anaphylaxis[2,31] (Figure 61-3). Plasma histamine levels are elevated for only 15 to 60 minutes after symptom onset. Special handling of the blood sample is required; specifically, it must be obtained through a large-bore needle, kept cold at all times, centrifuged immediately, and the plasma or serum must be frozen promptly. Histamine and its metabolite N-methylhistamine can also be measured in a 24-hour urine sample.[2,54]

Plasma or serum total tryptase levels (pro,pro', and mature forms of α- and β-tryptases) should be measured from 15 minutes to 3 hours after symptom onset. No special handling of the blood sample is required. Normal tryptase values in children are similar to those reported in adults.[55] Tryptase is seldom elevated in food-induced anaphylaxis,[18] even if the blood sample is

Table 61-1 Symptoms and Signs of Anaphylaxis in Infants

Anaphylaxis Symptoms that Infants Cannot Describe	Anaphylaxis Signs that May be Difficult to Interpret/ Unhelpful in Infants, and Why	Anaphylaxis Signs in Infants
General		
Feeling of warmth, weakness, anxiety, apprehension, impending doom	Nonspecific behavioural changes such as persistent crying, fussing, irritability, fright, suddenly becoming quiet	
Skin/Mucus Membranes		
Itching of lips, tongue, palate, uvula, ears, throat, nose, eyes, etc.; mouth-tingling or metallic taste	Flushing (may also occur with fever, hyperthermia, or crying spells)	Rapid onset of hives (potentially difficult to discern in infants with acute atopic dermatitis; scratching and excoriations will be absent in young infants); angioedema (face, tongue, oropharynx)
Respiratory		
Nasal congestion, throat tightness; chest tightness; shortness of breath	Hoarseness, dysphonia (common after a crying spell); drooling or increased secretions (common in infants)	Rapid onset of coughing, choking, stridor, wheezing, dyspnea, apnea, cyanosis
Gastrointestinal		
Dysphagia, nausea, abdominal pain/ cramping	Spitting up/regurgitation(common after feeds), loose stools (normal in infants, especially if breast-fed); colicky abdominal pain	Sudden, profuse vomiting
Cardiovascular		
Feeling faint, presyncope, dizziness, confusion, blurred vision, difficulty in hearing	Hypotension (need appropriate size blood pressure cuff; low systolic blood pressure for children is defined as less than 70 mm Hg from 1 month to 1 year, and less than (70 mm Hg + [2 × age in yr]) from 1-10 years; tachycardia, defined as >140 beats per minute from 3 months to 2 years, inclusive; loss of bowel and bladder control (ubiquitous in infants)	Weak pulse, arrhythmia, diaphoresis/ sweating, collapse/unconsciousness
Central Nervous System		
Headache	Drowsiness, somnolence (common in infants after feeds)	Rapid onset of unresponsiveness, lethargy, or hypotonia; seizures

(Adapted from Simons FER. J Allergy Clin Immunol 2007;120:537–540.)

BOX 61-3

Differential Diagnosis of Anaphylaxis in Infants

Skin

Acute episode of urticaria, urticaria pigmentosa/mastocytosis, hereditary angioedema

Respiratory (Upper or Lower Respiratory Tract)

Acute onset of symptoms due to obstruction which can be congenital (e.g. laryngeal web, vascular ring, malacias) or acquired (e.g. aspiration of foreign body, croup, bronchiolitis, asthma); asphyxiation/suffocation, breath-holding

Gastrointestinal Tract

Acute onset of symptoms due to obstruction, which can be congenital (e.g. pyloric stenosis, malrotation) or acquired (e.g. intussusception); food protein-induced enterocolitis syndrome

Central Nervous System

Seizure, postictal state, stroke, trauma, child abuse, increased intracranial pressure

Shock

Hypovolemic, cardiogenic, septic

Other

Metabolic disorders

Infectious diseases: pertussis, gastroenteritis, meningitis

Ingestion of: drug overdose, poison, or toxin (e.g. food, chemical, plant)

Munchausen syndrome by proxy

Apparent life-threatening event/sudden infant death syndrome

(Adapted from Simons FER. J Allergy Clin Immunol 2007;120:537–540.)

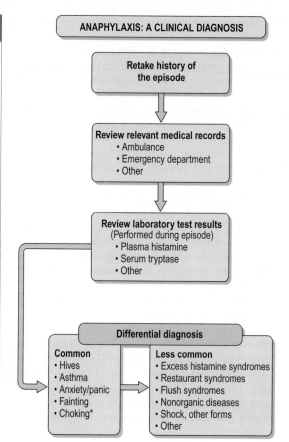

Figure 61-3 Algorithm for confirming the diagnosis of anaphylaxis. Details about the supreme importance of the history, the role of laboratory tests, and the differential diagnosis are found in the text. (Adapted from Simons FER, Frew AJ, Ansotegui IJ, et al. J Allergy Clin Immunol 2007;120:S2–S24.)

obtained in a timely manner, and food is by far the most common trigger in the pediatric population.[26–30] In addition, tryptase is seldom elevated in anaphylaxis episodes characterized chiefly by respiratory symptoms, and respiratory symptoms rather than hypotension or shock are typical of anaphylaxis in the pediatric population. Neither a normal histamine level nor a normal tryptase level can be used to refute the clinical diagnosis of anaphylaxis.[2]

Serial measurements of tryptase levels have been reported to increase the sensitivity and specificity of the test; however, this approach has not yet been studied in the pediatric population. Other potential biomarkers of mast cell activation include measurement of serum mature β-tryptase, mast cell carboxypeptidase A3, platelet-activating factor, bradykinin, and cytokines such as IL-2, IL-6, IL-10, and TNF-receptor I.[2,31,56,57] Some studies of these potential markers that have included children have also included appropriate control groups such as patients with acute asthma,[56] but others have not.[57] Measurement of a panel of different biomarkers might be more useful than measurement of a single biomarker for two reasons: mediators of anaphylaxis are released at different times from activated mast cells and basophils after exposure to the trigger, and patients experiencing anaphylaxis in community settings arrive at the emergency department at different times after symptom onset.[2]

Comorbidities and Concomitant Medications

Severity of concomitant atopic diseases is a predictor of life-threatening allergic reactions.[58] Persistent asthma, especially if not optimally controlled, is an important risk factor for death in young people with anaphylaxis.[18–21] The possibility of systemic mastocytosis or a clonal mast cell disorder should be considered; children with urticaria pigmentosa who have extensive skin involvement, or those with bullous mastocytosis of the skin are at particularly high risk of anaphylaxis, even if no specific trigger for the episode can be identified.[59] Other factors that are potentially implicated in increasing the risk and severity of an anaphylaxis episode include exercise, adverse ambient conditions such as extremes of temperature or humidity, concurrent upper respiratory tract infection or other acute infection, psychologic stress, menses (premenstrual or ovulatory phase), and concurrent use of a medication such as an NSAID. Most of these potential co-factors have not been systematically studied in patients of any age.[2,3,31]

Ingestion of a sedating H_1-antihistamine such as diphenhydramine, or any other central nervous system-active medication or chemical, including recreational drugs and ethanol, potentially impairs recognition of anaphylaxis symptoms and signs by those at risk, or by their care-givers.[3]

Risk Assessment: Confirmation of the Anaphylaxis Trigger

Patients with a history of anaphylaxis benefit from assessment by an appropriately trained and certified allergy/immunology specialist who will take the time required to obtain a meticulous history of the episode as the basis for interpretation of allergen skin tests and serum allergen-specific IgE levels measured using

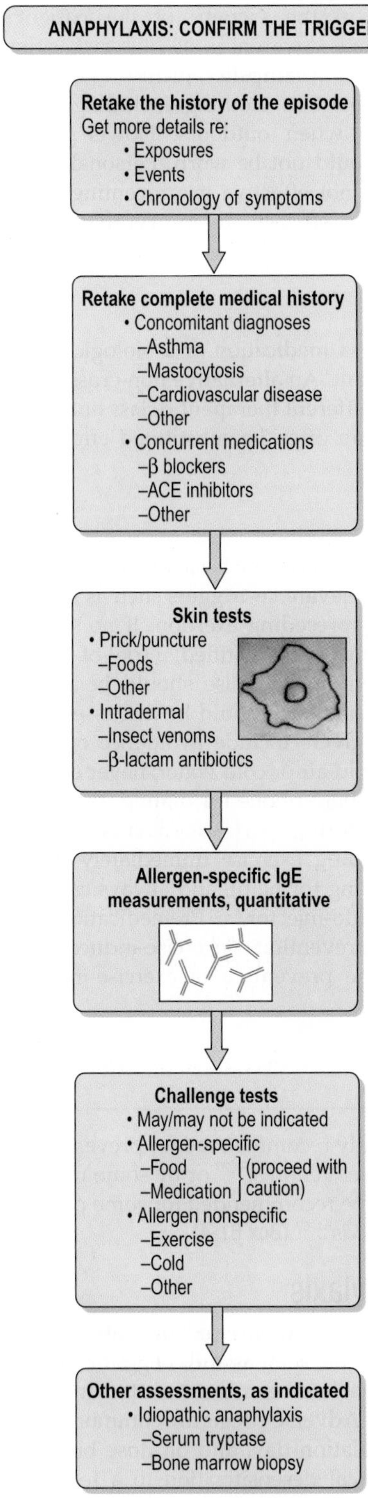

ANAPHYLAXIS: CONFIRM THE TRIGGER

Retake the history of the episode
Get more details re:
- Exposures
- Events
- Chronology of symptoms

Retake complete medical history
- Concomitant diagnoses
  - Asthma
  - Mastocytosis
  - Cardiovascular disease
  - Other
- Concurrent medications
  - β blockers
  - ACE inhibitors
  - Other

Skin tests
- Prick/puncture
  - Foods
  - Other
- Intradermal
  - Insect venoms
  - β-lactam antibiotics

Allergen-specific IgE measurements, quantitative

Challenge tests
- May/may not be indicated
- Allergen-specific
  - Food ⎤ (proceed with
  - Medication ⎦ caution)
- Allergen nonspecific
  - Exercise
  - Cold
  - Other

Other assessments, as indicated
- Idiopathic anaphylaxis
  - Serum tryptase
  - Bone marrow biopsy

Figure 61-4 Algorithm for confirming the anaphylaxis trigger. Details about the importance of the history, and about skin testing and specific IgE measurements to determine allergen sensitization are found in the text. In some patients, physician-monitored challenge tests are needed to determine the clinical relevance of sensitization. (Adapted from Simons FER, Frew AJ, Ansotegui IJ, et al. J Allergy Clin Immunol 2007;120:S2–S24.)

a quantitative test such as ImmunoCap (Pharmacia Diagnostics, Upsala, Sweden)[2,31,60] (Figure 61-4). Standardized allergen extracts are preferred for skin testing; however, they are not commercially available for most common allergens that potentially trigger anaphylaxis, such as foods, fire ant venom, biting insect saliva, medications, and natural rubber latex.[2] Allergen-specific IgE levels

obtained using different immunoassays are not necessarily equivalent, and this can potentially affect management decisions.[60]

Although a positive skin test and/or an increased serum IgE level to a specific allergen document sensitization to that allergen, these tests are not diagnostic of anaphylaxis because sensitization to one or more allergens is extremely common in the general pediatric population. For example, 50–60% of teenagers in the general population have a positive test to one or more foods; yet most of them are unlikely to experience anaphylaxis. Moreover, although children with strongly positive skin test responses to the allergen and/or high levels of allergen-specific IgE in serum have an increased probability of clinical reactivity to the allergen, the degree of positivity of these tests does not necessarily predict the severity of, or risk of fatality in, future anaphylaxis episodes.[2,61]

In some patients, physician-monitored challenge tests are needed to determine the clinical relevance of positive allergen skin tests or allergen-specific IgE levels. Challenges should be conducted in an appropriately equipped health-care facility staffed by professionals who are trained and experienced in selecting patients, conducting the challenge tests, and in recognizing and treating anaphylaxis.[2]

Pediatric patients with a convincing history of anaphylaxis to a specific food and evidence of sensitization to that food should not undergo oral food challenge/provocation tests because of the high risk of anaphylaxis from such tests. The caveat 'First, do no harm' should be kept in mind. Others, for example, those with an equivocal history and minimal evidence of sensitization might benefit from an oral food challenge test. A positive (failed) challenge provides a sound basis for continued avoidance of the food. A negative (passed) challenge allows introduction or re-introduction of the specific food into the diet. An extensive review of oral food challenge testing has recently been published.[2,62]

Eventually, the need for potentially risky challenge tests might diminish, because in vitro tests are being developed to distinguish reliably between sensitization and risk, i.e. between patients who are sensitized yet clinically tolerant to an allergen, and those who are sensitized but at risk of anaphylaxis from an allergen. Potentially useful tests include: assessment of sensitization by using recombinant or dialyzed allergens, basophil activation markers, peptide microarray-based immunoassays to map IgE and IgG$_4$ binding to sequential allergen epitopes, and assessment of allergen-specific cytokine or chemokine production.[2,31]

Idiopathic anaphylaxis is uncommon in the pediatric population. Before making this diagnosis, physicians should ensure that: (1) a hidden or previously unrecognized trigger of anaphylaxis has not been missed,[23,24,31,33–35,37,38,41,45,46,48,50] and (2) a comorbidity such as mastocytosis, urticaria pigmentosa, or a clonal mast cell disorder has not been missed.[59]

Long-Term Risk Reduction: Preventive Measures

Long-term risk reduction measures are an important strategy in preventing anaphylaxis and decreasing the impact of anaphylaxis. These preventive measures include trigger avoidance, immunomodulation, optimal management of asthma and other comorbidities, and preparation for recurrence of anaphylaxis[1,5,31,32,36,39,63–69] (Figure 61-5). Except where noted, recommendations for prevention of anaphylaxis are based on expert opinion and consensus, rather than on randomized controlled trials.

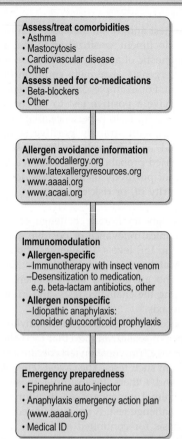

Long-Term Risk Reduction (Community Settings)

Assess/treat comorbidities
• Asthma
• Mastocytosis
• Cardiovascular disease
• Other
Assess need for co-medications
• Beta-blockers
• Other

Allergen avoidance information
• www.foodallergy.org
• www.latexallergyresources.org
• www.aaaai.org
• www.acaai.org

Immunomodulation
• **Allergen-specific**
  – Immunotherapy with insect venom
  – Desensitization to medication,
    e.g. beta-lactam antibiotics, other
• **Allergen nonspecific**
  – Idiopathic anaphylaxis:
    consider glucocorticoid prophylaxis

Emergency preparedness
• Epinephrine auto-injector
• Anaphylaxis emergency action plan
  (www.aaaai.org)
• Medical ID

Figure 61-5 Summary of the approach to long-term risk reduction. Optimal management of comorbidities such as asthma decreases the risk of severe or fatal anaphylaxis. Avoidance measures are allergen-specific. Immunomodulation is currently used for those at risk for anaphylaxis from insect stings, for some medications, and for those with frequent episodes of idiopathic anaphylaxis. ID, medical identification (e.g. bracelet, wallet card). (Adapted from Simons FER. J Allergy Clin Immunol 2008;121:S402–407.)

Avoidance of Specific Triggers

Written or printed, personalized information about avoidance of specific trigger(s) should be provided and reviewed at regular intervals.[31]

Food

Complete avoidance of exposure to some foods such as milk, egg, or peanut is easier said than done and is easier done than maintained over years or decades. Unintentional exposures are common.[63] The constant vigilance required to avoid hidden, cross-contacting, and cross-reacting food triggers every day, year-round, potentially has a negative effect on the quality of life for those at risk for anaphylaxis episodes and for their care-givers.[6-8]

The Food Allergy and Anaphylaxis Network (*www.foodallergy.org*) is a reliable source of up-to-date, consistent, practical information. For pediatric patients with multiple dietary restrictions necessitated by confirmed food allergies, a licensed nutritionist can provide helpful information about essential nutrients, basic food groups, and relevant food substitutes and recipe adaptations.[32]

Stinging Insects

For anaphylaxis triggered by stinging insects, avoidance of exposure involves several approaches. Yellow jacket or wasp nests or fire ant mounds in the vicinity of the patient's home should be exterminated. Awareness of high-risk situations, such as open food sources at campsites, picnics, or outdoor barbecues, is important. Protective clothing including shoes and socks should be worn when outdoors. Flower-printed clothing and floral scents should not be worn. Personal insect repellents such as DEET are not effective in preventing insect stings, in contrast to their efficacy in preventing insect bites.[36]

Medication

For anaphylaxis triggered by a medication or a biologic agent, avoidance is critically important. An alternative non-cross-reacting agent, preferably from a different therapeutic class but sometimes from the same class, can often be substituted effectively and safely.[39]

Exercise

For anaphylaxis triggered by exercise, the basic preventive strategy consists of avoidance of relevant co-triggers such as food or medication for several hours preceding exertion. If no specific food or medication co-trigger can be identified, a trial of fasting for 4 to 6 hours before strenuous exercise should be recommended. Additional precautions that should be discussed with those at risk and their care-givers include avoidance of other relevant co-triggers such as cold air or cold water; never exercising alone; carrying a cell (mobile) phone for dialing 911/emergency medical services (EMS) during sports such as cross-country running or skiing, discontinuing exercise immediately if any symptom develops (not running for help), and always carrying one or more epinephrine auto-injector/s. Premedication and warm-up are less effective in prevention of exercise-induced anaphylaxis than they are in the prevention of exercise-induced bronchospasm.[3,31]

Immunomodulation

Immunomodulation is currently recommended for prevention of anaphylaxis triggered by insect venoms,[36,70] or by some medications.[39] In the future, it might be recommended for some patients with food-triggered anaphylaxis[64-69] (Box 61-4).

Food-Triggered Anaphylaxis

In carefully selected and carefully monitored patients, clinical desensitization to a specific food such as milk, egg, or peanut presented to the oral mucosa has been documented in randomized controlled trials.[32,64-66] Adverse effects are common, especially on the initial dose-escalation day, and on dose build-up days.[67] In some studies, clinical desensitization to a food has been accompanied by long-term immunologic changes.[32,64-66] Food desensitization is currently a research procedure, and because of safety concerns, it should be conducted only in appropriately equipped centers specializing in food allergy research, by physicians who are trained and experienced in diagnosing and treating anaphylaxis.[32,64-67]

Treatments that are not specific for a particular food allergen also appear promising. Food Allergy Herbal Formula-2 (FAHF-2), an oral formulation of nine Chinese herbs that potentially provides long-term protection against food-induced anaphylaxis, has entered human trials.[32,68] Regular subcutaneous injections of anti-IgE antibody potentially increase the margin of protection against anaphylaxis from food and other triggers, although they are not curative.[32,69]

BOX 61-4

Prevention Strategies for Anaphylaxis in Community Settings

Avoid Confirmed Allergen Triggers

Foods, including additives, e.g. spices, colorants, and vegetable gums

Insect stings and bites

Medications

Biologic agents

Natural rubber latex

Inhalants (rare)

Previously unrecognized allergens*

Exercise-induced anaphylaxis†

Avoid Relevant Nonimmune Triggers

Cold air, cold water

Heat

Sunlight/radiation

Medications, e.g. opioids

Ethanol

Immunomodulation

Insect venoms: allergen-specific immunotherapy

Medications, e.g. beta-lactam antibiotics: desensitization

Idiopathic Anaphylaxis (If Episodes are Frequent)

Oral glucocorticoid, e.g. prednisone and H$_1$-antihistamine, e.g. cetirizine

---

*Save the allergen, e.g. food or insect, and save the patient's serum.
†Avoid relevant co-triggers such as food, medication, cold air or cold water.
(Adapted from references 1, 31, 32, 37, 39, 47, 49, 51, 52 and 74.)

Insect Sting-Triggered Anaphylaxis

As documented in randomized placebo-controlled, double-blind trials, anaphylaxis from bee, yellow jacket, wasp, and hornet venom(s) can be almost entirely prevented by a 3- to 5-year course of subcutaneous injections of the relevant stinging insect venom(s), under the supervision of a trained and certified allergy/immunology specialist. Venom immunotherapy provides protection in 97–98% of treated children. The effect lasts 10 to 20 years after venom injections are discontinued. For prevention of anaphylaxis from fire ant stings, subcutaneous injections with whole body fire ant extract are indicated.[36,70]

Medication-Triggered Anaphylaxis

Desensitization in a physician-monitored health-care setting is effective for anaphylaxis triggered by a medication such as a beta-lactam antibiotic, or an antineoplastic agent, for example, L-asparaginase. This strategy is effective during regular administration; however, long-lasting immunologic tolerance is not achieved, and symptoms recur when the medication is discontinued and then restarted.[39,71]

Idiopathic Anaphylaxis

For rare pediatric patients with frequent episodes of idiopathic anaphylaxis (≥6 per year, or ≥2 per 2 months), prophylaxis with an oral glucocorticoid such as prednisone and a nonsedating H$_1$-antihistamine such as cetirizine is recommended for 2 to 3 months. Recently, omalizumab has been reported to be an effective mast cell stabilizer in a child with likely idiopathic anaphylaxis.[72,73]

Long-Term Risk Reduction: Emergency Preparedness

Anaphylaxis episodes sometimes recur despite best efforts at prevention.[63] Those at risk (where age-appropriate) and their care-givers should therefore be prepared to recognize and treat recurrences in the community.[1,3,5,74] One or more epinephrine auto-injectors should be available at all times for them, and coaching in when and how to use the auto-injector should be provided along with a written, personalized anaphylaxis emergency action plan. Age-appropriate medical identification should be worn (Figure 61-5). These recommendations, including those for pharmacologic treatment of acute anaphylaxis episodes, are based on expert opinion rather than on randomized controlled trials,[75–77] although it is possible that such trials will be conducted in the future.[78]

Self-Injectable Epinephrine

Epinephrine injection is the initial treatment of choice in anaphylaxis. There is no absolute contraindication to this treatment.[79–82] Epinephrine's α_1 adrenergic vasoconstrictor effects prevent and relieve mucosal edema, upper airway obstruction, and shock. Its β_1 adrenergic effects lead to increased inotropy and chronotropy. Its β_2 adrenergic effects lead to increased bronchodilation and decreased release of mediators such as histamine and tryptase from mast cells and basophils[1,3,5,83–85] (Table 61-2).

Epinephrine should be injected intramuscularly in the mid-anterolateral thigh in order to achieve peak plasma and tissue concentrations rapidly.[83–85] Failure to inject an adequate dose of epinephrine in a timely manner potentially increases the risk of death in anaphylaxis, as documented in all case series fatalities published during the past two decades,[18–21] and failure to inject an adequate dose of epinephrine may increase the risk of a biphasic anaphylactic reaction.[86] Those at risk for anaphylaxis in the community (where age-appropriate), and their care-givers, should be taught how to use an epinephrine auto-injector correctly and safely[87,88] (Figure 61-5) and supplied with written instructions and a DVD or a website link showing a demonstration of the correct technique. Their understanding of when, why and how to use the auto-injector correctly and safely should be rechecked at regular intervals.

In most countries, only two premeasured fixed doses of epinephrine, 0.15 mg and 0.3 mg, are currently available in auto-injector formulations. The 0.15 mg dose is too high for infants and young children who weigh <15 kg.[89,90] The 0.3 mg dose is too low for many children and adolescents, especially those who are overweight or obese. The needle length on currently available auto-injectors (about 1.43 cm) is too short to permit intramuscular injection of epinephrine in many children and teens.[91,92] Reasons for failure to inject epinephrine promptly and reasons for occasional apparent failure of response to epinephrine injection are listed in Box 61-5.[93–96]

In many countries, life-saving epinephrine auto-injectors are not available for residents and travelers at risk of anaphylaxis.[93] Existing alternatives cannot be depended on to produce high plasma and tissue concentrations of epinephrine rapidly.[84] These include use of a needle and syringe by a lay person to draw up and measure an epinephrine dose from an ampule, use of an unsealed syringe prefilled with the epinephrine dose, or use of a chlorofluorocarbon-containing epinephrine metered-dose inhaler.[84]

Improved design of epinephrine auto-injectors will help to optimize ease and safety of use.[88,97] Noninjectable formulations of epinephrine, including sublingual formulations, are in development.[98]

Anaphylaxis Emergency Action Plan

Epinephrine should be prescribed in the context of broader anaphylaxis educational interventions, including a written, personalized, and regularly updated anaphylaxis emergency action plan, for example, the one developed by the American Academy of Allergy, Asthma, and Immunology (download from *www.aaaai.org*). Such plans should list the most common symptoms and signs of anaphylaxis, and emphasize the need for simultaneous, prompt, life-saving injection of epinephrine, activation of 911 or EMS, and transportation to the nearest hospital emergency department for further assessment and monitoring.[3,5,74,98] Biphasic anaphylaxis, defined as recurrence of symptoms up to 72 hours after the initial symptoms, despite no further exposure to the trigger, occurs in up to 6% of pediatric patients with anaphylaxis.[86,99] Up to 20% of patients with food-induced anaphylaxis in the community require more than one dose of epinephrine.[100] Anaphylaxis emergency action plans should include a reminder that H_1-antihistamines are not life-saving in anaphylaxis because they do not prevent or relieve airflow obstruction or shock;[3,101] in addition, sedation and other potential adverse effects of first-generation H_1-antihistamines are a concern[101,102] (Table 61-2). Evaluation of anaphylaxis emergency action plans in randomized controlled trials is needed.[98]

Medical Identification

Those at risk for anaphylaxis should be equipped with accurate, up-to-date medical identification listing their confirmed trigger(s), relevant comorbidities, and concurrent medications. Available options include medical identification jewelry, e.g. Medic-Alert (Turlock, CA, *www.medicalert.org*), and cards (available at *www.aaaai.org*) suitable for carrying in a wallet, purse, or backpack. For at-risk infants or very young children, age-appropriate options include t-shirts or clothing badges with allergy alert messages, as well as medical identification bracelets made of fabric.[3,53,74] Risk factors for anaphylaxis, including sensitization to allergens and severity and control of asthma, evolve throughout infancy, childhood and adolescence. It is therefore important that the patient's medical identification and health records are updated regularly.

Anaphylaxis Education

Education of those with anaphylaxis and their care-givers helps to reduce anxiety and fear, and to instill confidence in their ability to cope by preventing anaphylaxis episodes and by recognizing and treating them promptly if prevention fails. The current anaphylaxis epidemic is a relatively recent phenomenon[11-17] and it should not be assumed that all health-care professionals have up-to-date knowledge and skills with regard to the assessment and treatment of anaphylaxis in community settings.[87,88] Anaphylaxis education for health-care professionals, patients, care-givers, and the general public should include information about prevention of anaphylaxis in the community by allergen avoidance and the availability of immunomodulation. It should emphasize recognition and treatment of an acute anaphylaxis episode, specifically, when, why, and how to inject epinephrine promptly, call 911 or EMS for assistance, and implement the patient's anaphylaxis emergency action plan.[3,5,74]

Prevention of anaphylaxis in schools, and preparedness for recognizing it and treating it in schools, is a critically important

Table 61-2 Rationale for Epinephrine as the First-Aid Treatment of Choice for Anaphylaxis in the Community*†

Medications and Routes of Administration	Epinephrine (Injection)	β₂-Adrenergic Agonists (Inhalation)	H₁-Antihistamines (Oral)
Pharmacologic effects	At α_1 receptor ↑ vasoconstriction ↑ peripheral vascular resistance ↑ blood pressure ↓ mucosal edema, e.g. in larynx At β_1 receptor ↑ heart rate ↑ force of cardiac contraction At β_2 receptor ↓ mediator release ↑ bronchodilation ↑ vasodilation	At β_2 receptor ↑ bronchodilation	At H_1-receptor ↓ itch (skin, mucus membranes) ↓ flush ↓ hives ↓ sneezing ↓ rhinorrhea
Potential adverse effects when given in usual doses by the routes stated above	Transient anxiety, pallor, restlessness, tremor, palpitations, headache, dizziness	Tremor, tachycardia, dizziness, jitteriness	First-generation H_1-antihistamines (e.g. diphenhydramine) cause sedation and impaired cognitive/psychomotor function, also dry mouth and other antimuscarinic effects
Current recommendations	Treatment of first choice	Not life-saving; ancillary treatment for relief of wheezing, in addition to epinephrine	Not life-saving; ancillary treatment for relief of hives and itching, in addition to epinephrine

*Epinephrine is the initial treatment of choice in community settings, where health-care professionals are not available, and children and their care-givers are 'on their own' with regard to recognition and first-aid treatment of anaphylaxis.
†Glucocorticoids are not included in this Table because they are not recommended for the first-aid treatment of anaphylaxis in community settings.
(Adapted from references 74, 83 and 84.)

BOX 61-5

Epinephrine in Anaphylaxis: Issues

Why Health-Care Professionals, Patients and Care-Givers Fail to Inject Epinephrine Promptly

Lack of recognition of anaphylaxis symptoms/failure to diagnose anaphylaxis

Episode appears mild, or there is a history of a previous mild episode

H_1-antihistamine is given, although it is not life-saving

Prescription for epinephrine auto-injectors not given by physician

Prescription not obtained from pharmacy by patient or care-giver

Epinephrine auto-injectors are not available or affordable

Inappropriate concern about transient pharmacologic effects of epinephrine, e.g. tremor

Lack of awareness that serious adverse effects are almost always attributable to overdose, e.g.:

intravenous bolus of epinephrine

rapid intravenous infusion of epinephrine

intravenous infusion of 1:1000 solution instead of dilute 1:10000 solution of epinephrine

Reasons for Occasional Apparent Failure of Response to Epinephrine Injection

Patient-related factors:

extremely rapid progression of anaphylaxis

concurrent use of medications such as β-adrenergic blockers

Physician-related factors:

error in diagnosis

propping up the patient, leading to the empty inferior vena cava/ empty ventricle syndrome

Epinephrine-related factors:

injected too late

dose too low on mg/kg basis

dose too low because epinephrine is past the expiration date

injection route or site not optimal

(Adapted from references 31, 93–96.)

BOX 61-6

Anaphylaxis in Schools

Student's Responsibilities*

Avoid his or her confirmed trigger(s), e.g. if food-allergic:

do not trade food with others

do not eat anything containing unknown ingredients

Notify an adult immediately if inadvertently exposed to trigger or if symptoms develop

Wear medical identification jewellery and carry an anaphylaxis identification card in a backpack or wallet

Carry self-injectable epinephrine, if age-appropriate, and if permitted by local regulations

Family's Responsibilities*

Notify the school in writing of the student's risk for anaphylaxis and confirmed trigger(s)

Educate the student about trigger avoidance

Provide medical documentation from the student's physician, including an anaphylaxis emergency action plan

Provide a properly labelled epinephrine auto-injector

Replace epinephrine auto-injector after use, or if past the expiry date

Provide emergency contact information for parents/care-givers

Work with the staff to make the student's emergency action plan school-specific

Physician's Responsibilities*

Provide an accurate assessment of the student's risk of anaphylaxis recurrence

Recommend risk reduction measures (e.g. allergen avoidance, venom immunotherapy if relevant)

Prescribe self-injectable epinephrine

Train the student to use an epinephrine auto-injector, if age-appropriate

Recommend medical identification jewellery and an anaphylaxis identification card

Develop an anaphylaxis emergency action plan with the student, if age-appropriate, and the parents/care-givers

Provide medical information to the student and parents/care-givers

Provide medical documentation to the school

If the student has asthma, achieve and maintain optimal control of symptoms

School's Responsibilities*

Review health records of at-risk students

Identify a team, e.g. teachers, school nurse, principal, to prevent, recognize, and treat anaphylaxis

Designate school personnel who are trained to administer epinephrine injections

Rehearse the response to an anaphylaxis episode:

1. Give epinephrine promptly
2. Contact 911 or emergency medical services (EMS)
3. Contact parents/care-givers

*All information should be reviewed annually before the start of the school year and at additional intervals as needed, e.g. if an episode of anaphylaxis occurs, or if a student's allergen triggers change.
(Adapted from references 3, 74, 87, 88, 104 and www.foodallergy.org)

issue involving the student, the family, and the student's physician, as well as the school[74,103–107] (Box 61-6). In the school setting, as in other settings, prompt administration of epinephrine is life-saving.[106] Many children at risk of anaphylaxis have limited access to their epinephrine auto-injector(s) at school, and consequently might experience a delay in treatment.[107] The first episode of anaphylaxis can be fatal.[18–21] Therefore, not only teachers, but also coaches, camp directors, childcare providers, food industry workers, restaurant workers, and members of the general public need to be aware that anaphylaxis is a killer allergy and not a trivial lifestyle problem.[3]

Acute Anaphylaxis in the Physician's Office

Anaphylaxis in the physician's office or facility is most commonly triggered by a medical procedure such as a food or medication challenge/provocation test, or allergen-specific immunotherapy. Less commonly, it can be triggered by administration of a medication or biologic agent, by allergen skin tests, especially if the intradermal route is used or if large numbers of tests are performed, or by a vaccination to prevent infectious disease. In this setting, prevention of anaphylaxis involves awareness of patient- and procedure-related risk factors, careful selection of patients for diagnostic or therapeutic interventions, and careful reassessment immediately before each intervention. If, for example, a patient has had a recent asthma exacerbation, or has an FEV_1 of $\le 70\%$ predicted, an acute upper respiratory tract infection, or seems to be unduly stressed, consideration should be given to deferring the intervention.[1,39,47–49,62,82,108]

Anaphylaxis in the physician's office or facility differs from other anaphylaxis episodes in the community in that the trigger is usually obvious, the time of exposure has likely been recorded, and the patient's comorbidities, concurrent medications, and body mass (weight) are usually known to the health-care professionals involved. Mild anaphylaxis symptoms such as hives and cough can worsen with astonishing rapidity, and progress to fatality in anaphylaxis within minutes to hours. Therefore, as soon as the diagnosis is suspected, the patient's airway, breathing, circulation, etc. should be assessed, and the skin should be examined[1,75–78] (Box 61-7, Figure 61-6). He or she should be placed on the back or in a position of comfort with the lower extremities elevated, and epinephrine 0.01 mg/kg (to a maximum of 0.3 mg in a child or 0.5 mg in a teenager) should be injected intramuscularly in the midanterolateral thigh. A call for help should be placed to 911 or EMS in a community office, or to the resuscitation team in a multispecialty clinic or a hospital facility. This epinephrine dose of 0.01 mg/kg for first-aid treatment is effective when injected promptly; however, it is a low dose compared to the epinephrine dose required for resuscitation, and it therefore needs to be injected *before* anaphylaxis has progressed to cardiorespiratory failure.[31,78] Delaying injection is risky, because the severity of the anaphylaxis episode is difficult to predict at its onset.[78] If indicated, the physician should repeat the epinephrine dose every 5 to 15 minutes, administer supplemental high-flow oxygen and IV fluid resuscitation, and give additional medications.[75–78] Prompt recognition and aggressive treatment of anaphylaxis episodes, even those that initially appear to be mild, saves lives.

Essential medications, supplies and equipment for emergency use should be readily accessible. The medications should be within the expiration date. The responsibilities of individual staff members should be outlined in a posted, printed protocol, which should be rehearsed at regular intervals. The staff members responsible for calling for help promptly (911, EMS, or resuscitation team) should be predesignated.[78]

In the interests of patient safety, specific wait times after various diagnostic and therapeutic interventions in the physician's office or facility are suggested; for example, 30 minutes after allergen immunotherapy,[47] 1 hour after completion of a food challenge,[62] and 30 minutes to 2 hours after omalizumab injections.[108] Patients and their care-givers sometimes consider these wait times to be an unnecessary inconvenience and try to leave the office or facility early. Physicians should therefore prepare patients leaving their office or facility early after a diagnostic or therapeutic intervention to recognize and treat anaphylaxis in the community,[108,109] as described on pages 657–8. Anaphylaxis education messages should be reinforced on a regular basis. The SAFE Program for the management of anaphylaxis (download from *www.acaai.org*)[110] has been developed as a communication tool for use with emergency medicine colleagues.

Conclusions

The incidence rate of anaphylaxis is increasing, particularly during the first two decades of life. In the pediatric population,

---

BOX 61-7

Acute Management of Anaphylaxis in the Physician's Office

In this setting, the anaphylaxis trigger is usually obvious, the time of administration is likely to have been recorded, and the patient's risk factors (e.g. asthma) and weight are likely to be known; therefore act promptly!

Rapidly check airway, breathing, circulation, and assess skin and weight (body mass)

Place patient recumbent and elevate lower extremities*

Inject epinephrine (adrenaline) 0.01 mg/kg (up to a maximum dose of 0.3 mg [child] or 0.5 mg [teenager]) intramuscularly; repeat dose every 5 to 15 minutes if no improvement*†

Call for help (911, emergency medical services, or resuscitation team)*

If appropriate:

 Administer high-flow oxygen (6–8 L/min) by face mask or oropharyngeal airway

 Give IV fluid challenge, if indicated (child: 0.9% [isotonic] saline, up to 30 mL/kg in first hour;‡ teen: 0.9% [isotonic] saline, 1–2 L rapidly [5–10 mL/kg in first 5 min])‡

 Give ancillary medications, if indicated:

  diphenhydramine IV, 1 mg/kg (maximum 50 mg) to relieve itch/hives persisting despite epinephrine

  methylprednisolone IV, 1–2 mg/kg/day (maximum 60 mg, single dose)

  nebulized albuterol 1.25–2.5 mg every 20 min for 3 doses or continuously to relieve bronchospasm persisting despite epinephrine

 Start continuous monitoring of:

  heart rate and function (ECG)

  blood pressure

  oxygen saturation (pulse oximetry)

*Simultaneous steps: positioning the patient, injecting epinephrine, and calling for help.
†The epinephrine solution for intramuscular injection is 1:1000 (1 mg/mL). Intravenous administration of epinephrine is recommended only in specialist pediatric settings where continuous hemodynamic monitoring, and titration of the dose according to the hemodynamic response, is possible. In such settings, a *dilute* solution of 1:10000 (0.1 mg/mL) should be given by *slow* intravenous infusion.
‡Titrate the rate of volume expansion to the heart rate and to the blood pressure; monitor for volume overload.
(Adapted from references 79–82.)

---

the pathogenesis of anaphylaxis usually involves IgE and high-affinity IgE receptors (FcɛR1 receptors) on mast cells and basophils. Food is by far the most common trigger, however, any trigger is possible. New triggers of anaphylaxis are recognized from time to time. Diagnosis is based on a meticulous history of the episode. Negative laboratory test results cannot be used to refute the clinical diagnosis. Confirmation of an anaphylaxis trigger suggested by the history is important; however, finding one or more positive allergen skin tests, or one or more elevated allergen-specific IgE levels is not diagnostic of anaphylaxis because most children in the general population are sensitized to one or more allergens.

Long-term risk reduction measures in anaphylaxis potentially reduce the impact of anaphylaxis on children and their caregivers. Optimal management of asthma and other relevant comorbidities is an important aspect of risk reduction. Specific preventive treatment focuses on avoidance of the relevant specific allergen(s). For stinging insect venom triggers or some medication triggers, immunomodulation is indicated. Emergency

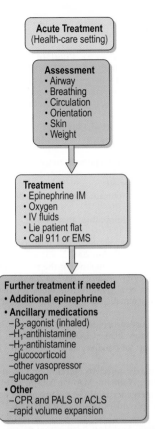

Acute Treatment
(Health-care setting)

Assessment
• Airway
• Breathing
• Circulation
• Orientation
• Skin
• Weight

Treatment
• Epinephrine IM
• Oxygen
• IV fluids
• Lie patient flat
• Call 911 or EMS

Further treatment if needed
• **Additional epinephrine**
• **Ancillary medications**
  – β_2-agonist (inhaled)
  – H_1-antihistamine
  – H_2-antihistamine
  – glucocorticoid
  – other vasopressor
  – glucagon
• **Other**
  – CPR and PALS or ACLS
  – rapid volume expansion

Figure 61-6 Acute treatment of anaphylaxis in the physician's office or facility. In addition to the assessment of airway, breathing, and circulation, the skin should be inspected, and the weight (body mass) should be estimated. Simultaneously and promptly, epinephrine should be injected intramuscularly, the patient should be placed in the recumbent position with legs elevated, and 911 or EMS (or resuscitation team) should be called. If indicated, the epinephrine dose should be repeated every 5 to 15 minutes, and supplemental oxygen, IV fluid resuscitation, and additional medications should be given. *ACLS*, Advanced Cardiac Life Support; *CPR*, cardiopulmonary resuscitation; *IV*, intravenous; *PALS*, Pediatric Advanced Life Support. (Adapted from Simons FER. J Allergy Clin Immunol 2008; 121:S402–407.)

preparedness for anaphylaxis includes availability of one or more epinephrine auto-injector/s, and knowledge of when, why, and how to inject epinephrine. Those at risk should have a written, personalized anaphylaxis emergency action plan, and should wear appropriate up-to-date medical identification.

Anaphylaxis in the physician's office or facility is probably inevitable; however, it is not a random event. Health-care professionals need to be aware of procedure-related risk factors and patient-related risk factors, and aim to prevent anaphylaxis as far as possible. If anaphylaxis occurs despite preventive efforts, the keys to successful outcomes include having a posted, printed protocol for treatment, rehearsing it regularly, and remembering to simultaneously and promptly inject epinephrine, position the patient appropriately, and call for assistance.

References

1. Simons FER. Anaphylaxis. 2008 Mini-primer on allergic and immunologic diseases. J Allergy Clin Immunol 2008;121:S402–7.
2. Simons FER, Frew AJ, Ansotegui IJ, et al. Risk assessment in anaphylaxis: current and future approaches. J Allergy Clin Immunol 2007;120:S2–24.
3. Simons FER. Anaphylaxis, killer allergy: long-term management in the community. J Allergy Clin Immunol 2006;117:367–77.
4. Young MC. General treatment of anaphylaxis. In: Leung DYM, Sampson HA, Geha RS, Szefler SJ, editors. Pediatric allergy: principles and practice. St. Louis, MO: Mosby, Inc; 2003. p. 643–54.
5. Sampson HA, Munoz-Furlong A, Campbell RL, et al. Second symposium on the definition and management of anaphylaxis: summary report: Second National Institute of Allergy and Infectious Disease/Food Allergy and Anaphylaxis Network symposium. J Allergy Clin Immunol 2006;117:391–7.
6. Oude Elberink JN. Significance and rationale of studies of health-related quality of life in anaphylactic disorders. Curr Opin Allergy Clin Immunol 2006;6:298–302.
7. Marklund B, Ahlstedt S, Nordstrom G. Food hypersensitivity and quality of life. Curr Opin Allergy Clin Immunol 2007;7:279–87.
8. Akeson N, Worth A, Sheikh A. The psychosocial impact of anaphylaxis on young people and their parents. Clin Exp Allergy 2007;37:1213–20.
9. Monga S, Manassis K. Treating anxiety in children with life-threatening anaphylactic conditions. J Am Acad Child Adolesc Psychiatry 2006;45:1007–10.
10. Greenhawt MJ, Singer AM, Baptist AP. Food allergy and food allergy attitudes among college students. J Allergy Clin Immunol 2009;124:323–7.
11. Clark S, Camargo CA Jr. Epidemiology of anaphylaxis. Immunol Allergy Clin North Am 2007;27:145–63.
12. Lieberman P, Camargo CA Jr, Bohlke K, et al. Epidemiology of anaphylaxis: findings of the American College of Allergy, Asthma and Immunology Epidemiology of Anaphylaxis Working Group. Ann Allergy Asthma Immunol 2006;97:596–602.
13. Decker WW, Campbell RL, Luke A, et al. The etiology and incidence of anaphylaxis in Rochester, Minnesota: a report from the Rochester Epidemiology Project. J Allergy Clin Immunol 2008;122:1161–5.
14. Simons FER, Sampson HA. Anaphylaxis epidemic: fact or fiction? J Allergy Clin Immunol 2008;122:1166–8.
15. Lin RY, Anderson AS, Shah SN, et al. Increasing anaphylaxis hospitalizations in the first 2 decades of life: New York State, 1990–2006. Ann Allergy Asthma Immunol 2008;101:387–93.
16. Sheikh A, Hippisley-Cox J, Newton J, et al. Trends in national incidence, lifetime prevalence and adrenaline prescribing for anaphylaxis in England. J R Soc Med 2008;101:139–43.
17. Liew WK, Williamson E, Tang MLK. Anaphylaxis fatalities and admissions in Australia. J Allergy Clin Immunol 2009;123:434–42.
18. Sampson HA, Mendelson L, Rosen JP. Fatal and near-fatal anaphylactic reactions to food in children and adolescents. N Engl J Med 1992;327:380–4.
19. Bock SA, Munoz-Furlong A, Sampson HA. Fatalities due to anaphylactic reactions to foods. J Allergy Clin Immunol 2001;107:191–3.
20. Bock SA, Munoz-Furlong A, Sampson HA. Further fatalities caused by anaphylactic reactions to food, 2001–2006. J Allergy Clin Immunol 2007;119:1016–8.
21. Pumphrey RSH, Gowland MH. Further fatal allergic reactions to food in the United Kingdom, 1999–2006. J Allergy Clin Immunol 2007;119:1018–9.
22. Peavy RD, Metcalfe DD. Understanding the mechanisms of anaphylaxis. Curr Opin Allergy Clin Immunol 2008;8:310–5.
23. Zanoni G, Puccetti A, Dolcino M, et al. Dextran-specific IgG response in hypersensitivity reactions to measles-mumps-rubella vaccine. J Allergy Clin Immunol 2008;122:1233–5.
24. Kishimoto TK, Viswanathan K, Ganguly T, et al. Contaminated heparin associated with adverse clinical events and activation of the contact system. N Engl J Med 2008;358:2457–67.
25. Dibs SD, Baker MD. Anaphylaxis in children: a 5-year experience. Pediatrics 1997;99:E7.
26. Novembre E, Cianferoni A, Bernardini R, et al. Anaphylaxis in children: clinical and allergologic features. Pediatrics 1998;101:e8.
27. Mehl A, Wahn U, Niggemann B. Anaphylactic reactions in children: a questionnaire-based survey in Germany. Allergy 2005;60:1440–5.
28. Braganza SC, Acworth JP, McKinnon DRL, et al. Paediatric emergency department anaphylaxis: different patterns from adults. Arch Dis Child 2006;91:159–63.
29. de Silva IL, Mehr SS, Tey D, et al. Paediatric anaphylaxis: a 5 year retrospective review. Allergy 2008;63:1071–6.
30. Simons FER, Chad ZH, Gold M. Anaphylaxis in children: real-time reporting from a national network. Allergy Clin Immunol Int: J World Allergy Org 2004;(Supp. 1):242–4.
31. Simons FER. Anaphylaxis: Recent advances in assessment and treatment. J Allergy Clin Immunol 2009;124:625–36.
32. Sicherer SH, Sampson HA. Food allergy: recent advances in pathophysiology and treatment. Ann Rev Med 2009;60:261–77.
33. Moore LM, Rathkopf MM, Sanner CJ, et al. Seal and whale meat: two newly recognized food allergies. Ann Allergy Asthma Immunol 2007;98:92–6.
34. Kuehn A, Hilger C, Hentges F. Anaphylaxis provoked by ingestion of marshmallows containing fish gelatin. J Allergy Clin Immunol 2009;123:708–9.
35. Wassenberg J, Hofer M. Lupine-induced anaphylaxis in a child without known food allergy. Ann Allergy Asthma Immunol 2007;98:589–90.

36. Freeman TM. Clinical practice: hypersensitivity to hymenoptera stings. N Engl J Med 2004;351:1978–84.

37. Peng Z, Beckett AN, Engler RJ, et al. Immune responses to mosquito saliva in 14 individuals with acute systemic allergic reactions to mosquito bites. J Allergy Clin Immunol 2004;114:1189–94.

38. Shkalim V, Herscovici Z, Amir J, et al. Systemic allergic reaction to tree processionary caterpillar in children. Pediatr Emerg Care 2008;24: 233–5.

39. Celik W, Pichler WJ, Adkinson NF Jr. Drug allergy. In: Adkinson NF Jr, Bochner BS, Busse WW, et al, editors. Middleton's Allergy: principles and practice. 7th ed. St. Louis, MO: Mosby, Inc; (an affiliate of Elsevier Science), 2009. p.1205–26.

40. Novembre E, Mori F, Pucci N, et al. Cefaclor anaphylaxis in children. Allergy 2009;64:1233–5.

41. Perez-Calderon R, Gonzalo-Garijo MA. Anaphylaxis due to loperamide. Allergy 2004;59:369–70.

42. Soyer OU, Aytac S, Tuncer A, et al. Alternative algorithm for L-asparaginase allergy in children with acute lymphoblastic leukemia. J Allergy Clin Immunol 2009;123:895–9.

43. Harper NJN, Dixon T, Dugue P, et al. Suspected anaphylactic reactions associated with anaesthesia. Anaesthesia 2009;64:199–211.

44. Kimata H. Latex allergy in infants younger than 1 year. Clin Exp Allergy 2004;34:1910–5.

45. Kolho K-L, Ruuska T, Savilahti E. Severe adverse reactions to infliximab therapy are common in young children with inflammatory bowel disease. Acta Paediatr 2007;96:128–30.

46. Limb SL, Starke PR, Lee CE, et al. Delayed onset and protracted progression of anaphylaxis after omalizumab administration in patients with asthma. J Allergy Clin Immunol 2007;120:1378–81.

47. Rezvani M, Bernstein DI. Anaphylactic reactions during immunotherapy. Immunol Allergy Clin North Am 2007;27:295–307.

48. Rodriguez-Perez N, Ambriz-Moreno M de J, Canonica GW, et al. Frequency of acute systemic reactions in patients with allergic rhinitis and asthma treated with sublingual immunotherapy. Ann Allergy Asthma Immunol 2008;101:304–10.

49. Kelso JM, Li JT, Nicklas RA, et al. Adverse reactions to vaccines. Ann Allergy Asthma Immunol 2009;103:S1–14.

50. Slade BA, Leidel L, Vellozzi C, et al. Postlicensure safety surveillance for quadrivalent human papillomavirus recombinant vaccine. JAMA 2009;302:750–7.

51. Du Toit G. Food-dependent exercise-induced anaphylaxis in childhood. Pediatr Allergy Immunol 2007;18:455–63.

52. Fernando SL. Cold-induced anaphylaxis. J Pediatr 2009;154:148.

53. Simons FER. Anaphylaxis in infants: can recognition and management be improved? J Allergy Clin Immunol 2007;120:537–40.

54. Schwartz LB. Diagnostic value of tryptase in anaphylaxis and mastocytosis. Immunol Allergy Clin North Am 2006;26:451–63.

55. Komarow HD, Hu Z, Brittain E, et al. Serum tryptase levels in atopic and nonatopic children. J Allergy Clin Immunol 2009;124:845–8.

56. Vadas P, Gold M, Perelman B, et al. Platelet-activating factor, PAF acetylhydrolase and severe anaphylaxis. N Engl J Med 2008;358:28–35.

57. Stone SF, Cotterell C, Isbister GK, et al. For the Emergency Department Anaphylaxis Investigators. Elevated serum cytokines during human anaphylaxis: identification of potential mediators of acute allergic reactions. J Allergy Clin Immunol 2009;124:786–92.

58. Summers CW, Pumphrey RS, Woods CN, et al. Factors predicting anaphylaxis to peanuts and tree nuts in patients referred to a specialist center. J Allergy Clin Immunol 2008;121:632–8.

59. Brockow K, Jofer C, Behrendt H, et al. Anaphylaxis in patients with mastocytosis: a study on history, clinical features and risk factors in 120 patients. Allergy 2008;63:226–32.

60. Wang J, Godbold JH, Sampson HA. Correlation of serum allergy (IgE) tests performed by different assay systems. J Allergy Clin Immunol 2008;121:1219–24.

61. Pereira B, Venter C, Grundy J, et al. Prevalence of sensitization to food allergens, reported adverse reaction to foods, food avoidance, and food hypersensitivity among teenagers. J Allergy Clin Immunol 2005;116:884–92.

62. Nowak-Wegrzyn A, Assa'ad AH, Bahna SL, et al. Work Group report: oral food challenge testing. J Allergy Clin Immunol 2009;123:S365–83.

63. Boyano-Martinez T, Garcia-Ara C, Pedrosa M, et al. Accidental allergic reactions in children allergic to cow's milk proteins. J Allergy Clin Immunol 2009;123:883–8.

64. Skripak JM, Nash SD, Rowley H, et al. A randomized, double-blind, placebo-controlled study of milk oral immunotherapy for cow's milk allergy. J Allergy Clin Immunol 2008;122:1154–60.

65. Narisety SD, Skripak JM, Steele P, et al. Open-label maintenance after milk oral immunotherapy for IgE-mediated cow's milk allergy. J Allergy Clin Immunol 2009;124:610–2.

66. Jones SM, Pons L, Roberts JL, et al. Clinical efficacy and immune regulation with peanut oral immunotherapy. J Allergy Clin Immunol 2009;124:292–300.

67. Hofmann AM, Scurlock AM, Jones SM, et al. Safety of a peanut oral immunotherapy protocol in children with peanut allergy. J Allergy Clin Immunol 2009;124:286–91.

68. Leung DYM, Sampson HA, Yunginger JW, et al. Effect of anti-IgE therapy in patients with peanut allergy. N Engl J Med 2003;348:986–93.

69. Srivastava KD, Qu C, Zhang T, et al. Food Allergy Herbal Formula-2 silences peanut-induced anaphylaxis for a prolonged posttreatment period via IFN-gamma-producing CD8+ T cells. J Allergy Clin Immunol 2009;123:443–51.

70. Golden DBK, Kagey-Sobotka A, Norman PS, et al. Outcomes of allergy to insect stings in children, with and without venom immunotherapy. N Engl J Med 2004;351:668–74.

71. Castells MC, Tennant NM, Sloane DE, et al. Hypersensitivity reactions to chemotherapy: outcomes and safety of rapid desensitization in 413 cases. J Allergy Clin Immunol 2008;122:574–80.

72. Greenberger PA. Idiopathic anaphylaxis. Immunol Allergy Clin North Am 2007;27:273–93.

73. Warrier P, Casale TB. Omalizumab in idiopathic anaphylaxis. Ann Allergy Asthma Immunol 2009;102:257–8.

74. Simons FER. Anaphylaxis: evidence-based long-term risk reduction in the community. Immunol Allergy Clin North Am 2007;27:231–48.

75. Sheikh A, Shehata YA, Brown SGA, et al. Adrenaline for the treatment of anaphylaxis: Cochrane systematic review. Allergy 2009;64:204–12.

76. Sheikh A, Ten Broek V, Brown SGA, et al. H₁-antihistamines for the treatment of anaphylaxis: Cochrane systematic review. Allergy 2007;62: 830–7.

77. Choo KJL, Simons FER, Sheikh A. Glucocorticoids for the treatment of anaphylaxis. Cochrane Database Syst Rev 2010;3:CD007596.

78. Simons FER. Emergency treatment of anaphylaxis. Br Med J 2008;336:1141–2.

79. Simons FER, Camargo CA. Anaphylaxis: rapid recognition and treatment. In: Basow DS, editor. UpToDate. Waltham, MA: UpToDate; 2010.

80. Soar J, Pumphrey R, Cant A, et al. Emergency treatment of anaphylactic reactions–guidelines for healthcare providers. Resuscitation 2008;77: 157–69.

81. Joint Task Force on Practice Parameters, American Academy of Allergy, Asthma and Immunology, American College of Allergy, Asthma and Immunology, Joint Council of Allergy, Asthma and Immunology. The diagnosis and management of anaphylaxis: an updated practice parameter. J Allergy Clin Immunol 2005;115(Suppl.):S483–523.

82. Oswalt ML, Kemp SF. Anaphylaxis: office management and prevention. Immunol Allergy Clin North Am 2007;27:177–91.

83. McLean-Tooke APC, Bethune CA, Fay AC, et al. Adrenaline in the treatment of anaphylaxis: what is the evidence? Br Med J 2003;327:1332–5.

84. Simons FER. First-aid treatment of anaphylaxis to food: focus on epinephrine. J Allergy Clin Immunol 2004;113:837–44.

85. Kemp SF, Lockey RF, Simons FER. Epinephrine: the drug of choice for anaphylaxis: a statement of the World Allergy Organization. Allergy 2008;63:1061–70.

86. Lieberman P. Biphasic anaphylactic reactions. Ann Allergy Asthma Immunol 2005;95:217–26.

87. Mehr S, Robinson M, Tang M. Doctor, how do I use my EpiPen? Pediatr Allergy Immunol 2007;18:448–52.

88. Simons FER, Lieberman PL, Read EJ Jr, et al. Hazards of unintentional injection of epinephrine from auto-injectors: a systematic review. Ann Allergy Asthma Immunol 2009;102:282–7.

89. Simons FER, Gu X, Silver NA, et al. EpiPen Jr versus EpiPen in young children weighing 15-30 kg at risk for anaphylaxis. J Allergy Clin Immunol 2002;109:171–5.

90. Simons FER, Peterson S, Black CD. Epinephrine dispensing patterns for an out-of-hospital population: a novel approach to studying the epidemiology of anaphylaxis. J Allergy Clin Immunol 2002;110:647–51.

91. Stecher D, Bulloch B, Sales J, et al. Epinephrine auto-injectors: is needle length adequate for delivery of epinephrine intramuscularly? Pediatrics 2009;124:65–70.

92. Song TT, Nelson MR, Chang JH, et al. Adequacy of the epinephrine auto-injector needle length in delivering epinephrine to the intramuscular tissues. Ann Allergy Asthma Immunol 2005;94:539–42.

93. Simons FER, for the World Allergy Organization. Epinephrine auto-injectors: first-aid treatment still out of reach for many at risk of anaphylaxis in the community. Ann Allergy Asthma Immunol 2009;102:403–9.

94. Simons FER, Clark S, Camargo CA. Anaphylaxis in the community: learning from the survivors. J Allergy Clin Immunol 2009;124:301–6.

95. Sicherer SH, Simons FER. Quandaries in prescribing an emergency action plan and self-injectable epinephrine for first-aid management of anaphylaxis in the community. J Allergy Clin Immunol 2005;115: 575–83.

96. Johnson TL, Parker AL. Rates of retrieval of self-injectable epinephrine prescriptions: a descriptive report. Ann Allergy Asthma Immunol 2006;97:694–7.

97. Rawas-Qalaji MM, Simons FER, Simons KJ. Sublingual epinephrine tablets versus intramuscular injection of epinephrine: dose-equivalence

for potential treatment of anaphylaxis. J Allergy Clin Immunol 2006;117: 398–403.

98. Nurmatov U, Worth A, Sheikh A. Anaphylaxis management plans for the acute and long-term management of anaphylaxis: a systematic review. J Allergy Clin Immunol 2008;122:353–61.

99. Lee JM, Greenes DS. Biphasic anaphylactic reactions in pediatrics. Pediatrics 2000;106:762–6.

100. Jarvinen KM, Sicherer SH, Sampson HA, et al. Use of multiple doses of epinephrine in food-induced anaphylaxis in children. J Allergy Clin Immunol 2008;122:133–8.

101. Simons FER. Advances in H$_1$-antihistamines. N Engl J Med 2004;351: 2203–17.

102. Starke PR, Weaver J, Chowdhury BA. Boxed warning added to promethazine labeling for pediatric use. N Eng J Med 2005;352:2653.

103. Bansal PJ, Marsh R, Patel B, et al. Recognition, evaluation, and treatment of anaphylaxis in the child care setting. Ann Allergy Asthma Immunol 2005;94:55–9.

104. Munoz-Furlong A. Food allergy in schools: concerns for allergists, pediatricians, parents, and school staff. Ann Allergy Asthma Immunol 2004;93: S47–50.

105. Young MC, Munoz-Furlong A, Sicherer SH. Management of food allergies in schools: a perspective for allergists. J Allergy Clin Immunol 2009;124:175–82.

106. McIntyre CL, Sheetz AH, Carroll CR, et al. Administration of epinephrine for life-threatening allergic reactions in school settings. Pediatrics 2005;116:1134–40.

107. Ben-Shoshan M, Kagan R, Primeau MN, et al. Availability of the epinephrine autoinjector at school in children with peanut allergy. Ann Allergy Asthma Immunol 2008;100:570–5.

108. Cox L, Platts-Mills TAE, Finegold I, et al. American Academy of Allergy, Asthma & Immunology/American College of Allergy, Asthma and Immunology Joint Task Force Report on omalizumab-associated anaphylaxis. J Allergy Clin Immunol 2007;120:1373–7.

109. Scranton SE, Gonzalez EG, Waibel KH. Incidence and characteristics of biphasic reactions after allergen immunotherapy. J Allergy Clin Immunol 2009;123:493–8.

110. Lieberman P, Decker W, Camargo CA, et al. SAFE: a multidisciplinary approach to anaphylaxis education in the emergency department. Ann Allergy Asthma Immunol 2007;98:519–23.

I

Clinical Immunology Laboratory Values

BOX AI-1 Autoantibodies in Pediatric Rheumatologic Diseases

Autoantibodies Associated with Systemic Lupus Erythematosus

Antinuclear Antibody (ANA)

Indirect immunofluorescence on Hep-2 cells is the method of choice for detection of ANA. The sensitivity of ANA for SLE is very high with positive results in 98% of patients with systemic lupus erythematosus (SLE). The specificity of the test is low with positive results in 13.3% of the normal population at titer of 1:160. May also be positive in scleroderma, Sjögren's syndrome, rheumatoid arthritis, polyarteritis nodosa, dermatomyositis, polymyositis

Pattern of staining is helpful in determining particular type of antinuclear antibody (see below)

Homogeneous staining

Anti-double-stranded (ds) DNA

50% of patients with SLE, suggests more serious disease

Titer correlates with disease activity

Antihistone

Associated with drug-induced lupus

Speckled Pattern

Anti-Smith (anti-Sm)

25% of patients with SLE

Most specific antibody test for SLE

Antiribonucleo protein (anti-RNP, anti-U1-RNP)

25% of patients with SLE

Also associated with mixed connective tissue disease (MCTD)

Anti-Ro/SSA

30% of patients with SLE

Also associated with Sjögren's syndrome, neonatal lupus, photosensitivity

Anti-La/SSB

15% of patients with SLE

Occurs in association with SSA

Antiphospholipid, anticardiolipin, lupus anticoagulant, anti-β_2 glycoprotein I (β_2-GPI)

33% of patients with SLE

One third of patients with antiphospholipid antibodies have thrombotic/embolic events

Autoantibodies in Juvenile Rheumatoid Arthritis

ANA positivity in patients with pauciarticular juvenile rheumatoid arthritis (JRA) is associated with increased risk of uveitis

Rheumatoid factor positivity in polyarticular JRA is associated with more chronic disease course

Autoantibodies in Scleroderma

Anticentromere and anti-Scl-70 and others are associated with scleroderma

Autoantibodies Associated with Systemic Vasculitides

Antineutrophil Cytoplasmic Antibody (ANCA)

Cytoplasmic ANCA (c-ANCA), particularly those directed to proteinase 3 (PR3), is highly specific for Wegener's granulomatosis

Perinuclear ANCA (p-ANCA), especially those associated with myeloperoxidase (MPO), is associated with microscopic polyangiitis, Churg-Strauss syndrome, IBD-associated vasculitis, and other vasculitides

Antiglomerular Basement Membrane (GBM)

Associated with Goodpasture's syndrome

Autoantibodies Associated with Other Autoimmune Diseases

Addison's disease: antiadrenal antibodies

Celiac disease and dermatitis herpetiformis: antigliadin, anti-endomysial, antireticulin, and antitissue transglutaminase antibodies

Chronic active hepatitis: antismooth muscle antibodies

Diabetes mellitus type I: anti-islet cell antibodies

Myasthenia gravis: antiacetylcholine receptor antibodies

Pemphigoid: anti-BP230 and BP180 (bullous pemphigoid)

Pemphigus: antidesmoglein and antiplakoglobulin

Pernicious anemia: antiintrinsic factor antibodies

Primary biliary cirrhosis: antimitochondrial antibodies

Thyroid disease: antithyroid peroxidase, antithyroglobulin, and antithyrotropin receptor antibodies

Table AI-1 Relative Size of Lymphocyte Subpopulations in Blood*

Lymphocyte Subpopulations	Neonatal (N = 20)	1 wk–2 mo (N = 13)	2–5 mo (N = 46)	5–9 mo (N = 105)	9–15 mo (N = 70)	15–24 mo (N = 33)	2–5 yr (N = 33)	5–10 yr (N = 35)	10–16 yr (N = 23)	Adults (N = 51)
CD19+ B lymphocytes	12% (5–22)	15% (4–26)	24% (14–39)	21% (13–35)	25% (15–39)	28% (17–41)	24% (14–44)	18% (10–31)	16% (8–24)	12% (6–19)
CD3+ T lymphocytes	62% (28–76)	72% (60–85)	63% (48–75)	66% (50–77)	65% (54–76)	64% (39–73)	64% (43–76)	69% (55–78)	67% (52–78)	72% (55–83)
CD3+/CD4+ T lymphocytes	41% (17–52)	55% (41–68)	45% (33–58)	45% (33–58)	44% (31–54)	41% (25–50)	37% (23–48)	35% (27–53)	39% (25–48)	44% (28–57)
CD3+/CD8+ T lymphocytes	24% (10–41)	16% (9–23)	17% (11–25)	18% (13–26)	18% (12–28)	20% (11–32)	24% (14–33)	28% (19–34)	23% (9–35)	24% (10–39)
CD4/CD8 ratio per CD3+	1.8 (1.0–2.6)	3.8 (1.3–6.3)	2.7 (1.7–3.9)	2.5 (1.6–3.8)	2.4 (1.3–3.9)	1.9 (0.9–3.7)	1.6 (0.9–2.9)	1.2 (0.9–2.6)	1.7 (0.9–3.4)	1.9 (1.0–3.6)
CD3+/HLA-DR+ T lymphocytes	2% (1–6)	5% (1–38)	3% (1–9)	3% (1–7)	4% (2–8)	6% (3–12)	6% (3–13)	7% (3–14)	4% (1–8)	5% (2–12)
CD3-/CD16-56+ NK cells	20% (6–58)	8% (3–23)	6% (2–14)	5% (2–13)	7% (3–17)	8% (3–16)	10% (4–23)	12% (4–26)	15% (6–27)	13% (7–31)

From Comans-Bitter WM, de Groot R, van den Beemd R, et al. J Pediatr 1997;130:388–393.
*The relative frequencies are expressed within the lymphocyte population: median and percentiles (5th to 95th percentiles).

Table AI-2 Absolute Size of Lymphocyte Subpopulations in Blood*

Lymphocyte Subpopulations	Neonatal (N = 20)	1 wk–2 mo (N = 13)	2–5 mo (N = 46)	5–9 mo (N = 105)	9–15 mo (N = 70)	15–24 mo (N = 33)	2–5 yr (N = 33)	5–10 yr (N = 35)	10–16 yr (N = 23)	Adults (N = 51)
Lymphocytes	4.8 (0.7–7.3)	6.7 (3.5–13.1)	5.9 (3.7–9.6)	6.0 (3.8–9.9)	5.5 (2.6–10.4)	5.6 (2.7–11.9)	3.3 (1.7–6.9)	2.8 (1.1–5.9)	2.2 (1.0–5.3)	1.8 (1.0–2.8)
CD19+ B lymphocytes	0.6 (0.04–1.1)	1.0 (0.6–1.9)	1.3 (0.6–3.0)	1.3 (0.7–2.5)	1.4 (0.6–2.7)	1.3 (0.6–3.1)	0.8 (0.2–2.1)	0.5 (0.2–1.6)	0.3 (0.2–0.6)	0.2 (0.1–0.5)
CD3+ T lymphocytes	2.8 (0.6–5.0)	4.6 (2.3–7.0)	3.6 (2.3–6.5)	3.8 (2.4–6.9)	3.4 (1.6–6.7)	3.5 (1.4–8.0)	2.3 (0.9–4.5)	1.9 (0.7–4.2)	1.5 (0.8–3.5)	1.2 (0.7–2.1)
CD3+/CD4+ T lymphocytes	1.9 (0.4–3.5)	3.5 (1.7–5.3)	2.5 (1.5–5.0)	2.8 (1.4–5.1)	2.3 (1.0–4.6)	2.2 (0.9–5.5)	1.3 (0.5–2.4)	1.0 (0.3–2.0)	0.8 (0.4–2.1)	0.7 (0.3–1.4)
CD3+/CD8+ T lymphocytes	1.1 (0.2–1.9)	1.0 (0.4–1.7)	1.0 (0.5–1.6)	1.1 (0.6–2.2)	1.1 (0.4–2.1)	1.2 (0.4–2.3)	0.8 (0.3–1.6)	0.8 (0.3–1.8)	0.4 (0.2–1.2)	0.4 (0.2–0.9)
CD3+/HLA-DR+ T lymphocytes	0.09 (0.03–0.4)	0.3 (0.03–3.4)	0.2 (0.07–0.5)	0.2 (0.07–0.5)	0.2 (0.1–0.6)	0.3 (0.1–0.7)	0.2 (0.08–0.4)	0.2 (0.05–0.7)	0.06 (0.02–0.2)	0.09 (0.03–0.2)
CD3-/CD16-56+ NK cells	1.0 (0.1–1.9)	0.5 (0.2–1.4)	0.3 (0.1–1.3)	0.3 (0.1–1.0)	0.4 (0.2–1.2)	0.4 (0.1–1.4)	0.4 (0.1–1.0)	0.3 (0.09–0.9)	0.3 (0.07–1.2)	0.3 (0.09–0.6)

From Comans-Bitter WM, de Groot R, van den Beemd R, et al. J Pediatr 1997;130:388–393.
*Absolute counts (× 10⁹/L): median and percentiles (5th to 95th percentiles).

APPENDIX

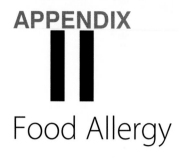

II

Food Allergy

A Functions and Food Sources of Vitamins

Vitamin Name	Chief Functions in the Body	Significant Sources
Vitamin A	Visual adaptation to light and dark, growth of skin and mucous membrane	Retinol (animal foods): liver, egg yolk, fortified milk, cheese, cream, butter, fortified margarine Carotene (plant foods): spinach, other dark leafy green vegetables, broccoli, deep orange fruits (apricots, cantaloupe), vegetables (squash, carrots, sweet potato, pumpkin)
Vitamin D	Absorption of calcium and phosphorus, calcification of bones	Self-synthesis from sunlight; fortified milk products, fortified eggs, liver, fish liver oils, fatty fish
Vitamin E	Antioxidant, stabilization of cell membranes, protection of polyunsaturated fatty acids and vitamin A	Polyunsaturated plant oils, green leafy vegetables, wheat germ, whole-grain products, nuts, seeds
Vitamin K	Normal blood clotting	Bacterial synthesis in the digestive tract; green leafy vegetables, cruciferous vegetables (cabbage, broccoli, Brussels sprouts), plant oils and margarine
Thiamine (B$_1$)	Coenzyme in carbohydrate and branched chain amino acid metabolism; normal function of the heart, nerves, and muscle	Pork, beef, liver, whole or enriched grains, legumes, nuts
Riboflavin (B$_2$)	Coenzyme in protein and energy metabolism	Milk, yogurt, cottage cheese, leafy green vegetables, whole or enriched grains and cereals
Niacin (B$_3$)	Coenzyme in energy production, health of skin, normal activity of stomach, intestines, and nervous system	Meat, fish, poultry, peanuts, legumes, and whole or enriched grains
Pyridoxine (B$_6$)	Coenzyme in amino acid metabolism, helps convert tryptophan to niacin, heme formation	Enriched and whole grains, seeds, liver, meats, milk, eggs, vegetables
Cyanocobalamin (B$_{12}$)	Coenzyme in synthesis of heme in hemoglobin, normal blood cell formation	Animal products (meat, fish, poultry, shellfish, milk, cheese, eggs), fortified cereals
Folic acid	Part of DNA, growth and development of red blood cells	Liver, leafy green vegetables, legumes, seeds, fortified grains
Pantothenic acid	Part of coenzyme A (used in energy metabolism); formation of fat, cholesterol, and heme; activation of amino acids	Meats, cereals, legumes, milk, tomato, potato, broccoli, egg yolk
Biotin	Part of coenzyme A (used in energy metabolism); involved in lipid synthesis, amino acid metabolism, glycogen synthesis	Liver, egg yolk, soy flour, cereals, tomatoes, yeast
Vitamin C	Collagen synthesis (strengthens blood vessel walls, forms scar tissue and matrix for bone growth), antioxidant, thyroxine synthesis, strengthens resistance to infection, helps with absorption of iron	Citrus fruits, tomatoes, dark leafy green vegetables, cruciferous vegetables, potatoes, peppers, cantaloupe, strawberries, melons, papayas, mangos

©2010 Elsevier Ltd, Inc, BV
DOI: 10.1016/B978-1-4377-0271-2.00063-8

B Functions and Food Sources of Minerals and Trace Elements

Mineral Name	Chief Functions in the Body	Significant Sources
Calcium	Bone and teeth formation; involved in normal muscle contraction and relaxation, nerve functioning, blood clotting, blood pressure	Milk and milk products, small fish (with bones), greens, legumes, calcium-fortified tofu, calcium-fortified juices, calcium-fortified alternative 'milk' beverage (rice, soy, oat, almond)
Chloride	Part of hydrochloric acid found in the stomach, necessary for proper digestion	Salt, soy sauce, moderate quantities in whole unprocessed foods, large amounts in processed foods
Chromium	Cofactor for insulin	Meat, fish, poultry, nuts, whole grains
Copper	Cofactor for enzymes; necessary for iron metabolism; cross-linking of elastin	Liver, shellfish, whole grain cereals, legumes, nuts, cocoa
Fluoride	Structural component in calcium hydroxyapatite of bones and teeth	Seafood, fluoridated water, fluoridated dental products
Iodide	A component of the thyroid hormone thyroxin, which helps regulate growth, development, metabolic rate	Iodized salt, processed foods, seafood
Iron	Structural component of hemoglobin (carries oxygen in the blood) and myoglobin (makes oxygen available for muscle contraction) and other enzymes necessary for the utilization of energy	Heme iron: meat, liver, fish, shellfish, poultry. Non-heme iron: enriched and whole grain products, legumes and dried fruits
Magnesium	One of the cofactors involved in bone mineralization, maintains electrical potential in nerves and muscle membranes, involved in building of proteins, enzyme action, normal muscular contraction, transmission of nerve impulses, maintenance of teeth	Widely distributed in most foods with nuts, fruits, vegetables, cereals as best sources
Manganese	Cofactor for enzymes	Whole grains, leafy green vegetables, wheat germ, legumes, nuts
Molybdenum	Cofactor for enzymes	Legumes, nuts, whole grains
Phosphorus	Bone and teeth formation, regulation of acid-base balance, present in cell's genetic material as phospholipids, in energy transfer, and in buffering systems	Milk and dairy products, poultry, fish, meat, eggs
Potassium	Regulation of osmotic pressure and acid-base balance, activation of a number of intracellular enzymes, nerve and muscle contraction	All whole foods; meats, milk, fruits, vegetables, grains, legumes
Selenium	Part of glutathione peroxidase (an enzyme that breaks down reactive chemicals that harm cells), works with vitamin E	Seafood, organ meats, muscle meats, grains and vegetables (depending on soil selenium content)
Sodium	Regulation of pH, osmotic pressure, and water balance; conductivity or excitability of nerves and muscles; active transport of glucose and amino acids	Salt, soy sauce, seafood, dairy products, processed foods
Zinc	Part of the hormone insulin and many enzymes; taste perception; wound healing, metabolism of nucleic acids	Red meat, seafood (especially oysters), beans, fortified grains

C Commercial Foods that Frequently Contain Unexpected Allergens

Foods Containing Milk Protein	Foods Containing Egg Protein	Foods Containing Wheat Protein	Foods Containing Soy Protein	Foods Containing Peanut Protein
Breads and bread crumbs	Egg substitutes (i.e. egg beaters®)	Barbecue-flavored potato chips	Bagel, breads, and bread crumbs	Cakes, cookies, muffins, and chocolate bars
English muffin	Baby food spaghetti	Cereals	Bouillon cubes and broths	Egg roll
Flavored crackers	Marshmallow pastry cream	Gluten-free products (wheat starch)	Chicken, turkey or reduced-fat hot dogs	Frozen desserts
Nondairy creamer	Pasta	Low-fat beef hot dogs	English muffins	Candies
Instant noodle cups	Waffles	Soy sauce and other condiments	Reduced-fat peanut butter	Sauces and chili
Sorbets	Shiny baked goods (egg wash)	'Spelt'	Waffles	
Soy cheese	Wine (fined or clarified with egg white)		Canned tuna fish	
Waffles				
Canned fish				
Baby foods with mixed ingredients				
Most mammalian milks cross-react with cow's milk (e.g. sheep, goat)				

D Label Ingredients/Terms That Indicate the Presence of Common Allergens

Milk

Milk is considered a major allergen. Any FDA-regulated product that contains milk or a milk derivative as an ingredient must list the word 'milk' on the product label

Artificial butter flavor, butter, buttermilk

Casein (rennet), caseinates (calcium, magnesium, potassium, and sodium)

Ghee

Hydrolysates (casein, milk, protein, and whey)

Lactalbumin, lactoglobulin, lactose (*may* contain), lactulose

Milk solids, milk powder, nonfat dry milk powder

Whey

Label ingredients that may indicate the presence of milk protein

Chocolate

Flavorings (artificial, caramel, and natural)

High-protein flour

Luncheon meats

Margarine

Egg

Egg is considered a major allergen. Any FDA-regulated product that contains egg or an egg derivative as an ingredient must list the word 'egg' on the product label

Albumin

Egg (white, yolk, dried, powdered, solids)

Mayonnaise

Label ingredients that may indicate the presence of egg protein

A shiny glaze or yellow baked goods

Flavorings (artificial and natural)

Lecithin

Wheat

Wheat is considered a major allergen. Any FDA-regulated product that contains wheat or a wheat derivative as an ingredient must list the word 'wheat' on the product label

Bran

Bread crumbs

Bulgur

Couscous

Cracker meal

Durum and durum flour

Farina

Flour (all-purpose, enriched, graham, high gluten, high protein, pastry, soft wheat)

Gluten

Kamut

Semolina

Spelt

Vital gluten

Whole-wheat berries

Whole-wheat flour

Label ingredients that may indicate the presence of wheat protein

Hydrolyzed protein

Flavorings (artificial and natural)

Modified food starch

Soy sauce

Starch (gelatinized, modified, vegetable)

Surimi

Soy

Soy is considered a major allergen. Any FDA-regulated product that contains soy or a soy derivative as an ingredient must list the word 'soy' on the product label

Hydrolyzed soy protein

Miso

Natto

Shoyu sauce

Soy (flour, grits, milk, nuts)

Soya

Soybean (granules, curd)

Soy protein isolate

Soy sauce

Tamari

Tempeh

Textured vegetable protein

Tofu

Label ingredients that may indicate the presence of soy protein

Flavorings (artificial and natural)

Vegetable broth, gum, starch

Peanut

Peanut is considered a major allergen. Any FDA-regulated product that contains peanut or a peanut derivative as an ingredient must list the word 'peanut' on the product label

Nuts (beer, ground, monkey, mixed)

Nu-Nuts flavored nuts

Peanut (butter, flour)

Peanut oil (cold pressed, expeller pressed, extruded)

Label ingredients that may indicate the presence of peanut protein

African, Chinese, Indonesian, Mexican, Thai, and Vietnamese dishes

Baked goods

Candy

Chili

Chocolate (candies, candy bars)

Egg rolls

Enchilada sauce

Flavorings (artificial and natural)

Marzipan

Nougat

 Modified from The Food Allergy and Anaphylaxis Network. How to read label cards. Fairfax, Va: The Food Allergy and Anaphylaxis Network; 2000.

E Suggestions for Early Nutritional Intervention for the Prevention or Delay of Onset of Allergic Disease in Infants at Risk of Atopy

Clinical Report Summary of the American Academy of Pediatrics Committee on Nutrition, 2008[1]*

This summary describes the means to prevent or delay atopic diseases through dietary intervention and is not intended for a child who has evidence of a food allergic disorder.

1. The documented benefits of nutritional intervention that may prevent or delay the onset of atopic disease are for the most part limited to infants at high risk of developing allergy. High risk is defined as an infant with at least one first-degree relative (parent or sibling) with allergic disease.
2. Current evidence does not support a major role for maternal dietary restrictions during pregnancy or lactation.
3. There is evidence that exclusive breast-feeding for at least 4 months, compared with feeding intact cow's milk protein formula, decreases the cumulative incidence of atopic dermatitis and cow's milk allergy in the first 2 years of life. Additionally, there is evidence that exclusive breast-feeding for at least 3 months protects against wheezing in early life. (However, the current evidence that exclusive breast-feeding protects against allergic asthma occurring beyond 6 years of age is not convincing.)
4. There is modest evidence that atopic dermatitis may be delayed or prevented by the use of extensively or partially hydrolyzed formulas, compared with cow's milk formula, in early childhood. Extensively hydrolyzed formulas may be more effective than partially hydrolyzed in the prevention of atopic disease.
5. There is no convincing evidence that the use of soy-based infant formula plays a role in allergy prevention.
6. Complementary foods should not be introduced prior to 4 to 6 months of age. There is no current convincing evidence that delaying the introduction of solid foods beyond 4 to 6 months of age has a significant protective effect.
7. For infants after 4 to 6 months of age, there is insufficient evidence to support a protective effect of any dietary intervention for the development of atopic disease.

*From The Commitee on Nutrition, American Academy of Pediatrics. Pediatrics 2008;121:183–191 (doi:10.1542/peds.2007-3022).

F Interpretation of Food-Specific Serum IgE Concentrations

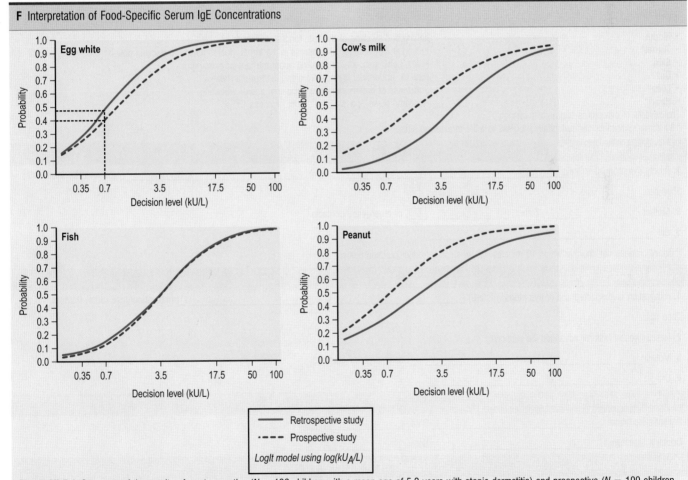

Figure AII-F-1 Summary of the results of a retrospective (*N* = 196 children with a mean age of 5.2 years with atopic dermatitis) and prospective (*N* = 100 children with a median age of 3.8 years, 61% with atopic dermatitis) study correlating the chance of an IgE-mediated clinical reaction (based upon blinded oral food challenges or convincing history) to the concentration of food-specific IgE antibody (measured in kU/L using the Pharmacia CAP System FEIA, Pharmacea & UpJohn Diagnostics, Uppsala, Sweden) for four foods. (From Sampson HA. J Allergy Clin Immunol 2001;107:891–896.)

It is important to recognize that the clinical history is paramount, that allergen prick skin tests may add additional important predictive information, and that the curves may be shifted significantly to the left for patients younger than those studied (e.g. for infants, a concentration equal to and over 2 kU/L to egg, and 5 kU/L to milk, is 95% predictive of a reaction).[2,3] Based upon these studies, suggestions were made as summarized in Table AII-F-1.

Table AII-F-1 Food-Specific IgE Concentration Clinical Decision Points

	Egg	Milk	Peanut	Fish	Soy	Wheat
Reactive if ≥ (no challenge needed)	7	15	14	20	65	80
Possibly reactive (physician challenge*)	↓	↓	↓	↓	↓	↓
Unlikely to be reactive if less than (home challenged*)	0.35	0.35	0.35	0.35	0.35	0.35

*In patients with a strongly suggestive history of an IgE-mediated food allergic reaction, food challenges should be performed with physician supervision, regardless of food-specific IgE value. If the food-specific IgE level is less than 0.35 kU/L and the prick skin test is negative, the food challenge can be performed at home unless there is a compelling history of reactivity. ↓ = values between. (From Sampson HA. J Allergy Clin Immunol 2001;107:891–896.)

G Food Allergy Action Plan for Schools/Camps

[Place child's picture here]

Allergy To: _____

Student's Name: _____ DOB: _____ Teacher: _____

Asthmatic: Yes*   No   *High risk for severe reaction

Signs of an Allergic Reaction

Systems

- **Mouth**
- **Throat***
- **Skin**
- **Gut**
- **Lung***
- **Heart***

Symptoms

Itching and swelling of the lips, tongue, or mouth
Itching and/or a sense of tightness in the throat, hoarseness, and hacking cough
Hives, itchy rash, and/or swelling about the face or extremities
Nausea, abdominal cramps, vomiting, and/or diarrhea
Shortness of breath, repetitive coughing, and/or wheezing
'Thready' pulse, 'passing out', pale, blueness

The severity of symptoms can quickly change
*All above symptoms can potentially progress to a life-threatening situation

Action for Minor Reaction

1. If only symptom(s) is(are): _____, give _____ (medication/dose/route)

Then call:

2. Mother: _____, Father: _____, or emergency contacts

3. Dr: _____ at _____

If condition does not improve within 10 minutes, follow steps for major reaction below

Action for Major Reaction

1. If ingestion is suspected and/or symptom(s) is(are) _____, give _____ (medication/dose/route) IMMEDIATELY!

Then call:

2. Rescue squad (ask for advanced life support)

3. Mother: _____, Father: _____, or emergency contacts

4. Dr: _____ at _____

Do Not Hesitate to Call Rescue Squad!

Patient's signature: _____ Date: _____

Doctor's signature: _____ Date: _____

Emergency Contacts

1. _____

Relation: _____ Phone: _____

2. _____

Relation: _____ Phone: _____

3. _____

Relation: _____ Phone: _____

Trained Staff Members

1. _____

Room: _____

2. _____

Room: _____

3. _____

Room: _____

G Food Allergy Action Plan for Schools/Camps—cont'd

EPI-Pen and EPI-Pen JR Directions

1. Pull off gray activation cap (Figure AII-G-1)
2. Hold black tip near outer thigh (always apply to thigh) (Figure AII-G-2)
3. Swing and jab firmly into outer thigh until Auto-injector mechanism functions. Hold in place and count to 10. The Epi-Pen unit should then be removed and taken with you to the emergency room. Massage the injection area for 10 seconds

For children with multiple food allergies, use one form for each food

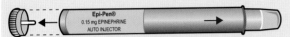

Figure AII-G-1 Pulling off gray activation cap of Epi-Pen.

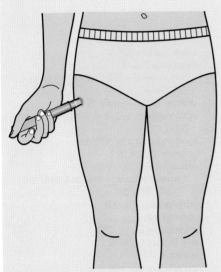

Figure AII-G-2 Applying Epi-Pen to outer thigh.

From Furlong AM, ed. The School Food Allergy Program. Fairfax, Va: The Food Allergy and Anaphylaxis Network; 1995.

H Example of a 'Chef Card' That Can Be Fashioned for Use in Restaurants. (From The Food Allergy and Anaphylaxis Network. The food allergy training guide for restaurants and food services. Fairfax, Va: The Food Allergy and Anaphylaxis Network; 2001.)

To the Chef:

WARNING! I am allergic to PEANUTS. In order to avoid a life-threatening reaction, I must avoid eating all foods that might contain peanuts, including:

Peanut	Ground nuts
Peanut butter	Mandelonas
Peanut flour	Nu-Nuts® or other artificial nuts
Peanut oil	Nut pieces
Artificial nuts	Monkey nuts
Beer nuts	Mixed nuts

Even a tiny amount of peanut can be dangerous to me. Please ensure any utensils and equipment used to prepare my meal, as well as prep surfaces, are thoroughly cleaned prior to use. Thanks for your cooperation.

References

1. Greer FR, Sicherer SH, Burks AW, American Academy of Pediatrics Committee on Nutrition; American Academy of Pediatrics Section on Allergy and Immunology. Effects of early nutritional interventions on the development of atopic disease in infants and children: the role of maternal dietary restriction, breastfeeding, timing of introduction of complementary foods, and hydrolyzed formulas. Pediatrics 2008;121:183–91.
2. Garcia-Ara C, Boyano-Martinez T, Diaz-Pena JM, et al. Specific IgE levels in the diagnosis of immediate hypersensitivity to cow's milk protein in the infant. J Allergy Clin Immunol 2001;107:185–90.
3. Boyano MT, Garcia-Ara C, Diaz-Pena JM, et al. Prediction of tolerance on the basis of quantification of egg white specific IgE antibodies in children with egg allergy. J Allergy Clin Immunol 2002;110:304–9.

Index

Note: page numbers in **bold** refer to figures, those in *italic* to tables and/or boxes

Index